pediatric chiropractic

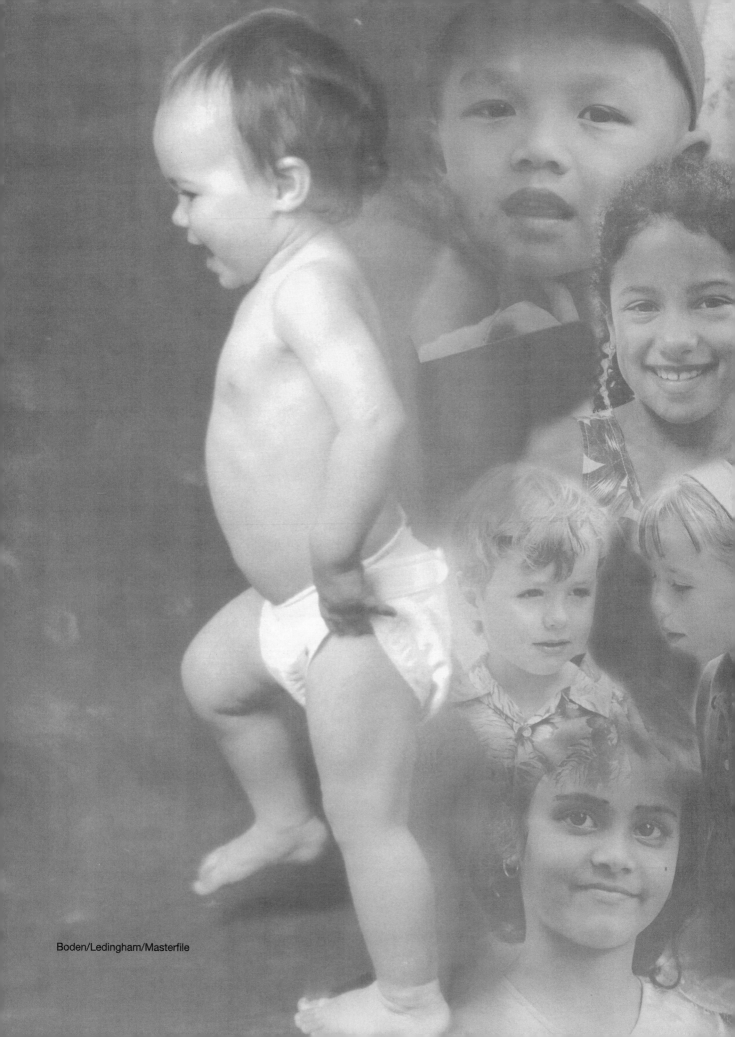

pediatric chiropractic

Editors

Claudia A. Anrig, D.C.
Private Practice, Fresno, California
Postgraduate Faculty, Life University, Marietta, Georgia
Life Chiropractic College West, San Lorenzo, California
Palmer College of Chiropractic, Davenport, Iowa
Parker College of Chiropractic, Dallas, Texas

Gregory Plaugher, D.C.
Associate Professor, Life Chiropractic College West, San Lorenzo, California
Director of Research, Gonstead Clinical Studies Society, Mt. Horeb, Wisconsin

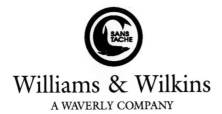

Williams & Wilkins
A WAVERLY COMPANY

BALTIMORE • PHILADELPHIA • LONDON • PARIS • BANGKOK
HONG KONG • MUNICH • SYDNEY • TOKYO • WROCLAW

Editor: Rina Steinhauer
Managing Editor: Susan Kimner
Marketing Manager: Christine Kushner
Production Coordinator: Carol Lindley Eckhart
Designer: Books By Design
Illustration Planner: Ray Lowman
Cover Designer: Studio Montage
Typesetter: Graphic World, Inc.
Printer & Binder: RR Donnelley & Sons Company

Copyright © 1998 Williams & Wilkins

351 West Camden Street
Baltimore, Maryland 21201-2436 USA

Rose Tree Corporate Center
1400 North Providence Road
Building II, Suite 5025
Media, Pennsylvania 19063-2043 USA

Accurate indications, adverse reactions and dosage schedules for drugs are provided in this book, but it is possible that they may change. The reader is urged to review the package information data of the manufacturers of the medications mentioned.

Printed in the United States of America

Library of Congress Cataloging-in-Publication Data

Pediatric chiropractic / editors, Claudia A. Anrig, Gregory Plaugher.
     p.   cm.
     Includes bibliographical references and index.
     ISBN 0-683-00136-1
     1. Children—Diseases—Chiropractic treatment. I. Anrig, Claudia
A. II. Plaugher, Gregory.
     [DNLM: 1. Chiropractic—in infancy & childhood. WB 905 P371
1997]
RZ263.P43   1997
615.5'34'083—dc21
DNLM/DLC
for Library of Congress   97-26950
                                             CIP

The publishers have made every effort to trace the copyright holders for borrowed material. If they have inadvertently overlooked any, they will be pleased to make the necessary arrangements at the first opportunity.

To purchase additional copies of this book, call our customer service department at **(800) 638-0672** or fax orders to **(800) 447-8438.** For other book services, including chapter reprints and large quantity sales, ask for the Special Sales department.

Canadian customers should call **(800) 665-1148,** or fax **(800) 665-0103.** For all other calls originating outside of the United States, please call **(410) 528-4223** or fax us at **(410) 528-8550.**

Visit Williams & Wilkins on the Internet: **http://www.wwilkins.com** or contact our customer service department at **custserv@wwilkins.com**. Williams & Wilkins customer service representatives are available from 8:30 am to 6:00 pm, EST, Monday through Friday, for telephone access.

98 99 00 01 02
2 3 4 5 6 7 8 9 10

Dr. Larry Webster
1937-1997

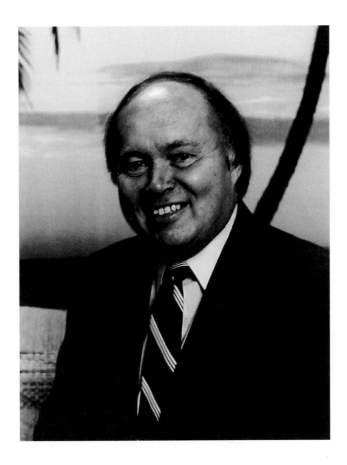

Known as the Grandfather of Pediatric Chiropractic, Dr. Larry Webster left his legacy as a chiropractor, author, teacher, researcher, and inventor. Dr. Webster was a 1959 graduate of Logan Chiropractic College and served his fellow man for thirty-eight years.

Founder of the International Chiropractic Pediatric Association (ICPA), Dr. Webster wanted to provide an association to assist field doctors. The ICPA has been a source of information for chiropractors and parents, as for national and state associations.

An advocate for children, Dr. Webster was an expert witness during the Wilk vs. AMA case in 1979. Dr. Webster was considered an authority in pediatric chiropractic and made himself responsible for increasing the general public's view of the growing demand for family chiropractic care by appearing on behalf of the profession.

During his service as Clinic Director at Life Chiropractic College as well as the college pediatric instructor, he influenced thousands of chiropractic students, sharing with future doctors his clinical experience and teaching them to detect and correct spinal subluxations.

Concerned about the constrained position of the fetus in the last semester of pregnancy, he developed the Webster In-Utero Constraint Procedure, a chiropractic analysis to detect the problem and a specific adjusting protocol. He taught this procedure for two decades and has helped thousands of chiropractors and their pregnant patients. Dr. Webster also was the inventor of the pediatric toggle headpiece board.

Although the "Grandfather of Pediatric Chiropractic" has departed, the thousands of doctors who were his "Children in Chiropractic" will honor his life by moving forward and dedicating our chiropractic efforts to the betterment of humanity. One candle lights the way, and as the torch bearer for pediatric chiropractic, Dr. Larry Webster instilled in all of us a passion and the commitment for serving children. He will continue to be an undying mentor to those of us who were graced and inspired by his life's work.

foreword

When invited to write a foreword for this ground-breaking text on chiropractic care for children, I accepted with both gladness and trepidation. Gladness because I firmly believe that such a serious compilation of work, meant primarily for students, teachers, and clinicians of chiropractic, advances the theory and practice of a field that fundamentally promotes health for children. Trepidation because I am a pediatrician, who has been indoctrinated to totally reject chiropractics and chiropractors, and who overcame prejudice and fear only two decades ago through my own direct experience. Overcoming prejudice and fear was not easy; I was prodded by extreme pain. I came into chiropractic care as most Americans do, by word of mouth. I came in pain and with a bad prognosis from my medical colleagues. I recovered pain-free function and complete well-being over a short period of several months. Since then, throughout my career I have supported chiropractic care as an adjunct to medical care for adults and for children whenever I believed that it was indicated.

As in allopathic medicine, chiropractic care ranges from excellent to poor. And, as in allopathic medicine, we can only approach excellence by continuing study, practice, and research. Throughout my years in clinical pediatrics, I have been fortunate to associate with excellent clinicians among the chiropractors who treated my friends, my referred patients, and me. I have known chiropractors who diagnosed medical conditions that had been missed by allopathic colleagues and who did not hesitate to refer patients to appropriate medical or surgical treatment.

The vehement opposition of medical physicians, individually and in their organizations, to chiropractic, has for too long kept chiropractors working in isolation and margined from access to research support and opportunities. The chiropractors' antitrust suit against the AMA that was definitively won in 1990 cleared the ground for a new foundation of collaboration. That, and the wide public demand for chiropractic health services acted on by at least 10% of Americans, brought the field into broad acceptance. Since 1974 Medicare has been required to pay for chiropractic services and currently about 85% of insurance companies provide some sort of coverage.

Research support for chiropractic has lagged far behind public acceptance. As an example, the National Institutes of Health first allocated two million dollars in 1974 for the scientific study of the biomechanics of the chiropractic adjustment. It was a definite step forward, but compare it to the billions spent on pharmacological research over a few years. The establishment of a chiropractic research center funded by the Office of Alternative Medicine is a further step in the right direction. There is fertile ground for research on the effects of chiropractic adjustments on physiological, biochemical, immunologic, hormonal and other body responses. There is fertile ground for research into the role of chiropractic care in promoting and enhancing healing and health.

Chiropractic care for infants and children is now coming of age. The publication of this text climaxes the achievement of a body of knowledge and of a budding collaboration of pediatric chiropractors with allopathic pediatricians. There are tantalizing collaborative research results already, some in common conditions such as infantile colic and middle ear infections that have baffled pediatricians for decades. From such collaboration, without bias and in a true spirit of support for optimal health for children, we may achieve the knowledge base for the holistic pediatrics of the future.

Helen Rodriguez-Trias, M.D., FAAP
Fellow, American Academy of Pediatrics
Co-Director, Pacific Institute for Women's Health/Public
 Health Institute
Los Angeles, California
Past President, American Public Health Association
Washington, D.C.

For the children

acknowledgments

This textbook was like a pregnancy in many respects; the conception of an idea among friends, then giving life to a story that needed to be told. The book brought on a unique type of morning sickness; but this was a blessing in disguise. During the first trimester, a number of top practitioners and internationally known educators came forward to complete key chapters, often putting their personal and professional lives on hold. Finally, as one would expect from a chiropractic birth, the labor process was quite natural but did not come without some pains. In the end, the contributors to this work can consider themselves proud parents. They are Dr. Mark Werking, Dr. Darrell Barnes, Dr. Stephen Collins, Dr. Gerald Waagen, Ms. Alana Callender, Dr. Phillip Ebrall, Dr. Neil Davies, Dr. Ron Lanfranchi, Dr. Joel Alcantara, Dr. Dan Murphy, Dr. Judy Forrester, Dr. Debra Levinson, Dr. Monica Buerger, Dr. Christopher Kent, Dr. David Borges, Dr. Karen Borges, Dr. David Steiner, Dr. Carol Phillips, Dr. Susan St. Claire, Dr. Ron Picardi, Dr. Mark Lopes, Dr. David Cichy, Dr. Steven Tanaka, Dr. Charles Martin, Dr. Peter Thibodeau, Dr. Peter Fysh, Dr. Raymond Brodeur, Dr. Rick Elbert, Dr. Charles Lantz, Dr. Shahinaz Soliman, Dr. Cheryl Goble, Dr. David Rowe, Dr. Christopher Hart and Dr. Larry Troxell.

An editorial review board, composed of experts in their respective fields, reviewed early drafts of manuscripts and assisted the individual authors with chapter content. We thank all that helped in this sometimes painful process of constructive criticism.

A number of other individuals helped in the creation of this book. Their efforts ranged from retrieving clinical files and radiographs to performing literature searches for the chapter authors or serving as models for illustrations. Some individuals simply provided the support or helpful guidance necessary for chapter authors to complete their work. These individuals include Dr. Anita L. Wubbena, Dr. Eric S. Osterberg, Dr. Ted J. Paquin, Dr. James A. Hicks, Dr. John L. Zozzaro, Dr. Ken J. Pieratti, Dr. Terry D. Tesar, Dr. Daniel D. Lyons, Dr. Kurt P. Huemmer, Dr. Joseph E. Martin, Amanda Nicole Cichy, Alyssa Shelsey, Dr. Mark and Mary Heal, Dr. Eddie Chevalier, Dr. Barbara Scheyer, Dr. Frank Costa, Dr. Nancy Abram, Dr. Susi Anrig, Dr. Larry Webster, Lee Sinclair, Robin Young, Marie Windrim, Michael Windrim, Sonia Courtney, Jane Hansen, Jacqueline Moffat, Dr. Steve Watson, Evelyn Forrester, Diane and David Krochko, Carla and Max Nealon, and Kathy and Christy Jaycock. Savannah and Jena Avalon provided the inspiration for Dr. Forrester.

Mr. Bong Mo Yeun was the chiropractic illustrator for this text and his commitment to the project is greatly appreciated. Mr. John Culp produced the photographic illustrations for the hundreds of radiographs used throughout the book.

Dr. Anrig extends deep gratitude and love to several individuals close to this project: Dr. Ernst and Huldy Anrig, her parents, who always embraced Claudia's deep passion for her dreams; her sister, Dr. Susi Anrig, who provided encouragement during the difficult times and kept Claudia on track; her brother and sister-in-law, Dr. Daniel and Karlin Anrig, who committed themselves to the project by always answering in the affirmative to the latest request; and to her nephews and niece, Keane, Jachin and Alyssa, who modeled endlessly for the perfect adjusting set-ups. Dr. Claudia also thanks kindred spirits, Drs. Forrester and Goble, and the endless numbers of colleagues who provided support throughout the process.

Dr. Plaugher extends his thanks to the many anonymous individuals who helped bring the project to a close; secretaries, staff, students, and doctors. He also acknowledges the professional support provided by Palmer College of Chiropractic West and the Gonstead Clinical Studies Society, without which none of this would have been possible. Sophia Elisabetta, Dr. Plaugher's baby daughter, provided the personal inspiration for bringing this work to the light of day. It's time to be more of a parent than a writer.

To the countless pioneers who preceded us in bringing chiropractic care to the children of the world, we salute you. Dr. Larry Webster, the grandfather of pediatric chiropractic, will be sorely missed.

Finally, we would both like to thank our life partners, Mr. Gary Janzen and Dr. Pamela Plaugher who bring joy and serenity to our lives. We send our love.

Claudia A. Anrig, D.C.
Gregory Plaugher, D.C.

editorial review board

contributors

Joel Alcantara, D.C.
Instructor
Palmer College of Chiropractic West
San Jose, California

Claudia A. Anrig, D.C.
Private Practice and Post Gradute Faculty
Life Chiropractic College, Life Chiropractic College West,
Palmer College of Chiropractic and Parker College of
Chiropractic
Fresno, California

David Borges, D.C.
Private Practice
South Lake Tahoe, California

Karen M. Borges, D.C.
Private Practice
South Lake Tahoe, California

Raymond R. Brodeur, D.C., Ph.D.
Assistant Professor
Michigan State University
East Lansing, Michigan

Monika A. Buerger, D.C.
Private Practice
Livermore, California

Alana K. Callender, M.S.
Director
Palmer Foundation for Chiropractic History
Davenport, Iowa

David L. Cichy, D.C.
Private Practice
Research Associate, Gonstead Clinical Studies Society
Providence, Rhode Island

Neil J. Davies, D.C.
Private Practice and Lecturer in Chiropractic,
RMIT University
Bundoora, Victoria
Australia

Phillip S. Ebrall, B. App. Sc. (Chiropractic)
Research Fellow, Foundation for Chiropractic Education
and Research
Private Practice and Senior Lecturer in Chiropractic
Head, The Chiropractic Unit
RMIT University
Bundoora, Victoria
Australia

Richard A. Elbert, D.C.
Private Practice
Ames, Iowa

Judy Forrester, D.C.
Private Practice
Calgary, Alberta
Canada

Peter N. Fysh, D.C.
Private Practice
Professor, Palmer College of Chiropractic West
San Jose, California

Cheryl E. Goble, D.C.
Private Practice
Winamac, IN

Christopher R. Hart, D.C.
Private Practice
Chadstone, Melbourne
Australia

Christopher Kent, D.C.
Private Practice
Post Graduate Faculty, Life University and
    Life Chiropractic College West
Paterson, New Jersey

Debra W. Levinson, D.C.
Private Practice and Post Graduate Faculty, Life University
Alpharetta, Georgia

Ronald G. Lanfranchi, D.C., Ph.D.
Private Practice and Post Graduate Faculty of New York
Chiropractic College
New York, New York

Mark A. Lopes, D.C.
Private Practice
Fremont, California

Charles J. Martin, D.C., D.A.C.A.N.
Private Practice
Monterey, California

Daniel Murphy, D.C., D.A.B.C.O.
Private Practice and Post Graduate Faculty
Life Chiropractic College West
Auburn, California

Carol J. Phillips, D.C.
Private Practice and Post Graduate Faculty of Northwestern
College of Chiropractic, Parker College of Chiropractic,
Canadian Memorial Chiropractic College, National College
of Chiropractic, and Los Angeles College of Chiropractic
Minneapolis, Minnesota

Ronald J. Picardi, D.C.
Private Practice
Bardonia, New York

Gregory Plaugher, D.C.
Associate Professor
Life Chiropractic College West
San Lorenzo, California
Director of Research
Gonstead Clinical Studies Society
Mount Horeb, Wisconsin

David J. Rowe, D.C.
Private Practice
New York, New York

Shahinaz E. Soliman, M.D.
Assistant Professor
Palmer College of Chiropractic West
San Jose, California

Susan M. St. Claire, D.C., M.S.
Associate Professor
Palmer College of Chiropractic West
San Jose, California

David M. Steiner, D.C.
Private Practice
Miramar, Florida

Steven T. Tanaka, D.C., D.A.C.A.N.
Private Practice
Watsonville, California

Peter Thibodeau, D.C., D.A.C.A.N.
Private Practice
Soquel, California

J. Larry Troxell, D.C.
Private Practice
Clinton, Iowa

contents

Foreword..vii
Acknowledgments xi
Editorial Review Board...xiii
Contributors...xv

Part I   **Contemporary Issues in Chiropractic Pediatrics** I

    1.   Introduction to Chiropractic Pediatrics...I
       Alana K. Callender, Gregory Plaugher, Claudia A. Anrig

    2.   Non-Accidental Injury and Child Maltreatment 14
       Phillip S. Ebrall, Neil J. Davies

    3.   Vaccination Issues 24
       Ronald Lanfranchi, Joel Alcantara, Gregory Plaugher

    4.   Children In Motor Vehicle Collisions 51
       Daniel J. Murphy

Part II   **Pregnancy, Birth, and Neonatal Assessments** 75

    5.   The Prenatal and Perinatal Period..75
       Judy A. Forrester, Claudia A. Anrig

    6.   Exercise During Pregnancy 162
       Debra W. Levinson, Judy A. Forrester

Part III   **Clinical and Radiological Assessments** 179

    7.   History and Physical Assessment 179
       Monika A. Buerger

8. Diagnostic Imaging **202**
Christopher Kent, Gregory Plaugher, David Borges, Karen M. Borges, David M. Steiner

Part **IV**   Clinical Techniques and "Dis—ease" Prevention **323**

9. The Spinal Examination and Specific Spinal and Pelvic Adjustments...................**323**
Claudia A. Anrig

10. Craniosacral Therapy...**424**
Carol J. Phillips

11. Pediatric Nutrition..**455**
Susan M. St. Claire and Ronald J. Picardi

Part **V**   Case Management **466**

12. Spinal Subluxation **466**
Joel Alcantara, Gregory Plaugher, Mark A. Lopes, David L. Cichy

13. Clinical Neurology **479**
Steven T. Tanaka, Charles J. Martin, and Peter Thibodeau

14. Orthopedics **612**
Peter N. Fysh

15. Scoliosis **642**
Raymond R. Brodeur, Gregory Plaugher, Richard A. Elbert, Charles A. Lantz

16. The Febrile Child **671**
Shahinaz E. Soliman, Gregory Plaugher, Joel Alcantara

17. The Challenged Child..**697**
Cheryl E. Goble

18. Care of the Adolescent **707**
Phillip S. Ebrall

19. **Adolescent Patients with Acute Spinal Fractures** **730**

Gregory Plaugher, David J. Rowe, David L. Cichy, Cheryl E. Goble, Richard A. Elbert, Christopher R. Hart, J. Larry Troxell, Peter Thibodeau

Index...**777**

Contemporary Issues in Chiropractic Pediatrics

1 Introduction to Chiropractic Pediatrics

Alana Callender, Gregory Plaugher, and Claudia A. Anrig

Pediatrics as a defined area in allopathic medicine did not emerge on the American scene until 1887 when it was one of the separate sections at the AMA sponsored International Congress of Medicine (1,2). The AMA Section on the Diseases of Children was the first national pediatric organization, but it was supplanted in importance by the formation the following year of the American Pediatric Society (APS), a group independent of the AMA. The founders of the APS included many of the leaders of the AMA Section. Over the next three decades, the focus of the APS was on research. "The unwillingness or inability of the APS to act on political and social issues made another pediatric forum inevitable," and the American Academy of Pediatrics (AAP) was formed in 1930. The members of the AAP concerned themselves with "education, public health, and social issues affecting children (1)."

Specialism

Definitions of specialism conflict. The first is when a practitioner limits practice to a certain population of patients, such as pediatrics or geriatrics. The second is limiting practice to a part of the whole, as in dermatology or extremities. When family practice became a medical specialty, a third concept needed to be added, as it would seem that a family practitioner is a generalist, or the opposite of a specialist. Therefore, a specialty can be defined as a group of practitioners who acquire advanced training and qualifications, have a learned society,

and produce at least one peer-reviewed journal for its practitioners and others.

As in chiropractic history, the history of allopathic medicine in America began with almost all physicians working as general practitioners. Rural areas were predominant and small communities were lucky to obtain the services of even one physician.

As the country moved from a rural population to a metropolitan population, specialism became practical. Metropolitan areas, with densely packed physician and patient populations, allowed for abundant referrals for those who wanted to limit their practices to areas of interest or expertise (3). This may be the best theory on the cause of the recent advent of specialties in chiropractic. As chiropractors become more abundant and the physician population becomes more densely packed, there is the opportunity for limiting practices to areas of interest. If the general population is served, then there is not only room for specialism—it may become necessary for survival in a very competitive market.

Another theory for specialism in allopathic medicine is the growth of science and technology (4). Although technology does not play as prominent a role in chiropractic as in medicine, big-ticket visualizing equipment such as CT scans and MRIs may lead to chiropractic specialties.

In 1970, with the inception of a specialty board, family practice was given a new status in allopathic medicine (5). A general hue and cry went up for more family physicians, and government support attempted to mandate generalists.

The specialist-technologist revolution was the "medical analogy to the industrial revolution." The attention that specialists were able to lavish on their areas of specialty led to a vast increase of knowledge in pharmacologic and surgical treatment of diseases. A hundred years later, the benefits of the specialist revolution may have run their course and the emphasis on specialism is now seen by some medical observers as the cause for the imminent collapse of the present medical care system (5). "Our leaders have noted that we now have 38,000,000 uninsured patients; explosive, uncontrollable health care costs; a disproportionate concentration of wealth in certain specialties; 'turf wars'; refusal to treat patients who cannot pay; overspecialization; increasing public dissatisfaction; and poor relations between physicians and other professionals and between allopathic and nonallopathic physicians" (5).

Chiropractic Specialties

As allopathic medicine moves away from specialism and toward general practice, chiropractors have begun to enter the era of specialism by limiting their practices to select groups of patients. The long-established Diplomates in orthopedics and radiology are being joined by specialists in nutrition, sports chiropractic, neurology, and pediatrics. Today's Diplomate of the American Board of Chiropractic Radiology can trace roots back to the Universal Spinographic Association founded in 1923 at the Palmer School Lyceum (6). Discussion on the future Diplomate of the American Board of Chiropractic Orthopedics began in 1964 with the introduction of graduate extension orthopedics training by the American Chiropractic Association (7).

The first examinations for the Diplomate in nutrition (DACBN) were offered in 1985. In 1987, the certificate for team physicians became a certificate for chiropractic sports physicians (8), and the Diplomate for Chiropractic Sports Physicians was approved at the 1989 ACA convention (9).

The ACA Board of Governors approved the formation of the Council on Neurology in 1971. The Diplomate in neurology has its own checkered history, culminating in the American Chiropractic Neurology Board awarding its first Diplomates in 1995 (10).

The chiropractic care of infants and children is that which would happen in any chiropractic practice and has been happening since the beginnings of chiropractic. After one hundred years of chiropractic care of infants and children, chiropractic pediatrics is emerging as a specialty.

Daniel David Palmer validated the adjusting of children in his 1910 Chiropractor's Adjustor [p.579] when he responded to M. Kueck of South Bend, Indiana. In a 1908 letter, Kueck wrote, "I think I have all Chiros beat on the youngest patient. Our daughter was adjusted when she was one day and two hours of age. That one adjustment corrected her of diarrhea."

The Founder replied, "B.J's child was adjusted by his grandfather when he was four days old - you get the persimmon." B.J. Palmer's child, Daniel David Palmer II (Dave), was born in 1906, so his adjustment by the founder of chiropractic predated that of the Kueck child. We have no

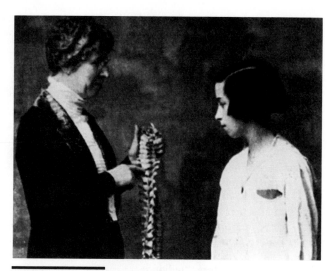

Figure 1.1.   An advertisement placed by a chiropractor, Cora Jacobsen, circa 1910. Courtesy Palmer College of Chiropractic Archives, Davenport, Iowa.

reason to believe that these were the first adjustments of children, just that they were the first recorded.

Pediatrics was offered in the curriculum at the West Coast Chiropractic College in Oakland, California, as early as 1915 (11). In 1918, Eastern College of Chiropractic (Newark, NJ) issued a patient education brochure. It proposed that the minor falls and bumps of childhood could produce subluxations that would manifest as adult diseases. For preventive measures, the brochure advocated 6-month checkups for all children. "One adjustment in the child is worth fifty in the adult (12)." Los Angeles College of Chiropractic offered 50 hours of course material in pediatrics by 1919. A chiropractor is shown explaining to a child the role of the spine in health in Figure 1.1 (c. 1910).

John H. Craven opened the pediatrics portion of his 1924 text, Chiropractic Hygiene and Pediatrics, "Chiropractic has nothing to do with obstetrics..."(13) He thus set the limitations of chiropractic care as accepted by the Palmer School at that time. His text was published on the Palmer campus as part of the Green Book series and covered the chiropractic treatment of such childhood maladies as convulsions, nocturnal enuresis, colic, and foreign bodies lodged in the nose (refer the patient out).

At many of the colleges for which a long run of catalogs is available, the introduction of pediatrics into the curriculum can be placed in the late 1920s, coinciding with the release of Craven's text. Whether Craven's work was written in response to demand for a chiropractic pediatrics text, or the availability of the text made teaching of chiropractic pediatrics a more reasonable proposition, or exterior factors motivated both the publication and addition of courses is impossible to tell. Minnesota Chiropractic College added pediatrics to its curriculum sometime between 1912 and 1937; National Chiropractic College between 1912 and 1933; Palmer School of Chiropractic between 1927 and 1930; Texas Chiropractic College between 1922 and 1948; and the Standard School of

Chiropractic (New York) between 1922 and 1937. Pinpointing the exact dates of curricular changes is problematic because many schools did not publish catalogs during the Depression.

A search of chiropractic periodical literature over the middle decades of chiropractic's history yielded little information on special treatment for pediatric patients. In fact, it was almost as if children did not exist with one exception. Chiropractic Home, "The Voice of the Layman," was published by Drs. Katherine and Chandler Bend from c.1936-1965. It included children's concerns and conditions as a regular part of its coverage, and often featured children who had benefited from chiropractic care on its cover (Fig. 1.2).

Dr. Leo L. Spears, of Denver, Colorado, opened a free clinic and dairy to meet the needs of Denver's children during the Depression. "In 1933, he incorporated his private practice as the non-profit Spears Free Clinic and Hospital for Poor Children." Although non-profit status was seen as a tax dodge by his detractors, "public records show that the clinic amply lived up to its name, at times treating up to 900 children in a week without charge" (14). His great contributions to the children of Denver were seldom recognized by a press that was focused on his battles with the Veterans' Administration.

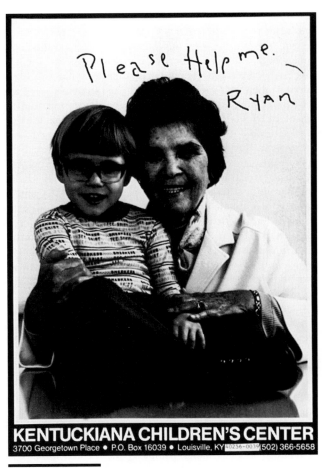

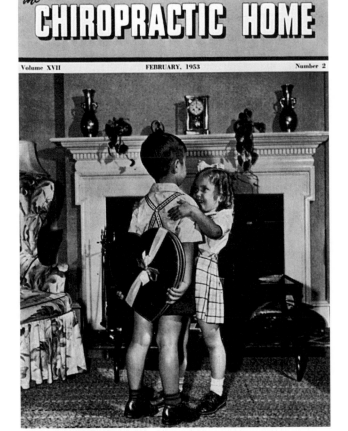

Figure 1.2. The February 1953 cover of Chiropractic Home. Courtesy Palmer College of Chiropractic Archives, Davenport, Iowa.

Figure 1.3. A fund-raising piece featuring Dr. Lorraine Golden (Palmer 1942) and a young patient. Courtesy Kentuckiana Children's Center, Louisville, Kentucky.

The first pediatric practice to take center stage has held it since its debut. Lorraine M. Golden, D.C., a general chiropractic practitioner in 1954, has dedicated her practice since then to serving physically and mentally handicapped, emotionally disturbed, and learning disabled children. Golden's practice is probably the best-known pediatric practice in the United States. The Kentuckiana Center for Education, Health and Research, Inc., serves not only a special group of children, it does so as a private, non-profit, non-sectarian, charitable organization, thus reaching those without means for specialized care (15) (Fig. 1.3).

The Children's Chiropractic Center was established in Oklahoma City in August 1963 by a group of chiropractors who volunteered their services. In 1977, Dr. Bobby Callahan Doscher joined the center as its director. Oklahaven Children's Center offers chiropractic care to indigent and severely handicapped children (16) (Fig. 1.4).

Clarence S. Gonstead, D.C., taught infant adjusting as part of his seminars at Mt. Horeb, Wisconsin. A chapter on spinal examination and specific adjustments is included in Herbst's 1968 description of the Gonstead technique (17).

The International Chiropractic Pediatrics Association (ICPA) was founded in 1975 by Larry Webster, D.C. (1937-

1997) to stimulate research and coordinate information. An advocate for children, Dr. Webster was an expert witness during the Wilk et. al. v. AMA case in 1979. Considered by many to be a leading authority on pediatric chiropractic, Dr. Webster represented the chiropractic profession as a spokesperson when the national media requested an opinion. He was also the originator of a pediatric toggle headpiece board and an in-utero constraint chiropractic technique (18). Beginning in 1993, the ICPA has offered a certificate course in pediatrics with venues in both the U.S. and Canada. The graduates of the certificate course will be eligible to enter the Life Chiropractic College pediatric diplomate program in 1998. The ICPA produces a regular newsletter received by 1400-1500 practitioners and frequently provides expert testimony in states where chiropractic is being denied to children. The ICPA is governed by a seven person board of directors and has non-profit status. Scholarships are awarded at its annual convention and a dedicated research facility is being planned. The ICPA is independent of any national professional association (19).

Dennis D. Stierwalt, D.C., introduced his 1976 text, "Since there are no known texts on children adjusting procedures, I felt compelled to write this text."(20) Gonstead's chapter focuses on infants, so the text to precede Stierwalt's on adjusting children would have been Craven's, 54 years earlier.

In the same year, Roy Hildebrandt, D.C. compiled an anthology of Joseph Janse's work. In the short chapter on pediatrics, Janse warned against specialism that would cause the practitioner to lose sight of the holistic concept. He justified adjusting children whose subluxation had not "as yet been established as a mechanical pathology and the likelihood of its actual existence could well be questioned" thus: "The chiropractic adjustment is one of the most effective forms of stimulation to the central nervous system via its effect on the cellular element..." (21).

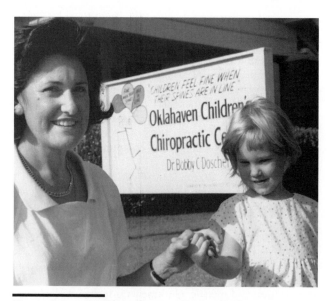

Figure 1.4. Dr. Bobby Doscher (Palmer 1977) has earned international recognition as president and chief executive of Oklahaven since 1977.

The International Year of the Child was 1979. Chartered in California that same year as a non-profit corporation, the American Chiropractic Pediatric Association envisioned regional clinics and at least one free children's hospital. It was the first attempt at a learned society for chiropractic pediatricians. A certificate program in pediatrics was planned, as was the production of patient education media. William Cockburn, a faculty member of Northern California College of Chiropractic (Sunnyvale, CA), was one of the leaders of the association. By 1984, the Association was focusing on the shortage of "documentation and professional literature on the subject of chiropractic pediatrics (22)," but shortly thereafter, the Association faded away.

An infant adjusting table was mentioned by Craven in 1924 so the first design for one must have predated his text. However, the history of the early tables seems to be lost (Fig. 1.5). The special needs of pediatric patients were recognized in late 1984 by J.P. Migliore, D.C., a faculty member at Life Chiropractic College, and Bill Perks, a toolmaker. They patented the PoneeTM table. It is a drop-release table designed for children and decorated like a wooden pony. It was followed by competing bench tables, also designed like woodland creatures (23).

To keep pace with growing demand, several chiropractors began postgraduate continuing education programs in the late 1980s. Many continue to this day, such as those by Dr. Peter Fysh of Palmer West (24) and Drs. Forrester and Anrig's Peter Pan Potential.

In 1985, Northwestern College of Chiropractic convened a pediatrics symposium that produced proceedings addressing various issues in chiropractic pediatrics. Between 1985 and 1991, Life College's Today's Chiropractic had four issues (v.14, n.5; v.15, n.6; v19, n.1; v.20, n.1) with pediatric themes. In 1989, the *Journal of Manipulative and Physiological Therapeutics* carried three articles discussing childhood complaints (v.12, nos.4 and 5). These were followed in 1990 by three issues of the ICA Review dedicated to pediatrics (v.46, nos.2–4). These issues set the stage for the announcement in March/April 1991 for the ICA's national conference of chiropractic and pediatrics.

The International Chiropractors Association, along with the Foundation for the Advancement of Chiropractic Tenets and Sciences presented a National Conference on Chiropractic and Pediatrics in San Diego, in November 1991. Twenty-two sessions were presented by 18 expert instructors. Approximately 400 chiropractors attended. The success of that conference resulted in the ICA Board of Directors establishing the Council on Chiropractic Pediatrics, whose focus would be postgraduate education.

The Council developed the curriculum of 360 classroom hours and three interim examinations that would be required by candidates. A research paper is also required before the candidates can be certified as board eligible. The first candidates entered the program in Chicago in 1993 and in May 1996 completed the classroom portion of the training (25).

This is the first Diplomate to be offered to the profession by the Council on Chiropractic Pediatrics, and to be sponsored by the ICA. In January 1996 the first issue of the *Journal of Clinical Chiropractic Pediatrics* (JCCP), a new original peer-reviewed

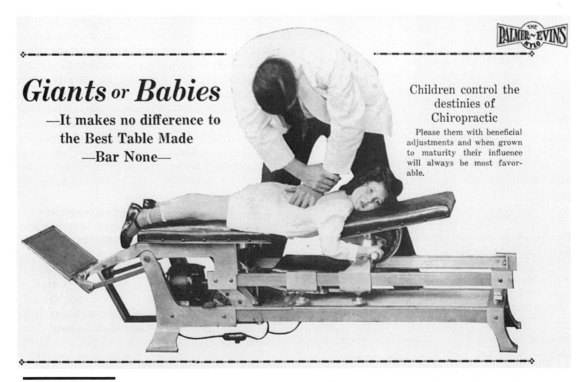

Figure I.5.   The Palmer-Evins Hylo was advertised as suitable for treating any size of patient, from baby to giant. Courtesy of Palmer College of Chiropractic Archives, Davenport, Iowa.

publication was presented by the ICA. It is planned as a quarterly and proposes to "provide the chiropractic practitioner with information that will foster clinical excellence, encourage dialog and research among academicians and researchers, and be a credible resource for those seeking information on the efficacy and appropriateness of chiropractic for infants, children, and mothers" (26).

With additional training and board certification and now a scholarly journal, chiropractic pediatrics has completed the journey to becoming a specialty within chiropractic. When asked for the genesis for chiropractic pediatrics, Maxine McMullen, D.C., Chair of the ICA Council on Chiropractic Pediatrics, did not refer to the national conference or to the meeting of those who would design the Diplomate program. Instead, she referred to D.D. Palmer's adjusting his grandson, as recorded in 1910 in The Chiropractor's Adjustor. The chiropractic treatment of children has been an integral part of the chiropractic profession since its beginning.

Philosophical and Scientific Principles

Chiropractic is a health care discipline that emphasizes the inherent (or innate) recuperative power of the body to heal itself without the use of drugs or surgery (27). Since the body's innate recuperative power is affected by and integrated primarily through the nervous system, chiropractors have a particular focus on disorders of the spinal column, especially subluxation. A subluxation or sprain (28) of a vertebral joint is a complex injury with both functional and structural manifes-

tations that compromise neural integrity thus influencing organ system function and general health (27). One modern descriptor for this spinal pathology is *vertebral subluxation complex* (See Chapter 12).

Several philosophical principles are inherent in the practice of chiropractic. These principles help to guide the art and science of chiropractic and provide an overall paradigm unique among health care providers. Eight principles or metaphors for a philosophy of science of chiropractic health care have been put forth by Keating et. al. (29) (Table 1.1). For a thorough discussion of these principles, the reader is referred to their original source (29).

Prenatal Spinal Development and Asymmetry

Graham and Dunne (30,31) have presented the factors that are associated with a fetal constraint position held over a sufficient period, which then influences the outcome of physical form. It is these physical alterations that can then lead to abnormal function. In the skeletally adult spine, the structure primarily dictates function with regards to joint movement. For the developing pediatric spine, the functional demands drive the formation of bones and joint surfaces.

The human fetus develops more quickly than the infant. Because of this rapid growth, the fetus is more susceptible to biomechanical forces that lead to constraining pressures and molding (31,32). Extrinsic factors may play a role in morpho-

Table 1.1. Principles and Metaphors of a Philosophy of the Science of Chiropractic

Clinical conservatism (first, do no harm) (primum non nocere)

Disease (reliable clustering of signs and symptoms)

Epistemology of science (scientific method)

Holism

Homeostasis and the self-healing capacity ("Innate Intelligence")

Professional autonomy

Structure-function reciprocity

Supremacy of the nervous system (strategic role of the nervous system)

Reprinted with permission from Keating JC, Plaugher G, Lopes MA, Cremata EE. Introduction to clinical chiropractic. In: Plaugher G, ed. Textbook of clinical chiropractic: a specific biomechanical approach. Baltimore: Williams & Wilkins, 1993:2.

genesis, which then influences the genetically predetermined shape of bone. An abnormal position occurs when the fetus does not move into the vertex position at the seventh month. In-utero constraint is the most common cause of extrinsic deformation.

Osseous development (i.e., longitudinal growth) may be adversely influenced by the excessive compression forces that are placed on the perpendicular growth plates (31). Unequal compression loading and stretching of a growth plate can alter deposition of bone thus leading to asymmetry of the osseous elements. The growth plate is also susceptible to torsional forces that may cause rotational alterations (31,33). Extrinsic forces that affect the musculoskeletal system include: strong muscles producing tensile loading, gravity (abnormal weight bearing affecting the force on bone), and dynamic stressors (31). The forces of shearing, stretching, compression, torsion, and bending are all extrinsic factors that may influence the growth and shape of the musculoskeletal system. These developmental factors can then lead to asymmetrical loading (34), subluxation, and/or degeneration of the motion segment later in life. Because many spinal abnormalities can be due to in-utero constraint factors, the care of the pregnant patient where indicated may be necessary to prevent these adverse osseous outcomes.

Post-Natal Spinal Development and Asymmetry

Excluding the sacrum, the average length of the spine of the neonate is approximately 20 cm. Within the first 24 months of life, the length of the spine will grow to approximately 45 cm (35). The pediatric vertebral column is largely composed of cartilaginous material up to about the age of 6 years. It is therefore sensitive to morphogenic alterations during this period (30,31,35,36).

The neonate's vertebrae consist of the centrum and the two halves of the neural arch. Joining all parts is hyaline cartilage. Although the spine consists of cartilaginous elements, it does not contraindicate carefully applied specific adjustments. Posterior synchondrosis (uniting of the vertebral arches) ordinarily occurs first. The closure begins at C1 during the first year, and the process is concluded by approximately the eighth year at the lumbar spine. The process of neurocentral synchondrosis (centrum ossification) is completed at approximately the third through the fifth year in the lumbar spine and by the fifth through the eighth year in the cervical spine. The sacrum and ilia do not completely ossify until the earlier half of the third decade of life.

Osseous development is influenced by nerve and circulatory factors (36). These two factors control chemical and cytologic function. The modeling of bone and the joint surfaces is contingent on whole body motion. Motion constraint will lead to developmental asymmetries.

The transitional areas (e.g., CO–C1, L5–S1) of the spine are more susceptible to biomechanical stresses. These regions are frequently affected more when asymmetrical loads or abnormal movements are encountered (36,37).

The infant or toddler developing the muscular coordination for standing or walking will encounter numerous falls to the sitting or lateral recumbent position. Symmetry and balance unfortunately does not exist for the pediatric spine as they progress through their developmental stages. Micro and macro trauma, postural and repetitive habits, and unilateral activities and sports are all considered a part of the normal childhood (35–41).

The role of left-right hand dominance is well documented to affect the structure of the spine (39,40). This extrinsic influence can further contribute to postural (e.g., idiopathic scoliosis and muscular imbalance) and osseous asymmetry. The role of chiropractic care in improving or preventing developmental spinal abnormalities is not well understood and merits further investigation.

In-Utero Constraint and Subluxation Injuries

In-utero constraint occurring in the last trimester of pregnancy may be one of the extrinsic factors that causes abnormal biomechanical stresses on the cartilaginous spine of the fetus (42). Lumbar or pelvic subluxation of the mother's spine may also alter the ligament attachments to the uterus, leading to asymmetrical forces on the fetus. Alterations in the position of the lumbar spine, pelvis, and birth canal may play a role in the development of in-utero constraint and certain constraints during passage through the canal. A large proportion of fetuses with breech positioning have scoliosis and/or hip dislocations.

Birth Trauma

The birth process may be another source of spinal trauma (See Chapters 5 and 10). Forces applied to the spine during the birthing process can cause spinal and neurologic trauma (42).

Cesarean, forceps, and vacuum extraction methods can also be injurious to the cervical and thoracic regions.

Accidental Injury

The leading cause of death in the United States under the age of 25 is accidents (38). Automobile injuries are the leader in accidental deaths from the ages of 1 to 25 years. When hyperextension and hyperflexion trauma occurs, spinal traction and cord compression or impingement can occur from acceleration/deceleration trauma. Careful examination must be made of the spine, cranium, and neurological aspects of the patient after motor vehicle accidents.

The home or day care center is the primary site for 2- or 3-year-old toddlers to receive injuries. For 5- to 18-year-old patients, the school playground is the most frequent place for accidents to occur (38). Sports, physical education, and unorganized activities play a role in the occurrence of these injuries.

Another source of head and neck trauma is bicycle accidents (43). Advocating the use of a helmet does reduce the number of head injuries, but unfortunately does little to protect the delicate cervical spine. Playground equipment (e.g., slides, swings, monkey bars, etc) is responsible for 118,000 accident-related injuries a year to children. The majority of these accidents will be falls, with half resulting in head and cervical trauma (38).

Sudden hyperflexion or hyperextension of the neck, or vertical compression of the head or onto the buttocks from falls, can cause spine and/or spinal cord injury (41). Recreational activities that are commonly associated with injury include skate boarding, roller-blading, horseback riding, trampoline jumping, water slides, and diving into shallow water.

Infants of physical abuse can sustain injuries to the spinal cord due to violent shaking of the head (Shaken Baby Syndrome) (41,44,45) (see Chapter 2). Another possible source of injury to the infant is a fall from a high place (e.g., sofa, bed). Diaper changing is a common activity that is performed at a high place (e.g., changing table). In a study conducted by the National Safety Council (43), 47.5% of the infants were discovered to have fallen head first from a high place during their first year of life.

Goldthwait and Coe (46) postulated that faulty body mechanics could alter the development of bone, eventually leading to adult functional disorders. Maigne (46) reports that head and cervical trauma could create irritation to the cervical sympathetic fibers and may cause a variety of dysfunctional states; headaches; auditory, vestibular and visual problems; vasomotor and secretional problems; pharyngolaryngeal and psychic disturbances. He reports positive results with these disorders when cervical adjustments are performed (46).

Pediatric Subluxation and Chiropractic Care

Heilig (36) indicates that the longer the duration of osseous development, during which asymmetrical forces are acting, the greater the occurrence, duration, and extent of spinal damage. If aberrant spinal function could be recognized and improved early on, the greater the opportunity for normal developmental patterns to be established. Addressing the osteopathic profession, Heilig appeals to his colleagues to consider spinal manipulation for children because developmental changes can be most easily affected at an early age. Lewit (37) discusses the possible ramifications of blockage (vertebral subluxation complex) if left untreated in the child.

If accidents are the leading cause of death and severe injuries to children in the United States, the potential for spinal injuries (subluxation) is also apparent. The consequences of vertebral subluxation may appear negligible, with the exception of occasional transitory pain or irritability. If the subluxation is left uncorrected, compensatory reactions can develop at adjacent motion segments, further concealing the effects of the original lesion. Long-term biomechanical strain deprives the disc tissue of needed nutrition, eventually leading to internal reabsorption and degeneration. Both hypomobile (subluxation) and hypermobile (compensation) segments will undergo degeneration.

The chiropractor has an opportunity to normalize, if not minimize, the effects of the vertebral subluxation complex. Thorough analysis and specific adjustments to the pregnant female and pediatric spine may have a far-reaching impact on whole body health.

Case Mix and Demographics

The case mix for the practicing chiropractor can vary, but usually involves a predominance of neuromusculoskeletal complaints (e.g., low back pain, neck pain, headache, etc.) and primarily involves patients in the 30- to 50-year range. A study by Ebrall (47) of Australian practitioners found that children (0–11 yr) constituted 4.6% of patient visits and adolescents (12–24 yr) accounted for 12.8% of visits. Although there is substantial variability among different countries, a survey of European chiropractors found that children account for a significant proportion of the case mix of chiropractic practice (48). In Denmark, children aged 0–14 yr represented approximately 10% of visits. Adolescents (15–24 yr) accounted for about 15% of patient visits. Children accounted for approximately 5% of visits to chiropractors. Neuromusculoskeletal complaints was the majority category for which chiropractic care was sought. The above results are similar to that of Nyiendo and Olsen (49), who analyzed the visit characteristics of 217 children attending a chiropractic college teaching clinic in the U.S. They found that of children (<18 yr) attending the clinic, 42% had musculoskeletal complaints, 20% had complaints that were not of a musculoskeletal nature, and 33% attended the clinic for a general physical examination. Patients who were members of the immediate family of the student intern were more likely to visit the clinic for a general physical examination or a nonmusculoskeletal complaint. These patients may be more likely to view chiropractors as primary health care providers

A survey in Canada of pediatric patients who visit alternative care practitioners found that the majority consulted chiropractors and that nonmusculoskeletal complaints (e.g., respiratory or ENT conditions) constituted the majority of reasons for visits to alternative care providers (50).

Wellness, Dis-ease, and Disease Models of Health Care

Chiropractors serve several models of health care. In the acute injury phase, emphasis is often placed on pain reduction and functional restoration. As care progresses, patients are often moved to a less acute phase of treatment with the patient gradually assuming more responsibility for his or her health. This may take the form of specific therapeutic exercise or dietary modifications as adjunctive treatment to the chiropractic adjustment.

Wellness or health is not simply the absence of disease but a state of optimal physical, emotional, and social well being. Dis-ease refers to a lack of ease within the body. Chiropractors believe that spinal subluxations have a tremendous impact on dis-ease, through the intimate relationship between the spine and nervous system. Adjustments of subluxation take on a therapeutic role in the case of the reduction of disease (i.e., the pathology of subluxation), but also a preventive function, minimizing the development of certain disease processes that result from uncorrected spinal subluxations.

Health promotion is also an integral component to chiropractic practice, with emphasis on regular chiropractic visits (depending on the individual patient's needs) to check for spinal subluxation and providing adjustments where indicated, but also with regards to certain "generic" aspects such as lifestyle changes (e.g., smoking cessation, exercise, diet, etc.).

What Are We Teaching Children About Health and Disease?

Children in kindergarten understand the cause of illness to be something magical or a result of their transgression of the rules. In the fourth grade, children believe all illness to be caused by germs whose very presence is sufficient to make a child sick (51). So much for telling children that they are strong and that their bodies can fight the germ.

In most patients, it is the host's susceptibility that is the primary problem, not the germ, especially in terms of the severity and complications that result from a particular illness. Children need to be taught to get adequate rest, to eat properly, and to exercise. Telling children that their bodies are weak and that they should be afraid of germs that are around them all the time seems of little use and may be counterproductive.

Where is the discussion of spinal health and neurological health in our public schools? Back pain alone is a significant public health problem, with about one-third of adolescents reporting back pain. Headache is also increasing in prevalence, affecting more and more children. Postural patterns due to different functions and spinal problems begin gradually at a very early age.

There needs to more public health awareness about spinal hygiene including the effects of certain sports trauma, back pain, headache, and other common childhood ailments.

Chiropractic examination should be performed on a regular basis for children due to the high incidence of spinal trauma, and children should report falls and other types of trauma. Teachers need to be aware when a child needs to have their spinal column examined. Most school health officials are unfamiliar with the complexity of spinal orthopedic disorders, indicating a need for further education in this area. Chiropractors may facilitate this educational process.

"Alternative," "Complementary," or "Unconventional"

Perhaps none of the above apply. Although chiropractors have seen expanded utilization of their services over the past two decades, this fact appeared to go largely unnoticed by most in the medical profession. It was not until the seminal study by Eisenberg et. al. (52) did the medical profession realize that consumers of health care used alternative practitioners at all. To the surprise of many, the number of visits to alternative care practitioners was calculated to be approximately 425 million in 1990. In contrast, the number of visits to primary care practitioners (i.e., MDs) was 388 million. One can entertain the question of who is alternative and who is conventional. Chiropractors, by and large, shiver at the notion of being called "alternative medicine" or "complementary medicine" or "unconventional" practitioners because many rightfully assume the role of primary contact providers and practice a form of health care (i.e., chiropractic) that in many ways substitutes for conventional medical practices. To many patients, chiropractic is the conventional form of care they rely on first, and medical (or surgical) care is only used in instances when their primary form of health care has no answers. The surveys of Spigelblatt (50) and Drs. van Breda (53) tend to confirm the usage of chiropractors as a largely primary form of health care, that is, for health conditions that are also typically addressed by pediatricians.

Chiropractic Science

Chiropractic's primary defining feature in its contribution to the health care delivery system is the importance that is placed on the health of the spinal column and by extension, the integrated nervous system. Although chiropractors use a variety of techniques for health promotion, such as exercise prescription or dietary advice, the majority of chiropractors use the adjustment as their key therapeutic approach for the reduction of a subluxation. Spinal trauma (with and without both fracture or dislocation; see Chapter 19) subluxates the joints from ligamentous stretch and sprain resulting in a disease or pathological disorder known as the vertebral subluxation complex (54) or subluxation (54). Chiropractors have adhered to the clinical importance and practical application of adjusting the spinal column and extravertebral articulations since the inception of the profession, over 100 years ago.

Although the importance of the nervous system in immune function is well established in both adults (55) and children (56–58), the various mechanisms of these complex interactions are only beginning to be understood. Studies on the effects of chiropractic care on immune function have been reviewed by Allen (59). Although only a few studies exist on this topic, there is basic biological plausibility for the impact of spinal nervous system function and host resistance. Allen (59) has called for prospective large-scale clinical trials in this area.

Because a large proportion of children who visit chiropractors do so for so-called "somatovisceral" problems (e.g., otitis media) (50), researchers should include children as well as adults, as subjects for experiments with respect to nervous system activity and immune responses.

Clinical Research

At the time of this writing, a number of randomized clinical trials were ongoing with respect to the effects of chiropractic adjustments in patients with a variety of health problems. These studies represent the evolution of the chiropractic sciences towards the evaluation of clinical efficacy. They build on the results from small scale, preliminary, or pilot projects, large-scale cohort investigations, case reports, and basic science data. The authors present a few of the current lines of investigation in the following sections. They by no means represent the entirety of the chiropractic research frontier.

SUBLUXATION

Subluxation or sprain of a joint occurs commonly when excessive loads are placed on the spinal column. A child's everyday activities or specific types of sports or recreational activities can lead to damage to the spinal joints. The signs of subluxation include pain, limitation of motion, point tenderness, edema, and neurological changes (joint proprioception, nerve irritation, etc.). Recent research has begun to elucidate the many pathological changes that occur at spinal joints in adolescents. Erkintalo et. al. (60) studied the development of degenerative changes in lumbar intervertebral discs. This prospective randomized study of 31 subjects with back pain and 31 subjects without the complaint was obtained from an original sample of 1,503 14-year-old schoolchildren. Their conclusion was that degenerative changes including dehydration, protrusion, and Scheuermann's changes emerge rapidly following the adolescent growth spurt. The degenerative process occurred in many asymptomatic as well as symptomatic patients. However, the signs associated with degeneration appeared more commonly in children with back pain, and they also occurred at an earlier age.

A 25-year study of 640 14-year-old children followed from 1965 through 1990, attempted to determine risk factors for the development of low back pain in adulthood (61). Low back pain occurring during the growth period and familial occurrence were both associated with an increased risk. The lifetime prevalence for back pain was 84% for this cohort. Radiologic findings of lumbar or thoracic Scheuermann's disease were also evaluated, occurring in 13% of subjects. Irregular end-plates occurred in 11% and disc degeneration occurred in 12% of subjects. Four subjects had spondylolisthesis, one subject a structural scoliosis combined with Scheuermann's changes, and one had a congenital block formation between T7 and T8. The proportion of subjects (out of 640) having radiographic

abnormalities was 36%. The studied radiographic changes were not associated with an increased incidence of back pain in adulthood. The investigators also found that there was a higher frequency of mental problems (e.g., fear, depression) in the group with x-ray findings in the T11–L2 area. The study authors offer no explanation for this finding. They also found that the presence of low back pain in the first months after childbirth was associated with radiological abnormalities of the T11–L2 region.

Salminen et al. (62) studied the association of disc abnormalities and low back pain in adolescents. Subjects were followed for 3 years. Nineteen percent of 15-year-old teens without back pain has degenerated discs. This rose to 26% of the asymptomatic group by age 18. In subjects with back pain, 42% had degenerated discs at age 15, increasing 58% by age 18. Disc protrusions had a similar pattern. No subject without back pain had a disc protrusion at age 15. By age 18, 16% of the asymptomatics had signs of disc protrusion. Disc protrusion occurred in 65 of the 15-year-old teens with back pain. Twenty-six percent of 18-year-old teens with back pain had disc protrusions.

Although spinal manipulation, including specific adjustments directed at sites of subluxation, decreases back pain in adults, little information is available with regard to children, or if preventive aspects potentially seen in adults, occur as a result of earlier treatment interventions. Objective parameters of subluxation such as radiological findings, motion abnormalities, edema, and tenderness, as well as subjective reports of pain or disability should be used in randomized clinical trials of chiropractic efficacy. Use of as many outcome measures that accurately depict the disorder will hopefully lead to further understanding of the modes of action and refinement of various chiropractic adjustive or rehabilitative techniques. The objective signs of subluxation and their relative clinical utility will need further research. Technology assessment remains a critical line of research chiropractic. Although not capable of producing the pizzazz seen in the results of a randomized clinical trial, refinement of examination procedures will enhance the assessment of patient outcomes and the internal validity of large-scale clinical trials.

In terms of causes and prevention, further research can lead to a better understanding of in-utero constraint and its prevention, as well as birthing practices that sometimes lead to injury and subluxation. Prevention-oriented research should be a high priority for the chiropractic profession.

HEALTH STATUS

Van Breda and van Breda (53) did a comparative study of the health status of children raised under the health care models of chiropractic and allopathic medicine. Two hundred chiropractors and 200 pediatricians participated in this random survey. Usable responses were obtained in 35% of chiropractors and 36% of pediatricians, including a low response rate. Although preliminary in nature, the findings from this study should stimulate more large-scale investigations in this area. For example, children of medical doctors reported more otitis media and tonsillitis than children raised by chiropractors. On the other hand, children of medical doctors reported decreased frequency of infections such as mumps, RUBEOLA, and rubella (see also Chapter 3) when compared with the children of chiropractors. Approximately 44% of chiropractic children were not vaccinated, compared with approximately 6% of MD children. Antibiotics were never used by approximately 50% of DC children compared with approximately 12% of children raised by pediatricians.

INFANTILE COLIC

Infantile colic is persistent crying (often violently) for no apparent reason. It usually begins at 1 to 4 weeks of age and ends spontaneously at 3 to 4 months. This disorder can have a tremendous impact on both the child and parent.

Klougart et al. (63) have presented the results of a large scale cohort of 316 infants treated using manual chiropractic methods. In this prospective multicenter study from Denmark, successful results were obtained in 94% of patients. At the time of this writing, a randomized clinical trial was nearing completion by the same group of Danish researchers.

ASTHMA

Asthma is the most common chronic illness in childhood and is characterized by variable airflow obstruction with airway hyperresponsiveness. In the US, asthma affects an estimated 14–15 million persons, including 4.8 million younger than 18 years of age. In 1993, asthma accounted for an estimated 198,000 hospitalizations and 342 deaths among persons younger than 25 years. Asthma-related mortality and hospitalization rates are increasing among persons younger than 25 years of age (64). African Americans appear to be particularly afflicted. Asthma mortality for whites remained stable from 1968 through 1991. In contrast the mortality rate increased by 337% during the same period in African Americans (65). The side effects (66) and long-term effectiveness (67) associated with current drug-treatment strategies combined with the increasing incidence of the disorder over the past decade, give cause for concern.

Nielsen et al. (68) studied the effects of spinal manipulation in 31 adults who were taking anti-asthma medications. Sham manipulation was compared with manipulation in a 4-week crossover design. No changes in forced expiratory volume were noted. Although objective lung function did not change, non-specific bronchial hyperactivity improved by 36% and patient-rated asthma severity decreased by 34%, indicating the need for further investigation in this area.

Menon et al. (69), in a pilot study of 22 subjects, have reported changes in airway function in non-asthmatics using the Gonstead technique. The exact implications of the results of this study are unknown. Future projects will need to involve symptomatic patients to assess the clinical significance of this form of spinal adjustment.

At the time of this writing, there was a practice-based large scale randomized clinical trial ongoing in Canada (i.e., CHILD Study). Treating doctors used diversified technique (short lever arm HVLA thrusts) and based the locus for the adjustment(s) on the palpatory findings of the patient. Conclusions on the question of efficacy with this methodology should be forthcoming in 1998.

Treatments that have proven effectiveness combined with minimal side effects will need to be discovered for patients with asthma. Chiropractic care may make an important contribution in this area if the clinical experiences of doctors are any guide. Most chiropractors are unaware that even a study that could prove treatment capable of keeping children out of the hospital during the year would significantly impact public health. Due to the nature of asthma and the potential for life-threatening complications without drug-treatment, multidisciplinary cooperative research projects should be performed to minimize any potential risks to subjects from drug withdrawal, if part of a study protocol.

HEADACHE

Sillanpaa and Anttila (70) studied the prevalence of headaches in 7-year-old school children. The overall prevalence of present headache (having occurred in the previous 6 months) increased from 14.4% in 1974 to 51.5% in 1992. The prevalence of migraine also increased from 1.9% to 5.7% during the same period.

A large (n=900) study of adolescents (10–18 yr) in Australia by King and Sharpley (71) found that lifetime prevalence for headache was 63.2%. About one third had headaches 1–2 times per month, 24.8% suffered every few days or once a week and 4.6% had constant headaches. One study of 11–14-year-old teens found the point prevalence for migraine with or without aura to be about 3% (72).

A randomized clinical trial on the efficacy of chiropractic adjustments compared with amitriptyline in adults with headache has been conducted by Boline et. al. (73) Their results indicated a lasting reduction in headache intensity, frequency, and over-the-counter medication usage in those subjects receiving adjustments. Side effects were common in the amitriptyline group (82.1%) and rare (4.3%) in those receiving chiropractic adjustments.

We are currently unaware of any ongoing studies specific to headache in children and the effects of chiropractic care. The data currently available on the efficacy of chiropractic care in adults with headache is encouraging (74). Studies involving children should be a high priority for the chiropractic profession given the significant level of functional impairment, pain, and disability (school absence) (75) caused by this disorder.

BACK PAIN

Back pain is a highly prevalent condition in children. A large scale survey (76) of 1178 schoolchildren found the cumulative prevalence of back pain was 51.2%. Lumbar, leg, and thoracic pain were the most common forms. Multivariate analysis showed that age, previous back injury, volleyball, female sex, and time spent watching television were positive correlations for the presence of back pain. Findings of a significant impact of low back pain among adolescent schoolchildren have been confirmed by other researchers (77,78).

Low back pain is even more common among adolescent athletes. The excessive spinal loading that accompanies many sporting activities (e.g., gymnastics, ice hockey, etc.) involves additional risk for acute low back injuries during the growth spurt, which is harmful to the lower back (79).

Recent independent evaluations of the effectiveness of chiropractic care in the management of adult patients with low back pain have been presented (80). For the questions of pain reduction, loss time from work, and patient satisfaction, chiropractic methods have continually shown to be of greater benefit to patients compared with medical or physiotherapeutic treatments. We can think of no biological explanation for why these benefits, apparently evident in adults, would not also be applicable to adolescents, especially since the adult patient usually begins showing signs of back problems (e.g., pain) during adolescence. Further research in this area will help to determine which chiropractic methods are the most effective for which particular patient and help to refine certain chiropractic adjustive techniques and examination procedures.

OTITIS MEDIA

In July 1994, the Agency for Health Care Policy and Research released clinical practice guidelines for otitis media with effusion (OME) (81). There were some 821,700 cases of OME in 1991 alone. The average cost of treatment was $1,330.00 per case. The total direct and indirect costs was estimated at $1.09 billion. The guideline recommendation for not performing certain surgeries or the prescription of medications runs counter to current medical practice in which antibiotics are frequently prescribed for an initially self-limiting disorder in many cases.

Froehle (82) studied a cohort of 5-year-old and younger patients with acute otitis media presenting to a chiropractic outpatient facility. Forty-six children were followed. Ninety-three percent of patients improved. Young age, no history of antibiotic use, initial episode (vs. recurrent), and designation of the episode as discomfort rather than an ear infection were associated with improvement in the fewest treatments. Treatments consisted primarily of adjustive care to the cervical spine. A typical treatment regimen consisted of three treatments in the first week and two in the second week. Treatment was terminated when there was clinical improvement.

Experimental studies (i.e., RCT) are much needed in the area of OME. It is the one of the most frequent reasons for presentation to a chiropractor by a pediatric patient, which should help in obtaining sufficient sample sizes for clinical trials. The associated morbidity and disability associated with the disease, combined with the increasing prevalence of drug-resistant strains as infectious agents due to inappropriate antibiotic use, should help provide the impetus for further clinical trials in this arena.

SCOLIOSIS

The effects of chiropractic care in patients with scoliosis have been largely documented in case reports (83–86). Lantz has recently completed a long-term analysis of a cohort of juveniles and adolescents with scoliosis who received chiropractic care. Preliminary reports of the cohort's results have been encouraging (87). Outcomes appear to be most favorable in children with mild curves and in those of a younger age. Randomized clinical trials are needed to compare the efficacy of chiropractic methods to that of medical treatments, or the natural history of the disorder.

DYSMENORRHEA

Primary dysmenorrhea (not due to organic pelvic disease, e.g., endometriosis) occurs in up to 50% of women of child-bearing age (88). The incidence is higher in adolescents. One study reported an incidence of 79% by age 18 (89).

Liebl and Butler (90) have presented a case report on the treatment of a patient with dysmenorrhea. The efficacy of chiropractic treatment in this area has been investigated by a team from National College of Chiropractic. Kokjohn et al. (91) have presented a pilot study using 45 adult women randomized into one of two treatment groups. Sham manipulation was compared with side posture high velocity thrust techniques to indicated dysfunctional motion segments from T10 through L5–S1, including the sacroiliac joints. Their results were suggestive of a potentially beneficial effect in those patients receiving spinal manipulation. A follow-up large-scale study has recently been completed and results should be forthcoming in 1998 (92).

Study in this area needs to be continued given the high level of disability caused by the disorder. In addition to dysmenorrhea, noncyclic pelvic pain and the effects of chiropractic intervention, have shown promising results in a recent feasibility study (93), also indicating the need for a randomized clinical trial in this area.

PREGNANCY AND LABOR

Back pain during pregnancy is common. A prospective cohort study of 200 consecutive women attending a prenatal clinic were followed throughout their pregnancy (94). Seventy-six percent reported back pain at some time during their pregnancy.

Diakow et al. (95) performed a retrospective study of 400 pregnancies and deliveries of 170 consecutive patients presenting to five outpatient chiropractic clinics. A subset of 170 patients who had painful pregnancies was divided into those receiving chiropractic care (i.e., manual manipulation) and those who did not. The group that received spinal adjustments experienced significantly less pain during labor.

Studies on the effectiveness of chiropractic care in patients with back pain during pregnancy and the reduction of pain during delivery are needed. Patients who receive chiropractic care during their pregnancy tend to have a shorter period of labor time before delivery (96). This hypothesis could also be tested.

ATTENTION DEFICIT HYPERACTIVITY DISORDER

Attention deficit hyperactivity disorder (ADHD) is a complex syndrome involving a variety of behavioral criteria including varying degrees of inattentiveness, impulsiveness, restlessness, and engagement in dangerous activities, etc. (See also Chapter 18). The syndrome is largely overdiagnosed and treated in the US. Ritalin is the most popular medical treatment method.

A hypothesis for how this disorder may be produced by the presence of spinal subluxation and subsequent autonomic hyperactivity has been presented by Giesen et al. (97). They used a multiple "n of 1" time series design in seven subjects to determine the effect of chiropractic adjustive care. The authors concluded from the results of the small-scale study that chiropractic treatment had the potential to become an important nondrug intervention for children with hyperactivity disorders.

Brzozowske and Walton (98) have published details of a compelling study on the effect of chiropractic care in students with learning and behavioral impairments, arising from neurological dysfunction. Following a pilot study, the researchers embarked on a comparison clinical trial of chiropractic treatment (e.g., adjustments, nutrition) vs. conventional medical treatment (e.g., Ritalin, depressants, etc.). The results, although based on a small sample size (n=12 in each group), offer evidence of a superior benefit using chiropractic treatment, without the side effects associated with medical intervention (50% of medically treated patients had side effects). The researchers provide guidelines for the diagnosis of hyperactivity/behavioral disorders and patient management.

The results of the these studies indicate a need for RCT research in this area. Investigators should use sufficient sample sizes to draw more definitive conclusions regarding chiropractic efficacy and effectiveness.

REFERENCES

1. Pearson HA. Pediatric history: the American Pediatric Society. Pediatrics 1995; 95(1):147-151.
2. King LS. Medical practice: specialization. JAMA 1984; 251:1333-1338.
3. Luce JM, Byyny RL. The evolution of medical specialism. Perspect Biol Med 1979; 22:377-389.
4. Adams DP. Evolution of the specialty of family practice. J Florida Med Assoc 1989; 76:325-329.
5. Garrison RL. The five generations of American medical revolutions. J Family Pract 1995;40:281-287.
6. Canterbury R, Krakos G. Thirteen years after Roentgen. Chiropractic History 1986; 6:24-29.
7. Watkinson WA. Introduction of graduate extension orthopedics training. ACA J Chiro 1964; 1(6):28-29.
8. Council reports. ACA J Chiropractic 1987; 24(6):66.
9. ACA approved diplomate. Chiropractic Sports Physician 1989;26 (8):76.
10. Taylor S. President, Board of Examiners, American Board of Chiropractic Neurology. Telephone interview, April 12, 1996.
11. West Coast Chiropractic College, Oakland, California. Catalog. 1915.
12. Whitleigh GA. "Consider the Children." (Newark, NJ) Eastern College of Chiropractic, 1918.
13. Craven JH. Chiropractic Hygiene and Pediatrics. Davenport, Palmer School of Chiropractic, 1924. p.277.
14. Rehm WS. Price of dissension: the private wars of Dr. Leo L. Spear, 1921-1965. Chiropractic History 1995; 15(1):31-37.
15. Kentuckiana Children's Center: a dream come true. J Chiropractic 1982;19(7):32.
16. Oaklahaven Children's Center. Today's Chiropractic 1985;14(5):67.
17. Herbst RW. Gonstead Chiropractic Science and Art. Chapter 19. Mt. Horeb, WI: Sci-Chi Publications 1968:261-268.
18. Anrig CA. Chiropractic approaches to pregnancy and pediatric care. In: Plaugher, G ed. Textbook of clinical chiropractic-a specific biomechanical approach. Baltimore: Williams & Wilkins, 1993:383-432.
19. Webster L. Telephone interview, March 21, 1996.
20. Stierwalt DD. Adjusting the child. Davenport, IA, Stierwalt 1976.
21. Hildebrandt RW. J. Janse principles and practice of chiropractic. Lombard, Illinois, National College of Chiropractic, 1976.
22. Cockburn W. Chiropractic pediatrics. Am Chiro 1984; Jan/Feb:14.
23. Maycroft T. Ponee, Inc.. Telephone interview, March 5, 1996.
24. Fysh P. Postgraduate seminar: Kids Need Chiropractic Too!, San Jose, CA.
25. Rangnath M. ICA. Telephone interview, March 6, 1996.
26. ICA presents a new original peer-reviewed publication. Dynamic Chiropractic 1996;14(7): 4.
27. Consensus Statement. Association of Chiropractic Colleges. Dynamic Chiropractic 1997; 15(5):[insert].
28. Oxford English dictionary. Oxford University Press, 1989.
29. Keating JC, Plaugher G, Lopes MA, Cremata EE. Introduction to clinical chiropractic. In: Plaugher G, ed. Textbook of clinical chiropractic: a specific biomechanical approach. Baltimore: Williams & Wilkins, 1993: 1-11.
30. Graham JM. Smith's recognizable patterns of human deformation. 2nd Ed. Philadelphia: W.B. Saunders Co., 1988.
31. Dunne KB, Clarren SK. The origin of prenatal and postnatal deformities. Pediatric Clin North Am 1986; 33:1277-1279.
32. Dunn PM. Congenital postural deformities. Br Med Bull 1976;32:71-76.
33. Moreland MS. Morphological effects of torsion applied to growing bone. J Bone Joint Surg 1980; 62B:230-237.
34. Panjabi MM, Krag MH, Chung TQ. Effects of disc injury on mechanical behavior of the human spine. Spine 1984; 9:707-713.
35. Lecture Notes. Congenital and developmental spinal biomechanics. Applied Spinal Biomechanical Engineering 1987 Postgraduate Seminar, Manchester, NH 03104.
36. Helig D. Osteopathic pediatric care in prevention of structural abnormalities. J Am Osteopath Assoc 1949; 48:478-481.
37. Lewit K. Manipulative therapy in rehabilitation of the locomotor system. London: Butterworth & Co, Ltd., 1985:23-29.
38. Paulson J. Accidental injuries. In: Behrman R, Vaughan VC, Nelson WE, eds. Nelson's textbook of pediatrics, 13th ed. Philadelphia, PA: WB Saunders Co., 1987:211-214.
39. Jirout J. Einfluss der einseitigen Grosshrndominanz auf das Rontgenbild der Halswirbelsaule. Radiologe 1980; 20:466-469.
40. Goldberg C, Dowling FE. Handedness and scoliosis convexity: a reappraisal. Spine 1990;15:61.
41. Menkes JH, Batzdorf U. Postnatal trauma and injuries by physical agents. In: Menkes JH, ed. Textbook of child neurology. 3rd ed. Philadelphia: Lea & Febiger, 1985:493-496.
42. Anrig C. Chiropractic approaches to pregnancy and pediatric care. In: Plaugher, G ed. Textbook of clinical chiropractic-a specific biomechanical approach. Baltimore: Williams & Wilkins, 1993:383-388.
43. Educational literature. National Head Injury Foundation. Wash., DC 20036.
44. Fielding JW. Cervical spine injuries in children. In: Sherk HH, Dunn EJ, Eismont FJ, eds. The cervical spine. 2nd ed. Philadelphia: JB Lippincott, Co. 1989; 199:422-435.
45. Pang E, Wilberger JE. Spinal cord injury without radiographic abnormalities in children. J Neurosurg 1982; 57:114-129.
46. Hinwood JA, Hinwood JA. Children and chiropractic: a summary of subluxation and its ramifications. J Aust Chiro Assoc 1981; 11:18-21.
47. Ebrall PS. A descriptive report of the case-mix within Australian chiropractic practice, 1992. Chiro J Aust 1993; 23:92-7.
48. Pedersen P. A survey of chiropractic practice in Europe. Euro J Chiro 1994; 42:3-27.
49. Nyiendo J, Olsen E. Visit characteristics of 217 children attending a chiropractic college teaching clinic. J Manipulative Physiol Ther 1988; 11:78-84.
50. Spigelblatt L, Laine-Ammara G, Pless B, Guyver A. The use of alternative medicine by children. Pediatrics 1994; 94:811-814.
51. Perrin EC, Gerrity PS. There's a demon in your belly: children's understanding of illness. Pediatrics 1981; 67:841-849.
52. Eisenberg DM, Kessler RC, Foster C, et. al. Unconventional medicine in the United States: prevalence, costs, and patterns of use. N Engl J Med 1993; 328:246-52.
53. van Breda WM, van Breda JM. A comparative study of the health status of children raised under the health care models of chiropractic and allopathic medicine. J Chiro Res 1989; Summer:101-103.
54. Gatterman MI, Hansen DT. Development of chiropractic nomenclature through consensus. J Manipulative Physiol Ther 1994; 17:302-309.
55. Ader R, Cohen N, Felten D. Psychoneuroimmunology: interactions between the nervous system and the immune system. Lancet 1995; 345:99-103.
56. Birmaher B, Rabin BS, Garcia MR, et. al. Cellular immunity in depressed, conduct disorder, and normal adolescents: role of adverse life events. J Am Acad Child Adolesc Psychiatry 1994; 33:671-8.
57. Biondi M, Peronti M, Pacitti F, et. al. Personality, endocrine and immune changes after eight months in healthy individuals under normal daily stress. Psychother Psychosom 1994; 62:176-84.
58. Boyce WT, Chesney M, Alkon A, et. al. Psychobiologic reactivity to stress and childhood respiratory illnesses: results of two prospective studies. Psychosom Med 1995; 57:411-22.
59. Allen JM. The effects of chiropractic on the immune system: a review of the literature. Chiro J Aust 1993; 23:132-5.
60. Erkintalo MO, Salminen JJ, Alanen AM, Paajanen HEK, Kormano MJ. Development of degenerative changes in the lumbar intervertebral disk: results of a prospective MR imaging study in adolescents with and without low-back pain. Radiology 1995; 196:529-533.
61. Harreby M, Neergaard K, Hesselsoe G, Kjer J. Are radiologic changes in the thoracic and lumbar spine of adolescents risk factors for low back pain in adults? A 25-year prospective cohort study of 640 school children. Spine 1995; 20;2298-2302.
62. Salminen JJ, Erkintalo M, Laine ML, Pentti J. Low back in the young. Spine 1995;20:2101-2108.
63. Klougart, Nilsson N, Jacobsen. Infantile colic treated by chiropractors: a prospective study of 316 cases. J Manipulative Physiol Ther 1989; 12:281-288.
64. MMWR 1996;45:350-353.
65. Targonski PV, Persky VW, Orris P, Addington W. Trends in asthma mortality among African Americans and whites in Chicago, 1968 through 1991. Am J Public Health 1994; 84:1830-1833.

66. Tinkelman DG, Reed CE, Nelson HS, Offord KP. Aerosol Beclomethasone Dipropionate compared with Theophylline as primary treatment of chronic, mild to moderately severe asthma in children. Pediatrics 1993; 92:64-77.

67. Cheung D, Timmers MC, Zwinderman AH, et. al. Long-term effects of a long-acting B2-adrenoceptor agonist, Salmeterol, on airway hyperresponsiveness in patients with mild asthma. N Engl J Med 1992; 327:1198-1203.

68. Nielsen NH, Bronfort G, Bendix T, Madsen F, Weeke B. Chronic asthma and chiropractic spinal manipulation: a randomized clinical trial. Clin Exp Allergy 1995; 25:80-88.

69. Menon M, Plaugher G, Jansen R, Sutowski J, Dhami MSI. Effect of spinal adjustment on peripheral airway function in normal subjects: a pilot study. Proceedings 1995 International Conference on Spinal Manipulation, Washington DC: Foundation for Chiropractic Education and Research, Arlington, VA.

70. Sillanpaa M, Anttila P. Increasing prevalence of headache in 7-year old schoolchildren. Headache 1996; 36:466-470.

71. King NJ, Sharpley CF. Headache activity in children and adolescents. J Paedtr Child Health 1990; 26:50-4.

72. Raieli V, Raimondo D, Cammalleri R, Camarda R. Migraine headaches in adolescents: a student population-based study in Montreal. Cephalgia 1995; 15:5-12.

73. Boline PD, Kassak K, Bronfort G, Nelson C, Anderson AV. Spinal manipulation vs. amitryptyline for the treatment of chronic tension-type headaches: a randomized clinical trial. J Manipulative Physiol Ther 1995; 18:148-54.

74. Vernon H. The effectiveness of chiropractic manipulation in the treatment of headache: an exploration in the literature. J Manipulative Physiol Ther 1995; 18:611-617.

75. Carlsson J, Larsson B, Mark A. Psychosocial functioning in schoolchildren with recurrent headaches. Headache 1996; 36:77-82.

76. Troussier B, Davoine P, deGaudemaris R, Fauconnier J, Phelip X. Back pain in school children: a study among 1178 pupils. Scan J Rehabil Med 1994; 26:143-146.

77. Olsen TL, Anderson RL, Dearwater SR, et. al. The epidemiology of low back pain in an adolescent population. Am J Public Health 1992; 82:606-608.

78. Balague F, Dutoit G, Waldburger M. Low back pain in school children. Scand J Rehab Med 1988; 175-179.

79. Kujala UM, Taimela S, Erkintalo M, Salminen JJ, Kaprio J. Low back pain in adolescent athletes. Med Sci Sports Exerc 1996; 28:165-170.

80. Manga P, Angus D, Papadopoulos C, Swan W. The effectiveness and cost-effectiveness of chiropractic management of low-back pain. Ottawa: Pran Manga & Associates, 1993.

81. Stool SE, Berg AE, et. al. Otitis media with effusion in young children. Rockville, MD: U.S. Dept. of Health and Human Services, Public Health Service, Agency for Health Care Policy and Research, 1994; AHCPR publication no. 94-0622.

82. Froehle RM. Ear infection: a retrospective study examining improvement from chiropractic care and analyzing for influencing factors. J Manipulative Physiol Ther 1996; 19:169-77.

83. Sallahian CA. Reduction of a scoliosis in an adult male utilizing specific chiropractic spinal manipulation: a case report. Chiropractic: J Chiropractic Res Clin Invest 1991; 7:42-45.

84. Mawhiney RB. Chiropractic proof in scoliosis care. Dig Chiro Econ 1984; Mar/Apr:65-70.

85. Aspergren DD, Cox JM. Correction of progressive idiopathic scoliosis utilizing neuromuscular stimulation and manipulation: a case report. J Manipulative Physiol Ther 1987; 10:147-156.

86. Betge G. Scoliosis correction. Euro J Chiro 1985; 33:71-91.

87. Lantz CA. Study on chiropractic care for adolescent scoliosis is encouraging. Dynamic Chiropractic 1997; 15(3):1,33.

88. Dawood MY. Dysmenorrhea. Clin Obstet Gynecol 1990; 33:168-178.

89. Teperi J, Rimpela M. Menstrual pain, health and behaviour in girls. Soc Sci Med 1989; 29:163-9.

90. Liebl NA, Butler LM. A chiropractic approach to the treatment of dysmenorrhea. J Manipulative Physiol Ther 1990; 13:101-106.

91. Kokjohn K, Schmid DM, Triano JJ, Brennan PC. The effect of spinal manipulation on pain and prostaglandin levels in women with primary dysmenorrhea. J Manipulative Physiol Ther 1992; 15:279-285.

92. Backman JA, Hondras MA, Burke M, Brennan PC. Recruitment and accrual of women with primary dysmenorrhea in a randomized controlled trial. Proceedings American Public Health Association 124th Annual Meeting, New York, 1996.

93. Hawk C, Long C, Azad A. Chiropractic care for women with chronic pelvic pain: a prospective single-group intervention study. J Manipulative Physiol Ther 1997; 20:73-79.

94. Kristiansson P, Svardsudd K, von Schoultz B. Back pain during pregnancy. A prospective study. Spine 1996; 21:702-709.

95. Diakow PRP, Gadsby TA, Gadsby JB, et. al. Back pain during pregnancy and labor. J Manipulative Physiol Ther 1991; 14:116-118.

96. Fallon JM. Chiropractic and pregnancy: a partnership for the future. Int'l Rev Chiro 1990; Nov/Dec:39-42.

97. Giesen JM, Center DB, Leach RA. An evaluation of chiropractic manipulation as a treatment of hyperactivity in children. J Manipulative Physiol Ther 1989; 12: 353-363.

98. Brzozowske WT, Walton EV. The effects of chiropractic treatment on students with learning and behavioral impairments resulting from neurological dysfunction. ACA J Chiro 1977; 11:S127-S140.

2 Non-accidental Injury and Child Maltreatment

Phillip S. Ebrall and Neil J. Davies

Non-accidental injury and child maltreatment are serious concerns for all primary health care professionals, especially those who regularly deal with infants, children, and adolescents. Over the last 20 years, the clinical flags of such trauma have become well established (1). Given the estimate that some 100,000 children suffering from abuse or neglect annually pass through the doors of chiropractors' offices in the United States (2), it is not surprising that the chiropractic literature has started to address the issue (2–5).

The issues surrounding non-accidental injury and child maltreatment, however, are not as simplistic as the general term "child abuse" might imply. Children suffer more victimizations than do adults, including more conventional crimes, more family violence, and some forms virtually unique to children such as family abduction. Victimizations have been grouped into three categories: the pandemic, such as sibling assault, affecting most children (6); the acute, including physical abuse, affecting a small but significant percentage of children; and the extraordinary, such as homicide, affecting a very small number (7). This latter point is notwithstanding the fact that 1 out of 5 teenage and young adult deaths in the United States was gun related in 1988, and firearm death rates for both black and white teenagers exceed the total for all natural causes of death combined (8).

This chapter deals with acute victimization and will demonstrate the nature of the non-accidental injury and the other manifestations of maltreatment that can be expected to be seen in chiropractic practice.

The Nature of the Problem

In Western societies the highest rates of substantiated abuse and neglect occur with children age 13 and 14 years (5.1 and 5.2 children per 1000, respectively), followed by children younger than 1 year (4.6 per 1000), and those age 3 years (4.5 per 1000) (9). Ninety percent of fatal child abuse and neglect occurs among children younger than 5 years, and 41% occurs among infants (10). In the United States, the highest rates of abusive violence towards children were found among families located in the East; families whose annual income was below the poverty line; families in which the father was unemployed; families in which the caretakers held blue collar jobs; families with four or more children; caretakers who used drugs at least once; families with male children; and children age 3 to 6 years (11).

Rates of substantiated sexual abuse increase with age up to 14 and 15 years, whereas rates of substantiated emotional abuse and neglect were highest for those age 1 and younger (9). Girls are the subjects in the majority (75%) of sexual abuse cases; both sexes were the subjects in a nearly equal number of cases of neglect, physical abuse, and emotional abuse (9). In the Netherlands, where voluntary notification exists, an "extraordinary increase" was found in cases of emotional maltreatment over the 10-year period of 1974 and 1983, and sexual abuse was more recognized during the period, accounting for 7.2% of detected cases of maltreatment in 1983 (12).

Reports of child abuse and neglect come mainly from friends or neighbors (17% of finalized cases), or parents (14%), however, the reports of friends and neighbors have one of the lowest rates of substantiation. Importantly, although the child is one of the sources reporting least often, it provides one of the highest rates of substantiation (9).

The long-term effects of child maltreatment are becoming evident. A history of abuse among adolescent males is predictive of serious drinking problems (13). Identifying high-risk youths and their families can effectively address the youth's problems and troubled behavior before drug use and delinquent careers become firmly established (14). Early detection and reduction of some forms of abuse can produce long-term cost benefits within the public health system. Female patients older than age 15 who experienced childhood sexual abuse reported more problems in respiratory, gastrointestinal, musculoskeletal, neurological, and gynecological functions than a control group (15). Further, 65% of women outpatients with chronic mental illness reported a history of some type of abuse or neglect as a child (16).

Exposure to physical or sexual abuse has been associated with a significantly increased risk of suicide attempts for chemically dependent male adolescents, but not for females (17). Among the general Australian population, men between the ages of 15 and 24 are more likely to take their own lives, and in Tasmania, the Australian state with the highest suicide rate (20.7 per 100,000), just under 11% of telephone calls to a "Kids Help Line" involved physical or sexual abuse (18,19). Although we do not yet know how many of the suicides among a normative population are preceded by a history of maltreatment, abused children are at specific risk of developing depression, suicide (20), and borderline personality disorder (21). There is also an increased risk of subsequent substance abuse in maltreated children. A study of psychiatrically hospitalized, dually diagnosed, adolescent substance abusers found 61% had a history that warranted suspicion of past or current maltreatment, most commonly physical abuse, followed by sexual abuse, and neglect (22).

Types of Maltreatment

In broad terms, the abuse of children may be physical, sexual, or deprivational, or may take the form of neglect (23). In specific terms, child abuse may take a variety of forms ranging from extreme physical violence to nutritional deprivation. Further, abuse is rarely a single incident, but rather a pattern of behavior that is repeated over time. The longer it continues, the more serious the effects on the child, the family, and the community.

On the surface, that which constitutes child abuse may seem obvious, but in fact, the diversity of opinion as to definition at the "lesser end of the scale" contributes to a significant diagnostic dilemma. The definition of what constitutes abuse varies widely from culture to culture, making a "standard international" approach to the problem enigmatic. Nevertheless, an excellent broad definition has been formulated by the South Australian Police Department for use by their Victims of Crime Section (24). The definition states:

> *"Child abuse is any non-accidental act of omission or commission that endangers or impairs a child's physical or emotional health and development."*

Although this definition incorporates the widest possible characteristics of child abuse, greater specificity is required for each category of abuse for there to be useful guidelines for health care providers faced with the invidious task of deciding whether to initiate the intervention process.

Physical Abuse

Physical abuse is any non-accidental physical injury inflicted on a child by a parent or caregiver. Non-accidental injuries may include beatings, burns, scalds, ruptured spleens, hematomas, retinal hemorrhages, fractures, poisoning, bruises, welts, brain damage, and suffocation.

Emotional Abuse

This form of abuse may be defined as the continual rejection or scapegoating of a child through humiliation, name-calling, coldness, or open hostility. Emotional abuse may range from ignoring the child to the induction of psychopathology through verbal threats and psychologic terrorism.

Psychological maltreatment has been defined by Garbarino in terms of caregiver behavior that thwarts the meeting of the needs of the child. Garbarino demonstrates that psychological maltreatment can be evident in five forms: rejecting by sending messages of rejection to the child; ignoring by being psychologically unavailable to the child; terrorizing by using intense fear as a weapon against the child; isolating by removing the child from normal social relationships; and corrupting by missocializing the child into self-destructive and antisocial patterns of behavior (25).

Sexual Abuse

Child sexual abuse happens when an adult or someone bigger and/or older than a child involves a child in sexual activity by using his or her power over a child or taking advantage of the child's trust. Often tricks, bribes, threats, or coercion and sometimes physical force are used to make a child participate in the activity.

Child sexual abuse includes a range of sexual activity, including exhibitionism, fondling genitals, oral sex, and vaginal or anal penetration by a finger, penis or other objects, and even coercion into prostitution.

Neglect

Neglect is a failure on behalf of the caregiver to provide a child with adequate nutrition, medical care, clothing, shelter, or supervision to such an extent that the child's health and development are impaired or placed at serious risk. A child may further be defined as neglected if left uncared for or unsupervised over long periods, either inside or outside the home. Neglect is usually a "sin of omission" rather than an overt act of commission, but this depends on jurisdiction.

Physical neglect, in comparison to the other types of abuse, is the most predictable and distinguishable (26). Although the general rule of thumb is that non-accidental injury and child maltreatment know no social, economic, or racial boundaries, recent studies using exploratory logistic regression models suggest that physical neglect is most clearly related to economic factors such as low income and Aid to Families with Dependent Children (AFDC) status, regardless of race (26).

Other Abuse

Unusual and bizarre forms of child abuse have been reported, including the extraction by parents of their children's permanent incisors as a punishment for misdemeanors (27). Also, sadistic ritual abuse, including satanic cult abuse, is now emerging as a syndrome among people with severe dissociative disorders, including multiple personality disorder. Sadistic ritual abuse remains highly controversial but should not be dismissed as a possible clinical differential in cases of adolescent and child victimization (28).

Non-accidental injury and maltreatment is accepted as being inflicted within the family situation, however as recent evidence from Romania demonstrates, devastating victimization of children can occur within government-operated institutions. A health team working in an institution for intellectually challenged children in Romania diagnosed many children with under-nourishment, retarded growth, skin infections, injuries, and untreated physical deformities. Some of these children were in urgent need of medical attention and, sadly, children with cerebral palsy and motor, auditive, and visual challenges were not given attention (29). This type of maltreatment is social neglect and resulted in children who displayed signs of deprivation, anxiety, and behavioral maladjustment. Further tragic cases of social neglect will be uncovered as more chiropractors commit their professional services to third world countries.

It can also be a mistake to think the "out-of-home" placement system in Western societies is always safe for children and adolescents. Cases of physical abuse, sexual abuse; and neglect in foster homes, group homes, residential treatment centers, and institutions have been reported (30). In these environments, physical abuse is the most frequent cause of injury, and reports of sexual abuse are most likely to be confirmed. Prior allegations of abuse or neglect regarding the perpetrator were indicated in 27% of reports (30).

Third world countries have further, unique types of abuse, however the literature tends to be based on studies of Western society, and reliable, peer-reviewed, and indexed reports of problems in other societies are only now becoming available. For example, a study of child abuse and neglect in northern Nigeria, a third world state, has shown that some children are exploited by poor families for street begging, perhaps because the laws that exist to protect minors and prevent street begging by children are seldom enforced (31).

Self-inflicted intentional injury (as assault or suicide attempts) is also a form of abuse that must be considered in clinical practice, particularly with adolescent patients. The average annual incidence of intentional injuries treated in the hospital was 76.2 per 10,000 person years, and 11.4% of these were self-inflicted (32). The chiropractor needs to be aware that self-inflicted injury does not always result in hospital attendance; for example, a 16-year-old female in the practice of one of the authors presented with multiple small, circular lesions on her forearms. A directed history revealed these were the result of her burning herself with a cigarette in an attempt to balance out the pain her behavior during early adolescence had caused her mother, a history that was confirmed by her older sister. This type of adolescent behavior is usually transient; however, a small percentage will repeatedly inflict injury on themselves.

Characteristics of Non-accidental Injury and Maltreatment

Child maltreatment is the outcome of many interacting factors that affect parental capabilities, including stress (6). However, given the continuum along which maltreatment ranges, from mild sibling violence to child murder, it is challenging to try to determine what degree of physical injury is necessary before an act is determined to be abusive (33). In some jurisdictions, if abuse is *suspected*, it is to be reported.

Some sociological indicators may be of assistance. For example, in Finland, severe violence was perpetrated more frequently by fathers, and the highest incidence of severe violence was found in youth living in families with a stepfather (34). Unemployment within a family tended to increase both mild and severe violence. However, aside of studies that suggest a higher incidence of abuse in certain populations, the astute clinician will realize that non-accidental injury and maltreatment can affect a child regardless of his or her age, sex, socioeconomic class, or geographic location (35).

Although maltreatment crosses all social boundaries, there are some risk factors (36). These include young maternal age, an unwanted pregnancy, a history of family disturbance, foster care, and poverty (36). Some knowledge of stressors within the family environment of the child patient may assist the clinician who suspects maltreatment. Three stress indicators, namely "trouble with teenagers," "violence and separation," and "public assistance" were identified in a study of 151 parents of abused children (37).

Notwithstanding the frank effects of physical abuse on the musculoskeletal system, which are discussed in this chapter, the chiropractor is also likely to detect the sometimes subtle neurological signs that attend abuse by nutritional deprivation. Vitamin B12 deficiency has been related to maltreatment by abnormal eating habits. Of two reported cases from The Netherlands, one was a 2-year-old girl with neurodevelopmental regression and macrocytic anemia, as a result of the combination of maternal deficiency and inadequate feeding after birth, and the other was a 14-year-old obese girl with severe polyneuropathy and mild macrocytic anemia, as a result of a bizarre feeding pattern adopted subsequent to being the victim of child abuse (38).

The injuries associated with physical abuse may involve any anatomic focus and organ system, although most of these injuries cannot serve as definitive evidence of maltreatment. It is vital to retain a high index of suspicion and an awareness of the patterns of injury commonly observed in abused infants and children. The less familiar intracranial and abdominal injuries must be thoroughly evaluated for possible abuse when circumstances suggest maltreatment or when no plausible explanation is given for the radiologic findings (39).

Of 1248 cases of child maltreatment on file at a major county hospital in the US, physical abuse cases (41%) outnumbered sexual abuse (35.4%) and neglect episodes (23.6%). Of all cases, 37.5% presented with head injuries; however, when only physical abuse cases were considered, head injuries doubled to 75.5%, and included intraoral injury such as tooth fracture, tongue and tongue frenulum lacerations, lip frenulum lacerations, lesions to the oral mucosa and palate, and fractures of the mandible or maxilla (40). More than half (52.9%) of all children were in the birth to 4 years age range. The face is typically the region with the most abnormal findings, and soft-tissue findings will be the most numerous (41).

Approximately 50–70% of abused children manifest skeletal trauma (42); therefore, chiropractors, with their clinical focus on the musculoskeletal system, will detect radiographic findings that are suggestive of physical abuse, either incidentally or through directed investigation.

Complicated skull fractures, such as multiple, bilateral or diastatic fractures, in children younger than 3 years of age are indicative of abuse, whereas skull fractures from unintentional injury are typically linear fractures of the parietal bone (43,44). Linear fracture alone may not indicate abuse, and the clinician must assess the history for appropriateness. Typical falls by babies, such as from a bed onto a carpeted floor, rarely result in skull fracture (43). Additional characteristics that lead to a suspicion of abuse are multiple, depressed, wide or growing fractures.

Given that most babies are only beginning to walk at around 1 year of age, a high index of suspicion is warranted with nonsupracondylar humerus fractures in infants, and femoral shaft fractures in the first year of life (45). Humeral fractures are typically of the shaft or metaphysis in the abused child, as opposed to typically supracondylar when unintentional (43). Femoral fractures are more indicative of abuse in children younger than 1 year of age (43). An analysis of 80 femoral fracture episodes in children younger than 4 years of age found 30% were related to child abuse (46). Fractures at the subtrochanteric level and chip fracture of the distal metaphysis were more common in abused children (46).

The chip fracture or bucket handle fracture is a sign that is virtually diagnostic of abuse. It is visualized as a metaphyseal "corner" fracture in long bones, typically the distal femur, tibia, fibula, humerus, radius, or ulna (42,47) (Fig. 2.1). The usual mechanism is a sudden, twisting motion of the limb that

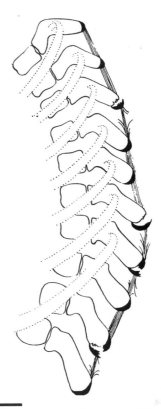

Figure 2.2.   Spinous process fractures and ligamentous hyperflexion injury from physical abuse. Adapted from Kleinman PK, Zito JL. Avulsion of the spinous processes caused by infant abuse. Radiology 1984; 151:390.

stretches the metaphyseal ligaments, resulting in the subsequent fracture and avulsion of one or both of the metaphyseal corners due to the traction, stretching, and shearing, acceleration-deceleration stresses on the periosteum and articular capsules (42,47). Often, bones on both sides of a single joint are affected, especially at the knee (47).

Rib fractures in children, although rare, are a marker of severe trauma and have a high mortality rate, 42% (48), which increases as the number of ribs fractured increases. When combined with head injury, the mortality rate becomes 71%. In Gareia's study, physical abuse accounted for nearly two thirds of children younger than 3 years of age with rib fractures (48).

With respect to head injury, the combination of any two of the following three factors was associated with inflicted head injury: an inconsistent history and/or physical examination; retinal hemorrhages; or parental risk factors (alcohol or drug abuse, previous social service intervention within the family, or a past history of child abuse or neglect) (49).

The heavy infantile head is poorly supported by the weak cervical musculature and the upper spine is highly vulnerable to the repeated shaking (Fig. 2.2) that may occur in physical abuse; however, spinal column fractures in children are unusual. They affect the cervical spine in cases of abuse or battering but rarely require operational intervention (50). A 1969 study, while acknowledging that the incidence of spinal trauma was not as high as the incidence

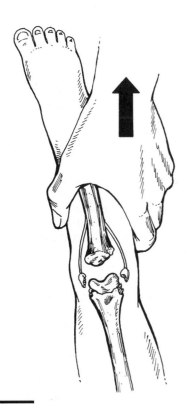

Figure 2.1.   Metaphyseal corner fracture. Adapted from Deltoff M. Non-accidental pediatric trauma: radiographic findings in the abused child. J Can Chiro Assoc 1994; 38:100.

of trauma to the extremities and skull, reported six cases of spinal trauma and one case with associated spinal cord injury in children 2 years of age and younger (51). The specific spinal abnormality in four of those cases consisted of intervertebral disk-space narrowing and anterior vertebral notching at the thoracolumbar junction. Two other subjects showed simple vertebral body compression fractures, and there was one fracture-dislocation (51). An important clinical observation was that, in spite of the radiographic evidence of spinal change, symptoms specifically referable to the area were minimal or absent. Further, vertebral notching was also noted in apparently normal, asymptomatic children. Symptoms associated with that type of spinal trauma were either absent or so minimal that they were not brought to the attention of the parents or physician (51). Kleinman and Zito (52), in a survey of 19 abused infants younger than 5 months, reported an incidence of 16% (3 infants) for spinous process avulsion injury (Fig. 2.2).

A more insidious injury results with the shaken impact syndrome (Fig. 2.3), in which intracranial injury and intraocular hemorrhage may exist in the absence of external signs of direct head trauma (53). A high index of suspicion is warranted with every child younger than age 1 who presents with altered consciousness (54). The child victim will usually be younger than 1 year of age (often younger than 6 months), and the caretaker will often give a history of no predisposing event (50%), a minor fall (30%), a seizure (10%), or a respiratory arrest (10%) (54). The reports of a seizure

or altered consciousness are key findings in the history as the custodian often puts the child down to rest after inflicting the injury in the hope they will recover, and during this period, the elevated intracranial pressure leads to seizure or respiratory arrest (54). The violent shaking also tears the delicate blood vessels servicing the eye, resulting in retinal and subconjunctival hemorrhages, detectable through simple observation or by ophthalmoscope.

The cardinal findings of shaken-impact syndrome therefore include (1) an uncertain history or one that seems to be at odds with your physical findings, (2) the new onset of seizures in association with (3) retinal hemorrhages, and (4) intradural hemorrhages seen on the CT scan or MRI (1). Potentially pathogenic whiplash-shaking is practiced commonly in a variety of ways, under a variety of circumstances, by a variety of persons, for a variety of reasons (47).

Secondary symptoms include vomiting, irritability, listlessness, lethargy, bradycardia, apnea, poor feeding response, failure to thrive, and other vague symptoms suggestive of other conditions (55). When shaken impact syndrome is suspected, any ocular findings should be clearly documented. These include orbital and lid ecchymosis, hyphema, anisocoria, disconjugate eye movement, papilledema, sixth-nerve palsy, and retinal detachment as well as subconjunctival hemorrhage, and the classic retinal hemorrhages that are bilateral in most cases (44,55,56). Regrettably, the severity of retinal hemorrhage has a significant correlation with the severity of acute neurological findings (53). These include a decreasing level of consciousness, focal or generalized weakness, seizure activity, head circumference greater than the 90th percentile or bulging fontanelle, and CT findings such as subarachnoid hemorrhage, subdural hematoma, and cerebral oedema (53).

Birth trauma may result in retinal hemorrhages but these should resolve within 1 month of birth. Otherwise, retinal hemorrhage in children younger than age 4 is highly suggestive of the shaken-impact syndrome (55). Similarly, spontaneous subconjunctival hemorrhages are rare in normal, healthy children; however, they too may occur during birth or may be associated with whooping cough, but usually resolve in 2 weeks (57). Subconjunctival hemorrhage may not be suspicious if small, and if not accompanied by other unexplained injuries, and, as opposed to retinal hemorrhage, requires the clinician to rule out a self-inflicted injury, such as a fall by a mobile infant onto a heavy object (57).

In summary, the shaken-impact or whiplash-shake syndrome must be clinically suspected in the presence of retinal hemorrhages, an uncertain or inappropriate history, and the new onset of seizures. The additional presence of new or healing extremity and/or rib fractures appears to be pathonomic for non-accidental injury (1).

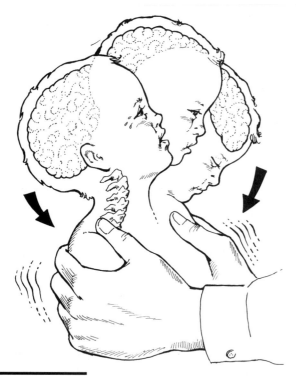

Figure 2.3.   Vigorous shaking produces acceleration/deceleration of the infant's head and spinal column "whiplash injury." Adapted from Coody D, Brown M, Montgomery D, Flynn A, Yetman R. Shaken baby syndrome: identification and prevention for nurse practitioners. J Pediatric Health Care 1994; 8:51.

Clinical Indicators of Abuse and Neglect

Given the published statistics on abuse and neglect (58,59), chiropractic clinicians all over the world are rendering pediatric and family care to both offenders and abused children, without ever being conscious of the fact.

The clinical indicators of abusive and neglectful behavior patterns fall into three categories: physical, behavioral, and non-specific. These indicators vary according to the form of maltreatment the child is suffering. Parents of abused children tend to use a different health practitioner each time to prevent a "paper trail" of charts on the child.

Physical Abuse

Physical abuse will most likely be identified by the clinician on examination, but there are also some behavioral indicators.

PHYSICAL INDICATORS

- Bruises on areas of the body not usually subject to trauma (i.e., thighs, back, torso). The bruises may have the shape of an instrument and be in various stages of healing, thus indicating ongoing, multiple event trauma. The parent or guardian usually provides an inappropriate history to explain the trauma, such as "he fell off a swing" or "she ran into a tree in the park."
- Fractures to the skull, face, and spine with a disproportionate explanation. Any fracture to this area in a child younger than 2 years of age should seriously raise the index of suspicion for physical abuse.
- Pattern-shaped burns. The sort of patterns seen include burns from cigarettes and electric hot plates or irons, and sock or glove-like shapes from immersion in hot water.

BEHAVIORAL INDICATORS

The clinician should consider the possibility of physical abuse if a child:

- Says someone has injured or hurt them;
- Offers an explanation at history that is inconsistent with the injury sustained;
- Displays behavioral extremes, either very aggressive or withdrawn;
- Appears afraid of parents or guardians. Close observation of the dynamics of this relationship should be made during the history and physical examination;
- Appears to express no emotion in what would normally be a frightening situation to a child;
- Expresses either a fear to go home, or wants to stay away from the home. In particular, the child may be hesitant to leave the clinic.

Emotional Abuse

There is seldom any physical evidence on a child who is being victimized by emotional abuse. The behavioral signs are often subtle and therefore in need of careful probing during the history taking before any conclusions can be drawn. The following are significant (60).

BEHAVIORAL INDICATORS

Low self-esteem

Sudden onset of pathophysiological conditions such as asthma, constipation, secondary enuresis, and others

Behavioral changes such as passivity, excessive compliance, fearfulness, aggression, being demanding and assertive, apathy

Depression and/or extreme anxiety

Poor social and interpersonal skills

Developmental delays

Persistent habit disorders such as sucking, biting, and rocking

Sudden change in temperament

Self-destructive behavior

Unexplained poor academic achievement

Sexual Abuse

The following indicators are not always obvious, and one should explore them in a fairly oblique way if they are being hinted at or inadvertently suggested. Importantly, if a child tells you what happened, you must believe them, as children do not lie about such experiences.

PHYSICAL INDICATORS

- Irritation or infection of the genital area
- Inadequately explained trauma to the anogenital area
- Persistent vaginal discharge
- Pregnancy in young adolescents
- Difficulty walking
- Recurrent urinary tract infections

BEHAVIORAL INDICATORS

- Preoccupation with symptoms based around the anogenital region (24)
- Excessive and inappropriate sexual activity in young children, including activities such as masturbation with an object, rubbing genitals against adults, or game playing echoing a sexual event
- Sexual knowledge or behavior inappropriate for the child's developmental age
- Fear of having the diaper or nappy changed, or of being bathed
- Sudden avoidance of familiar adults or places
- Delinquent and aggressive behavior in adolescence
- Regressive behavior, such as the onset of secondary bedwetting or speech loss
- Sleep disturbances and "night terrors"
- Depression or suicidal behavior or attempts at suicide
- Drug or alcohol abuse (61)
- Prostitution or sexual promiscuity (62)

The following signs and symptoms may be in evidence during history taking and should, when interpreted in conjunction with a pattern of physical and/or behavioral signs, alert the clinician to the possibility of sexual abuse. These include the following.

NON-SPECIFIC INDICATORS

- Sudden change in behavior or temperament
- Sleep disorders
- Constant complaint of headache and/or abdominal pain
- Difficulties at school or a sudden change of performance at school
- Serious difficulties relating to peers or adults
- Self-destructive behaviors
- Persistent habit disorders such as sucking, biting, and rocking
- Excessive concerns about physical privacy
- Reluctance to go home from school, your clinic, or other regularly attended places

The clinician should look for a pattern of indicators rather than individual indicators, particularly in the behavioral area.

Neglect

Physical and sexual abuse is a very definable, identifiable, and dramatic phenomenon (64). Neglect, however, while it may prove fatal, is typically insidious, chronic, and private. In Australia, the entries made into the Victorian Children At Risk Register are identified into one or more of seven categories of neglectful abuse, as follows:

1. Abandonment/desertion. The child is left destitute or without adequate support.
2. Medical neglect. The lack of adequate medical or dental treatment. There is no direct reference to mental health conditions.
3. Environment neglect. Unhygienic and unsafe living conditions.
4. Failure to provide adequate clothing. Lack of minimum clothing to protect the child from the elements.
5. Failure to ensure safety. The placing of a child in a situation in which there is no or insufficient adult supervision to protect the child from real and significant risk and harm.
6. Failure to provide adequate food/fluid. Lack of food or fluids adequate to sustain normal functioning.
7. Failure to thrive (inorganic). Failure to thrive is presented as a likely harmful outcome as a result of neglect, whereas the other subtypes are presented primarily as parental or caretaker omissions. Failure to thrive is directly associated in this type with failure to provide

food/fluid partly or entirely as a result of underlying interactive concerns, which contribute to the failure to thrive syndrome (65).

Evidence of neglectful abuse are diffuse and in many instances non-specific in nature. The clinician needs to carefully consider the "sum total" of the evidence before reaching a conclusion that neglect is occurring (65).

Knowledge of the child in question, their family circumstances, and experience in practice will aid in coming to the conclusion that a particular child has become the subject of abuse by neglect. The principal signs are as follows.

PHYSICAL INDICATORS

- Constant hunger
- Failure to thrive or malnutrition
- Lack of subcutaneous tissue
- Poor hygiene that may result in health problems or ostracism by peers
- Inappropriate dress for the climatic conditions
- Consistent lack of supervision, especially in dangerous activities or for long periods
- Unattended physical problems or medical needs
- Abandonment
- Health or dietary practices that endanger health development, such as fad diets

BEHAVIORAL INDICATORS

- Stealing food
- Extending days at school
- Constant fatigue, listlessness, or falling asleep in class
- Alcohol or drug abuse
- Statements from the child that there is no caregiver
- Aggressive or inappropriate behavior
- Isolation from peer group
- Prolonged absenteeism or school refusal

Techniques for History Taking

There is no substitute in clinical practice for a thorough and sound knowledge base. All health care providers who deal with children should be aware of the clinical indicators of child maltreatment. Abused children often present with behavioral dysfunctions; therefore, any physical signs or symptoms should be checked for consistency and probability against the explanation offered by the historian.

An awareness of family background is most helpful. One should obtain as much family/social history as possible in a tactful, non-threatening manner. Accurate, dated documentation is of the utmost importance, particularly if the case becomes a legal matter. Documentation should include relevant data with your impression of:

- Clinical symptoms
- Developmental status
- Emotional state of the child

The use of drawings or if possible, photographs and radiographs, is a valuable addition to clinical notes.

When talking to a child about what is happening, use a very gentle and reassuring manner because you might be the first person the child has ever told. Despite how difficult it may be for you to believe what is being said, particularly if you know the family, remain calm and detached, accepting at face value what the child is saying. Children rarely lie about abuse.

When abuse is disclosed, never blame the child or cause them to feel pressured for information. Remember, it is not the role of clinicians to prove that abuse is occurring, but only to recognize it and initiate intervention that will benefit the child. Inform the child that you are going to make an appropriate report to help stop the abuse.

A Raised "Index of Suspicion"

During a patient consultation, the following may raise your "index of suspicion" of the possibility of abuse and thus cause you to look carefully into the case, framing questions within the parameters of the known signs and symptoms of child abuse:

- Direct disclosure of abuse by the child. Remember, children rarely lie about such matters. Allow the child to tell you whatever details they want without feeling pressured
- Someone other than the child tells you of the abuse
- Statements like "I know of someone who is being abused" often mean the person telling you may be the one being abused
- Your impression of the child's behavior or the nature of injuries being inconsistent if you have prior knowledge of the family background
- Significant change in the demeanor of the child, particularly from being temperamentally sanguine to introverted or shy
- Symptoms such as secondary enuresis, encopresis, constipation, or recurrent abdominal pain suddenly appear
- An infant with failure to thrive syndrome who has evidence of hygienic neglect, rampant skin conditions, thin extremities, narrow face, prominent ribs or gluteal atrophy
- Flattened occiput, which may indicate a child who has been left unattended for long periods
- Marks on the body at examination not adequately explained by the caregiver

Initiating Intervention

As stated earlier, intervention will to some extent be community specific and related to the degree to which facilities exist to cope with an abusive situation. It is your responsibility as a primary health care provider to be fully aware of both your legal responsibility and the mechanisms that exist to initiate intervention in cases of suspected abuse in the jurisdiction in which you practice. However, whether or not the reporting of child abuse is mandatory in your jurisdiction, all clinicians have a moral obligation to do so to protect the child from further abuse. You must ultimately be prepared to testify at any subsequent hearing into claims of maltreatment (66).

The overriding principle for the chiropractic clinician is recognition that maltreatment exists, followed by referral to the appropriate agency. This will only be possible in the first instance when the abuse has been frankly admitted. In the majority of instances, you will be in the position of suspecting maltreatment and therefore in need of protocols to effect the appropriate referral. The protocols that have been suggested for use in Australia are to recommend in a concerned manner to the parents that the condition their child has is "perplexing" and needs further, more expert diagnosis at a children's hospital. Great care should be taken to not alert the parents to your suspicions, but instead to give the deliberate impression that the child needs immediate, further expert attention.

An appointment should be arranged by telephone in the presence of the parents and a statement like "please let me know how you get on" is made to them as they leave your clinic to confirm the impression of concern for the child's condition. After the parents leave, the hospital should again be called and the admitting officer informed of the reasons why abuse is suspected. This procedure will ensure that the child is protected and placed into the system at the most effective level from the outset.

In the event that the abuse is either obvious or has been admitted during your consultation, the parents should be asked to voluntarily enter a program provided by a local government authority. If they refuse, a report should be made to either the police or a child protection authority, who will take immediate action.

Because of the distressing circumstances necessarily surrounding a case of child abuse, chiropractic care should be offered to all those affected by the situation once proper "agency management" has commenced. Not only the child, but the immediate relatives and loved ones may be adversely affected by an episode of abuse and thus could benefit from the application of chiropractic care for the resulting stress-related spinal problems.

Chiropractors as Primary Health Care Providers

While the great majority of children who attend your office for treatment, or attend while their parents or caregiver are treated, will be well loved and cared for, it is an unfortunate fact that some will be the object of abusive or neglectful behavior.

The role of the chiropractor at the doctor-patient interface is one of recognition of maltreatment and initiation of intervention. To be maximally effective in this role, the chiropractic clinician must be fully conversant with the physical, behavioral and clinically non-specific signs that may signify an underlying problem of abuse or neglect when such an admission by the caregiver is not forthcoming. Because much of the evidence of abuse and neglect will only be detected by a careful and thoughtful clinical history, the continuing development of professional skills in this area cannot be overemphasized. Further, an appreciation of the many myths that permeate the abuse and neglect spectrum is most important for information given by a child to be accurately interpreted.

In addition to recognition, a functional and effective model for initiating the intervention process must be developed. While some very worthwhile generalizations have been made in this chapter, models of intervention are, by necessity, specific to the jurisdiction of your practice. It is your responsibility, as a primary health care practitioner, to be aware of these strategies and facilities as they exist in the area in which you practice.

The typical response of a practitioner to the issue of maltreatment is a heightened awareness for signs and symptoms among their adolescent, child, and neonatal patients. The greater challenge comes from the realization that many adult patients may well carry a secret history of childhood maltreatment, and, in fact, every chiropractor will consult with a female patient who is a survivor of child sexual abuse, with reported incidences ranging from 8–10% of Swedish women (67) to 26% of American women (15).

Some two-thirds of a sample of 535 young women from the state of Washington who became pregnant as adolescents had been sexually abused (and in many cases, physically abused as well) (68), and a study of 668 middle class females in a gynecologic practice, which investigated the long-term health effects of physical, sexual, and emotional abuse during childhood, found half (53%) of the sample reported some form of childhood abuse. Although 28.9% reported exposure to one type of abuse, a smaller proportion (5.4%) reported being exposed to all three kinds of abuse (69).

Further, given the results of one study that found female survivors of child sexual abuse are more likely to report multisystemic medical complaints than nonabused patients (15) and another that found that women who experienced violent sexual abuse were almost four and one half times more likely to report high depressive symptoms (70), there would reasonably be an expectation to obtain a thorough sexual history when working with women's health or when a female patient has multisystemic complaints. The sad irony is that the greater the number of childhood abuses, the poorer one's adult health and the more likely one is to experience abuse as an adult (69). However, the perpetuation of the maltreatment habit is worse. A study of 352 pregnant teenagers found that 7% reported use of illicit substances after conception was confirmed (71).

The rule of thumb for clinical practice is to ensure that a thorough and complete examination is made of every young patient for whom a suspicion of maltreatment exists. Of a total of 5181 children brought to a health agency for evaluation before placement into foster care, 44% had some medical problem, including anemia, otitis media, sexually transmitted diseases, and lead poisoning (72).

Several guidelines stem from the realization that, among one's patient base, there will be a number of patients with a positive history of maltreatment and abuse. When dealing with a patient one suspects may have such a history, the guidelines, as explained to the chiropractic profession by Gier (4), are: (1) approach the patient with slow, gentle movements, avoiding all quick and abrupt moves; (2) explain what you will be doing in the form of manipulation; and (3) be especially sensitive when examining and treating vulnerable areas such as the neck, chest, and face.

Chiropractors are well placed within the primary health care arena to detect and identify victims of non-accidental injury and maltreatment and to initiate intervention for the benefit of the child. To do so can only be seen as a privilege of clinical practice.

REFERENCES

1. Luerssen TG, Bruce DA, Humphreys RP. Position statement on identifying the infant with non accidental central nervous system injury (the whiplash-shake syndrome). Pediatric Neurosurg 1993; Jul/Aug:170.
2. Nash EM. Child abuse: recognizing and reporting. ICA Int Rev Chiropr 1990;Mar/Apr:19-23.
3. Stierwalt DD. Child abuse and the chiropractor. Dig Chiropr Economics 1976;Jul/Aug:138.
4. Gier JL. Recognizing and treating the abuse victim. J Am Chiropr Assoc 1987; Apr:39-41.
5. Davies NJ. Recognising the abuse and at-risk child. Chiropr J Aust 1992; 22:27-30.
6. Christoffel KK. Violent death and injury in US children and adolescents. AJDC 1990;144:697-706.
7. Finkelhor D, Dziuba-Leatherman J. Victimization of children. Am Psychol 1994; 49(3):173-83.
8. Richters JE, Martinez P. The NIMH community violence project: I. Children as victims of and witnesses to violence. Psychiatry 1993; 56(1):7-21.
9. Australian Institute of Health and Welfare. Child abuse and neglect 1991-92. Austral Health Rev 1994; 17(2):120-1.
10. McClain PW, Sacks JJ, Froehlke RG, Ewigman BG. Estimates of fatal child abuse and neglect, United States, 1979 through 1988. Pediatrics 1993; 91:338-43.
11. Wolfner GD, Gelles RJ. A profile of violence toward children: a national study. Child Abuse Negl 1993; 17(2):197-212.
12. Pieterse JJ, Van Urk H. Maltreatment of children in The Netherlands: an update after 10 years. Child Abuse Negl 1989; 13:263-9.
13. Hernandez JT, Lodico M, DiClemente RJ. The effects of child abuse and race on risk-taking in male adolescents. J Natl Med Assoc 1993; 85:593-7.
14. Dembo R, Williams L, Wothke W, Schmeidler J, Brown CH. The role of family factors, physical abuse, and sexual victimization experiences in high-risk youths' alcohol and other drug use and delinquency: a longitudinal model. Violence Vict 1992; 7:245-66.
15. Lechner ME, Vogel ME, Garcia-Shelton LM, Leichter JL, Steibel KR. Self-reported medical problems of adult female survivors of childhood sexual abuse. J Fam Pract 1993; 36:633-8.
16. Muenzenmaier K, Meyer I, Struening E, Ferber J. Childhood abuse and neglect among women outpatients with chronic mental illness. Hosp Community Psychiatry 1993; 44:666-70.
17. Deykin EY, Buka SL. Suicidal ideation and attempts among chemically dependent adolescents. Am J Publ Health 1994; 84:643-9.
18. Miranda C. Tasmania nation's suicide leader. The Mercury. Hobart: Tasmania. 1994: Oct 12: 10(col 4-6).
19. Prismall B. Help line to be manned every day. The Examiner. Launceston, Tasmania. 1994: Sep 3: 3(col 5,6).
20. Stone N. Parental abuse as a precursor to childhood onset depression and suicidality. Child Psychiatry Hum Dev 1993; 24(1):13-24.
21. Salzman JP, Salzman C, Wolfson AN, Albanese M, Looper J, Ostacher M, Schwartz J, Chinman G, Land W, Miyawaki E. Association between borderline personality structure and history of childhood abuse in adult volunteers. Compr Psychiatry 1993; 34:254-7.
22. Van Hasselt VB, Ammerman RT, Glancy LJ, Bukstein OG. Maltreatment in psychiatrically hospitalized dually diagnosed adolescent substance abusers. J Am Acad Child Adolesc Psychiatry 1992; 31:868-74.

23. Altieri MF. Child abuse. When to be suspicious and what to do then. Postgrad Med 1990; 87(2):153-6, 161-2.
24. Task force on child abuse. Adelaide, Australia. South Australian Police Force, 1989.
25. Garbarino J. Psychological child maltreatment, a developmental view. Prim Care 1993; 20:307-15.
26. Jones ED, McCurdy K. The links between types of maltreatment and demographic characteristics of children. Child Abuse Negl 1992; 16:201-15.
27. Carrotte PV. An unusual case of child abuse. Br Dent J 1990; 168:444-5.
28. Young WC. Sadistic ritual abuse. An overview in detection and management. Prim Care 1993; 20:447-58.
29. Indredavik MS, Skranes J, Skranes J, Sundt NP. Assistance work in Romania. A multidisciplinary study of institutionalised children. Tidsskr Nor Laegeforen. 1991; 111:2109-13.
30. Rosenthal JA, Motz JK, Edmonson DA, Groze V. A descriptive study of abuse and neglect in out-of-home placement. Child Abuse Negl 1991; 15:249-60.
31. Ojanuga DN. Kaduna beggar children: a study of child abuse and neglect in northern Nigeria. Child Welfare 1990; 69:371-80.
32. Guyer B, Lescohier I, Gallagher SS, Hausman A, Azzara CV. Intentional injuries among children and adolescents in Massachusetts. N Engl J Med 1989; 321: 1584-9.
33. Roscoe B. Defining child maltreatment: ratings of parental behaviors. Adolescence 1990; XXV(99):517-28.
34. Sariola H, Uutela A. The prevalence and context of family violence against children in Finland. Child Abuse Negl 1992; 16:823-32.
35. Muram D. Child sexual abuse. Curr Opin Obstet Gynecol 1993; 5:784-90.
36. Christoffel KK. Intentional injuries: homicide and violence. In: Pless IB. ed. The epidemiology of childhood disorders. New York. Oxford University Press 1994:392-411.
37. Barton K, Baglio C. The nature of stress in child-abusing families: a factor analytic study. Psychol Rep 1993; 73(3 Pt 1):1047-55.
38. Prakken AB, Veenhuizen L, Bruin MC, Waelkens JJ, can Dijken PJ. Vitamin B12 deficiency due to abnormal eating habits. Ned Tijdschr Geneeskd 1994; 138:474-6.
39. Merten DF, Carpenter BL. Radiologic imaging of inflicted injury in the child abuse syndrome. Pediatr Clin North Am 1990; 37(4):815-37.
40. da Fonseca MA, Feigal RJ, ten Bensel RW. Dental aspects of 1248 cases of child maltreatment on file at a major county hospital. Pediatr Dent 1992; 14:152-7.
41. Leavitt EB, Pincus RL, Bukachevsky R. Otolaryngologic manifestations of child abuse. Arch Otolaryngol Head Neck Surg 1992; 118:629-31.
42. Deltoff M. Non-accidental pediatric trauma: radiographic findings in the abused child. J Canadian Chiropr Assoc 1994; 38:98-105.
43. Leventhal JM, Thomas SA, Rosenfield NS, Markowitz RI. Fractures in young children. AJDC 1993; 147:87-92.
44. Brown JK, Minns RA. Non-accidental head injury, with particular reference to whiplash shaking injury and medico-legal aspects. Dev Med Child Neurology 1993; 35:849-69.
45. Oestreich AE. Imaging of the skeleton and soft tissues in children. Curr Opin Radiol 1992; 4(6):55-61.
46. Beals RK, Tufts E. Fractured femur in infancy: the role of child abuse. J Pediatr Orthop 1983; 3:583-6.
47. Caffey J. On the theory and practice of shaking infants. AJDC 1972; 124:161-69.
48. Garcia VF, Gotschall CS, Eichelberger MR, Bowman LM. Rib fractures in children: a marker of severe trauma. J Trauma 1990; 30:695-70.
49. Goldstein B, Kelly MM, Bruton D, Cox C. Inflicted versus accidental head injury in critically injured children. Crit Care Med 1993; 21:1328-32.
50. Crawford AH. Operative treatment of spine fractures in children. Orthop Clin North Am 1990; 21:325-39.
51. Swischuk LE. Spine and spinal cord trauma in the battered child syndrome. Radiology 1969; 92:733-8.
52. Kleinman PK, Zito JL. Avulsion of the spinous processes caused by infant abuse. Radiology 1984; 151:389-391.
53. Wilkinson WS, Han DP, Rappley MD, Owings CL. Retinal hemorrhage predicts neurologic injury in the shaken baby syndrome. Arch Ophthalmol 1989; 107: 1472-74.
54. Bruce DA, Zimmerman RA. Shaken impact syndrome. Pediatric Ann 1989;18(8): 482-94.
55. Coody D, Brown M, Montgomery D, Flynn A, Yetman R. Shaken baby syndrome: identification and prevention for the nurse practitioner. J Pediatr Health Care 1994; 8:50-6.
56. Munger CE, Peiffer RL, Bouldin TW, Kylstra JA, Thompson RL. Ocular and associated neuropathologic observations in suspected whiplash shaken infant syndrome. Am J Forensic Med Pathol 1993; 14:193-200.
57. Rose SJ. Recognition of child abuse and neglect. London: Gower Medical Publishing, 1985.
58. Dwyer K, Strang H. Violence against children. Series title: Violence Today. Australian Institute of Criminology. Woden, 1989.
59. Young L, Brooks R. The profile of child abuse and neglect in NSW. Sydney, New South Wales Department of Family and Community Services, 1989.
60. Nelson WE. Nelson Textbook of Pediatrics. 13th Ed. Philadelphia. WB Saunders, 1987.
61. Oates K. Sexual abuse of children. Australian Family Physician 1986; 15:786.
62. Child Protection Unit: Preventing and reporting child abuse Adelaide. South Australian Department of Community Welfare, 1990:14-5.
63. Abel G, Mittelman M, Becker JV, Cunningham-Rathner J, Wcas I. The characteristics of men who molest children. Presented to World Congress of Behaviour Therapy. Washington DC, 1983.
64. Polansky NA, Gavdin JM, Ammons PM, Davis KB. The psychological ecology of the neglectful mother. Child Abuse Negl 1978; 9:265-75.
65. Helfer RE. The neglect of our children. Pediatr Clin North Am 1990; 37:923-42.
66. Halverson KC, Elliott BA, Rubin MS, Chadwick DL. Legal considerations in cases of child abuse. Prim Care 1993; 20:407-16.
67. Bengtsson O. Child and adolescent psychiatry and child abuse. Arctic Med Res 1994; 53 Suppl 1:57-62.
68. Boyer D, Fine D. Sexual abuse as a factor in adolescent pregnancy and child maltreatment. Fam Plan Perspect 1992; 24(1): -11, 19.
69. Moeller TP, Bachmann GA, Moeller JR. The combined effects of physical, sexual, and emotional abuse during childhood: long-term health consequences for women. Child Abuse Negl 1993; 17:623-40.
70. Hall LA, Sachs B, Rayens MK, Lutenbacher M. Childhood physical and sexual abuse: their relationship with depressive symptoms in adulthood. Image J Nurs Sch 1993; 25:317-23.
71. Bayatpour M, Wells RD, Holford S. Physical and sexual abuse as predictors of substance use and suicide among pregnant teenagers. J Adolesc Health 1992; 13(2):128-32.
72. Flaherty EG, Weiss H. Medical evaluation of abused and neglected children. Am J Dis Child 1990; 144:330-4.

3 Vaccination Issues

Ronald Lanfranchi, Joel Alcantara, and Gregory Plaugher

The topic of vaccination is controversial and sensitive (1,2). Our impetus in writing this chapter and addressing these issues, was in part motivated by a study by Fitzgerald and Glotzer (3). They undertook a study to assess the informational needs of parents regarding childhood immunizations and their satisfaction with the vaccine information pamphlets (VIPs). The VIPs were developed to satisfy a Congress mandated program that each child's legal representative receive an informational brochure to communicate 10 specific points regarding vaccination. These points are as follows:

1. Frequency, severity, and potential long-term effects of the disease to be prevented by the vaccine

2. Symptoms or reactions to the vaccine that, if they occur, should be brought to the immediate attention of the health care provider

3. Precautionary measures legal representatives should take to reduce the risk of any major adverse reactions to the vaccine that may occur

4. Early warning signs or symptoms as possible precursors to such major adverse reactions to which the legal representative should be informed

5. Description of the manner in which legal representatives should monitor such adverse reactions, including a form on which reactions can be recorded to assist legal representatives in reporting information to appropriate authorities

6. Specification of when, how, and to whom legal representatives should report any major adverse reaction

7. Contraindications to (and bases for delay of) the administration of the vaccine

8. Identification of the groups, categories, of characteristics of potential vaccine recipients who may be at significantly higher risk of major adverse reaction to the vaccine

9. Summary of:
   a) Relevant federal recommendation concerning a complete schedule of childhood immunizations
   b) Availability of the program

10. Other relevant information as determined by the secretary (3)

The VIPs were a component of the National Vaccine Injury Compensation Program, established by Congress in 1986. Of 227 parents or guardians surveyed, given the open-ended question: "What information do you want to be given before giving permission for your child to receive their 'shots'?," the majority of the respondents indicated they would like information about side effects. The other top responses included the purpose of the vaccine and the safety/risk of vaccination. The study was performed at three different sites and the majority of respondents in all three sites also indicated as "very important" the following: to receive information regarding the disease for which the immunization is given; the common side effects, the rare, serious side effects; and the contraindications to vaccination.

Measles Virology

The measles virus belongs to the paramyxovirus group of the morbillivirus genus. It is considered a large virus with pleomorphic and spherical morphology composed of an outer lipoprotein envelope and an internal helical nucleocapsid composed of RNA and protein. The RNA genome is a negative-sense single-strand RNA, and the virus replicates via an RNA-dependent RNA polymerase. The genome of the Edmonston strain encodes for six major structural proteins.

Two types of transmembrane proteins are found in the envelope; the hemagglutinin protein (H) and the fusion (F) protein. An M protein is found on the inner surface of the virion envelope and functions for the successful generation of new viral particles (4).

Clinical Features

Measles infection in a compromised host results in an acute, febrile, and exanthematous illness. The primary site of infection is the respiratory epithelium of the nasopharynx. Transmission of the virus occurs via respiratory secretions and the virus undergoes multiplication in the epithelium and lymphatic tissue of the upper respiratory tract. During the multiplicative phase, the virus disseminates to the various lymphoid tissues after viremia. After incubation for a period of 10-12 days, viral replication in the upper respiratory tract occurs, resulting in the prodromal symptoms characterized by coryza, conjunctivitis, dry cough, sore throat, headache, low grade fever, and enanthem or Koplik spots (bluish-white spots on a red background). Towards the end of the prodromal stage, a second viremic phase occurs with the virus disseminating to the skin and lymphoid tissue. This results in the characteristic maculopapular rash associated with the measles. The rash is initially maculopapular but becomes confluent and disappears within 5-7 days in order of appearance. Substantial quantities of the virus are shed in respiratory secretions, tears, and urine during the prodromal stage before any symptoms appear and the diagnosis of measles may be made from cell cultures of the virus. However, this is often difficult and more conventional diagnosis of measles involves assays for the measles antibodies such as complement fixation, immunofluorescence, neutralization, hemagglutination inhibition and last but most popularly used, enzyme immunoassays that are commercially available (5,6).

Measles Vaccine

Currently, the measles vaccine in the United States is the live attenuated measles vaccine called Moraten. Since licensing in 1971, the measles vaccine is administered as a trivalent vaccine along with the mumps and rubella vaccine. Moraten, along with measles vaccines used worldwide were derived from the Edmonston strain. Attenuation and derivation of the vaccine strains involve the multiple passages of the virus through foreign host cell cultures (i.e., chick embryo cells, human diploid cells) and different incubation temperatures. Other measles vaccines are developed from strains isolated from Russia (vaccine Leningrad-16), China (vaccine Shanghai 191), and Japan (vaccine CAM-70).

Success and Failures of Measles Control

EFFICACY

According to the medical community, the efficacy of the measles vaccine has been demonstrated within the United States and around the world by the decrease in incidence of the disease. Serious childhood diseases such as measles have either been eradicated or have become negligible disease entities as a result of massive immunization programs and routine immunizations of infants and children.

The World Health Organization's (WHO) Expanded Program on Immunization (EPI) had a global measles vaccination program to reduce reported measles incidence by 90% and measles mortality by 95% from prevaccination levels by 1995 (7). In developed countries like the United States, enforcement of school vaccination laws (8) have helped to achieve measles eradication. Since 1979, more than 95% of those entering school have histories of receiving the measles vaccine (9). According to some studies (10–11), the measles vaccine is highly effective, and at least 90% or greater of vaccine recipients are protected. No vaccine is 100% effective, and some

proportion of vaccinees (10% or less) will remain susceptible to the disease (12). The incidence of measles in the United States declined from more than 400,000 reported cases annually before vaccination to less than 1% of prevaccinated levels. In 1983, measles elimination appeared close when only 1497 cases were reported (13).

VACCINE FAILURES

After 1983, major outbreaks occurred, especially among highly vaccinated school age populations. Measles cases reached a peak of 6,282 cases in 1986 and more than 14,000 cases in 1989 (14–15). The sustained outbreaks in highly vaccinated populations were attributed primarily to vaccine failures. Vaccine failures can be divided into two major causes; primary, which is due to lack of seroconversion (failure to develop immunity to the vaccine) and secondary, defined as loss of immunity after initial seroconversion (waning immunity). Because seroconversion is rarely checked or established after immunization, it is difficult to distinguish the two causes. Field trial conditions according to some studies show primary failure rates to be less than 5% (11,16,17). According to some authors, secondary vaccine failures do not play a significant role in measles outbreaks (14,18). However, 5% experience seroconversion 10 years after vaccination (19). Cases of secondary vaccine failures have been documented (20–22), and important questions remain unanswered regarding the role and effect of waning immunity as a factor for measles eradication. Questions such as the ability to transmit the virus after secondary vaccine failure and successful revaccination and its sustainability after secondary vaccine failure remain unanswered (22).

In 1978, the Centers for Disease Control (CDC) set out to eradicate measles within 5 years. Although this goal was overly ambitious and not achieved, the incidence of measles decreased by 90% (23). The pattern of reasoning is to eliminate the measles virus like that of smallpox. However, the eradication of measles posed a far more substantial obstacle than did smallpox (24,25). For the 10 years from 1979 to 1988, an average of fewer than 4 deaths from measles occurred annually. This trend was altered in 1983 when the number of reported measles cases doubled for all age groups over the next 5 years, and in 1989–1990, the U.S. experienced the worst epidemic of measles in nearly 20 years with more than 46,000 cases by 1991. The measles vaccine efficacy in the 1989–1990 epidemic is similar to those in previous years and indicates that this measles epidemic occurred despite high vaccine effectiveness (26).

Measles outbreaks in the United States include the following reported incidents. Between March 3 and April 18, 1984, an outbreak of measles occurred in a high school in Massachusetts with a documented school immunization level of 98% (12). According to Nkowane et al. (12), vaccine failures may perpetuate an outbreak even in highly vaccinated population, depending on how they are dispersed in the population and the extent of exposure. A case of more than a dozen outbreaks among students in junior and senior high schools occurred despite greater than 95% documented immunization on or after their first birthday. In 1985, at Corpus Christi, Texas, a measles outbreak occurred, even though vaccination requirements were fully enforced for school attendance. According to Gustafson et al. (27), outbreaks occurred even though more than 99% of the students had been vaccinated. From January 4 to May 13, 1985, an outbreak of 137 cases of measles occurred in children in Montana despite a 98.7% vaccination coverage of the students (28). Between January 1 and September 1, 1986, a sustained outbreak of 235 cases of measles-like rash illness occurred in Dade County, Wisconsin (29). The mean age of persons with measles was 13 years. An audit of 13 of the 30 schools where measles occurred showed that more than 96% of the enrolled students had prior measles vaccination. According to Edmonson et al. (29), the paradox of supposedly high measles vaccine efficacy and occurrence of measles outbreak in a highly vaccinated population can be explained in two ways. One, "the measles virus is so contagious, particularly because of airborne spread from point sources that measles elimination will require that both vaccine efficacy and vaccination coverage be higher than previously estimated. Second, cases of measles outbreak must take into account the occurrence of secondary measles vaccine failure (*i.e.,* waning immunity)."

To further define measles epidemiology in the US and explore possible reasons why measles has not been eliminated, Markowitz et al. (14) analyzed outbreaks that occurred in 1985 and 1986. They examined measles outbreaks among preschool-age, school-age and post–school-age persons. A large majority of the outbreaks occurred in school-age children. Outbreaks are attributed to failure to primary and secondary vaccines, but they also challenge the concept of herd immunity. Herd immunity is the resistance of a group to infectious attack by microbes due to immunity by a large proportion of its members. Mathematical modeling asserts that vaccine efficacy of 95 to 97 percent is required to interrupt measles transmission and to prevent outbreaks should the measles virus be introduced to the population. One of the models assumes a contact rate of 14 to 18 persons; that is, an infected person would come into contact with an average of 14 to 18 susceptible people. In school settings, the contact rate may be much higher. Airborne transmission (30), if it is a factor, may also increase the contact rate. An increased contact rate in the mathematical modeling would require higher vaccination levels than that which presently exists. The authors of this chapter question whether this is possible to achieve and question the cost. This also raises the question of the efficacy of herd immunity for vaccination strategies. As Fine and Zell (31) commented, herd immunity thresholds for disease eradication are based on the assumption that immune and susceptible individuals are randomly distributed. However, they assert that vaccines (and hence immune individuals) are not randomly distributed. Also, vaccine failures are not randomly distributed and susceptible individuals may be clustered, isolating them from indirect protection by immune members of the population. Socioeconomics may also be a factor; infection may be introduced into communities with poor nutrition, lack of hygiene, health care, etc. at a higher rate than those in communities with better nutrition and health care.

Measles outbreaks are not exclusive to the United States. An increase in incidence of measles was observed in other well immunized countries such as Canada, the Caribbean, and Central America (32,33). High case mortality rates are seen only in developing countries (34).

In the sub-Saharan Africa, with an immunization rate of 82% in 1987 and 83% in 1988 for children 9-23 months, they experienced periodic epidemics. In 1983, 1986, and 1988, 265, 4522, and 4424 measles cases were reported, respectively.

Antigenic Variability

A potential factor in the resurgence of measles in the United States and globally may be due to antigenic changes in the wild type virus. Several strains of wild type measles viruses have genetic and antigenic variability (35–40).

Tamin et al. (41) performed an analysis of current wild type and vaccine strains of the measles virus and showed that recent strains of wild type had antigenic changes detectable by monoclonal antibodies. The degree of antigenic shift correlated well with predicted amino acid substitutions in the H protein. The study also showed that the new and modified epitopes on the wild type strains are not present in the vaccine strains. Although the wild type strains are currently neutralized by vaccine-induced antibodies, antigenic changes, when combined with waning immunity, may increase infection and transmission within highly vaccinated populations.

Bellini et al. (42) analyzed the genetic sequences of the H, F, and N genes of the Edmonston-derived vaccine strains and vaccine strains derived from independent isolates of the measles virus. Their findings showed that even though the vaccine viruses had a diverse geographic origin and different attenuation procedures, their sequences differed by no more than 0.5–0.6% at the nucleotide levels. The F gene was very stable but the degree of variability was greater in the vaccine strains compared with the wild type. This was attributed to cell culture adaptation and/or attenuation. The N sequences were highly conserved in the vaccine strains and highly variable in the wild types. The H gene was most susceptible to positive selective pressures during cell culture adaptation and/or attenuation in the vaccine strains. Analysis of wild type isolates of their N, H, P and M genes indicate distinct lineage. According to Bellini et al. (42), isolated measles virus strains from the United States contain the greatest number of overall genetic diversity to date. From 1954–1989, the average rate of nucleotide change in the H gene is 0.08% per year, whereas the wild type isolates from 1977–1989, are 0.13% per year. The accelerated rates for the more recent isolates are within an order of magnitude of the rates calculated for the Influenza type A virus, a virus that evolves in response to immunologic pressure (43). Sera from recently infected individuals neutralize the current wild type viruses 4-8 times better than they neutralized the vaccine strains. Again, possible differences may exist between wild type strains of the measles virus and vaccine strains. The wild type may have at least one unique or sufficiently modified region on the H protein that is immunodominant than that in the vaccine strain.

A genetic study by Rota et al. (44) of wild type strains of measles virus isolated from recent epidemics showed that the greatest degree of genetic change were those from the wild type viruses isolated from the United States, Canada, and the United Kingdom. Rota et al. (44) doubt that antigenic drift played a role in the resurgence of measles during the last 5 years, but they do suggest that, "before the widespread use of measles vaccines in the 1960s, measles viruses were genetically homogenous and a single lineage of measles virus may have existed." The vaccine pressure may have driven virus evolution a step forward and at a faster rate. With respect to long term effects, future variants may accumulate enough mutations that vaccine-induced immunity may no longer prevent so-called vaccine-preventable diseases.

Side Effects

Side effects after measles vaccination are fever of 39.4 degrees Celsius or higher in 5–15% of recipients and transient rash (45,46). The fever and rash last 1–2 days and occurs between the 5th and 12th day after vaccination.

In the 1960s, formalin-inactivated measles vaccine were given, and initial reports showed high antibody titer response in immunized individuals. Several years later, these individuals presented with fever, pneumonia with pleural effusions, and severe petechial or hemorrhagic rash that had an atypical distribution over the skin during outbreaks of natural measles. In addition, some of these individuals exhibited an Arthus-type skin lesion when reimmunized with live measles vaccine (47,48).

As stated, the killed measles vaccine was derived from the Edmonston strain. The component antigen was the virus inactivated by formalin and precipitated in alum. Although the vaccine was used for 4 years (1963–1967), it was abandoned when the vaccine provided only short-lived immunity, and vaccinated children developed severe reactions called "atypical measles" (49).

Adverse Reactions

Soon after the administration of the measles vaccine, children began contracting a new form of measles termed, "atypical measles." Three hundred eighty-six Cincinnati children received three doses of the killed measles vaccine. Nine cases of atypical measles were reported. One hundred twenty-five had been exposed to the measles, and the disease developed in 54 children (50). Ten children who had received the killed measles vaccine 5 to 6 years earlier had atypical measles. Pneumonia that resisted all medical treatments developed in 9 of these children (51). Despite these disturbing results, researchers published articles on the benefits of this measles vaccine (52). To this day, it is unknown whether the problem is inherent to the killed measles viruses or due to the vaccine processing (53).

Live attenuated Edmonston–Zagreb (EZ) vaccine, which was developed at the Institute for Immunology in Yugoslavia and produced in human diploid cells (HDC), was suitable for immunization in children before the age of 9 months (54–56). The EZ vaccine was immunogenic at ages 4–6 months in several countries. In 1989, the World Health Organization (WHO) recommended its use in countries where measles was a substantial cause of death before the age of 9 months (57). This recommendation was then reversed after data from three

countries (Guinea-Bissau, Senegal and Haiti) demonstrated increased mortality among children who received the high titer vaccine compared with recipients who received the standard vaccine at 9–10 months of age (58). The EZ vaccine was protecting these children against the measles but they were dying of other diseases (pneumonia, diarrhea, parasitic infections) at a rate of 20% in the years to follow. Researchers cannot explain the excess mortality linked to the EZ and Schwartz vaccines, although they do suspect immune suppression. Compared with children who receive low-titer vaccines, high-titer recipients had a lower percentage of circulating CD4+ lymphocytes and consistently lower mitogen-induced lymphoproliferation and delayed type hypersensitivity (DHT) response (59). Following the reduced survival of recipients of the EZ vaccine in several studies (60–62), WHO recommended that vaccines with a titer of 104-107 plaque-forming units (PFU) should no longer be used in routine immunization programs (63).

Infant mortality caused by vaccines such as the EZ vaccine is an example of just how vaccines in the market place are actually "experimental." It may take years of close clinical observation to uncover an adverse consequence of a particular vaccine, which initially appears beneficial. Is immune suppression vs. immune activation a normal course for viral infections? Scientists know very little about the measles virus (64). A prevailing observation was discovered with the EZ vaccine. The increased mortality did not occur until the second year of life or later, a considerable time after vaccination. A demonstration contrary to the arbitrary "reasonable" time of 24–48 hours allotted by vaccine proponents for an adverse reaction to be causally related to a particular vaccine. An accurate period of post-inoculation should be scientifically demonstrated for the incidence of an adverse effect of a particular vaccine. Without this period being defined, vaccine reporting systems such as the Vaccine Adverse Effects Reporting System (VAERS) will continue to be biased toward underreporting and correspondingly distorted.

Since the licensure of the measles vaccine 25 years ago, the number of measles cases has declined by 98–99% (65). In 1981, the number of reported measles cases annually in the United States averaged 3000. However, frequent periodic outbreaks occurred among the vaccinated population. In 1986, 6282 cases were reported (65). Between 1989 and 1991, 55,000 measles cases and 132 associated deaths occurred (66). In 1989, the Centers for Disease Control received reports in the first 4 months of the year of 56 outbreaks, which accounted for more than a 300% increase in the incidence of measles. Interestingly, more than half of the cases occurred in those older than 10 years of age, with 32% being college students, an abnormal age distribution for the measles (14,67). Only a minority (13%) of the measles cases appeared in unvaccinated people. An increased risk of adverse effects may exist in individuals already immune to measles and/or rubella when they receive additional doses of the antigens (68-70). The long-term efficacy of the vaccine is still in question.

In the first 26 weeks of 1989, 13 States reported at least 100 cases and accounted for 6588 (89.8%) of all reported cases of measles. Again, more than half occurred among the appropriately vaccinated children. In 1985–1986 most of the cases occurred in persons who either had been appropriately vaccinated (60%) or in children not old enough to receive routine vaccination at 15 months of age (27%) (71,72). In 1985 and 1986, 101 outbreaks (67%) primarily occurred among vaccinated school age children. In contrast, only 27% occurred in unvaccinated preschool children (14). Of the 256 students at Maryland State College who were evaluated, 43 (21%) were seronegative for measles alone, 13 (5%) were seronegative to rubella alone, and 5 (2%) were seronegative to both. Among those seronegative to measles, 86% were vaccinated previously (33).

The side effects and adverse reactions of MMR are associated with clinical manifestations in approximately 5–20% of the vaccine's recipients (74). Interestingly, although there are frequent measles outbreaks, many North American physicians have never seen a case of measles (65,75). Failure of the measles vaccine to immunize infants less than 12 months of age correlated serologically with the presence of maternal antibodies in the infant, which interfered with successful vaccination (27). At the time of these studies, most women of childbearing age acquired measles immunity naturally. Consequently, they exhibited a higher antibody titer. In contrast with mass vaccination today, most mothers have acquired measles artificially.

In the United States, the definition of vaccine failure has been expanded to include not only inadequate/waning immunity but also measles vaccination before the 15th month of age (76). The occurrence of measles outbreaks among the vaccinated population have stimulated interest in the mechanism of vaccine failures and the reason for inadequate immunity. Individuals vaccinated with the measles virus despite previous vaccination had a normal capacity to generate a humoral and cellular immune response to the vaccine. Vaccine failure in these individuals was said to be due to the host's inability to generate an enhanced cellular immune response thereby increasing the vaccine recipients' susceptibility to measles infection (77). In areas free from natural measles, antibody levels for MMR are likely to decline with advancing age. Revaccination would be needed to boost decreasing antibody titers (78), unlike natural disease, which confers life-long immunity (12).

Alterations in immune cell function can be detected in most individuals after vaccination (12,79–86). The MMR vaccine will suppress polymorphonuclear neutrophil function (87), the initial defense response of the immune system.

Vaccine-induced immunity is shorter lived than the life-long immunity conferred by natural disease (12,88). This raises the question as to the long-term effects in most of the population of individuals who are without any immunologic contact with the naturally occurring wild-type measles virus, a virus that increases antibody concentrations (89,90). The recommended age for initial measles vaccination has been modified twice in the United States. In 1965, the vaccination age was increased from 9 months to 12 months, and in 1976 it was again increased to 15 months. These alterations were due to persistent maternal antibodies (91,92). Studies have indicated that infants vaccinated at 12 through 14 months of age may have an elevated risk of contracting measles later in childhood (93–96). Are infants more susceptible in recent years

to the measles because of an early decline in maternal antibodies now induced by vaccines rather than natural infection? Do vaccines deplete retinoids and/or other antioxidants thus increasing the risk of autoimmunity? The answers to these questions remain unknown and a reassessment of the measles vaccine is needed (97–98). This discussion illustrates the possibility that vaccination against measles in one generation may open a window of opportunity for infection in infants of the next generation.

One argument against vaccinating against measles is that measles is a mild disease with rarely a serious complication and negligible rate of fatalities in healthy children. More than half of the deaths occur in persons with serious chronic disease or disability (99). The degree of immunity and the length of time of "protection" still remains controversial. On one hand, the efficacy of a single dose of measles vaccine appears to give 90% protection for at least 15 years (100). On the other hand, a properly administered vaccine will, in most cases, provide life-long immunity (101). This is assumed, not confirmed.

Several groups of central nervous system diseases complicate measles virus infection/vaccination (102–104). The first incident of measles and/or mumps causing encephalitis or encephalopathy was a report of 23 cases of neurologic disease after measles vaccination in the United States from January 1965–February 1967, 3 to 24 days post-inoculation. Curiously, it was concluded that, "no single clinical or epidemiological characteristic appears consistent in the reports of cases of possible neurologic sequela of measles vaccine" (105). Eighty-four cases of neurologic disorders occurring within 30 days of vaccination against measles were reported to the CDC over the 9-year period from 1963 to 1971. Fifty-nine patients with extensive neurologic disorders, which included encephalomyelitis, were reported (106). A study based in Canada reported a rate of 1.1 cases of meningitis per 100,000 doses of MMR, a statistically significant finding (107). Several reports of encephalopathy following measles vaccination can be found in the Vaccine Adverse Effects Reporting System between November 1990 and July 1992. Seventeen cases were suggestive of encephalopathy or encephalitis from vaccines (mostly MMR) from age 5 to 16 years of age. Encephalitis is thought to occur in 1 in a million doses of measles vaccine (108).

The Institute of Medicine concluded that there is inadequate evidence to accept or reject a causal relationship between measles or mumps vaccination and encephalitis or encephalopathy (109). We suggest, however, there is a literature base (as discussed above) for the biological correlation between measles vaccine and encephalopathy.

Subacute sclerosing panencephalitis (SSPE) is characterized by a long latent period after infection/vaccination. The clinical manifestations are progressive mental retardation and involuntary movements over several months or years (110–112). Laboratory and epidemiologic studies have linked SSPE to measles infection/vaccination. The first report of SSPE in a patient with a negative history of measles but a positive history of vaccination with live attenuated measles vaccine was reported in 1968 (113). The child received a measles vaccine 3 weeks before the onset of the symptoms and died 18 months postinoculation. Newly diagnosed cases of SSPE occurring in children identified by their medical histories as being vaccinated against measles increased approximately threefold from 1967-1974 (114). SSPE is a recognized sequela of measles infection, and it is biologically plausible that it could occur after administration of the live attenuated vaccine. The Institute of Medicine suggests that the issue is still in question and has concluded that the evidence is inadequate to accept or reject a causal relationship between measles vaccine and SSPE (115).

The National Collaborative Perinatal Project followed nearly 54,000 pregnant women living in 13 cities in the United States, between 1959 and 1966 (132). Among the children born to these women, 2,766 children (19.5%) experienced at least one seizure within the first 7 years of life. Forty children experienced seizures within 2 weeks following immunization. Ten seizures occurred following measles vaccination. After a 7 year follow-up, the study concluded that the children who received the measles vaccine "did well with no (overt) neurologic sequela."

THROMBOCYTOPENIA

Recent data suggest that the MMR vaccine can cause thrombocytopenia purpura. The United States administered an MMR similar to that used in Finland. Finnish researchers discovered 23 cases out of approximately 700,000 children immunized with MMR developed thrombocytopenia purpura in 1992. The children developed thrombocytopenia purpura between 7 and 59 days post-inoculation (117-118). On the basis of the data from Finland and Sweden, the incidence appeared to be in the order of 1:30,000-40,000 vaccinated children. The Institute of Medicine concluded that the evidence establishes a causal relationship between MMR vaccine and thrombocytopenia (119).

Measles and mumps viruses are grown in cell cultures of chicken embryo fibroblasts. Concerns have been acknowledged regarding the safety of egg-derived vaccines in individuals who are sensitive to egg protein since there is an undefined portion of the population who are biologically sensitive to it (116). The suspected correlation between measles and mumps vaccines and anaphylaxis are based on reports following administration of measles, measles-mumps vaccines or MMR (120-125).

In 1981 there were reports of immediate reactions 30 minutes following administration of a live attenuated measles vaccine in three Australian children. Fifteen reports of reactions occurring within 30 minutes of vaccination with the live attenuated measles virus were acknowledged by the Adverse Drug Reaction Advisory Committee in Australia from February 1980 to March 1982 (126). Nine cases of possible anaphylactic reactions were reported in the United States by VAERS between November 1990 and July 1992 following administration of the MMR vaccine (116).

Several citations in the literature describe safe measles vaccines and MMR vaccination in patients with varying degrees (including severe reactions) of allergic symptoms to egg protein (127-128). Skin testing with the MMR vaccine itself has been evaluated. A case series of 140 children with egg hypersensitivity were evaluated. The authors of the study concluded that MMR skin testing was not helpful in predicting an adverse reaction to the MMR vaccine (129). It must be noted that these studies are limited to only Type 1 IgE mediated reactions. The authors did not address the viability of Types II, III and IV hypersensitivity reactions and what effects and/or reactions were plausible. The evidence establishes a causal relation between MMR and death from anaphylaxis or complications of severe thrombocytopenia (130).

In 1989, the measles case fatality rate for admissions to Grouch Base Hospital (GBH) in New Guinea was 17%, the highest level recorded in 20 years. It appears that measles infection changed from being a disease of apparently minor importance to a major killer of children admitted to GBH. Reviewing the history of infectious diseases there is the suggestion that viruses alter their virulence when their environment is altered. Is it possible that the practice of vaccination over the past 25 years has caused the measles virus to mutate? This appears to be a more likely explanation than spontaneously magnified virulence (see Antigenic Variability of Wild type and Vaccine Strains of the Measles Virus above). This would be analogous to bacterial resistance selected for by antibiotic therapy.

Vaccination Recommendations and Contraindications

INFORMED CONSENT

The question as to whether a parent chooses to have his/her child vaccinated is a personal one. Herein lies the controversy since many municipalities/schools require compulsory vaccination. As in any health care procedure or decision, it is our position that informed consent should always be required and that ultimately the parent or legal guardian is the decision maker. Many jurisdictions in the United States allow exemptions to compulsory vaccination for either religious, cultural or scientific reasons (131-134). The parents should be provided information by their health care provider about both the benefits and short and long term risks of any vaccine so that an informed decision could be made. Depending on the attitude of a particular health care provider, the information regarding vaccines and whether to immunize or not can be presented in a negative or positive frame. Positive framing regarding vaccines would emphasize the public health benefits (e.g. reduce risk of disease) while negative framing would emphasize the possible adverse effects. O'Connor et al. (135), found that framing does not influence patient's vaccination decisions, possibly due to the stronger influence of perceived risk and subjective norms. The medical literature frames the vaccination program in a positive light. In order for there to be informed consent, the adverse effects and risks of vaccination should also be provided to the parent/guardian. Shortly after the VIP's were introduced in 1992, there were severe criticisms from the medical community regarding the brochure. The two major concerns were that they were too long and difficult to read in an office setting, and that the cost of the purchase and/or duplication was too significant (136). Another concern against the VIPs was that they presented a barrier to the timely immunization of children (137).

MEDICAL RECOMMENDATIONS

For the parent who chooses the standard recommendation, we offer the following. The rate at which an individual will seroconvert following vaccination depends on the age at which the vaccination is applied. Passively acquired antibodies by newborns such as from breastmilk may interfere with the development of an active immune system. The presence of maternal antibodies persist at different age groups and therefore the optimal seroconversion rates will also vary in different age groups. In the United States, the maternal antibodies have been shown to persist beyond 12 months of age (92). In developing countries, the age of successful seroconversion can be less than 1 year (138). For example, a high-titer Edmonston-Zagreb (EZ) vaccine was shown to be immunogenic in 4 to 6 month old infants (139,140). Based on these findings, the Expanded Programme on Immunization (EPI) of the World Health Organization recommended its use in developing countries where high morbidity and mortality from measles exist in children less than 9 months (141). Subsequent studies suggested however that children receiving high-titer vaccines at an early age compared to those receiving standard titer vaccines at older age groups had a higher mortality. This resulted in the withdrawal of the recommendation for early vaccination (142). In the United States, the Committee of Infectious Diseases of the American Academy of Pediatrics recommend that the MMR vaccine should be administered at 15 months of age and the second dose at 11-12 years (143).

The two-dose schedule was recommended to reduce the number of primary vaccine failures and potentially raise the immunity levels above 95 percent. This strategy is costly. According to Markowitz et al. (14), at a 1989 CDC contact price of $9.19, $35 million more would be required each year for the single-antigen measles vaccine. For a two-dose schedule given at 15 months and the other at school-entry age, a doubly-vaccinated cohort would not be achieved for another 10-14 years. In 10-14 years, one must take into account the possibility that the wild-type virus may mutate and that these future variants are such that vaccine induced immunity may no longer be possible with the present vaccines presently being used.

A study by Cohn et al. (144) was undertaken to assess the antibody responses of measles-seronegative adolescents and young adults after revaccination. They found that only 58% of sample seronegative individuals between the ages of 10 and 30 years developed measles specific antibodies that remained for at least 1 year after revaccination. Approximately 30% developed only a transient response and 12% never developed a positive titer. Vaccine histories were confirmed from the subjects' physicians or from physician-completed records. This study shows that even after the two-dose recommended vaccination schedule, some adolescents and adults still lack protective titers of measles-specific antibody.

Controversies in measles immunization recommendations exist. Three influential groups involved in the prevention, control and eradication of the measles virus are the Immunization Practices Advisory Committee (ACIP) of the US Public Health Service, the Committee on Infectious Dis-

eases of the American Academy of Pediatrics (AAP) and the US Preventive Task Force (USPSTF). Their recommendations for the MMR vaccination for routine circumstances, endemic areas are as follows (145):

Routine:

ACIP: 2 doses of MMR; the 1st at 15 months of age, the 2nd at school age entry

AAP: 2 doses of MMR; 1st at 15 months, 2nd at junior high entry

USPSTF: single dose of MMR at 15 months

Endemic Areas:

ACIP: same as for routine

AAP: 2 doses of MMR; 1st at 12 months, 2nd at 4-6 yrs

USPSTF: 2 doses of vaccine; 1st with monovalent measles at 9 months, 2nd with MMR at 15 months

Post Secondary Institutions:

ACIP: dose of MMR if unable to show proof of vaccination

AAP: same as ACIP

USPSTF: no specific recommendations

VACCINATION CONTRAINDICATIONS

Vaccination should be postponed in individuals suffering from severe febrile illnesses; in persons who have received IG, whole blood or other antibody-containing blood products for 3 months to prevent or avoid possible seroconversion failure; to pregnant women and to people with a history of anaphylactic hypersensitivity to neomycin and eggs; to people with immunosuppressed or compromised immune responses due to illness or medication (14).

Mumps Vaccination

Mumps has classically been considered a disease of children and young adults with the highest incidence in persons between the ages of 5 to 9 years. The disease is more severe in older children and adults and a single attack, clinical or subclinical, confers lifelong immunity. With vaccination, a marked decline in reported cases in all age groups has been observed with an all-time low of 2982 cases reported in 1985. This represents a 98% decline in the disease when compared to that of 1968. In 1986-1987, there was a resurgence with the disease. This affected all groups but more so those in ages 10-19, showing a 7-8 fold increase compared to 1985. Provisional data from 1988 showed an incidence of 1.4 per 100,000 in states with kindergarten to grade law vaccination laws, a 1.0 per 100,000 in states with partial laws and 3.2 per 100,000 in states with no state laws regarding vaccination (146).

Mumps Virology

The mumps virus belongs to the paramyxovirus family. Its genome consists of a negative sense single stranded RNA located in a helical nucleocapsid along with an RNA-dependent RNA polymerase and a nucleoprotein. The virus lipid layer is derived from the host cell wall and contains glycosylated proteins with hemagglutinating and neuraminidase activities and a fusion (F) protein.

CLINICAL FEATURES

Infection in a susceptible host by the mumps virus occurs through the respiratory system either by droplets or droplet-spread from saliva or fomites. The incubation lasts an average of 18 days and the virus replicates in the nasopharyngeal mucosa and regional lymph nodes. The parotid glands are distinctively involved as well as the central nervous system (CNS), the gonads, pancreas, mammary glands, meninges, myocardium, kidneys and other glands.

Parotid gland enlargement is the most commonly recognized manifestation. Mumps is more severe in older children and adults. Epididymo-orchitis is the most common nonsalivary manifestation, present in 15-29 year old males 30-38% of the time (147). Testicular atrophy may occur more commonly unilaterally but sterility rarely results. Meningoencephalitis occurs commonly. CNS involvement results in headache, mental confusion, a stiff neck and CFS lab abnormalities.

Mumps Vaccine

In 1950, a formalin killed vaccine was introduced which was only 80% protective in outbreak situations; it produced short-lived IgG antibodies directed against the hemagglutinating and neuraminidase proteins but not against the fusion protein and required yearly booster shots (148). Mumps virus isolated from a child (Jeryl Lynn B strain) was attenuated by 17 passages through embryonated hens' eggs and 10 passages through chick embryo and was licensed in 1967. The vaccine is given as a trivalent along with measles and rubella vaccines known as the measles-mumps-rubella (MMR) vaccine. After administration of the vaccine, it was shown to produce protective neutralizing antibodies in 97% of children and 93% of adults. The antibody levels are of a lower level and are produced more slowly but have been shown to have efficacy in households and schools at 95%. In other studies, they were shown to have efficacies in the order of 75-91% (149-151).

Success and Failures of Mumps Control

VACCINE EFFICACY

In 1977, the Immunization Practices Advisory Committee (ACIP) recommended the use of the attenuated mumps vaccine along with measles and rubella (MMR) in children after the age of 12 months. A significant decline in the incidence of reported mumps cases hit an all-time low in all age groups in 1985 with 2982 cases—a decline of 98% when compared to cases reported in 1968 (146).

VACCINE FAILURE

In 1986-1987, there was a resurgence of mumps. All age categories were affected but more so the 10-19 age groups

where there was a 7 to 8 fold increase compared to 1985 and the age group with the highest risk shifted from 5-9 years of age to older groups. This shift to an older age group was similar but less marked than what was observed in measles and rubella cases. This raised concerns about the efficacy of the vaccine (146).

SIDE EFFECTS AND ADVERSE REACTIONS

Vaccine side effects have been found to be mild parotitis, fever and rash. The vaccine has been shown to infect the placenta when given to pregnant women (152).

Mumps has been associated with aseptic meningitis. Nottingham (UK) Public Health Laboratories isolated mumps virus from the cerebral spinal fluid (CSF) of eight children following administration of Urabe-containing MMR vaccine (153). Seven of the isolates resembled the vaccine strain (the eighth sample could not be typed). The rate was virologically confirmed and suspected MMR-associated meningitis was calculated to be 1 case per 3,800 doses. The authors of the study also reviewed laboratory records for approximately a 3-year period and determined that there were excess cases of lymphocytic meningitis in the group that was recently vaccinated with MMR compared with those that were not.

In 1989 a nationwide surveillance of neurologic complications after administration of the mumps vaccine was conducted in Japan. This was based on the notification of cases and the testing of the mumps virus isolated from cerebral spinal fluid for their relatedness to the vaccine by nucleotide sequence analysis. Among 630,157 recipients of MMR vaccine containing Urabe Am9 mumps vaccine, there were at least 311 meningitis cases (154).

In 1986, soon after vaccination with MMR in Canada, an increase a number of mumps meningitis cases began to appear. A study at Montreal's Children's Hospital of 4 patients with meningitis that appeared within 19 to 26 days after receiving the Urabe-containing vaccine, mumps virus was isolated from the patients' cerebral spinal fluid. It was confirmed that these patients had no previous contact with any persons contracting with naturally occurring mumps virus (155-156).

Introduction of the vaccination for measles, mumps and rubella in Japan in 1989 coincided with reports of mumps vaccine-associated meningitis (157). There were 35 cases of aseptic meningitis within 8 weeks of vaccination with MMR. The patients had no history of contact with individuals with natural viral mumps infection. An extended nationwide survey of the neurological complications after mumps vaccine administration revealed 311 cases of vaccine-related meningitis among 630 (49%) individuals vaccinated with MMR. There is a strong biological evidence that the mumps virus could cause aseptic meningitis. The incidence appears to be 1 in a few thousand recipients of the Urabe strain (158). In the United States where the Jeryl Lynn strain is used the occurrence of "atypical" mumps has developed. Symptoms include fever, loss of appetite, nausea, malaise and a 24-hour erythematosus papular rash (159). Six schools in Atlantic County, New Jersey reported 63 cases of the mumps (a 40% increase over the previous year). Vaccination compliance was

95% and was given as not the reason for the outbreak. An outbreak in 1983 in the Egg Harbor Township school district in Atlantic City, N.J. represented a 40% increase incidence of the mumps compared with the previous year (160). Nineteen cases of serious neurological sequela possibly associated with the Jeryl Lynn mumps strain was reported in Sweden from 1982-1984 (161). Interestingly, the live virus mumps vaccine was licensed in 1967 but the vaccine's presence took a decade before it was endorsed as a routine vaccine and even then it was slowly accepted. The reason for the vaccine's deferring acceptance was due to the benign nature of mumps as well as the high cost of the vaccine (162). In lieu of its slow acceptance, mumps was on the decline. Since 1986 there has been a resurgence of mumps among middle and high school students (163). As mumps vaccination compliance increased, substantial outbreaks began to occur. Mumps is complicated by orchitis in one-fifth of all cases of mumps occurring in males after puberty (164). It appears that the age distribution of the mumps has been altered from 4 to 10 year-olds to over 10 years of age by the vaccine. Is this a cyclic change or is it possible that the advocates of vaccination, in trying to direct the natural course of the mumps, has transposed a low incidence of orchitis in childhood to a greater incidence in the prepubescent population where these complications are more devastating?

Neurological complications occurring in children vaccinated with Jeryl Lynn or Rubini mumps strains do not appear to occur at a higher frequency compared to those who are unvaccinated (165-166).

A nationwide surveillance of neurological complications after mumps vaccine administration in Japan during 1989 revealed 311 vaccine-related cases of meningitis among the 630,157 vaccines administered (167). The incidence rates of meningitis was reported to be 1 in 2,026. A 7 year-old girl developed unilateral deafness 11 days after receiving MMR vaccine (168-169). Nineteen cases of serious neurological complications possibly associated with the Jeryl Lynn mumps strain were reported in Sweden (170).

Three cases of insulin dependent diabetes mellitus (IDDM) 10 days to 2 weeks after inoculation with a mumps vaccine in a 2, 3 and 16 year old, respectively have been reported (171). One hundred twelve parents of diabetic children in Erie County, New York were interviewed. The parents noted that in 11% of those affected, they had received the mumps vaccine, with a median lag time of 3 years (172).

Vaccination Recommendations

As with the measles vaccine, our stance on informed consent as discussed above remains. For those who choose to vaccinate their child, the first dose of the vaccine is given to children as part of the MMR vaccine schedule. A second dose, as in measles, is recommended. Again, the second dose schedule contains much controversy. The Public Health Service Advisory Committee on Immunization Practices (ACIP) recommends that the vaccine (MMR) should be given prior to school entry. The Committee on Infectious Diseases of the Academy of Pediatrics suggest the second dose schedule at the sixth grade level.

Vaccination Contraindications

Vaccination should be postponed in persons who have received IG, whole blood or other antibody-containing blood products for 3 months to prevent or avoid possible seroconversion failure; to pregnant women and to people with immunosuppressed or compromised immune responses due to illness or medication (122).

Rubella Vaccination

Like mumps, rubella occurs most commonly in 5-9 year olds. Prior to vaccination, it was seen in both epidemic and endemic forms in the United States. Clinical and subclinical entities of rubella confer lifelong immunity to the disease. However, it has been found that chances of reinfection are much greater with vaccine-induced immunity as compared to infection with the wild-type. Rubella can be distinguished into two types, postnatal rubella which is mild and self-limiting and congenital rubella—a more severe, disseminated and chronic disease.

Rubella Virology

The Rubella virus belongs to the genus Rubiviridae of the Togaviridae group of viruses. The virus has an outer envelope as in the measles and mumps virus and a single stranded RNA core.

CLINICAL FEATURES

Rubella is an illness characterized by a nondescript maculopapular rash of short duration of 2-3 days. The incubation period for rubella is 14-25 days, during which time viremia results in the spread of the virus throughout the body. The prodromal stage is characterized by fever, malaise, cervical and occipital lymphadenopathy. During this time and for 1 to 2 days after the rash appears, the virus can be cultured from the blood. There is no pathological lesion characterized by rubella (173-174). The primary concern regarding rubella infection is in the first trimester of pregnancy which carries the highest fetal mortality due to the increased placental transmission of the virus. Congenital rubella syndrome can be manifested by fetal death, deafness, cataracts, cardiac abnormalities, microcephaly, motor defects, thrombocytopenia purpura, hepatosplenomegaly, anemia and low birth weight.

Rubella Control

Over 83 million doses of rubella have been administered since 1969 and there are still periodic upswings in incidence. Essentially, we have controlled the disease in persons 14 years of age and younger but have given a free hand in those 15 or older. The point of the rubella vaccine is not the prevention of rubella but the prevention of "congenital rubella syndrome" (175). Over 1,000 cases of rubella were reported between January and May of 1971 in Casper, Wyoming. This occurred nine months after a rubella vaccination program in which 83% of elementary school children and 52% of pre-school children were inoculated (176).

The persistence of antibodies 10 years after rubella vaccination with three different vaccines in some 5,153 children on the islands of Kauai and Hawaii has been studied. The report demonstrated that within four years, the level of antibodies decreased by one-half as compared to the original levels immediately after vaccine injection (177).

Australian army recruits with confirmed lack of immunity to rubella were given the rubella (Cendevax) vaccine. The population was sent to a camp which had periodic outbreaks of rubella. Three to four months after vaccination, 80% of the men acquired rubella. Another similar trial on an institutionalized population resulted in a similar lack of immunity (178). It appears that the rubella vaccine may afford temporary protection to some but not all individuals vaccinated.

Acute arthralgia and arthritis following vaccination have been documented since the earliest studies of the rubella vaccine (179-182). These acute events have been associated to varying degrees with all rubella vaccine strains and occur more frequently in adult women than in men or prepubertal children of either sex (183). The literature suggests a causal relationship between the currently used rubella vaccine (RA 27/3) and acute arthritis (184).

There have been reports of numerous cases of paresthesia following rubella vaccination (185-187). At this time the Institute of Medicine concludes that there is insufficient evidence to indicate a causal relationship between the currently used rubella vaccine (RA 27/3) and neuropathies (188).

An investigation of vaccine failure in 13 Canadian adults was carried out. Seven of the recipients were partially immunized and six were fully immunized against rubella. These patients had a significant medical history: chronic inflammatory joint syndrome (n=3), recurrent parotiditis (n=1), variable hypogammaglobulinemia (n=1), chronic lymphocytic thyroiditis (n=1) (189).

Two cases of congenital rubella were found after previously presumed maternal immunity, one of which was vaccinated. The authors concluded that the quality of antibody produced in women where seroconversion has occurred after vaccination may be inadequate for total protection compared with natural infection. There were significant differences in rubella specific IgG, IgA and IgM responses on subsequent challenge with rubella vaccine between vaccinated and the naturally immune (190-191).

SIDE EFFECTS FROM VACCINATION

Side effects from vaccination may include fever, rash, and lymphadenopathy as well as depression of platelet count. Optic neuritis, transverse myelitis, arthralgia and arthritis may also be seen, particularly in adult women after vaccination. One group of scientists has isolated rubella virus from children with long standing arthritis long after vaccination (192).

VACCINE RECOMMENDATIONS AND CONTRAINDICATIONS

As discussed previously, for those who choose to have their child vaccinated, the vaccination recommendations and contraindications are generally similar to the measles and mumps vaccine as is our stance on informed consent.

Polio Virology

The viruses that cause polio are classified as enteroviruses belonging to the picornaviridae family. The virion is a 27nm diameter icosohedron structure composed of 60 copies each of the four virion protein subunits—VP1, VP2, VP3 and VP4. Contained within the icosohedral capsid is a single-stranded RNA genome. This RNA is identical with the mRNA except for the presence of a 22 amino acid protein (V Pg) linked to the 5′ end and a polyA tail attached to the 3′ terminus. The three major viral proteins VP1, VP2 and VP3 are surface proteins and are the major viral antigens for the induction of neutralizing antibodies. The VP4 protein appears to be internal and does not function in antibody response. The three-dimensional structure of the antigenic sites on the capsid proteins must be intact in order for a reaction to occur with neutralizing antibodies (193).

Polio Vaccine

There are 3 types of poliomyelitis virus: Types 1, 2 and 3. Each type is capable of infecting humans. There appears to be a lack of cross-immunity; therefore, exposure to Type 1 does not confer immunity to Types 2 and/or 3. The virus enters the body via the nasal/oral route and multiplies within the intestines. Within a week or two, multiplication and excretion of the virus ceases and the episode is over without the child or its parents having noticed any ill effects (194). If the virus passes into the blood and if it reaches the nervous system, a variety of symptoms may occur ranging from headache, fever, non-paralytic and paralytic polio with the most extreme manifestation being death.

Infection from the poliovirus can manifest in several forms: subclinical infection, mild infection, non-paralytic polio and paralytic polio. It is estimated that 4 to 8 percent of all wild-type polio infections result in non-paralytic polio (195). When the viral replication invades the nervous system of the susceptible host and destroys sufficient numbers of neurons, paralysis occurs. This develops in less than 1 percent of all polio cases (196).

Poliomyelitis occurs worldwide, year-round, in the tropics and during the summer and fall in the temperate zones. Winter outbreaks are rare. By far the most common course of a poliovirus infection is a mild and silent episode. Severe paralytic polio is uncommon (197).

Poliovirus survived for many centuries in an endemic manner, infecting a continuous supply of new susceptible infants. In this pattern, women of childbearing age almost universally possessed antibodies to all three types of polio, and passive immunity transferred to the infant. The shift from endemic to an epidemic phase of poliovirus was first seen in societies that had advanced systems of hygiene and sanitation and were located in cooler climates. In the latter part of the 19th century, Northern Europe and the United States began to have epidemics of paralytic polio that became larger, more frequent, and more widely spread. Hence, more people encountered poliovirus for the first time in later childhood/ adulthood, the ages when polio is more likely to take the paralytic form (198–199).

In the United States in early 1954, at about the onset of the inactive polio vaccine, approximately 21,000 cases of paralytic polio were present. In this epidemic scenario, the peak incidence was in children 5 to 9 years of age. One-third of the cases and two-thirds of the deaths were reported in persons older than 15 years (200–202). This pattern differed markedly from what was seen in the 1916 epidemic, in which 80% of the cases were in children younger than 5 years of age (203).

The rarity of reporting of clinical paralytic poliomyelitis from tropical and subtropical areas led many investigators to believe that no polio virus infections were present. However, the reverse was true. Poliovirus was highly endemic, but immunizing exposure occurred early in life, and the majority of the cases were subclinical in nature (204). The administration of vaccines may be displacing the incidence of paralytic polio from infancy (when paralysis is uncommon) to adolescence/adulthood in whom paralysis is more prominent. Because most infections with the polio virus are subclinical, the practice of mass vaccination may be upsetting nature's intent to safely and effectively immunize the infant population against paralytic polio (205).

Inactive oral polio vaccine (IPV) was developed in 1953 by Jonas Salk (206–207). Oral polio vaccine (OPV) was developed by Koprowski et al. (208), and Albert Sabin was the first to use it (209). An enhanced-potency IPV was developed in the late 1970s and is currently used in the United States. IPV and OPV are both available in the United States but the OPV is the vaccine that is recommended.

Polio represents an example of an infectious disease in which the lack of susceptibility to the disease is so widespread that only under particular environmental conditions does it ever assume epidemic proportions. An example is the polio outbreak in Brooklyn where it was impossible to establish contact with a previous case in 469 of 500 cases (93%) (210).

At the University of Michigan, more than 1 million children were inoculated with three doses of the Salk vaccine between May 1 and December 1, 1954. One hundred twenty nine "suspected" cases of poliomyelitis occurred during this period, including 3 weeks after the third and final inoculation. Ninety cases occurred in the vaccinated group and 39 in the placebo group. Of the 90 "suspected" cases occurring during the vaccine trial period, these cases were omitted from the calculations. Of the 749,236 unvaccinated group, 428 developed poliomyelitis. Of the 1,080,680 vaccinated group, 585 developed polio. The incidence as stated is 57/100,000 among the vaccinated and 54/100,000 among the unvaccinated (211).

The association between live polio virus vaccine and associated paralytic polio dates back 60 years to the first live attenuated vaccine tested by Kolmer in 1936. One hundred twenty-three cases classified as paralytic poliomyelitis, which occurred within 30 days after vaccination with OPV were reported to the Centers for Disease Control (CDC) between 1962–1964. The CDC evaluated them and decided 57 cases (47%) were vaccine induced. Fifteen of the cases occurred after receiving Type 1 vaccine, 2 cases occurred after vaccination of Type 2, 36 cases occurred after vaccination with Type 3 vaccine. The remaining four occurred after administration of the trivalent vaccine. Also described were 3 cases of poliomyelitis due to contact with recipients of Type 3 vaccine (212). Sabin's assumption that whether or not the virus was recovered from the central nervous system (CNS) or the stool of the paralytic polio victims did not indicate the vaccine was responsible for the illness. Scientists sided with Sabin as they presented coincidence and highly theoretical explanations for the occurrence of vaccine-induced polio (213).

During the search for the "optimal" strains for vaccine use, Sabin and colleagues found that motor neurons in the spinal cord of humans were more resistant to poliovirus than those of the spinal cords of monkeys. However, the reverse is true for the alimentary tract (214). This finding may support the hypothesis that a virus sufficiently attenuated to prevent neurovirulence in humans may successfully infect the alimentary tract and induce immunity to the wild type polio virus.

From the beginning, experimental trials in humans (215) causing extensive excretion of the virus by the vaccine recipients and the spread of the virus to close contacts has been documented. One important study in 1958 was of families living under normal conditions in Louisiana. Among the 61 persons who were successfully infected, fecal excretion was the most sensitive indicator. Pharyngeal excretion could be detected in 20–30 persons who received a high dose of 107 plaque-forming units (PFU) (216).

All poliovirus strains, regardless of how attenuated, retain the property of multiplying and destroying cells in the monkey spinal cord. The degree to which this property is retained varies over an enormous range as one progresses from virulent strains to the attenuated ones used in vaccines (217).

A critical question arises relating to the progeny of the vaccine virus after it has multiplied in the alimentary tract of humans. Is the virus genetically stable or can it revert to increased virulence? With the obvious recognition of the spread of the polio virus among family contacts with vaccinees, the answer to this question becomes imperative. One hundred twenty three cases of paralytic poliomyelitis occurring in less than 30 days after the administration of the oral polio vaccine have been reported (218).

The oral polio virus (OPV) originated from live attenuated viruses of Types 1, 2, and 3 polio strains grown in Earle's salt solution containing amino acids, antibiotics (streptomycin and neomycin), and calf serum. The virus multiplies in the intestinal tract and may transform back into the more virulent form, causing the actual disease. In addition, the vaccine recipients excrete the live virus in both saliva and feces for 6–8 weeks postinoculation.

The CDC data for the years 1975–1984 revealed the reported incidence of 1 case of vaccine-associated paralytic polio per 3.22 million doses of OPV distributed. When all cases were factored in (including the immunodeficient recipients and contacts with patients), the incidence increased to 1 in 2.64 million doses distributed (219). Although the OPV virus is attenuated, the incidence of paralytic polio is 1/1,000,000 (220).

The concept of "reporting" is significant. The general and chronic under-reporting of infectious disease after the introduction of any vaccine in the United States is well known. The disclosed number of cases of "vaccine failures" on record is not an absolute aggregate since the true sum will be higher than reported. Curiously, the Monitoring System for Adverse Effects Following Immunization (MSAEFI) does not list poliomyelitis as a separate adverse incident, although it may be included in "other neurological symptoms," "other reactions," or "serious events." The reasons for the most feared disease of the 40s and 50s not having its separate incident category and the accuracy of this reporting system are questionable.

Despite intensive study over the century, many basic points of the epidemiology of polio infections remain obscured and unknown. One of the most interesting findings was the significant upward trend in age but no upward trend in incidence occurred between 1910 and 1954 in Northern Europe and the U.S. before mass vaccination began (221).

RISK MODIFIERS

Immune integrity of the recipient or contact of the vaccine recipient modifies the risk of polio as a sequela of the OPV. Typically cited are patients with hypogammaglobulinemia, non-Hodgkin's lymphoma, and agammaglobulinemia (222–224). The aforementioned citations are examples of an apparent clinical immune-compromising condition. It has not been reported or suggested that an undetectable (by current laboratory methods) but significant dysfunction of the immune system may allow a subject to have greater susceptibility to disease.

GUILLAIN BARRÉ SYNDROME

The annual incidence of Guillain Barré Syndrome (GBS) appears to be 1 per 100,000 adults and children younger than 5 years of age. In children older than 5 years of age, it is lower (225). Data from the MSAEFI noted 14 cases of GBS after OPV from 1979–1990. In most of the cases, OPV was given in combination with DTP, MMR, or both. VAERS listed two cases of GBS between November 1990 and July 1992 after administration of OPV in combination with DTP and either MMR or Haemophilus influenza type b vaccine.

An observational study on the incidence of GBS was performed in Uusimaa, Finland. The surveillance of GBS from 1981–1986 uncovered a large incidence of GBS after a nationwide immunization program using IPV. The outbreak of 10 cases of poliomyelitis between August 1984 and January 1985 prompted Finland to carry out a mass vaccination campaign using the OPV with 94% of the population vaccinated between February 10 and March 15. During and shortly after the OPV vaccine campaign, hospitals in the southern province of Uusimma (population 1.17 million) received an unusually high volume of patients with GBS (226).

Shortly after polio vaccine licensing in 1955, the vaccine manufactured by Cutter was found to cause paralytic poliomyelitis. The vaccine contained a residual infectious virus. At the time the dynamics of the viral inactivation process were not fully understood, and the U.S. government's requirement for vaccine production was ambiguous. (227). In lieu of the industry's inexperience with the advent of vaccine manufacturing, mass vaccination continued.

During the course of diphtheria inoculation, which began in 1942, sporadic cases of paralysis were reported after injection. The paralysis had been frequently associated with the limb of the injection site. In a majority of cases, a diagnosis of poliomyelitis was made (228).

Not surprisingly, an American study of similar conjointment discounted any similar association between diphtheria and pertussis inoculation and their possible association to poliomyelitis. However, the authors cautioned against administration of any inoculations during the polio season. In another study, the authors stated that there was a high degree of correlation between the injection site and the site of paralysis for poliomyelitis patients who had received some "antigen" during the month before the onset. Such cases show a different distribution and more severe paralysis (229–230). Seventeen cases of paralysis after diphtheria inoculations occurred in one limb within 28 days of injection. In almost all cases, poliomyelitis was confirmed (231).

The literature establishes a causal relationship between OPV and paralytic poliomyelitis; however, the causal relationship between OPV and GBS remains controversial, and the causal relationship between the polio vaccine and sudden infant death syndrome (SIDS) has been scarcely studied. At this time, the evidence is inadequate to accept or reject a causal relationship between polio and SIDS (232).

Contraindications

Vaccination of children with congenital and acquired immunodeficiency status may decrease vaccine efficacy and increase vaccine-induced side effects, and in people such as an HIV-infected child, may increase the spread of the HIV during the vaccination process. The use of the OPV is contraindicated in children with cellular and humoral immunodeficiency states. The efficacy of IPV in these children is questionable. Vaccination with IPV or OPV is also contraindicated in pregnant patients (193,233–235).

The Present State of Polio Vaccination

On June 20, 1996, the Advisory Committee for Immunization Practices (ACIP) of the CDC revised their proposal for the polio vaccination schedule to two doses of IPV at 2 and 4 months of age, followed by two doses of OPV at 12 to 18 months and 4 to 6 years of age (236). This change in policy and the recommendation arose from two facts: (1) the dramatic decrease in incidence of polio from the Western hemisphere and in the rest of the world, and (2) since 1979, the only poliomyelitis acquired in the United States has been the 8-10 cases of vaccine-associated paralysis (VAP) attributable to the OPV (237). The merits of both OPV and IPV have been debated by proponents of both vaccines; however, Plotkin (236) and Paradiso (237) place the controversy in its current context.

The OPV was first used in the United States due to its ease of administration. Because it is a live vaccine, it may induce a greater immunological response. As a secondary advantage, the virus is excreted rapidly and may cause secondary infection to others and hence increase the immunization rate. This is especially advantageous in countries with poor immunization rates. The problems associated with the OPV are as follows. In tropical countries, the vaccine strain must compete with other agents (possibly the normal microflora) in the intestine, and as many as 10–12 doses of OPV are required to obtain 100% seroconversion. When the attenuated polio strains multiply in the intestinal tracts of individuals, there is reversion to virulence. That is, the virus mutates with altered characteristics, one of these being an increase in neurovirulence.

With major technological advances in molecular biology, a new IPV has been developed. This new IPV has enhanced potency such that there is 100% seroconversion in vaccinees after only two doses. The major objection to the use of the IPV seems to be the threat of importation of the polio virus from individuals from one of the polio-endemic countries in the world, and this can only be controlled with continued use of OPV. The WHO estimates that approximately 70,000 to 100,000 paralytic polio cases occur around the world based on passive reporting (238) and that there is a 10-fold estimate of underreporting. The use of IPV to prevent VAP still remains uncertain; and that there are still too many unknown variables to determine the exact efficacy of IPV in preventing VAP. As Paradiso concluded, the sequential use of an IPV/OPV schedule to eliminate VAP and maintain coverage against polio looks attractive on the surface. However, the worldwide experience with sequential IPV/OPV schedules is too small to be instructive, and the schedule proposed by the U.S. has never been used anywhere else in the world. There are too many questions in this regard that must be answered "before we embark on a major experiment with our immunization program and ultimately our children" (237).

Haemophilus Influenza Type B Influenza (Hib)

Haemophilus influenza type B influenza (Hib) is the major cause of bacterial meningitis to susceptible children in the United States, the etiologic agent of most cases of epiglottitis, and an important cause of pneumonia, septic arthritis, cellulitis, and bacteremia (239). The incidence of Hib is inversely related to age; the attack rate per 100,000 for the 1984 U.S. birth cohort was estimated to be 451, 284, 56, 47, and 24 in the first, second, third, fourth, and fifth years of age, respectively (240).

In the 1970s, a Hib vaccine was developed having ribose, ribitol, and phosphate (PRP). This polysaccharide was immunogenic in adults and older children. However, responsiveness to the PRP vaccine was highly dependent on age. The vaccine did not protect children younger than 18 months of age and had a variable efficacy when given to children at 2 years of age

(241–244). In addition, several investigators noted that vaccine efficacy varied. Numerous researchers noted an increase incidence of the disease (< 7 days) postinoculation (244–246).

In the 1980s, investigators developed a Hib polysaccharide-protein conjugate vaccine. The immunogenicity of the carbohydrate antigens was enhanced by chemical conjugation with proteins, which had been reported in 1929 (247). The United States' licensure of this vaccine was based on a Finnish trial, but the efficacy data came from a randomized clinical trial involving 16,000 children 2 months to 5 years of age (248). The study demonstrated a 69% efficacy rate for the vaccine. A trial of 48,977 children 3 months to 5 years of age were injected with the vaccine, while the same number of children served as controls. The vaccine was 90% effective, but not in the 3–18-month-old infants (249). Of the 100,000 children studied, only 1,000 were included in follow-up for adverse reactions and 500 for serum antibody levels. One child experienced an anaphylactic reaction and was treated with adrenaline. The authors of this study claimed no serious side effects.

A postlicensure follow-up study was performed studying 152 recorded cases, excluding the vaccine failures and what was termed "concurrent infections." Newly observed immediate reactions included convulsions, serum-sickness "type" reactions, and vomiting (250).

In three of the four postlicensure case-control studies of the performance of PRP in the U.S., the risk of invasive Hib disease unexpectedly increased in the immediate period after inoculation (251–255) (Table 3.1).

Due to the lack of consistency in immune response of the PRP vaccine, another improved version of the PRP termed the PRP-D was developed and licensed by the FDA in December 1987. Approval was based again on a Finnish study (256), in which 30,000 children were inoculated with the PRP-D vaccine along with 3 DTP vaccines and 1 polio. The control consisted of 30,000 children inoculated with 3 DTP vaccines and 1 polio group. Follow-up antibody response was performed on only 99 children. The efficacy of the vaccine was considered 83% with 20 potentially serious adverse reactions. In the follow-up group (n=99), increased irritability was reported in 41% of the DTP-polio-PRP-D recipients and 23% in the DTP-polio only recipients.

Routine immunization of infants with Hib conjugate vaccine in a multiple-dose schedule is currently recommended in the United States (257). A new and improved version of the Hib conjugate vaccine, PRP conjugated with tetanus toxoid (PRP-T), was licensed on March 30, 1993 by the CDC and was approved by the FDA for use of a new Haemophilus b conjugate vaccine combined with diphtheria-tetanus-pertussis for infants and children (258). The immunogenicity of this vaccine in infants immunized at ages 2, 4, and 6 months was similar to that of previously licensed Hib conjugate vaccines (259). Although control trials on the PRP-T in the United states have been halted, no cases of immediate invasive disease has been reported in approximately 100,000 children receiving two or more doses (260–261).

Vaccination with the first generation of Hib polysaccharide, or purified PRP vaccine stimulates production of anti-PRP

Table 3.1. Postlicensure Studies of Hib Polysaccharide Vaccine

Investigator	Reference	Study Location	Efficacy %	Efficacy at 10 Years After Vaccination
Harrison et al. 1988	238	MO, NJ, OK, TN, WA, Los Angeles (day-care based)	45	?
Harrison et al. 1989	239	MO, NJ, OK, TN, WA, Los Angeles (no day-care)	62	?
Black et al. 1988	240	Kaiser-N CA	62	?
Shapiro et al. 1988	241	CT, Pittsburgh, Dallas	88	?
Osterholm et al. 1988	242	MN	55	?

Modified from Cryz SJ. Vaccines and Immunotherapy. Elmsford, NY: Pergamon Press, 1991:59.

antibody in the same manner as natural infection (262–267). Two hundred twenty eight reports of Hib disease in vaccinated children were submitted to the FDA between May 1985 and September 1987. The vaccine was proclaimed to be effective in greater than 90% of the affected children older than 24 months. The vaccine did not alter the expected frequency of the disease. Alaskan (2,202) children were vaccinated with the PRP-D vaccine. "No significant" protective capability was achieved with the vaccine. The incidence of Hib actually decreased in children not participating in the study. Aseptic meningitis and sudden infant death syndrome (SIDS) were greater in the vaccinated group than the control group (268).

In 1989, three cases of Guillain Barré Syndrome (GBS) were reported after inoculation with the Hib conjugate vaccine PRP-diphtheria toxoid (PRP-D). Two children received the PRP-D vaccine alone, the third received a DTP and OPV as well (269).

Five thousand Navajo Indian infants were inoculated from July 1988–August 1990. Two thousand, five hundred and eighty eight infants were inoculated with Hib together with DTP and OPV; 2602 infants were given DTP, OPV and placebo. The first dose was given at 42–90 days after birth and again at days 70–146. An independent committee was appointed to advise investigators if and when the study should be discontinued. The trial was stopped after 4,161 (80%) of the infants received a second dose of the vaccine or placebo. The vaccinated group essentially had the equivalent rates of death and convulsions as the placebo group. There were 16 deaths reported within the vaccinated group; however, the committee considered them "unrelated to the vaccine" (270).

In conducting vaccine efficacy trials for Hib vaccines, investigators expected to observe a certain number of vaccine "failures." For calculation of efficacy, the definition of "immunization" is defined as, "receipt of a vaccine more than 14 days prior to the onset of the disease." According to the authors, 14 days is considered a reasonable time period for antibody development. In studies of vaccine efficacy for the unconjugated PRP vaccine, a range of estimates of vaccine efficacy were observed (243–244, 271). This observation is not easily interpreted due to discrepancies in study design, vaccine potency, or genetic variations among the study populations. In several case-control studies, the incidence of disease increased in the immediate (less than 7 days) postinoculation period (244,272–273).

PRP vaccines contain purified capsular protein, so early-onset Hib infection is probably not due to infectious material in the vaccine unless contaminated with another microbe (299). Several investigators have postulated that the increased susceptibility to infection in the immediate post-inoculation period may be due to a transient decrease in preexisting antibody production caused by the formation of antigen-antibody complexes or by transient suppression of antibody synthesis. With clustering of early cases in the first week after vaccination and the "absence" of cases in the second and third week after vaccination, vaccination may shorten the incubation period of Hib in children already destined to become ill (275–276). Although there are no apparent "infectious agents" in the PRP vaccine, foreign proteins may be present with it which are highly antigenic. Unlike natural infection by HIB, the high dose exposure of the virus, other immunogenic proteins as well as the altered route of exposure (injection) of the vaccine may overwhelm the immune system thereby making the recipient more susceptible to the disease.

Has Haemophilus influenza been resolved with mass vaccination? The number of cases of invasive infection (including meningitis) has not diminished, but instead of being associated with capsular Hib, they are now associated with non-capsular Hib in vaccinated children (277).

Diphtheria, Tetanus, and Pertussis (Dtp)

Diphtheria

Diphtheria is an acute respiratory infection caused by Corynebacterium diphtheria. The organism colonizes in the throat of susceptible individuals and produces mild pharyngitis. However, when the bacteria also contains the bacteriophage carrying the structural gene for biosynthesis of the toxin responsible for clinical disease, classic diphtheria results.

The first vaccine against diphtheria contained active toxin and antitoxin prepared from horses and was administered as a mixture. Fatalities occurred in the children who were given these mixtures. After the introduction of toxin neutralization by formalin, a report of incomplete detoxification appeared in the literature. In Kyoto, Japan, 606 children were inoculated with the formalin-detoxified vaccine. Sixty-eight of the child recipients died (278). Currently, licensed toxoids produced in the United States are tested by procedures set forth by the Code of Federal Regulation. There have been no reported cases of death since 1948.

Diphtheria toxoid absorbed with aluminum hydroxide or phosphate was highly immunogenic and produced fewer local reactions than fluid toxoid. The schedule for children was three doses, with the first two doses spaced by 1–2 months, the third dose given 6-12 months later. Booster shots are necessary every 10 years, particularly in countries where widespread immunization markedly decreased the opportunity for asymptomatic infection (279–283).

Tetanus

Clostridium tetani produces two exotoxins, tetanolysin and tetanospasmin. Classic tetanus is the result of tetanospasmin, one of the most potent toxins known (384). Tetanus toxin enters the nervous system at the peripheral nerve endings. It binds to a receptor, is internalized by receptor-mediated endocytosis, and is transported to the cell bodies of neurons, primarily motor neurons in the central nervous system (285).

Diphtheria and Tetanus Toxoids

Diphtheria toxin causes a toxic peripheral neuropathy in approximately 20% of individuals exposed (286), but diphtheria toxin has not been proven to be associated with central nervous system diseases such as encephalopathy. Tetanus is a neurologic disease characterized by lower motor neuron hyperexcitability with concomitant muscle spasm produced by the neurotoxin tetanospasmin (284). The neurologic sequelae of tetanus includes irritability, sleep disturbances, myoclonus, postural hypotension, and abnormal electroencephalograms (287). The symptoms may take within 2 years to disappear for complete recovery. The neurologic sequela of diphtheria is peripheral neuropathy.

In The North West Thames Study (288), of the 400,500 doses of diphtheria /tetanus (DT) and oral polio virus (OPV), given to 133,500 children completing a primary series of three doses of vaccine and 221,000 single booster doses of diphtheria and tetanus (DT) given at school entry, seven children had seizures, three children with other neurologic sequela were identified, one child had infantile spasms, another had seizures with hemiplegia (1 day after their DT vaccination, but was "normal" upon follow-up), and hemiparesis developed in another child 14 days postinoculation.

A prime case-controlled study that provides information about immunization with DT and associated neurologic illness is the National Childhood Encephalopathy Study (289). The study identified children ages 2–36 months who were admitted to the hospital for neurologic illness during the 3-year period from July 1976 through June 1979 in England, Scotland and Wales. The first 1,000 for the 1,182 identified were used in the study. The study concluded that there was "no statistically significant association with DT immunization and neurologic adverse events compared with controls." Interestingly, the control group was defined as two "at home" controls matched for age, sex, and area of residence.

The injection of a microbe, either live or attenuated, may induce an autoimmune response to the peripheral nerves and/or nerve roots in a susceptible host. This may occur either by dysregulation of the immune system, non-specific activation of T-cells directed against myelin proteins, or by autoimmunity triggered by sequence similarities to host proteins such as those of myelin. The latter mechanism might evoke a response to a self-antigen, the so-called phenomenon of molecular mimicry (290).

Twenty-nine instances of diphtheria or tetanus toxoid-induced Guillain Barré syndrome (GBS) or polyneuritis have been cited in the medical literature (291-297). The majority of these cases occurred in adults who received either tetanus toxoid alone (n=21) or tetanus toxoid and anti-tetanus toxin serum (n=4). Anti-tetanus toxoid induces GBS by itself (298). According to the Institute of Medicine, the evidence favors a causal relationship between tetanus toxoid, DT, TD and GBS (299).

Anaphylaxis

There are numerous reports of anaphylactic reactions after administration of tetanus or diphtheria toxoid (300–311). Two deaths occurred in association with tetanus toxoid administration as a single antigen. A 20-year-old man died 2 hours after receiving his third tetanus injection. The patient had a history of collapse and convulsions after receiving his second dose of tetanus toxoid (312). In the reported death of a 24-year-old woman 30 minutes after receiving an injection of tetanus toxoid, the cause of death was thought to be due to an anaphylactic reaction. A postmortem examination revealed pulmonary emphysema with bronchial hypersecretion and peribronchial infiltration with eosinophils, findings consistent with anaphylaxis (313).

Pertussis

Pertussis, a.k.a. whooping cough, a.k.a. "Hundred Day Disease," is a respiratory infection caused by Bordetella pertussis. This disease is characterized by a paroxysmal, spasmodic cough that ends in a prolonged inspiratory high-pitched crowing ("whoop") (314–316). Children are most commonly affected, although there are indications of an adult form of pertussis (317–319).

The incubation period of pertussis averages 7–14 days, with a maximum of 21 days. Clinically, pertussis can be divided into three stages: catarrhal, paroxysmal, and convalescent. The onset of pertussis in the early catarrhal stage is subtle and is usually indistinguishable from a minor upper-respiratory infection. The individual is most infectious during this period, which then gradually declines. Rhinorrhea, sneezing, lethargy, anorexia, and a nocturnal cough slowly develops. In 7–10 days, the cough becomes explosive and episodic, which begins the paroxysmal stage. The paroxysmal stage lasts 1–4 weeks and is exhibited by severe episodes of coughing. The convalescent stage usually begins 4 to 6 weeks after the onset of the disease and is characterized by diminishing frequency and severity of the cough.

PERTUSSIS VACCINE DEVELOPMENT

When the description of the Bordet-Gengou technique for isolating the pertussis bacterium was published (Bordet and Gengou) in 1906, numerous researchers began to experiment with vaccines from killed whole cells of B. pertussis. Such vaccines were developed and administered to children by Bordet and Gengou in 1912, Nicholle of the Pasteur Institute in Tunis in 1913 and Madsen of the Danish State Serum Institute in 1914, to name a few (320). In 1942, Kendrick combined killed vaccine with diphtheria and tetanus toxoids for the DTP combination vaccine (321–322). Science has made it possible in recent years to develop a vaccine that is theoretically limited to the components that are thought to be responsible for natural immunity. The well-known reactivity of the whole-cell vaccine made it an unpopular practice (323). This reactivity led to the belief that the whole-cell pertussis vaccine was responsible for frequent permanent neurologic disabilities and/or death. However, these concerns were unreasonable to some (324). Pertussis mortality declined in the United States, United Kingdom, Sweden, and among other developed countries during the first half of this century before the implementation of a "preventative therapy" or therapeutic measures (325–328).

Vaccines were ineffective because no significant difference was observed in the incidence or severity of whooping cough between the vaccinated and unvaccinated (329). The pertussis vaccine was always controversial. In the Oxford City trial, 12.5% (n=327) vaccinated and 14.1% (n=305) unvaccinated children developed pertussis. In the residential nurseries in which pertussis developed, 55% of the 33 vaccinated (n=18) and 63% of the 30 (n=19) unvaccinated children developed pertussis.

In the Faroe Island epidemic, vaccination was completed after the first pertussis epidemic. Of the 1,832 vaccinated children, 458 (25%) did not contract pertussis compared with 8 (> 2%) among the 446 unvaccinated children. In both epidemics, 6 patients of the 3,926 vaccinated (<0.01%) died and 26 among the 1,073 unvaccinated (28%) cases died. The study population of vaccinated vs. unvaccinated were so different that the conclusion (as it appears superficially) that the vaccine affords protection has questionable validity (330).

Acellular vaccines were developed in Japan due to the deleterious experiences with the whole-cell vaccine (331). Japan made pertussis vaccination mandatory in 1948, but it was not until 1950 that nationwide immunization, using the whole-cell vaccine, took place (332).

Within a 2-month period in 1974–1975, two Japanese infants died less than 24 hours after receiving the DTP vaccine (333–334). Although the investigators concluded the

whole-cell component of the DTP vaccine had not caused the deaths, the vaccine policies were affected with noncompliance.

Sweden stopped vaccinating with the whole cell pertussis vaccine in 1979. Despite general immunization, pertussis returned to Sweden after more than a 10-year absence (335). Pertussis became endemic. In 1978, 127 bacteriologically verified cases of whooping cough were reported to the National Bacteriological Laboratory in Stockholm. Investigation revealed 620 cases in 1–6-year-old children with pertussis; 521 (84%) had received a full series of three pertussis vaccines. Discontinuation of the pertussis vaccine resulted in 3 years of low endemic levels. Thereafter, the incidence gradually increased with two outbreaks in 1983 and 1985 (336). Outbreaks appeared in Sweden in 1977–1978 despite high immunization (80%) compliance. There was no mention of the severity of the "natural" form of the disease, an issue that deserves worthwhile documentation and further research.

Sweden experimented with the Japanese acellular vaccines developed by the Japanese National Institute of Health (JNIH). One of these vaccines JNIH-6 was a two component vaccine containing formaldehyde-detoxified lymphocytosis-promoting factor and filamentous hemagglutinin used in Japan for children less than 2 years of age. JNIH-7 was an experimental monocomponent vaccine manufactured for this experiment. Three thousand eight hundred and one children 6–11 months of age were divided into two groups of approximately 1,400 each. They were inoculated with either JNIH-6 or JNIH-7 acellular vaccines. Nine hundred fifty four babies were given placebo, which interestingly consisted of formalin, thiomersol (mercury preservative) and aluminum phosphate in a final preparation of 0.15 mg of aluminum, each of these substances being immunotoxins. This study was lacking as it did not address the late phase systemic reactions (Table 3.2). Due to the toxicity of the "placebo," this study substantiates the fact that not only is Bordetella pertussis a valid argument for a serious systemic reaction but also the solvents, fixatives, and preservative in the vaccine preparation itself.

Another interesting observation about this study was the increased incidence of secondary bacterial infections. Eleven children in the two vaccine groups contracted invasive bacterial infections associated with Haemophilus influenza, Klebsiella pneumonia, Staphylococcus aureus, Streptococcus pneumonia, and Meningococcus. Four of the children died, and neuroblastoma developed in one child.

A two-part study conducted on Alaskan children was performed to evaluate the potential risk of invasive bacterial disease and the occurrence of minor illnesses after immunization with DT and whole-cell pertussis vaccine. Although there were high rates of invasive bacterial disease, the authors of the study concluded that, "there was no consistent relationship that could be demonstrated between DTP immunization and susceptibility to infectious disease (337)." However, the highest incidence of invasive disease occurred after the third DTP vaccination. This occurrence parallels the well-documented pattern of sensitization after repeated exposure to antigens. The authors also set an arbitrary 30-day cut-off limit and hypothesized that the cause-and-effect reaction would develop within this time period. However, prevalent invasive bacterial disease occurred 31–60 days post-inoculation.

INFANTILE SPASMS

A report of one of the largest series of infantile spasm following pertussis immunization was published in 1987. Six children varying in age from 2 to 9 months were included. The time interval from inoculation to the onset of spasm was 6.5 hours to 5 days. Except for one child who experienced monoclonic seizures at birth, there was no history of seizures in the children before vaccination. The investigators' postulated mechanism for pertussis related seizures are (1) neurotoxic effect, (2) immediate immune reaction, (3) delayed hypersensitivity, and (4) vaccine-induced activation of a latent neurotropic virus infection (338).

Another study considered the frequencies of epilepsy, febrile seizures, infantile spasm, and CNS infections (bacterial and aseptic meningitis) in children ages 1 month to 2 years. Two time periods, 1967 to 1968 and 1972 to 1973 were selected for comparison. Exact dates of pertussis inoculation were known in 372 (1967–1968) and 432 children (1972–1973). Comparison of the distribution of the ages at the time of vaccination for the two time intervals revealed a marked difference in the frequency of vaccination at different ages, corresponding to the ages at which vaccinations were recommended. In the period 1967–1968, the peak ages of vaccination were 5, 6, 7, and 15 months, while in 1972–1973 vaccination peaked at 5 and 9 weeks and 10 months. The authors concluded that the study was not consistent with the hypothesis that pertussis vaccination is associated with the risk of infantile spasm. The reasoning was that there was no change in the distribution of ages at the time of onset of spasm when the ages of vaccination varied. Only 80% of the cases were included in the study; given this small sample size, the study had a low statistical power to detect a difference in the age distribution (339).

The North West Thames Study describes vaccine reactions from 1975 through 1981 and a separate review of hospitalized cases of neurologic disorders in children for 1979. During the 7-year study, approximately equal numbers of children completed regimes of DTP (134,700) and DT (133,500). There were 1,172 reports of "vaccine-associated" events. Of these, 926 (79%) were "considered simple" reactions. Of the remaining 246 reports, 114 (10%) experienced anaphylaxis or collapse, convulsions, neurologic disorder, or death. Forty-five (35%) of the more serious reactions were observed after administration of DTP or monovalent pertussis, 20 (18%) occurred after DT administration, and 37 (32%) occurred after the measles vaccine. The remaining 12 (11%) followed vaccination of rubella or another infectious disease (340). Five of the 114 children with the more serious vaccine-associated reactions were diagnosed with infantile spasm. Four of the children received DTP 8 days to 6 weeks before the onset of spasms. One had received DT.

Table 3.2. Systemic Reactions within the First 24 Hours Post-inoculation

Ailment	JNIH-6 %	JNIH-7 %	"Placebo"	Late Phase Effects JNIH-6	Late Phase Effects JNIH-7	Late Phase Placebo
Twitching/spasm						
(dose 1)	0.3	0.5	0.4	?	?	?
(dose 2)	0.1	0.5	0.0			
Anorexia						
(dose 1)	7.1	6.2	6.1	?	?	?
(dose 2)	6.1	5.8	7.5			
Vomiting						
(dose 1)	5.6	4.1	5.0	?	?	?
(dose 2)	4.7	3.2	4.1			
Persistent crying						
(dose 1)	1.1	2.1	0.8	?	?	?
(dose 2)	1.4	1.4	1.1			
Fever 3–6 hr after vaccine						
(dose 1)	6.1	6.7	4.0	?	?	?
(dose 2)	4.9	6.0	5.2			
Drowsiness (no fever)						
(dose 1)	7.0	6.8	6.0	?	?	?
(dose 2)	6.6	6.7	6.7			
Pallor						
(dose 1)	1.3	0.8	1.3	?	?	?
(dose 2)	0.5	0.4	0.6			

Modified from: Scheibner V. Vaccination: The medical assault on the immune system. 1993:35-36.

Table 3.3.   **National Childhood Encephalopathy Study: Estimated Relative Risks of Specific Acute Neurologic Conditions After DTP Inoculation within the Previous 7 Days**

Category	Total Cases (No.)	DPT Within 7 Days (No.) Cases	DPT Within 7 Days (No.) Controls
All except infantile spasm	904	30	23
Seizures	515	18	12
Encephalopathy	389	12	11
All except infantile spasm and viral	773	28	23
Seizure and encephalopathy in previously normal children	770	26	?
Previously normal: died or neurologically impaired at age 12 months	241	7	3★

★Reprinted from Madge et al National Childhood Encephalopathy Study: 10-Year Follow-up. DHHS Pub. No. (FDA) 90-1162. Bethesda, MD. U.S. Dept. of Health.
Modified from: Miller et al Severe neurological illness: further analyses of the British National Childhood Encephalopathy Study. J Exper Clin Med (Suppl.):145-155.

ASEPTIC MENINGITIS

A variety of factors have been identified as causes of aseptic meningitis. These include viruses such as mumps, herpes, and infectious hepatitis; bacterial (tuberculosis and syphilis); other agents (toxoplasma); parainfectious processes (varicella, measles and rubella), and vaccine injections (306,341).

Data from Rochester, Minnesota, for the period 1950-1981 indicates that evidence of a virus was obtained in 12% of the aseptic meningitis cases (342). Based on the results of animal studies, pertussis immunization may affect susceptibility to other infections, thereby increasing the risk of aseptic meningitis (343).

ENCEPHALOPATHY

No signs of CNS inflammation have been observed in the majority of cases of whooping cough encephalopathy. Findings are nonspecific and include cerebral edema, eosinophilic degeneration, multiple petechiae, lymphocytic plugs in veins and capillaries, and small subarachnoid hemorrhages (344).

Two reviews of suspected deaths after pertussis vaccination have been conducted. One of the reviews is based on 12 previous reports of vaccine-associated deaths. The second is based on a retrospective review on infant or child deaths associated with pertussis, which occurred in England and Wales between 1960 and 1980 (345). The authors identified 40 deaths and obtained information that included details of a general postmortem examination for 29 of them. The 29 deaths were categorized into one of two groups: "acute group" infants dying within 3 weeks of immunization (n=18) and "chronic group" children dying 6 months to 12 years after vaccination (n=11). The review of both acute and chronic groups indicated no specific findings that were consistently observed after pertussis vaccination. These inconsistencies may be due to bioindividuality and need to be considered. The authors conclude neither the cerebral changes in the present study nor those abstracted from the previous literature have provided evidence of a pattern of damage in the brain identifiable as a specific reaction to immunization against whooping cough. However, the authors do acknowledge deficiencies in the neuropathologic data and inadequate documentation. A more careful and complete collection of such data should be reviewed in the future.

The National Childhood Encephalopathy Study (NCES) was conducted in England, Wales and Scotland from July 1, 1976–June 30, 1979. During this study period, 1,182 children were hospitalized with acute neurological illness. DTP vaccination was administered more frequently within 72 hours and the first 7 days after vaccine injections in children with neurological illness than the controls in the same time period. A similar analysis for DT also showed an increase in relative risk of neurologic illness in affected children compared with control subjects. The estimated risk of serious neurologic disorder within 7 days post-DTP inoculation in previously healthy children was demonstrated to be 1:110,000. The rate of permanent brain damage 1 year later was estimated to be 1:310,000 (Table 3.3).

OTHER ADVERSE COMPLICATIONS

The earliest report of adverse events after administration of pertussis vaccine was reported in 1933 when two cases of sudden death occurred. One case occurred after second immunization and was characterized by contractions of the arms and legs, cyanosis, hiccups, convulsions, and death within 30 minutes (346).

A 10-month-old infant experienced generalized hypotonia and weakness with increased deep tendon reflexes in the lower extremities after his third pertussis vaccination. Similar episodes occurred 2 weeks after his first vaccination and 1 week after his second vaccination. A fourth episode occurred spontaneously at 25 months. Neurologic disability persisted.

At 43 months, the child received a fourth pertussis vaccination, and within 25 minutes, the child became lethargic. Flaccid paralysis developed within 12 hours, and the child died of bronchopneumonia 7 weeks later (347).

Despite these reports, it was not until a larger observational group was reported that the possibility of adverse consequences of the pertussis vaccine was entertained. Fifteen cases occurred between 1939–1947 in children 5 to 18 months. The children presented with fever, irritability, convulsions, and coma occurring within 12 hours after being vaccinated with pertussis (348).

One hundred eight cases of neurologic illness occurred after the pertussis vaccination. These neurologic illnesses followed usually within 48 hours after one of the four pertussis vaccinations (349).

Reports of 149 infants experiencing adverse effects after pertussis vaccination were disclosed to the vaccine manufacturers. Thirteen (9%) of the infants died, 59 (40%) experienced severe manifestations including convulsions, shock, persistent screaming, and "various involvement of the central nervous system." The remaining 77 (51%) experienced "local reactions." Fatalities and local reactions were more common after the second pertussis dose inoculation (350).

Neurologic symptoms within 72 hours after DTP immunization were reported in 46 children. No other cause of these symptoms were found. Seventy four percent (74%) occurred between 4 and 24 hours postinoculation with pertussis with symptoms ranging from encephalopathy (2 cases); SIDS (2 cases); hypotonia, hyporesponsiveness (1 case); possible hypoglycemia (1 case), and seizures (40 cases). Of the surviving children, 58% were moderately or severely retarded and 72% had uncontrolled seizures (351) (Table 3.4). A total of 2,531 cases of reported febrile seizures (combined ICD 9 codes 780.3 [idiopathic convulsions] plus 780.5 [fever]) and 344 cases of afebrile seizures/idiopathic convulsions (ICD 9 code 780.3) occurring within 28 days of DTP immunization were also reported through the MSAEFI system from 1978 to 1990. A total of 1,284 (75%) of the 2,531 cases of febrile seizures and 258 (75%) of the 433 cases of afebrile seizures/convulsions also received at least one other vaccine at the time of DTP immunization. No follow-up of the cases were made, and a physician's diagnosis was not required (352). Cody and colleagues compared the reactions that occurred in the first 48 hours after vaccination in 15,752 children receiving DTP vaccine and in 784 children receiving DT vaccine. The children's ages ranged from 0 to 6 years. Nine seizures were reported following receipt of DTP vaccine, whereas no seizures were reported after DT. No cases of diagnosed encephalopathy, permanent neurologic damage, or death were observed in the first 48 hours after innoculation. The cases of seizures occurred after any one of the three primary series or the first booster DTP vaccination. All cases reported the onset of symptoms within 24 hours postinoculation. Two children had histories of febrile seizures and no children had a history of seizure activity or neurologic illness (353). A follow-up examination of nine seizure cases was performed 7 years later. Eight of the nine children were given a complete neurologic and psychometric evaluation consisting of the Wechsler Intelligence Scale for Children. Verbal IQ scores were less than 80 in two of the seven children tested and overall IQ was less than 80 in one child (354). The National Childhood Encephalopathy Study (NCES) was a large case-control study in 1976 in response to concerns about declining levels of DTP in Great Britain. The objective of the study was to assess the risks of certain serious neurologic disorders associated with immunization in early childhood and to identify factors that may cause or predispose to such disorders (355). The results of this study state that DTP immunization is associated with an increased risk, within 7 days, of seizures and encephalopathy.

Discussion

The topic of vaccination and the decision to immunize is complex. Despite the current medical opinion of the success of vaccines in reducing risks of contracting diseases, current vaccination policies are still controversial. The phenomenal reduction in the risk of contracting diseases such as measles, mumps and rubella, diphtheria and pertussis, especially in the developed countries, has renewed public interest and concern about vaccine safety. Issues such as the risks of contracting so-called vaccine-preventable diseases, vaccine side effects (especially the serious side effects), vaccine efficacy, and vaccine failures take on greater weight, especially for the parent or guardian who must ultimately decide whether to

Table 3.4.   **Studies of Acute Neurologic Events Occurring Within 48 Hours of DTP Vaccination in Defined Populations**

Reference	Years	Age	Vaccine	Children (No.)	Vaccinated (No.)	Encephalopathy (No.)	Seizures (No.)
Harker 1977	1972–1975	0–5 years	DPT	~11,028	~32,000	NA*	0
Hirtz 1983	1959–1966	0–7 years	DPT	~54,000	NA*	NA*	8
Feery 1985	1983	>1 year	DPT	1,075	2,041	NA*	2
Long 1990	1984–1985	2–20 months	DPT	538	1,771	0	0

*NA, Not available.
†Within 1 week post-inoculation.
Modified from: Institute of Medicine. Effects of Pertussis and Rubella Vaccines. pp 96, 1991.

vaccinate the child. A dramatic example of this is the case of polio. In the mid-1950s, the benefit to the individual child from vaccination with the readily available Salk vaccine in reducing the possibility of contracting polio far outweighed the small risk of serious side effects of the vaccine. Today, the certainty of contracting the wild polio virus for a child born in America is rare. Yet, 8-10 people each year will develop paralytic polio, as a result of vaccination or as a result of coming into contact with someone vaccinated with the oral polio vaccine (356).

According to Nelson (357), chiropractors should embrace immunization. He frames the issue in a series of arguments. We would like to address some of these arguments. Anti-immunization proponents argue that immunizations are not effective. Nelson distills the arguments into the common elements of: 1) Cyclical patterns of disease: The naturalistic chiropractic argument is that some diseases (e.g., polio) follow a cyclical pattern that is independent of vaccination and that the incidence of polio was already on the decline before the introduction of vaccines. Nelson argues that in the case of polio as an example; after the introduction of the polio vaccine, the incidence of polio took on an acyclic quality and that the incidence of polio the last two decades has been less than 10 per year, an incidence rate several hundred times lower than the lowest preimmunization rates; and 2) improved sanitation and hygiene: Anti-immunization critics point out that the incidence of diseases declined dramatically as a result of improved sanitation, hygiene, nutrition, working conditions, etc. Nelson attacks this assertion based on unsubstantiated arguments from anti-immunization individuals.

With respect to the cyclical or acyclical patterns of disease and the role of vaccine (or lack of it) in the decline of the incidence of disease, we offer that both arguments are too rigid and overly simplistic. There is a lack of credible scientific evidence that vaccination alone causes diseases to disappear or that diseases follow a cyclical pattern and are self-limiting. The eradication of smallpox has often been attributed to the success of vaccination while an argument for the self limitation of disease can be made with measles. Before vaccination, from 1915–1958, the U.S. and Great Britain experienced a greater than 95% decline in the measles death rate and the death rate after the introduction of the measles vaccine was the same as it had been in the pre-vaccination era (Anderson M. Facts on File. International mortality statistics, Washington, DC 1981, p 182-183). Only through a controlled experiment can one decipher the respective roles of such factors as vaccination, nutrition, hygiene, or the natural history of a particular disease. The crux of the question is fundamentally whether chiropractors should advocate to enhance the host response to illness through conservative means (e.g., nutrition, hygiene, chiropractic adjustments, etc.) or are these components of a health care program relegated to a secondary or a nonexistent role. Reports have questioned the role of antibodies as essential for recovery from acute measles infection (358). In this article, two pediatric residents, frequently exposed to measles, were tested for measles complement fixation antigen. Both residents had never had clinical measles or atypical measles and had negative HIA titers. Their lymphocyte responsiveness to measles were strong and correlated well with their clinical protection against

measles via the cell-associated immune response. Again, the question remains as to the contribution of proper nutrition, rest, chiropractic care, hygiene, etc. to the combating of disease. On the other hand, should chiropractors tell an inner city school child living in poverty with poor hygiene and poor nutrition that they should not be vaccinated? We certainly do not advocate such a position in so much as the types of factors that could influence the child's health are not being addressed. Conversely, to advocate mass vaccination of high risk populations without paying attention to socioeconomic, hygienic, and nutritional factors is an equally irresponsible position. In 1989 and 1990, a measles epidemic in the Los Angeles region was concentrated among low income, minority preschool children. For example, Latino children were 9.6 times and African-American children were 7.2 times more likely as Caucasian preschoolers to contract measles (359). In a study by Wood et al. (360), immunization rates among inner-city Latino and African-American 2-year-old children were found to be very low in 1992.

The subject of herd immunity merits reiteration. Non-vaccinated individuals are protected by those that are vaccinated due to herd immunity. There are flaws to this argument. In the case of polio, the risk of contracting polio in the herd from those individuals that have been vaccinated increases. This infection occurs mainly from direct contact or fecal contamination (361). We reiterate the following argument: Mathematical modeling asserts that vaccine efficacy of 95 to 97 percent is required to interrupt the transmission of disease and to prevent outbreaks should the disease be introduced to the population. One of the models assumes a contact rate of 14 to 18 persons; that is, an infected person would come into contact with an average of 14 to 18 susceptible people. In school settings, the contact rate may be much higher. Airborne transmission (30), if it is a factor, may also increase the contact rate. An increased contact rate in the mathematical modeling would require higher vaccination levels than that which presently exist. The authors of this chapter question whether this is possible to achieve and at what cost. As Fine and Zell (31) commented, herd immunity thresholds for disease eradication are based on the assumption that immune and susceptible individuals are randomly distributed. However, they assert that vaccines (and hence immune individuals) are not randomly distributed. Also, vaccine failures are not randomly distributed and susceptible individuals may be clustered isolating them from indirect protection by immune members of the population. Socioeconomics may also be a factor such that infection may be introduced into communities with poor nutrition and hygiene, health care, etc. at a higher rate than those in communities with better nutrition and health care.

Vaccine Failures

We have cited examples and cases of vaccine failures (primary or secondary), especially with the measles vaccine. Our contention is not to question the impact of vaccination on the natural course of an epidemic as anti-immunization critics have been quoted by Nelson, since we do not know its exact role. We do, however, bring up the following issue. Despite evidence of vaccine failures, flaws in the herd immunity argument for vaccination and in the case of polio, contracting the disease is more likely from the vaccine than through natural infection; why advocate universal immunization, especially in the developed countries? This question is significant, as in the case of measles and polio, when one considers the argument of the possibility that vaccine pressure can drive virus evolution and make existing vaccines essentially useless. Although this issue was raised with respect to the measles vaccine, antigenic drift in the polio virus has already produced a different strain not fully covered by the vaccine (and can also lower the herd immunity to the wild-type) as was demonstrated in Finland with an outbreak in 1984–1985 (362–364).

Nelson and anti-immunization individuals point out that vaccines are not 100% effective and not 100% safe. However, Nelson advocates that the protection offered to many through vaccination is an acceptable trade-off to the small risk of having an adverse reaction, even a serious one. As an example, Nelson asserts that it is acceptable to have a few cases caused by a polio vaccine because thousands of cases would occur without vaccination. However, this assertion maintains that there are predictable patterns of susceptibility to disease and that naturalistic or other forces (e.g., hygiene) have no influence on the course of the disease. This assertion is flawed in that one simply does not know. We have shown, based on the scientific literature, that adverse reactions and side effects (with respect to the specific vaccines addressed) from immunization can be harmful. With respect to the notion that these are rare and acceptable, we offer this: to the parent that has a child suffering from the adverse reaction to a vaccine, it is not rare.

With respect to multiple vaccine or combination vaccines, one must be cautious (365–366). The safety and immunogenicity of combined or multiple vaccines have been reported (367–371); other considerations should be made. The immune system may be able to handle all the antigens from such combination vaccines when administered sequentially but if administered simultaneously, antigenic competition and reduction in immunogenicity (365,372–375) as well as suppressor T-cell production (365,376) may occur.

In closing, we have raised many issues regarding vaccination in this chapter. The issue is complex and deserves a robust debate. Ultimately, the funding of well-controlled studies will be needed to sort out the plethora of issues involved. To further question conventional wisdom will be constructive to our understanding of the treatment and prevention of disease. We should not be so short sighted in our evaluation of efficacy and must consider also the long-term consequences of a vaccination program. Our emphasis on presenting the adverse consequences of certain vaccines is healthy, and it may allow parents to make more informed decisions. Parents may choose to live entirely under the rubric of the medical model, they may choose to integrate conventional medicine with alternative approaches (e.g., nutritional, chiropractic, naturopathic, homeopathic), or they may choose to care for their children through an entirely non-conventional approach. Health care providers should provide as much accurate information as possible so that the patient can make the most informed choice regarding the health and well being of their child. Ultimately,

regardless of what any doctor may believe, the patient's right to self-determination should always be preserved (377).

REFERENCES

1. Colley F, Haas M. Attitudes on Immunization: a survey of American chiropractors. J Manipulative Physiol Ther 1994; 17:584-590.
2. Cashley MAP. Letter to the editor: attitudes on immunization: a survey of american chiropractors. J Manipulative Physiol Ther 1994; 18:420-421.
3. Fitzgerald TM, Glotzer DE. Vaccine information pamphlets: More information than parents want? Pediatrics 1995; 95:331-334.
4. Markowitz LE, Orenstein WA. Measles vaccine. Pediatr Clin North Am 1990;37: 603-625.
5. Ray CG. Viruses of mumps and childhood exanthems. In: Sherris JC, ed. Medical microbiology: an introduction to infectious diseases. Norwalk, Connecticut: Appleton & Lange, 1990.
6. Volk WA, Benjamin DC, Kadner RJ, Parsons JT. Orthomyxoviridae and paramyxoviridae. In: Volk WA, Benjamin DC, Kadner RJ, Parsons JT, eds. Essentials of Medical microbiology, 4th ed. Philadelphia: JB Lippincott Co.,1991.
7. World Health Organization. EPI for the 1990's. Geneva: World Health Organization. 1992; publication WHO/EPI/GEN/92.2
8. The National Childhood Vaccine Injury Act of 1986. 42 USC Sec 300aa-1-33 (Supp 1987).
9. Centers for Disease Control: Measles Surveillance Report No. 11, 1977-1981. Atlanta: CDC, 1982.
10. Brunnel PA, Weigle K, Murphy MD, Shehab Z, Cobb E. Antibody response following measles-mumps-rubella vaccine under conditions of customary use. JAMA 1983; 250:1409-1412.
11. Cooperative study. Extensive evaluation of a highly attenuated live measles vaccine. JAMA 1967; 199:26-30.
12. Nkowane BM, Bart SW, Orenstein WA, Baltier M. Measles outbreak in a vaccinated school population; epidemiology, chains of transmission and the role of vaccine failures. Am J Pub Health 1987;77:434-438.
13. Centers for Disease Control. Elimination of indigenous measles: United States. MMWR 1982;31:517-519.
14. Markowitz LE, Preblud SR, Orenstein WA, et al. Patterns of transmission in measles outbreaks in the United States, 1985-1986. N Engl J Med 1989; 320:75-81.
15. Centers for Disease Control. Cases of specified notifiable diseases. MMWR 1990; 38:888.
16. Schwartz AJ. Immunization development and evaluation of a highly attenuated live measles vaccine. Ann Pediatr (Basel) 1964; 202:241-252.
17. Hilleman MR, Buynak EB, Weikel RE, Stokes J, Whitman JE, Leagus MB. Development and evaluation of the Moraten measles virus vaccine. JAMA 1968; 206:587-590.
18. Frank JA, Orenstein WA, Bart KJ, El-Tantawy N, Davis RM, Hinman AR. Major impediments to measles elimination: the modern epidemiology of an ancient disease. Am J Dis Child 1986; 139:881-888.
19. Mathias RC, Meekison WG, Arcand TA, Schecter MT. The role of secondary vaccine failures in measles outbreaks. Am J Public Health 1989; 79:475-478.
20. Reyes MA, Franky de Borro M, Roa J, Bergonzoli G, Saravia NG. Measles vaccine failure after documented seroconversion. Ped Infect Dis 1987; 6:848-851.
21. Chen RT, Markowitz LE, Albrecht P, Stewart JA, Mofenson LM, Preblud SR, Orenstein WA. Measles antibody: reevaluation of protective titers. J Infect Dis 1990; 162:1036-1042.
22. Markowitz LE, Preblud SR, Fine PE, Orenstein WA. Duration of live measles vaccine-induced immunity. Ped Infect Dis J 1990; 9:101-110.
23. Centers for Disease Control. Summary of notifiable disease. United States, 1991. MMWR 1991d;40 (53).
24. Kenya PR. Measles and mathematics; "control or eradication." East Africian Med J 1990;Dec:846-863.
25. Cheah D, Lane JM, Passaris I. Measles vaccine efficacy study in a Canberra high school: a study following a measles outbreak. J Pediatr Child Health 1993; 29:455-458.
26. King GE, Markowitz LE, Patriarca P, Dales LG. Clinical efficacy of measles vaccine during the 1990 measles epidemic. Ped Infect Dis J 1991;10:883-887.
27. Gustafson TL, Lievens AW, Brunnel PA, Moellenberg RG, Buttery CMG, Sehulster LM. Measles outbreak in fully immunized secondary-school population. N Engl J Med 1987; 316:771-774.
28. Davis RM, Whitman ED, Orenstein WA, Preblud SR, Markowitz LE, Hinman AR. A persistent outbreak of measles despite appropriate prevention and control measures. Am J Epidemiol 1987;126:438-449.
29. Edmonson MB, Addiss DG, McPherson JT, Berg JL, Circo SR, Davis JP. Mild measles and secondary vaccine failure during sustained outbreak in a highly vaccinated population. JAMA 1990; 263:2467-2471.
30. Remington PL, Hall WN, Davis IH, Herald A, Gunn RA. Airborne transmission of measles in a physician's office. JAMA 1985; 253:1574-1577.
31. Fine PEM, Zell ER. Outbreaks in highly vaccinated populations: implications for further studies of vaccine performance. Am J Epidemiol 1994; 139:77-90.
32. Gindler JS, Atkinson WL, Markowitz LE, Hutchins SS. Epidemiology of measles in

the United States in 1989 and 1990. Pediatr Infect Dis J 1992; 11:841-846.

33. McLean ME, Walsh PJ, Carter AO, Lavinge PM. Measles in Canada - 1989 CDWR 1990; 16:213-218.

34. Markowitz LE, Orenstein WA. Measles vaccines. Pediatric Clinics of North America 1990;37(3):603.

35. Baczko K, Brinckmann U, Pardowitz I, Rima B, ter Muelen V. Nucleotide sequences of the genes encoding the matrix protein of two wild type measles virus strains. J Gen Virol 1991; 72:2279-2282.

36. Baczko K, Pardowitz I, Rima B, ter Muelen V. Constant and variable regions of measles protein encoded by the nucleocapsid and phosphoprotein genes derived from lytic and persistent viruses. Virology 1992; 190:469-474.

37. Giraudon P, Jacquier MF, Wild TF. Antigenic analysis of African measles virus field isolates:identification and localization of one conserved and two variable epitope sites on the NP protein. Virus Res 1988; 18:137-152.

38. Rota JS, Hummel KB, Rota PA, Bellini WJ. Genetic variability of the glycoprotein genes of current wild type measles isolates. Virology 1992; 188:135-142.

39. Rota PA, Bloom AE, Vanchiere JA, Bellini WJ. Evolution of the nucleoprotein and matrix genes of wild type strains of measles virus isolated from recent epidemics. Virology 1994; 198:724-730.

40. Schultz TF, Hoad JG, Whitby D, Tizard EJ, Dillon M, Weiss R. A measles isolate from a child with Kawasaki disease: sequence comparison with contemporaneous isolates from "classical" cases. J Gen Virol 1992; 72:83-88.

41. Tamin A, Rota PA, Wang Z, Heath JL, Anderson LJ, Bellini WJ. Antigenic analysis of current wild type and vaccine strains of measles virus. J Infect Dis 1994; 170:795-801.

42. Bellini WJ, Rota JS, Rota PA. J Infect Dis Virology of measles virus. 1994; 170:S15-31.

43. Almond JW. The attenuation of poliovirus neurovirulence. Ann Rev Micro 1991;8:737-771.

44. Rota PA, Bloom AE, Vanchiere JA, Bellini WJ. Evolution of the nucleoprotein and the matrix genes of wild type strains of measles virus isolated from recent epidemics. Virology 1994; 198:724-730.

45. Lerman SL, Bollinger M, Brunken JM. Clinical and serologic evaluation of measles, mumps and rubella (HPV-77, DEA5 and RA/3) virus vaccines, singly and in combination. J Pediatrics 1981; 68:18.

46. Petola H, Heinonen O. Frequency of true adverse reactions: measles-mumps-rubella vaccine. Lancet 1986; 1:939.

47. Centers for Disease Control. Measles : United States,1988. MMWR 1989; 38:601.

48. Buser F. Side reaction to measles vaccination suggesting the Arthus phenomenon. N Engl J Med 1967; 277:251.

49. CDC Recommendations of the Public Health Service Advisory Committee on Immunization Practices: Measles Vaccine MMW 1967; 16:169-271.

50. Raul LW, Schmidt R. Measles immunization with killed virus vaccine. Am J Dis Child 1965; 109:232-237.

51. Fulginiti VA, Eller JJ, Downie AW, Kempe CH. Altered reactivity to measles virus. Atypical measles in children previously immunized with inactivated measles virus vaccines. JAMA 1967; 202 (12): 1075-1080.

52. Witte JJ, Axnick NW. The benefits of 10 years of measles immunization in the United States. Publ Health Rep 1975; 90 (3):205-207.

53. Weiss R. Measles battle loses potent weapon [news]. Science 1992;258:546-547.

54. Albrecht P, Klutch M. Sensitive hemagglutination inhibition test for mumps antibody. J Clin Microb 1981;13:870-876, 52.

55. Sabin AB, Arechiaga AF, Castro JF, Albrecht P, Sever JL, Shekarachi. I: Successful immunization of infants with and without maternal antibody by aerosolized measles vaccine. II: Vaccine comparison and evidence for multiple antibody response. JAMA 1984; 251:2363-2371.

56. Pongrithsukda V, Gluck S, Suwatanapongched S, Kaewmalung P, Muyakul J. Trial of Edmonston-Zagreb measles vaccine in infants under nine months. Southeast Asian J Trop Med Publ Health 1991; 22(3):347-350.

57. Rogers S, Sanders RC, Alpers MP. Immunogenicity of standard dose Edmonston-Zagreb measles vaccine in Highland Papua New Guinean children from four months of age. J Trop Med Hygiene 1991 94;88-91.

58. Wkly Epidemiol Rec 1992; 67:357-61 in: Br Med J 1993;20:307.

59. Leon ME, Ward B, Kanashiro R, Hernandez H, Berry S, Vaisberg A, Escamilla J, Campos M, Bellomo S, Azabache V, Halsey N. Immunolologic parameters 2 years after high-titer measles immunization in Peruvian children. J Infect Dis 1993; 168:1097-1104.

60. Aaby P, Knudsen K, Whittle H, et al. Long term survival after Edmonston-Zagreb measles vaccination; increased female mortality. J Pediatrics 1993; 122:904-908.

61. Aaby P, Samb B, Simondon F, Knudsen K., Seck AME, Bennett J, Whittle H. Divergent mortality for male and female recipients of low-titer and high titer measles in rural Senegal. Am J Epidemiol 1993; 138:746-755.

62. Halsey N. Increased mortality following high titer measles vaccines: too much of a good thing. J Pediatr Infect Dis 1993; 12:462-465.

63. Expanded Programme on Immunization. Consultation of studies involving high titer measles vaccines. Weekly Epidemiol Rec 1992; 67:357-361.

64. Weiss R. Measles battle loses potent weapon. Science 1992;258:546-547.

65. Committee on Infectious Diseases. Measles: reassessment of the current immunization policy. Pediatrics 1989;84(6):1110-1114.

66. Centers for Disease Control. MMRW 1993;42:378-381.

67. Centers for Disease Control - United States. MMWR 1987; 36; 301-305.

68. Krause PJ, Cherry JD, Deseda-Tous J, Champion JG, Strassburg M, Sulliva, C, et al. Epidemic measles in young adults. Ann Intern Med 1979; 90:873-876.

69. Tingle AJ, Yang T, Allen M, Kettyls GD, Larke RPB, Schulzer M. Prospective immunologic assessment of arthritis induced rubella vaccine. J Infect Immunol 1983; 40:22-28.

70. Coyle PK, Wolinsky JS, Buimovici-Klien E, Moucha R, Cooper LZ. Rubella-specific immune complex after congenital infection with vaccination. J Infect Immunol 1982; 36:498-503.

71. Pabst HF, Spady DW, Marusyk RG, Carson MM, Chui LW-L, Joffres MR, Grimsrud KM. Reduced measles immunity in infants in a well vaccinated population. Ped Infect J 1992;11:525-529.

72. Preblub SR, Markowitz L.E, Orenstein WA. Update on measles vaccine effectiveness. Twenty-First Immunization Conference Proceedings, New Orleans, La. June 8-11, 1987.

73. Conte TR, Siverston D, Horan JH, Lindergren M, Dwyer D. Evaluation of a two dose measles, mumps and rubella vaccination schedule in a cohort of college athletes. Publ Health Rep 1993; 108(4):431-435.

74. Robertson CM, Bennett VJ, Mayon-White RT. Serological evaluation of a measles, mumps and rubella vaccine. Arch Dis Child 1988; 63:612-616.

75. Orenstein WA, Hinman AR, Preblub SR, et al. Additional strategies for measles elimination. Twenty-First Immunization Conference Proceedings, New Orleans, LA June 8-11, 1987.

76. Fescharek R, Quast U, Merkle W, Schwartz S. Measles-mumps vaccination in the FGR: an empirical analysis after 14 years of use. I. Efficacy and analysis of vaccine failures. Vaccine 1990; 8:333-336.

77. Wu VH, McFarland H, Mayo K, Hanger L, Griffin D, Dhib-Jalbut S. Measles virus-specific cellular immunity in patients with vaccine failure. J Clin Micro 1993; 31(1):118-122.

78. Lichenstein R, Feigelman S, Luna C, Permutt T, Patel J. Measles, mumps and rubella antibodies in vaccinated Baltimore children. Am J Dis Child 1993; 147:558-560.

79. Hildreth EA, Frederic MW, Randall P. Alterations in delayed hypersensitivity produced by live attenuated measles virus in man. Trans Am Clin Climatolol Assoc 1963; 75;37-51.

80. Fireman P, Friday G, Kumate J. Effect of measles virus vaccine on immunologic responsiveness. Pediatrics 1969; 43;264-272.

81. Zweiman B, Pappagianis D, Maibach H, Hildreth E.A. Effect of measles immunization on tuberculin hypersensitivity and in vitro lymphocyte reactivity. Int Arch Allergy Immunol 1971; 40;834-841.

82. Munyer TP, Mangi RJ, Dolan T, Kantor FS. Depressed lymphocyte function after measles-mumps-rubella vaccination. J Infect Dis 1975; 132:75-78.

83. Hirsch RL, Mokhtarian F, Griffin DE, Brooks BR, Hess J, Johnson RT. Measles virus vaccination of measles seropositive individuals suppress lymphocyte proliferation and chemotactic factor production. Clin Immunol Immunopathol 1981; 21; 341-350.

84. Mellman WJ, Wetton R. Depression of the tuberculin reaction by attenuated measles virus vaccine J Lab Clin Med 1963; 61:453-458.

85. Brody JA, McAlister R. Depression of tuberculin sensitivity following measles vaccination. Am Rev Respir Dis 1964; 90;607-611.

86. Starr S, Berkovich S. Effects of measles gamma-globulin modified measles and vaccine measles on the tuberculin test. N Engl J Med 1964; 270:386-391.

87. Toraldo R, Tolone C, Catalanotti R, Iannielo R, D'Avanzo M, Canino G, Galdiero F, Iafusco F. Effects of measles-mumps-rubella vaccination on polymorphonuclear neutrophil function in children. Acata Paediatr 1992; 81:887-890.

88. Lennon JL, Black FL. Maternally derived measles immunity in an era of vaccine-protected mothers. J Pediatr 1986;108:671-676.

89. Jenks PA, Caul EO, Roome PHC. Maternally derived measles immunity in children of naturally infected and vaccinated mothers. Epidemiol Infect 1988; 101:473-476.

90. Eghafona NO, Ahmad AA, Ezeokoli PBM, Emejuaiwe SO. Haemagglutination inhibition antibody levels one year after natural measles infection and vaccination. Microbios 1991; 68:33-36.

91. Yeager AS, Davis JH, Ross LA, Harvey B. Measles immunization: successes and failures JAMA 1977; 237:347-351.

92. Albrecht P, Ennis FA, Saltzman EJ, Krugman S. Persistence of maternal antibody in infants beyond 12 months; mechanism of measles vaccine failure. J Pediatr 1977; 91:715-718.

93. Hersh BS, Markowitz LE, Hoffman RE, et al. A measles outbreak at a college with a prematriculation immunization requirement. Am J Publ Health 1991; 81: 360-364.

94. Mast EE, Berg JL, Hanrahan LP, Wassell JT, Davis JP. Risk factors for measles in a previously vaccinated population and cost-effectiveness of revaccination strategies. JAMA 1990; 264:2829-2833.

95. Shelton JD, Jacobson JE, Orenstein WA, Schultz KF, Donnell HD. Measles vaccine efficacy; influence of age at vaccination vs. duration of time since vaccination. Pediatrics 1978; 62:961-964.

96. Hutchins SS, Markowitz LE, Mead P, et al. A school-based measles outbreak; the effect of a selective revaccination policy risk factors for vaccine failure. Am J Epidemiol 1990; 132:157-168.

97. Lennon JL, Black FL. Maternally derived measles immunity in an era of vaccine-protected mothers. J Pediatr 1986; 108:671-676.

98. Jenks PA, Caul EO, Roome PHC. Maternally derived measles immunity in children of naturally infected and vaccinated mothers. Epidemiol Infect 1988; 101:473-476.

99. Miller DL. Frequency of complications of measles, 1963. Report of a national inquiry by the Public Health Laboratory Service in collaboration withy the Society of Medical Officers. Health BMJ 1963;2;75-78.

100. Park JE. Measles. Textbook of Prevention and Social Medicine. 12th ed 1989: 118-120.

101. Cryza SJ. Vaccines and Immunotherapy. Elmsford, New York: Pergamon Press, 1991.

102. Kipps A, Dick G, Moodie JW. Measles and the central nervous system. Lancet 1983; 2:1406.

103. Billeter MA, Cattaneo R, Schmid A. Host and viral features in persistent measles virus infection of the brain. In: Mahy BWJ, Kolakofsky D, eds. Genetics and pathogenicity of negative strand viruses. Amsterdam: Elsevier,1989:356.

104. Kipps A, Dick G, Moodie JW. Measles and the central nervous system. Lancet 1983; 2;1406.

105. Nadler PR, Warren RJ. Report neurologic disorders following live measles vaccine. Pedriatrics 1968; 41:997-1001.

106. Landrigan PJ, Witt JJ. Neurological disorders following live measles-virus vacci-nation. JAMA 1973; 223:1459-1462.

107. Kochm J, Leet C, McCarthy R, Carter A, Cuff W. Adverse events temporally associated with immunizing agents -1987 report / Manifestations facheuses associees dans le temps a des agents immunisants-rapport de 1987. Canada Diseases Weekly Report/Rapport Hebdomadaire des Maladies au Canada 1989; 15:151-158.

108. Carter H, Campbell H. Rational use of measles, mumps and rubella (MMR) vaccine. Drugs. 1993; 45 (5):677-683.

109. Institute of Medicine Adverse Events Associated with Childhood Vaccines. 1994;130.

110. Dunn RA. Subacute sclerosing panencephalitis. Pediatr Infect Dis J 1991;10:68.

111. Dyken PR. Subacute sclerosing panencephalitis. Current status. Neurol Clin 1985; 3:179.

112. Jabbour JT, Garcia JH, Lemmi H. Subacute sclerosing panencephalitis. a multidis-ciplinary study of eight cases. JAMA 1969; 207:2248.

113. Schneck SA. Vaccination with measles and central nervous system disease. Neurology 1968;18:78-82.

114. Moldlin JF, Jabbour JT, Witte JJ, Halsey NA. Epidemiological studies of measles, measles vaccine, and subacute sclerosing panencephalitis. Pediatrics 1977; 59:505-512.

115. Institute of Medicine. Adverse events associated with childhood vaccines 1994:142.

116. Hirtz DG, Nelson KB, Ellenberg JH. Seizures following childhood immunizations. J Pediatr 1983; 102:14-18.

117. Nieminen U, Peltola H, Syrjala MT, Makipernaa A, Kekomaki R. Acute thrombo-cytopenia purpura following measles, mumps and rubella vaccination: a report of 23 patients. Acta Paediatr 1993; 782:267-270.

118. Rejjal AL, Britten G. Thrombocytopenia purpura following MMR vaccination (letter). Ann Trop Paediatr 1993; 13:103-104.

119. Institute of Medicine. Adverse events associated with childhood vaccines. 1994:169.

120. Aukrus L, Almeland TL, Refsum D, Aas K. Severe hypersensitivity or intolerance reactions to measles vaccine in six children: clinical and immunological studies. Allergy 1980; 35:581-587.

121. Fescharek R, Quast U, Maass G, Merkle W, Schwartz S. Measles-mumps vaccination in the FRG: an empirical analysis after 14 years of use. II. Tolerability and analysis of spontaneous reported side effects. Vaccine 1990; 8:446-456.

122. Herman JJ, Radin R, Schneiderman R. Allergic reactions to measles (rubeola) vaccine in patients hypersensitive to egg protein. J Pediatr 1983; 102:196-199.

123. McEwen J. Early-onset reaction after measles vaccination: further Australian reports. Med J Austral 1983; 2:502-505.

124. Pollack TM, Morris J. A 7-year survey of disorders attributed to vaccination in North West Thames region. Lancet 1983: 1;753-757.

125. Ewen J. Early-onset reaction after measles vaccination: further Australian reports. Med J Austral 1983;2:503-505.

126. Van Asperen PP, McEniery J, Kemp AS. Intermediate reactions following live attenuated measles vaccine. Med J Austral 1981; 2:330-331.

127. Bruno G, Giampietro PG, Grandolfa ME, Milita O, Businco, L. Safety of measles immunization in children with IgE mediated egg allergy (letter). Lancet 1990; 335:739.

128. Kemp A, Van Asperen P, Mukhi A. Measles immunization in children with clinical reactions to egg protein. Am J Dis Child 1990; 144:33-35.

129. Fasano MB, Wood RA, Cooke SK, Sampson HA. Egg hypersensitivity and adverse reactions to measles, mumps and rubella vaccine. J Pediatr 1992; 120:878-881.

130. Institute of Medicine Adverse Effects Associated with Childhood Vaccinations 1994:177.

131. Frankel DH. New US laws on childhood vaccines [news]. Lancet, 1993 Sep 4, 342(8871):607.

132. Jackson BM, Payton T, Horst G, Halpin TJ, Mortensen BK. An epidemiologic investigation of a rubella outbreak among the Amish of northeastern Ohio. Publ Health Rep 1993 Jul-Aug, 108(4):436-9.

133. Rodgers DV, Gindler JS, Atkinson WL, Markowitz LE. High attack rates and case fatality during a measles outbreak in groups with religious exemption to vaccination. Pediatr Infect Dis J 1993;12(4):288-92.

134. McGrath D, Swanson R, Weems S, Mack D, Barbour SD. Analysis of a measles outbreak in Kent County, Michigan in 1990. Pediatr Infect Dis J 1992;11(5):385-9.

135. O'Connor AM, Pennie RA, Dales RE. Framing effects on expectations, decisions, and side effects experienced:the case of influenza immunization. J Clin Epidemiol 1996;49(11):1271-6.

136. Goldsmith MF. Vaccine information pamphlets here, but some physicians react strongly. JAMA 1992;267:2005-2007.

137. Crozier K. VIP's: just another barrier to vaccination? Infect Dis Child 1993;6:12.

138. Halsey NA, Boulos R, Mode F, et al. Response to measles vaccine in Haitian infants 6 to 12 months old: Influence of maternal antibodies, malnutrition and concurrent illness. N Engl J Med 1985; 313:544.

139. Job JS, Halsey NA, Boulos R, et al. Successful immunization of infants at 6 months of age with high dose Edmonson-Zagreb measles vaccine. Pediatr Infect Dis J 1991;10:303-311.

140. Markowitz LE, Sepulveda J, Diaz-Ortega JL,et.al. Immunization of six-month-old infants with different doses of Edmonson-Zagreb and Schwarz measles vaccines. N Engl J Med 1990; 322:580-587.

141. Expanded Programme on Immunization. Measles immunization before 9 months of age. Wkly Epidemiol Rec 1990; 65:8.

142. Expanded Programme on Immunization. Safety of higher titer measles vaccines. Wkly Epidemiol Rec 1992; 67:357-361.

143. Bellanti JA. Basic Immunologic principles underlying vaccination procedures. Pediatr Clin North Am 1990;37:513-533.

144. Cohn ML, Robinson ED, Faerber M, Thomas D, Geyer S, Peters S, et.al. Measles vaccine failures: lack of sustained measles-specific immunoglobulin G responses in revaccinated adolescents and young adults. Pediatr Infect Dis 1994; 13: 34-38.

145. Robbins AS. Controversies in measles immunization recommendations. West J Med 1993;158:36-39.

146. Philip RN, Reinhard KR, Lackman DB. Observations on a mump epidemic in a "virgin" population. Am J Hygiene 1959; 69:91.

147. Weibel RE, Buynak EB, McLean AA. Persistence of antibody after administration of monovalent and combined live measles, mumps and rubella virus vaccines. Pediatrics 1978;61:5.

148. Lewis JE, Chernesky MA, Rawls ML, et al. Epidemic of mumpsin a partially immune population. Can Med Assoc J 1979; 121:751.

149. Sullivan KM, Halpin TJ, Marks JS, et al. Effectiveness of mumps vaccine in a school outbreak. Am J Dis Child 1985;3:109.

150. Wharton M, Cochi SL, Hutcheson RH, et al. A large outbreak of mumps in the post vaccine era. J Infect Disease 1988; 158:1253.

151. Bakshi SS, Cooper LZ. Rubella and mumps vaccines. Pediatr Clin North Am 1990;37:651-669.

152. Yamanishi K, Takahashi M, Ueda S, et al. Transmission of live attenuated mumps virus to the human placenta. N Engl J Med 1973; 290:710.

153. Coville A, Pugh S. Mumps meningitis and measles, mumps and rubella vaccine. Lancet 1992; 340:786.

154. Sugiura A, Yamada A. Aseptic meningitis as a complication of mumps vaccination. Pediatr Infect Dis J 1991; 10:209-213.

155. McDonald JC, Moore DL, Quennec P. Clinical and epidemiological features of mumps meningoencephalitis and possible vaccine related disease. Pediatr Infect Dis J 1989; 751-755.

156. Maguire HC, Begg NT, Handford SG. Meningoencephalitis associated with MMR vaccine. CRD (London England Review) 1991;1(6):R60-1 May 24.

157. Fujinaga T, Motegi Y, Tamura H, Kuroume T. A nation-wide survey of mumps meningitis associated with the measles, mumps and rubella vaccine. Pediatr Infect Dis J 1991; 10:204-209.

158. Sugiura A, Yamada A. Aseptic meningitis as a complication of mumps vaccination. Pediatr Infect Dis J 1991; 10:209-213145.

159. Gunby P. Atypical mumps may occur after immunization. JAMA 1980; 243(23): 2374-2375.

160. Chaiken BP, Williams NM, Preblud SR, Parkin W, Altman R. The effect of a school entry low on mumps activity in a school district. JAMA 1987; 257;18:2455-2458.

161. Bottiger M, Christenson B, Romanus V, Taranger J, Strandell A. Swedish experience of two dose vaccination program aiming at eliminating measles, mumps and rubella. Br Med J 1987; 295:264-267.

162. Pless IB. The epidemiology of childhood disorders. Oxford: University Press, 1994.

163. Cochi SI, Preblud SR, Orienstein WA. Perspectives of the relative resurgence of mumps in the United States. Am J Dis Child 1988; 142:449-507.

164. Werner CA. Mumps orchitis and testicular atrophy. I. Occurrence. Ann Intern Med 1950a; 32:1066-1074.

165. Hockin JC. Mumps meningitis, possibly vaccine-related. Canada Dis Wkly Rep 1988; 144:209-211.

166. Thomas E. A case of mumps meningitis: a complication of vaccination. Can Med Assoc J 1988; 138:135.

167. Sugiura A, Yamada A. Aseptic meningitis as a complication of mumps vaccination. Pediatr Infect Dis J 1991; 10:209-213.

168. Nabe-Nelson J, Walter B. Unilateral deafness as a complication of the mumps, measles and rubella vaccination. Scand Audiol 1988a; 30:69-70.

169. Nabe-Nelson J, Walter B. Unilateral deafness as a complication of the mumps, measles and rubella vaccination. Br Med J 1988b; 297:489.

170. Bottinger M, Christenson B, Romanus V, Taranger J, Strandell A. Swedish

experience of two dose vaccination programme aiming at eliminating measles, mumps and rubella. Br Med J 1987; 295:264-267.

171. Otten A, Helmke K, Stief T. Mueller-Eckhard G, Willems WR, Federlin K. Mumps, mumps vaccine, islet cell antibodies and the first manifestation of diabetes mellitus Type 1. Behring Institute Mitteilingen 1984; 75:83-88.

172. Sulz HA, Hart BA, Zielezny M, Schlesinger ER. Is mumps virus an etiologic factor in juvenile diabetes mellitus? J Pediatr 1975; 86:654-656.

173. Cooper LZ. History and medical consequences of rubella. Rev Infect Dis 1985; 7(suppl):S2-S9.

174. Davis B, Dulbecco R, Eisen HN, Ginsberg HS. eds. Microbiology. Philadelphia: Harper and Roe Publishers, 1983:1149-1154.

175. Cherry JD. The "new"epidemiology of measles and rubella. Hosp Practice 1989(July):49-57.

176. Rachelfsky GS. Failure of rubella herd immunity during an epidemic. N Engl J Med 1973; 288(2):69-72.

177. Hermann KL, Halstead SB, Wienbenga NH. Rubella antibody persistence after immunization. JAMA 1982; 7(2):193-196.

178. Allan B. Rubella immunisation. Aust J Med Tech 1973;4:26-27.

179. Horstman DM, Liebhaber H, Kohorn EL. Post-partum vaccination of rubella-susceptible women. Lancet 1970; 2:1003-1006.

180. Lerman SJ, Nankervis GA, Heggie AD, Gold E. Immunologic response, virus excretion, and joint reactions with rubella vaccine: a study of adolescent girls and young women given live attenuation virus vaccine (HPV-77:DE-5). Ann Intern Med 1971; 74;67-73.

181. Spruance SL, Smith CB. Joint complications associated with derivatives of HPV-77 rubella virus vaccine. Am J Dis Child 1971; 122;105-111.

182. Thompson GR, Ferreyra A, Brackett RG. Acute arthritis complicating rubella vaccination. Arthritis Rheumatism 1971; 14:19-26.

183. Polk BF, Modlin JF, White JA, DeGirolami PC. A controlled comparison of joint reactions among women receiving one of two rubella vaccines. Am J Epidemiol 1982; 115:19-25.

184. Institute of Medicine. Adverse effects of pertussis and rubella. 1991;197.

185. Tingle AJ, Chantler JK, Pot KH, Paty DW, Ford DK. Postpartum rubella immunization: association with development of prolonged arthritis, neurological sequela and chronic rubella viremia. J Infect Dis 1985; 152:606-612.,

186. Chin J, Werner SB, Kusumoto HH, Lennette EH. Complications of rubella immunization in children. West Med J 1971; 114:7-12.

187. Morton-Kute L. Rubella vaccine and facial paresthesias (letter) Ann Intern Med 1985; 102;563.

188. Institute of Medicine. Adverse effects of pertussis and rubella. 1991;199.

189. Joncas J. Preventing the congenital rubella syndrome by vaccinating women at risk. Can Med Ass J 1983; 129(12):110-112.

190. Tingle AJ, Chantler JK, Kettyls GD, Bryce Larke RP, Schulzer M. Failed rubella immunization in adults: association with immunologic and virological abnormalities. J Infect Dis 1985; 151(2):330-336.

191. Das BD, Lakhani P, Kurtz JB, Hunter N, Wartson BE, Cartwright, KAV, Caul EO, Rome APCH. Congenital Rubella after previous maternal immunity. Arch Dis Child 1990; 65:545-546.

192. Chantler JL, Tingle AJ, Petty RE. Persistent rubella infection associated with arthritis in children. N Engl J Med 1985; 313:1117-1123.

193. Kimpen JLL, Ogra PL. Poliovirus vaccines. Pediatr Clin North Am 37; 3:627-649.

194. Burnet M, White D. The natural history of infectious disease. Cambridge: University Press, 1972:94.

195. Institute of Medicine. Adverse events associated with childhood vaccines. 1994;189.

196. Raciniello VR. Poliovirus vaccines. Biotechnology 1992; 20:205-222.

197. Peabody FW, Draper G, Dochez AR. A Clinical study of acute poliomyelitis. Monograph No.4 New York, Rockefeller Institute for Medical Research, 1912.

198. Melnick JL, Ledinko N. Social serology: antibody levels in a normal young population during an epidemic of poliomyelitis. Am J Hyg 1951; 54:354-382.

199. Melnick JL, Paul JR, Walton M. Serologic epidemiology of poliomyelitis. Am J Publ Health 1955; 45: 429-437.

200. McCarroll JR, Melnick JL, Horstmann DM. Spread of poliomyelitis infection in nursery school. Am J Publ Health 1955; 45;1541-1550.

201. Melnick JL, McCarroll JR, Horstmann DM. A winter outbreak of poliomyelitis in New York City. The complement-fixation test as an aid in rapid diagnosis. Am J Hyg 1956; 63;95-114.

202. Nolan JP, Wilmer BJ, Melnick JL. Poliomyelitis: its highly invasive nature and narrow stream of infection in a community of high socioeconomic level. N Engl J Med 1955; 253:945-954.

203. Lavinder CH, Freeman AW, Frost WH. Epidemiologic studies of poliomyelitis in New York City and Northeastern United States during the year 1916. Publ Health Bull 1918; 91(July).

204. Plotkin SA, Mortimer E. Vaccines. Philadelphia:W.B. Saunders Co 1988:119.

205. Melnick JL, Paul JR, Walton M. Serologic epidemiology of poliomyelitis. Am J Publ Health 1955; 45:429-437.

206. Salk JE. Recent studies in immunization against poliomyelitis. Pediatrics 1953; 12:471-482.

207. Salk JE, Bennett BL, Lewis LJ, Ward EN, Youngner JS. Studies in human subjects on active immunization against poliomyelitis. 1. A preliminary report of experiments in progress. JAMA 1953; 151:1081-1098.

208. Koprowski H, Jervis GA, Norton TW. Immune responses in human volunteers upon oral administration of a rodent-adapted strain of poliomyelitis virus. Am J Hygiene 1952;55:108-126.

209. Sabin AB. Immunization of chimpanzees and human beings with avirulent strains of poliomyelitis virus. Ann NY Acad Sci 1956;61:1050-1056.

210. Jungebult CW, Engle ET. Resistance to poliomyelitis. The relative importance of physiologic and immunologic factors. JAMA 1932; 99(25):2091-2097.

211. Francis T, Korns RF, Voight RB, Boisen M, Hemphill FM, Napier JA, Tolchinski A. Evaluation of the 1954 poliomyelitis vaccine trials. Poliomyelitis Vaccine Evaluation Center: University of Michigan, Ann Arbor, Michigan 12 April 1955;50.

212. Henderson DA, Witte JJ, Morris L, Langmuir AD. Paralytic disease associated with oral polio vaccines. JAMA 1964; 190:41-48.

213. Sabin AB. Is there an exceedingly small risk associated with oral polio vaccine? JAMA 1963; 183(4): 268-271.

214. Sabin AB, Hennessen WA, Winsser J. Studies on variants of poliomyelitis virus. I. Experimental segregation and properties of avirulent variants of three immunologic types. J Exp Med 1954; 99:551-576.

215. Pan American Sanitary Bureau: Line Poliovirus Vaccines, Special Publication of the Pan American Sanitary Bureau, No.44, 1959. Pan American Health Organization: Live Poliovirus Vaccines, Special Publication of the Pan American Health Organization No. 50. 1960.

216. Gelfand HM, Potash L, LeBlanc DR, Fox JP. Revised preliminary report on the Louisiana observations of the natural spread within families of living vaccine strains of poliovirus. In: Live Poliovirus Vaccines, Papers Presented and Discussions Held at the First International Conference on Live Poliovirus Vaccines. Special Publication No. 44. Washington, D.C., Pan American Sanitary Bureau, 1959.

217. Plotkin SA, Mortimer EA.. Vaccines. Philadelphia: W.B. Saunders. 1988:125.

218. Henderson DA, Witte JJ, Morris L, Langmuir AD. Paralytic disease associated with the oral polio vaccines. JAMA 1990; 1:41-48.

219. Nkowane BM, Wassilak SG, Orenstein WA, Bart KJ, Schonberger LB, Hinman AR, et al. Vaccine associated paralytic poliomyelitis, United States: 1973 through 1984. JAMA 1987; 257:1335-1340.

220. Institute of Medicine. Adverse events associated with childhood vaccines. 1994; 194.

221. Nathansin N, Martin JR. The epidemiology of poliomyelitis:enigmas surrounding its appearance, epidemiology and disappearance. N Engl J Med 1979; 110; 6:672-692.

222. Chang TW, Weinstein L, MacMahon HE. Paralytic poliomyelitis in a child with hypogammaglobulinemia: probable implications of type 1 vaccine strain. Pediatrics 1966;37:630-636.

223. Loffel et al. Vaccine poliomyelitis in an adult undergoing chemotherapy for non-Hodgkin's lymphoma. Schweiz Medizinische Wochenschrift 1982; 112: 419-421.

224. Sanko et al. Vaccine-associated poliomyelitis in an infant with agammaglobulinemia. Acta Paediatr Scand 1980;69:549-551.

225. Anderson O, Eeg-Olofsson E. A perspective study of paraparesis in western Sweden. Acta Neurol Scand 1976; 54:312-320.

226. Kinnunen E, Farkkila M, Hovi T, Juntunen J, Weckstrom P. Incidence of Guillain Barré syndrome during a nationwide oral poliovirus vaccine campaign. Neurology 1989; 39:1034-1036.

227. Stratton KR, et.al. eds. Institute of Medicine: Adverse effects of childhood vaccines. National Academic Press, 1994:188.

228. Hii BA, Knowelden J. Inoculation and poliomyelitis -a statistical investigation in England and Wales in 1949. Br Med J 1950; 1: 6-7.

229. Strobile PM, Ion-Needled N, Bahamian RW, Butter RW, Cochi SL. Intramuscular injections within 30 days of immunization with oral polio vaccine. A risk factor for vaccine associated poliomyelitis. N Engl J Med 1995;332:500-506.

230. Anderson GW, Skaar AE. Poliomyelitis occurring after antigen injection. Pediatrics 1994; 7(6):741-759.

231. Martin JK. Local paralysis in children after injections. Arch Dis Child 1950; 25:1.

232. Stratton KR, et al, eds. Institute of Medicine: Adverse effects of childhood vaccines. National Academic Press, 1994:205-206.

233. Wyatt HV. Poliomyelitis in hypogammaglobulinemics. J infect Dis 1973; 128: 802-806.

234. Ogra PL, Sinks LF, Karzon DT. Poliovirus antibody response in patients with acute leukemia. J Pediatr 1971;79:444-449.

235. Onorato IM, Markowitz LE, Oxtoby MJ. Childhood immunization, vaccine-preventable diseases and infection with human immunodeficiency virus. Pediatr Infect Dis J 1988; 7:588-595.

236. Paradiso PR. The future of polio immunization in the United States: are we ready for change? Pediatr Infect Dis J 1996; 15:645-649.

237. Plotkin SA. Inactivated polio vaccine for the United States: a missed vaccination opportunity. Pediatr Infect Dis J 1995; 14:835-839.

238. Hull HF, Ward NA, Milstein JB, deQuadros C. Paralytic poliomyelitis: seasoned strategies, disappearing disease. Lancet 1994; 343:1331-1337.

239. Broome CV. Epidemiology of Haemophilus influenza type B infections in the United States. Pediatr Infect Dis J 1987; 6:779-782.

240. Cochi SL, Broome CV, Hightower AW. Immunization of U.S. children with Haemophilus influenza type B polysaccharide vaccine. JAMA 1985; 253; 521-529.

241. Petola H, Kayhty H, Virtanen M, Makela PH. Prevention of Haemophilus influenza

type B bacteremia infections with the capsular polysaccharide vaccine. N Engl J Med 1984; 310:1561-1566.

242. Osterholm HT, Rambeck JH, White KE, Jacob JL, Pierson LM, Neaton, JD, et al. Lack of efficacy of Haemophilus B polysaccharide vaccine in Minnesota. JAMA 1988; 260:1423-1428.

243. Black SB, Shinefield HR, Hiatt RA, Fireman BH, Beekly M, Callas ER, et al. Efficacy of Haemophilus influenza type B capsular polysaccharide vaccine. Pediatr Infect Dis J 1988; 7:149-156.

244. Shapiro ED, Murphy TV, Wald ER, Brady CA. The protective efficacy of Haemophilus B polysaccharide vaccine. JAMA 1988; 260:1419-1422.

245. Black SB, Shinefield HR, Hiatt RA, Fireman BH, Beekly M, Callas ER, et al. Efficacy of Haemophilus influenza type B capsular polysaccharide vaccine. Pediatr Infect Dis J 1988; 7:149-156.

246. Osterholm HT, Rambeck JH, White KE, Jacob JL, Pierson LM, Neaton JD, et al. Lack of efficacy of Haemophilus B polysaccharide vaccine in Minnesota. J AMA 1988; 260:1423-1428.

247. Avery OT, Goebel WF. Chemo-immunological studies on conjugate carbohydrate-proteins II. Immunological specificity of synthetic sugar-protein antigens. J Exp Med 1929; 50:533-550.

248. Parke JC, Schneerson R, Robbins JB, et al. Interim report of a controlled field trial of immunization with capsular polysaccharide of Haemophilus type B and group C Neisseria meningitides in Mecklenburg County, North Carolina. J Infect Dis 1977; 136:S51-S56.

249. Peltola H, Kayhty H, Sivonen A, Makela HP. Haemophilus influenza type B capsular polysaccharide vaccine in children; double-blind field study of 100,000 vaccinees 3 months to 5 years of age in Finland. Pediatrics 1977; 60:730-737.

250. Milstien JB, Gross TP, Kuritsky JN. Adverse reactions reported following receipt of Haemophilus influenza type B vaccine: an analysis after 1 year of marketing. Pediatrics 1987; 80(2);270-274.

251. Sood SK, Daum RS. Haemophilus influenza type B disease in the immediate period following homologous immunization: Immunologic investigation. Pediatrics 1990; 85:698-704.

252. Harrison LH, Broome CV, Hightower AW, Hoppe CC, Makintubee S, Sitze SL, Taylor JA, Gaventa S, Wenger JD, Facklam RR. Haemophilus vaccine efficacy study group: a daycare-based study of the efficacy of Haemophilus B polysaccharide vaccine. JAMA 1988; 260:1413-1418.

253. Harrison LM, Broome CV, Hightower AW, Efficacy study group. Haemophilus influenza type B polysaccharide vaccine: An efficacy study. Pediatrics 1989; 84:255-261.

254. Black SB, Shinefield HR, Hiatt RA, Fireman BH, Kaiser Permanente Pediatric Vaccine Study group. Efficacy of Haemophilus influenza type B capsular polysaccharide vaccine. Pediatr Infect Dis 1988;7:149-156.

255. Osterholm MT, Rambeck JH, White KE, Jacobs JL, Pierson LM, Neaton JD, Hedburg CD, MacDonald KL, Granoff DM. Lack of efficacy of Haemophilus B polysaccharide vaccine in Minnesota. JAMA 1988; 260:1423-1428.

256. Eskola J, Peltola H, Takala AK, et. al. Efficacy of Haemophilus influenza type B polysaccharide - Diptheria-toxoid conjugate vaccine in infancy. N Engl J Med 1987; 317(12):717-722.

257. American Academy of Pediatrics, Committee on Infectious Diseases. The Red Book. Report of the Committee of Infectious Disease, 22nd ed Peter G. ed, Elk Grove, Il American Academy of Pediatrics.

258. Centers for Disease Control - United States MMWR 1993;42:296-298.

259. Decker MD, Edwards KM, Bradley R, Palmer P. Comparative trial in infants of four conjugate Haemophilus influenza type B disease: serologic response to conjugate vaccine. Am J Dis Child 1989; 143:31-33.

260. Greenberg DP, Vadheim CM, March SM, Ward JI. Kaiser-UCLA Hib Vaccine Study Group. Evaluation of Safety, immunogenicity, and efficacy of Haemophilus B (Hib) PRP-T conjugate vaccine in a prospective, randomized, and placebo-controlled trial in young infants. Program abstracts of the 32nd Interscience Conference on Antimicrobial Agents and Chemotherapy. Abstract 65:100. Washington, D.C. American Society of Microbiology.

261. Fritzell B, Plotkin S. Efficacy and safety of a Haemophilus influenza type B capsular polysaccharide-tetanus protein conjugate vaccine. J Pediatr 1992; 121:355-362.

262. Trollfors B, Lagergard T,Claesson BA, Thornberg E, Martinell J, Schneerson R. Characterization of serum antibody response to the capsular polysaccharide Haemophilus influenza type B in children with invasive infections. J Infect Dis 1992; 166:1335-1339.

263. Norden CW, Michaels RH, Melish M. Serological responses of children with meningitis due to Haemophilus influenza type B. J Infect Dis 1976; 134:495-499.

264. Granoff DM, Cates KL. Haemophilus influenza type B polysaccharide vaccines. J Pediatr 1985; 107:330-336.

265. Steinoff MC, Auerbach BS, Nelson KE, Vlahov D, Becker RL, Graham NMH, et al. Antibody responses to Haemophilus influenza type B vaccines in men with human immunodeficiency virus infection. N Engl J Med 1991; 325:1837-1842.

266. Weinberg GA, Granoff DM. Polysaccharide-protein conjugate vaccines in the prevention of Haemophilus influenza type B disease. J Pediatr 1988;113:621-631.

267. Robbins JB, Schneerson R. Polysaccharide-protein conjugates: a new generation of vaccines. J Infect Dis 1990; 161:821-832.

268. Ward JI, Brenneman G, Lepow M, Lum M, Burkhart K, Chiu CY. Haemophilus influenza type B anticapsular antibody responses to PRP-pertussis and PRP-D vaccines in Alaska native infants. J Infect Dis 1988; 158:719-723.

269. D'Cruz OF, Shapiro ED, Spiegelman KN, Leicher CR, Breningstall GN, Khatri BO, et al. Acute inflammatory demyelinating polyradiculoneuropathy (Guillain Barré Syndrome) after immunization with Haemophilus influenza type B conjugate vaccine. J Pediatr 1989; 115:743-746.

270. Decker MD, Edward KM, Bradley R, Palmer P. Comparative trial in infants of four conjugated Haemophilus influenza type B vaccines. J Pediatr 1988; 120:184-189.

271. Osterholm MT, Rambeck JH, White KE, Jacobs JL, Pierson LM, Neaton JD, Hedburg CD, MacDonald KL, Granoff DM. Lack of efficacy of Haemophilus B polysaccharide vaccine in Minnesota. JAMA 1988:260:1423-1428.

272. Osterholm MT, Rambeck JH, White KE, Jacobs JL, Pierson LM, Neaton JD, Hedburg CD, MacDonald KL, Granoff DM. Lack of efficacy of Haemophilus B polysaccharide vaccine in Minnesota. JAMA 1988:260:1423-1428.

273. Harrison LH, Broome CV, Hightower AW, Hoppe CC, Makintubee S, Sitze SL, Taylor JA, Gaventa S, Wenger JD, Facklam RR. Haemophilus vaccine efficacy study group: a daycare-based study of the efficacy of Haemophilus B polysaccharide vaccine. JAMA 1988; 260:1413-1418.

274. Stratton KR, et al, eds. Institute of Medicine: Adverse effects of childhood vaccines. National Academic Press, 1994:251.

275. Marchant CD, Band E, Froeschle JE, McVerry PH. Depression of anticapsular antibody after immunization with Haemophilus influenza type B polysaccharide-diphtheria conjugate vaccine. Pediatr Infect Dis J 1989; 8:508-511.

276. Sood SK, Daum RS. Disease caused by Haemophilus influenza type B in the immediate period after homologous immunization: immunologic investigation. Pediatrics 1990; 85:698-704.

277. Peltola HH. Influenza in the post-vaccination era. Lancet 1993; 341:864-865.

278. Dittman S. Diptheria immunization. Beitrage zur Hygiene und Epidemiologie 1981; 25:237-239

279. Rappouli R, Perugini M, Falsen E. Molecular epidemiology of the 1984-1986 outbreak of diphtheria in Sweden. N Engl J Med 1988; 318:12-14.

280. James G, Longshore WA, Hendry JL. Diphtheria immunization studies of students in an urban high school. Am J Hygiene 1951; 53:178-201.

281. Karzon D, Edwards K. Diphtheria outbreaks in immunized populations. N Engl J Med 1988; 318:41-43.

282. Christenson B, Bottiger M. Serological immunity to diphtheria in Sweden in 1978 and 1984. Scand J Infect Dis 1986; 18:227-233.

283. Bjorkholm B, Bottinger M, Cristenson B. Antitoxin antibody levels and the outcome of illness during an outbreak of diphtheria among alcoholics. Scand J Infect Dis 1986; 18:235-239.

284. Wassilak SG, Oreinstein WA. Tetanus. In: Plotkin SA, Mortimer EA, eds. Vaccines. Philadelphia: W.B. Saunders, 1988.

285. Fishman PS, Carrigan DR. Motorneuron uptake from the circulation of the binding fragment of tetanus toxin. Arch Neurol 1988; 45:558-561.

286. Mortimer EA. Diphtheria toxoid. In: Plotkin SA, Mortimer EA, eds. Vaccines. Philadelphia:W.B. Saunders,1988.

287. Illis LS, Taylor FM. Neurological and electroencephalographic sequela of tetanus. Lancet 1971; 1826-1830.

288. Pollock TM, Morris J. A 7-year survey of disorders attributed to vaccination in North West Thames region. Lancet 1983; 1:753-757.

289. Alderslade R, Bellman MH, Rawson NSB, Ross EM, Miller DL. The National Childhood Encephalopathy Study: a report on 1,000 cases of serious neurological disorders in infants and young children from the NCES research team. In: Whooping Cough: Reports from the Committee on the Safety of Medicine and the Joint Committee on Vaccination and Immunisation. Department of Health and Social Security, London: Her Majesty's Stationary Office, 1981.

290. Fujinami PS, Carrigan DR. Molecular mimicry as a mechanism for virus-induced autoimmunity. Immunol Res 1989; 8:3-15.

291. Hopf HC. Guillain Barré Syndrome following tetanus toxoid administration: survey and report of a case. Aktuelle Neurologie 1980; 7:195-200.

292. Holliday PL, Bauer RB. Polyradiculoneuritis secondary to immunization with tetanus and diphtheria toxoids. Arch Neurol 1983; 40:56-57.

293. Quast U, Hennessen W, Widmark RM. Mono-and polyneuritis after tetanus vaccination (1970-1977). Develop Biol Standardization 1979; 43:25-32.

294. Onisawa S, Sekine I, Ichimura T, Homma N. Guillain Barré syndrome secondary to immunization with diphtheria toxoid. Dokkyo J Med Sci 1985; 12:227-229.

295. Reinstein L, Pargament JM, Goodman JS. Peripheral neuropathy after multiple tetanus toxoid injections. Arch Physical Med Rehab 1982; 63:332-334.

296. Robinson IG. Unusual reaction to tetanus toxoid (letter). NZ Med J 1981; 94:359.

297. Rutledge SL, Snead OC. Neurologic complications of immunizations. J Peds 1986; 109:917-924.

298. Miller HG, Stanton JB, Neurological sequela of prophylactic inoculation. Q J Med 1954; 23:1-27.

299. Stratton KR, et al eds. Institute of Medicine: Adverse effects of childhood vaccines. National Academic Press, 1994:89.

300. Willingham HE. Anaphylaxis following administration of tetanus toxoid. Br Med J 1940; 1:292-293.

301. Parish HG, Oakley CL. Anaphylaxis after injection of tetanus toxoid. Br Med J 1940; 1:294-295.

302. Lleonart-Bellfill R, Cistero-Bahima A, Cerda-Trias MT, Olive-Perez A. Tetanus toxoid anaphylaxis. DICP Ann Pharmacother 1991; 25:870.

303. Ratcliff DA, Burns-Cox CJ. Anaphylaxis to tetanus toxoid. Br Med J 1984; 228:114.

304. Zaloga GP, Chernow B. Life-threatening anaphylactic reaction to tetanus toxoid. Ann Allergy 1982; 49:107-108.

305. Chanukoglu A, Fried D, Gotlieb A. Anaphylactic shock due to tetanus toxoid. Harefauh 1975; 89:456-457.

306. Fischmeister M. Acute reaction following injection of tetanus toxoid (letter). Deutsche Medizinsche Wochenschrift 1974; 99:850.

307. Bilyk MA, Dubchik GK. Anaphylactic reaction following subcutaneous adminis-tration of tetanus antitoxin. Klinicheskaia Medistina 1978; 56:137-138.

308. Mansfield LE, Ting S, Rawls DO, Federick R. Systemic reactions during cutaneous testing for tetanus toxoid hypersensitivity. Ann Allergy 1986; 757: 135-137.

309. Ovens H. Anaphylaxis due to vaccination in the office. Can Med Assoc J 1986;134:369-370.

310. Mandel GS, Mukhopadhyay M, Bhattacharya AR. Adverse reactions following tetanus toxoid injection. J Indian Med Assoc 1980; 74:35-37.

311. Werne J, Garrow I. Fatal anaphylactic shock occurrence in identical twins following second injection of diptheria toxoid and pertussis antigen. JAMA 1946; 131:730-735.

312. Regamey RH. Tetanus immunization in Handbook of Immunization. In: Herrlick, A., ed. Hanbuch der Schutz- impfungen. Berlin: Springer,1965.

313. Staak M, Wirth E. Anaphylactic reactions following active tetanus immunization. Deutsche Medizinische Wochenschrift 1973; 98:110-111.

314. American Academy of Pediatrics. The Red Book. Report of the Committee on Infectious Disease, 20th edition. Peter G, ed. Elk Grove Village, IL, 1986.

315. American Academy of Pediatrics. Cherry JD, Brunell PA, Golden GS, Karzon DT. Report of the task force on pertussis and pertussis immunization. Pediatrics 1988; 81(6, part 2):939-984.

316. Mortimer EA. Pertussis vaccine. In: Plotkin SA, Mortimer EA, eds. Vaccines. Philadelphia: W.B. Saunders Co., 1988.

317. Aoyama T, Goto R, Iwai H, Murase Y, Iwata T. Pertussis in the adult. In: Manclark, C.R., ed. Sixth International Symposium on Pertussis, Abstracts. DHHS Publica-tion No. (FDA) 90-1162. Bethesda, MD: Public Health Service, U.S. Department of Health and Human Services, 1990.

318. Farzio KM, Cochi SL, Zell R, Patriarca PA, Wassilak S, Brink EW. Perspectives on the epidemiology of pertussis in the United States, 1980-1988. In: Manclark, CR, ed. Sixth Internation Symposium on Pertussis, Abstracts. DHHS Publication No. (FDA) 90-1162. Bethesda, MD: Public Health Service, U.S. Dept. of Health and Human Services.

319. Nelson JD. Their changing epidemiology of pertussis in young infants: the role of adults as reservoirs of infection. Am J Dis Child 1978; 132:371-373.

320. Chase A. Magic shots: A human and scientific account of the long and continuing struggle to eradicate infectious diseases by vaccination. New York: William Morrow and Company, Inc. 1982.

321. Kendrick P. The use of alum-treated pertussis vaccine, and the alum-precipitate combined pertussis vaccine and diptheria toxoid, for active immunization. Am J Publ Health 1942; 32:615-626.

322. Wardlaw AC, Parton R, eds. Pathogenesis and immunity in pertussis. New York: John Wiley & Sons Ltd., 1988.

323. Cody CL, Baraff LJ, Cherry JD, Marcy SM, Manclark CR. Nature and rates of adverse reactions associated with DTP and DT immunization in infants and children. Pediatrics 1981; 68:650-660.

324. Howson CP, Fineberg HV. Adverse events following pertussis and rubella vaccines. Summary of the report of the Institute of Medicine. JAMA 1992; 267:392-396.

325. Cherry JD. The epidemiology of pertussis and pertussis vaccine in the United Kingdom and the United States; a comparative study. In: Lockheart JD, eds. Current Problems in Pediatrics. Chicago. Year Book Medical Publishers, 1984.

326. Kimura M, Kuno-sakai H. Developments in pertussis immunisation in Japan. Lancet 1990; 336:30-32.

327. Romanus V, Jonsell R, Berquest S-O. Pertussis in Sweden after the cessation of general immunization in 1979. Pediatr Infect Dis J 1987; 6:664-671.

328. Mortimer EA, Jones PK. An evaluation of pertussis vaccine. Rev Infect Dis 1979; 1:927-932.

329. McFarlan AM, Topley E, Fisher M. Trial of whooping cough vaccine in city and residential nursery groups. Br Med J 1945; 2:105-108.

330. Scheibner V. Vaccination: The medical assault on the immune system. 1993:15.

331. Stratton KR, et.al. eds. Institute of Medicine: Adverse effects of childhood vaccines. National Academic Press, 1994:18.

332. Kanai K. Japan's experience in pertussis epidemiology and vaccination in the past thirty years. Japan J Med Sci Biol 1980; 33:107-143.

333. Hinman AR, Oranato IM. Acellular pertussis vaccines. Pediatr Infect Dis J 1987; 6:341-343.

334. Sato Y, Kimura M, Fukumi H. Development of a pertussis component vaccine in Japan. Lancet 1984; 1(8369):122-126.

335. Trollors B, Rabo E. Whooping cough in adults. Br Med J 1981; 283:696-697.

336. Romanus V, Jonsell R, Bergquist SO. Pertussis in Sweden after the cessation of general immunisation in 1979. Pediatr Infect Dis J 1987; 6:364-371.

337. Black SB, Cherry JD, Shinefield HR, Fireman B, Christensen P, Lambert D. Apparent decreased risk of invasive bacterial disease after heterologous child-hood immunization. Am J Dis Child 1991;145(7):746-749.

338. Millicap JG. Etiology and treatment of infantile spasm: current concepts, including the role of DTP immunization. Acta Paediatr Japonica 1987; 29:54-60.

339. Shields WD, Nielson C, Buch D, Jacobsen V, Christenson P, Zachau-Christiansen B, Cherry JD. Relationship of pertussis immunization to the onset of neurologic disorders: a retrospective epidemiologic study. J Pediatr 1988; 113:801-805.

340. Pollock TM, Morris J. A 7-year survey of disorders attributed to vaccination in North West Thames region. 1983; 1:753-757.

341. Berkow R. ed. Pertussis. Merck Manual of Diagnosis and Therapy, 15th edition. Rahway NJ: Merck Sharpe & Dohme Research Laboratories, 1987.

342. Beghi E, Nicolosi AN, Kurland LT, Mulder DW, Hauser WA, Shuster L. Encephalitis and aseptic meningitis, Olmsted County, Minnesota, 1950-1981. I Epidemiology. Ann Neurol 1984; 16;283-294.

343. Cavanagh NPC, Brett EM, Marshall WC, Wilson J. The possible adjuvant role of Bordetella pertussis and pertussis vaccine in causing severe encephalopathic illness: a presentation of three case histories. Neuropediatrics 1981;12:374-381.

344. Dogopol VP. Changes in the brain in pertussis with convulsions. Arch Neurol Psychiatr 1941;46:477-503.

345. Corsellis JAN, Janota I, Marshall AK. Immunization against whooping cough: a neuropathological review. Neuropathology and Neurobiology 1983;9:261-270.

346. Madsen T. Vaccination against whooping cough. JAMA 1933;101:187-188.

347. Brody M, Sorley RG. Neurologic complications following the administration of pertussis vaccine. NY State J Med 1947;47:1016-1017.

348. Byers RK, Moll FC. Encephalopathies following prophylactic pertussis vaccination. Pediatrics 1948; 1:437-457.

349. Berg JM. Neurological complications of pertussis immunization. Br Med J 1958; 2:24-27.

350. Institute of Medicine. Adverse effects of pertussis and rubella. 1991;92-93.

351. Mentes JH. Neurologic complications of pertussis vaccination (abstract). Ann Neurol 1990;28:426-427.

352. Stratton KR, et al, eds. Institute of Medicine: Adverse effects of childhood vaccines. National Academic Press, 1994:94.

353. Cody CL, Baraff JL, Cherry JD, Marcy MD, Manclark MR. Nature and rates of adverse reactions associated with DTP and DT immunization in infants and children. Pediatrics 1981 68:650-660.

354. Baraff LJ, Shields D, Beckwith L, Strome G, Marcy SM, Cherry JD, Manclark CR. Infants and children with convulsions and hypotonic-hyporesponsive episodes following DTP immunization; follow-up evaluation. Pediatrics 1988; 81:789-794.

355. Alderslade R, Bellman MH, Rawson NSB, Ross EM, Miller DL. The National Childhood Encephalopathy Study; a report on 1,000 cases of serious neurological disorders in infants and young children from the NCES research team. In: Whooping cough: Reports from the Committee on the Safety of Medicines and the Joint Committee on Vaccination and Immunisation. Department of Health and Social Security. London: Her Majesty's Stationery Office, 1981.

356. Prevots DR, Sutter RW, Stickel PM, et al. Completeness of reporting for paralytic poliomyelitis, United States, 1980-1991. Arch Pediatr Adolesc Med 1994;148: 479-485.

357. Nelson CF. Why chiropractors should embrace immunization. Chiropractic Technique 1993;68-74.

358. Ruckdeschel JC, Graziano KD, Mardiney, MR. Additional evidence that the cell-associated immune system is the primary host defense against measles (rubeola). Cell Immunol 1975;17:11-18.

359. Centers for Disease Control. Measles-Los Angeles County, California, 1988. MMWR 1989a;38:49-53.

360. Wood D, Donald-Sherbourne C, Halfon N, Tucker MB, Ortiz V, Hamlin JS, Duan N, et al. Factors related to immunization status among inner-city Latino and African-American preschoolers. Pediatrics 1995;96:295-301.

361. Deshpande JM, Rao VK, Karnataki MV, Nadkarni SS, Saxena VK, Karambelkar RR, Ramdasi SG, Patil KS, Rodrigues JJ. Absence of wild poliovirus circulation among healthy children in a rural area with high oral poliovirus vaccination coverage. Indian J Med Res 1996;103:289-293.

362. Hovi T, Huovilainen A, Kuronen T, et al. Outbreak of paralytic poliomyelitis in Finland: widespread circulation of antigenically altered poliovirus type 3 in a vaccinated population. Lancet 1986;1:42—72

363. Huovilainen A, Hovi T, Kinnunen L, et.al. Evolution of poliovirus during an outbreak: sequential type 3 poliovirus isolates from several persons shows shifts of neutralization determinants. J Gen Virol 1987;68:1373

364. Huovilainen A, Kinnunen L, Ferguson M, et.al. Antigenic variation among 173 strains of type 3 poliovirus isolated in Finland during the 1984 to 1985 outbreak. J Gen Virol 1988;69:1941-1948.

365. D'Angio CT, Maniscalco WM, Pichichero ME. Immunologic response of ex-tremely premature infants to tetanus, Haemophilus influenzae and polio immu-nization. Pediatrics 1995;96:18-22.

366. Plotkin SA, Fletcher MA. Combination vaccines and immunization visits. Pediatr Infect Dis J 1996;15:103-105.

367. Watson BM, Laufer DS, Kuter BJ, Staehle B, White CJ. Safety and immunogenicity of a combined live attenuated measles, mumps, rubella and varicella vaccine (MMRIIV) in healthy chilldren. J Infect Dis 1996;173:731-734.

368. Arbeter AM, Baker L, Starr SE, et al. Combination measles, mumps, rubella and varicella vaccine. Pediatrics 1986;78(suppl):74-747.

369. Arbeter AM, Baker L, Starr SE, Plotkin SA. The combination of measles, mumps, rubella and varicella vaccine in healthy children. Dev Biol Stand 1986;16:275-279.

370. Taylor-Wiedeman J, Novelli VM, Brunnel P, et al. Combined measles, mumps, rubella and varicella vaccine in children. Pediatr Res 1985;19:306A.

371. Dennejhy PH, Saracen CL, Peter G. Seroconversion rates to combined measles-mumps-rubella-varicella vaccine of children with upper respiratory tract infection. Pediatrics 1994;94:514-516.

372. Clemens JD, Ferrecio C, Levine MM, et al. Impact of Haemophilus influenza type b polysaccharide-tetanus protein conjugate on responses to concurrently administered diphtheria-tetanus-pertussis vaccine. JAMA 1992;267:673-678.

373. Scheifele D, Bjornson G, Guasparini R, Meekison W. Is Haemophilus influenza type B conjugated vaccine (meningococcal protein conjugate) compatible with diphtheria-pertussis-tetanus vaccine in young infants? Pediatr Infect Dis J 1993; 12:952-954.

374. Haplperin SA, Eastwood BJ, Langley JM. Immune responses to pertussis vaccines concurrently administered with viral vaccines. Ann NY Acad Sci 1995;754:89-96.

375. Insel RA. Potential alterations in immunogenicity by combining or simultaneously administering vaccine components. Ann NY Acad Sci 1995;754:35-47.

376. Johansson BE, Moran RM, Kilbourne ED. Antigen-presenting B cells and helper T cells cooperatively mediate intravirionic antigenic competition between influenza A virus surface glycoproteins. Proc Natl Acad Sci USA 1987;84:6869-6873.

377. Margareta A. Respect for the patient's integrity and self determination-an ethical imperative called upon in the Swedish Health and Medical Care Act. Med Law 1996;15:189-193.

4 Children In Motor Vehicle Collisions

Daniel J. Murphy

*W*orldwide through 1986 approximately 2 million persons have died and 100 million have been injured from motor vehicle collisions. Between 1984 and the year 2000, it is expected that at least 6 million more people will die and 350 million more will be injured subsequent to vehicle collisions throughout the globe (1).

Motor vehicle collisions cause between 4 and 5 million injuries each year in the United States (2). Motor vehicle collision survivors lost 11 million work days in 1985 as the result of their injuries (3). A recent review reported that 2.3 million children were involved in motor vehicle collisions over a 2-year period (4).

Motor vehicle-related deaths were the fourth leading cause of mortality in the United States in 1987, killing more than 47,000 people. An additional 1.8 million individuals sustained disabling injuries (5). Motor vehicle collisions resulted in 40,300 deaths in 1992, making them the seventh leading cause of death overall in the United States, and the first leading cause of death from ages 1–30 years (6).

Pathomechanics of Injury

Early research on motor vehicle collisions and its biological effects have used a variety of experimental designs. These have included the use of anthropomorphic dummies (7,8), primates (9–11), rabbits (12), mathematical modeling (13), unembalmed human cadavers (14), and human volunteers (7,8,15).

In 1955, Severy et al. (7,8) performed a series of controlled rear-end collisions using both anthropomorphic dummies and human volunteers. The subject vehicle was struck from behind by a vehicle that was traveling between 7 and 20 miles per hour. These studies are considered one of the earliest attempts to quantify the forceful effects of rear-end motor vehicle collisions on a vehicle's occupants.

These early research studies and more contemporary writings reveal several concepts regarding motor vehicle collisions.

Force of Impact

The forces produced by motor vehicle collisions are high. An 8 mile per hour rear-end collision results in a 2 G acceleration acting on the impacted vehicle and a 5 G force acting on the occupant's head (16–18). Rear-end collision speeds between 7 and 20 miles per hour can create head accelerations as great as 11.4 G (7,8,19,20). According to Barnsley et al. (21), an impact speed of 20 miles per hour causes the human head to reach a peak acceleration of 12 G during extension. A 5 G force of acceleration acting on the heads of primates results in a 50% probability of brain stem injury, cerebral concussion, and cranial nerve stretch (10,17). During frontal impacts at speeds of approximately 40 miles per hour the vehicle decelerates at a force of 90 G while the head of an occupant is subjected to a deceleration force of 46 G (22).

Collision Time Sequence

The mechanism of a motor vehicle collision and its associated injury occur in a very short span of time. Various studies indicate a range from .25 seconds (23,24) to .5 seconds (25) from impact to completion of the flexion / extension motions of the cervical spine. Consequently, because of this short time sequence even low-speed rear-end collisions may result in significant injury (25).

Vehicle Damage and Personal Injury

Vehicle speed and damage are not reliable indicators of injury to the occupants. This is supported by the writings and research of Macnab (19), Carroll (26), Ameis (27), Hirsch (16), Navin (28), Morris (29), Emori (30), and Sturzenegger (31). Macnab (19) has created a scenario in which a vehicle is stuck in concrete and badly damaged by a collision impact yet the occupants are not injured because their vehicle could not move forward, and a scenario in which a vehicle on ice is undamaged by a collision impact yet the occupants sustain significant injury because of the rapid accelerations permitted.

Emori (30) concludes that an individual can sustain ligamentous injury to the cervical spine from rear-end collisions at impact speeds as low as 2 miles per hour (2.5 km/hr). Morris (29) indicates that rear-end impacts of as little as 5 miles per hour increase significant patient symptoms.

Mechanism of Injury

The principle of inertia was first described by Sir Isaac Newton more than 300 years ago. Inertia is the tendency of an object at rest to want to remain at rest, and to resist change in its resting status. Unfortunately, different parts of a human body, adult or child, will have different inertias. As an example, the human head will function inertially differently than will the human torso. Specifically, if the torso is suddenly moved, the inertially independent head will tend to remain at rest. This creates mechanical stress on the tissue that is responsible for attaching these two functionally different inertial masses to one another, the cervical spine.

Inertia is also the tendency of an object in motion to want to remain in motion, and to resist change in its motion status. Again, unfortunately, different parts of a human body, adult or child, will have different inertias. Specifically, if the human body is in motion, and the torso is suddenly stopped, the inertially independent head will continue in motion. This will once again create mechanical stress on the cervical spine, as it is responsible for attaching these two functionally independent inertial masses to one another.

Velocity is the changing of position as a function of time. An example would be driving one's automobile 55 miles per hour. This would mean that one's position would change 55 miles if that velocity was maintained for 1 hour. Velocity alone will not injure or adversely affect the tissues of the human body. Velocity is frequently not noticed by human consciousness as long as all the parts of one's body are traveling at the same velocity (speed and direction). Planet earth with an approximate circumference of 24,000 miles makes one complete revolution every 24 hours. This means that all of us are traveling at an approximate velocity of 1,000 miles per hour, yet we remain consciously unaware of this motion. In an airplane, one may be traveling at a speed of 500 miles per hour, yet the conscious perceptions are not that different than sitting in a chair on the ground.

Changes in velocity are perceptible. This occurs when one experiences an increase or a decrease in speed. Recall the sensations of increasing speed when merging onto a freeway, or the sensations of decreasing speed experienced when an airplane lands on a runway. This increasing or decreasing speed over a period is referred to as acceleration or deceleration.

The most common cause of bodily injury during motor vehicle collisions occurs when change in the velocity of a vehicle (acceleration or deceleration) occurs rapidly, which results in different acceleration / deceleration between the different inertial masses of the occupant's bodies. Therefore, the basic mechanism of injury during motor vehicle collisions involves inertia acceleration differences between the different inertial parts of the occupant's body (19,20,22,23,32).

Soft Tissue Injury

The basic injury is considered to be a soft tissue injury. This is supported by the writings of Macnab (19), Dunn (20), Hirsch (16), Chester (17), Barnsley et al. (22), Jonsson et al. (33), and Barnsley et al. (34), to name but a few. Fractures of the spine do occur, but they are rare. Yet, Walter et al. (35) notes that approximately 80% of all cervical spine fractures are the result of motor vehicle accidents (See Chapter 19). Occult fractures that do not demonstrate on standard radiographs are also noted. These occult fractures may not even manifest on high resolution CT scanning (22).

Injury Repair

The soft tissue injury reported from motor vehicle collisions and their subsequent pathologies are slow to resolve. Ameis (27) notes that mild motor vehicle collision soft tissue injuries achieve symptom-free status about 6 months post injury. He also notes that moderate category soft tissue injury reaches maximum improvement between 12 and 36 months post injury. Ameis claims that 50% of injured patients recover by the end of the first year after injury, 75% recover at 18 months post injury, and 85–90% recover between 2–3 years, although some patients report recovery up to 5 years later.

Parmar et al. (36) reported that 50% of patients who have soft tissue neck injuries from rear impacts have significant pain 8 months after injury; 44% have significant pain at 12 months post injury; 22% have significant pain at 2 years; 18% have significant pain at 3 years; and 14% have significant pain at 8 years.

Schofferman and Wasserman (37) treated patients with low back and neck pain after motor vehicle accidents with an aggressive physical therapy stabilization program. Their patients reached maximum improvement between 8 and 108 weeks, with a mean duration of treatment being 29 weeks.

Residual Injury

Motor vehicle collisions are associated with a high percentage of residual chronicity of symptoms. Ameis (27) notes that 40–70% of injured patients endure permanent mild symptom persistence.

A study by Hodgson (38) involving 40 patients indicated that 62% of those injured in automobile accidents still have significant symptoms caused by the accident 12.5 years after being injured.

Nunn and Greenwood (39) write that follow-up studies on whiplash have shown that with standard treatment, up to 50% of the patients have significant pain at 5 years post injury.

Gargan and Bannister (40) reviewed 43 patients who had sustained soft-tissue injuries of the neck. They note that 10.8 years after injury only 12% of patients completely recovered. Residual symptoms were intrusive in 28% of patients, and severe in another 12%.

Watkinson et al. (41) reviewed 35 patients and reported that after more than 10 years after soft-tissue cervical spine injury, residual symptoms were found in 86% of patients and were significant in 23%.

In an extensive review of published studies on motor vehicle collision patients, Barnsley et al. (22) state that chronic neck pain develops in approximately 14–42% of patients with whiplash injuries, and approximately 10% have constant severe pain indefinitely.

Permanent Functional Impairment

Motor vehicle collisions are associated with a high percentage of residual permanent functional impairments. Ameis (27) indicates that 10–15% of patients never functionally recover after moderate category whiplash soft tissue injury.

Hodgson (38) has reported that 62% of those injured in automobile accidents were still having symptoms 12.5 years after being injured; and of the symptomatic 62%, 44% changed to lighter work activities permanently, and 62.5% modified their leisure activities to avoid exacerbation of symptoms.

Inertial Acceleration Injuries

The five classic inertial acceleration injured regions associated with motor vehicle collisions are as follows:

1. Inertial acceleration injuries between the head and the trunk, which primarily injures the cervical spine (19)
2. Inertial acceleration injuries between the skull and the brain, which injures the brain (10,12,13)
3. Inertial acceleration injuries between the skull and the mandible, which injures the temporomandibular articulation (19,42–44)
4. Inertial acceleration injuries between stapes bone in the inner ear and adjacent structures, which disturbs the vestibular apparatus and its concomitant balance / postural mechanisms (17)
5. Inertial acceleration injuries between the pelvis and the trunk, which injuries the lower back

These inertial injuries are often magnified by lap seat belts and are detailed later.

Chronicity of Symptoms and Functional Impairment

Leading explanations for the probability of long-term recovery, residual subjectivity, and for residual functional impairments are based on recent advances in neuroanatomy, histology, histopathology, and empirical responses to patients during various invasive clinical studies. Culprit tissues in patients with problems are not the usual muscular strain or ligamentous sprain, but rather it is damage to the facet joint capsules and/or to the intervertebral disc. Barnsley et al. (22) note that a significant proportion of patients with post-whiplash injury have chronic and unremitting symptoms reflecting serious damage to the zygapophyseal joints or the intervertebral disc.

Several contemporary authors have identified the anulus of the intervertebral disc as the source of chronic spine pain, including Nachemson (45), Mooney (46), and Kuslich (47). Barnsley (21) summarizes that injuries to the intervertebral disc from motor vehicle accidents have repeatedly been reported from a number of sources. Taylor (48) gave histological proof that the anulus of the disc is injured in motor vehicle collision neck sprains. Jonsson et al. (33) reported a high number of discoligamentous injuries when reviewing a series of 50 patients with whiplash distortion.

Other contemporary authors have identified the zygapophyseal joints as the source of chronic post-traumatic spine pain. Barnsley (21) notes that the cervical zygapophyseal joints are damaged in whiplash injuries; there is remarkable consistency among experimental data from cadavers, radiographic findings operative findings, and postmortem studies. Lord (24) notes that in experimental studies using animals or cadavers subjected to whiplash motions, injuries

to the cervical zygapophyseal joints are among the most common and most consistent lesion produced. Postmortem studies of victims of motor vehicle accidents reveal that zygapophyseal joint injuries are present in 86% of the necks examined. In a rare double blind study, Barnsley et al. (34) further confirmed the high incidence of chronic post-traumatic whiplash pain arising from the cervical zygapophyseal joints, with up to 68% probability.

In 1993, Bogduk and April (49) concluded that in post-traumatic neck pain, 41% of the patients had both a symptomatic zygapophyseal joint and a symptomatic disc at the same level; that 20% of the patients had a symptomatic disc alone; and 23% had a symptomatic zygapophyseal joint alone. Addition of these numbers indicates that of patients with post-traumatic chronic neck pain, 61% have intervertebral disc involvement and 64% have zygapophyseal joint involvement. Only 17% of the patients in this study did not have a symptomatic disc or a symptomatic zygapophyseal joint.

Head Restraints

A properly fitted head restraint minimizes the extension injuries and dampens rebound flexion injuries that occur as a result of being struck from the rear (19,23,29,50–52). A properly fitted headrest is one that is sufficiently high enough to avoid accentuated head restraint fulcrum injuries, and close enough to effectively minimize posterior head rotation and compression injuries. The head restraint must be at least as high as the center of mass of the skull and within one inch (25 mm) from the back of the skull (29,51,52). The majority of head restraints in current automobile models do not meet either criterion (23,50–52).

Seat Belts

Seat belts minimize certain types of injuries, especially serious injuries and death (53,54). Lap/shoulder belts when worn correctly reduce the risk of fatal injury by 45% (5,6) and the risk of moderate to critical injury by 50% to front seat passengers. A study by Newman (55) concluded that the incidence of serious injury and death in frontal impacts is dramatically reduced by the use of seat belts. Orsay et al. (3) reported a 60.1% reduction in the severity of injury, a 64.6% reduction in hospital admissions, and a 66.3% reduction in hospital charges in seat belt wearers. Lap belts without shoulder harness in the rear seating positions reduced fatalities 18–40%. Therefore, the installation of lap-shoulder seat belts in rear seating positions should be implemented (56). Worldwide vehicle occupant fatalities have been reduced by an average of 40% in front seat occupants and 70% in rear seat occupants, if restrained. With the universal use of vehicle restraints, fatal collision statistics would decrease by approximately 50% (57). However, seat belts increase other types of injuries (58,59), including the following:

1. Neck sprains occur more often in belted occupants than in non-belted occupants (16,52,60–63).
2. There are more fractures to the sternum in belted passengers (60).

3. Chest wall and breast injuries (64–67) occur more often.

4. There are more abdominal viscera injuries (60).

This increased incidence of other injuries occurs because, at the time of impact, the belt serves as a fulcrum, increasing belt-fulcrum injuries (58,59,68–70). Pre-pubertal children are particularly vulnerable.

Sato (71) states that seat belt users are likely to sustain injury with frontal impact at 18 km/hr; non seat belt users are likely to be injured in the same accident at only 5 km/hr.

Improper use of seat belts increases injury. The two most noted improper uses are listed:

1. Wearing a belt that is too loose. This would increase probability of submarining beneath the belt, injuring the abdomen and the head by the shoulder harness portion of the belt. Motorists should not put more than 2 inches of slack in the shoulder belt (72).

2. Placing the belt too high on the abdomen. In a crash, the belt may impose a load 20–50 times greater than the body weight. The only part of the body that can withstand this heavy load is the bony pelvis.

Lumbar Spine Injury

Lumbar spine injuries occur in approximately 50% of those involved in motor vehicle collisions (73). Many of the lumbar spine injuries are related to belt fulcrum trauma.

Air Bags

Air bags reduce overall motor vehicle collision injuries, especially when used in conjunction with lap and shoulder belts. They minimize serious injuries from sudden deceleration events. Alone, they reduce fatalities by 40%, and when used with belt restraints, they reduce fatalities by 66% (56). The United States Department of Transportation estimates that the installation of air bags in all motor vehicles would save approximately 8,800 lives per year (74). Airbags do not inflate inadvertently, are reliable for years, require no maintenance, and when used with the lap-shoulder restraint, provide the best possible occupant protection (75).

Air bags are associated with certain types of injuries. They have occasionally been implicated in abrasions to the face, neck, and chest. They may injure the eye, cause facial bruising, and temporomandibular joint injury (76). Skin burns have been observed from escaping gas (63). Rare cervical spine fractures have been documented (77). Serious injuries to infants in rear facing restraint buckets have been observed (78).

Optimum Safety

Occupant safety during motor vehicle collisions is probably greatest with adequate head restraint, adequate belt restraint, and air bags (77).

Prognosis Factors

Other factors are frequently related to increased injury, slower recovery, and worse prognosis for individuals involved in motor vehicle collisions. These factors include the following:

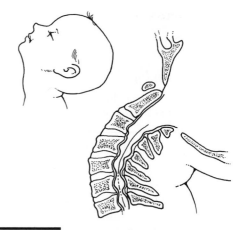

Figure 4.1.   Demonstration of pinching of the spinal cord, during extension, between the bulging ligamentum flavum and the posterior aspect of the vertebral body. Modified from Regenbogen VS, Rogers LF, Atlas SW, Kim KS. Cervical spinal cord injuries in patients with cervical spondylosis. AJR 1986; 146:282.

1. The occupant being unaware of impending collision before impact; i.e., the occupant is caught by surprise (24,25,30,31). This is an important factor to consider when assessing children, as most children are unprepared for any collision. Sturzenegger claims that the patient's state of preparedness is the most significant factor with respect to injury.

2. The occupant's head being turned at the moment of impact, or there being an oblique line of impact causing head rotation during the collision (18, 31,34,79,80). There is a natural compromise of the intervertebral foramen and its neurovascular contents, as well as to the intervertebral disc and to the capsules of the zygapophyseal articulations when the head is turned. Additionally, when in this rotated position, certain accident mechanisms cause increased rotation before flexion or extension mechanisms, resulting in magnified compromise to the disc, facet capsules, and the contents of the intervertebral foramen, etc.

3. Pre-accident degenerative joint disease (16,20,27–41,52,73,79–82). These degenerated articulations and tissues are less capable of adequately handling and dispersing the forces of a traumatic event, resulting in greater injury, more required care, increased chronicity, and accelerated degenerative joint disease (51).

4. Pre-accident central neural canal spinal stenosis (73,83,84). The pre-collision narrowing of the central neural canal reduces the space tolerance of the spinal cord and its coverings. This compromise and subsequent injury are greatest during extension/hyperextension movements, as the central neural canal narrows in extension while the ligamentum flavum bulges anteriorly into the spinal cord creating additional space impairment (Fig. 4.1). Some children have congenital central neural canal stenosis (51).

Litigation and Outcome

Litigation or its absence does not influence the long-term clinical outcome. Patients are not "cured by verdict." Reviews of long-term clinical outcomes for patients after motor vehicle collision injuries show high incidences of residual chronicity and impairment years after settlement of the injury claims, and when no possible additional monetary compensation was available (22,51,85). Using a different approach but arriving at the same conclusion, Schofferman (37) undertook a follow-up study of a group of litigants injured in motor vehicle collisions and noted that the majority improved or resolved with treatment, despite their ongoing litigation. Many of the preceding principles also apply to children in crashes.

Summary

Individuals are injured in motor vehicle collisions. The nature of the injury falls under the rubric "soft tissue injury." Fractures are rare, but they do occur, occult and otherwise. The type and severity of the injuries sustained cannot be determined by evaluating the damage to the patient's vehicle or by understanding the speeds of the involved vehicles.

Seat belts minimize serious injury and fatalities, but increase other injuries, such as neck sprain, abdominal viscera injury, lumbar spine belt fulcrum injury, and chest wall injuries. Seat belts do not reduce extension cervical spine injuries.

Proper head restraints minimize extension cervical spine injuries and dampen rebound flexion cervical spine injuries. A proper head restraint is close to the back of the occupant's head (approximately one inch), and at least as high as the center of mass of the skull. If the head restraint is too low, it may increase the patient's extension injuries by functioning as a fulcrum.

Air bags prevent serious flexion or rebound flexion injuries. Air bags minimize the flexion of the head and cervical spine; something that shoulder harness seat belts will not do. Air bags will also minimize belt-induced chest wall, abdominal viscera, and lumbar fulcrum trauma. Air bags are not a panacea. They have been implicated in injuries to the temporomandibular joints, face, certain cervical spine fractures, and burns. However, injuries created by air bags are minor compared with those that occur without an air bag.

The extent of injury and the patient's prognosis for recovery are influenced adversely when the patient is caught by surprise, when the head is rotated at the moment of impact, if the patient has congenital or acquired central canal spinal stenosis, and if there is pre-accident degenerative joint disease.

When the injured patient's symptoms resolve in 2–3 months, the soft tissue injuries were probably to the muscles and noncapsular ligaments. When the injured patient requires many months to years to reach maximum improvement, the soft tissue injuries were probably to the zygapophyseal joint tissues or to the intervertebral disc, or to a combination of the two. When maximum improvement is achieved, residual symptomatology is the rule. This residual symptomatology varies from a minor annoyance to severe enough to require a permanent alteration of work and leisure activities. Ten to fifteen percent of motor vehicle collision patients with soft tissue injury have indefinite constant severe pain and never achieve a full functional recovery. Litigation or its absence does not appear to influence the long-term clinical outcome or the patient's eventual functional status.

Pediatric Injuries

Many of the concepts that pertain to adults in motor vehicle collisions also apply to children, including the basic principles of inertial acceleration/deceleration injuries, patient preparedness before impact, and rotation of the head or trunk before impact. Other concepts will be modified because of the uniqueness of child safety seats, the increased size of the pediatric head as a proportion of the overall body mass, the child's ability to be restrained while facing rearward, the use of seat belts that are designed for adults, the use of lap belts without shoulder harnesses, the reduced height of the developing pediatric pelvis, the underdevelopment of the pediatric anterior superior iliac spine, the higher center of gravity for the pediatric body, the diminished development and strength of various spinal musculoskeletal components, and the ability to sit on the lap of adults when traveling in a vehicle. Overall, the pattern of injury among children in motor vehicle collisions is similar to those of the general population (86), excepting the differences noted below.

Injuries are the leading cause of death in children older than 1 year (4,87,88). Fifty percent of children between 1 and 14 years of age who died in the United States in 1980 died of injuries. Once a child is older than 12 months, injury becomes the leading cause of children's doctor visits and the most common reason for admittance to the emergency department of hospitals (87,89). Motor vehicle accidents are the most frequent cause for these injuries to children and young adults (88).

The 1993 edition of Accident Facts by the National Safety Council indicates that in 1992, 40,300 deaths and 2,200,000 disabling injuries occurred from motor vehicle accidents, with the total associated costs estimated to be $156.6 billion. Eight thousand three hundred students were injured from school bus accidents from 1991–1992. In 1990, 40.8% of all reported automobile occupant injuries were contusions; 17% were lacerations; 12.7% were abrasions; 11.8% were strains; 7.4% were fractures; 4.2% were concussions. Of the strains, 66.9% were to the neck, and 25.1% were to the back. Of the 40,300 deaths related to motor vehicle collisions in 1992, 5.1% were children younger than 5 years; 4.9% were children between ages 5–14 years.

Accidental injury overshadows all other causes of death among children. North American statistics consistently show that over the past 35 years, motor vehicle collisions are the leading cause of mortality and morbidity among children 1–14 years (4,90). In the 1970s, before childhood restraint laws, 16,820 children 0–4 years were killed in motor vehicle accidents (91). Motor vehicle collisions account for 37–50% of the deaths among children and lead to significant morbidity among those who survive the collision (92,93). Each year twice as many children are injured or killed while inside automobiles as are injured or killed outside automobiles (94). More children die from automobile trauma than from any disease in the United States (75). One in every 48 children born in the United States will die in a motor vehicle collision before the age of 25 and one in every 20 children born in the United States will be seriously injured in a motor vehicle collision (75).

In children, motor vehicle collisions contribute to an even greater proportion of injuries and deaths than in adults. Motor vehicle occupant-related injury is the major cause of mortality among the pediatric population in the United States (4,5,95,96), resulting in approximately 2000 fatalities per year before the enactment of most state child restraint laws (97). Alcoff (95) notes that it has been estimated that a young child is 40 to 50 times more likely to die from injuries sustained in a car crash than from all the common childhood diseases against which children are immunized. He notes that in 1973, 116 Americans of *all* ages died of measles, mumps, rubella, polio, diphtheria, pertussis and tetanus combined, while that same year 1,988 children younger than 5 years were killed in vehicular collisions. Even after the enactment of child restraint laws, still more than 600 infants younger than 5 years were killed in motor vehicle collisions in 1989 in the United States (75). The rate of children involvement in vehicle collisions is 21.4 per 1000 per year. The rate of child injury from vehicle collisions is 4.76 per 1000 per year, with the highest rate of injury in 3-year-old infants (4).

Approximately 700 infants and toddlers were killed in automobile accidents in 1994, and another 75,000 were injured. Only about 60% of children consistently ride in car seats and as many as 25% of them are not buckled in properly (98).

Most of the collisions that injure or kill children occur when someone else hits a vehicle driven by the child's mother in good weather, without the influence of alcohol, and within a few miles of their home (91). A collision does not have to occur for a child to be injured or killed while being an occupant of a motor vehicle; sudden swerves, stops, and turning corners cause movements of children in a vehicle and subsequent injury (74). One third of fatal pediatric injuries occur at speeds of 40 mph or less (99). The percentage of children being injured in speeds of 0–34 mph, 35–54 mph, and 55 mph and over is essentially the same (4).

Anthropometric and Positioning Variables for Children

HEAD SIZE

The increased size of the pediatric head as a proportion of the overall body mass influences the location and type of injuries sustained by children involved in motor vehicle collisions (74, 100–102). At birth, the head is proportionately larger and accounts for approximately 25% of the body length as compared with 15% in the adult. Consequently, in motor vehicle collisions, it is the head and cervical spine of the newborn that are most likely to be injured (74).

Toddlers 0–3 years of age continue to have a disproportionately large head size and high center of gravity, and therefore, also tend to sustain head injuries. Rear-facing child safety seats tend to restrict forward head movement and prevent young heads from striking the interior of the vehicle (100, 103).

PELVIC HEIGHT

The reduced height of the developing pediatric pelvis predisposes this patient population to unique injury (104). Each anatomical part of a child is reduced in size as compared with the adult, including the height of the pelvis. This reduced height increases the probability for a lap belt to slip over the top of the brim of the pelvis during a motor vehicle collision, resulting in more serious abdominal visceral and lumbar spine fulcrum injuries.

ANTERIOR SUPERIOR ILIAC SPINE

The underdevelopment of the pediatric anterior superior iliac spine increases the probability for unique injury for young patients (54, 70, 94, 100–102, 105). Children younger than 10 years of age have less development of the anterior superior iliac spine as compared with the adult. This increases the probability for a lap belt to slip over the top of the brim of the pelvis during a motor vehicle collision, resulting in more serious abdominal viscera and lumbar spine fulcrum injuries.

CENTER OF GRAVITY

The higher center of gravity for the pediatric body changes the nature and location of injury (54, 70, 94, 100–102). Children have a relatively higher center of gravity and a greater tendency for the lap belt to ride cephalad to across the abdomen as compared with adults. This elevated position allows the child to submarine forward under the belt, increasing injury to the abdomen and/or the spine (106) (Figs. 4.2, 4.3).

Four to 9-year-old children have a relatively lower center of gravity in contrast to infants and toddlers, closer to the umbilicus but still above the lap belt. Yet the iliac crests are underdeveloped in this age group, and the lap belt tends to slip over the bony pelvis and onto the abdomen. With rapid deceleration, with a greater proportion of body mass above the lap belt and with the lap belt already in contact with the abdomen, "jackknifing" occurs with compression and injury

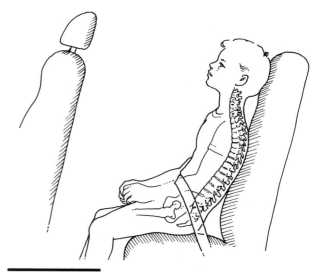

Figure 4.2. Child restrained with a lap seatbelt.

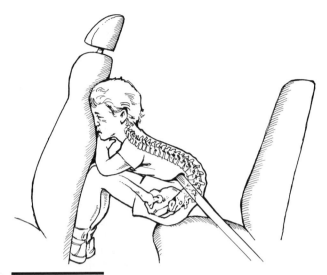

Figure 4.3.   Submarining of the pelvis under the lap belt. Modified from Johnson DL, Falci S. Diagnosis and treatment of pediatric lumbar spine injuries caused by rear seat lap belts. Neurosurgery 1990; 26:438.

of the abdominal viscera (Figs. 4.4, 4.5). The hallmark indicator of abdominal viscera and mid-lumbar spine injury is abdominal or flank ecchymosis (100, 103).

TISSUE INJURY

The diminished development and strength of various spinal musculoskeletal components increase the probability of significant tissue injury. Children have less well-developed muscle and connective tissue, which increases probabilities for spinal joint and neurological injury.

SUBMARINING

Primarily because of the shortness of the pelvis and underdevelopment of the anterior superior iliac spine, children, especially those between ages 4–9, have a higher probability of having the torso slip under the lap belt during a motor vehicle collision and sustaining associated injuries. This is termed *submarining* (101, 102, 105, 107). Ten to 14-year-olds have a better developed anterior superior iliac spine, a "taller" pelvis, and consequently experience submarining less often (56).

CHILD ON AN ADULT LAP

A parent should never hold an infant or child on his or her lap while riding in a motor vehicle. In a front end collision at 25 miles per hour at impact, the forces on the baby may reach 20 G. If the weight of the baby is 7.5 pounds, its effective weight increases to 150 pounds (7.5 lb × 20 G = 150 lb). If the weight of the child is 25 pounds, its effective weight increases to 500 pounds (25 lb × 20 G = 500 lb). It is impossible for the adult to hold the baby under those circumstances (75). To hold a 10 pound infant at 30 mph, the adult strength required would be roughly that needed to lift 300 pounds one foot off the ground (108).

If the adult is also unrestrained, his or her body may crush the baby against the dashboard or the back of the front seat (75). When the adult is not restrained, the infant is crushed by a force equal to the mass of the adult multiplied by the square of the speed and divided by two (108). When the child is held in the arms of an adult and neither is using belt restraints, the weight of the adult is added to the child's weight as they are thrown forward (Fig. 4.6A–C). The adult will crush the child with an incredible force. An example from Lipe (74) would be: (15 pound child + 170 pound adult) × (20 mph) = 3700 pounds of force, or nearly two tons.

Sitting on an adult's lap decreases the risk of minor injury but increases the risk of serious injury (109). As many as 40% of infants younger than age one traveling in cars are carried on adult laps (88).

UNRESTRAINED CHILDREN

Careful observation of anthropomorphic video graphically demonstrates that even though the principles of inertia apply

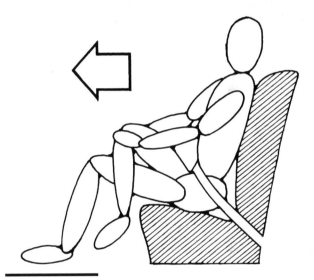

Figure 4.4.   Lap belt restraint.

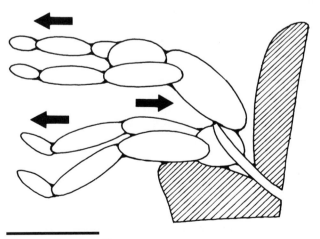

Figure 4.5.   Jacknifing.

correctly used child safety seats reduce the risks of fatalities by 71% and serious injury by 67%. Children not in safety restraint devices are 11 times more likely to die in a motor vehicle collision than children placed in restraints (113). Unrestrained children are three times more likely to sustain a brain injury than restrained children (114). Children not wearing restraints are more likely to be seriously injured in vehicle collisions. Restraint by either adult harnesses or by vehicle safety seats undoubtedly prevents both injuries and fatalities. However, restraint devices are frequently used incorrectly (115).

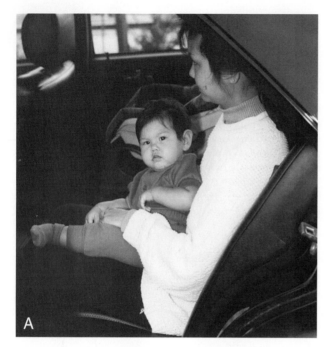

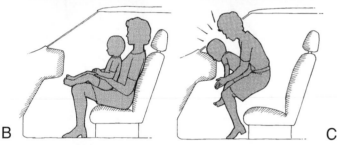

Figure 4.6.   A. Infant on an unrestrained adult's lap. B. Infant on adult's lap while at rest. C. Infant on adult's lap during a frontal collision.

to children, they are different, especially when the child is less than 40 lbs. When these young children are unrestrained, their entire body functions as a single piece of inertial mass and will fly through the air during motor vehicle collisions (Fig. 4.7A,B); Burg (110) refers to such events as "human projectiles." This includes crashing through the glass and being thrown from the vehicle, as well as colliding with the inside of the vehicle. In a moving vehicle that is stopped suddenly by an impact, an unrestrained smaller child will continue to move at the original vehicle speed until stopped by the interior of the vehicle (108). Even in low speed collisions, an unrestrained child becomes a human projectile (90).

Children run more risk of injury or death traveling unrestrained in a vehicle than by being hit by a vehicle as a pedestrian (86). It is estimated that disabling to fatal injuries to these children would decrease by 78–91% if the child was using a restraint system during motor vehicle collisions (86). Still (111) states that 49% of child passenger deaths from motor vehicle collisions could have been prevented with appropriate child restraint use. Chorba and Klein (112) indicate that

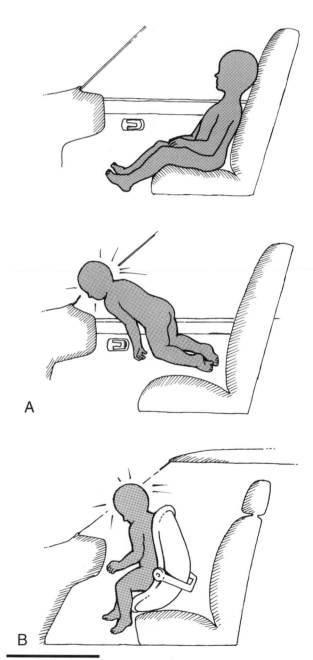

Figure 4.7.   A. Unrestrained child acting as a human projectile. B. Unrestrained safety seat with toddler, acts as a projectile during a collision.

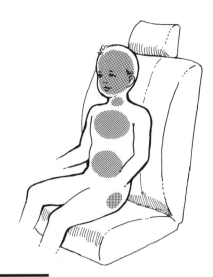

Figure 4.8.   Common sites for serious injury in an unrestrained occupant in a motor vehicle accident include the head, face cervical spine, chest, abdomen, and pelvis. Modified from Hendey GW, Votey SR. Injuries in restrained motor vehicle accident victims. Ann Emerg Med 1994; 24:79.

The approximate force of impact for an unrestrained child in a frontal impact against the dash or windshield equals the child's weight multiplied by the speed of the vehicle. An example from Lipe (74) would be: (15 pound child) × (20 mph vehicle speed) = 300 pounds of force crushing the child. Most motor vehicle collision injuries in unrestrained children occur in the cervical or mid thoracic spinal regions (116). Injuries to the face, chest, abdomen, and pelvis also occur (Fig. 4.8).

CHILDREN IN RESTRAINTS

Before 1968, children were not restrained when riding in vehicles. In 1968, seat belts were required in all new vehicles in the United States. The first preschool child passenger restraint law went into effect in Tennessee in 1978. The 50th state passed its preschool child passenger restraint law in 1984. Compliance with these laws has increased dramatically to approximately 82.5% of 0-4 year olds by 1989 (117). Yet, as many as 74% of child safety seats are used improperly (118).

Mandatory seat-belt use legislation for children minimizes both injuries and fatalities (119). In a 6-year study in Michigan (120), mandatory child restraint laws revealed a 36% decline in hospitalization, a 25% decrease in head injuries, and a 20% decrease in extremity injuries for children younger than 4 years. Use of restraints in this age group increased from 12% to 51% with mandatory use legislation.

Numerous studies have detailed the overall and optimal use of restraint devices for children. Wagenaar (121,122) noted that 75% of children ride in restraints but only 63% were optimally restrained. In 1984, 66% of infants, 50% of toddlers, 15% of preteens (ages 5–12 yr), and 7% of teens (ages 13–19 yr) were restrained while in a motor vehicle. By 1987, 78% of infants, 85% of toddlers, 36% of preteens (ages 5–12 yr), and 25% of teens (ages 13–19 yr) were restrained while in a motor vehicle (56). Thompson (123) found that only 42% of local children in the United Kingdom were appropriately restrained. By 1993, 80% of all small children were restrained while in vehicles (112).

A study reported in 1994 (4) indicated that optimal car seat restraint use by children 0–14 years was only 40%, suboptimal restraint use was found in 29%, and 31% were unrestrained. The optimal use of car seats for infants 0–12 months was 76%. The optimal use of car seats for toddlers 1–4 years was 41%. The nonuse of belt restraints was greatest for teens 10–14 years at 43%. Although 68% of children 5–9 years were restrained, only 35% were optimally restrained with a lap and shoulder harness.

REDUCTION IN INJURIES

The use of car seats and seatbelts reduces morbidity and mortality (4, 124, 125) in children involved in motor vehicle collisions. Yet even with increased use of child safety seats, the leading cause of death among 1 to 4-year-old children in the United States continues to be injuries to them while they are occupants of motor vehicles (126).

Sherz (91) claims that proper use of child restraints prevents 95% of deaths and 60% of injuries from motor vehicle collisions. He notes that a child younger than 4 years is 10 times more likely to die if unrestrained.

Wagenaar and Webster (127) note that the risk of death or serious injury from motor vehicle collisions is reduced by at least 50% when children are properly restrained in approved child restraint devices or adult seat belts. Partyka (109) estimates that child restraints decrease the occurrence of injury by more than 80%, and adult belts prevent injury in 60% of young children.

Agran (56) indicates that restrained children (all groups) sustain significantly fewer intracranial and facial injuries but significantly more spinal strains than unrestrained children.

Osberb and Scala (128) note that belted pediatric survivors were overall less severely injured, were hospitalized for shorter periods, were less likely to be discharged with residual impairments, and less likely to require health services after hospital discharge.

Ruffin and Kantor (129) found the prevalence of child restraint devices to be low, noting only 10–30% of children riding in motor vehicles are restrained by these devices, and incorrect use occurs 30–75% of the time.

Walter and Kuo (99) note that child restraint devices are 71% effective at preventing death, 67% effective in reducing hospitalizations, and 50% effective in preventing minor injury.

In the United States in 1990, the estimated use of child safety seats was 83% of infants and 84% of toddlers, as compared with 60% and 38%, respectively in 1983. Seventy percent of fatally injured children younger than 5 years in 1990 were not restrained. The use of child safety seats reduces the likelihood of fatal injury by approximately 69% for infants, 47% for toddlers, and 36% for toddlers that are in adult safety belts (126). These figures contradict a 9-year analysis of crash data from 4 states by Chorba and Klein (112). They found that fatalities among occupants younger than 5 years have increased, even though the percentage of restraint use for this age group dramatically increased.

Johnson et al. (4) indicates the use of car seats reduced injuries by 60% in the 0–4 age group. Lap shoulder harnesses were only 38% effective at preventing injury in the 5–14 age group. A high of 49% of unrestrained 10–14-year-olds were injured. A low of 17% of restrained toddlers in car seats were injured. An overall average of 31% of those children in crashes sustained injury. A fatality occurred in 1 in 288 collisions for those unrestrained, and 1 in 1000 collisions for those who were restrained. Five to 14-year-old children had a 70% higher injury risk as compared with the 0–4 age group restrained in car seats. The authors claim that 59% of toddlers are not restrained when involved in vehicle collisions. Toddlers have an 83% chance of not being injured in a collision if restrained, but this chance reduces to 57% if unrestrained. One hundred thousand children are injured unnecessarily in motor vehicle collisions because of no or suboptimal restraint use.

The greatest probability of both morbidity and fatality is noted in front impacts. Restraint use was effective in all collision directions, but the highest level of effectiveness, 40%, was reached only in frontal collisions (104). Consequently for infants and toddlers, the best protection is to have the child restraint seat facing the rear (Fig. 4.9). This distributes the forces of a frontal collision impact over the child's back and pelvis, avoiding the hyperextension or hyperflexion of the cervical spine that would occur in the forward facing position. Child restraint seats should remain in the rearward facing direction for as long as possible as the child grows, ideally until a minimum of 18–20 lbs is reached, and if possible to age 4. As many as 33% of infant seats are installed facing the wrong way for best child protection (92). This forward direction dramatically increases the probability of serious cervical spine fractures and neurologic deficits (118).

Childhood restraints are often discussed in categories because of differences related to the fit of the restraint device; 0 to 4-year-olds are restrained in a car safety seat. New studies by Drongowski et al. (130) indicate that in this age group, there were no differences in mean trauma severity between restrained and unrestrained children. Older children did benefit from the use of restraint devices.

Infants must be facing the rear of the vehicle because of the potential for neck injury during a motor vehicle collision even when restrained. For infants, the most safe seating position is the rear-center facing backwards. For toddlers too large to face the rear, the most safe seating position is the rear-center, facing forward. Most adults surveyed do not know basic child restraint safety principles (129). Basic guidelines for safe seating are presented in Table 4.1.

Four to 9-year-old children are different because of the underdevelopment of the anterior superior iliac spine, which increases the probability of the child slipping under a lap belt during a collision, especially if the child is using a lap belt alone. These children are a special group because they have outgrown the child safety seat and are placed in a restraint system designed for the adult body. The addition of a shoulder harness may adversely affect the neck or face (Fig. 4.10). In this

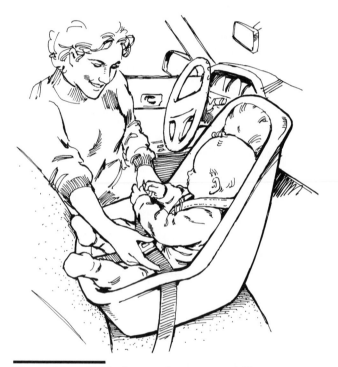

Figure 4.9.   Child safety seat facing rearward. This position should not be used if the vehicle is equipped with air bags.

Table 4.1.   Basic Guidelines for Child Positioning in Automobiles

	Infant	Toddler	Ages 4–9	Ages 10–14
Device	Safety seat	Safety seat	Booster cushion with head restraint	"Child safe" restraint belt device
Position	Rear center	Rear center	Rear seat	Rear seat
Direction	Facing backward	Facing forward	Facing forward	Facing forward
Instructions	Child properly restrained in safety seat. Safety seat properly anchored to vehicle.		Booster cushion and child properly restrained by adult lap and shoulder harness. Shoulder harness across chest and clavicle, not across neck/face, or under the arm or behind the back.	

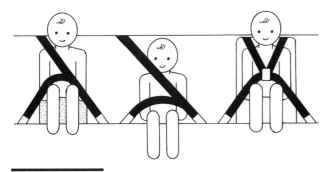

Figure 4.10. Children in adult restraints.

age group, most injuries occur in frontal impacts as compared with rear-end impacts, and because of the restraint devices, they occur primarily in the lower torso (131). Spinal strain injuries were seen primarily in rear-end collisions, and more often in front seat passengers (42%) than back seat passengers (22%) (131). Belt restraint systems do not provide adequate protection in side impacts. A large percent of restrained children in this age group receive head and face injuries, as these anatomical parts are not restrained (131). All authors reviewed agree that adult restraints are not optimal for children in this age group (4, 54). The optimal protection system for pediatric motor vehicle protection has not yet been designed, but any restraint system is better than no restraint (128).

Tingvall (104) reports that children under a certain age or size cannot safely use adult restraint systems without modifications. His recommendations for optimal safety include the following:

1. Newborns to 9-month-infants should be placed in rearward-facing child seats in the front passenger position; the seat should be anchored by the adult seat belt to the vehicle. He cautions to not use the instrument panel as part of the restraint system;

2. Children ages 9 months–4 years should be placed in rearward-facing child seats, using the instrument panel as part of the restraint system (Fig. 4.11) only when air bags are not present.

3. For children 5–10 years who have outgrown the safety seat, use a forward-facing booster cushion that is restrained by the adult seat belt and the cushion is also anchored to the vehicle by the adult seat belt. This booster cushion should have a seatback and a head restraint (Fig. 4.12).

Tingvall (104) also reports that common problems encountered when there is injury to children include the following:

1. Child restraint not suitable for its purpose
2. Child restraint not properly anchored to the vehicle
3. Child not properly anchored to the child restraint

Of the children in Tingvall's (104) study, 1.2% using a rearward-facing child restraint were injured, 6.9% using a forward-facing child seat were injured, 8.9% of those using an adult restraint belt were injured, and 15.6% of unrestrained children were injured. The use of restraints prevented or reduced injuries to the head and extremities, but for injuries to the neck, chest, and abdomen, no effectiveness was established. Forward-facing child seat restraints, booster cushions, and the use of adult restraints were not as effective in reducing mortality and injury because of their low effectiveness on neck injuries.

INJURIES FROM RESTRAINTS

The leading cause of morbidity and mortality in children is trauma, and the most frequent mechanism is motor vehicle collisions. Restraining children decreases their chance of

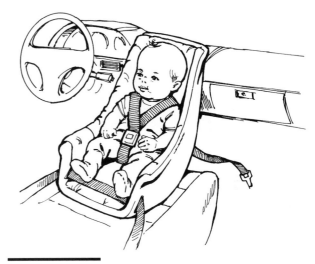

Figure 4.11. Rearward facing child safety seat using the instrument panel as part of the restraint system to be used only when air bags are not present. Modified from Tingvall C. Children in cars: some aspects of the safety of children as car passengers in road traffic accidents. Acta Paediatr Scand Suppl 1987; 339:7.

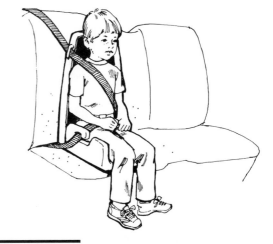

Figure 4.12. Child in booster seat. Modified from Tingvall C. Children in cars: some aspects of the safety of children as car passengers in road traffic accidents. Acta Paediatr Scand Suppl 1987; 339:7.

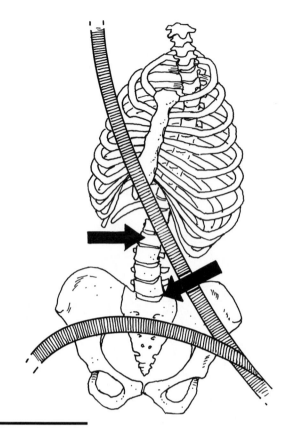

Figure 4.13. Restraints can accentuate abdominal injuries.

injury or death. Seat belts prevent ejections and reduce impact between the child and the interior of the vehicle (105). Yet serious injury can still occur even when restraining belts are used. The belts themselves can cause harm and injury. The belt systems have their own unique pattern of injury as they change the distribution of forces, especially to the abdominal viscera in a deceleration event (Fig. 4.13). Violent hyperflexion of the child's torso over the lap belt applies flexion-distraction forces to the spine. Submarining, or slipping of the child underneath the lap belt, can occur and predispose the child to additional abdominal trauma. Children at maximum risk are those too large to be in a safety seat, yet too small for the available restraint belt system that are designed for adults (101,102). Despite the drawbacks, adult seat belts are recommended over no restraint since they reduce injury and death.

There are reports of injuries being caused by the restraint systems. Agran (100) cites studies that indicate an increase in facial, intra-abdominal, and lumbar spine injuries in children restrained with a lap belt alone. She also notes studies that indicate an increase of minor and moderate neck injuries and chest injuries in children restrained with shoulder harnesses. Similar results were reported by Hoffman et al. (132). Tingvall (104) notes that non-contact injuries caused by the restraint were common. Among children using an adult restraint only, the restraint was the cause of most of the injuries discovered. Tingvall (104) further claims that injuries to the head and extremities were less common while injuries to the neck and abdomen were more common among restrained than among

unrestrained children. In Australia, 10% of passengers presenting to a hospital after a frontal impact motor vehicle collision have injuries directly related to the wearing of a seat belt (107).

Agran (100) notes that 81% of restrained but injured 0–3-year olds incurred injury from striking against some portion of the vehicle. These injuries were primarily to the head after the infant or toddler "jackknifed" forward over the seatbelt and struck a portion of the vehicle. This motion is promoted by the child's proportionately larger head size and higher center of gravity. Eleven percent of these restrained children sustain whiplash strain injuries, and 6% sustain seat belt strain injury.

Agran (107) reports that 50% of restrained but injured 4–9-year-old children incurred injury from striking against some portion of the vehicle; 9% sustained whiplash strain injuries and 12% sustained seat belt strain injury. Twenty-one percent sustained abdominal injuries from straining against the seat belt, as the belt would ride up over the immature iliac crest in this age group. Seat belts cause certain injuries, particularly in the 4–9-year-old group, in which children are too big for child safety seats and too small for adult belts. Injuries associated with seat belt use in these children include chest and abdominal injuries, cervical spine injury, and cardiac contusions (128).

Agran (100) notes that 67% of restrained but injured 10-14 year olds incurred injury from striking against some portion of the vehicle; 33% sustained whiplash strain injuries, and 13% sustained seat belt strain injury. This information shows a significant number of whiplash spinal strain types of injuries in this group as compared with the others. Of this entire group of restrained 0–14 year olds evaluated after motor vehicle accident, only 17% were determined medically to be uninjured (100).

Seat belts may cause injuries from the neck to the pelvis. The probability of seat belt-induced injuries increases when the restraint device is not used properly. Common errors in restraint use include the following:

1. The child is placed in a restraint not designed for his/her size or weight.
2. The child restraint is not properly anchored to the vehicle.
3. The restraint is not properly applied to the child (133).

Current restraint systems for the pediatric population are suboptimal, and further improvement in safety design is necessary (63). Injuries occurring among restrained children are mainly located in the head and the neck. Neck injuries constitute the most severe problem (Fig. 4.14). Consequently, prevention or mitigation of injuries to the neck among children should have a high priority in future research and development of child restraints (104).

LAP BELT INJURIES

When lap belts were initially used, fatality rates declined due to reduced ejections and reduced severity of head trauma. However, lap belt wearers still suffered head, face, and chest injuries due to contact with the dashboard or steering wheel. Also, up to 58% of injured occupants received abdominal injuries, especially when the lap belt slipped over the top of the anterior superior iliac spine (105) (Fig. 4.15). Lumbar spine injuries and Chance fractures were much more common among lap belt wearers (Figs. 4.16, 4.17). Of those patients with Chance fracture, 63% also suffered intestinal injuries (63) (Fig. 4.18). The probability of Chance fracture and abdominal injury increases in the pediatric population wearing lap seatbelts during motor vehicle collision (134).

Lap belt injuries are usually associated with children between ages 4–9 years because these children are too large to use restraint seats and are too small to safely use adult lap belts. Children in this age group have special and unique anatomical characteristics that increase their vulnerability to lap belt injuries. Children have larger heads and less well developed spinal musculature than adults, putting children at greater risk of hyperflexion injuries. The immature pelvis is more likely to slip below the seat belt creating fulcrum load injuries to the abdomen.

Conventional lap restraints do not properly restrain or protect children because the anterior superior iliac spine is under developed in this population. The belt rides up onto the abdomen and chest and may itself cause significant injury. If the vehicle rapidly decelerates, the child may whip forward with increased force than an adult because of the child's higher center of gravity and greater body mass above the waist (94). Children have greater probability of lap belt-induced abdominal and spinal injuries because of their greater percentage of body mass above the umbilicus, the poorly developed anterior superior iliac spine, the frequent lack or misuse of the shoulder harness for children, and the immature spinal support structures (54, 70, 94, 100, 101, 104, 105). Anderson (54) indicates that 90% of restrained children with seat belt abdominal injuries also sustained lumbar spine flexion injuries. Children lap belt syndrome injuries typically have an abrasion or contusion across the abdomen, created by the lap belt. These

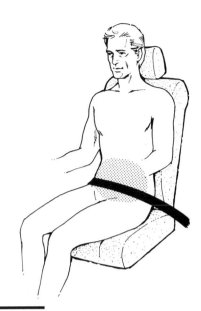

Figure 4.15. Abdominal injury can occur if the lap belt slips over the ASIS during a collision. Modified from Johnson DL, Falci S. Diagnosis and treatment of pediatric lumbar spine injuries caused by rear seat lap belts. Neurosurgery 1990; 26:438.

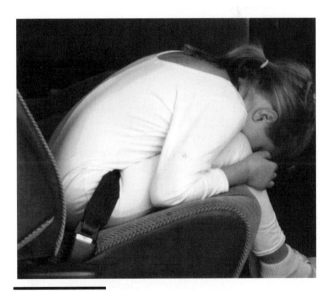

Figure 4.16. A 7-year-old demonstrates the mechanism of injury for the Chance fracture.

children suffer from fracture, dislocations, neurologic damage, and significant intra-abdominal injuries (105, 116). Because of the high probability of serious abdominal visceral injury, Newman et al. (106) recommends children presenting with 'lap belt' ecchymosis and injury to the lumbar spine after a car crash should receive routine diagnostic peritoneal levage.

Lap belts that remain below the anterior superior iliac spine in accidents can transfer loads up to 2000 pounds of force to the body without serious visceral injury. If the lap belt is placed above the bony pelvis or if submarining occurs, this amount of

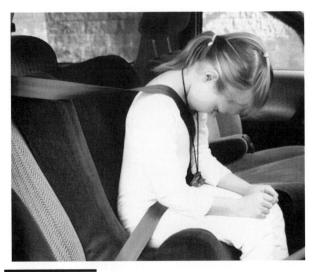

Figure 4.14. Properly restrained 7-year-old remains susceptible to cervico-thoracic injuries.

force will cause serious or fatal visceral trauma, including damage to the intestines, mesentery, liver, kidneys, and aorta (72). Lap belts become a fulcrum creating significant hyperflexion injury (70, 135).

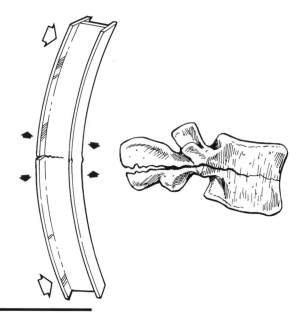

Figure 4.17. Associated bony vertebral injuries in the Chance fracture. Modified from Smith WS, Kaufer H. A new pattern of spine injury associated with lap-type seatbelts: a preliminary report. Univ Michigan Med Center J 1966; 33:247.

Frontal impact is responsible for the majority of serious and fatal injuries in restrained occupants (100, 105). As the forward velocity of a vehicle is sharply stopped in a frontal collision, the occupants continue to move forward with considerable inertial force, depending on the magnitude of the deceleration. If the child is restrained, the belt acts as the fulcrum of a first class lever system, increasing the forces to the pelvis, spine, and abdominal viscera (105).

The usual sitting posture of a child is slouched rather than upright with the lap belt resting across the abdomen. Even if the lap belt is properly placed on the pelvis, the poorly developed anterior superior iliac spine will allow the lap belt to slip up over the iliac crest and onto the abdomen as the child slides forward and under the belt during an accident. The child's relatively large head and higher center of gravity above the waist accentuate the bending moment about the lumbar spine and abdominal viscera (105).

Of injured children in motor vehicle collisions, none of the children restrained with shoulder harnesses sustained lumbar spine Chance-type flexion-distraction fractures, whereas 11% of those with lap belts alone did (136). Frequently the mid lumbar spinal injuries associated with children in lap belts are only visible on lateral lumbar radiograph. These injuries include facet subluxations and horizontal fractures (See Chapter 19). These types of trauma findings are often missed on CT scans. The clinical presentation of these children may be acute back pain or delayed onset back pain (70).

A report from the National Transportation Safety Board (137) suggested that the use of rear seat lap belts may be more harmful than no seat belt use at all, stating, "In many cases, the

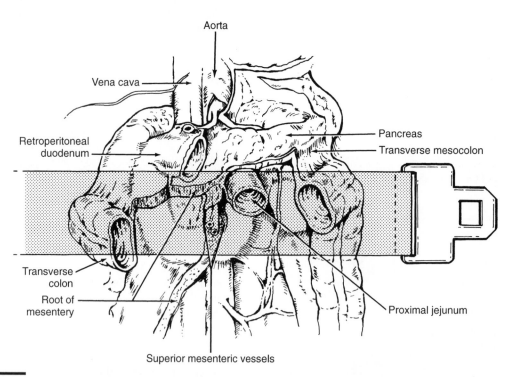

Figure 4.18. Intraabdominal structures that are fixed in the retroperitoneum at the midlumbar region are vulnerable to lap belt injuries. Modified from Johnson DL, Falci S. Diagnosis and treatment of pediatric lumbar spine injuries caused by rear seat lap belts. Neurosurgery 1990; 26:439.

lap belts induced severe to fatal injuries that probably would not have occurred if the lap belts had not been worn." Although rear seat lap belts do not meet the special needs of children (105), restraining a child with a lap belt is preferable to having no restraint at all (135, 138).

SHOULDER HARNESS INJURY

Children between ages 4–9 years are too large to use a restraint seat and too small to safely use an adult shoulder harness restraint. If such children use an improperly fitting adult shoulder harness across their neck or face, serious and fatal injuries have been reported (74). Because the neck/face position for the shoulder harness is uncomfortable for these children, they often modify its placement by putting the shoulder harness behind their back or under their arm (Fig. 4.19).

Newman (106) notes that the National Highway Traffic Safety Administration recommends that children not use the shoulder belt component of a three-point restraint if it falls across their neck or face. The shoulder belt must be placed so that it rests on the anterior surface of the chest and on top of the clavicle. Although clavicle and rib fractures and low neck injuries do occur in this position, without the shoulder harness more severe head, spine, and chest injuries will occur in these same crashes without the use of the shoulder harness.

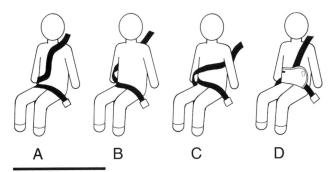

Figure 4.19. A. Shoulder harness too loose. B. Shoulder harness behind the back. C. Shoulder harness under the arm. D. Correct placement of the shoulder harness across the clavicle.

SHOULDER HARNESS BEHIND THE BACK

The use of the adult shoulder harness in this position renders the child vulnerable to the lap belt injuries noted earlier (54).

SHOULDER HARNESS UNDER THE ARM

Because of their shorter stature, children will often place a shoulder belt under their arm. Yet loads far in excess of the tolerance for injury of the upper abdomen and lower chest are imposed by the shoulder belt being placed in the underarm position. Lacerations of the liver, spleen, intestines, mesentery, diaphragm and aorta, as well as spinal injuries can occur. States et al. (72) warn that the use of the shoulder harness in the underarm position is hazardous and causes fatal injuries in otherwise survivable collisions. Placing the shoulder belt under the arm is considered to be a dangerous misuse of the restraint (72). Shoulder belt placement below the arm concentrates the load on the abdomen and causes injuries similar to those resulting from lap belt placement above the bony pelvis. In addition, the risk of cardiac, pulmonary, and diaphragm injury is increased.

INFANTS AND AIR BAGS

The deployment of air bags occurs at high velocity and creates a serious hazard for children as a result of "bag slap" (74, 139). The air bag mushrooms out in a fraction of a second, reaching speeds up to 200 mph. Because the rear of the infant child restraint seat is close to the air bag compartment, it will receive a tremendous force from air bag deployment, resulting in serious head injuries to the child (Fig. 4.20). Therefore, rear-facing infant seats should be used only in the back seat of vehicles that have front passenger air bags.

Types of Injuries to Children

According to Margolis et al. (120), 10% of children involved in motor vehicle collisions require hospitalization. A 10-year study (140) of 479 automobile accidents in Finland with 796 children younger than 16 years revealed that 26% died, 22% were severely injured, 34% were mildly injured, and 18% were uninjured.

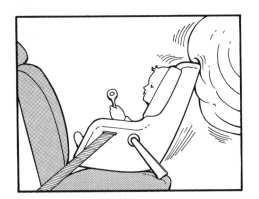
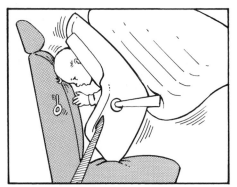

Figure 4.20. Deflection of the restrained child by an airbag.

The authors estimated that a child safety seat would have saved 50% of the children younger than 5 years from dying and would have reduced injury 60%; a seat belt would have saved 28% from dying and reduced injury for 42%. Twenty-six percent of these children required physical therapy rehabilitation for their injuries. Seven percent of the children sustained permanent various pains, and 4% sustained permanent psychological problems. Psychological symptoms were reported in 58% of the injured children and in 43% of the uninjured children. The most common psychic disorder was the fear of traffic (38%) and nightmares (27%). Thirty percent of these children reported some kind of permanent harmful effects in their lives.

BRAIN INJURY

Studies indicate that the number one cause (27.5%) of closed head injury in the pediatric population is motor vehicle collision. During these collisions 25% of the children are restrained, and 75% are unrestrained in the vehicle. The unrestrained group is also more seriously injured including significantly more fatalities (114). A study published in 1986 indicated that 24% of pediatric brain injuries reported to hospitals in San Diego County were caused by motor vehicle collisions (87). Because the head of the child is proportionally heavier, it tends to be the first body part to be impacted (74). Unrestrained children are three times more likely to sustain a brain injury than restrained children (114).

Most injuries sustained to unbelted vehicle occupants are from hitting the interior of the vehicle or from being ejected. The head, face, and chest are the most common and serious injuries sustained, and fatalities are caused by head trauma (63).

FACIAL FRACTURES

Seventeen to fifty percent of facial fractures in children are from motor vehicle collisions (94), with speculation that the higher end is the result of increasing use of protective child restraints and other safety measures that improve childhood motor vehicle collision survival.

CERVICAL SPINE INJURIES

Children can injure their cervical spine even though they are properly restrained (141). The injury results from hyperflexion of the cervical spine while the torso was securely restrained. The injuries occurred even when the children were wearing a 3- or 4-point restraint belt.

Improved torso restraints increases stress loads to the cervical spine and head, especially because younger children have larger heads (142).

Injuries to the neck were more common in children in forward facing car seats or in adult seat belts as compared with unrestrained children (118). Two thirds of disabilities in injured restrained children are neck injuries (104).

Tingvall (104) notes that neck injuries causing strain and pain for children using forward-facing restraint systems occurred often. Approximately 20% of the children restrained in the forward direction sustained neck injury. These neck injuries may lead to permanent disability and long-term

consequences, even among young car occupants. Children should use head restraints if they are sitting in such a way that the head is above the highest point of the car seat.

UPPER CERVICAL INJURY

Pang and Wilberger (143) have reported that the infantile atlanto-occipital junction to be inherently unstable, and that extension events can injure the vertebral arteries. Spine injuries in children are usually in the upper cervical spine, whereas spine injuries to adults are in the lower cervical spine (143, 144). Injuries of the upper cervical spine are more frequent in younger children than older children regardless of the restraint used because of the relative weakness of the upper cervical spine in infants (145). Because of this increased upper cervical mobility and more horizontal facet angulation, radiographic appearance of injury is rare in children younger than 8 years and extremely rare in infants younger than 26 months. Rachesky et al. (144) have reported that there is a high probability that a radiographic abnormality will be found when a child both complains of neck pain and has a history of motor vehicle collision in which they received a head trauma.

CERVICAL DISC INJURY

As noted, intervertebral disc injury is common in adults subsequent to motor vehicle collisions and is associated with chronic symptomatology and dysfunction. Disc problems are rare in children, but do occur, and are usually preceded by trauma (146). Jackson (147) notes that the cervical spine is subjected to many traumatic experiences in childhood, and these minor injuries begin the process of disc degeneration; occasionally resulting in enough degeneration that a pathological fusion results which may be interpreted as being of congenital origin when discovered. Figure 4.21 demonstrates early signs of degenerative joint disease in a 13-year-old child who sustained a cervical injury from a motor vehicle collision at the age of seven.

APOPHYSIS INJURY

In adolescents, the ununited ring apophysis of the vertebral body is an inherently weak junction. It is more susceptible to injury than the disc itself after motor vehicle collision hyperextension or axial distraction distortions. Subsequent injuries occur at the cartilaginous end plate. Consequently, MR imaging may reveal normal disc signals, as the discs are structurally intact in these avulsion injuries (33).

CERVICAL SPINAL CORD INJURY

During the extremes of flexion in the child, the nucleus pulposus might protrude backwards and injure the spinal cord, and then spontaneously retract back inside the anulus (143). Pang and Wilberger (143) report on spinal cord injury without radiographic abnormalities in children, caused primarily from motor vehicle collisions. They suspect that this occurs because of the increased elasticity of the spinal soft tissues in this group. These injuries can be caused by either flexion or extension mechanisms. The child's neurologic signs can be delayed from between 30 minutes to as long as 4 days. In children, because

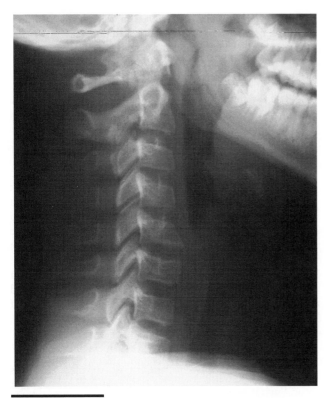

Figure 4.21. The lateral cervical radiograph demonstrates early degenerative changes at C5 with anterior osteophyte formation and compression of the superior endplate of C6.

the capsular ligaments are more elastic than adults and the facet joint planes are more horizontal, they are very susceptible to injury in hyperextension. In infants and children younger than age 10, the flatness of the uncinate processes cannot resist flexion and rotational forces. These factors combined with the proportionally heavier head and relatively underdeveloped cervical spine musculature, constitute an increased susceptibility for flexion and extension injuries. Pang and Wilberger (143) note that because of increased upper cervical mobility in infants and children younger than 8 years, the spinal cord is primarily injured in this region. Overall increased injury is noted in younger children, reflecting a relevant inherent instability and weakness of musculoskeletal tissues of the spine in this age group.

SEAT BELT SYNDROME INJURIES

Seat belt syndrome injuries refer to serious spinal injuries and fracture that are caused by the seat belt acting as the fulcrum of a first class lever (70). One study (141) indicated that 5.4% of injured children received lumbar seat belt syndrome injuries, and that 1.3% received cervical seat belt syndrome injuries. Stylianos and Harris (135) indicated that children wearing lap belts sustained abdominal injuries but no head injuries, whereas unrestrained children sustained head injury but no abdominal injuries. Tso et al. (102) noted that belted children still sustain head, face, and chest injuries, indicating that the upper body is not well protected by belts during a crash. The

authors emphasize that doctors must maintain a high degree of suspicion for abdominal viscera / spinal injuries when evaluating a child who has been restrained during a motor vehicle collision even when there is no seat belt signs on the child's body.

Two point belts were designed to reduce head and face injuries. They also increased the number of chest injuries, rib injuries that further lacerated the liver and spleen, sternal injuries, and clavicle fractures. Cervical spine fractures have occurred as the occupant slides under the belt and is caught by the neck. Decapitations have also been reported (63) (Fig. 4.22).

Three point lap and shoulder belts reduced deaths by 45% and moderate to critical injuries by 50%. Yet chest wall and cervical spine soft tissue injury increased (63) (Figs. 4.23, 4.24).

PSYCHOLOGICAL INJURY

Thompson and McArdle (148) have suggested that up to 30–50% of children exposed to psychic trauma show signs of post-traumatic stress reaction; this includes those suffering from the psychological sequelae of motor vehicle collisions. Symptoms can include nightmares, separation anxiety, fear of the dark, sleep disturbance, reluctance to cross roads or travel by vehicle, and a preoccupation with road safety. Similar findings were noted by Karttunen and Karkola (140).

SEATING POSITION

For adults, there is no significant difference in the type of injury, the incidence of permanent disability, or on the mortality rate based on the location of the injured occupants (front or rear seat) within vehicles involved in collisions (149). In contrast, risk of injury to restrained children is greater in the front seat position than for the rear seat position, and the incidence is primarily due to neck injuries (104).

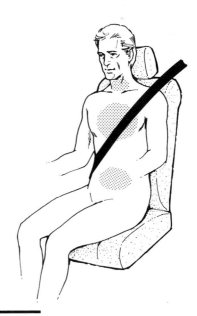

Figure 4.22. Injury sites with a two-point shoulder restraint. Modified from Hendey GW, Votey SR. Injuries in restrained motor vehicle accident victims. Ann Emerg Med 1994; 24:80.

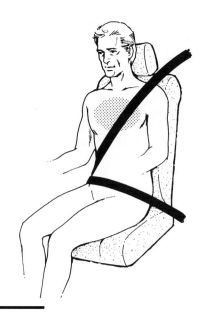

Figure 4.23. The chest and cervical spine can be injured while wearing a three-point seat belt. Modified from Hendey GW, Votey SR. Injuries in restrained motor vehicle accident victims. Ann Emerg Med 1994; 24:81.

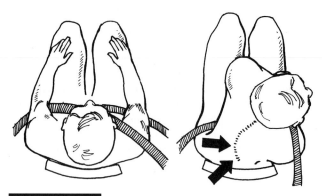

Figure 4.24. The roll-out phenomenon can lead to thoracic and lumbar spine injuries including anterolateral compression fractures (See Chapter 19).

RESTRAINT MISUSE

Misuse of child restraint seats results in 7% of trauma hospital visits for the infant and toddler age group (150). For a restraint to be effective, it must be anchored to the vehicle securely, and the child must be attached by belts to the restraint device. If one or both of these conditions is not achieved, the child restraint seat may become a child launch pad during a collision or when the child safety seat is not secured to the vehicle, the seat, with the child in it, will become a projectile in a crash (108, 118).

Conry and Hall (115) give an example of an infant in a safety seat in which the crotch strap was not properly locked. The result was a submarining of the infant and an odontoid fracture from impact with the buckle (Fig. 4.25).

Placing the shoulder harness belt behind a child age 4–9 is considered to be misuse and is associated with increased injury (54,56). With this type of misuse, the child is prone to the lap seat belt injury syndrome. Placing the shoulder harness belt under their arm for these children is also considered misuse and results in serious thoracic cage, cardiac, and pulmonary injury (72).

Redesigning the child safety seat to allow children to face the rear until 2–4 years of age would reduce head and neck injuries to toddler passengers (117). Booster seats are needed to improve positioning in older children with shoulder harnesses (102).

SUMMARY

Children are injured in motor vehicle collisions; it is a huge problem. Motor vehicle collisions are the number one reason for both mortality and morbidity in children younger than 14 years of age.

The bodies of children younger than 1 year function as a single piece of inertial mass during motor vehicle collisions. Children in this age group have a proportionately larger head size as compared with overall body mass. Consequently, when they are unrestrained during a motor vehicle collision, they tend to "lead" with their head. Their heads and bodies collide with the interior of the vehicle, and ejections of their bodies occur. Such unrestrained children sustain serious head, brain, and cervical spinal cord injuries, leading to death and significant lifelong disabilities.

When children younger than 1 year of age are restrained in a child restraint seat and the child restraint seat is not securely attached to the vehicle seat with the appropriate

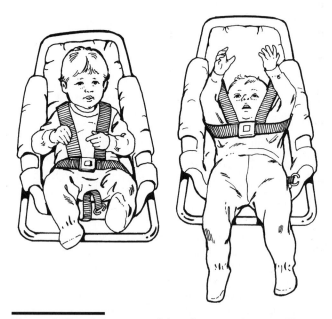

Figure 4.25. Submarining of the infant in a safety seat. The middle strap is unlocked, either inadvertently or due to a malfunction of the locking mechanism. Modified from Conry BG, Hall CM. Cervical spine fractures and rear car seat restraints. Arch Dis Child 1987; 62:1268.

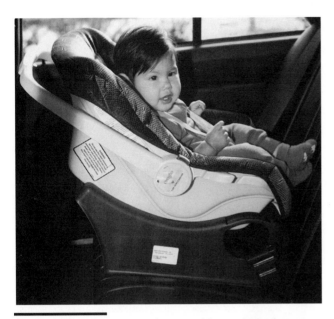

Figure 4.26.   Proper use of rearward facing child safety seat.

adult restraint belt, the child's body and the restraint seat together will function as a single piece of inertial mass. Once again, the child will sustain serious head and brain injuries. Not securing the child safety seat to the vehicle is a misuse of the safety device.

When children younger than 1 year of age are properly restrained in a *forward facing* child safety seat and the child safety seat is properly secured to the vehicle with the adult restraint belt, serious head, brain, and cervical spinal cord injuries are largely avoided. Yet, in this forward facing position, the properly restrained child has increased vulnerability to cervical spine injury, especially in frontal impacts. This is because the restraints immobilize the child's body, yet the head can move. With this young child's proportionately larger head size as compared with overall body mass, and with the child's poorly developed strength of the cervical spine musculoskeletal tissues, significant cervical spine soft tissues occur.

Most serious injuries to restrained children younger than 1 year of age are incurred during a frontal impact collision. These serious injuries can be reduced by placing the child restraint seat in a rearward facing direction, and then properly securing this child restraint seat to the vehicle using the adult restraint belts (Fig. 4.26). Serious injuries are reduced as the forces of the frontal impact are dispersed over a broader surface area of the child; over the back of the skull, the thoracic cage, and the pelvis. A child of this age group who is properly restrained in the rearward facing position has the best chance of avoiding injury in a motor vehicle collision, especially in serious frontal impact collisions.

When a child younger than 1 year of age is restrained in a safety seat that is properly secured to the vehicle by the adult belt, but the crotch strap of the child safety seat is not properly attached, the child's body will "submarine" under the waist strap, catching the child under the chin. The

results are serious cervical spine injury, including fracture of the odontoid process or a bipedicular (hangman's) fracture of C2. An adult must always properly secure the crotch strap portion of the child restraint seat for children in this age group.

Children younger than 1 year of age should not be restrained in a child safety seat in the rearward facing position in the front seat of a vehicle that has a passenger side air bag. In this position, the closeness of the child to a rapidly outwardly exploding air bag can launch the safety seat and child at an extremely high velocity, resulting in serious head and brain injury.

Children between 1–4 years of age are similar to children younger than age one in that their heads are proportionately larger as compared with overall body mass and the strength of their musculoskeletal spinal tissues are not as developed as those of the adult. When they are unrestrained, they tend to "lead" with their heads sustaining serious head, brain, and cervical spinal cord injuries after colliding with the interior of the vehicle, and are at risk of ejection. Children in this age group are least injured when they are properly restrained in a child safety seat facing the rearward direction. When children in this age group are properly restrained and facing the forward direction, they sustain significant cervical spine soft tissue injury during frontal collisions. Contrary to common practice, children should remain in child restraint seats facing the rearward position for as long as possible as they age, ideally to approximately age 4.

Caution should be used when restraining children between 1–4 years of age in an adult lap belt. The pelvis of children in this age group is much shorter in height, and the anterior superior iliac spine is grossly underdeveloped as compared with that of the adult, increasing the tendency for the lap belt to slip up over the top of the pelvis rim and to be in contact with the abdomen and its contents. Because of the shorter stature of these children, in a frontal impact, their face or chest will not collide with the dashboard or with the seat in front of them. This results in a serious rapid flexion of the child's torso around the adult lap belt, or "jackknifing." Serious and fatal abdominal viscera and mid lumbar spinal injuries result.

Children between ages 4–9 years have the greatest difficulty with motor vehicle collision safety. Children in this age group face forward nearly always and are restrained in the adult seat belt. Unfortunately, adult seat belts do not meet the special needs of this group of children. Often they are riding in the rear seat of the vehicle, and at the time of this writing, the majority of vehicles do not have shoulder harness restraints available for rear seat passengers. As the developing pelvis remains short in height with an underdeveloped anterior superior iliac spine in this age group, it is once again common for the adult lap belt restraint to slip over the rim of the pelvis and to come into contact with the abdomen and its contents. The center of gravity for these children is higher as compared with that of the adult, superior to the lap belt. This proportionately increases the fulcrum stress above the lap belt in a frontal impact or during a rebound flexion after a rear impact. Again, this results in serious injuries to the abdominal viscera and mid lumbar spine,

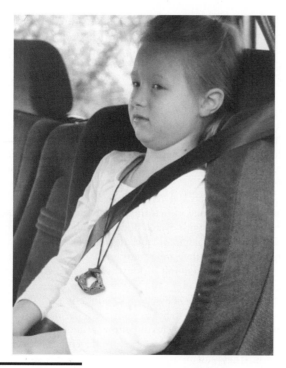

Figure 4.27.   Proper positioning by use of a booster seat.

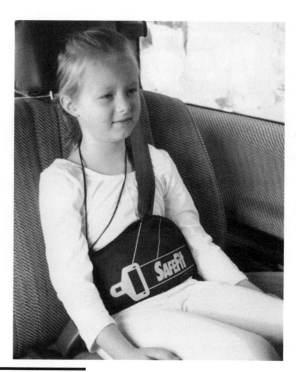

Figure 4.28.   Safety device for positioning of a three-point harness on a child.

including Chance fractures. Depending on the stature of these children, their face/head may impact the dashboard or the seat in front of them, resulting in significant face, head, brain, and cervical spinal cord injuries. Whenever possible, children of this age group should be restrained in a lap belt/shoulder belt combination.

Children between ages 4–9 years also have unique problems when using the recommended adult lap belt with shoulder harness combination. Because of their short stature, the shoulder harness does not fit their body adequately. For many children in this age group, the shoulder harness will cut across their cervical spine or face rather than their chest. When left in this position, the shoulder harness can cause serious and fatal cervical spine and facial injuries. Also, because of the uncomfortable annoyance of the shoulder belt crossing the neck or face, many children of this age group will simply place the shoulder strap behind their back, rendering them susceptible to the lap belt injuries noted earlier. Other children will place the shoulder harness under the arm. This position is also dangerous, as the thoracic cage is not capable of handling the forces of a frontal collision during this age of skeletal maturation that are generated by the shoulder harness. The stresses imparted to the child can seriously injure the thoracic cage, including imparting cardiac and pulmonary trauma. The proper shoulder harness placement for this age is across the chest, over the clavicle, but remaining off the cervical spine and face. This is best accomplished by using a booster seat that effectively increases the height of the child (Fig. 4.27), or by using a device that lowers the shoulder harness away from the face and neck and into the proper position and secures it in place by attaching to the lap belt (Fig. 4.28).

REFERENCES

1. Sleet DA. Motor vehicle trauma and safety belt use in the context of public health priorities. J Trauma 1987; 27:695-702.
2. Sewell CM, Hull HF, Fenner J, Graff H, Pine J. Child restraint law effects on motor vehicle accident fatalities and injuries: the New Mexico experience. Pediatrics 1986; 78:1079-84.
3. Orsay EM, Turnbull TL, Dunne M, Barrett JA, Langenberg P, Orsay CP. Prospective study of the effect of safety belts on morbidity and health care costs in motor-vehicle accidents. JAMA 1988; 260:3598-603.
4. Johnson C, Rivara FP, Soderberg R. Children in car crashes: analysis of data for injury and use of restraints. Pediatrics 1994; 93:960-5.
5. Agran PF, Castillo DN, Winn DG. Comparison of motor vehicle occupant injuries in restrained and unrestrained 4 to 14-year olds. Accid Anal Prev 1992; 24: 349-55.
6. Baker SP, O'Neill B, Ginsburg MJ, Li G. Injury fact book. 2nd ed. New York: Oxford University Press, 1992.
7. Severy DM, Mathewson JH, Bechtol CO. Controlled automobile rear end collisions, an investigation of related engineering and medical phenomena. In: Medical Aspects of Traffic Accidents: Proceedings of Montreal Conference. Montreal: Traffic Accident Foundation for Medical Research, 1955:152-184.
8. Severy DM, Mathewson JH, Bechtol CO. Controlled automobile rear-end collisions: an investigation of related engineering and medical phenomena. Can Serv Med J 1955; 11:727-59.
9. Macnab I. Acceleration injuries of the cervical spine. J Bone Joint Surg 1964; 46A:1797-9.
10. Ommaya AK, Hirsch AE. Tolerances for cerebral concussion from head impact and whiplash in primates. J Biomech 1971; 4:13-21.
11. Unterharnscheidt F. Traumatic alterations in the Rhesuus monkey undergoing -GX impact accelerations. Neurotraumatology 1983; 6:151-67.
12. Wickstrom J, Martinez J, Rodriquez R. Cervical strain syndrome: experimental acceleration injuries of the head and neck. In: Selzer ML, Gikas PW, Huelke DF, eds. Prevention of Highway Injury: Proceedings of a Symposium held April 19-21, 1967, in the honor of the University of Michigan's Sesquicentennial Celebration and sponsored by the University's Medical School and Highway Safety Research Institute. Ann Arbor: Highway Safety Research Institute, University of Michigan, 1967:182-7.
13. Martinez JL, Garcia DJ. Model for whiplash. J Biomech 1969; 1:23-32.
14. Clemens HJ, Burrow K. Experimental investigation on injury mechanisms of cervical spine at frontal and rear-front vehicle impacts. In: Proceedings of the Sixteenth Stapp Car Crash Conference: November 8-10, 1972, Detroit, Michigan. New York: Society of Automotive Engineers, 1972:76-104.

15. Ewing CL, Thomas DJ. Human head and neck response to impact acceleration. NAMRL monograph ed. v. 21. Pensacola, Fla: Naval Aerospace Medical Research Laboratory, Naval Aerospace Medical Institute, Naval Aerospace and Regional Medical Center, 1971.

16. Hirsch SA, Hirsch PJ, Hiramoto H, Weiss A. Whiplash syndrome. fact or fiction? Orthop Clin North Am 1988; 19:791-5.

17. Chester JB Jr. Whiplash, postural control, and the inner ear. Spine 1991;16:716-20.

18. Havsy SL. Whiplash injuries of the cervical spine and their clinical sequelae: part I. Am J Pain Manag 1994; 1:23-31.

19. Macnab I. Acceleration extension injuries of the cervical spine. In: The Spine. Rothman RH, Simeone FA, eds. W.B. Saunders 1982:647-660.

20. Dunn EJ, Blazar S. Soft-tissue injuries of the lower cervical spine. Instr Course Lect 1987; 36:499-512.

21. Barnsley L, Lord S, Bogduk N. Pathophysiology of whiplash. In: Teasell RW, Shapiro AP, eds. Spine: State of the Art Reviews. v. 7. Philadelphia: Hanley & Belfus, 1993:329-53.

22. Barnsley L, Lord S, Bogduk N. Whiplash injury. Clinical review. Pain 1994; 58:283-307.

23. White AA, Panjabi MM. Clinical biomechanics of the spine. 2nd ed. Philadelphia: J B Lippincott Company, 1990.

24. Lord S, Barnsley L, Bogduk N. Cervical zygapophyseal joint pain in whiplash. In: Spine: State of the Art Reviews. v. 7. Philadelphia: Hanley & Belfus, 1993:355-72.

25. Teasell RW, McCain GA. Clinical spectrum and management of whiplash injuries. In: Tollison CD, Satterthwaite JR, eds. Painful cervical trauma: diagnosis and rehabilitative treatment of neuromusculoskeletal injuries. Baltimore: Williams & Wilkins, 1992:292-318.

26. Carroll C, McAfee PC, Riley LH. Objective findings for diagnosis of 'whiplash'. J Musculoskel Med 1986; 3:57-76.

27. Ameis A. Cervical whiplash: considerations in the rehabilitation of cervical myofascial injury. Can Fam Physician 1986;32:1871-6.

28. Navin FPD, Romilly DP. Investigation into vehicle and occupant response to low-speed rear impacts. In: Proceedings of the Multidisciplinary Road Safety Conference IV. New Brunswick, 1989.

29. Morris F. Do head-restraints protect the neck from whiplash injuries? Arch Emerg Med 1989; 6:17-21.

30. Emori R. Whiplash at low speed collisions. New York: SAE, 1990:103-8.

31. Sturzenegger M, DiStefano G, Radanov BP, Schnidrig A. Presenting symptoms and signs after whiplash injury: the influence of accident mechanisms. Neurology 1994; 44:688-93.

32. McKenzie JA, Williams JF. Dynamic behavior of the head and spine during whiplash. J Biomech 1971; 4:477-90.

33. Jonsson H, Cesarini K, Sahlstedt B, Rauschning W. Findings and outcomes in whiplash-type neck distortions. Spine 1994; 19:2733-2743.

34. Barnsley L, Lord S, Wallis BJ, Bogduk N. The prevalence of chronic zygapophysial joint pain after whiplash. Spine 1995; 1:20-26.

35. Walter J, Doris P, Shaffer M. Clinical presentation of patients with acute cervical spine injury. Ann Emerg Med 1984; 13:512-5.

36. Parmar HV, Raymakers R. Neck injuries from rear impact road traffic accidents: prognosis in persons seeking compensation. Injury 1993; 24:75-8.

37. Schofferman J, Wasserman S. Successful treatment of low back pain and neck pain after a motor vehicle accident despite litigation. Spine 1994; 19:1007-10.

38. Hodgson SP, Grundy M. Whiplash injuries: their long-term prognosis and its relationship to compensation. Neuro-Orthopedics 1989; 7:88-91.

39. Nunn PJ, Greenwood MT. Whiplash syndrome-a transformational approach. Pain 1990; 5 (suppl):S324.

40. Gargan MF, Bannister GC. Long-term prognosis of soft-tissue injuries of the neck. J Bone Joint Surg1990; 72B:901-3.

41. Watkinson A, Gargan MF, Bannister GC. Prognostic factors in soft tissue injuries of the cervical spine. Injury 1991; 22:307-9.

42. Kaplan AS, Assael LA, eds. Temporomandibular disorders. Philadelphia: W.B. Saunders, 1991:202-205.

43. Epstein JB. Temporomandibular disorders, facial pain and headache following motor vehicle accidents. J Can Dent Assoc 1992; 58:493-5.

44. Brooke RI, LaPointe HJ. Temporomandibular joint disorders following whiplash. In: Teasell RW, Shapiro AP, eds. Spine: State of the Art Reviews. v. 7., Philadelphia: Hanley & Belfus, 1993:443-54.

45. Nachemson AL. Lumbar spine. an orthopaedic challenge. Spine 1976; 1:59.

46. Mooney V. Presidential address. International Society for the Study of the Lumbar Spine. Dallas, 1986. Where is the pain coming from? Spine 1987; 12:754-9.

47. Kuslich SD, Ulstrom CL, Michael CJ. Tissue origin of low back pain and sciatica: a report of pain response to tissue stimulation during operations on the lumbar spine using local anesthesia. Orthop Clin North Am 1991; 22:181-7.

48. Taylor JR, Twomey LT. Acute injuries to cervical joints. An autopsy study of neck sprain. Spine 1993; 18:1115-22.

49. Bogduk N, Aprill C. On the nature of neck pain, discography and cervical zygapophysial joint blocks. Pain 1993; 54:213-7.

50. O'Neill B, Haddon W Jr, Kelley AB, Sorenson WW. Automobile head restraints-frequency of neck injury claims in relation to the presence of head restraints. Am J Public Health 1972; 62:399-406.

51. Sherk HH. Developmental anatomy. In: Cervical Spine Research Society. Editorial Committee, ed. Cervical Spine. 2nd ed. Philadelphia: J B Lippincott Company, 1989:1-10.

52. Porter KM. Neck sprains after car accidents. BMJ 1989; 298:973-4.

53. Christian MS, Bullimore DW. Reduction in accident injury severity in rear seat passengers using restraints. Injury 1989; 20:262-4.

54. Anderson PA, Henley MB, Rivara FP, Maier RV. Flexion distraction and chance injuries to the thoracolumbar spine. J Orthop Trauma 1991; 5:153-60.

55. Newman RJ. Prospective evaluation of the protective effect of car seatbelts. J Trauma 1986; 26:561-4.

56. Agran PF, Castillo D, Winn D. Childhood motor vehicle occupant injuries. Am J Dis Child 1990; 144:653-62.

57. El-Nour S, Mufti MH. Seat belt legislation and the experience of the world. J Traffic Med 1992; 20:83-8.

58. Garrett JW, Braunstein PW. Seat belt syndrome. J Trauma 1962; 2:220-38.

59. Gertzbein SD, Court-Brown CM. Flexion-distraction injuries of the lumbar spine: mechanisms of injury and classification. Clin Orthop 1988; 227:52-60.

60. Rutherford WH, Greenfield T, Hayes HRM. Medical effects of seat belt legislation in the United Kingdom. Research Report 13. London: Great Britain. Department of Health and Social Security, 1985.

61. Krafft M, Nygren C, Tingvall C. Rear seat occupant protection. A study of children and adults in the rear seat of cars in relation to restraint use and car characteristics. J Traffic Med 1990; 18:51-60.

62. Hargarten SW, Karlson T. Motor vehicle crashes and seat belts: a study of emergency physician procedures, charges, and documentation. Ann Emerg Med 1994; 24:857-60.

63. Hendey GW, Votey SR. Injuries in restrained motor vehicle accident victims. Ann Emerg Med 1994; 24:77-84.

64. Murday AJ. Seat belt injury of the breast-a case report. Injury 1982; 14:276-7.

65. Newman RJ, Jones IS. Prospective study of 413 consecutive car occupants with chest injuries. J Trauma 1984; 24:129-35.

66. Dawes RF, Smallwood JA, Taylor I. Seat belt injury to the female breast. Br J Surg 1986; 73:106-7.

67. Arajarvi E, Santavirta S. Chest injuries sustained in severe traffic accidents by seatbelt wearers. J Trauma 1989; 29:37-41.

68. Smith WS, Kaufer H. New pattern of spine injury associated with lap-type seat belts: a preliminary report. Univ Mich Med Cent J 1967; 33:99-104.

69. Greenbaum E, Harris L, Halloran WX. Flexion fracture of the lumbar spine due to lap-type seat belts. Calif Med 1970; 113:74-6.

70. Taylor GA, Eggli KD. Lap-belt injuries of the lumbar spine in children: a pitfall in CT diagnosis. AJR 1988; 150:1355-8.

71. Sato TB. Effects of seat belts and injuries resulting from improper use. J Trauma 1987;27:754-8.

72. States JD, Huelke DF, Dance M, Green RN. Fatal injuries caused by underarm use of shoulder belts. J Trauma 1987; 27:740-5.

73. Foreman SM, Croft AC. Whiplash injuries, the cervical acceleration/deceleration syndrome. Baltimore: William & Wilkins, 1988.

74. Lipe HP. Prevention of nervous system trauma from travel in motor vehicles. J Neurosurg Nurs 1985; 17:77-82.

75. ACOG technical bulletin number 151: automobile passenger restraints for children and pregnant women. Int J Gynecol Obstet 1991; 37:305-8.

76. Garcia R. Air bag implicated in temporomandibular joint injury. Cranio 1994; 12:125-7.

77. Traynelis VC, Gold M. Cervical spine injury in an air-bag-equipped vehicle. J Spinal Disord 1993; 6:60-1.

78. Moriarty G. How airbags can kill your baby. Good Housekeeping 1994 Feb; 218:160.

79. Cailliet R. Neck and Arm Pain. Philadelphia: F.A. Davis Company, 1981.

80. Webb MN, Terrett AGJ. Mechanisms and patterns of tissue injury. J Aust Chiropractors' Assoc 1985; 15:60-9.

81. Maimaris C, Barnes MR, Allen MJ. 'Whiplash injuries' of the neck: a retrospective study. Injury 1988; 19:393-6.

82. Hohl M. Soft-tissue neck injuries. In: Cervical Spine Research Society. Editorial Committee, ed. Cervical Spine. 2nd ed. Philadelphia: J B Lippincott Company, 1989:436-41.

83. Bland J. Disorders of the cervical spine: diagnosis and medical management. Philadelphia: W.B. Saunders, 1987.

84. Torg JS. Risk factors in congenital stenosis of the cervical spinal canal. In: Cervical Spine Research Society. Editorial Committee, ed. Cervical Spine. 2nd ed. Philadelphia: J B Lippincott Company, 1989:272-85.

85. Mendelson G. Not cured by a verdict. Effect of legal settlement on compensation claimants. Med J Aust 1982; 2:132-4.

86. Al-Saleh MS, Alam MK, Abdul Kareem AM, Wong S. Pediatric injuries due to road traffic accidents a cause for concern. In: Dunbar JA, El-Nour S, Pikkarainen J, eds. Proceedings of International Symposium on Road Traffic Accidents, 9-12 February 1992: organized and held at Security Forces Hospital, General Administration for Medical Services, Ministry of Interior, Riyadh, Kingdom of Saudi Arabia. Stockholm, Sweden: International Association for Accident and Traffic Medicine, 1992:180-5.

87. Kraus JF, Fife D, Cox P, Ramstein K, Conroy C. Incidence, severity, and external causes of pediatric brain injury. Am J Dis Child 1986;140:687-93.

88. O'Shea JS. Childhood accident prevention strategies. Forensic Sci Int 1986; 30:99-111.

89. MacKellar A. Head injuries in children and implications for their prevention. J Pediatr Surg 1989; 24:577-9.

90. Stulginskas JV, Pless IB. Effects of a seat belt law on child restraint use. Am J Dis Child 1983; 137:582-5.

91. Scherz RG. Fatal motor vehicle accidents of child passengers from birth through 4 years of age in Washington State. Pediatrics 1981;68:572-5.

92. Diekema DS. Odontoid fracture in a child occupying a child restraint seat. Pediatrics 1988; 82:117-8.

93. Waller AE, Baker SP, Szocka A. Childhood injury deaths: national analysis and geographic variations. Am J Public Health 1989; 79:310-5.

94. Kaban LB. Diagnosis and treatment of fractures of the facial bones in children 1943-1993. J Oral Maxillofac Surg 1993; 51:722-9.

95. Alcoff JM. Car seats for children. Am Fam Physician 1982; 25:167-71.

96. Baker SP, Waller AE. Childhood injury state-by-state mortality facts. Washington, D.C.: National Maternal and Child Health Clearinghouse, 1989.

97. Chang A. Car passenger injuries and child restraints. West J Med 1983; 139:362.

98. Martinez R. Car seat misuse is killing kids. National Highway Traffic Safety Administration, in USA Today by Healy M. May 17, 1995.

99. Walter RS, Kuo AR. Taxicabs and child restraint. Am J Dis Child 1993; 147: 561-4.

100. Agran PF, Dunkle DE, Winn DG. Injuries to a sample of seatbelted children evaluated and treated in a hospital emergency room. J Trauma 1987; 27:58-64.

101. Rumball K, Jarvis J. Seat-belt injuries of the spine in young children. J Bone Joint Surg 1992; 74B:571-4.

102. Tso EL, Beaver BL, Haller JA Jr. Abdominal injuries in restrained pediatric passengers. J Pediatr Surg 1993; 28:915-9.

103. Statter MD, Coran AG. Appendiceal transection in a child associated with a lap belt restraint: case report. J Trauma 1992; 33:765-6.

104. Tingvall C. Children in cars: some aspects of the safety of children as car passengers in road traffic accidents. Acta Paediatr Scand Suppl 1987; 339:1-35.

105. Johnson DL, Falci S. Diagnosis and treatment of pediatric lumbar spine injuries caused by rear seat lap belts. Neurosurgery 1990; 26:434-41.

106. Newman KD, Bowman LM, Eichelberger MR, et al. Lap belt complex: intestinal and lumbar spine injury in children. J Trauma 1990; 30:1133-40.

107. Taylor TKF, Henderson JJ, Trinca GW. Seat-belt injuries of the spine in children and young adolescents-an increasing cause for concern. Med J Aust 1990; 152:447-8.

108. Robertson LS. Motor vehicles. Pediatr Clin North Am 1985; 32:87-94.

109. Partyka SC. Papers on child restraints-effectiveness and use. Washington, DC: US Department of Transportation, National Highway Traffic Safety Administration, 1988 DOT HS 807 286.

110. Burg FD, Douglass JM, Diamond E, Siegel AW. Automotive restraint devices for the pediatric patient. Pediatrics 1970; 45:49-53.

111. Still A, Roberts I, Koelmeyer T, Vuletic J, Norton R. Child passenger fatalities and restraint use in Auckland. N Z Med J 1992; 105:449-50.

112. Chorba TL, Klein TM. Increases in crash involvement and fatalities among motor vehicle occupants younger that 5 years old. Pediatrics 1993; 91:897-901.

113. Fuller AK, Fuller AE, Yates LE Jr. Use of child restraint devices in vehicles [letter]. JAMA 1986; 255:614.

114. Henry PC, Hauber RP, Rice M. Factors associated with closed head injury in a pediatric population. J Neurosci Nurs 1992; 24:311-6.

115. Conry BG, Hall CM. Cervical spine fractures and rear car seat restraints. Arch Dis Child 1987; 62:1267-8.

116. Moskowitz A. Lumbar seatbelt injury in a child: case report. J Trauma 1989;29: 1279-82.

117. Christoffel KK. Child passenger safety: past, present, and future [editorial]. Am J Dis Child 1989;143:1271-2.

118. Fuchs S, Barthel MJ, Flannery AM, Christoffel KK. Cervical spine fractures sustained by young children in forward-facing car seats. Pediatrics 1989; 84:348-54.

119. Chorba TL, Reinfurt D, Hulka BS. Efficacy of mandatory seat-belt use legislation: the North Carolina experience from 1983 through 1987. JAMA 1988; 260:3593-7.

120. Margolis LH, Wagenaar AC, Liu W. Effects of a mandatory child restraint law on injuries requiring hospitalization. Am J Dis Child 1988; 142:1099-103.

121. Wagenaar AC, Molnar LJ, Buzinski KL, Margolis LH. Correlates of child restraint use. Ann Arbor: University of Michigan, Transportation Research Institute, 1986.

122. Wagenaar AC, Webster DW. Preventing injuries to children through compulsory automobile safety seat use. Pediatrics 1986; 78:662-72.

123. Thompson A. Child safety in cars: implications for health authorities. J Traffic Med 1989; 17:29-35.

124. SriVatsa LP. Dangers in restraining seats [letter]. J Traffic Med 1989; 17:57-8.

125. Ruta D, Beattie T, Narayan V. Prospective study of non-fatal childhood road traffic accidents: what can seat restraint achieve? J Public Health Med 1993; 15:88-92.

126. Klein TM, Walz MC. Child passenger restraint use and motor-vehicle-related fatalities among children-United States, 1982-1990. MMWR 1991; 40:600-2.

127. Wagenaar AC, Webster DW, Maybee RG. Effects of child restraint laws on traffic fatalities in eleven states. J Trauma 1987; 27:726-31.

128. Osberg JS, Di Scala C. Morbidity among pediatric motor vehicle crash victims: the effectiveness of seat belts. Am J Public Health 1992; 82:422-5.

129. Ruffin MT 4th, Kantor R. Adults' knowledge about the use of child restraint devices. Fam Med 1992; 24:382-5.

130. Drongowski RA, Coran AG, Maio RF, Polley TZ Jr. Trauma scores, accident deformity codes, and car restraints in children. J Pediatr Surg 1993; 28:1072-5.

131. Agran PF, Winn DG, Dunkle DE. Injuries among 4 to 9-year old restrained motor vehicle occupants by seat location and crash impact site. Am J Dis Child 1989; 143:1317-21.

132. Hoffman MA, Spence LJ, Wesson DE, Armstrong PF, Williams JI, Filler RM. Pediatric passenger: trends in seatbelt use and injury patterns. J Trauma 1987; 27:974-6.

133. Bodenham A, Newman RJ. Restraint of children in cars: education not just legislation. BMJ 1991; 303:1283-4.

134. Reid AB, Letts RM, Black GB. Pediatric chance fractures: association with intra-abdominal injuries and seatbelt use. J Trauma 1990; 30:384-91.

135. Stylianos S, Harris BH. Seatbelt use and patterns of central nervous system injury in children. Pediatr Emerg Care 1990; 6:4-5.

136. Glassman SD, Johnson JR, Holt RT. Seatbelt injuries in children. J Trauma 1992; 33:882-6.

137. Goldman PA. Safety Recommendations H86-44 through 47. Washington DC: National Transportation Safety Board, 1986.

138. Sripathi V, King PA. Mid-ileal stricture and spinal injury sustained by a 7-year-old child restrained by a lap seat belt involved in a motor vehicle accident. Aust NZ J Surg 1991; 61:640-1.

139. Patrick LM, Nyquist GW. Airbags effects on the out-of-position child. Society of Automotive Engineers, 1972.

140. Karttunen P, Karkola K. Children in traffic accidents- a follow-up study. J Traffic Med 1992; 20:115-20.

141. Hoy G, Cole WG. Paediatric cervical seat belt syndrome. Injury 1993; 24:297-9.

142. Keller J, Mosdal C. Traumatic odontoid epiphysiolysis in an infant fixed in a child's car seat. Injury 1990;21:191-2.

143. Pang D, Wilberger JE Jr. Spinal cord injury without radiographic abnormalities in children. J Neurosurg 1982; 57:114-29.

144. Rachesky I, Boyce T, Duncan B, Bjelland J, Sibley B. Clinical prediction of cervical spine injuries in children: radiographic abnormalities. Am J Dis Child 1987; 141:199-201.

145. Bohn D, Armstrong D, Becker L, Humphreys R. Cervical spine injuries in children. J Trauma 1990;30:463-9.

146. Kozlowski K. Anterior intervertebral disc herniations in children. Report of four cases. Pediatr Radiol 1977; 6:32-5.

147. Jackson R. Cervical syndrome. 4th ed. Springfield, IL: Charles C Thomas Company, 1977.

148. Thompson A, McArdle P, Dunne F. Children may be seriously affected [letter]. BMJ 1993; 307:1282-3.

149. Mucci SJ, Eriksen LD, Crist KA, Bernath LA, Chaudhuri PK. Pattern of injury to rear seat passengers involved in automobile collisions. J Trauma 1991; 31: 1329-31.

150. Graham CJ, Kittredge D, Stuemky JH. Injuries associated with child safety seat misuse. Pediatr Emerg Care 1992; 8:351-3.

SUGGESTED READING

Agran PF, Winn DG, Anderson CL. Differences in child pedestrian injury events by location. Pediatrics 1994;93:284-8.

Baker SP. Motor vehicle occupant deaths in young children. Pediatrics 1979; 64:860-1.

Cameron BH. Injuries in children wearing seat belts [letter]. Can Med Assoc J 1986; 134:308-9.

Campbell BJ. Safety belt injury reduction related to crash severity and front seated position. J Trauma 1987; 27:733-9.

Carette S. Whiplash injury and chronic neck pain [editorial]. New Engl J Med 1994; 330:1083-4.

Chronicle Wire Services. Crashes hurt toddlers more than infants. San Francisco Chronicle June 9, 1994, Sec A, p.10.

Davis D, Bohlman H, Walker E, Fisher R, Robinson R. Pathological findings in fatal craniospinal injuries. J Neurosurg 1971; 34:603-13.

Dehkordi F, Mueller BA, Rivara FP. Risk of injury to restrained children in motor vehicle crashes. Am J Dis Child 1988; 142:401-2.

El-Khoury GY, Clark CR, Gravett AW. Acute traumatic rotatory atlanto-axial dislocation in children. J Bone Joint Surg 1984;66A:774-7.

Evans L. Fatality risk reduction from safety belt use. J Trauma 1987;27:746-9.

Fields M, Weinberg K. Coverage gaps in child-restraint and seat-belt laws affecting children. Accid Anal Prev 1994; 26:371-6.

Fleming A, ed. Children in Crashes. Rev. ed. Washington, D.C.: Insurance Institute for Highway Safety, 1986.

Foss RD. Evaluation of a community-wide incentive program to promote safety restraint use. Am J Public Health 1989; 79:304-6.

Gallup BM, Newman JA. Assessment of facial injury to fully restrained drivers through full-scale car crash testing. J Trauma 1987; 27:711-8.

Gloag D. Compulsory rear seat belts for adults? BMJ 1990; 300:1225-6.

Guthkelch AN. Infantile subdural haematoma and its relationship to whiplash injuries. BMJ 1971; 2:430-1.

Hildingsson S, Hietala O, Toolanen G. Scintigraphic findings in acute whiplash injury of the cervical spine. Injury 1989; 20:265-6.

Huelke DF, Sherman HW. Seat belt effectiveness: case examples from real-world crash investigations. J Trauma 1987; 27:750-3.

Knapp JF, Dowd MD, O'Conner T, Sharp R. Case 01-1993: a six-year old girl with respiratory distress following involvement in a motor vehicle crash. Pediatr Emerg Care 1993; 9:116-20.

Lestina DC, Williams AF, Lund AK, Zador P, Kuhlmann TP. Motor vehicle crash injury patterns and the Virginia seat belt law. JAMA 1991; 265:1409-13.

Mason MA. Restraining infants in cars. BMJ 1988; 296:1345-6.

National Safety Council. Accident Facts. 1993 ed. Itasca, IL: Author, 1993.

Newman RJ. Chest wall injuries and the seat belt syndrome. Injury 1984; 16:110-3.

Nitecki S, Karmeli R, Ben-Arieh Y, Schramek A, Torem S. Seatbelt injury to the common iliac artery: report of two cases and review of the literature. J Trauma 1992; 33:935-8.

Nygren A, Tingvall C, Turbell T. Misuse of child restraints in cars and potential hazards from such misuse: road traffic observations and barrier sled tests. Acta Orthop Scand Suppl 1987; 339:V:1-19.

Penry-Jones K, Boswell DR, Tongue R. Restraint of babies in cars. BMJ 1986;292:591.

Petrucelli E. Seat belt laws: the New York experience-preliminary data and some observations. J Trauma 1987; 27:706-10.

Richmond PW, Skinner A, Kimche A. Children's car-restraints: use and parental attitudes. Arch Emerg Med 1989; 6:41-5.

Ritchie WP, Ersek RA, Bunch WL, Simmons RL. Combined visceral and vertebral injuries from lap type seat belts. Surg Gynecol Obstet 1970; 131:431-5.

Ross DJ, Gloyns PF. Failure of child safety seat to prevent death. Br Med J [Clin Res Ed] 1986; 292:1636.

Schaaf K. Child auto restraints. Alaska Med 1983; 25:76-8.

Seletz E. Whiplash injuries. JAMA 1958; 168:1750-5.

Sprigg SJ. Passenger safety in cars. Arch Dis Child 1985; 60:678-9.

Vandersluis R, O'Connor HMC. Seat-belt syndrome. Can Med Assoc J 1987; 137:1023-4.

Williams AF. Children killed in falls from motor vehicles. Pediatrics 1981; 68:576-8.

Williams JS, Kirkpatrick JR. Nature of seat belt injuries. J Trauma 1971;11:207-18.

Pregnancy, Birth, and Neonatal Assessments

5 The Prenatal and Perinatal Period

Judy A. Forrester and Claudia A. Anrig

*A*t no time in human life are there more critical and influential developments than in the pre and perinatal period. The massive growth encountered during this epoch is unparalleled by any other. The far-reaching consequences of healthy anatomical and physiological maturation during an individual's evolution are established even as conception is taking place and as the germinal tissues are being synthesized. The complexities of the incipient processes of specialization and differentiation are well documented, yet our comprehension of most of the contributory developmental mechanisms is destitute at best. Still, the rapid, relentless, innate unfolding of embryological cells, tissues and systems comprising an intricate reticulum lends itself to the manifestation of the ultimately complex functional structure that we call a human being.

The chiropractor has a pivotal role to play in the health care of the maternity patient, her pregnancy, and the neonate. A successful neonatal outcome will be more easily achieved when chiropractic care is established as an essential element in the aggregate pre and perinatal period.

The prenatal period describes the processes that transpire before birth. These are depicted from both a maternal and fetal mien.

The perinatal period encompasses the interval shortly before and after birth. In specific terms, it exists from week 29 of gestation until 1 to 4 weeks after birth of the neonate.

First Trimester

Maternal Anatomy and Development

The duration of pregnancy is calculated from the first day of the last normal menstrual period. This assumes a regular 28-day cycle and that ovulation occurred 14 days after bleeding commenced. Therefore, the duration of pregnancy (the actual period of amenorrhea) is between 37 and 42 weeks (259–293 days). Full-term delivery occurs between 37 and 42 weeks from the date of the last normal menstrual period.

Gestation is segmented into three trimesters, each one lasting approximately 3 months. In the first trimester, the maternal uterus undergoes massive preparatory transformations. Initially, the endometrium of the uterus becomes thicker and increasingly vascular to sustain embryologic growth and development through its rich source of nourishment. The primitive placenta is constructed at the end of the first gestational month by the chorionic villi extending into the endometrium. Fetal circulation extends through the roots of this formation while the maternal blood circulates through the intervillous spaces. A thin membrane separates the fetal and maternal circulation, typically not mixing.

Through a complex process of cell division and differentiation, the embryo, placenta, and amniotic sac and fluid are formed. The amniotic sac envelops the blastocyst. The enclosed amniotic fluid provides for temperature regulation, facile embryologic and fetal movement, and shock absorption from extrinsic movements and bumps.

The maternity patient will frequently experience overwhelming fatigue, largely due to the increased physiological demands and the consequent metabolic shift. Nausea and vomiting is encountered in approximately 80% of pregnant women in the first trimester. Although this is generically termed "morning sickness," it is more frequently present at random periods throughout the day. The etiology is hypothesized to be an effect of human chorionicgonadotropin produced by the placenta.

The breast tissue is influenced by the augmented levels of circulating estrogen and progesterone as pregnancy advances. Breast enlargement, prominent veins, and a subjective tenderness and a tingling sensation in the nipples are common signs of hormonal activity during the first trimester. In addition, the areola enlarges and darkens, and the Montgomery glands proliferate and enlarge to assist in lubricant production.

The superior border of the uterus remains just immediately above the pubic symphysis; however, the moderate enlargement of this organ creates pressure on the bladder and therefore stimulates more frequent urination. The vagina and cervix become bluish – (Chadwick's sign), the cervix softens, and vaginal secretions increase.

Emotional volatility and extreme fatigue are often pathognomonic signs of early pregnancy.

PELVIC STRUCTURES

The bony pelvis is comprised of four osseous structures, namely the two innominate bones, the sacrum and the coccyx (Fig. 5.1 A-B). The four joints uniting these bones are the symphysis pubis, the sacrococcygeal joint, and the bilateral sacroiliac joints. These pelvic structures function as the foundational and functional support for the spinal column and upper body, and transmit the weight bearing and gravitational forces of the lower extremities.

The female pelvis adapts for childbearing during adolescent growth. The pre-adolescent pelvis is of anthropoid configuration, growing to a larger gynecoid pelvis through the adolescent growth spurt. Fetopelvic disproportion occurs with greater frequency in teenage girls than in osseously mature women (1).

THE INNOMINATE BONES

The two innominate bones are formed by the fusion of the ilium, the ischium, and the pubis around the acetabulum. The ilium portion is found on the superior innominate. The ilial body fuses with the ischial body, the ilial ala is aligned superiorly and laterally. On the ilium, the following anatomical landmarks are noted: the anterior superior iliac spine, which provides attachment for the inguinal ligament; the posterior superior iliac spine, which lies on a horizontal line with the second sacral segment; and the iliac crest, which extends from the anterior superior iliac spine to the posterior superior iliac spine.

The ischium is comprised of the ischial body in which the superior and inferior rami merge. On the ischium, some salient anatomical landmarks are displayed, including the acetabulum, which is formed in part by the ischial body, the superior ramus located posteriorly and inferior to the body, the inferior ramus, which fuses with the inferior ramus of the pubis, and the ischial spine, separating the greater sciatic from the lesser sciatic notch. The ischial spine provides for attachment of the levator ani muscle. The ischial tuberosity is located on the lower part of the ischium and is described as the "sitting bone."

The pubis is comprised of two rami and the body. The eminent anatomical landmarks noted here are the body of the pubis, which has a rough surface on its medial aspect uniting to the corresponding area on the opposite pubis to create the symphysis pubis. The levator ani muscles also attach to the pelvic part of the pubis. The pubic crest represents the superior border of the body, and the pubic tubercle, or pubic spine, designates the lateral portion of the pubic crest. It provides for attachment of the inguinal ligament and the conjoined tendon. The superior ramus joins the body of the pubis at the pubic spine and the ilial body at the iliopectineal line, forming a part of the acetabulum. The inferior ramus coalesces with the inferior ramus of the ischium.

Additional anatomical pelvic landmarks include the iliopectineal line extending from the pubic tubercle posteriorly to the sacro-iliac joint. This line forms the greater part of the boundary of the pelvic inlet. The greater sacrosciatic notch is located between the posterior inferior iliac spine above and the ischial spine below. The lesser sacrosciatic notch is bounded by the ischial spine superiorly and the ischial tuberosity inferiorly. The obturator foramen is created by the acetabulum, the ischial rami, and the pubic rami.

THE SACRUM

The sacrum is a triangular bone with the base above and the apex below. It consists of five vertebral segments fused together at osseous maturity. The sacrum is located between the innominate bones and is attached to them by the sacro-iliac joints.

Superiorly, the first sacral segment articulates with the inferior surface of the fifth lumbar vertebra, separated by an intervertebral disc. The anterior or pelvic surface of the sacrum is concave and the posterior surface convex. At the anterior superior border of the first sacral segment is the sacral promontory. This structure protrudes slightly into the cavity of the pelvis, reducing the anteroposterior diameter of the inlet. According to Barge (2), the sacral promontory exhibits a greater percentage of a sacral "plateau" in the female. He describes its radiographic appearance "like a ¼″ of a vertebral body attached to the top of the sacrum." He further states that this type of sacrum often displays unequal development in height from one side to the other. These findings were supported by Bautch et al. (3) with the suggestion that this plateau incidence in the female contributed to the higher incidence of scoliosis due to the biomechanical instability.

THE COCCYX

The coccyx, commonly termed the "tailbone," is composed of three to five rudimentary vertebrae. The superior surface of

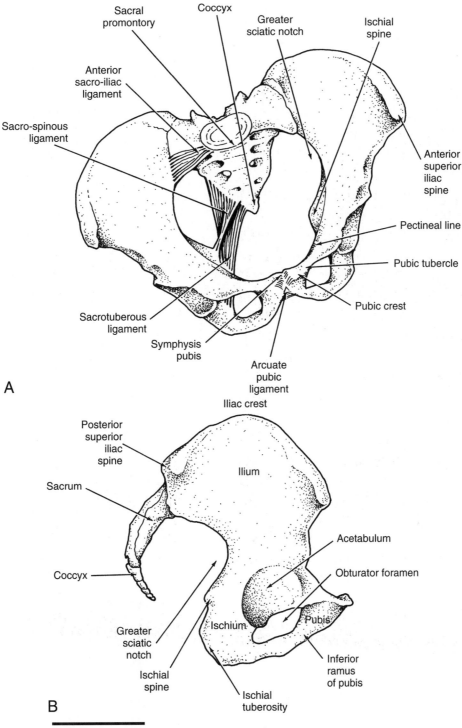

Figure 5.1.   A, Anatomical structures of the pelvis. Anteroposterior view.
B, Anatomical structures of the pelvis. Lateral view.

the first coccygeal segment articulates with the inferior surface of the fifth sacral vertebra to form the sacrococcygeal joint. The coccygeus muscle, the levator ani muscles, and the sphincter ani externus are attached to the coccyx from above downward.

PELVIC JOINTS

The symphysis pubis is a cartilaginous joint with no capsule and no synovial membrane. There is minimal movement at this joint. The posterior and superior ligaments are weak. The strong anterior ligaments are reinforced by the tendons of the rectus abdominous and the external oblique muscles. The strong inferior ligament in the pubic arch is known as the arcuate pubic ligament. It extends between the rami and leaves a small space in the subpubic angle.

The sacrococcygeal joint is a synovial hinge joint located between the fifth sacral and the first coccygeal segments. It allows both flexion and extension. Extension, by increasing the anteroposterior diameter of the outlet of the pelvis, plays an important role in parturition. Overextension during delivery may break the small cornua by which the coccyx is attached to the sacrum. This joint has a weak capsule, which is reinforced by anterior, posterior, and lateral sacrococcygeal ligaments.

The sacroiliac joints are found between the articular surfaces of the sacrum and the ilium. These joints transmit the weight of the body to the pelvis and further to the lower extremities. These joints are synovial joints and each permits a small degree of measurable movement (4). The capsule is somewhat weak, and stability is provided particularly by the muscles around it as well as by four primary and two accessory ligaments.

The primary ligaments observed normally are the anterior sacroiliac ligaments, which are short and transverse and run from the preauricular sulcus on the ilium to the anterior aspect of the sacral ala; the interosseous sacroiliac ligaments, which are short, strong transverse bands that extend from the rough area behind the auricular surface on the ilium to the adjoining area on the sacrum; the short posterior sacroiliac ligaments, which are strong transverse bands that lie behind the interosseous ligaments; and the long posterior sacroiliac ligaments that are attached to the posterior superior spine on the ilium and to the tubercles on the third and fourth sacral segments.

The accessory ligaments include the sacrotuberous ligaments, which are attached on one side to the posterior superior iliac spine, the posterior inferior iliac spine, the third, fourth and fifth sacral tubercles, and the lateral border of the coccyx. On the other side, the sacrotuberous ligaments are attached to the pelvic aspect of the ischial tuberosity. The sacrospinous ligament is triangular. Its base is attached to the lateral parts of the fifth sacral and first coccygeal segments, and the apex is attached to the ischial spine.

The Obstetric Pelvis

The bony pelvis during pregnancy is described largely as the obstetric pelvis and is characterized by a number of delineations specific to the changes occurring to it during the early and later stages of maternal development.

The linea terminalis separates the false pelvis from the true pelvis (Fig. 5.2), the true pelvis being situated entirely below the pelvic brim. The false pelvis is anatomically defined by the lumbar vertebrae posteriorly, the iliac fossae laterally, and the anterior abdominal wall anteriorly. Its function during pregnancy is to sustain the uterus throughout pregnancy. The true pelvis is the bony canal through which the fetus will pass during the birth process and is divided into the pelvic inlet, the pelvic cavity, and the pelvic outlet (Fig. 5.3).

The pelvic inlet is defined by the pubic crest and spine anteriorly, the iliopectineal lines on the innominate bones laterally, and by the anterior borders of the ala and promontory of the sacrum posteriorly. The pelvic cavity is a curved passage bordered by the straight and shallow wall comprised of the pubis, the deep, concave posterior wall bounded by the sacrum, and by the anterior borders of the sacral ala and promontory posteriorly. The pelvic outlet is formed by the arcuate pubic ligament and the pubic arch anteriorly, by the ischial tuberosity and sacrotuberous ligament laterally, and by the apex of the sacrum posteriorly.

Pelvic inclination (Fig 5.4) is evaluated in the standing, weight-bearing position. The plane of the pelvic brim illustrates an approximate sixty degree angle with the horizontal. The pubic spine and the anterior superior iliac

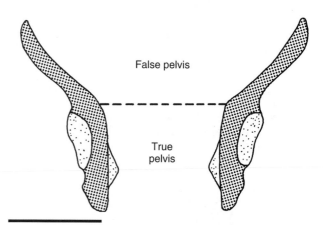

False pelvis

True pelvis

Figure 5.2.   The obstetric pelvis. A/P view. Modified from Oxom H. Human Labor and Birth. 1980:23.

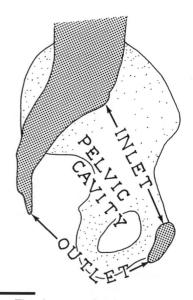

INLET

PELVIC CAVITY

OUTLET

Figure 5.3.   The obstetric pelvis. Lateral view. Pelvic cavity. Modified from Oxom H. Human labor and birth. 1980:23.

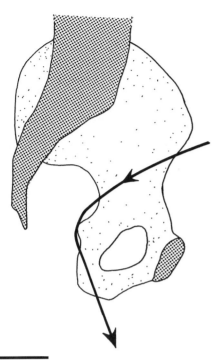

Figure 5.4. The obstetric pelvis. Lateral view. The measurement of pelvic inclination. This is assessed with the gravid patient in an upright position. Modified from Oxom H. Human labor and birth 1980:23.

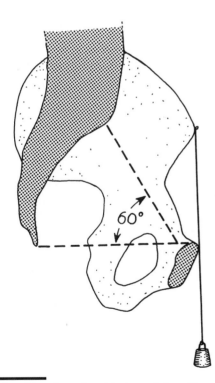

Figure 5.5. The obstetric pelvis. Lateral view. The axis of the birth canal. This is the course of the presenting fetal part as it travels downward through the pelvic structures. Modified from Oxom H. Human labor and birth. 1980:23.

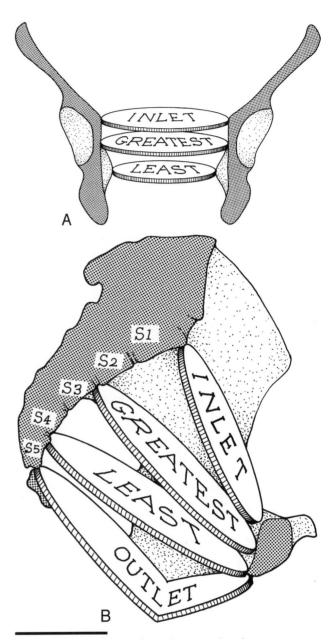

Figure 5.6. A, Planes of the obstetric pelvis. Anteroposterior view. Modified from Oxom H. Human labor and birth, 1980:25. B, Planes of the obstetric pelvis. Lateral view. Modified from Oxom H. Human labor and birth, 1980:25.

spine are in the same vertical plane. The axis of the birth canal (Fig 5.5) is the path taken by the presenting fetal part as it progresses downward through the pelvis. Initially, it advances inferiorly and posteriorly to the level of the ischial spines, then alters its direction to inferior and anterior.

The planes of the pelvis are hypothetical flat surfaces that extend across the pelvic structures at different levels (Fig. 5.6 A–B). These pelvic planes are used for obstetrical description only and are classified as follows:

1. The plane of the pelvic inlet, or the superior strait
2. The planes of the pelvic cavity, the most significant two are known as the plane of greatest dimensions and the plane of least dimensions
3. The plane of the pelvic outlet, or the inferior strait

Obstetric diameters specify the distances between depicted anatomical points. The diameters of greatest significance are the anteroposterior diameters, the transverse diameters, the left and right oblique diameters, the posterior sagittal diameter, and the anterior sagittal diameter.

There are three different anteroposterior diameters extending from anterior pelvic points to posterior pelvic points. The most important of these diameters is the obstetric conjugate i.e., the one through which the fetus must pass and extend from the middle of the sacral promontory to the posterior superior margin of the pubic symphysis. The transverse diameter is the widest distance between the iliopectineal lines. The left oblique diameter lies between the left sacroiliac joint and the right iliopectineal eminence, where the right oblique diameter lies between the right sacroiliac joint and the left iliopectineal eminence.

Pelvic Classifications

Due to a diversity of anatomical presentations, the female pelvis is classified according to its conforming and non-conforming characteristics. The pelvis varies greatly with reference to each of the pelvic planes, being predominantly of the female type in one, and the male type in another. The pelvis is classified germane to its structure at the pelvic inlet, with its nonconforming characteristics referred to at the midpelvis and pelvic outlet. Table 5.1 describes the Caldwell and Moloy classifications of the pelvis.

The four illustrations viewed in Figure 5.7 A–D illustrate the pelvic classifications at the pelvic inlet. Figure 5.8 A–D exhibits the same four pelvic classifications where they present at the midpelvis. It becomes obvious upon study of these renderings how the variety of pelvic shapes can affect the prognosis for a safe and healthy delivery. The female pelvis, when viewed radiographically on pre-conception films, can be revealing in facilitating determination of the various pelvic types.

Differentiation of Primipara Versus Multipara

Classifications of maternal obstetrical situations can be described in nomenclature of term pregnancies, premature births, abortions, and living children.

Gravidity is the term referring to the total number of pregnancies of a woman of any duration. During pregnancy, the woman is described as a gravida. A woman pregnant for the first time is described as a primigravida, for the second time as a secundigravida, and for the third and subsequent pregnancies as a multigravida.

Parity is the term referring to the number of previous pregnancies that have been viable and delivered. This term does not recognize the number of delivered babies, as in the case of multiple births, rather the number of pregnancies solely. Therefore, para refers to past, viable pregnancies. A woman who has delivered one viable pregnancy is called a primipara. This description is applied regardless of whether the infant is alive or stillborn. A woman who has had two or subsequent viable pregnancies is called a multipara. Examples of gravida and para are as follows:

Gravida 1, Para 0 : Primigravida, or a woman pregnant for the first time

Gravida 1, Para 0 : If abortion occurs prior to a viable delivery

Gravida 1, Para 1 : Primipara, or a woman who has delivered a viable fetus, whether or not the infant is alive or stillborn

Gravida 2, Para 1 : Second pregnancy

Gravida 2, Para 2 : Following the delivery of the second child

Gravida 2, Para 0 : Two abortions and no viable infants

Gravida 1, Para 1 : Viable triplets following a first pregnancy

Developmental Assessment

Numerous methods can assess the integrity of the fetoplacental unit. These include, but are not limited to, assessing the integrity of the fetoplacental unit, diagnosing fetal abnormality, monitoring fetal growth, and evaluating well-being.

Clinical assessment of maturity depends on measurement of fundal height. This is most accurate in the first 10 weeks of pregnancy and can be very unreliable later in pregnancy or in obese women.

Fetal quickening can help in dating the duration of the pregnancy; in primiparous women movements are felt at approximately 20 to 21 weeks, and in multiparous women at approximately 18 weeks.

Ultrasound as a measurement of embryological and fetal development in patients with no known risk factors is controversial in some circles. Traditionally, medicine utilizes a number of ultrasonic measurements that correlate with gestational age in the first trimester. These include crown–rump length, biparietal diameter (BPD), and femur length. The BPD measurement is among the best of all methods for assessing duration of pregnancy.

Fetal radiography is also used to visualize the appearance of various fetal ossification centers to aid in the assessment of maturity. The talus ossifies at approximately 26 weeks, and the lower femoral epiphysis appears at 37 weeks. Variations can occur, and fetal radiology is of limited practical value. Radiography of the fetus is now rarely used as a method of establishing maturity due to the damaging effects of ionizing radiation.

Human placental lactogen (HPL) is less helpful than estriol excretion estimations because HPL reflects placental function and weight only.

Table 5.1.   **Caldwell and Moloy Classifications of the Pelvis**

	Gynecoid	Android	Anthropoid	Platypelloid
Pelvic inlet				
Sex type	Normal female	Male	Ape-like	Flat female
Prevalence	50 percent	20 percent	25 percent	5 percent
Shape	Round or transverse oval; transverse diameter is a little longer than the anteroposterior	Heart or wedge shaped	Long anteroposterior oval	Transverse oval
Antero-posterior diameter	Adequate	Adequate	Long	Short
Transverse diameter	Adequate	Adequate	Adequate, but relatively short	Long
Posterior sagittal diameter	Adequate	Very short and inadequate	Very long	Very short
Anterior sagittal diameter	Adequate	Long	Long	Short
Posterior segment	Broad, deep, roomy	Shallow; sacral promontory indents the inlet and reduces its capacity	Deep	Shallow
Anterior segment	Well-rounded forepelvis	Narrow, sharply angulated forepelvis	Deep	Shallow
Pelvic cavity: midpelvis				
Antero-posterior diameter	Adequate	Reduced	Long	Shortened
Transverse diameter	Adequate	Reduced	Adequate	Wide
Posterior sagittal diameter	Adequate	Reduced	Adequate	Shortened
Anterior sagittal diameter	Adequate	Reduced	Adequate	Short
Sacrum	Wide, deep curve; short; slopes backward; light bone	Flat; inclined forward; long; narrow; heavy	Inclined backward; narrow; long	Wide, deep curve; often sharply angulated with enlarged sacral fossa
Sidewalls	Parallel, straight	Convergent; funnel pelvis	Straight	Parallel
Ischial spines	Not prominent	Prominent	Variable	Variable
Sacrosciatic notch	Wide; short	Narrow; long; high arch	Wide	Short
Depth: iliopectineal eminence to tuberosities	Average	Long	Long	Short
Capacity	Adequate	Reduced in all diameters	Adequate	Reduced

Table 5.1.   *(continued)* **Caldwell and Moloy Classifications of the Pelvis**

	Gynecoid	Android	Anthropoid	Platypelloid
Outlet				
Antero-posterior diameter	Long	Short	Long	Short
Transverse diameter (bituberous)	Adequate	Narrow	Adequate	Wide
Pubic arch	Wide and round; 90 degrees	Narrow; deep; 70 degrees	Normal or relatively narrow	Very wide
Inferior pubic rami	Short; concave inward	Straight; long	Long; relatively narrow	Straight; short
Capacity	Adequate	Reduced	Adequate	Adequate
Effect on labor				
Fetal head	Engages in transverse or oblique diameter in slight asynclitism; good flexion; OA is common	Engages in transverse or posterior diameter in asynclitism; extreme molding	Engages in antero-posterior of oblique; often occiput posterior	Engages in transverse diameter with marked asynclitism
Labor	Good uterine function; early and complete internal rotation; spontaneous delivery; wide pubic arch reduces perineal tears	Deep transverse arrest is common; arrest as OP with failure of rotation; delivery is often by difficult forceps applica	Delivery and labor usually 'easy' birth face to pubis is common	Delay at inlet
Prognosis	Good	Poor	Good	Poor; disproportion; delay at inlet; labor often terminated by caesarean section

Genetic Testing Procedures and Prenatal Diagnosis

The use of prenatal diagnosis for the prediction of genetic disorders and birth defects in the fetus continues to increase in parallel with technological and genetic advances, and, as such, is a continually evolving field.

Genetic indications for prenatal diagnosis can be summarized as follows:

A. Increased risk for chromosomal abnormalities
   1. Maternal age
   2. Biochemical markers
      i.   Maternal serum alpha fetoprotein
      ii. Maternal serum unconjugated estriol
      iii. Maternal human chorionic gonadotropin

   3. Family history
      i.   Previous stillbirth/livebirth with a trisomy or other chromosome abnormality
      ii. Parent with a potentially transmissible chromosome rearrangement
      iii. Relatives (other than offspring) with Down syndrome or other trisomies
      iv. Genetic disorders with an identifiable chromosome marker or abnormality
      v.   Other X-linked disorders
      vi. Maternal or paternal therapeutic irradiation
   4. Abnormal ultrasound scan
B. Morphologic abnormalities
   1. Neural tube defects
   2. Other morphologic malformations

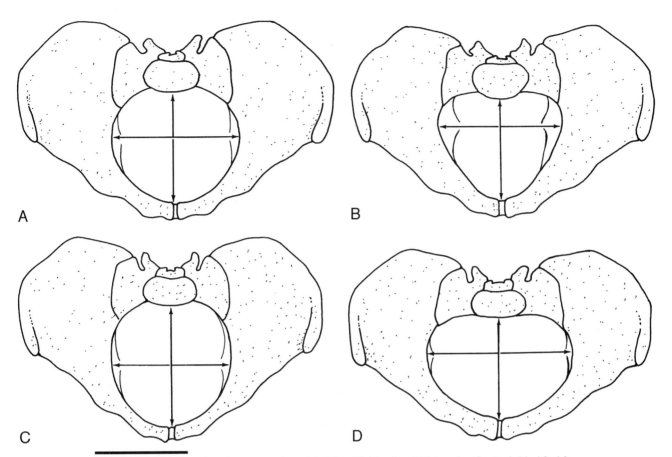

A

B

C

D

Figure 5.7. Pelvic classifications at the pelvic inlet. (Caldwell and Moloy classification). Modified from Oxom H. Human labor and birth, 1980:33. A, Gynecoid. B, Android. C, Anthropoid. D, Platypelloid.

C. Biochemical and molecular disorders

D. Carrier (heterozygote) screening

Prenatal genetic testing is not available to all women. Guidelines to testing are an attempt to balance genetic risks against procedural risks and economic considerations. Recommendations are based on the concept of increased genetic risk. A variety of screening techniques is currently employed to determine whether a couple is at an increased risk to produce a child with a chromosomal abnormality.

The techniques available to monitor fetal genotype and development include amniocentesis, chorionic villus sampling (CVS), cordocentesis (PUBS), fetal tissue sampling, radiography, fetoscopy, embryoscopy, and diagnostic ultrasound. Some diagnostic results may be obtained by more than one technique (fetal karyotype can be obtained with cells from amniocentesis, CVS, or fetal blood sampling), but some prenatal diagnostic techniques will have specific indications for their use.

Amniocentesis

Amniocentesis is a second-trimester prenatal diagnostic procedure usually performed after 14 weeks from the last menstrual period. The indications for this procedure include advanced maternal age, history of a stillborn or liveborn child with a chromosomal abnormality, parental chromosome translocations, history of specific congenital abnormalities (neural tube defects), and other biochemical or molecular genetic diseases in which results can be obtained from amniocytes or amniotic fluid (See Chapter 17).

Ultrasound is performed before amniocentesis to determine fetal gestational age, location of placenta and amniotic fluid, fetal cardiac activity, and the number of fetuses.

In most centers, amniocentesis is done with continuous ultrasound guidance. The technique is usually performed with a 22-gauge spinal needle; 15 to 30 ml of amniotic fluid is removed. Obtaining the fluid takes less than 1 minute; the patient may experience some mild uterine cramping and describe a mild pressure sensation.

The risks of amniocentesis are considered in three categories. The most important is fetal loss after amniocentesis, with or without infection. This is estimated to be 1 pregnancy loss for every 200 amniocenteses (5–7).

Other complications after amniocentesis include continued leakage of amniotic fluid, bleeding, and infection. The risk of infection after the procedure is very low. Fetal injuries at the

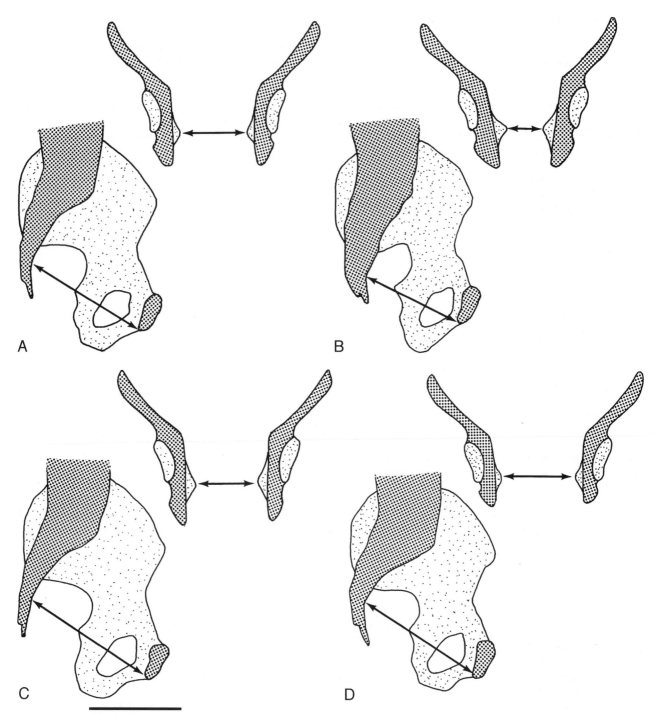

Figure 5.8. Pelvic classifications at the midpelvis. (Caldwell and Moloy classification). Modified from Oxom H. Human labor and birth, 1980:35. A, Gynecoid. B, Android. C, Anthropoid. D, Platypelloid.

time of amniocentesis have been reported but, with continuous ultrasound guidance, are very rare.

Increased risks are present when the patient has experienced bleeding before the procedure. Amniotic fluid is normally similar in color to white wine. If the patient has previously had a history of antepartum bleeding, the amniotic fluid may be brown or dark red due to

blood pigments being absorbed across the chorionic membranes. This type of discolored fluid is associated with an increased risk of pregnancy loss due to the previous bleeding episode (8).

The main advantage of amniocentesis is that accurate analysis of the fetal karyotype or other genetic disease can be obtained from the cultured amniocytes or by measurement of specific substances in the amniotic fluid. Results can be obtained before 20 weeks gestational age.

Since the early 1990s, some research clinics have lowered successively the gestational age limit for routine diagnostic amniocentesis, first to 14 and then to 13 weeks of gestation with no problems encountered (9). Recent clinical trials indicate that early amniocentesis (11–15 weeks) is also feasible (10).

The major disadvantage of amniocentesis is that the results of the prenatal diagnosis are not available until 19 to 20 weeks of gestational age. If genetic abnormalities are identified and the patient requests termination of the pregnancy, the techniques of pregnancy termination carry a greater emotional and physical risk than techniques used for gestational age up to 15 weeks.

Chorionic Villus Sampling

Chorionic villus sampling (CVS) is an ultrasound guided technique that is carried out in the first trimester between 9 and 12 weeks of gestational age. CVS was initially developed as a transcervical technique, but more recently, both transcervical and transabdominal techniques have become available. The upper gestational age of 12 weeks is usually considered for the transcervical technique, but as more experience is gained with the transabdominal technique, gestational age may not be a consideration in that a placental specimen may be obtained at any time during pregnancy.

Chorionic villi can be used for chromosome analysis, metabolic studies, and DNA analysis. CVS should not be used for prenatal diagnosis of congenital malformations including neural tube defects, which have no known metabolic or molecular basis.

When considering the risks of CVS, two large collaborative studies (11,12) have indicated that transcervical CVS, when performed by expert technicians, is a relatively safe procedure and may be considered an acceptable alternative to mid-trimester genetic amniocentesis.

According to the above trial (11), a woman who chooses to have CVS instead of an amniocentesis has a 0.6 per cent higher loss rate. The background rate for spontaneous abortion in the advanced maternal age population is estimated at 4 to 6 percent when the pregnancy is viable by ultrasound at 10 weeks from the last menstrual period (13, 14). Other factors that increase the risk of the procedure are vaginal bleeding before the procedure and an increased number of attempts (greater than one) to obtain the chorionic tissue. Uterine and placental locations may be additional risk factors depending on the CVS technique that is used (12).

The major advantage of CVS is the early gestational age at sampling so that if a chromosomal or DNA abnormality is detected and pregnancy termination is requested, both the physical and emotional aspects of pregnancy are less than terminations after amniocentesis. A second advantage is that a large amount of DNA can be extracted directly from the villi, allowing an early result for molecular analysis of many genetic disorders.

The major disadvantages of CVS involve placental mosaicism and maternal contamination, which may require that two tissue culture procedures be carried out to achieve an acceptable accuracy: a short-term culture (cytotrophoblast cells) and a long-term culture (mesenchymal core of villus). Also, additional screening at a later gestational age is necessary to test for neural tube defects. The latter is usually achieved by a 16- to 20-week detailed ultrasound study and/or maternal serum AFP measurement. Gestational age for ultrasound assessment varies in different centers. Local consultation is recommended.

An increased risk for a facial-limb malformation sequence due to CVS may be present at a gestational age of less than 9 weeks from the last menstrual period (15, 16). The risk of limb malformations for the fetus exposed to CVS sampling after 10 weeks from last menstrual period is not known. The incidence of limb malformations in various CVS populations is 1 per 1,000 to 1,500 with background estimates (non-CVS exposed population) from 1 per 2,000 to 1 per 10,000 (17). Placental trauma in CVS may be the likely cause of hypoperfusion and hypoxia in the embryo (18).

A Workshop on CVS was convened by the National Institute of Child Health and Human Development (NICHD) and the American College of Obstetricians and Gynecologists at the National Institutes of Health in April 1992 to discuss recent reports of an increased occurrence of malformations of the upper and lower limbs and oral structures among CVS-exposed infants (19). The report on the NICHD Workshop summarizes the defects described in CVS-exposed infants. The findings were controversial regarding the conclusions of whether CVS caused limb defects, although all agreed that the frequency of the syndrome of oromandibular-limb hypogenesis was more common among CVS-exposed infants. This appeared to correlate with, but was not necessarily limited to, CVS performed at or earlier than 7 weeks postfertilization.

Whether CVS caused a distinctive type of limb defect could not be determined from the information available, nor could it be determined whether the CVS-exposed infant had an increased frequency of other malformations, including cavernous hemangiomas. The report recommended that the prevalence of all types of limb deficiencies in unexposed and CVS-exposed infants should be evaluated more thoroughly, including determining whether the limb deficiency in CVS-exposed infants is unique or specific in any way.

Nutrition

Maternal nutrition has a profound effect on the developing embryo and fetus, on labor and delivery, and on postpartum recovery (See Chapter 11). Despite an expanding cognizance of nutrition by health practitioners and lay people alike, the question of what the pregnant mother should consume still provokes debate. A basic understanding of human physiology during the gestational period provides a foundation for an adequate nutritional program.

Dynamic changes occur in the maternal body that determine the outcome for a successful pregnancy, delivery, and infant. The three physiological changes of paramount consequence are the development of the placenta, the expansion of

Table 5.2.   **Increase in Maternal Blood Volume**

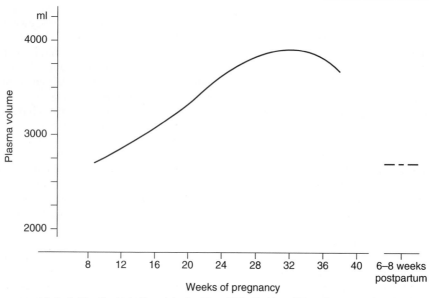

Plasma volume in normal women pregnant for the first time. Reprinted with permission from Hytten F. The Physiology of Human Pregnancy, 2nd ed. Philadelphia: J.B. Lippincott Co., 1971.

the maternal blood volume and the increased demand on maternal liver function. Any pregnancy diet recommendation should regard the significance of these consequent requirements, and a nutritional profile should adjust to circumvent problems for both the mother and the baby.

The placenta is an organ unique to pregnancy. It begins developing early in embryonic life to provide function for the transfer of nutrients, oxygen, and waste products between the mother and baby. The placenta most often implants on the superior posterior wall of the uterus to prevent an obstruction to the emergence of the fetus during labor. As the baby's requirements for nutrients increase, the placenta responds with astronomical growth. By the termination of the full-term pregnancy, a normal placenta is the size and shape of a dinner plate, approximately one inch thick, and weighs between 1 and 3 pounds. It is exclusively a fetal organ, therefore, after delivery of the neonate and its function is fulfilled, the placenta is expelled along with the membranous sac that the baby has been enclosed in during gestation. Expulsion of the placenta is considered to be the third stage of labor.

Placental Function

The placenta facilitates the vascular circulations of the mother and fetus to meet intrinsically, yet never combine. The baby's capillaries are continually bathed in a "lake" of maternal blood. When necessary nutrients are at a more elevated level in the maternal blood than in the baby's, they diffuse through the one-cell thickness of the baby's capillaries, then proceed to the fetal liver to synthesize into proteins and additional building blocks essential to fetal growth. Similarly, when toxic waste products reach a higher level in the fetal circulation, they

diffuse back through the capillary network into the maternal circulation and are eventually eliminated from the vascular system by the maternal liver and excreted by the maternal kidneys.

The process of oxygen and carbon dioxide exchange functions in a similar manner. Keeping placental function healthy throughout pregnancy is one of the most important tasks the maternal physiology must accomplish. If the placenta begins to fail, fewer nutrients are available to the fetus over any given period, subsequently creating a retardation in the growth and development of the fetus.

Maternal Blood Volume

Sustaining the reservoir of blood necessary to service the ever-enlarging placenta requires a dramatic modification in the blood volume in the maternal circulation. At the placental site, it additionally involves a variation in the way the maternal circulation functions. Unlike the closed capillary system of the fetus, the maternal circulation is open. With each maternal heartbeat, jets of blood are pushed from the arteries against the surface of the placenta. Blood drains away from the placenta through the venous system through a process called the arteriovenous (AV) shunt. Because quantities of blood are free at all times in the AV shunt, the maternal blood volume must expand by 40 to 60 percent to provide enough for optimal placental perfusion and to keep all the other maternal organs well supplied.

Fetal size escalates dramatically at the beginning of the fifth gestational month. According to the chart illustrated in Table 5.2, the increase in maternal blood volume also has a sudden upsurge during that same month and continues to increase until just before birth. Any reduction in the amount of blood servicing the placenta impairs its ability to function and, ultimately, imperils the baby.

Nutrition becomes of pre-eminent significance when the problem of maintaining such an expanded blood volume is considered. The maternal physiology requires its salt-retaining mechanisms of reabsorption of sodium by the kidneys and an increased taste for salt through the taste buds, as salt assists in maintaining water in the circulation.

A second factor is an increase in the synthesis of albumin by the liver, which attracts water into the circulation. A maternal blood volume subordinate to the levels necessary to meet the demands of pregnancy is a critical problem, becoming a condition known as hypovolemia. Not only is placental function threatened, but the built-in maternal safeguard against dehydration and shock in the circumstance of excess blood loss during labor and delivery is destroyed. Hypovolemia is exclusively preventable when the maternal diet is adequate for pregnancy, particularly with regard to salt and protein intake.

The liver's contribution toward a viable and healthy pregnancy has an exceptional impact on the well-being of the mother and the baby; notably, the metabolic functions of albumin synthesis, hormone metabolism, and vascular cleansing of the colon.

Albumin synthesis is one of the most complicated of the liver-governed physiological processes, involving the selective combining of specific amino acids into protein molecules that maintain an appropriate amount of fluid in the vascular circulation. Should the liver become damaged, albumin synthesis is one of the initial functions to be affected. If albumin levels in the circulation decrease, water that should be present in the circulation leaks out into the tissues causing pathological edema, and leaving the blood volume contracted below the needs of pregnancy (hypovolemia). If the liver malfunction is severe, and the blood volume continues to be diminished, organs throughout the body are adversely affected by the reduction in blood flow. In the kidneys, a reduced blood volume elevates blood pressure.

Removal from the body of a staggering load of female hormones manufactured continually by the placenta requires that the liver attach fat-soluble hormones to other molecules, thus making them water soluble. The kidneys can then excrete them in the urine. If the liver does not maintain this task of hormone clearance, they can accrue in the vascular circulation and tissues and reach toxic levels.

Accordingly, the liver must additionally cleanse the bloodstream of toxins originating in the colon. As a deceleration in the process of digestion is a well-known phenomenon in pregnancy, these substances have a more favorable environment in which to develop, thus increasing the stress on the liver.

The singular means to confront the stress imposed by this increased metabolic activity is by rigorous attention to nutrition and diet. The stress on the liver increases as pregnancy advances, therefore there is an incremental requirement for protein, calories, vitamins, sodium, and other minerals in the last two trimesters of pregnancy. The liver functions overtime in the second half of pregnancy to meet the physiological demands and adjustments necessary to both the maternal and fetal health.

Inadequate nutrition, primarily lack of high-quality protein, during this critical period can result in severe metabolic derangement and disease. Metabolic toxemia of pregnancy (MTLP) and placenta abruptio are life-threatening complications of pregnancy that result from hypovolemia and liver dysfunction created by malnutrition.

Pregnant and nursing women require a greater amount of every vitamin and mineral than in a pre-pregnant stage. There is an essential need for substantially increased protein during pregnancy — between 75 and 100 grams per day. Protein is the building block of new tissue, vital to both the baby and to prevent MTLP. Brewer's (20) research on toxemia has revealed it as a disease resulting from metabolic disturbance, chiefly in the liver tissue, and that it is primarily caused by malnutrition, principally protein deficiency.

Misunderstanding of the role played by malnutrition in the onset of these and other obstetrical and pediatric problems has blocked efforts to establish standards of nutritional management in pregnancy. Antiquated dietary regimens, usually featuring low-calorie, low-salt diets, and the use of diuretics to combat edema, actually establish the conditions supposedly prevented by inducing malnutrition in pregnant women. In addition to MTLP and placenta abruptio, severe infections, anemia, hemorrhage, and delayed and compromised post-partum healing are common obstetrical problems when mothers are malnourished. Lower birth weight and resulting neurological deficits in children also directly depend on the quality of the maternal diet. Infants who are underweight at birth have a significantly higher incidence of a broad spectrum of developmental problems including mental retardation, epilepsy, cerebral palsy, hyperactivity, and learning disabilities (21). Neonates who die within the first 28 days of life are 30 times more likely to have been underweight at birth (20).

Maintaining a sufficient supply of nutrients available to the growing fetus is critical during the last 8 weeks of pregnancy when the fetal brain is growing at its most rapid rate. Neurological cells are proliferating, and synapses are being created. British reports spanning the last 20 years have illustrated that even mild degrees of maternal undernutrition in the last few weeks of pregnancy can adversely affect this phase of fetal brain and central nervous system development (20). The crucial nutritional elements during pregnancy are described in the following sections.

Iron

Because iron is required for the manufacture of hemoglobin, and blood volume increases by approximately 50% during pregnancy, the need for hemoglobin increases, as well as other important blood constituents. During the last 6 weeks of gestation, the fetus stores enough iron in the liver to supplement its needs for the first 3 to 6 months of postnatal life. Breast milk and formula only partially fulfill an infant's requirements for iron during this period.

The normal pregnancy requirement is 800 mg daily. Of this, 300 mg contributes to the developing fetus, and 500 mg functions to prevent anemia in maternal blood, which increases in volume by at least a quart during pregnancy.

Many mothers experience digestive tract disturbances as a result of iron ingestion. Nausea, heartburn, and diarrhea occur, and iron can cause constipation. These symptoms are related to the amount of elemental iron consumed and individual reactions, as opposed to the type of preparation. These effects can be counteracted by taking supplements with meals. If the body does not absorb iron well, small doses should be taken more frequently. Alternatively, time-released iron may be suggested. Iron absorption can be enhanced by eating vitamin C-rich foods such as citrus fruits or tomatoes, or by calcium-rich nondairy foods, such as broccoli and almonds (21). If this is not successful, simultaneous consumption of 100 mg of vitamin C may facilitate iron absorption.

Iron is most effectively assimilated into the body through consumption of iron-rich foods. Iron is found in liver and other organ meats, red meats, egg yolks, dried fruits, prune and apple juices, almonds, walnuts, oysters, lentils, dried peas and beans, and blackstrap molasses.

It is of extreme importance for the mother to avoid anemia, as an anemic condition can compound post partum hemorrhage, result in fetal distress in labor, and cause maternal weakness after the birth process. The mother should have her blood tested at the initial prenatal visit and again in the seventh or eighth month of pregnancy.

Folic Acid

Folic acid is a water-soluble vitamin in the B complex. This important component is essential for normal growth of all cells and is involved in the crucial synthesis of RNA and DNA. The body requires double its normal amount during pregnancy; therefore, any prenatal vitamins should contain the proper dosage. The National Research Council's Committee on Maternal Nutrition recommends a daily supplement of 400 micrograms during the last half of pregnancy (22). Its deficiency is associated with hemorrhage and placenta abruptio.

Folic acid can be found in liver and organ meats, nuts, nutritional yeast (torula), leafy green vegetables, oysters, salmon, whole grains, and mushrooms.

Vitamin B$_{12}$

Vitamin B$_{12}$ is acquired from cheese, milk, milk products, fish, organ meats, and eggs. This vitamin is integral because its deficiency causes anemia. This may be lacking in a prolonged vegan diet. Vegetarian diets should incorporate yeast which has been specifically prepared to contain B$_{12}$. Alternately, the use of vitamin B$_{12}$ tablets may be suggested. Vitamin B$_{12}$ is also found in a soy product known as tempeh.

Calcium

Calcium cultivates the mineralization of the fetal skeleton and teeth. The fetus requires approximately 66% more calcium than normal during the last trimester of pregnancy, when the teeth are undergoing formation and skeletal growth is the most rapid. Calcium is also stored in the maternal bones to be used as a reserve for lactation.

The requirement for calcium during pregnancy is 1200 mg per day. Calcium must be accompanied by vitamin D to be adequately assimilated into the body. In recommending supplementation, advise a calcium product with half as much magnesium as calcium.

Calcium is naturally occurring in dairy products, almonds, cracked sesame seeds or tahini, canned fish with bones, tofu, soybeans, and garbanzo beans. High caffeine intake can interfere with the assimilation of calcium.

Protein

All fetal cells are constructed from protein. With the rapid growth encountered during pregnancy and the increased blood volume and amniotic fluid, maternal protein requirements increase by approximately 16 grams above the normal requirement.

Protein is primarily concentrated in meats, poultry, fish, whole grains, legumes (peas, beans, lentils, etc.), seeds, nuts, dairy products (milk, yogurt, cheese, cottage cheese), and eggs. Food products or protein supplements are the sole sources of protein; prenatal vitamins and mineral supplements do not supply any. Examples of complementary proteins are outlined in Table 5.3.

Along with careful monitoring of adequate dietary intake, a cognizance of substances to avoid during pregnancy is essential. Among the most crucial are alcohol, medications and other drugs, caffeine, and tobacco.

Alcohol

Alcohol quickly crosses the placenta entering the fetal circulation in the same concentration as in the maternal circulation, and indisputably affects the fetus (23). Although up to two alcoholic drinks per day may not have any lasting effect on either the fetus or the mother, even moderate alcohol consumption can cause the fetus to develop a series of birth defects described as *fetal alcohol syndrome* (FAS) (See also Chapter 17). FAS describes an array of disabilities including mental and physical retardation, tremors, and facial deformations. Birth weight is significantly lower in babies whose mothers have

Table 5.3. **Examples of Complementary Proteins**

Wheat and milk	Soybeans and millet
Rice and milk	Peanuts and sunflower seeds
Rice and legumes	Beans and corn
Wheat and legumes	Beans and milk
Rice and sesame seeds	Peanuts and milk

consumed alcohol than in those born to nondrinking mothers. It is best to recommend complete abstinence during the full gestational period.

Drugs

No drug has been demonstrated to be safe for all fetuses under all circumstances. All drugs cross the placental "barrier." Antibiotics cross it rapidly. Some sulfa drugs can disturb fetal liver function. Tetracycline may cause discoloration of the permanent teeth and may affect fetal bone growth and development. Aspirin taken daily results in a higher rate of complications during pregnancy, labor and delivery, most notably increasing the risk for hemorrhage, infection, and anemia (24).

Some medications cause birth defects, and some are the antecedent for slow growth, developmental or mental retardation, or aberration of visceral development (25). The effects on the fetus are similar to and potentially greater than their effect on the mother due to the small size of the fetus and its rapid development and growth.

All medications should be under a physician's strict and conscientious supervision. The optimal course to pursue when considering the benefit of a drug is to weigh the possible and known risks against the necessity.

The services of an herbalist, a naturopathic, or a homeopathic practitioner may offer a customarily safer alternative to many prescription medications.

Tobacco

The existing evidence strongly suggests elimination or reduction of tobacco. Nicotine is not the only perpetrator — cigarette smoke contains tars, carbon monoxide, lead, and other dangerous elements. Pregnant women who smoke give birth to infants of smaller average size and have an increased propensity for premature rupture of the membranes, premature birth, perinatal death, placental abnormalities, and gestational hemorrhage (26). These conditions are directly proportional to the amount of smoking during the course of pregnancy. The more inhaled smoke, the greater the chance of the fetus encountering these complications. Passive smoking is also under close scrutiny and is currently suggested to be harmful to the fetus.

Caffeine

Caffeine causes birth defects when animals are exposed to moderately high levels (27), levels similar to which some women in pregnancy may expose themselves. Caffeine has been implicated in miscarriages occurring in the last, first, and second trimesters (28) and with low birth weight in term infants (29).

According to the National Academy of Sciences, pregnant women consume an average of 200 milligrams of caffeine per day, the equivalent of one and a half to three cups of coffee or two to four cups of tea. Physiologically, caffeine increases urinary excretion of calcium and decreases the available circulating amount. The elimination of caffeine from the maternal system in pregnancy is reduced from non-pregnant values. Therefore the fetal and maternal effects exist longer. Caffeine also causes an increased production of epinephrine and norepinephrine, which constrict peripheral vessels, including those in the uterus and create a temporary decrease in the amount of oxygen and other nutrients available to the fetus. If caffeine is present in the fetal circulation, it takes much longer to be eliminated than in the adult (30).

Caffeine is present in coffee, black and green teas, colas and other soft drinks, chocolate, and some over-the-counter medications.

Additional research is necessary on the possible role of caffeine in human birth defects, miscarriages, and infertility. It should be recommended that the mother limit caffeine intake.

Other Chemicals

Foods containing artificial colors, flavors, additives, preservatives or artificial sweeteners, particularly aspartame should be strictly avoided. Aspartame is a combination of two amino acids, phenylalanine and aspartic acid, both of which are toxic at high levels. The FDA has not yet addressed the issue of safe levels of aspartame for pregnant women and the embryo/fetus. Nitrates and nitrites present in hot dogs, luncheon meats, and bologna have also displayed deleterious effects on the developing fetal unit.

Foods high in calories and low in nutritional value should be replaced with foods containing potent nutritional value and nutrients essential to optimal fetal development and growth.

Spontaneous Abortion

A miscarriage, or spontaneous abortion is defined as the loss of the products of conception from the uterus before the fetus is viable. It is experienced as an unanticipated and involuntary expulsion of the embryo or fetus before the twentieth week of pregnancy. Another parameter of measurement of spontaneous abortion is when the fetus-neonate is delivered weighing less than 500 grams. Although the etiology is most often idiopathic, some genetic aberrations can interfere with embryological development. Infrequently the etiology of miscarriage can be of severe physical shock, uterine abnormalities, or acute infectious process endocrine abnormalities, including diabetes mellitus. Smoking of tobacco has been associated with an increased risk of abortion of chromosomally normal abortuses, as well as moderate alcohol consumption (23). Coffee consumption greater than four cups daily appears to elevate the risk of spontaneous abortion (28). The risk increases with escalating amounts.

Radiation is clinically acknowledged to be an abortifacient. It is therefore incumbent upon the chiropractor who performs diagnostic radiography to adhere to the absolute 10-day rule used in the x-ray examination of all females of childbearing years. This describes the administration of a radiographic examination only in the first 10 days after the onset of menstrual flow. Despite the use of birth control methods, a woman may be in the early stages of pregnancy without her knowledge. The responsibility for competent care in all radiography remains solely with the practitioner.

The clinical signs of a threatened or potential abortion are vaginal bleeding and possible intermittent abdominal or pelvic pain. When pain is present, it is characteristically experienced as mild cramping discomfort resembling that encountered with a menstrual period or as diffuse, low back pain. Commonly, bleeding appears initially, followed by cramping abdominal pain a few hours or days later. One of every four or five pregnant women exhibits signs of vaginal spotting or heavier bleeding throughout the first trimester. Of the women who bleed spontaneously in early gestation, approximately half will abort. Despite conjecture otherwise, it is not apparent that the risk of abortion of a malformed embryo or fetus is increased.

If a spontaneous abortion is suspected, immediate referral should be made to the physician or obstetrican for evaluation. The prognosis for pregnancy continuation in the presence of bleeding and pain is poor, although some women displaying these symptoms successfully carry a baby to term.

Second Trimester

Fetal Development

The resemblance to the adult human form is obvious at the end of 12 weeks gestation. By the end of 12 weeks, and sometimes earlier, the sexual differences in genitalia between male and female are recognized in abortuses. The fetal structures and organs, which have undergone extraordinary evolution in the first trimester, now enlarge and mature. The first appearance of lanugo (fine, downy hair) develops on the arms, legs, and back of the fetus. Head hair, eyelashes and eyebrows also appear. The cardiovascular system is functioning, and the fetal heartbeat is easily auscultated by the seventeenth or eighteenth week. At the conclusion of the twenty-fourth week, the fetus measures approximately 12 inches in length and 1.5 pounds in weight. The skin is wrinkled and sheathed with the vernix caseosa, a creamy, protective coating to protect the integument as it undergoes refinement.

The fifteenth to twenty-seventh gestational weeks mark the second trimester of pregnancy. The most profound development during this period is the growth at the latter part of the second trimester, as fetal growth is greatest during the sixth and seventh months of intrauterine life.

Quickening (the perception by the pregnant woman of fetal movements in utero) occurs between the sixteenth and twentieth weeks of pregnancy. The time of quickening is too variable to be of value in determining the expected date of confinement or when term has been reached. Active intestinal peristalsis is the most common phenomenon mistaken for quickening.

Maternal Development

The second trimester is experienced by the mother as a period of well-being. The nausea and fatigue indigenous to the first trimester usually disappears or at the very least declines. The uterus expands into the abdominal cavity in response to the enlarging fetus, placenta, and increased amniotic fluid. By the conclusion of the fifth gestational month, the uterine fundus reaches the level of the umbilicus, and fundal height measurement is routinely evaluated by the physician to ensure adequate fetal growth and confirm the length of the pregnancy. The gestational length can be approximated by measuring the interval in centimeters between the pubic symphysis and the uterine fundus.

Some subjective complaints of diaphragmatic compromise and abdominal crowding may arise in this trimester, particularly in women of shorter status.

Colostrum, the yellowish precursor to breastmilk, is found in the mammary glands by mid pregnancy. Stimulated by massive hormonal changes, the nipples and areola take on a darker pigment, as do other areas of integument. Some women exhibit the linea nigra, a dark vertical line between the pubic symphysis and the umbilicus. Chloasma, the so-called mask of pregnancy, often surfaces as patchy, darkening of the skin surrounding the nose and eye.

Third Trimester

Maternal Development

During the third trimester, the uterine fundus expands to a level immediately below the xiphoid process of the sternum. Uterine crowding coupled with high levels of circulating progesterone often incite maternal indigestion and heartburn. Furthermore, with uterine compression of the diaphragm and ribs, the mother may endure dyspnea, or thorax and rib discomfort. Varicose veins in the legs, hemorrhoids, and edematous ankles often appear due to increased abdominal pressure, decreased venous return from the lower extremities, and the relaxing effect of progesterone on the circulatory vessel walls.

Maternal weight gain is also most significant during this gestational period. This contributes largely to the profound biomechanical compromise of the lumbosacral spine. With a drastic shift in the gravitational weight bearing of the mother, pelvic musculoskeletal function, principally of the sacroiliac and hip joints, is imperiled. This leads to often significant soft tissue structure changes such as hypertonicities or ligament laxity, which in turn creates biomechanical instability. Not just the lumbosacral spine, but compensatorily, the thoracic and even cervical spine acquire a diversity of combinations of aberrant segmental and global motion. The unfortunate typical short radius sacral curve of later pregnancy provides the foundational imbalance for thoracic hyperkyphosis and cervical kypholordosis (Fig. 5.9). Cellular edema and inflammation, along with anatomical yielding of the intervertebral foraminae, generate neuropathophysiology of the important spinal nerve tissues with resultant cellular and aggregate tissue malfunction. Summarily, the potential for extensive vertebral subluxation complex in the maternity patient is physiologically inherent for the last 3 gestational months.

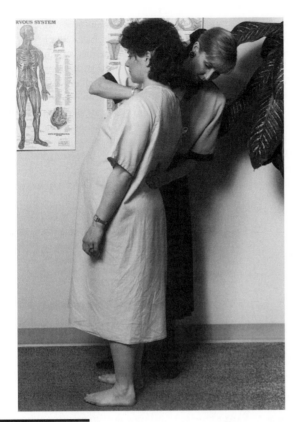

Figure 5.9.   Standing evaluation of the third trimester patient. Notice the short radius sacral curve with the compensatory thoracic hyperkyphosis and cervical kypholordosis.

The prevalence of low back pain during pregnancy can be as low as 42.5% (31) and as high as 90% (32). The most common cause of low back pain in pregnancy is sacroiliitis (32). The chief mechanism of etiology for sacroiliitis encountered in pregnancy is the circulation of relaxin and its consequent effect on the pelvic articulations (33,34).

Mantero and Crispini (35) found from their radiographic and radiopelvimetry studies of 20 expectant women that the constitutional alterations of the lumbosacral region observed at gestational term were consistent for pelvic inclination alteration, sacrofemoral measurement alterations, sacral inclination alteration, lumbar hyperlordosis and retrolisthesis of L5 on the sacrum. They concluded that a preventive and therapeutic regimen for correction of the described alterations was necessary for symptomatic resolution. Their consequent treatment objectives were to restore the abdominal musculature tone, to improve the tone of the pelvic floor to prevent such disturbances as uterine prolapse and urinary incontinence at a distance, to avoid lower extremity venous circulation alterations, and to correct altered posture. They cited the main concern of their investigation as being the mechanical postural aspect of a bone structure, which undergoes altered stresses of gravitational origin. They further stated that the mechanical alterations caused by altered postures can produce functional alterations of the articular motion, and that if the alterations of the normal

physiological articular motion are not corrected, that they are one of the major causes of the onset of painful symptomatologies, local or reflexed, on the vertebral areas of the nerves involved, and in time they can determine arthrosic alterations. After scrutiny of the chiropractic treatment of these pregnancy-induced conditions, they concluded that chiropractic is "by far the most indicated treatment for painful spinal symptomatologies caused by mechanical alterations due to pregnancy" (35).

Some of the variables established as contributory to low back pain in pregnancy are maternal weight gain, fetal weight, the number of previous pregnancies, and the number of prior children (35).

Fetal Development

At the advent of the third trimester of gestation, the fetus is undergoing its most rapid growth. The fetal head continues to be notably large in proportion to the body, the hair on the head grows, and the eyebrows and eyelashes are now discernible. A refinement of the fetal features occurs during these last 3 months of pregnancy: the fat is deposited under the skin and the skin takes on a distinctive wrinkled appearance, the permanent teeth buds are laid down behind the milk teeth buds, the pupillary membrane disappears from the eyes, the fingernails reach the fingertips, and the lanugo (the fine, downy hair covering the body of the fetus) begins to disappear.

The fetus now experiences periods of wakefulness and sleep and responds to bright light. Loud noises may elicit a reaction in utero. The baby's hearing becomes more acute, and it displays familiarity to the maternal voice, exhibiting definite preference to the mother's over a stranger's voice immediately after birth. The fetus repeatedly displays, on ultrasonic examination, the ability to suck the thumb, practicing the activity that will ensure its survival postnatally. A series of rhythmic jolts experienced subjectively by the mother indicates fetal hiccups. The fetal limbs move energetically, although as fetal growth and weight gain continues, activity diminishes as there is less room for it to move. The fetus gains approximately three and a half pounds and grows about five and a half inches during this later third of gestation.

Babies born during this trimester have a high chance of survival, although their chances for both survival and an easier transition to independent life are enhanced as they approach the full term due date. Late in pregnancy, antibodies transfuse through the placenta to the fetus, contributing short-term resistance to the disease processes to which the mother maintains immunity. The premature infant having received less of this protection is increasingly predisposed to contagious illness.

At some interval during the early part of the last trimester, the fetus assumes a favorite in-utero position, usually head down, known as vertex. In the third trimester, the most important obstetrical component of the fetus is the head. Optimally, the vertex is the presenting part of the baby and is the largest and least compressible structure. This presentation occurs in 96% of deliveries (37). After delivery of the head in a vertex birth, there is little delay or difficulty in the delivery of the balance of the baby.

The Fetal Skull

The cranial vault of the skull is comprised of several bones. Obstetrically, there are seven bones of significance, namely the frontal bones, the parietal bones, the temporal bones, and the occipital bone. These are united by sutures that are membranous between the bones (Figs. 5.10, 5.11). The sutures allow for cranial molding during the descent of the fetus through the birth canal and are integral structures to assist in the identification of the fetal head upon vaginal examination. At the time of birth, the cranial bones are poorly ossified, thin and easily compressible to facilitate passage of the fetal head. The overlapping of these bones during the descent of the baby through the birth canal is permitted by the looseness of union of the skull bones. Subsequently the fetal head adapts its shape to fit the maternal pelvis. This is designated as cranial molding.

The sutures are labeled as the sagittal suture between the parietal bones, the lambdoidal sutures sequestering the occipital bone from the parietal bones, the coronal sutures between the frontal and parietal bones, and the frontal suture between the frontal bones (Fig. 5.10). The frontal suture is a continuation of the sagittal suture.

The fontanelles are the membranous intersections of the cranial sutures. The anterior fontanelle, also called the bregma, is located at the intersection of the frontal, coronal, and sagittal

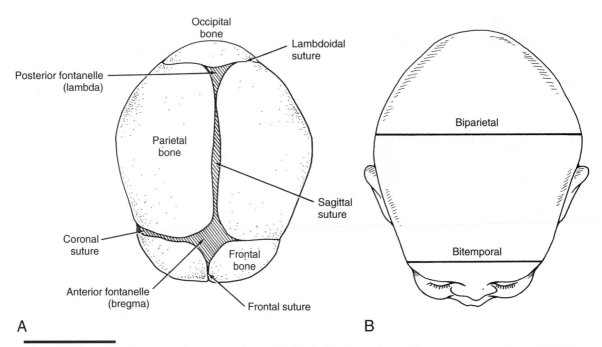

Figure 5.10.   Cranial bones and sutures of the fetal skull. Modified from Oxom H. Human labor and birth, 1980:39.

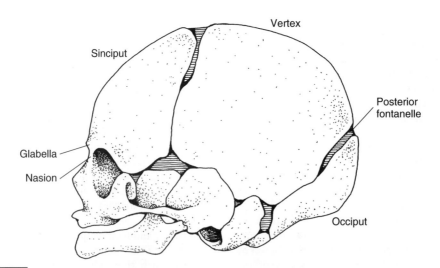

Figure 5.11.   Cranial bones and fontanelles of the fetal skull. Modified from Oxom H. Human labor and birth, 1980:43.

Table 5.4.   Fetopelvic Relationships According to Fetal Position

Presentation	Attitude	Presenting Part	Denominator
Longitudinal lie (99.5%)			
Cephalic (96 to 97%)	Flexion	Vertex (posterior part)	Occiput (O)
	Military	Vertex (median part)	Occiput (O)
	Partial extension	Brow	Forehead (frontum) (Fr)
	Complete extension	Face	Chin (mentum) (M)
Breech (3 to 4%)			
Complete	Flexed hips, knees	Buttocks	Sacrum (S)
Frank	Flexed hips, extended knees	Buttocks	Sacrum (S)
Footling: single, double	Extended hips; flexed knees	Knees	Sacrum (S)
Kneeling: single, double	Extended hips	Knees	Sacrum (S)
Transverse or oblique lie (0.5%)			
Shoulder	Variable	Shoulder, arm, trunk	Scapula (Sc)

sutures. It measures approximately 2 x 3 cm and is most often described as diamond-shaped. This fontanelle undergoes full ossification by 18 months post-natally. An important function of this fontanelle is to facilitate cranial molding during delivery, and its responsibility after birth is to accommodate the rapid growth of the brain.

The posterior fontanelle, also called the lambda, is situated at the intersection of the lambdoidal and sagittal sutures. It is considerably smaller than the anterior fontanelle and forms a "Y" configuration with the sagittal suture as the base and the lambdoidal sutures as the arms. This fontanelle undergoes its final ossification by 8 weeks of age.

The bones that comprise the base of the skull are not easily compressible as they protect the integral centers in the brain stem.

Fetopelvic Relationships

The descriptive terms of the fetopelvic relationships referred to during pregnancy and labor are of crucial significance to the chiropractor in acknowledging and understanding the potential for both in-utero constraint and birth trauma. They are characterized as follows and presented in Table 5.4.

The fetal lie is depicted as the relationship of the long axis of the fetus to the long axis of the mother, assuming the mother to be in the standing position. There are two succinct obstetrical lies. The first is designated as the longitudinal lie where the long axes of the mother and the fetus are parallel. The second is classified as the transverse or oblique lie which is perceived when the long axis of the fetus is either perpendicular or oblique to the long axis of the mother. An oblique lie is perennially unstable because of the 45 degree angle of the fetal and maternal axes. Due to its instability, the oblique lie always becomes longitudinal or transverse during the labor process. Longitudinal lies are observed in approximately 99.5% of pregnancies at term.

A longitudinal lie is further categorized as either a cephalic presentation, where the head is presenting at the cervical os, found in 96–97% of longitudinal lies; or as a breech presentation, where any combination of the lower limbs or the buttocks present at the cervix, occurring as 3–4% of longitudinal lies. Therefore, the fetal presentation describes the part of the fetus that lies most proximate to the pelvic inlet. A shoulder presentation would describe a transverse lie where the shoulder is the presenting part.

The presenting part is the part of the fetal anatomy that is in closest approximation to the birth canal. This describes the structure that is first perceived by the examining finger upon vaginal or rectal examination.

Fetal attitude pertains to the relationship of the fetal parts to each other. The primary attitudes are flexion and extension. The fetal head is in flexion when the chin approximates the chest and in extension when the occiput approaches the back. The primary fetal attitude is in flexion, with the head flexed forward in front of the chest and the arms and legs gathered in front of the body (Fig. 5.12A). The spine will be curved in slight forward flexion, rendering the spine convex. A neutral position of the fetal head being in neither flexion or extension is termed a military attitude (Fig. 5.12B). This attitude is not considered to be optimal and can delay and complicate the birth process. If the fetal head becomes increasingly extended backward upon the neck, a brow or facial presentation becomes apparent, depending on the degree of extension (Fig. 5.12 C, D). The progressive change in fetal attitude as a result of a facial presentation results in a concave profile of the fetal spinal column.

The denominator specifies an arbitrarily chosen landmark on the presenting fetal part. The denominator aids in describing fetal position. Every presentation has a unique denominator.

Position refers to the relationship of the denominator to the right or left sides of the maternal birth canal. Hence, there may be either a right or left described position with each fetal presentation.

Examination of the Third Trimester Patient

ABDOMINAL INSPECTION AND PALPATION

The chiropractor should be thoroughly familiar with abdominal inspection and palpation to assist in determining in-utero constraint. Because of the extraordinarily skilled palpation that most doctors of chiropractic have practiced and perfected, this is a relatively uncomplicated skill to acquire.

The position of the baby in-utero is determined by inspecting and palpating the mother's abdomen, with some salient questions to be methodically answered for the fetal position to be accurately assessed.

Primarily the lie, whether longitudinal, transverse or oblique is determined. Consequent to this discernment, the fetal part that is presenting at or in the pelvic inlet is assessed. The fetal spine and the small parts belonging to the extremities can then be evaluated. Once the presenting part has been ascertained, the structure occupying the uterine fundus can also be palpated and labelled. Concomitant with this step, the fundal height can be estimated. At this point, the side that the cephalic prominence is on can be discovered.

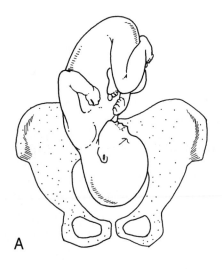

A

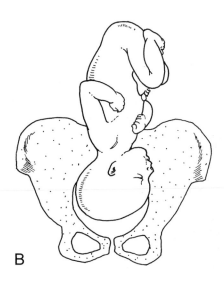

B

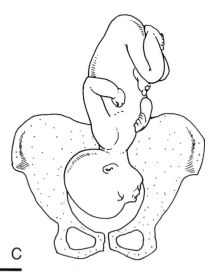

C

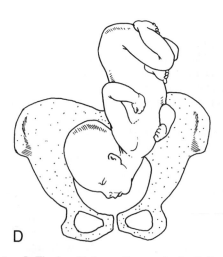

D

Figure 5.12. Fetal attitude. Modified from Cunningham FG, MacDonald PC, Gant NF, Leveno KJ, Gilstrap LC. Williams' Obstetrics, 19th ed. 1993:274. A, The head is in an attitude of flexion. B, The head is in a military attitude. C, Partial extension of the head in a brow presentation. D, Full extension of the head in a facial presentation.

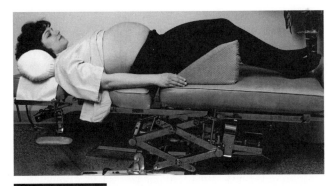

Figure 5.13.   Patient position for examination of fetal lie, presentation, attitude, and position. The shoulders should be slightly raised and the knees supported up to assist the abdominal muscles in relaxing.

The first maneuver is designed to determine the presenting fetal part (Fig. 5.14). The practitioner should stand at the patient's side and gently, but firmly grasp the lower uterine segment between the thumb and fingers of the inferior hand to palpate the presenting part (Fig. 5.15). The superior hand should then be placed on the fundus to steady the uterus and apply slight counterpressure (Fig. 5.16). This maneuver is best performed initially, as the head is the part of the fetus that can be identified with the most certainty. The head is palpated as hard, round and regular-shaped, and is easily ballottable when it is located in the uterine fundus. It is occasionally possible to palpate the neck as a furrowed structure, however, the depth at which the baby is positioned may make it more difficult to ascertain. It is usually a simple procedure to align the glabella under one of the examining fingers and the external occipital protuberance under the other; this facilitates the examiner in moving the fetal head. The fetal head can also be pushed posteriorly in the pelvic cavity, where the amniotic fluid buoys

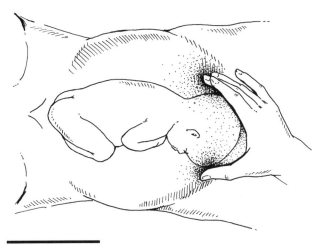

Figure 5.14.   External fetal examination: first maneuver. Modified from Cunningham FG, MacDonald PC, Gant NF, Leveno KJ, Gilstrap LC. Williams' Obstetrics, 19th ed. 1993:279.

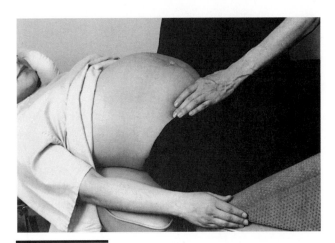

Figure 5.15.   First maneuver: locating the fetal part at the lower uterine segment.

Additionally, it is of value to evaluate whether engagement has taken place and perhaps to estimate the size of the baby. To examine the third trimester patient, she should be instructed to lie on her back with the abdomen exposed (Fig. 5.13). To facilitate relaxation of the abdominal wall muscles, the shoulders should be raised slightly, and the knees are flexed up, comfortably supported. If the patient is in labor, the examination can be performed between contractions.

Obstetrically, there is a menu of methods used to diagnose fetal presentation and position. These comprise any combination of the following: vaginal examination, auscultation, and location of fetal heart, ultrasonography or radiography, and abdominal palpation. It is unusual for an obstetrician to rely solely on abdominal palpation to confirm fetal presentation and position. Abdominal palpation easily reveals to the experienced chiropractor the nature of the fetal situation. There are a series of maneuvers used in abdominal examination of the fetus.

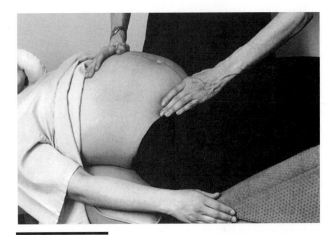

Figure 5.16.   First maneuver: slight counterpressure at the uterine fundus.

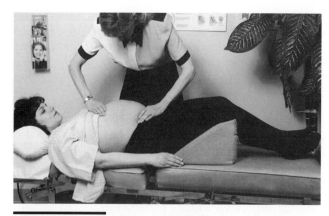

Figure 5.17. First maneuver: ballotment of the fetal head at the lower uterine segment.

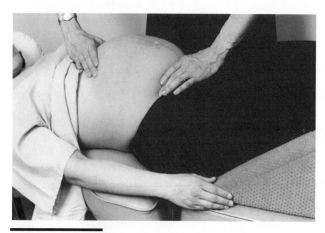

Figure 5.18. External fetal examination: second maneuver. Locating the fetal part at the uterine fundus.

the head. When this type of pressure on the fetal head is released, the head rises back and abuts against the examiner's hand or fingers (Fig. 5.17).

Because the fetal head is at or in the pelvis in more than 90% of pregnancies, the rational thing to do first is to look for the head in its most frequent location. When it has been confirmed that the fetal head is at the inlet, two important facts are discovered. Chiefly, that the lie is longitudinal, and that the presentation is cephalic.

An attempt should be made to gently maneuver the head from side to side to see whether it is still outside the pelvis and floating or in the pelvis and fixed or engaged.

In administration of the second maneuver, the inferior examining hand is applied to the presenting part, while the superior examining hand palpates the uterine fundus (Fig. 5.18). The breech is most often located here and feels softer, more irregular, less globular and less like a defined structure than the head. The breech is not as easily movable as the head and is continuous with the spinal column. When it is attempted to ballot the breech, the body moves laterally with it. A description by the mother of fetal movement such as kicking

and pummeling assists in diagnostic confirmation. Moreover, palpation of mobile, small parts in the proximity of the breech aids in detection.

This step is sequentially significant because a comparison can be made between the fetal structures perceived in a longitudinal lie by the simultaneous palpation of the two examining hands. Both hands may palpate a suspected structure at either the fundus or the pelvic inlet in the course of evaluation. This process assists in positive confirmation of the presenting part.

The third maneuver to be performed is to confirm the location of the fetal spinal column. This is best accomplished by placing the hands on either side of the abdomen (Figs. 5.19, 5.20). It is best if one hand feels the fetus while the other secures the uterus (Figs. 5.21, 5.22).

The fetal spine is perceived as firmer, smoother, and somewhat ridged. It should form a gradual convex arch, and as pressure is applied toward the maternal umbilicus, there is uniform resistance to the palpating fingers.

On the contralateral side, there is uneven resistance to examining pressure, with the fingers burrowing more deeply in some areas than in others. Any palpation of moving appendages facilitates diagnosis.

The fourth maneuver concludes the abdominal examination by locating the cephalic prominence. The cephalic prominence can be palpated through the abdomen by placing both hands on the side of the lower part of the uterus with the fingers aligned inferiorly, and moving them gently toward the pubis (Fig. 5.22 A, B). When there is a cephalic prominence, the examining fingers abut against it on that side, and on the contralateral side, meet with little or no resistance. The location of the cephalic prominence aids in diagnosing attitude.

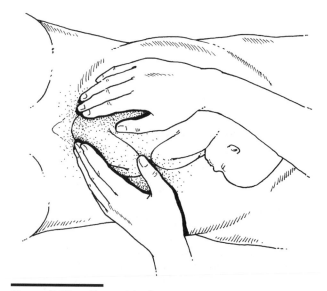

Figure 5.19. External fetal examination: third maneuver. Location of the fetal spine and the fetal extremities. Palpation can start at the uterine fundus. Modified from Cunningham FG, MacDonald PC, Gant NF, Leveno KJ, Gilstrap LC. Williams' Obstetrics, 19th ed. 1993:279.

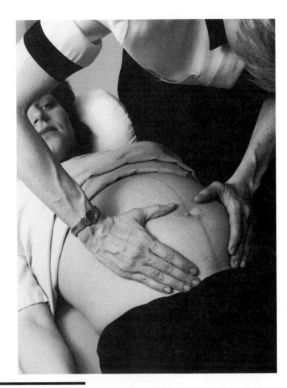

Figure 5.20. External fetal examination: third maneuver. Palpation has moved down the lateral walls of the uterus to the cervical area.

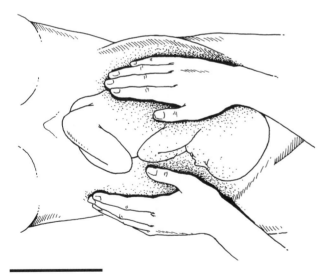

Figure 5.21. Third maneuver: examiner's hand palpates the fetus while the other hand secures the lateral wall of the uterus. Modified from Cunningham FG, MacDonald PC, Gant NF, Leveno KJ, Gilstrap LC. Williams' Obstetrics, 19th ed., 1993:279.

The cephalic prominence is produced by flexion or extension of the fetal head on the neck. When the head is well flexed, the occiput is lower than the sinciput and the forehead is the cephalic prominence (Fig. 5.24 A, B). When there is

extension, the occiput is higher than the sinciput and the occiput or back of the head is the cephalic prominence (Fig. 5.25 C, D). When the cephalic prominence and the back are on opposite sides, the attitude is termed as flexion. When the cephalic prominence and the back are on the same side, the attitude is that of extension. When no cephalic prominence is palpable, there is neither flexion nor extension and the head is in a neutral position described as the military attitude.

Fetal presentation may be confirmed by fetal heart auscultation, which is best performed with the use of an obstetrical fetoscope (Fig. 5.25 A, B).

In-utero Constraint and Biomechanical/Subluxation Premises

In-utero constraint provides the premise for pre-natal chiropractic care as it relates to biomechanical stress of the fetus conceivably leading to the vertebral subluxation complex (See Chapter 12). This axiom is derived from an acknowledgment of the perinatal concerns in a diversity of fetal malpresentations encountered during the last trimester of pregnancy, and supported by considerable evidence represented in the scientific literature.

It is normal up to the seventh month of gestation to be in a breech or any other intrauterine position. After the seventh month, throughout the third trimester, any position other than vertex in an attitude of flexion is considered to create constraint of the fetus to one degree or another.

Any existing abnormal biomechanical stresses to the fetal vertebrae may cause abnormal developmental effects of the hypertrophied cartilage and early articular structures, and therefore be the precursor of spinal asymmetry and the vertebral subluxation complex with resultant long-standing consequences.

The more apparent etiologic factors of in-utero constraint may be classified into maternal and fetal determinants. From a maternal perspective, the most important factor is of the

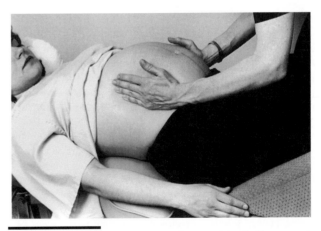

Figure 5.22. Third maneuver: palpation of the fetal spine and extremities located on the opposite side.

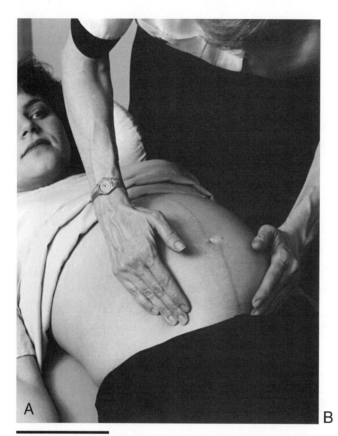

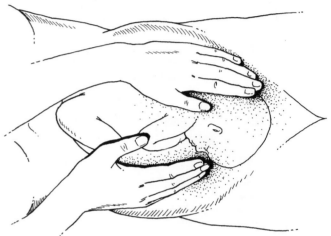

Figure 5.23. A, External fetal examination: fourth maneuver. Location of the cephalic prominence. B, Fourth maneuver: moving the fingers down to locate the cephalic prominence.

Modified from Cunningham FG, MacDonald PC, Gant NF, Leveno KJ, Gilstrap LC. Williams' Obstetrics, 19th ed., 1993:279.

existence of a contracted pelvis. This may be anatomically demonstrated at the pelvic inlet, the midpelvis or the pelvic outlet. Any of these areas may present with difficulty when there is a reduction in the normal measurements of the pelvic diameters or pelvic planes as discussed at the beginning of this chapter. There are a number of pre-existing elements of etiology with a contracted pelvis, among them rickets, poor osseous and articular development of the maternal pelvis, a rigid perineum encountered at the level of the pelvic outlet, and most pivotal to the chiropractor, any degree of pelvic compromise, either structural or functional. From this awareness, the onus is on the chiropractor to maintain an optimal degree of biomechanical spinal and pelvic function in the maternity patient from the onset of pregnancy. The ultimate goal would be to have a biomechanically stable maternal pelvis and spine long before the advent of conception and pregnancy.

Additional components of maternal conditions influencing in-utero constraint are uterine abnormalities, particularly in a bicornuate uterus where the nonpregnant horn may prejudice fetal position. This is a common catalyst in breech positions. Abnormalities of placental location or size may contribute to unfavorable fetal positions; placenta previa is often an implicating factor. When a pendulous maternal abdomen is observed, there is an increased propensity of the uterus and fetus to fall forward, creating a positional shift.

Fetal determinants consist of excessive fetal size, inborn errors in fetal polarity as evidenced in breech presentation and transverse lie, abnormal internal occipital rotation, fetal attitude where there is extension instead of normal flexion, multiple pregnancy, polyhydramnios where an excessive amount of amniotic fluid permits fetal freedom of activity, and fetal anomalies such as hydrocephaly and anencephaly.

In-utero constraint may be caused in some cases by sacral subluxation (positional dyskinesia). The sacral subluxation may have several etiologies: pre-existing maternal sacral subluxation before conception, micro or macro trauma inducing subluxation during pregnancy, or pelvic malformation disorders. Specifically, sacral rotation causes an anterior torquing mechanism on the uterine ligaments and musculature, decreasing space and altering the environment for the fetus. Therefore, at the third trimester when the fetus is expected to position itself into the vertex position, it is unable to due to in-utero constraint caused by the adverse sacral rotation. When correction of the sacral subluxation occurs, the structure and therefore the function of the uterine structures are improved allowing the fetus to position itself properly. The same would be true for the base posterior sacrum seen in the breech presentation. The angulation of the sacrum causes a vertically imposed stress on the uterus creating this constraint position. The chiropractic adjustment, specifically the posterior to

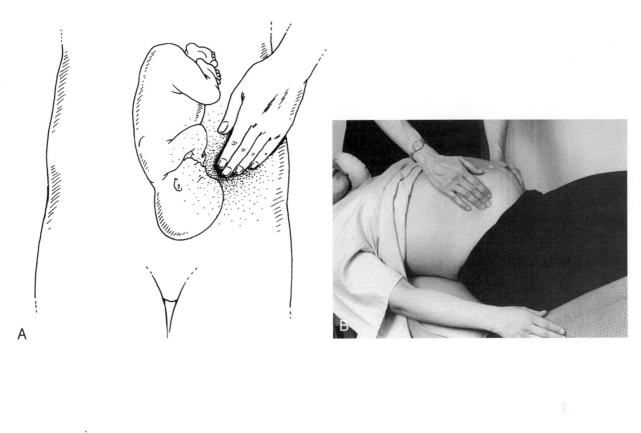

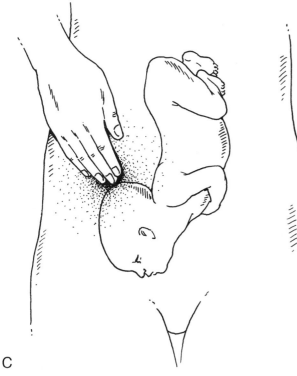

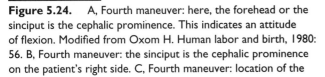

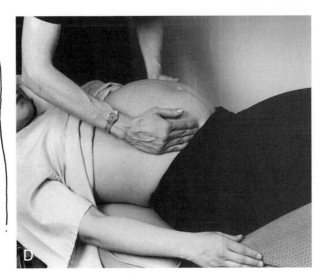

Figure 5.24. A, Fourth maneuver: here, the forehead or the sinciput is the cephalic prominence. This indicates an attitude of flexion. Modified from Oxom H. Human labor and birth, 1980: 56. B, Fourth maneuver: the sinciput is the cephalic prominence on the patient's right side. C, Fourth maneuver: location of the occiput as the cephalic prominence indicating fetal head extension. Modified from Oxom H. Human labor and birth, 1980:56. D, Fourth maneuver: the occiput is the cephalic prominence on the patient's right side.

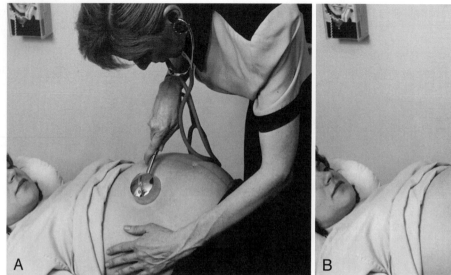

Figure 5.25.   A, Auscultation of the fetal heart in the upper fundal segment of the uterus. This may indicate a breech presen-   tation. B, Auscultation of the fetal heart in the lower cervical segment of the uterus. This may indicate a vertex presentation.

anterior and superior to inferior arc corrects the positional and dyskinetic stress placed on the uterus and fetus.

The critical effects of in-utero constraint involve the biomechanical considerations on fetal development, the potential for a reduced efficiency in labor resulting in a longer, harder labor process with an increased incidence of anoxia, brain damage, asphyxia, prolapse of the umbilical cord and intrauterine death and a greatly elevated propensity toward operative delivery which exacerbates the danger of trauma to the neonate. Excessive cranial molding is also of concern.

Breech Presentations

The optimal in-utero fetal position is described as a longitudinal lie, cephalic presentation with the vertex as the presenting part in an attitude of flexion. Any position other than this can manifest with in-utero constraint. The breech or pelvic presentation, while still in a longitudinal lie, is classified according to the attitudes presenting at the hips and knees. There are four classifications of breech presentations described obstetrically. They are the complete breech (Fig. 5.26A), in which both the thighs and knees of the fetus are maintained in flexion; the frank breech (Fig. 5.26B), which illustrates flexion at the thighs and extension at the knees. This is the most customary type of breech position, comprising approximately two-thirds of breech presentations. The third breech presentation is a footling, either single (Fig. 5.26C) or double with the foot as the presenting part. Here, there is extension at the thighs and the knees. Last, and least encountered, is the kneeling breech (Fig. 5.26D), either single or double with extension at the thighs and flexion at the knees. Here, the knee is the presenting part.

A routine fetal attitude in breech presentation is of head hyperflexion. If this breech position is maintained in-utero for even a brief period, there is an increased predilection for a fetal

attitude of head rotation through one right angle with the face looking to one side and inclined so that the ear approximates to the chest wall. This attitude has been described by Trillat (38) and observed by Gibberd (39) on pre-natal radiography. They suggest that because this attitude (Trillat's attitude) is observed only in cases of breech presentation, it is the result of constraint due to the fetal head experiencing difficulty accommodating itself in a symmetrical position where it is tightly tucked under the maternal costal margin. Gibberd extrapolates that "if it were the result of forces arising in the fetus itself (*viz.* inequality of muscular action on the two sides of the neck) one would not expect to find it confined to breech presentations (39)."

Fetal skull hyperextension in the breech presentation is reported extensively in the literature as severely compromising to the upper cervical spinal cord and brain stem structures. Unique descriptions of in-utero breech presentations with hyperextension of the neck and concomitant intrauterine dislocation of cervical vertebrae are recounted (40).

Often, the etiology of the fetal breech presentation is idiopathic. Acknowledged factors include prematurity, polyhydramnios, multiple pregnancy, placenta previa, contracted pelvis, hydrocephalus, macrosomia and fibromyomas. A habitual breech is also described. In this definition, some women deliver all their children in the breech position, which implies that the pelvic anatomy facilitates the breech rather than the vertex.

In a breech presentation, the patient seldom experiences the lightening sensation, and it is unusual for the fetus to engage before labor. The patient is likely to experience fetal movements of the small parts in the lower abdominal quadrants and may complain of painful kicking against the rectum or bladder.

Breech presentations account for 3-4% of all term deliveries and are affiliated with higher perinatal morbidity and mortality than term cephalic presentations.

The incidence is decreased as term is achieved, and increased in patients who enter into labor before full term. Approximately 15% of neonates in breech presentations are preterm.

A further prenatal deformation as a result of in-utero constraint is termed plagiocephaly, which is medically defined as "a bizarre distortion of the shape of the skull." This deformity usually implicates the occipital bones and predisposes to a shearing effect on the occiput, atlas and axis, affecting occipital condylar maldevelopment and asymmetry. The presenting clinical sign is observed to be a cervical torticollis. Torticollis can be readily resolved with immediate chiropractic attention (41).

The brow or facial presentation corollary to a hyperextended fetal attitude is of dire concern to the chiropractor and the obstetrician. Biomechanically, it produces an extension style trauma that can establish a compression mode lesion. This position, if prolonged for any period of time in-utero forces the occiput into varying degrees of extension on the cervical spine. The facial presentation transpires in approximately

1 of every 500 births, the brow presentation less commonly occurring. The biomechanical implication is greatest on the occipital-atlantal region where an anterior superior condyle listing is most frequently apparent. This is accompanied by a rather severe hyperlordotic cervical instability. Helstrom and Sallmander (42) describe the "intolerable stresses brought to bear on the infant's neck" as a result of this position.

The transverse or oblique lie exists when the long axis of the fetus is perpendicular or oblique to the long axis of the mother (Fig. 5.27). Because of the crowding from the uterine wall parameters, this malposition frequently forces the head into excessive extension upon the neck, promoting the brow or facial attitude. There is habitual evidence of the appearance of cervical torticollis here, often being labeled at birth as congenital torticollis. Furthermore, because the shoulder is often the presenting part at the cervix, torquing spinal compression may lead to a chronic thoracic or cervicothoracic fixation complex or a distortion of the sternoclavicular or costosternal joints. Certainly, the costovertebral joints of the upper thoracic

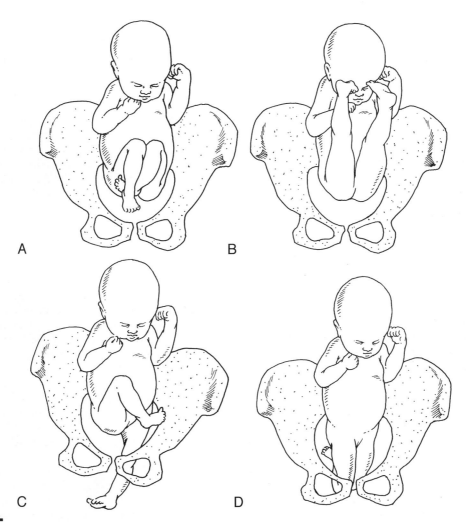

Figure 5.26.   Fetal breech presentations. Modified from Oxom H. Human labor and birth, 1980:53. A, Complete breech presentation. B, Frank breech presentation. C, Single footling breech presentation. D, Kneeling breech presentation.

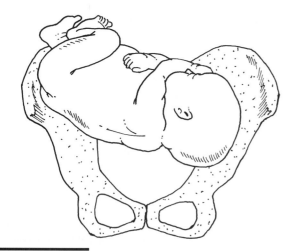

Figure 5.27. Fetal transverse lie. Modified from Oxom H. Human labor and birth, 1980:53.

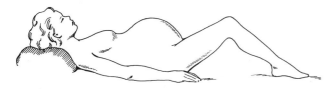

Figure 5.28. Abdominal examination of the maternity patient for in-utero constraint.

region are at risk in this instance. A transverse lie is detected in 1 of every 300–600 births (43) and is significantly increased with multiparity.

Burns (44), Knowlton (45), and Kobak (46) have reported cases of deflection attitudes in transverse presentations. The term "flying fetus" has been set forth by Knowlton (45) to describe this adverse fetal position.

Ensuring optimal pelvic and lumbo-sacral structure and function is the singular most effective technique the chiropractor can offer to the maternity patient. In the third trimester, the patient should be monitored regularly and evaluated chiropractically on a weekly basis. Fallon (47) outlines a treatment protocol supporting weekly chiropractic assessments from the twenty fourth week of pregnancy.

Chiropractic Management of In-utero Constraint

The contemporary chiropractic technique for altering adverse fetal presentation has been advanced by Webster (48). He reports effecting successful version in 97% of adverse in-utero presentations. This technique has been termed the "Webster In-Utero Constraint Turning Technique" (48). It is described in the following section.

It is imperative to confirm the diagnosis of a pernicious fetal presentation before proceeding. For this purpose, the abdominal examination of the third trimester patient should be studied and clinically perfected.

Acquiring a maternal history of the pregnancy and any

other relevant factors is mandatory from the outset. This is followed by the abdominal examination of the maternity patient in the supine position (Fig. 5.28). It may be difficult to assess what classification of in-utero presentation the fetus is postured in. This information is not imperative in applying Webster's technique. When it is corroborated that the fetus is in an unpropitious position, the patient is asked to assume a prone position on the examining/adjusting table (Fig. 5.29). A pelvic elevation or drop piece, or a hi-lo table ensures the optimal comfort of both the maternal and fetal patients. The patient should be comfortable without any undue stress over the uterine anatomy. In the initial procedure or Step 1, the chiropractor grasps the patient's ankles and flexes both knees approximating the buttocks with the feet (Fig. 5.30). Moderate, equally bilateral pressure is applied toward the buttocks to determine any disparity between leg resistances. Should there be an inequality in pressure perceived, this is hypothesized to be demonstrative of a posterior sacral rotation subluxation/fixation (ie. P-L or P-R) on the ipsilateral side of increased

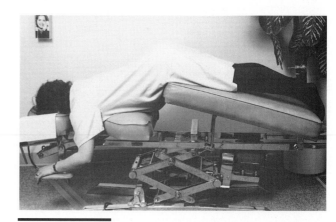

Figure 5.29. Initial patient position for in-utero constraint technique.

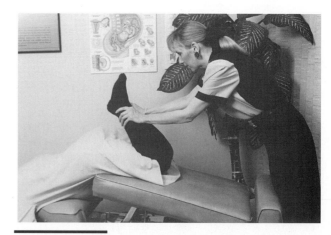

Figure 5.30. Step 1. Moderate, equally bilateral pressure is applied above the ankles approximating the feet towards the buttocks.

resistance (Fig. 5.31). This should be confirmed by static and motion palpation of the sacrum and adjacent articular and soft tissue structures.

In Step 2, the patient is positioned for a side posture adjustment of the side of sacral bala posterior rotation (i.e., P-L or P-R) (Fig. 5.32A). This involves placing the involved side up in most corrective techniques. The contact point of the chiropractor may be the pisiform (Fig. 5.32A), thenar, fingers, or thumb (Fig. 5.32B). The contact location is described as a specific point between the second sacral tubercle and the posterior superior iliac spine directly on the sacral ala. The thrust vector is from posterior to anterior (+Z) following the plane of the articulation.

In Step 3, the patient is placed in a supine position, with the chiropractor standing next to the patient's lower abdomen on the contralateral side of the sacral bala rotation (Fig. 5.33). The location of the fetus is determined in relationship to the umbilicus. A measurement is then performed, placing the "knife edge" of the inferior hand and angling it 45 degrees from the anterior superior iliac spine, from lateral to medial and from inferior to superior. The superior hand is then placed at a 45 degree angle from the umbilicus, from medial to lateral and from superior to inferior (Fig. 5.34). The intersecting point of the two hands should be located at a trigger point for the rectus abdominus muscle, immediately overlaying the broad ligament of the uterus (Fig. 5.35). The chiropractor then places the thumb directly over this contact point (Fig. 5.36). The pressure should be exerted gradually and evenly straight downward until the trigger point is palpated. The pressure should then be maintained, but shifted slightly cephalad to isolate the broad ligament. As little as 3 to 6 ounces of pressure may induce relaxation of the trigger point. Additional pressure may be necessary if fetal movement is not initiated and if the trigger point remains rigid and transfixed. The contact on the point is steadily maintained for a minimum of 1 to 2 minutes, being prolonged as necessary by the palpatory evaluation of the trigger release. One of the authors has observed that this contact point has been held in some instances as long as 35 minutes, although this is unusual. If little or no fetal movement is discerned during the trigger point pressure, some counter pressure with the chiropractor's opposite hand can be applied on the uterine wall opposite the side of the trigger point. One of the authors has also found that gentle intermittent medial pressure with this hand will initiate movement and motivate the trigger point to release more quickly.

After the adjustment, the patient is again placed in the prone position for the assessment of leg resistance. This is described as Step 4. In typical cases, the leg resistance will have equalized. If equalization has not been achieved, the patient should be placed again in the side posture position and the sacrum adjusted with augmented depth. The next phase of this technique should not be initiated until equal leg resistance has been established. If this is not the case, the patient should be re-examined on the subsequent day.

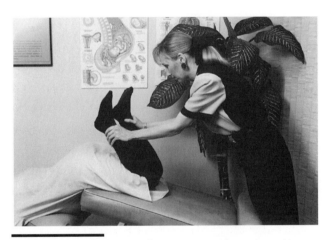

Figure 5.31. Evaluation of posterior sacral rotation subluxation. This is seen on the patient's right leg because of increased resistance.

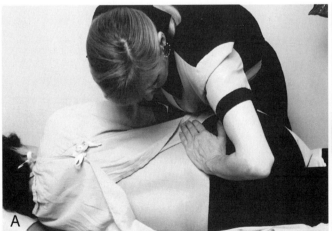
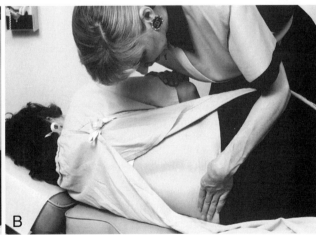

Figure 5.32. A, Step 2. Positioning of adjustment for right sacral base posterior rotation. Pisiform contact.

B, Step 2. Positioning of adjustment for right sacral base posterior rotation. Thumb contact.

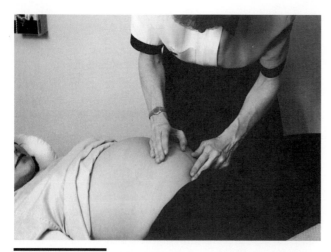

Figure 5.33. Step 3. Preparation for uterine trigger point includes palpation of the fetus in relationship to the umbilicus.

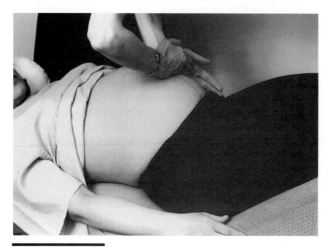

Figure 5.34. Step 3. Hand placement for determination of left trigger point overlying the rectus abdominus muscle and broad ligament of the uterus.

Anrig (48) has noted that in rare cases such as noted in the complete breech or ventral vertex posture, equal leg resistance may be displayed during the initial leg check or Step 1. She suggests that these patients be adjusted for a sacral base posterior. The contact site is the first or second sacral tubercle. The adjustive thrust is posterior to anterior with a superior to inferior arc. One of the authors recommends the application of gentle manual sacral traction (Fig. 5.37) before this adjustment. In these clinical circumstances, Step 3 will assess for bilateral trigger points, which should then be applied with bilateral and simultaneous pressure.

Additional adjustments should not be performed on the same day that the Webster technique is applied. Clinical experience provides wide parameters for the number of technique sessions required for the fetus to achieve version. As little as one procedure may effect the result, but typically the procedure may produce positive results within three to ten

sessions performed over a 2- to 3-week period. It is of tremendous benefit to initiate this technique as soon as possible after diagnosis of the breech presentation is made in the third trimester. Mechanically, it is more laborious for the fetus to achieve version close to term.

The authors have elaborated on this technique further by applying it to the transverse or oblique lie. In these fetal situations, Steps 1 and 2 of the Webster technique are followed, until the beginning of Step 3. At this stage, bilateral trigger points should be addressed in the same described locations with similar pressure (Fig. 5.38). The facial or brow presentation, where the cephalic prominence is the sinciput, responds to slight modification of Webster's technique. Specifically, the sacral assessment and adjustment (Steps 1 and 2) are performed in a similar manner as described; however, in Step 3, the trigger point is applied on the ipsilateral side of sacral rotation. Here, the cephalic prominence is determined as previously portrayed in the examination of the third trimester patient.

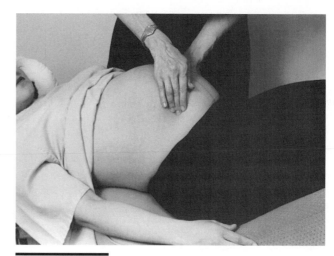

Figure 5.35. Step 3. Location of the trigger point, located here on the patient's right side.

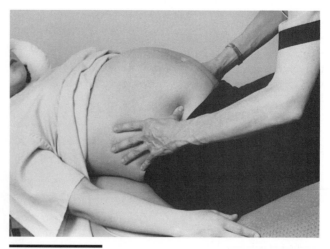

Figure 5.36. Step 3. Thumb contact over the right trigger point. The examiner's other hand stabilizes the uterus.

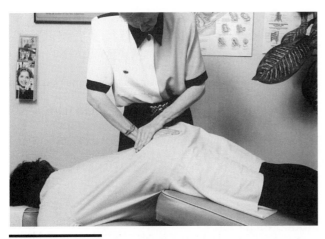

Figure 5.37. Manual sacral traction utilizing a gentle rocking superior to inferior posterior to anterior movement.

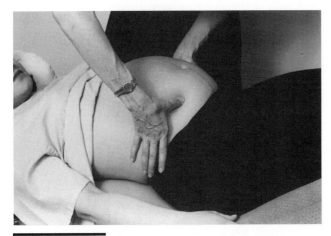

Figure 5.38. In-utero constraint. Bilateral trigger points applied for a diagnosis of a fetal transverse or oblique lie.

Obstetrical Management of In-utero Constraint

External cephalic version for breech presentations, performed at about thirty seven to thirty eight weeks gestationally, entails much higher risk and reduced success than the Webster technique in the authors' opinion. This is described as external manual manipulation of the fetus toward a vertex presentation. Most obstetricians skilled in this procedure report an approximate 50 percent success rate. Although there are several supportive studies in the medical literature, this procedure has not received widespread acceptance. The iatrogenic results of this procedure include uterine rupture, premature placental separation, fetal-maternal hemorrhage and failure.

The external version procedure is preceded by ultrasonic diagnosis to confirm fetal presentation and position and to visualize the site of placental attachment. A nonstress test is routinely performed before and following the version attempt to confirm the well-being of the fetus. A tocolytic drug such as ritodrine, terbutaline or relaxin is administered to the mother to relax the uterine muscle and reduce the risk of preterm labor contractions. Ultrasound examination is continued for guidance and to monitor the fetal heart rate, as the physician attempts to manipulate the fetus by pressing and pushing on the abdomen.

Should the fetus exhibit signs of distress, the procedure is immediately ceased. In the rare circumstance where the placenta begins to separate during the version attempt or when the fetus is in distress after the procedure is completed, an emergency caesarean section may have to be performed. A successful version does not guarantee the fetus remaining in the vertex position for the balance of the pregnancy. The benefit of the external version is that it lowers the caesarean rate for breech presentations.

The Webster technique does not convey any risk to the fetus or the mother, because it reinstates the proper pelvic biomechanics, it functions to stimulate the fetus to reposition itself, rather than forceful manipulation being applied. The Webster in-utero constraint technique is not recommended for the multiple fetus pregnancy (i.e. twins, triplets).

Scheduled caesarean delivery of the breech is frequently evaluated by the physician based upon risk deliberation. Some patients are legitimate candidates for caesarean breech delivery because of obstetrical factors. Others are scheduled for caesarean section simply because their obstetrician is skilled in this technique and prefers to deliver all breech babies surgically. Furthermore, some women attempting a vaginal breech birth develop problems in labor that necessitate a caesarean delivery. Consequently, the caesarean birth rate for the breech fetus is extremely high.

Obstetricians are becoming increasingly knowledgeable and skilled in vaginal delivery of the breech fetus. Their considerations for performing the procedure include the size and gestational age of the fetus, the type of breech presentation, the size of the maternal pelvis and other factors. Some doctors require that the patient has had a previously successful vaginal birth. The best candidate for a vaginal breech delivery is a term fetus estimated to weigh less than 8 pounds who is in a frank breech presentation with a well-flexed head within a roomy pelvis. Careful monitoring and medical interventions during labor are anticipated in this situation. This is most often an ultrasound guided technique. When the physician has been experienced in the management of vaginal breech births, outcomes have been illustrated to be much more successful with vaginal than with caesarean delivery (49, 50).

A fetus remaining in the transverse lie to term is almost always scheduled for caesarean delivery due to the potential for severe dystocia or cephalopelvic disproportion.

Additional Recommendations for Reduction of Breech Presentation

Simkin (51) recommends that the mother of a breech baby be taught to perform the "breech-tilt" position to encourage the baby to turn. She describes the position as tilting the body so that the hips are higher than the head. The patient is instructed to lie on her back with the knees flexed and the feet placed flat on the floor. The pelvis then should be slowly raised, and firm cushions slid underneath the buttocks to raise them 10-15 inches above the head. A tilt board or ironing board slanted with one end placed on a chair and the other on the floor may accomplish this same effect. This position should be performed for approximately ten minutes three times daily when the baby is discernably active. The mother should be advised to perform this technique with an empty bladder and stomach. The fetus will typically squirm as its head is compressed into the uterine fundus, and seeks a more comfortable position. The success rate of this technique is arbitrary; however it does not impair the fetus or the mother to attempt it.

The application of sound to turn the breech fetus is another benign technique (77). The earphones of a cassette tape or CD player should be placed by the mother immediately superior to the pubic bone. Soothing music is then played for the fetus during its active periods. The volume is maintained at a level that is comfortable for the mother to listen to. Sound travels well, although somewhat muted through the amniotic fluid to the fetal hearing apparatus. The rationale applied to the success of this procedure is that should the fetus hear pleasing sounds arising from low in the uterus, it might be motivated to move the head down to better hear them. Numerous women who have attempted this technique have reported that their babies have turned readily (51).

Subluxation Analysis and Adjustive Techniques

Observation

The postural alterations of the gravid female varies with each patient and each trimester. These normal postural changes must be carefully differentiated from postural abnormalities unrelated to the pregnancy that are clinically relevant.

From the lateral view, increased lumbar lordosis and sacral base angle are usually present by the second trimester. The thoracic and cervical spine may compensate for the lumbopelvic alterations. It is common for the thoracic region to translate posterior causing anterior translation of the head and cervical spine.

The innominates may flare outward ($\pm\theta Y$) to compensate for the developing fetus. This may cause a compensatory gait alteration (i.e., the "waddle"). This compensation does not indicate a bilateral "In" ilium fixation or a bilateral ilium adjustment.

The constantly changing posture and spinal biomechanical adaption of the gravid patient may present the doctor with a more complex and difficult palpation assessment. The doctor must be careful to differentiate from the examination findings of subluxation (e.g., fixation) from that of compensation (e.g., hypermobility).

The region of compensation (joint hypermobility) typically above the region of vertebral subluxation may manifest as more symptomatic than the site of joint fixation.

The sacroiliac joints may be symptomatic and reveal tenderness upon static palpation. However, the movement of these articulations will often be normal and thus not warrant an adjustment. The same symptomatic complaints may be found in transitional regions (e.g., C0-C1, C7-T1, T12-L1).

Static Palpation

Digital palpation for tenderness and edema (52) can be detected at the hypomobile segment although hypermobility at a joint can also create the same findings.

The gravid female is in a constant state of adaptation due to both hormonal and biomechanical factors. These include postural and spinal compensations typically above the region of the vertebral subluxation (hypomobile) site.

The doctor should thoroughly evaluate the patient and interpret findings correctly before deciding to deliver an adjustment to a tender and edematous region motion segment. It would be a contraindication to adjust a hypermobile articulation.

Motion Palpation

Intersegmental range of motion palpation (IRMP) is performed during passive and/or patient-assisted motion to detect intervertebral movement. The cervical and thoracic regions are usually palpated with passive motion. The lumbar and sacroiliac areas are typically palpated actively with the assistance of the patient (Fig. 5.39).

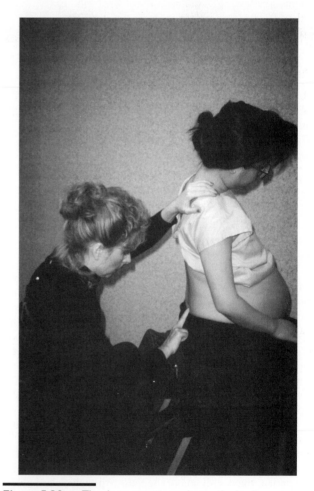

Figure 5.39.   The doctor motion palpates the lumbar spine with the assistance of the patient.

Intersegmental range of motion palpation (52) should be conducted at each visit. Modification of technique for the protruding abdomen (e.g., lumbopelvic flexion assessment) is constantly assessed at each visit.

The hormonal and weight-bearing changes to the spinal segments must be weighed in the overall assessment of the patient. The practitioner who adjusts based on apparent symptomatic signs alone without other examination findings, including review of pre-pregnancy radiographs if they are available, may not be providing the most optimal assessment, and therefore, the most optimal treatment.

Instrumentation

The procedure for performing a paraspinal skin temperature examination (e.g., Nervoscope) (52) is the same as in the adult non-gravid female. It is the authors' experience that the temperature patterns vary more in the gravid female than in the non-gravid patient. The regions of the spine that are compensating with increased hypermobility may manifest as increased temperature differentials. However, findings associated with hypomobility will likely continue to demonstrate a constant "break" in temperature symmetry on repeat scanning. Instrumentation findings should be correlated with the results of other examination procedures (e.g., motion palpation, static palpation, etc.).

Radiography

Radiographs, especially of the low back, are usually not obtained on the pregnant female because of the increased risk associated with fetal exposure to ionizing radiation (see Chapter 8). In the case of cervical trauma (e.g., whiplash, sports injury, fall), one may consider limited cervical views to determine the appropriate diagnostic and/or treatment options (48). A discussion with the patient, spouse, parents, and obstetrician may be necessary to answer any questions before the radiographic procedure. The involved parties should be informed of the safety precautions provided. This should include wearing a full-trunk lead apron and brain, eye, and thyroid shielding.

Any woman of child-bearing age should be required to answer on the case history form if there is a possibility of pregnancy. The patient should again be queried immediately before the radiographic examination. With the trend toward an earlier age at which females reach menarche as well as the initiation of sexual activity, the doctor should tactfully question the young adolescent about the possibility of pregnancy. The patient's response to the possibility of pregnancy should be noted in the records.

Adjustments

During the course of pregnancy, hormonal changes alter the function of musculature and other supporting structures. This alteration normally increases mobility of the spinal motion segments and sacroiliac articulations. If a motion segment is compensating for a lack of mobility at an adjacent level, then

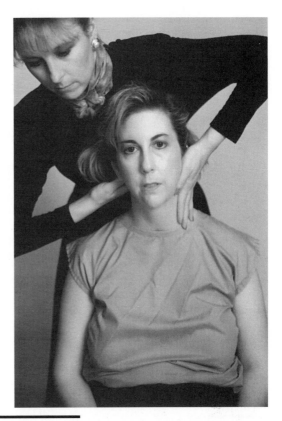

Figure 5.40.   The ASR atlas is contacted with the distal tip of the right thumb on the antero-superior aspect of the right transverse of atlas.

these segments may become more hypermobile. Therefore, forces should not be introduced into joints that exhibit increased mobility.

Before the delivery of the thrust, the practitioner should consider all issues relating to protection of both the mother and fetus. It is not necessary to introduce forces that move the patient into positions of Y-axis rotation and the extremes of flexion, extension, and lateral flexion during an adjustment.

Patient positioning is critical for the delivery of a safe and effective adjustment. The reader should review the adolescent patient set-ups in Chapter 9 for more information on short-lever arm adjustment positions.

CERVICAL CHAIR

The cervical chair is useful for adjusting cervical and upper thoracic segments (53). In the seated position, the surrounding segments may be effectively stabilized while allowing an inferior to superior pattern of thrust. Chapter 9 discusses thoroughly the set-up procedure.

ATLAS ASR ADJUSTMENT

Example. ASR (+Z), -θX, -θZ, (-X) listing (Fig. 5.40). The anterior tubercle of atlas has moved into a positon of extension (antero-superior), and the atlas is laterally flexed to the left.

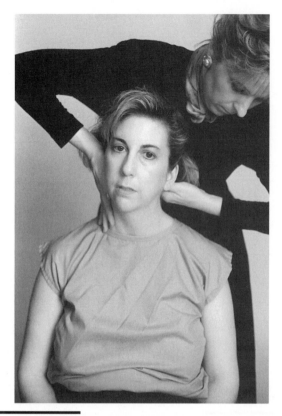

Figure 5.41.   To correct the atlas posterior rotational component, the head is slightly rotated away from the side of contact.

Contraindications. All other listings, hypermobility, normal
functional spinal unit, instability, lytic metastasis at or near the
area to be adjusted, transverse ligament rupture, spinal infection in the area to be adjusted.

Patient Position. The patient is placed in a seated position on
the cervical chair.

Contact Site. Antero-lateral aspect of the left transverse process
of the atlas.

Adjusting and Stabilizing Hand Contact. Distal tip of the left
thumb. To correct the rotational component (-θX), the head
is slightly rotated away from the side of contact. The amount
of prepositioned head rotation is in direct proportion to extent
of rotational malalignment and fixation. The stabilization hand
is cupping the opposite ear and stabilizing the C2-C3 articulation and the lateral musculature.

Supportive Assistance. The stabilization strap may be used.

Pattern of Thrust. Lateral to medial, inferior-ward arc toward
the end of the thrust.

Contraindications. All other listings, hypermobility, normal
functional spinal unit, instability, lytic metastasis at or near the
area to be adjusted, transverse ligament rupture, spinal infection in the area to be adjusted.

Patient Position. The patient is placed in a seated position on
the cervical chair.

Supportive Assistance. The stabilization strap may be used.

Contact Site. Antero-lateral aspect of the right transverse
process of the atlas.

Adjusting and Stabilizing Hand Contact. Distal tip of the right
thumb. The stabilization hand is cupping the opposite ear and
stabilizing the C2-C3 articulation and the left lateral musculature.

Pattern of Thrust. Lateral to medial, inferior-ward arc (+θX)
toward the end of the thrust.

ATLAS ASLP ADJUSTMENT

Example. ASLP (+Z), -θX, +θZ, (+X), +θY listing (Fig.
5.41). Antero-superior, lateral flexion to the right and left axial
rotation.

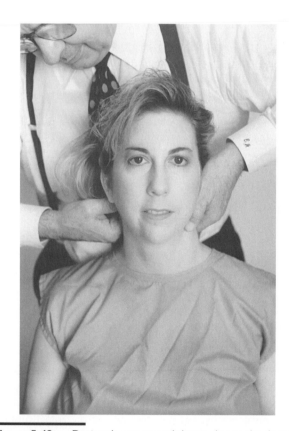

Figure 5.42.   During the set-up and thrust phases, the doctor
should avoid placing the cervical spine in excessive lateral
flexion.

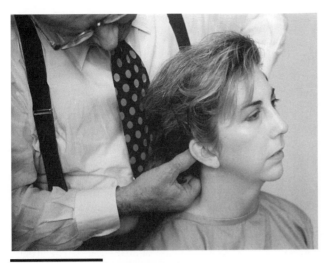

Figure 5.43. The distal end of the right second digit contacts the medial portion of the opposite lamina.

C5 PRS Adjustment

Example. PRS (-Z, +θY, -θZ) C5 listing (Fig. 5.42).

Contraindications. All other listings, normal functional spinal unit, instability, hypermobility, destruction or fracture of the spinous process or neural arch, or infection of the contact vertebra.

Patient Position. Patient is seated on the cervical chair.

Doctor Position. The doctor stands slightly to the right side.

Contact Site. The inferior right lateral aspect of the spinous process.

Adjusting and Stabilizing Hand Contact. The distal (and palmar) end of the right second digit is placed on the contact site. To increase adjusting hand stabilization, the third digit is placed next to the second digit. The contact hand thumb is placed on the ramus of the mandible. The contact thumb should not pull on the skin near the eye or be placed on the temporomandibular joint. The palmar surface of the stabilization hand is placed on the opposite lateral musculature of the cervical spine. The thenar eminence of the stabilization hand is below the ear and thumb along the angle of the jaw.

Supportive Assistance. The cervical strap may be used.

Set-up. The stabilization hand is first placed on the top of the patient's head. The head should be slightly flexed to separate the spinous process. The contact digit is placed on the contact site. The head is brought up to a neutral position by the stabilization hand and then positioned on the opposite lateral musculature of the cervical spine. To relax the posterior musculature, the chin is raised slightly. The cervical spine is laterally flexed slightly (10 to 15 degrees) to the right side. To reduce slack, pressure is applied posterior to anterior (+Z) with the contact digit. Head movement is restricted by the stabili-

zation hand during the thrust. The stabilization hand does not pull up during the thrust.

Pattern of Thrust. An arcing movement posterior to anterior and inferior to superior with a slight -θY rotation through the plane of the intervertebral disc and facet articulations. At the end of the thrust, a slight vector is applied through the center of mass of the segment that causes right lateral flexion of the vertebra.

C6 PLI-la Adjustment

Example. PLI-la (-Z, -θY, -θZ) C6 listing (Fig. 5.43).

Contraindications. All other listings, normal functional spinal unit, instability, hypermobility, destruction or fracture of the lamina or neural arch, or infection of the the contact vertebra.

Patient Position. The patient is seated on the cervical chair.

Doctor Position. The doctor stands slightly to the right side.

Contact Site. The medial portion of the right lamina.

Adjusting and Stabilizing Hand Contact. The distal (and palmar) end of the right second digit is placed on the contact site. To increase adjusting hand stabilization, the third digit is placed next to the second digit. The contact hand thumb is

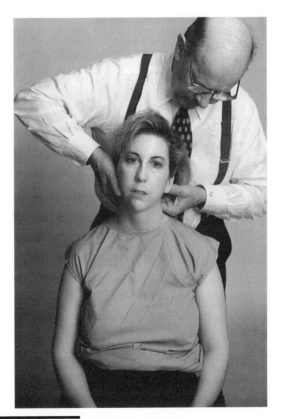

Figure 5.44. The doctor stands slightly to the lateral side of listing. Stabilization occurs with the palmar side of the opposite hand on the lateral cervical musculature.

placed on the ramus of the mandible or on the mastoid behind the ear. The contact thumb should not pull on the skin near the eye or be placed on the temporomandibular joint. The palmar surface of the stabilization hand is placed on the opposite lateral musculature of the cervical spine. The thenar eminence of the stabilization hand is below the ear and thumb along the angle of the jaw.

Supportive Assistance. The cervical strap may be used.

Set-up. The stabilization hand is placed on the top of the patient's head. The head should be slightly flexed to separate the spinous process. The contact digit is placed on the contact site. The head is brought up to a neutral position by the stabilization hand and then positioned on the opposite lateral musculature of the cervical spine. To relax the posterior musculature, the chin is raised slightly. The cervical spine is laterally flexed slightly (10 to 15 degrees) to the side of laterality. To reduce slack, pressure is applied by a posterior to anterior (+Z) with the contact digit. Head movement is restricted by the stabilization hand during the thrust. The stabilization hand does not pull up during the thrust.

Pattern of Thrust. An arcing movement posterior to anterior and inferior to superior with a slight $+\theta Y$ rotation through the plane of the intervertebral disc and facet articulations. At the end of of the thrust a slight clockwise torque is applied through the center of mass of the segment that causes left lateral flexion of the vertebra.

Contraindication to Thrust. The doctor is unable to prevent the following vectors: excessive lateral flexion, extension or rotation in the thrust phase.

C5 PL ADJUSTMENT

Example. PL (-Z, $+\theta Y$,) C5 listing (Fig. 5.44).

Contraindications. All other listings, normal functional spinal unit, instability, hypermobility, destruction or fracture of the spinous process and neural arch, or infection of the contact vertebra.

Patient Position. The patient is seated on the cervical chair.

Doctor Position. The doctor stands slightly to the side of laterality.

Contact Site. The inferior left lateral aspect of the spinous process.

Adjusting and Stabilizing Hand Contact. The distal (and palmar) end of the left second digit is placed on the contact site. To increase adjusting hand stabilization, the third digit is placed next to the second digit. The contact hand thumb is placed on the ramus of the mandible or on the mastoid behind the ear. The contact thumb should not pull on the skin near the eye or be placed on the temporomandibular joint. The palmar surface of the stabilization hand is placed on the opposite lateral

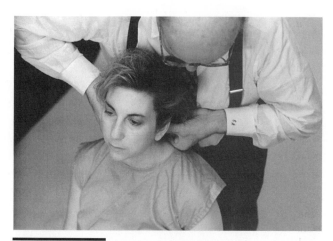

Figure 5.45.   Stabilization may be provided by the head of the patient resting against the chest or abdomen of the doctor.

musculature of the cervical spine. The thenar eminence of the stabilization hand is below the ear and thumb along the angle of the jaw. The doctor's forearms should follow the plane line of the joint.

Supportive Assistance. The cervical strap may be used.

Set-up. The stabilization hand is placed on the top of the patient's head. The head should be slightly flexed to separate the spinous process. The contact digit is placed on the contact site. The head is brought up to a neutral position by the stabilization hand and than positioned on the opposite lateral musculature of the cervical spine. To relax the posterior musculature, the chin is raised slightly. The cervical spine is laterally flexed slightly (10 to 15 degrees) to the side of laterality. To reduce slack, pressure is applied posterior to anterior (+Z) with the contact digit. Head movement is restricted by the stabilization hand during the thrust. The stabilization hand does not pull up during the thrust.

Pattern of Thrust. An arcing movement posterior to anterior and inferior to superior with a slight $+\theta Y$ rotation through the plane of the intervertebral disc and facet articulations. At the end of the thrust, a slight counterclockwise torque is applied through the center of mass of the segment that causes right lateral flexion of the vertebra.

Contraindication to Thrust. The doctor is unable to prevent the following vectors: excessive lateral flexion, extension or rotation in the thrust phase.

T1 PL ADJUSTMENT

Example. PL (-Z, $-\theta Y$) T1 listing (Fig. 5.45).

Contraindications. All other listings, normal functional spinal unit, hypermobility, instability, destruction or fracture of the neural arch or spinous process, infection of the contact vertebra.

Patient Position. The patient is seated on the cervical chair.

Doctor Position. The doctor stands slightly to the side of laterality.

Contact Site. Inferior and lateral aspect of the spinous process.

Adjusting and Stabilizing Hand Contact. The distal end of the left second digit (palmar and lateral aspect) is placed on the contact point. The second digit is supported by the third digit. The left thumb is placed on the ramus of the mandible or on the mastoid behind the ear. An arch is formed by the thumb and contact digit. The arch decreases unnecessary overlapping to the contact and adjacent vertebras. The stabilization hand (palmar aspect) contacts the opposite cervical musculature. A foundation for the adjustment is established by stabilizing the vertebra below and above the subluxation. Further stabilization may be provided by the head of the patient against the chest or abdomen of the doctor.

Supportive Assistance. The cervical strap may be used.

Set-up. The stabilization hand is placed on the top of the patient's head. The head should be slightly flexed to separate the spinous process. The contact digit is placed on the contact site. The head is brought up to a neutral position by the stabilization hand and then positioned on the opposite lateral musculature of the cervical spine. To relax the posterior musculature, the chin is raised slightly. The cervical spine is laterally flexed slightly (15 to 20 degrees) to the side of laterality. To reduce slack, apply posterior to anterior (+Z) pressure with the contact digit. Head movement is restricted by the stabilization hand during the thrust. The stabilization hand does not pull up during the thrust.

Pattern of Thrust. Posterior to anterior (+Z), lateral to medial (+θY).

Contraindication for the Adjustment. Doctor is unable to prevent the stabilization hand from thrusting.

T2 PRI-t Adjustment

Example. PRI-t (−Z, +θY, −θZ) T2 listing (Fig. 5.46).

Contraindication. All other listings, normal functional spinal unit, hypermobility, instability, destruction or fracture of the neural arch or transverse process, infection of the contact vertebra.

Patient Position. The patient is seated on the cervical chair.

Doctor Position. The doctor stands slightly to the side of laterality.

Contact Site. The left transverse process.

Adjusting and Stabilizing Hand Contact. The distal end of the left second digit (palmar and lateral aspect) is placed on the

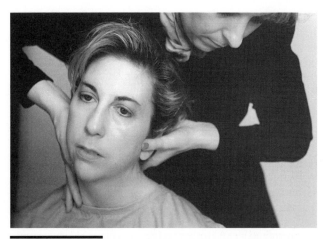

Figure 5.46. The doctor stabilizes the upper torso with a caudal pressure without introducing posterior rotation.

contact point. The second digit is supported by the third digit. The left thumb is placed on the ramus of the mandible. An arch is formed by the thumb and contact digit. The arch decreases unnecessary overlapping to the contact and adjacent vertebras. The stabilization hand (palmar) contacts the opposite cervical musculature. A foundation for the adjustment is established by stabilizing the vertebra below and above the subluxation. Further stabilization may be provided by the head of the patient against the chest or abdomen of the doctor.

Supportive Assistance. The stabilization strap may be used.

Set-up. The stabilization hand is placed on the top of the patient's head. The head should be slightly flexed to separate the spinous process. The contact digit is placed on the contact site. The head is brought up to a neutral position by the stabilization hand and then positioned on the opposite lateral musculature of the cervical spine. To relax the posterior musculature, the chin is raised slightly. The cervical spine is laterally flexed slightly (15 to 20 degrees) to the side of laterality. To reduce slack, apply posterior to anterior (+Z) pressure with the contact digit. Head movement is restricted by the stabilization hand during the thrust. The stabilization hand does not pull up during the thrust.

Pattern of Thrust. Posterior to anterior (+Z) through the disc plane line, lateral to medial (−θY), with an inferior-ward (+θZ) arcing motion toward the end of the thrust.

Contraindication for the Adjustment. Doctor is unable to prevent the stabilization hand from thrusting.

PELVIC BENCH

During the side posture set-up, the doctor should carefully stabilize the upper torso with cephalic pressure, without pressing the patient's shoulder posterior-ward toward the pelvic bench. As the abdominal region of the pregnant patient enlarges, the doctor must occasionally compensate the stance away from the abdominal region (Fig. 5.47). In the more advanced gravid female, no body-drop, nor pull moves during the thrust phase should occur. The patient may need to be assisted in raising herself off of the table during the last trimester.

L5 PLS Adjustment

Indications. Retrolisthesis of L5 with decreased anteriorward translation and flexion during forward bending. Fixation dysfunction in right spinous rotation (+θY) and left lateral flexion (-θZ) (Fig. 5.48).

Contraindications. All other listings, normal FSU, hypermobility, instability, destruction or fracture of the neural arch or spinous process infection of the contact vertebra.

Patient Position. Right side posture position.

Doctor Position. The doctor stands at a 45 degree angle facing cephalad to the patient. The doctor should compensate their stance for the gravid female. To prevent lumbar strain to the doctor, he or she should contract the abdominal musculature before the adjustment.

Contact Site. Posterior, inferior, left lateral border of the spinous process. The tissue pull for the lateral flexion positional dyskinesia should be from superior to inferior.

Adjusting and Stabilizing Hand Contact. The spinous process is contacted by the pisiform. The stabilization hand contacts the anterolateral portion of the shoulder and axilla region with a slight cephalad distraction.

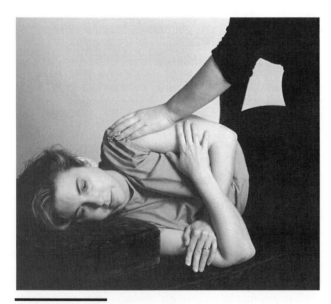

Figure 5.47.   The doctor may have to compensate their stance away from the larger gravid abdomen.

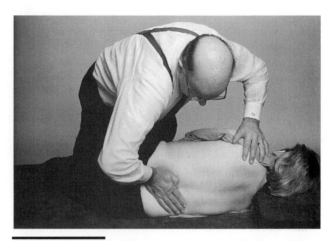

Figure 5.48.   The right pisiform contacts the spinous process for the PLS listing.

Pattern of Thrust. Posterior to anterior (+Z) vector along the sacral base angle. The sacral base angle is reduced when the patient lies in the side posture position. It is further reduced when the patient's thigh is flexed before the thrust. Lateral to medial (+θY), with an inferior-ward arcing motion (-θZ) toward the end of the thrust.

Contraindication for the Thrust. The involved segment should not receive a thrust if the possibility exists of placing rotation and/or flexion in the spine above the involved segment. The patient feels encroachment on the fetus.

PIIn (Left) Side Posture Adjustment

Indications. PIIn (-Z, -θX, +θY) left listing (Fig. 5.49).

Contraindications. All other listings, hypermobility, instability, lytic metastasis in the region, inability to lie in the side posture position, hip replacement on the involved ilium.

Doctor Position. The doctor stands in front and slightly inferior of the patient. The superior bent leg is straddled by the doctor's legs. The doctor should compensate the stance for the gravid female. To prevent lumbar strain to the doctor, he or she should contract the abdominal musculature before the adjustment.

Contact Site. The location is slightly inferior of the PI site and the medial border of the PSIS. With the stabilization hand, tissue pull is inferior to superior and medial to lateral.

Adjusting and Stabilizing Hand Contact. The right pisiform is placed on the contact site. The stabilization (cephalad) hand should be placed on the anterolateral portion of the axilla region.

Pattern of Thrust. The thrust is given in a posterior to anterior (+Z), inferior to superior (+θX), and medial to lateral (-θY) direction. There is no torque or body drop.

Contraindication for the Thrust. The patient is unable to be stabilized in the perpendicular position. The patient feels encroachment on the fetus. The doctor is unable to prevent or minimize rotation to the torso.

SIDE POSTURE SACRAL PUSH ADJUSTMENT

Indications. P (-Z) sacral (Fig. 5.50) subluxation.

Contraindications. All other listings, hypermobility, instability, lytic metastasis in the region, inability to lie in the side posture position, hip replacement on the involved side.

Patient Position. The P (-Z) sacral listing can be positioned either side up.

Doctor Position. The doctor adopts the side posture position for the pelvic bench. The doctor will straddle the superior bent leg. The doctor should compensate their stance for the gravid female. To prevent lumbar strain to themselves, the doctor should contract his or her abdominal musculature before the adjustment.

Contact Site. The first or second sacral tubercle for the posterior (P) listing. Tissue pull is performed by the stabilization hand from inferior to superior.

Adjusting and Stabilizing Hand Contact. The pisiform is placed on the sacral tubercle. The direction of the finger's of the

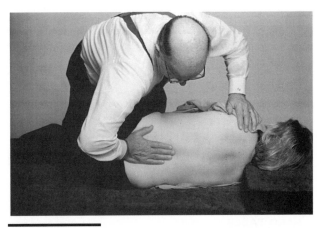

Figure 5.50. The direction of the fingers of the pisiform for the posterior sacrum listing is cephalad.

pisiform for the posterior listing is cephalad. The doctor's forearm should follow the plane line of correction for the involved joint. The stabilization (cephalad) hand contacts the anterolateral portion of the axilla region.

Pattern of Thrust. The thrust for the P listing is posterior to anterior (+Z). To improve the line of correction, the doctor leans over the patient to lower the elbow to the level of the plane of the sacroiliac joint.

Contraindication for the Thrust. The patient cannot be stabilized in a perpendicular position or feels encroachment to the fetus. The doctor is unable to minimize upper torso rotation.

P-L SIDE POSTURE ADJUSTMENT

Indications. P-L (-θY) sacral subluxation (Fig. 5.51).

Contraindications. All other listings, hypermobility, instability, lytic metastasis in the region, inability to lie in the side posture position, hip replacement on the involved side.

Patient Position. The patient is in the side posture position, with the involved side up, for the P-L listing on the pelvic bench.

Doctor Position. The doctor adopts the side posture position for the pelvic bench. The doctor will straddle the superior bent leg. The doctor should compensate his or her stance for the gravid female. To prevent lumbar strain to the doctor, the abdominal musculature should be contracted before the adjustment.

Contact Site. The left sacral alar is contacted. Tissue pull is performed by the stabilization hand from inferior to superior and medial to lateral.

Adjusting and Stabilizing Hand Contact. The pisiform is placed on the sacral alar. The direction of the fingers of the pisiform contact for the P-L listing is toward the table (resting across the

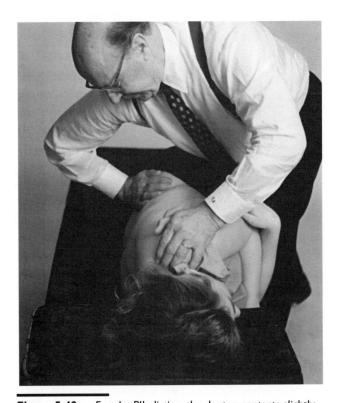

Figure 5.49. For the PIIn listing, the doctor contacts slightly inferior of the PI site and medial border of the PSIS.

sacrum and contralateral ilium). The doctor's forearm should follow the plane line of correction for the involved joint. The stabilization (cephalad) hand contacts the anterolateral portion of the axilla region.

Pattern of Thrust. The thrust is posterior to anterior (+Z) and slight medial to lateral (+θY). To improve the line of correction, the doctor leans over the patient to lower the elbow to the level of the plane of the sacroiliac joint.

Contraindication for the Thrust. The patient cannot be stabilized in a perpendicular position or feels encroachment to the fetus. The doctor is unable to minimize upper torso rotation.

HI-LO TABLE

The hi-lo table also can be used during the majority of the pregnancy. The hi-lo thoracic piece should be set in a locked position to avoid rebounding during the thrust.

As the stomach begins to protrude, the thoracic and lumbar pieces are separated (Fig. 5.52) to compensate for the fetus. As the thoracic section is raised, the face piece will eventually become out of reach for the patient. The patient's chin should remain in a neutral postion. If this position is uncomfortable, the knee-chest table should be used. The introduction of cervical rotation or flexion of the cervical spine will be counterproductive to a specific thoracic adjustment. Adjusting the cervical spine prone while the patient's face is away from the face piece is contraindicated. Prone pillows adapted to the early stages of pregnancy have been developed (Fig. 5.53).

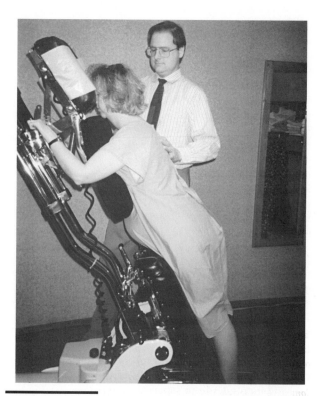

Figure 5.52.   As the abdomen begins to protrude, the thoracic and lumbar pieces are separated.

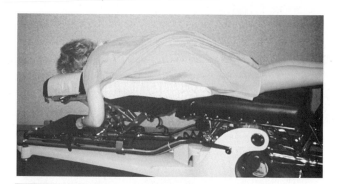

Figure 5.53.   A prone pillow designed for the expanding abdomen may be used during the early stages of pregnancy.

These pregnancy pillows should be used early in the pregnancy by the doctor who cannot separate the sectional pieces of the adjusting tables. A thrust is contraindicated in a gravid female who is unable to have a space provided for the protruding abdomen.

T5 PRS PRONE ADJUSTMENT

Indications. PRS (-Z, -θY, +θZ) T5 listing (Fig. 5.54).

Contraindications. All other listings, normal functional spinal unit, hypermobility, instability, destruction or fracture of the spinous process, infection of the contact vertebra.

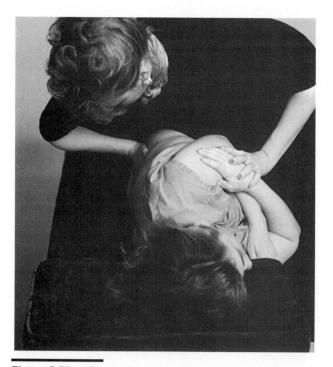

Figure 5.51.   For the P-L sacrum listing, the pisiform rests on the left sacral ala with the fingers resting across the sacrum and contralateral ilium.

Patient Position. The patient is positioned prone on the table. Depending on the size of the abdomen, the thoracic and lumbar sections are separated to provide space for the fetus. If the chin is unable to reach the facial section, the patient's chin must be maintained in a neutral position. The thoracic piece should be locked to prevent rebounding. The hands should rest on the hand plates. A second alternative is the use of an adapting abdomen pillow. Thrust to the spinal region of the pillow section is contraindicated in the advanced gravid patient.

Contact Site. The inferior and lateral portion of the spinous process. Tissue pull occurs with the stabilization hand from inferior to superior and medial to lateral.

Adjusting and Stabilizing Hand Contact. The fleshy portion of the right pisiform is placed on the contact site. The fingers do cross the spine. The stabilization hand rests on top of the adjusting hand for the pisiform contact. The adjusting forearm must follow the joint plane line.

Pattern of Thrust. Posterior to anterior (+Z) through the disc plane line, lateral to medial (−θY) with an inferior-ward (+θZ) arcing motion toward the end of the thrust.

Contraindication for the Thrust. The patient feels encroachment on the fetus.

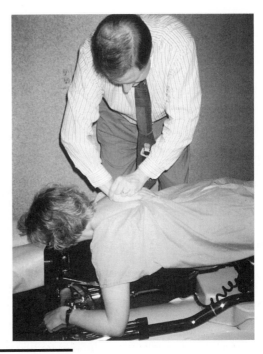

Figure 5.55.   The fingers do not cross the spine for a transverse process contact.

T6 PLI-t Prone Adjustment

Indications. PLI-t (−Z, −θY, −θZ) T6 listing (Fig. 5.55).

Contraindications. All other listings, normal functional spinal unit, hypermobility, instability, destruction or fracture of the transverse process, infection of the contact vertebra.

Patient Placement. The patient is positioned prone on the table. Depending on the size of the abdomen, the thoracic and lumbar sections are separated to provide space for the fetus. If the chin is unable to reach the facial section, the patient's chin must be maintained in a neutral position. The thoracic piece should be locked to prevent rebounding. The hands should rest on the hand plates. A second alternative is the use of an adapting abdomen pillow. Thrust into the spinal region of the pillow section is contraindicated in the advanced gravid patient.

Contact Site. The inferior and lateral portion of the right transverse process. Tissue pull occurs with the stabilization hand from inferior to superior and medial to lateral.

Adjusting and Stabilizing Hand Contact. The fleshy portion of the right pisiform is placed on the contact site. The fingers do not cross the spine. The stabilization hand rests on top of the adjusting hand for the pisiform contact. The adjusting forearm must follow the joint plane line.

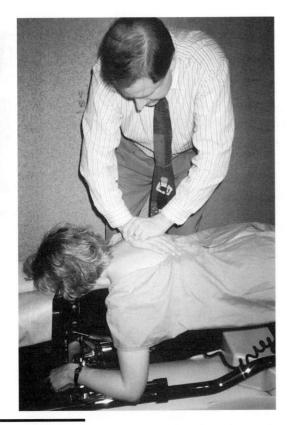

Figure 5.54.   The fleshy portion of the right pisiform is placed on the contact site. Fingers crossing the spine for the PRS listing.

Pattern of Thrust. Posterior to anterior (+Z) through the disc plane line, lateral to medial (+θY) with an inferior-ward (−θZ) arcing motion toward the end of the thrust.

Contraindication for the Thrust. The patient feels encroachment on the fetus.

KNEE-CHEST TABLE

The knee-chest table (Fig. 5.56) is very effective for adjusting the thoracic and lumbar spine in the pregnant female (54). The proper knee-chest procedure for patient placement, indications, contraindications, and thrust are thoroughly discussed in Chapter 10. Before the thrust, the set-up should reflect the appropriate motion segment planes in the different regions of the spine.

A double-thumb or thumb-pisiform contact can be performed on the mammillary process in the lumbar region. A toggle-recoil should not be performed at any time on the knee-chest table during the thrust stage. Rather, a set and hold (approximately 2 seconds) is recommended (see Chapter 9).

T3 PLI-t ADJUSTMENT

Indications. PLI-t (-Z, -θY, -θZ) T3 listing (Fig. 5.57).

Contraindications. All other listings, normal functional spinal unit, hypermobility, instability, destruction or fracture of the transverse process, infection of the contact vertebra.

Patient Position. The patient is positioned on the knee-chest table with the thoracic spine slightly higher than the lumbar spine. The knees should be positioned so the femurs can be perpendicular to the floor. The hands should rest on the hand plates.

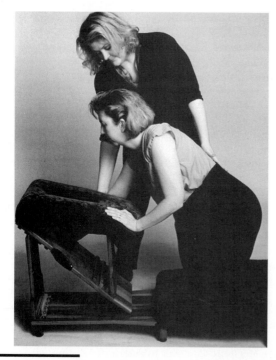

Figure 5.56.   In the last trimester, the gravid female may require doctor assistance to set up on the knee-chest table.

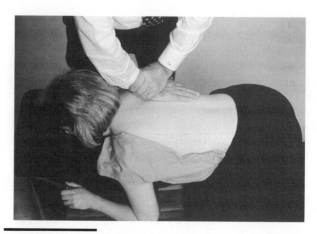

Figure 5.57.   The pattern of thrust for the listing of PLI-t is posterior to anterior, lateral to medial with an inferiorward arcing movement.

Contact Site. The inferior portion of the right transverse process. Tissue pull occurs with the stabilization hand from inferior to superior and medial to lateral.

Adjusting and Stabilizing Hand Contact. The fleshy portion of the right pisiform is placed on the contact site. The fingers do not cross the spine. The stabilization hand rests on top of the adjusting hand for the pisiform contact. The adjusting forearm must follow the joint plane line.

Pattern of Thrust. Posterior to anterior (+Z) through the disc plane line, lateral to medial (+θY) with an inferior-ward (+θZ) arcing motion toward the end of the thrust.

Contraindication for the Thrust. The patient feels abdominal discomfort. The doctor's thrust would end with a toggle-recoil.

T8 POSTERIOR DOUBLE-THUMB ADJUSTMENT

Indication. P (-Z) T8 listing (Fig. 5.58).

Contraindications. All other listings, normal functional spinal unit, hypermobility, instability, destruction or fracture of the mammillary process, infection of the contact vertebra.

Patient Position. The patient is positioned on the knee-chest table with the thoracic spine slightly higher than the lumbar spine. The knees should positioned so the femurs can be perpendicular to the floor. The hands should rest on the hand rests.

Contact Site. The medial portions of both transverse processes.

Doctor Position. The doctor stands posterior to the patient.

Adjusting and Stabilizing Hand Contact. The thumbs are placed on the contact site. The adjusting forearm must follow the disc plane line.

Pattern of Thrust. Posterior to anterior (+Z) through the disc plane line.

Contraindication for the Thrust. The patient feels abdominal discomfort. The doctor's thrust would end with a toggle recoil.

T11 POSTERIOR DOUBLE-THENAR ADJUSTMENT

Indication. P (-Z) T11 listing (Fig. 5.59).

Contraindications. All other listings, normal functional spinal unit, hypermobility, instability, destruction or fracture of the mammillary process, infection of the contact vertebra.

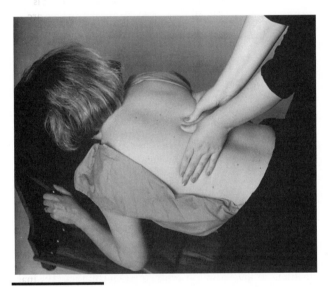

Figure 5.58. The doctor stands posterior to the patient contacting the medial portions of both mamillary processes for the double thumb contact.

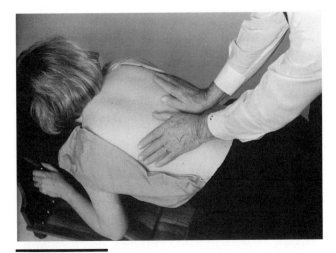

Figure 5.59. The medial portions of the mamillary process is contacted by the thenar eminence.

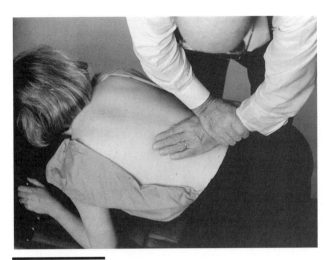

Figure 5.60. The fleshy portion of the pisiform contacts the spinous process.

Patient Position. The patient is positioned on the knee-chest table with the thoracic spine slightly higher than the lumbar spine. The knees should be positioned so the femurs can be perpendicular to the floor. The hands should rest on the hand rests.

Contact Site. The medial portions of both mamillary processes.

Doctor Position. The doctor stands posterior to the patient.

Adjusting and Stabilizing Hand Contact. The thenar eminence are placed on the contact site. The adjusting forearm must follow the disc plane line.

Pattern of Thrust. Posterior to anterior (+Z) through the disc plane line.

Contraindication for the Thrust. The patient feels abdominal discomfort. The doctor's thrust would end with a toggle recoil.

L5 PRS ADJUSTMENT

Indication. PRS (-Z, +θY, -θZ) L5 listing (Fig. 5.60).

Contraindications. All other listings, normal functional spinal unit, hypermobility, instability, destruction or fracture of the spinous process, infection of the contact vertebra.

Patient Position. The patient is positioned on the knee-chest table with the thoracic spine slightly higher than the lumbar spine. The knees are positioned so the femurs can be perpendicular to the floor. The hands should rest on the hand rests.

Contact Site. The lateral, posterior, inferior portion of the spinous process.

Doctor Position. The doctor stands on the side of spinous laterality.

Adjusting and Stabilizing Hand Contact. The fleshy portion of the right pisiform is placed on the contact site, the fingers crossing the spine. The inferior adjusting forearm must follow the disc plane line. The stabilization hand is placed on top of the adjusting hand, fingers resting on top or wrapped around the wrist.

Pattern of Thrust. Posterior to anterior (+Z) through the disc plane line, lateral to medial (-θY) with a slight inferior-ward (+θZ) arcing movement at the end of the thrust. There is a hold and set after the thrust.

Contraindication for the Thrust. The patient feels abdominal discomfort. The doctor's thrust would end with a toggle recoil.

L3 PL-m Thumb-pisiform Adjustment

Indication. PL-m (-Z, -θY) L3 listing (Fig. 5.61).

Contraindications. All other listings, normal functional spinal unit, hypermobility, instability, destruction or fracture of the mamillary process, infection of the contact vertebra.

Patient Position. The patient is positioned on the knee-chest table with the thoracic spine slightly higher than the lumbar spine. The knees are positioned so the femurs can be perpendicular to the floor. The hands should rest on the hand rests.

Contact Site. The medial portion of the right mamillary process.

Doctor Position. The doctor stands on the side opposite the spinous listing.

Adjusting and Stabilizing Hand Contact. The right thumb is

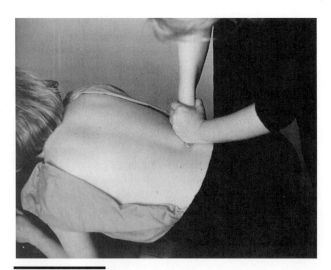

Figure 5.61.   The thumb contacts the right mamillary for the PL-m listing.

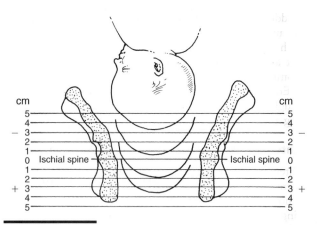

Figure 5.62.   Fetal station.

placed on the contact site. The left pisiform rests on top of the thumb nailbed. The adjusting forearm must follow the disc plane line.

Pattern of Thrust. Posterior to anterior (+Z), lateral to medial, through the disc plane line.

Contraindication for the Thrust. The patient feels abdominal discomfort. The doctor's thrust would end with a recoil.

Preparation for Labor

At some point during late pregnancy or during early labor, the fetus begins its downward movement into the bony pelvis. This process is termed "descent." When the fetus is described as "floating," its lowest or "presenting part" is still above the level of the pubic symphysis. In primigravidas, some descent, either gradual or sudden, typically occurs before the onset of labor. In multigravidas, it is common for labor to commence with the fetus still floating or positioned rather high in the bony pelvis. The majority of descent, both in primigravidas and multigravidas, transpires during labor.

As the fetus descends, its progress is measured in terms of "station," which refers to the location of the presenting part in relation to an imaginary line drawn between the ischial spines (Fig. 5.62). The location of the bony skull (not the caput succedaneum) in cephalic presentations, or the buttocks in breech presentations, at the level of the ischial spines, indicates that the station is 0. If the vertex of the fetal skull is at 0 station, this describes the head as descended to the midpelvis. When the head is floating, it is at a -4 (minus four) station (4 cm above the midpelvis). If it is at a -1 or -2 station, the top of the head is 1 or 2 cm above the midpelvis. When the head is at a +1 (plus one) or a +2 (plus two) station, it is 1 or 2 cm below the midpelvis. When the head is at the introitus and crowning, it is at a +4 station. In summary, descent connotes that the fetus moves from the highest station (-4) down to the lowest station (+4) and is then born. Many women commence labor at a -1 or 0 station, meaning that some descent has already taken place.

Additional terms used to describe the descent that takes place in late pregnancy include "lightening" and "dropping," which refer to the subjective relief of pressure in the mother's chest and upper abdomen, and to a noticeable change in abdominal contour.

"Engagement," which can be definitively determined only through a vaginal examination, refers to the presenting part as being engaged, or at 0 station, and fixed in the pelvis.

Lightening and Engagement

Lightening is the subjective sensation felt by the patient as the presenting part descends during the latter weeks of pregnancy. It is not synonymous with engagement, although both may be taking place at the same time. Lightening is caused by the tonus of the uterine and abdominal muscles and is part of the adaptation of the presenting part to the lower uterine segment and to the pelvis. Symptoms include less dyspnea, decreased epigastric pressure, a feeling that the baby is lower, increased pressure in the pelvis, low backache, urinary frequency, constipation, initial appearance or aggravation of already present hemorrhoids, varicose veins of the lower limbs, edema of the feet and legs, and increased difficulty in walking.

By definition, engagement has taken place when the widest diameter of the presenting part has passed through the inlet. In cephalic presentations, this diameter is the biparietal, between the parietal bosses. In breech presentation, it is the intertrochanteric diameter.

In most women, once the head is engaged, the bony presenting part (not the caput succedaneum) is at or nearly at the level of the ischial spines. This relationship is not constant, and in women with a deep pelvis, the presenting part may be as much as a centimeter above the spines even though engagement has occurred.

The presence or absence of engagement is determined by abdominal, vaginal, or rectal examination. It is easy as a chiropractor to determine engagement from an abdominal examination. This is of particular necessity if in-utero constraint occurs and needs to be addressed biomechanically. In primigravidas, engagement usually takes place 2 to 3 weeks before term. In multiparas, engagement may occur any time before or after the onset of labor. Engagement tells us that the pelvic inlet is adequate. It gives no information as to the midpelvis or the outlet. While failure of engagement in a primigravida is an indication to carefully examine the patient to rule out disproportion, abnormal presentation, or some condition blocking the birth canal, it is not necessarily a cause for alarm. The occurence of engagement in normal cases is influenced by the tonus of the uterine and abdominal muscles.

Risk Assessment

In the third trimester, a number of obstetrical procedures and tests can assess the fetal and placenta unit.

Ultrasonography

The use of ultrasonography can evaluate development of the fetus itself. Serial estimates of biparietal diameter (BPD) are used to monitor fetal growth, but the head is the last structure to cease growing when placental insufficiency occurs. Consequently, measurements of abdominal circumference and head to abdomen ratios may be more useful. Ultrasound can detect the position of the fetus in-utero, confirming presentation and position. It assists in the assessment of amniotic fluid volume. Diagnostic accuracy of ultrasound varies and depends on the quality of the equipment, the skill of the technician, and the gestational age of the fetus. Attempts to measure fetal weight by ultrasound are not yet widely accepted.

Fetal breathing movements can most easily be assessed by ultrasound. The benefit of ultrasound examination here is that it can show marked variability. Abnormalities include gasping type respiration, extreme irregularity of breathing in a term fetus, and complete cessation of breathing. This technique has not yet been fully evaluated, and its practical value is limited.

Doppler

Doppler flow velocity analysis measures doppler flow velocity waveforms of the fetal umbilical artery and/or the maternal uterine artery to provide information on blood flow resistance in the placenta. It is an ultrasonic technique. Reverse flow velocity during diastole is an ominous sign and is associated with imminent fetal demise. The significance of absent diastolic flow velocity is uncertain but may not be threatening. Also known as velocimetry, this procedure can assist in identifying a fetus at risk for an adverse outcome due to fetal-placental blood flow problems such as those in intrauterine growth retardation, gestational hypertension, and other problems. This technique is not recommended as a primary screening test in pregnancy, but is reserved for the evaluation of high-risk pregnancies. Its purpose during labor is to assist in evaluating the effect of labor or obstetric intervention on fetal-placental circulation. This technique is sometimes regarded to be an inappropriate intervention due to its unclear ability to predict maternal and fetal outcome.

Electronic Fetal Monitoring

Antepartum monitoring, also known as fetal non-stress testing, appraises the response of the fetal heart trace to naturally occurring Braxton Hicks contractions or fetal movements. This procedure provides information on fetal health during the third trimester. The fetal heart rate is recorded for 20 to 30 minutes with an external electronic fetal monitor, with the mother indicating the presence of fetal movements. The fetal heart trace is classified as reactive or non-reactive depending on whether there is a minimum of two accelerations of 15 beats per minute or more, lasting at least 15 seconds in response to fetal movements over a 20-minute observation period. A reactive diagnosis is normal and a sign of fetal well-being.

Nonstress tests are considered reliable only during the last weeks of pregnancy. The interpretation of results are considered to be somewhat subjective, and opinions may differ over the meaning from experts. Antepartum monitoring randomly produces false results.

Contraction Stress Test

The contraction stress test or oxytocin challenge test indicates the fetal heart rate response to uterine contractions and is considered reliable only during the latter weeks of pregnancy. The patient is administered intravenous Pitocin (a form of oxytocin) until she experiences three contractions in 10 minutes. An external electronic fetal monitor measures the fetal heart rate while the uterus continues contracting at that rate. When the heart rate remains normal during contractions, test results are classified as normal or "reassuring." When the test results are "nonreassuring" or "ominous," it evidences fetal distress. This procedure can cause preterm labor and intermittently produces false results, which may lead to unnecessary intervention.

Estriol Excretion Test

Estriol excretion studies may demonstrate efficiency of the placenta and the status of the fetus. It is best performed when deciding whether to induce labor or continue a pregnancy complicated by diabetes, maternal hypertension, or postmaturity. This technique is not regarded as accurate enough to be used to resolve whether to induce labor or perform a caesarean section because numerous factors other than fetal problems can cause low estriol excretion, and other tests are more reliable.

Fetal Biophysical Profile

The fetal biophysical profile (FBP or BPP) evaluates fetal physical functions. It consists of five components; FBP combines a nonstress test to check the fetal heart rate during movement with an ultrasound scan that allows assessment of fetal activity, muscle tone, respiratory movements, and amniotic fluid volume. Each component is scored with 0, 1, or 2 points, with the highest possible total of 10 points. This test is usually executed in the latter weeks of gestation.

Radiography

Traditional radiography is rarely performed on pregnant patients. Ultrasound has replaced it as a method of gestational diagnosis because it is safer, more reliable, and a more useful alternative. Early prenatal exposure to ionizing radiation is associated with leukemia and genetic mutations in the neonate. If used, radiography should never be performed until well into the second trimester. In the suspicion of maternal anatomical disproportion, pelvimetry may determine the shape and size of the pelvis. It may also assist in confirming fetal skeletal deformities.

Labor Education

It is not an easy task to dispel the age-old fear of pain during labor and delivery. From the initial awareness of pregnancy, a conscious effort should be made on the part of all health personnel to emphasize that labor and delivery are *normal physiologic processes*. The doctor of chiropractic has a significant role to play in this regard.

To eliminate the harmful influence of fear in labor, the advantages of "natural childbirth" or "physiological childbirth" should be emphasized. Natural childbirth means many different things to different parents, and it is important to determine what a patient is seeking when she or he speaks of natural childbirth. This concept entails antepartum education that emphasizes elimination of fear, exercises to promote relaxation, muscle and breathing control, perhaps visualization and meditation techniques to embellish the "mind-body connection" philosophy in childbirth education. Adroit management throughout pregnancy and labor by the attendance of professionals and birth advocates skilled in the reassurance of the mother is further suggested.

The physiologic reality is that with natural childbirth, most women experience pain, and every childbirth experience is as individual as the laboring mother. It is virtually impossible to describe to a primipara what she can subjectively expect in childbirth.

The purpose of training for childbirth is to prepare a woman for labor and delivery so that she approaches the end of her pregnancy with knowledge, understanding, and confidence rather than apprehension and fear.

One of the first modern advocates of natural childbirth was Grantly Dick-Read (55). He described the "fear-tension-pain" cycle and hypothesized that fears regarding labor produced tension in the circular muscle fibers of the lower part of the uterus. As a result, the longitudinal muscles of the upper part of the uterus act against resistance, causing tension and pain. His solution to this problem was to counteract the socially induced expectations regarding labor by providing mothers-to-be with information and assurance.

Velvovsky and his followers in the Soviet Union denied that labor was inherently painful (56). Based on the work of the physiologist Pavlov, they worked out a training procedure designed to inhibit the experience of pain at the cortical level. This is known as the psychoprophylactic method. Lamaze (57), originator of the Lamaze method, is the best known proponent in the Western world.

Great benefits can be obtained by women and their partners who attend childbirth preparation classes. There are a diversity from which to choose, including the Modified LaMaze, which no longer uses the eight levels of breathing, but has adopted a somewhat more relaxed and self-guided approach, the Bradley Method or husband-coached childbirth, and a method which is increasingly being labeled as Natural Childbirth using the MindBody Connection (58). This teaching is being heralded by childbirth educators universally as embracing the most instinctive psychology and resultant physiology of labor and delivery, thereby facilitating a successful and joyous birth experience.

Enhancing the Probability for a Vaginal Birth

There are a myriad of recommendations that can be made to the maternity patient to ameliorate the opportunities for a successful vaginal birth.

1. Maternal self-care through good nutrition, moderate exercise, stress management, avoidance of drugs and

tobacco so that the mother has the greatest potential for entering labor in the best possible health.

2. Use of a birthing facility that has low caesarean and infection rates and encourages their maternity patients to use self-help techniques that embrace the "mind-body connection" (58).

3. Preparation of a birth plan with a caregiver to ensure that the patient's priorities are respected.

4. Childbirth preparation classes that emphasize the patient's preparation in decision making and the use of nonpharmacologic methods to relieve pain and stress and to promote labor progress.

5. Plan to utilize medications and interventions only when clearly necessary because these alter the course of normal labor.

6. Use of a labor support person (in addition to the spouse) with the mother in labor, one who is familiar to the mother and knows and shares her priorities. Childbirth educators or experienced professional labor support people are often called doulas, monitrices, or birth assistants and are available in many rural and urban areas.

7. Attendance to a support group that promotes vaginal births after caesareans (VBACs) for mothers who have undergone previous caesarean section to assist psychological preparation and practical information.

Stimulation of Labor

Advice to stimulate labor originates when problems emerge for either the fetus or the mother during the last trimester. The indications to activate labor are predicated on results of maternal examination, lab testing, and investigation for fetal well-being and maturity.

The conventional grounds for initiating labor are a protracted pregnancy, long-standing ruptured membranes (36 to 48 hours), pregnancy-induced hypertension (PIH), a distressed fetus or one that is not continuing to thrive or develop, preeclampsia, maternal diabetes, or cardiovascular disease. If any of these circumstances are suspected or present, close monitoring of the fetus and mother are advised. If compromise of the well-being of either the fetus or mother is apparent, labor is activated.

Several diverse methods can induce labor. These incorporate artificial rupture of membranes (AROM), stripping the membranes, prostaglandin gel, and intravenous Pitocin. The method of induction is dictated by the philosophy of the obstetrical team and by the state of the cervix.

Pitocin infusion is the most common type of medical induction in North America (59). The most currently popular method is to apply prostaglandin gel, followed by a Pitocin drip. The reason for this synthesized approach is because the Pitocin drip is not as likely to be successful when the cervix is posterior, thicker, and unripe. The prostaglandin gel is applied in or around the cervix once or twice or more within a 1- or 2-day period. After this stage, intravenous Pitocin is administered. This approach is significantly gradual and successful, although it can be fatiguing for the mother.

Prostaglandin gel, although minimally invasive and considerably effective, is not available at all obstetrical facilities. The reason for this is that the U.S. Food and Drug Administration (FDA) has not approved it for the purpose of ripening the cervix. The FDA does not believe this substance to be unsafe, rather the pharmaceutical manufacturers are not asking the FDA to consider it. Prostaglandin gel has been studied in Canada and Europe and is a standard method of induction there. In the U.S., numerous physicians perceive the value and reasonable safety of prostaglandins and use the gel with confidence.

Stripping the membranes is also a relatively noninvasive procedure, although it exhibits a lower success rate.

Artificial rupture of the membranes (AROM) is seldom successful when the cervix is unripe, posterior, and thick. AROM is occasionally attempted before or concurrent with Pitocin administration, especially in instances in which the cervix is opportune for the procedure. Here, the cervix is anticipated to be ripe, anterior, and partially effaced and dilated.

Many mothers prefer to attempt to stimulate their labors without medical induction procedures. There are measured risks associated with medical inductions of labor. At the very least, the mother may be able to precipitate enough changes in the cervix to facilitate a medical induction.

Simkin (51), a childbirth educator and physical therapist, has published rational guidelines for non-medical labor stimulation. She cautions to consult the obstetrical health-care provider before attempting any of the suggested techniques. The techniques include incorporating lengthy walks of 30 minutes to several hours duration, acupressure, in particular the "Spleen 6" point located four fingerbreadths above the inner anklebone and maintained for 10 to 15 seconds for three repetitions, bowel stimulation through an enema or the ingestion of castor oil to increase the production of prostaglandins and initiate uterine activity, nipple stimulation to cause the release of oxytocin, sexual orgasm for prostaglandin action on the uterus to initiate contractions, and various herbal teas and tinctures to induce labor.

True versus false labor have different characteristics (Table 5.5).

Onset of Labor

Parturition is defined as the expulsion or delivery of the fetus, viable or stillborn, from the body of the maternal organism. In studying the uterine phases of parturition, Phase 1 may be described as the period of uterine preparedness for labor when functional changes in the uterine myometrium and cervix, which are necessary for natural labor induction, are implemented. This phase is routinely distinguished clinically during the last days of pregnancy by distinctive signs comprising ripening of the cervix, increasing prevalence of reasonably painless uterine contractions, maturation of the lower uterine segment and myometrial irritability.

The period of uterine smooth muscle contraction is designated as the prelude to Phase 1, termed Phase 0. This characterizes the time of uterine smooth muscle contractile tranquility and cervical rigidity. This phase is normally sustained from before implantation until late in gestation. Phase 0 is established by immobilizing the potential power of the uterus, by rendering this organ unresponsive to natural stimuli, and by imposing contractile paralysis against immense mechanical and chemical challenges to evacuate its contents.

The transition from uterine Phase 0 to Phase 1 of parturition is called the initiation of parturition. This is the period late in pregnancy when uterine latency is interrupted, facilitating the recovery of the contractile competency of the uterus preparatory to labor.

The active phase of labor is labeled Phase 2, when the uterine contractions initiate cervical dilatation, fetal descent, and delivery. This phase of parturition is divided into three or four stages of labor. The number is contingent on the author. Four stages will be described in this chapter. The fourth stage is synonymous with Phase 3 of parturition in which postpartum recovery occurs. This culminates in uterine involution. Although a woman may be considered to be "post-partum" from a uterine and hormonal attitude for 6 to 8 weeks after delivery of the neonate, she is truly post-partum on a musculoskeletal basis for as long as 12 months. A responsibility for "involution" and maintenance of normal maternal biomechanical structure and function is implicit for the first postpartum year.

Table 5.5.   True and False Labor Differential

True Labor	False Labor
Pains at regular intervals	Irregular
Intervals gradually shorten	No change
Duration and severity increase	No change
Pain starts in back and moves to front	Pain mainly in front
Walking increases the intensity	No change
Association between the degree of uterine hardening and intensity of pain	No relationship
Bloody show often present	No show
Cervix effaced and dilated	No change in cervix
Descent of presenting part	No descent
Head is fixed between pains	Head remains free
Sedation does not stop true labor	Efficient sedative stops false labor pains

In predicting the length of labor, keep in mind some basic definitions and concepts. First, obstetrical labor is the progressive effacement and dilatation of the cervix in the presence of regular contractions. Most of the information about the length of "normal" labors come from investigations by Friedman (60). Thus, the frequent references to the "Friedman curve." This curve establishes limits that are not averages but limits of normal.

Phenomena Preliminary to the Onset of Labor

Lightening occurs 2 to 3 weeks before term and is the subjective sensation felt by the mother as the baby settles into the lower uterine segment. Engagement universally takes place 2 to 3 weeks before term in primigravidas. Also before labor, vaginal secretions increase, a small loss of weight is caused by the excretion of body water, the mucous plug is discharged from the cervix, and a bloody show is noted. Internal examination reveals that the cervix has become soft and effaced. It is current standard obstetrical practice to avoid the procedure of internal examinations in the last trimester of pregnancy due to the risk of infection. Many women complain of a persistent backache, and false labor pains occur with variable frequency.

Contemporary thought (61) corroborates that the fetus governs the time of initiation of labor. The adrenal cortex is imputed to be the precipitating organ of involvement. Other theories of labor etiology have been set forth, among them uterine stretching, fetal presenting part pressure on the cervix and nerve plexuses around the cervix and introitus, and placental aging altering the production of enduring hormones or the secretion of new ones.

Stages of Labor

The first stage of labor begins with cervical effacement and dilatation and ends with complete dilatation. The first stage is further divided into a *latent phase* and an *active phase*. The latent phase begins with cervical change in the presence of regular contractions. The active phase that follows begins with an increasing rate of cervical dilatation. As with labor itself, these divisions of the first stage are retrospective diagnoses. In most women, the latent phase ends, and the active phase begins at 4 cm dilatation.

The second stage of labor begins with complete cervical dilatation of 10 cm and ends with the birth of the baby. This stage includes the processes termed "transition" and pushing. The third stage of labor commences immediately after the birth of the baby and is completed with the delivery of the placenta.

The fourth stage of labor begins when the placenta is delivered and continues until the maternal condition is stable as demonstrated by the blood pressure, pulse, lochia (the usual vaginal discharge of blood from the uterus), and uterine tone. This stage persists for 1 to 2 hours. It may be prolonged by a difficult or prolonged labor, application of anesthesia or surgical delivery by caesarean section.

Physiologic Processes of the First Stage

The first stage of labor lasts an average of approximately 6 to 18 hours in a primigravida and 2 to 10 hours in a multipara. This stage is characterized by contractions that are subjectively intermittent and painful, and the uterine hardening is felt easily by hand on the abdomen. The pains become more frequent and more severe as labor proceeds. As a rule, labor pains begin in the back and passes to the front of the abdomen and upper thighs. Many women describe them as feeling like intense menstrual cramps.

Effacement and dilatation of the cervix is a normal physiologic process of labor necessary for a successful first stage. During most of the pregnancy, the cervix uteri is approximately 2.5 cm in length and closed. Toward the end of the period of gestation, progressive changes occur in the cervix, including the softening, effacement (shortening), dilatation, and movement from a posterior to an anterior position in the vagina. The internal os starts to disappear as the cervical canal becomes part of the lower segment of the uterus. The extent to which these changes have taken place correlates with the proximity of the onset of labor and with the success of attempts to induce labor.

Ideally, the cervix should be ripe at the onset of labor. A ripe cervix is one that is soft, less than 1.3 cm in length, admits a finger easily, and is dilatable. When these conditions are present, induction of labor is feasible. During labor, the cervix further shortens, and the external os dilates. When the os has opened enough (average 10 cm) to permit passage of the fetal head, it is said to be fully dilated.

Most frequently, the membranes rupture near the end of the second stage, but this event can take place at any time during or before labor. When the membranes rupture, the fluid may come away with a gush or may dribble away. On occasion it is difficult to know whether the membranes are ruptured or intact.

In normal cases, after the membranes have ruptured (spontaneously or artificial) the uterine contractions are more efficient and labor progresses faster.

Obstetrical Procedures

Obstetrical interventions in labor and delivery are procedures executed by any member of the obstetrical team to provide diagnostic information, to alter the course of labor, or to prevent perceived complications of the birth process. All medical interventions sustain some disadvantages and should not be used unless they are clinically necessary. There is disagreement within the obstetrical community over how routine some of these intercessions should be.

The rationale for desirable routine interventions should be discussed between the patient and the obstetrical caregivers well in advance of labor and delivery and confirmed with the implementation of a birth plan. Many obstetrical procedures can be avoided by using applauded techniques advocated by childbirth educators, encompassing relaxation and breathing patterns, postural position changes, a diversity of comfort measures, the support of a labor coach or doula, and simply, time.

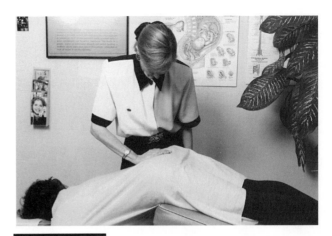

Figure 5.63.   Manual sacral traction of the full term patient.

Chiropractic Techniques

Many chiropractic techniques enhance comfort and facilitate progress during the birth process. Manual sacral traction or sacral pumping administered concurrently with uterine contractions provides immense relief to most patients during the first stage of labor (Fig. 5.63). Many mothers insist on a sustained tractional pressure on the sacrum to alleviate any lumbosacral discomfort, particularly concomitant with "back labor" or an occiput posterior fetus.

Trigger points applied to the piriformis musculature, either unilaterally or bilaterally can ease pelvic biomechanical tension (Fig. 5.64). Habitual contracture of either or both iliolumbar ligaments in labor responds favorably to directly applied pressure, intermittently implemented (Fig. 5.65). Paraspinal muscle circular massage reduces the apparent hypertonicities endured in labor due to prolonged concentration and intensity of uterine contractions. The "all-fours" position is frequently adopted in both the first and second stages of labor, rendering the posterior area of the pelvis accessible for these types of soft tissue techniques. The woman can place her elbows or hands on some stacked pillows or bed headboard, or perhaps stand with her arms supporting her on a windowsill or piece of furniture. Often, the birth partner can support her as she faces him/her and drapes her arms over his/her shoulders. In the chiropractic office, the tables should be elevated to accomodate the fully gravid uterus (Fig. 5.66).

Understanding of and respect for the natural process of birth provides for the greater outcome in most cases. The orthodoxy of the obstetrical specialities conforms to a heterogeneity of interventions.

Intravenous Fluids

In the first stage of labor, the mother may be recommended for the administration of intravenous fluids. These fluids are administered through a small gauge plastic tube or needle inserted into a vein in the back of the hand or forearm. On occasion, a heparin lock is used on admission to the obstetrical facility to maintain an open vein if the need for IV fluids is anticipated.

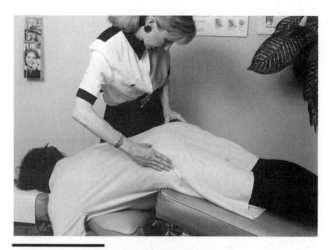

Figure 5.64.   Bilateral piriformis trigger points.

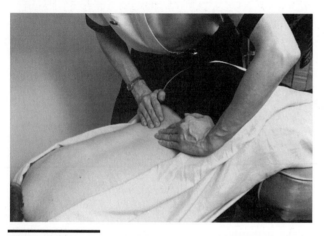

Figure 5.65.   Bilateral pressure over the iliolumbar ligaments.

The functions of the intravenous fluid administration are to maintain hydration when the mother is unable to drink adequate liquids, to assist in sustaining blood pressure in the event that regional anesthesia is used, or in the case of excessive bleeding, to permit immediate access to a vein if medications or a blood transfusion are necessary, to provide calories for energy, and to administer Pitocin if deemed necessary to augment or induce labor.

The disadvantages of IV application are that it restricts relaxed movement during labor — walking is more difficult unless a heparin lock is used; it may result in infiltration of fluids leaking into tissues surrounding the vein near the puncture site, causing tenderness and edema; and it is unnecessary if the mother is drinking sufficient fluids, receiving no medication or anesthesia, and labor is progressing normally.

Induction and Augmentation of Labor

Another obstetrical procedure is the induction and augmentation of labor. Induction is medically advised when any of the following clinical indications are present: when labor is not initiated within 24 hours after the spontaneous rupture of

membranes, notably if the pregnancy is within 2 weeks of term; for uncontrollable toxemia of pregnancy, heralded by maternal edema, sudden weight gain, abnormally elevated blood pressure of proteinuria; with polyhydramnios, when the resultant pressure symptoms and dyspnea of the accumulation of an excessive amount of amniotic fluid are so severe that the patient is unable to carry on; with uncontrollable antepartum bleeding, including cases of placenta previa and mild placenta abruptio or fetal death; intrauterine fetal death to prevent the development of afibrinogenemia; for permitting surgical, radiation or chemical treatment of cancer; with a history of precipitate labors to avoid the birth of the baby during transport to the birthing facility; and as an elective indication for the purported convenience of the patient, the doctor, or both.

Fetal concerns requiring the consideration of labor induction include rhesus incompatibility, when the fetus is being sensitized or where there has been previous fetal deaths; recurrent uterine death near term in past pregnancies; for excessive size of the fetus, significantly in the case of maternal diabetes — it is frequently suggested that the pregnancy be terminated at approximately the thirty seventh week, as it is cited that fetal death in-utero is common during the later weeks of gestational diabetes in pregnancy; and in post term pregnancies, in which there is some evidence that there is a progressive decrease in placental function and in the oxygen content of fetal blood as pregnancy proceeds past term. Artificial rupture of the membranes is associated with greater umbilical cord compression, molding of the fetal head, and decreases in fetal heart rate during contractions.

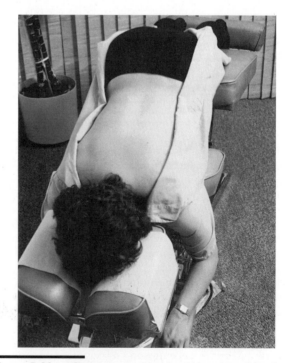

Figure 5.66.   Chiropractic tables should be adapted for the fully gravid uterus. This illustrates a pelvic elevation piece to accommodate a woman through full term.

Maternal concerns involve increasing intensity of uterine contractions, requiring greater maternal concentration and relaxation and breathing techniques, increased need for pain medications due to the intensity and therefore increased discomfort of the first stage of labor. All induction and augmentation procedures require close observation and monitoring of the mother and the fetus to avoid undesirable effects and therefore limit freedom of activity in labor.

Although the shortcomings of induction and augmentation are often inconsequential, for example, the procedure simply may not induce labor; it may cause a small amount of bloody or brownish vaginal discharge, often mistaken for bloody show; or it may rupture the membranes prematurely. These inherent dangers are of much greater importance. These perils consist of potential prolapse of the umbilical cord if artificial rupture of the membranes is performed when the presenting part is high or not well engaged, prolonged labor as a result of the domino effect of obstetrical interventions, genital and fetal infection after a long period of ruptured membranes, premature birth as a result of miscalculation of the expected date of confinement, and unexplained fetal death.

Failure of induction may be defined as occurring either when the uterus does not respond to stimulation at all or when the uterus contracts abnormally and the cervix does not dilate.

Contraindications for induction and augmentation of labor are a high presenting part, a fetal presentation other than vertex, an unripe cervix, and abnormal fetal heart rate.

Second Stage Labor

Physiologic Processes

The second stage of labor proceeds from the moment of full cervical dilatation and effacement to the birth of the baby. As the patient passes through the end of the first stage and into the second stage, the contractions become more frequent and are accompanied by some of the most intense pain of the entire labor.

This period is commonly termed *transition*. When the second stage is achieved, the subjective discomfort is considerably reduced.

The clinical indicators that the second stage has been initiated are described by a number of objective and subjective signs. There is typically an increase in the "bloody show" indicating increasing breakdown of the mucous plug. The patient expresses the need to "bear down" or push with each contraction. She perceives pressure on the rectum accompanied by the desire to defecate. Nausea and retching are frequent as the cervix approximates full dilatation. The patient's verbal noises become more guttural. An experienced midwife is easily able to determine the precise stage of labor simply by recognizing the types of sounds emitted by the laboring mother. These signs are not irrefutable. It may be necessary to confirm the condition of the cervix and station of the presenting part by rectal examination.

Normal Mechanism of the First and Second Stages of Labor

The process through which the neonate is delivered necessitates the baby adapting itself to and passing successfully through the maternal pelvis and birth canal.

Six movements outlining the mechanism of labor are obstetrically described (Fig. 5.67A-H). They comprise descent, flexion, internal rotation, extension, restitution, and external rotation. The anatomical and physiologic path of the delivery may be portrayed as tortuous, and certainly complex. This format describes the fetus in normal fetal position.

In primigravidas, considerable descent has occurred before labor (Fig. 5.67A). Descent is defined as incorporating engagement and, if there is no evidence of disproportion, descent should proceed during the actual process of engagement. In multiparous women, descent is more likely to be initiated during labor. The process of descent is stimulated by the downward pressure of the uterine contractions and the pushing efforts of the patient in the second stage of labor (Fig. 5.67B).

Flexion of the fetal head prevails before labor. Partial flexion is observed as the most natural fetal attitude in-utero. Increased fetal head flexion is caused by resistance to descent imposed by the osseous and articular pelvic structures. Normally, the occiput is anticipated to descend ahead of the sinciput, the posterior fontanelle should be inferior to the bregma and the fetal chin approximates its chest. This phase routinely occurs at the pelvic inlet, but may not resolve until the presenting part contacts the pelvic floor (Fig. 5.67C).

When the occiput reaches the pelvic floor of the levator ani muscles and fascia, the occiput rotates 45 degrees toward the midline. The sagittal suture of the fetal head turns from the oblique diameter to the anteroposterior diameter of the pelvis, either from ROA to OA or from LOA to OA. The occiput becomes proximate to the pubic symphysis and the sinciput to the sacrum. As the head rotates to the anteroposterior diameter of the maternal pelvis, the fetal shoulders remain in the oblique diameter. Therefore, the common relationship of the long axis of the head to the long axis of the shoulders is altered, and the neck undergoes a rotation of 45 degrees. This circumstance is sustained for the time period that the fetal head remains in the bony pelvis (Fig. 5.67D).

The etiology of the process of internal rotation is both osseous and soft tissue in nature. The ischial spines extend medially into the pelvic cavity. The lateral borders of the pelvis anterior to the ischial spines curve forward, inferior and medially. The pelvic floor, which is comprised of the levator ani muscles and associated fascia, inclines interior, anterior, and medial. The part of the fetal head that arrives first at the pelvic floor and ischial spines is rotated anteriorly by these structures. If the head is well flexed when it reaches the pelvic floor, the occiput encounters the pelvic floor first and is rotated anteriorly underneath the pubic symphysis. Summarily, the exact mechanism for internal rotation in labor is mostly anatomical conjecture. This stage is usually complete when the fetal head reaches the pelvic floor, or immediately

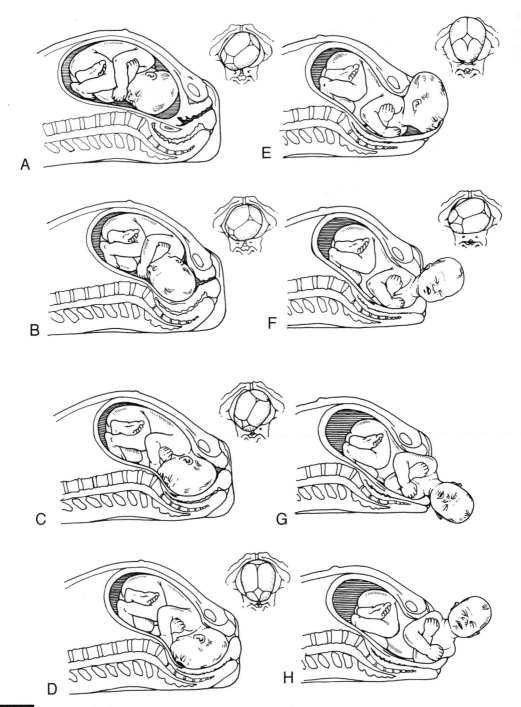

Figure 5.67. The labor and birth process. Modified from Cunningham FG, MacDonald PC, Gant NF, Leveno KJ, Gilstrap LC. Williams' Obstetrics, 19th ed., 1993:364. A, Onset of labor. B, Descent of the fetus. C, Flexion of the fetal head. D, Internal rotation of the fetal head. E, Extension of the fetal head. F, Restitution. The fetal head turns back toward the side. G, Delivery of the anterior shoulder. H, Delivery of the posterior shoulder.

following. Internal rotation occurs principally in the second stage of labor.

Extension may be viewed as the outcome of two forces. Here, the pelvic floor presents significant resistance as the uterine contractions relentlessly exercise downward pressure.

Because the posterior wall where the sacrum is located is much longer than the anterior wall at the pubic symphysis, the sinciput has a greater distance to proceed through than the occiput. With each contraction, the head advances and then recedes as the uterus relaxes in between contractions. Each time, a little advancement is gained. The introitus becomes an anteroposterior slit, then an oval, and finally a circular opening. The pressure of the fetal head thins out the perineum. Feces may be forced out of the mother's rectum. As the anus distends, the anterior wall of the rectum bulges through. With continued descent of the fetal head, the occiput comes to lie under the pubic symphysis. As the flexed head persists in its downward movement, the perineum bulges just before crowning. The occiput proceeds through the pelvic outlet, and the cervical curve pivots in the subpubic angle. At this point, the sinciput moves along the sacrum by a rapid process of head extension. Finally, a strong contraction forces the largest diameter of the head, usually the vertex through the vulva. This stage is called crowning. Once this has occurred there is no going back, and by a continued process of extension, the forehead, nose, mouth and chin appear over the perineum (Fig. 5.67E). At the stage where the head is passing through the introitus, the patient has the sensation of being torn apart. Laceration of the vulva sometimes occurs. To avoid tearing, the mother should pause at this point, to allow viscoelastic creep of the perineum. Massage is also helpful to stretch the perineum.

When the fetal head reaches the pelvic floor, the shoulders enter the pelvis. As the shoulders persist in the oblique diameter while the head rotates anteriorly, the neck becomes twisted. After delivery of the neonatal head, it then falls back toward the anus. Once it is out of the vagina, the head restitutes back 45 degrees as the neck untwists. The normal anatomical relationship of the head on the shoulders is attained (Fig. 5.67F).

A few moments after delivery of the head, external rotation takes place as the shoulders internally rotate from the oblique to the anteroposterior diameter of the pelvis. Generally, when the shoulders have been delivered, the rest of the neonate's body arrives rapidly. This process is summarized in Figures 5.67G and H. At this stage, full delivery of the baby is achieved.

Neonatology

Neonatology is defined as the art and clinical science of diagnosis, treatment, and care of the newborn infant. This section reviews the development and care of the infant from the moment of birth, through the consequential evolution of the neonatal first year.

Perinatology pertains to the specialty relating to the period shortly before and after birth. This is deemed to be from the twenty-ninth week of gestation to 1 to 4 weeks after birth.

Clinical Examination and Assessment of the Neonate

The newborn infant is routinely examined by a variety of people. The birth attendant will notice major congenital abnormalities, and the mother will closely scrutinize the baby for congenital defects, birthmarks, etc. Consequently most obvious defects will be detected shortly after birth. The newborn physical examination is the most valuable screening test performed at any time during life. The early detection of various occult abnormalities (congenital heart disease, hip dislocation, cataracts, etc.) can be made. This also includes the musculoskeletal, neurological and specifically vertebral subluxation or biomechanical complexes involving subluxation may allow early and effective treatment/correction before permanent damage or morbidity occurs.

The doctor of chiropractic has a crucial role in this assessment due to training and clinically acquired skills to determine problems otherwise undetected by the obstetric team.

The Apgar Score

The initial and most revealing assessment of the infant at birth uses the Apgar Score (Table 5.6). This appraisal was initially described by Apgar in 1953 (62).

The Apgar Score is a quantitative appraisal of the neonate, which is performed at 1 minute, 5 minutes, and if necessary, 10 minutes. This series of evaluations is considered to be the most current and optimal method of assessing the newborn infant's overall condition. Its reliability and reproducibility is based on accurate and objective performance of each of the five items at exactly 1 and 5 minutes. Herein lies its greatest value in assessing severity of asphyxia.

The recommended method for scoring the Apgar is by an equation of deleting points from 10 for a baby who appears healthy and in good condition at birth, and granting points from 0 for a baby who is depressed at birth.

The primary sign, which may be lost, and the last one to be regained after resuscitation, is muscle tone. Infant heart rate is considered to be the most singular sign of value in judging the need for resuscitation. The general sign of bradycardia of less than 100 beats per minute usually necessitates positive-pressure ventilation of the baby, performed by the neonatal team.

Table 5.6.   **Apgar Score**

Sign	0	1	2
Heart rate	Absent	<100 min	>100 min
Respiratory effort	Absent	Weak cry	Strong cry
Muscle tone	Limp	Some flexion	Good flexion
Reflex irritability	No response	Some motion	Cry
Color	Pale. Overall cyanosis	Centrally pink, periphery blue	Pink

An Apgar score, at 1 minute, of 7 to 10 is normal, 4 to 6 is moderately depressed, and 0 to 3 severely depressed. A significant number of infants can be successfully resuscitated despite an Apgar score of zero at birth and may sustain no long-term neurologic damage.

Although the Apgar is the most common test for assessing birth asphyxia, the doctor of chiropractic should be thoroughly familiar with the Apgar Score evaluation and its clinical implications. This is recommended as a routine question on the chiropractic case history to provide salient information regarding the functional status of the brain stem. Because a great body of research reveals the effects of birth trauma on the brain stem and upper spinal cord function, this is the singular most important initial assessment indicating the necessity for chiropractic evaluation and potential treatment.

Neonate Case History

The case history is of great value. The mandate to obtain all information indigenous to the pregnancy and birth history is inherent for all chiropractic professionals seeking to administer neonatal chiropractic care. A cursory modification of the typical adult case history is inadequate at best.

Accompanying the traditional format of information of the child's and parents' names, address and telephone, sex, date and place of birth, and ancillary information, it is vital to obtain the following detail. Procure the birth date and current age, the birth and current weight, and birth and current length, summarily to assist in assessing the infant's physical development and appraisal of whether it is thriving. The type of birth, either vaginal or by caesarean section, and whether forceps or ventouse extraction was used is relevant to understand the mechanisms of potential trauma to the baby. Also salient to this discernment is the presentation of the baby at birth, whether it was in a breech or vertex position, or in a transverse lie. If any sedation or anesthesia was applied, the type should be recorded. It is often of great benefit to inquire as to the place of birth; if a birthplace embraces more natural birthing philosophies, such as a birthing center or at a home, the propensity for resultant obstetrical interventions and subsequent birth trauma is highly diminished.

A detailed disclosure of the pregnancy, including a discussion of any problems encountered may be divided into the three trimesters for ease of assimilation of information. Such queries as to the duration of the pregnancy, the growth of the fetus and total maternal weight gain, maternal nutrition and exercise, ingestion of or exposure to any potentially harmful substances at any point during the pregnancy, the use of diagnostic techniques such as ultrasound or amniocentesis, the parity and gravidity of the mother, and any known fetal or maternal compromise or distress are of significance at this point. If there were Rh typing and serologic tests, pelvimetry, medications or radiographic procedures, these should be elaborated upon and noted. Conditions such as toxemia, gestational diabetes, elevated blood pressure, bleeding, vomiting, malnutrition and infectious processes should be more thoroughly questioned so that an intrinsic cognizance of the pregnancy in its entirety can be advanced.

After a fundamental understanding of the pregnancy, the labor and delivery should be reviewed in parallel detail. More important than the total length of the three stages of labor is an appreciation of the progress of the individual labor. How the labor was initiated (by contractions or membranes rupturing), what progress occurred during the first stage to full cervical dilation and effacement, what the symptoms of transition and the second stage involved, the fetal presentation and presenting part is important in overall elicitation. Any complications or concerns, particularly of fetal or maternal distress, what obstetrical procedures and interventions, if any, were employed, the state of the infant at birth, the need for resuscitation, the onset of respiration and the first cry, delivery of the placenta, and general management of the birth process are all questions of value that require specific explanations.

Apgar scores should be reviewed. In the instance in which a parent may not have knowledge of the actual scores, questioning as to how quickly the baby began to breathe on its own, how quickly it "pinked up," whether there were any emergent neonatal evaluations or procedures immediately after the birth process, when the infant was able to "latch on" to the breast and initiate the suckle reflex, etc. will provide clues as to the Apgar assessment. An inquiry as to the presence of either jaundice or cyanosis at birth is of assistance in determination of the infant's physiological function.

Any known congenital anomalies or defects should be considered before proceeding on to the physical examination. This includes the presence, suspected or confirmed, of any infectious process, neurologic disturbance, orthopedic condition, cardiovascular compromise, digestive disorders, kidney dysfunction, or immune function disturbance. The value of eliciting the greatest amount of information known to the parents or guardians and the caregivers cannot be overestimated because the neonate is unable to communicate on his or her own behalf.

Infant feeding, whether by breast or bottle, is relevant to the chiropractic examination to establish the probability for intact neurologic function. Critically, this knowledge also provides information as to spinal biomechanical efficiency. Because the physiology of infant feeding by the breast mandates symmetry, switching equally from side to side, there is a greater concern for potential vertebral subluxation complex in the bottle fed infant. This is due to the caregiver who will likely lapse into the prevalent one-sided feeding pattern and unintentionally lay the biomechanical framework for spinal compromise. Of course, nutritional considerations are also of consequence in any discussion of infant feeding. Any major changes in or allergies to formula should be registered. A chronicle of the infant's bowel and bladder habits is useful, including appearance, frequency, and any concerns. Young babies urinate frequently, the clinical parameters for the normal urine output of a newborn being 1–3 ml/kg/hr. As the normal newborn kidney has poor concentrating ability, this means that the neonate can urinate as frequently as 12 to 14 times in a 24-hour period. Two to four bowel movements and upward per day is considered to be healthy for the infant. The character of breastfed babies stool is mustard, very loose, and curd-like. Infants fed partially or completely on formula will exhibit darker, more formed stools with a noticeably stronger odor.

More important than the number of hours of sleep per night is the quality of sleep. This should be rated by the parent or guardian as good, fair, or poor, bearing in mind that it is customary and physiologically normal for the infant to have numerous periods of awakening for as long as it is being fed by the breast. Formulas currently being sold on the market exercise a tranquilizing effect on the infant (62). This effect is not noticed with the breastfed baby, therefore some deception of the sleeping pattern of the formula fed infant is apparent. Establishing so-called normal sleeping patterns is a complex act that is usually not completed until the child is between 4 and 6 years of age. It is unrealistic to expect a neonate, particularly younger than 1 year of age, to "sleep through the night."

The names and locations of the obstetrician or midwife, along with the pediatrician or family physician should be obtained, as well as the date of the most recent medical visit and the purpose. Inquiry as to the schedule of standard pediatric visitations is important, with specific questioning as to the quality of physical examinations already performed. This will facilitate the decision for any additional detailed examination procedures by the chiropractor such as hip joints evaluation or neurologic assessment. A knowledge of the standard and currently accepted pediatric testing procedures is imperative for interpretation and, if necessary, performance. If the infant has been treated on an emergency basis, this should be elaborated on at this time. Immunization history and public health nurse visits should be recorded if relevant.

If the infant is of an age in which developmental history is germane, it may be acquired at this juncture. This would encompass the age in weeks of response to sound, following an object with her/his eyes, holding the head up independently, sitting alone, crawling, standing, "cruising" (holding on to a piece of furniture while moving in an upright manner), and walking unassisted.

There should correspondingly be a section of the case history form where the parent or guardian can state whether the infant has experienced any subjective or objective complaints. These complaints or signs are derived from standard pediatric history protocol and can be summarized as follows:

1. Inability to suckle
2. Poor feeding
3. Regurgitation
4. Nasal congestion or discharge
5. Chest congestion or cough
6. Gasping, choking, or wheezing
7. Earaches
8. Poor sleeping patterns
9. Inconsolable crying
10. Inability or reluctance to move a limb
11. Digestive disorders
12. Vomiting
13. Constipation
14. Diarrhea
15. Poor weight gain
16. Colic
17. Allergies, including skin reactions
18. Hernia/ruptures
19. Heart condition
20. Respiratory condition
21. Orthopedic problems
22. Neurologic condition
23. Convulsions
24. Paralysis
25. Broken bones
26. Kidney dysfunction
27. Skin problems/rashes
28. Immunization reaction

Of greatest indulgence should be the detailed discussion of the presenting complaint, if any, following established protocol for case history investigation.

Some determination of socioeconomic status may be of benefit in assessing the infant's well-being. Be alert to any signs of child abuse (see Chapter 2), neglect, or psychological inability to cope on the part of the parents or guardians. The responsibility as primary health care practitioners mandates chiropractors to follow recommended guidelines and procedures for investigation and referral of potentially abusive situations.

Finally, any history of surgical procedures, medications, allergies to medications, accidents or traumatic injuries, and family history should be scrutinized.

Before administration of any pediatric examination or treatment procedures, a signed authorization for the care of a minor (i.e., informed consent) must be signed only by a parent or legal guardian, witnessed and dated. There are no legal jurisdictions in North America that would ignore the absence of this requirement in any legal circumstance.

Physical Examination

The neonate chiropractic clinical examination must be implemented in a logical sequence so that items are not omitted. A practical approach is the 'head to toe' technique. Whenever possible, the infant should be examined in the presence of at least one parent or guardian.

For a cogent examination to be performed, it is requisite to review the maternal and fetal history, labor and delivery process, and any known complications at birth. This is best accomplished through the taking of a thorough case history as described. It is critical to ensure that the infant is kept warm during the examination and that both the infant and parents are secure and comfortable with all clinical procedures. Explanation of all procedures prior to their performance and reassurance of the neonate's well-being is fundamental in a successful doctor-patient-parent relationship. The practitioner is presumably forging a long-term association with the infant, therefore the respect engendered by this goal is implicit. The infant should be treated as an individual whose feelings and sensibilities are well developed. A friendly, calm manner, quiet

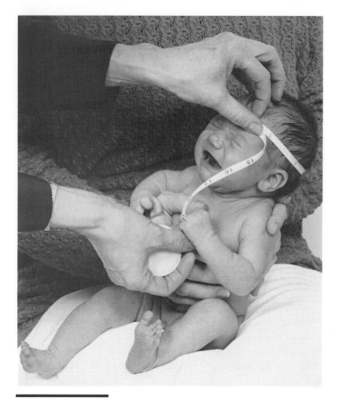

Figure 5.68.   Measurement of head circumference.

soothing voice, and slow and easy approach will facilitate a consonant initial introduction.

The infant should be held by the parent or guardian during the entire physical examination, with the exception of those tests that require the examiner to hold the baby solely. Being held in the primary caregiver's arms, either in a seated or supine position, assures the comfort of the young infant. The examination room temperature should be notably warm, as the neonate's ability to adapt to temperature changes is immature for the first few months of life. Flannel receiving blankets should be at hand to cover the baby when her/his clothes are removed for examination purposes.

Initial observation of the infant provides a great deal of information to the chiropractor. The comprehensive evaluation should include impressions from the time of initial introduction to the patient and not be solely based on the period during which the baby is being examined nor on specific tests that may occasionally be difficult to render. The opportunity to hold the baby provides further insight into assessment of muscular tone, strength, movements, and other activities. This should always be suggested respectfully, and only when the baby is calm and not exhibiting signs of fussiness. In addition, this is an opportune time to appraise the interaction between parent and child.

The Head

Note the shape of the head and determine the extent of cranial molding. Head circumference should be recorded as the maximum occipitofrontal circumference (Fig. 5.68). A num-

ber of measurements should be made and only the maximum or mean of the largest two measurements recorded.

Molding and caput succedaneum (edematous thickening of the scalp due to passage of through the vagina) is a normal, temporary asymmetry of the skull resulting from the birth process and prolonged engagement or labor. It is more common with vaginal delivery but may occur in caesarean delivery if labor was prolonged before delivery. This disappears within 2 to 3 days, and a completely normal shape is regained within 1 week. Cranial molding is largely influenced by the fetal position in the third trimester and during the birth process (Fig. 5.69).

Plagiocephaly (parallelogram head) is characterized by a flattening of the occipital region on one side. The etiology is suspected to be a result of the position the infant has been lying in-utero and is medically considered to have no pathologic significance. However, chiropractically, the significance is great due to remodeling of the occipital condyles. Anderson states that basioccipital angulation occurred in nearly 60% of the cases (64). Moreover, he suggests that right-handed dominance can impel the cervical spine toward permanent distortion with persistent tension of the left-sided musculature, corollary to structural deviation. When seen in older children, plagiocephaly presents with a cervical torticollis with biomechanical restriction of neck rotation on the ipsilateral side as the occipital flattening.

Scaphocephaly describes an elongated head with flattening of the bones in the temporoparietal regions. This condition is seen frequently in premature infants and dissipates somewhat with age, although the cranial configuration causes concern to

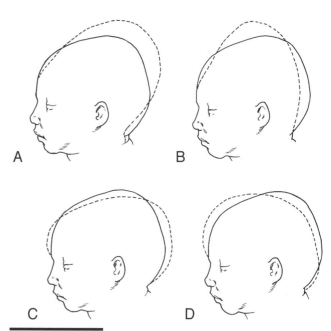

Figure 5.69.   Cranial molding according to fetal position A, Left occiput anterior [LOA]. B, Right occiput posterior [ROP]. C, Facial presentation (full extension). D, Brow presentation (partial extension).

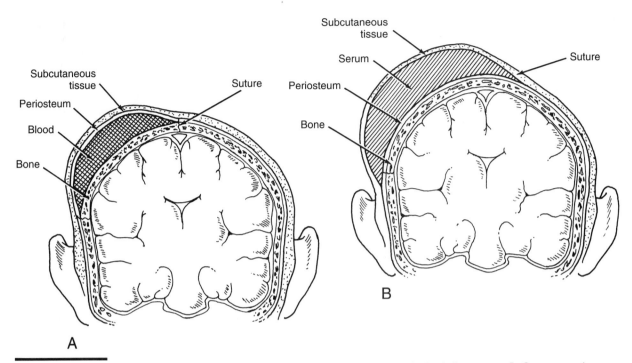

Figure 5.70. Differentiation between caput succedaneum and cephalhematoma. A, Cephalhematoma. B, Caput succedaneum.

practitioners of cranial therapies, and to a lesser degree, of biomechanical techniques.

Cephalhematoma is the term applied to a condition that transpires when there is bleeding over the outer surface of a skull bone elevating the periosteum. The hemorrhage causes a soft, fluctuant swelling confined to the limits of the bone. It is occasionally bilateral but only crosses the midline in the uncommon occipital variety. Figure 5.70 illustrates the distinctions between cephalhematoma and caput succedaneum.

The cranial fontanelles are the membrane-covered spaces located at the junction of the skull sutures observed at birth and into the neonate year. The anterior and posterior fontanelles vary in size and are normally soft and flat. Slight visible pulsations over the anterior fontanelle are considered a normal finding in infants. Fontanelle tension is best determined with the child calm and in a sitting position. Gentle palpation by the examiner's first two digits is performed over each of the fontanelles (Fig. 5.71 A, B). Slight pulsations over the anterior fontanelle may occur in normal neonates. When bulging of either fontanelle is observed, this may be due to raised intracranial pressure, meningitis, or hydrocephalus and should always be referred for neonatology examination. A large anterior fontanelle is also seen with hypothyroidism. Depressed or sunken fontanelles are seen with dehydration. In early neonatal development, the fontanels expand under normal tension as the brain's growth-rate transiently excels that of the skull. A positive Macewen sign may be evident normally until fontanelle closure. This is characterized by a "cracked pot" sound when the cranium is percussed with the examining finger. The anterior fontanelle usually closes at 9 to 12 months and the posterior fontanelle at 2 to 4 months. A third fontanelle between the anterior and posterior is present in approximately

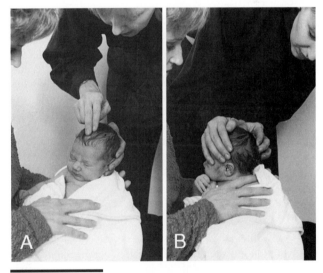

Figure 5.71. Palpation of the cranial fontanelles. A, Anterior fontanelle. B, Posterior fontanelle.

6% of infants and is more apt to occur in infants with various abnormalities.

Craniosynostosis refers to premature fusion of one or more of the sutures of the cranial bones. The sagittal suture is most commonly involved, although any of the skull bones may be affected. If facial bones are affected, dysmorphism is a usual sequel. This is seen in Crouzon's disease. Craniosynostosis should be considered in any neonate with an asymmetric cranium. The anterior fontanelle usually palpates as noticeably small with a ridged suture. It may be impossible to move the cranial bones freely. Craniosynostosis causes abnormal head growth; the head often becomes scaphocephalic when the sagittal suture is involved. Radiographic examination will confirm the synostosis upon suspicion of this condition. Medical treatment uses neurosurgical release of the fused bones.

The term craniotabes (ping-pong ball skull) is assigned to the softening of the skull bones, and where, with pressure the skull may be momentarily indented before springing out again. Slight indentation and recoil of the parietal bones is elicited by lightly pressing with the thumb. It is most commonly seen in preterm infants but also occurs in normal neonates for the first 2 to 4 months of life. Its major clinical significance is with congenital rickets. Rarely, osteogenesis imperfecta or congenital hypophosphatasia may be causes.

Persistent recumbence of the newborn in either lateral position commonly results in a flattening or skew of the facial or cranial bones, frequently coupled with cervical torticollis. This is often observed in the chiropractic office and should be addressed from a biomechanical mien. Manual cervical traction should be considered a valuable part of the treatment. The parents should be advised of the importance of ensuring that the baby is symmetrically balanced in all prolonged positions, whether recumbent, seated in a car seat, held, or fed.

Facies

Recognizable patterns of abnormalities based on facial features vary extensively. These are rare and not often seen in chiropractic offices. Such chromosomal disorders as trisomies 21 (Down Syndrome), 18 (Edward's Syndrome), and 13 (Patau's Syndrome) should be recognized. In addition, the following are often obvious: fetal alcohol syndrome, Crouzon's syndrome, Treacher-Collins' syndrome, and Potter's syndrome.

Because babies prefer to breathe through their noses, when respiratory distress is present, bilateral choanal atresia should be suspected. This is a clinical sign often indicative of a more severe syndrome, such as encountered in the rare Charge syndrome.

Color

Color is an integral assessment of the neonate's well-being. A uniform pinkness should be observed; however, acrocyanosis characterized by blueness of the hands and feet is not abnormal. Generalized or central cyanosis including the tongue and lips is caused by low oxygen saturation in the blood and may be associated with congenital heart disease or lung disease. This, as well as pallor, jaundice, plethora (brick-red color), bruises and petechial hemorrhages are abnormal and should be referred. Mottling or a lacy red pattern may be seen in a normal infant or in one with cold stress, hypovolemia, or sepsis.

Position

Overall posture and range of spontaneous movements should be observed and recorded throughout the examination. The neonate resting posture exhibits flexed, somewhat hypertonic extremities (Fig. 5.72). The fists are normally clenched until as

late as 2 months postnatally. Asymmetries of the skull, face, jaw or extremities may result from in-utero constraint. Limited movement, exaggerated or asymmetrical movements, hypotonia or stiffness must be investigated further. The Dubowitz Neurodevelopmental Protocol as described later in this chapter is helpful in evaluating infant position.

Cry

The infant's noise should be brisk, vigorous and sustained after stimulation, but consolability should be attained through comfort and cuddling. One should be alerted by a weak or high-pitched cry, which is usually considered abnormal. Hoarseness is also abnormal. Inconsolable crying is one of the pathognomonic signs of colic.

Skin

Contingent on gestational age, skin appearances vary greatly. Full or over-term babies often illustrate degrees of mild to moderate peeling. Milia is a rash in which tiny sebaceous retention cysts are evident. They appear as whitish, pinhead-sized concretions, most often found on the chin, nose, forehead, and cheeks. They are benign and disappear within a few weeks. The skin of the face should be washed with warm water only and a simple mineral oil applied if dryness persists.

Erythema toxicum describes numerous small areas of red skin, visualized with a yellowish white papule in the center. They are most observed at 48 hours but can appear as late as 7 to 10 days. The rash resolves spontaneously.

Macular hemangioma, commonly referred to as "stork bites" is normally seen on the occipital area, eyelids, and glabella. The lesions are of no clinical significance and most disappear spontaneously within the first year of life.

Mongolian spots are seen as flat, large, dark blue or purple macular spots resembling bruises, most frequently located over the lumbar spine sacrum. They are demonstrated in 90% of the black and oriental population and in 10% of caucasian infants. They disappear usually by 4 years of age and have no pathologic significance. Abnormal appearances, pigmentation and naevi may present and require referral.

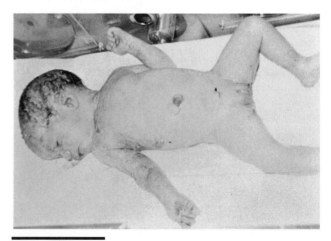

Figure 5.72. The neonate's normal resting posture with limbs flexed.

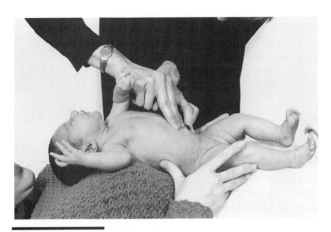

Figure 5.73. Abdominal palpation.

Chest

Symmetrical contours should be uniformly observed in the chest, and respiratory movements should be well perceived and equivalent. Of clinical note is pectus excavatum, which is observed as an alteration in the shape of the sternum. It is of no clinical significance, however, auscultation should be performed for confirmation of symmetric breath sounds. The breasts of a newborn are often abnormally enlarged secondary to the effects of maternal estrogen. This is also of no clinical concern and customarily lasts for less than 1 week.

In assessing the cardiovascular system, the normal neonate heart rate varies between 100 and 175 per minute and decreases normally to 90 per minute during restful sleep. Palpation of peripheral pulses includes radial and femoral pulses, which should be consistently steady and regular. Any alteration from normal pulse rhythm and intensity may indicate a congenital anomaly of the heart or aorta and require referral. The apical heart beat is positioned at the fourth intercostal space in the midclavicular line. Auscultation producing a systolic murmur is possibly normal within the first 24 hours of life. A gallop or triple rhythm is abnormal and should be referred.

Abdomen

A brief, but precise palpation of the abdomen can be succinctly revealing (Fig. 5.73). The examiner should start in the upper abdominal quadrants and work down to the lower abdominal quadrants, using both light and deep palpation. Any abdominal distention insinuates an intestinal obstruction or intra-abdominal mass. Umbilical hernias are commonly seen in the first 2 years of life and usually resolve spontaneously (Fig. 5.74). Detection of a hernia, unilateral or bilateral, warrants referral.

Lymphatic System

Lymph nodes should be palpated and noted for any irregular masses or swelling (Fig. 5.75). The axillary and femoral lymph nodes should be barely discernible. The posterior cervical lymph nodes will be present only with infection. There are

lymph nodes located above the superior nuchal line bilaterally on the occiput. These are considered to be normal, if small, and disappear spontaneously within the first year of life.

Neurological Examination

The neurological assessment is an essential component of the examination process and deserves to be thoroughly performed and assimilated into the comprehensive clinical understanding of the neonate's well being (see Chapter 13).

Initially, the infant's responses and movements should be annotated on observation of interaction with the parent and the examiner. Muscular tone may be assessed by the baby's resistance to passive movements or gravity. Sensory examination may be performed by pin prick or from pressure on the palms of the hands and soles of the feet. Fussiness or crying, then withdrawal of the legs is displayed. The overall state of alertness should be appraised by observing any evidence of hyper-irritability or lethargy. When per-

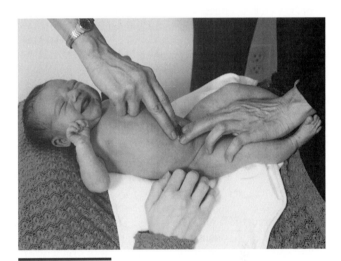

Figure 5.74. Examination for umbilical hernia.

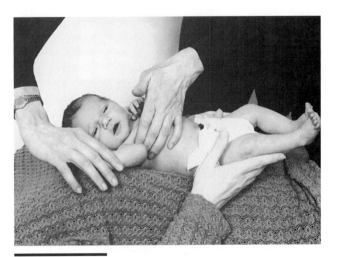

Figure 5.75. Palpation for axillary lymph nodes.

forming a neurologic evaluation, the behavioral condition of the infant will affect the neurologic signs elicited. The behavioral state of the neonate may be considered using the classification of Brazelton:

State 1. Quiet sleep. Regular breathing, eyes closed, no spontaneous movement.

State 2. Active sleep. Eyes closed, rapid eye movements, irregular respiration, some movement.

State 3. Semi-wakefulness. Eyes open or closed, variable activity, usually smooth muscular movements.

State 4. Awake and alert. Bright look, minimal motor activity.

State 5. Awake and eyes open but considerable motor activity. Less cooperative.

State 6. Crying.

It is best to assess neurobehavioral elements and tone in state 3, 4, or 5. Cerebral function is most efficiently tested through observation of general behavior, including but not limited to level of consciousness, orientation, spontaneous movements, cortical sensory interpretation, posture and character of cry. Resting tone should display flexion of the upper and lower extremities.

The tongue may be briefly examined for evidence of atrophy or fasciculations, which may suggest a lower motor neuron lesion.

CRANIAL NERVES

The cranial nerves are easy to assess in the neonate. The procedures used for testing each of these 12 nerves are much the same as in the adult. The examination should include observation for spontaneous extraocular movements and ptosis. Cognizance of crying and smiling movements is helpful in assessing the facial nerve. Healthy rooting, sucking, swallowing and gag reflexes demonstrate competence of cranial nerves V, VII, IX, X, and XII. The optic nerve or second cranial nerve requires adaptation of evaluation. The infantile reflex known as the blink response helps indicate visual acuity, and an opthalmoscopic examination may be performed to view the inner eye structures (Fig. 5.76). The eighth cranial nerve or the vestibulocochlear nerve is the most difficult to test. The acoustic blink infant response is of some value in ferreting out gross hearing loss, and an otoscopic examination can also be integrated into this portion of the examination (Fig. 5.77).

INFANT NEUROLOGIC REFLEXES

ROOTING

The rooting reflex is an excellent indicator of general central nervous system function. It is imperative to allow the infant to feed spontaneously to stimulate the sucking response. The examiner's finger should firmly stroke above the ramus of the

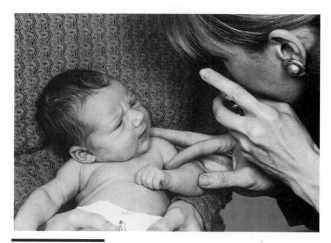

Figure 5.76.   Ophthalmoscopic examination of the neonate. This assists in evaluating the function of the second cranial nerve.

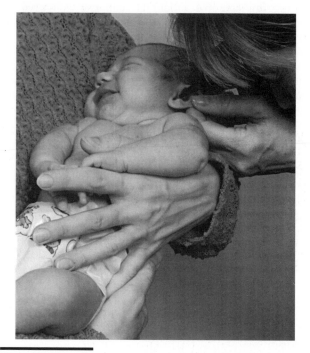

Figure 5.77.   Otoscopic examination of the neonate.

mandible from the zygoma towards the mouth. The infant should respond with a definitive "rooting" or movement of the mouth towards the finger (Fig. 5.78). The movement should be a gross movement with no hesitation or uncertainty. This is performed bilaterally. This reflex is present immediately after birth and usually disappears by the third to fourth month. Rooting may continue during sleep for the first 6 months of life.

SUCKING

The sucking response is also critical for spontaneous feeding of the new infant and is an assessment of central nervous system function. The examiner should insert a clean finger with the pad of the finger into the newborn's mouth. The finger should lightly touch the hard palate. The examiner should be feel an enthusiastic sucking response, with the finger being drawn inwards and upwards (Fig. 5.79). This reflex presents immediately after birth and is seen well into the third or fourth month of life.

BLINK

This response assesses a limited level of visual acuity. A bright light is shone into the eyes of the infant. The normal response is a tight shutting of the eyes (Fig. 5.80).

ACOUSTIC BLINK

This response tests auditory function to a limited degree. Absence of this response may indicate partial or total hearing loss. The examiner should create a sharp, loud noise away from the infant's visual gaze. This may be the shutting of a door or clapping the hands (Fig. 5.81). The neonate should respond by blinking the eyes bilaterally and/or "startling" which may produce a partial Moro response. This reflex is present immediately after birth and disappears gradually as the startle response starts to wane. This response is also known as the cochleopalpebral test.

MORO RESPONSE

This is considered to be the most critical of neonatal neurologic tests to evaluate. Often, performance of this singular assessment will provide comprehensive insight into the neonate's neurological status. This evaluation is the most complex of infant neurologic reflexes. The infant should be supported securely in a supine position with both of the examiner's hands underneath. The examiner's hands then bring or "drop" the infant quickly downwards to alter the position of the neonate's head by one to two centimeters. Initially, the examiner looks for symmetrical extension and full ab-

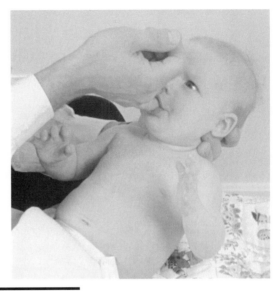

Figure 5.79. Sucking reflex. The examiner's finger should be drawn back and up toward the soft palate.

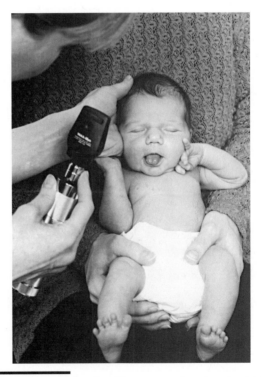

Figure 5.80. Blink reflex. The neonate shuts its eyes tightly in response to a concentrated light source directed at the eyes.

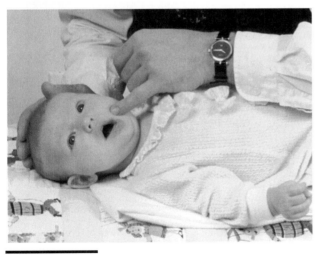

Figure 5.78. Rooting response. Enthusiastic rooting towards the stimulus is anticipated.

duction of the arms bilaterally, concomitant with extension of the trunk and flexion of the knees and hips (Fig. 5.82A). The hands should illustrate a prominent spreading or extension of the fingers. This will be followed shortly by adduction of the arms into an "embrace" position and, occasionally, crying (Fig. 5.82B). Lack or reduction of upper

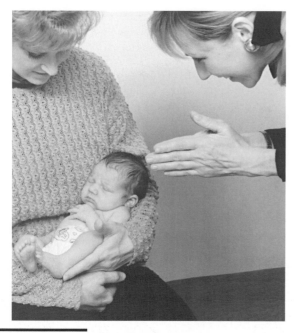

Figure 5.81.   The acoustic blink reflex. The neonate blinks in response to a loud noise.

extremity response, or asymmetry may indicate a hemiparesis or injury to the brachial plexus (Fig. 5.82C). Inappropriate response, particularly asymmetry in the lower extremities, may signify congenital hip dislocation or lower spinal cord injury. The Moro response should be observed from immediately after birth with gradual diminishment until 4 months of age. This test is also known as the "startle" reflex and should not be performed in an overexaggerated manner as it can be frightening for the baby. *Note*: It is within normal limits to witness an upgoing Babinski reflex and/or several beats of clonus.

GALANT'S TEST

This test is performed to assess for any presence of spinal cord lesion. The neonate should be held in a prone position supported securely from underneath the abdomen by the examiner's hands. The examiner should unilaterally stroke the paraspinal musculature from the cervical region to the iliac crest. The anticipated response is that of extension and lateral flexion of the head and trunk towards the ipsilateral side of the stimulus (Fig. 5.83). This should be executed bilaterally. This reaction is present from birth to 8 weeks of age. Another name for this test is the trunk incurvation test.

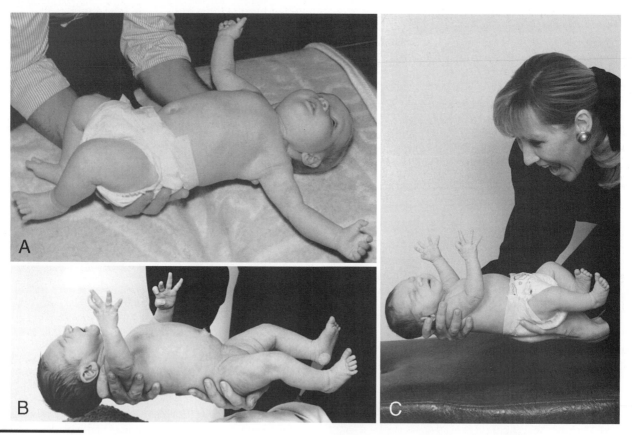

Figure 5.82.   A, Moro response. First phase of symmetrical abduction and extension of the upper extremities with extension of the trunk and flexion of the lower extremities. B, Moro response. Second phase illustrating the upper extremities returning to the thorax in adduction as "though in an embrace." C, An inappropriate Moro response would exhibit asymmetry of the upper extremities or lower extremities.

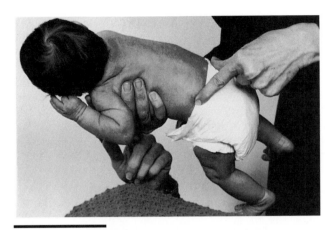

Figure 5.83. Galant's test or trunk incurvation test.

the contralateral side. This imitates the "fencing" posture. This test is performed bilaterally and should not always be reproducible with subsequent testings. An obligate or persistent tonic neck reflex is always abnormal. An obligate tonic neck reflex describes the abnormal maintenance of the tonic neck posture for the duration of head rotation. Asymmetry, which is consonant, may indicate hemiparesis of the ipsilateral side of persistent response. A test that is persistently present after 6 months of age is considered abnormal and may suggest cerebral dysfunction. The normal response is expected to appear from the second week through to the sixth month of age. This reflex is most conspicuous during the second month of life and infants may assume it extemporaneously.

NECK RIGHTING

This response is evaluated by rotating the head of the infant to one side. The neonate may be in either a supported upright or supine position. The anticipated reaction is ipsilateral rotation of the trunk. This reflex appears when the asymmetric tonic neck reflex (ATNR) disappears at approximately 4 months, when the infant starts to roll over on its own. Healthy infants display a neck righting reflex until 8 to 10 months of age, after which it becomes part of voluntary activity.

PLACING RESPONSE

The neonate is held in an upright position, supported by the examiner's hands around the torso. The dorsum of one foot is then lightly rubbed on the underside of a surface, such as an examining table. The infant should flex the knee and bring the foot up onto the surface (Fig. 5.84A). This is followed by the other foot replicating the response (Fig. 5.84B). Inadequate response may suggest paresis or hip dislocation. This reflex should be apparent from immediately after birth to approximately the sixth week.

PARACHUTE REFLEX

The neonate should be suspended in a prone position, supported securely around the torso by the examiner's hands (Fig. 5.85). The infant should be "plunged" downwards for 3–4 centimeters. The anticipated response is extension of the arms downwards, with hands and fingers extended, as though to "break a fall." This reflex appears at 6 to 8 months of age and is thoroughly developed by 1 year. This reflex is an excellent test of upper extremity pyramidal function. Asymmetry may be a sign of hemiparesis.

ASYMMETRIC TONIC NECK REFLEX

Also known as the ATNR, this test is performed with the infant in a supine position. The examiner gently rotates the head to one side, looking for a response of extension of the upper and lower extremity on the ipsilateral side of rotation, and flexion of the upper and lower extremity on

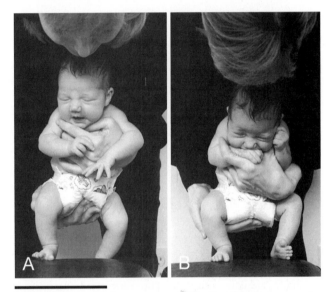

Figure 5.84. Placing response. A, The first foot steps up onto the surface. B, The second foot follows to place itself onto the surface.

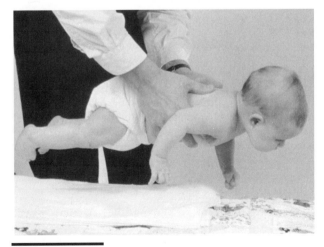

Figure 5.85. The parachute repines.

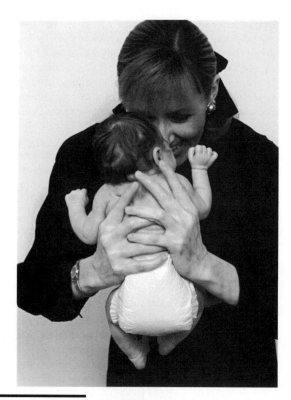

Figure 5.86.   Vertical suspension.

VERTICAL SUSPENSION

This procedure, also known as the Landau maneuver, evaluates the potential for hip joint dysfunction, hypotonia, and spastic paraplegia or diplegia (Fig. 5.86). The examiner should support the upright infant securely around the torso, then raise the baby suddenly upwards. The anticipated response is bilateral flexion of the hips and knees. When a diminished or absent response is noted, the examiner may observe scissoring or adduction of the lower extremities or fixed leg extension. This reflex is normally observed from birth to the sixth month of age.

PALMAR GRASP

The examiner should place a finger into the palm of the neonate's hand. The infant should respond by tightly curling the digits and thumb around the examining finger. The dorsal surface of the hand should never be touched. This response should be observed from immediately after birth and dissipates gradually over the first 6 months of life. A persistent "fistlike" presentation of the hands during waking hours beyond the second month may indicate a central nervous system disorder or cerebral lesion, such as cerebral palsy.

DIGITAL RESPONSE

The neonate's forearm is stroked over the ulnar nerve distribution from proximal to distal towards the hand. The anticipated response is a fistlike curling of the hand with slight extension of the thumb (Fig. 5.87). This response is expected

from birth through the first 6 months. The neonate should be able to grasp objects by 5 months of age. Opposition of the thumb and finger in a grasp commences at approximately 6 months of age, increasing until full development at 1 year. The infant is capable of transferring objects from one hand to the other at approximately 8 months of age. The predilection to become "one handed" is evident by 1 year of age. Any time earlier in the first year of life, the tendency to use one hand exclusively should provide suspicion of neurologic dysfunction.

TRACTION RESPONSE

The neonate is placed in the supine position. The examiner gently pulls the arms upwards to induce the infant towards a sitting position. The normal response is an initial head lag, followed by active flexion to the midline for a few seconds, then the head falls forward.

DEEP TENDON REFLEXES

This aspect of the neurologic test is diverse according to the state of reflex maturation. The deep tendon reflexes in the neonate may be tested with the reflex instrument applied over the examiner's thumb or finger overlying the tendon (Figs. 5.88, 5.89). The reflex response should be brisk and easily palpated under the examiner's thumb. A diverse response is anticipated because of immature development of the corticospinal tract in the neonate. A positive response should always be confirmed by repeated and comprehensive neurologic testing (Figs. 5.90, 5.91). The triceps reflex is difficult to elicit in the first 6 months of life due to predominance of flexor tone. A crossed adductor reflex may present with the patellar reflex. This reflex illustrates contraction of the hip adductors bilaterally when the stimulus is applied. This response is expected to disappear by 8 months of age. Presence beyond then may indicate pyramidal anterior cortical spinal tract dysfunction.

The superficial abdominal reflexes should be evaluated in all

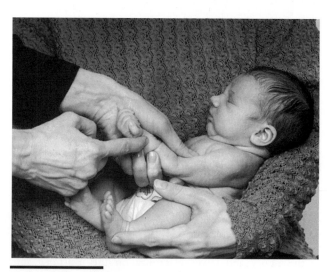

Figure 5.87.   Digital response.

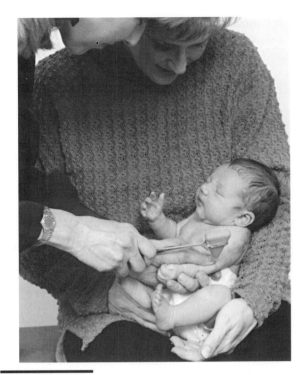

Figure 5.88. Elicitation of the biceps deep tendon reflex.

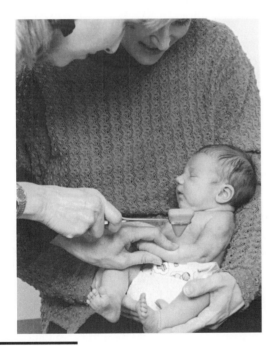

Figure 5.89. Elicitation of the coracobrachialis deep tendon reflex.

T10–T12 levels in the lower quadrants. A reduced or absent reflex may indicate a central motor lesion os spinal cord lesion of the involved vertebral/nerve segment.

Clonus may normally be present in the first 2 to 4 months of life. The Babinski response has received some scrutiny as to its validity, although it is considered by most authorities to be normal for the first year of life. This pathologic reflex is elicited by stroking the plantar surface of the foot from the heel towards the toes (Fig. 5.92). The anticipated response is extension and fanning of the toes with a flexor response of the big toe. If this response is asymmetrical, too easily elicited, or associated with other suspicious neurologic findings, further investigation is warranted.

DUBOWITZ NEURODEVELOPMENTAL PROTOCOL

The Dubowitz Neurodevelopmental protocol provides a concise method for documentation of the neurologic behaviors of

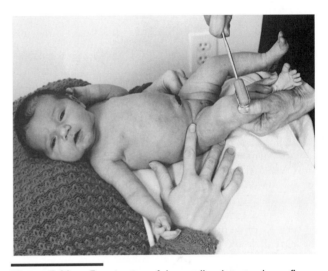

Figure 5.90. Examination of the patellar deep tendon reflex.

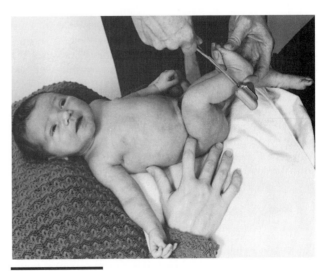

Figure 5.91. Achilles deep tendon reflex.

four quadrants. With the infant lying in a supine position, the examiner should firmly stroke from the lateral corner of each of the quadrants towards the umbilicus. A definitive deviation of the umbilicus towards the stimulation is anticipated. The T8–T10 spinal levels are tested in the upper quadrants, and the

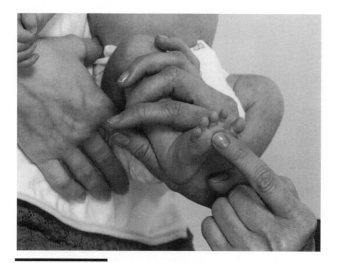

Figure 5.92.   Babinski response.

the neonate at specific intervals. The Dubowitz protocol chart details four groups of items (Table 5.7).

Habituation evaluates the infant's decrease in response to repetitive auditory and visual stimuli. The presence of habituation is not considered to be a reliable test of neurologic integrity on its own merit, but represents a cursory view into neurologic response.

Movement and tone assess the degree of resistance to passive movement. The presence of tremors, startles, or abnormal movements during testing should be noted appropriately. The diagram that corresponds to the neonate's pattern is ringed on the proforma. Irritable or colicky infants may display extensor posturing with arching of the back, opisthotonus, scissoring of the legs and thumbs tightly adducted across the palm, and need to be differentiated from true neurologic compromise.

Reflexes are classified according to the most fundamental relative to this protocol.

Neurobehavioral items are significant to evaluate higher cerebral function. The state of the infant as classified according to Brazelton becomes critical in appropriate assessment. A red woolen ball, held 15–25 cm from the infant's eyes is recommended as the visual stimulus. Consolability measures the ability of the infant to be consoled by the examiner if he/she has attained state 6.

In recording this protocol, responses to the left of the midline of the chart illustrate infants who tend to be floppy and apathetic. Responses to the right of the midline of the chart display hypertonic, irritable babies. The state of the infant must be recorded initially to establish parameters for anticipated normal reactions.

Spinal Examination

The patient should be unclothed and comfortably settled in a parent/caregiver's arms. Evaluation of the spine must encompass the entirety of examination procedures including obser-

vation, static palpation, motion palpation, range of motion, and spinal percussion.

Observation of symmetry of bone development and muscular tone provides the examiner with information salient to the potential for vertebral subluxation complex, as well as for other physical infirmities. Assessment of the level of development of the postural curves should be recorded; the secondary curves of the cervical and lumbar lordoses may be at early levels of evolution at birth. Scrutiny for webbed neck, spina bifida, tufts of hair, mongolian spots, and pilonidal dimple or cysts should be integrated into this portion of the examination. Palpation is best performed with the infant in a relaxed position against the chest of the parent, who may be seated or recumbent. Neonates consistently exhibit a definite preference of either the prone or supine position. It is advised to initiate the spinal examination in the position least favored and complete it in the position most favored. The infant will easily communicate which is the preferred position through restlessness of movements and fussiness.

Palpation should be initiated with static evaluation to establish the anatomical landmarks as a baseline for spinal assessment. Rigidity or unusual gross alignment should be perceived. Isolation of each vertebral segment and motor unit is requisite. Fulfilment of an acute biomechanical understanding of the structural and functional components must be attained. The examiner should use any combination of the first digits, or the thumbs and first digits as accurately as possible to determine the structures being palpated (Fig. 5.93). In the cervical spine, it is often most facile to have the patient in either a supported, seated position or prone position with the neck in slight anterior flexion to expose the vertebral articulations for static palpation. The thoracic spine best accommodates itself to palpation in the prone position, as the spinal postural muscles are not working to maintain the infant in an upright attitude (Fig. 5.94). This also applies to static palpation of the lumbar and sacral regions. If lying on the mother, the baby may often seek comfort in nursing while this portion of the examination is being carried out (Fig. 5.95). This does not compromise the quality of the examination in any way and ensures that the infant will cooperate throughout the balance of the spinal evaluation.

Motion palpation to assess spinal function is imperative; joint play must be arrantly noted. In the cervical spine, the parent should assist in stabilization of the infant by firmly but gently supporting the chest. When passive rotation or lateral flexion are introduced into the head and neck, there is a propensity for the infant to roll or move in the direction of motion. This is attributable to the neck righting reflex. The examiner's hands should embrace the infant's head and stabilize the cranium while the first digits introduce motion and joint play with bilateral, birotational and flexion/extension movements (Fig. 5.96). In the thoracic region, the parent may provide stabilization by holding the neonate's hands or buttocks. Joint movement must be elicited and discerned in a posterior to anterior manner, as this is the most commonly noted kinesiopathology in the pediatric vertebral subluxation complex. This should be performed with the tip of the index finger or the thumb, either singly or doubly. Lateral movement

Table 5.7. Dubowitz Neurodevelopmental Protocol

NAME _____ DOB/TIME _____ WEIGHT _____

NO. _____ DATE OF EXAM _____ HEIGHT _____

RACE _____ SEX _____ AGE _____ HEAD CIRC. _____

GESTATIONAL SCORE WEEKS
ASSESSMENT

STATES
1. Deep sleep, no movement, regular breathing.
2. Light sleep, eyes shut, some movement.
3. Dozing, eyes opening and closing.
4. Awake, eyes open, minimal movement.
5. Wide awake, vigorous movement.
6. Crying.

Columns: STATE | ASYMMETRY | COMMENT

HABITUATION (<state 3)

LIGHT Repetitive flashlight stimuli (10) with 5-sec gap. Shutdown = 2 consecutive negative responses	No response.	A. Blink response to first stimulus only. B. Tonic blink response. C. Variable response.	A. Shutdown of movement but blink persists 2–5 stimuli. B. Complete shutdown 2–5 stimuli.	A. Shutdown of movement but blink persists 6–10 stimuli. B. Complete shutdown 6–10 stimuli.	A. Equal response to 10 stimuli. B. Infant comes to fully alert state. C. Startles + major responses throughout.
RATTLE Response stimuli (10) with 5-sec gap	No response.	A. Slight movement to first stimuli. B. Variable response.	Startle or movement 2–5 stimuli, then shutdown.	Startle or movement 6–10 stimuli, then shutdown.	A B} Grading as above. C

MOVEMENT AND TONE

Undress infant.

POSTURE (At rest—predominant)

*

(hips abducted)   (hips abducted)   (hips adducted)

Abnormal postures:
A. Opisthotonus.
B. Unusual leg extension.
C. Asymm. tonic neck reflex.

Table 5.7.   *(continued)* **Dubowitz Neurodevelopmental Protocol**

					S C A
ARM RECOIL Infant supine. Take both hands, extend parallel to the body; hold approx. 2 sec. and release.	No flexion within 5 sec.	Partial flexion at elbow >100° within 4–5 sec.	Arms flex at elbow to <100° within 2–3 sec.	Difficult to extend; arm snaps back forcefully.	
ARM TRACTION Infant supine; head midline; grasp wrist, slowly pull arm to vertical. Angle of arm scored and resistance noted at moment infant is initially lifted off and watched until shoulder off mattress. Do other arm.	Arm remains fully extended.	Weak flexion maintained only momentarily.	Arm flexed at elbow to 140° and maintained 5 sec.	Arm flexed at approx. 100° and maintained.	Strong flexion of arm <100° and maintained.
LEG RECOIL First flex hips for 5 sec. Then extend both legs of infant by traction on ankles; hold down on the bed for 2 secs. and release.	No flexion within 5 sec.	Incomplete flexion of hips within 5 sec.	Complete flexion within 5 sec.	Instantaneous complete flexion.	Legs cannot be extended; snap back forcefully.

LEG TRACTION
Infant supine. Grasp leg near ankle and slowly pull toward vertical until buttocks 1–2″ off. Note resistance at knee and score angle. Do other leg.

No flexion.

Partial flexion, rapidly lost.

Knee flexion 140–160° and maintained.

Knee flexion 100–140° and maintained.

Strong resistance; flexion <100°.

POPLITEAL ANGLE
Infant supine. Approximate knee and thigh to abdomen; extend leg by gentle pressure with index finger behind ankle.

180–160°

150–140°

130–120°

110–90°

<90°

HEAD CONTROL (post. neck m.) Grasp infant by shoulders and raise to sitting position; allow head to fall forward; wait 30 sec.

No attempt to raise head.

Unsuccessful attempt to raise head upright.

Head raised smoothly to upright in 30 sec. but not maintained.

Head raised smoothly to upright in 30 sec. but maintained.

Head cannot be flexed forward.

HEAD CONTROL (ant. neck m.) Allow head to fall backward as you hold shoulders; wait 30 sec.

Grading as above.

Grading as above.

Grading as above.

Grading as above.

Table 5.7. (continued) Dubowitz Neurodevelopmental Protocol

						S	C	A
HEAD LAG Pull infant toward sitting posture by traction on both wrists. Also note arm flexion.	*							
VENTRAL SUSPENSION Hold infant in ventral suspension; observe curvature of back, flexion of limbs and relation of head to trunk.	*							
HEAD RAISING IN PRONE POSITION Infant in prone position with head in midline.	No response.	Rolls head to one side.	Weak effort to raise head and turns raised head to one side.	Infant lifts head, nose and chin off.	Strong prolonged head lifting.			
ARM RELEASE IN PRONE POSITION Head in midline. Infant in prone position; arms extended alongside body with palms up.	No effort.	Some effort and wriggling.	Flexion effort but neither wrist brought to nipple level.	One or both wrists brought at least to nipple level without excessive body movement.	Strong body movement with both wrists brought to face or "press-ups".			
SPONTANEOUS BODY MOVEMENT During examination (supine). If no spontaneous movement try to induce by cutaneous stimulation.	None or minimal. Induced.	A. Sluggish. B. Random, incoordinated. C. Mainly stretching.	Smooth movements alternating with random, stretching, athetoid or jerky.	Smooth alternating movements of arms and legs with medium speed and intensity.	Mainly: A. Jerky movement. B. Athetoid movement. C. Other abnormal movement.	1 2		

	1	2	3	4	5
TREMORS Fast (>6/sec.) or Slow (<6/sec.) Mark:	No tremor.	Tremors only in state 5–6.	Tremors only in sleep or after Moro and startles.	Some tremors in state 4.	Tremulousness in all states.
STARTLES	No startles.	Startles to sudden noise. Moro; bang on table only.	Occasional spontaneous startle.	2–5 spontaneous startles.	6+ spontaneous startles.
REFLEXES					
ABNORMAL MOVEMENT OR POSTURE	No abnormal movement.	A. Hands clenched but open intermittently. B. Hands do not open with Moro.	A. Some mouthing movement. B. Intermittent adducted thumb.	A. Persistently adducted thumb. B. Hands clenched all the time.	A. Continuous mouthing movement. B. Convulsive movements.
TENDON REFLEXES Biceps jerk Knee jerk Ankle jerk	Absent.		Present.	Exaggerated.	Clonus.
PALMAR GRASP Head in midline. Put index finger from ulnar side into hand and gently press palmar surface. Never touch dorsal side of hand.	Absent.	Short, weak flexion.	Medium strength and sustained flexion for several secs.	Strong flexion; contraction spreads to forearm.	Very strong grasp. Infant easily lifts off couch.
ROOTING Infant supine, head midline. Touch each corner of the mouth in turn (stroke laterally).	No response.	A. Partial weak head turn but no mouth opening. B. Mouth opening, no head turn.	Mouth opening on stimulated side with partial head turning.	Full head turning, with or without mouth opening.	Mouth opening with very jerky head turning.
SUCKING Infant supine; place index finger (pad towards palate) in infant's mouth; judge power of sucking movement after 5 sec.	No attempt.	Weak sucking movement: A. Regular. B. Irregular.	Strong sucking movement, poor stripping; A. Regular. B. Irregular.	Strong regular sucking movement with continuing sequence of 5 movements. Good stripping.	Clenching but no regular sucking.

Table 5.7.   *(continued)* Dubowitz Neurodevelopmental Protocol

					S	C	A
WALKING (state 4, 5) Hold infant upright, feet touching bed, neck held straight with fingers.	Absent.	Some effort but not continuous with both legs.	At least 2 steps with both legs.	A. Stork posture; no movement. B. Automatic walking.			S
MORO One hand supports infant's head in midline, the other the back. Raise infant to 45° and when infant is relaxed let his head fall though 10. Note if jerky. Repeat 3 times.	No response, or opening of hands only.	Full abduction at the shoulder and extension of the arm.	Full abduction but only delayed or partial adduction.	Partial abduction at shoulder and extension of arms followed by smooth adduction. A. Abd > Add B. Abd = Add C. Abd < Add	J		S

NEUROBEHAVIORAL ITEMS

					S	C	A
EYE APPEARANCES	Sunset sign. Nerve play.	Transient nystagmus. Strabismus. Some roving eye movement.	Normal conjugate eye movement.	A. Persistent nystagmus. B. Frequent roving movement. C. Frequent rapid blinks.			
AUDITORY ORIENTATION (state 3, 4) To rattle (Note presence of startle.)	A. No reaction. B. Auditory startle but no true orientation.	Brightens and stills; may turn toward stimuli with eyes closed.	Alerting and shifting of eyes; head may or may not turn to source.	Alerting; prolonged head turns to stimulus; search with eyes.	Turning and alerting to stimulus each time on both sides.		S
VISUAL ORIENTATION (state 4) To red woolen ball.	Does not focus or follow stimulus.	Stills; focuses on stimulus; may follow 30°; jerky; does not find stimulus again spontaneously.	Follows 30–60° horizontally; may lose stimulus but finds it again. Brief vertical glance.	Follows with eyes and head horizontally and to some extent vertically, with frowning.	Sustained fixation; follows vertically, horizontally, and in circle.		

ALERTNESS (state 4)	Inattentive; rarely or never responds to direct stimulation.	When alert, periods rather brief; rather variable response to orientation.	When alert, alertness moderately sustained; may use stimulus to come to alert state.	Sustained alertness; orientation frequent, reliable to visual but not auditory stimuli.	Continuous alertness, which does not seem to tire, to both auditory and visual stimuli.
DEFENSIVE REACTION A cloth or hand is placed over the infant's face to partially occlude the nasal airway.	No response.	A. General quieting. B. Non-specific activity with long latency.	Rooting; lateral neck turning; possible neck stretching.	Swipes with arm.	Swipes with arm with rather violent body movement.
PEAK OF EXCITEMENT	Low level arousal to all stimuli; never > state 3.	Infant reaches state 4–5 briefly but predominantly in lower states.	Infant predominantly state 4 or 5; may reach state 6 after stimulation but returns spontaneously to lower state.	Infant reaches state 6 but can be consoled relatively easily.	A. Mainly state 6. Difficult to console, if at all. B. Mainly state 4–5 but if reaches state 6 cannot be consoled.
IRRITABILITY (states 3, 4, 5) Aversive stimuli; Uncover; Ventral susp. Undress; Moro Pull to sit Walking reflex Prone	No irritable crying to any of the stimuli.	Cries to 1–2 stimuli.	Cries to 3–4 stimuli.	Cries to 5–6 stimuli.	Cries to all stimuli.
CONSOLABILITY (state 6)	Never above state 5 during examination, therefore not needed.	Consoling not needed. Consoles spontaneously.	Consoled by talking, hand on belly or wrapping up.	Consoled by picking up and holding; may need finger in mouth.	Not consolable.
CRY	No cry at all.	Only whimpering cry.	Cries to stimuli but normal pitch.	Lusty cry to offensive stimuli; normal pitch.	High-pitched cry, often continuous.

NOTES *If asymmetrical or atypical, draw in on nearest figure.
Record any abnormal signs (e.g., facial palsy, contractures, etc.) Draw if possible.

Record time after feed: _____

EXAMINER: _____

and rotational assessment may be executed with contact on the transverse processes (Fig. 5.96). The brown adipose tissue or "baby fat" must be moved well out of the way of the examining contact to sequester the structure being evaluated. In the lumbosacral spine, precise thumb contact should be made over the interspinous spaces and between the sacral tubercles while flexion/extension motion is controlled with the grasp of the other examining hand underneath the bilateral thighs (Fig. 5.98). Full range of motion should be introduced to assess the end of the motor unit range of motion and joint play. Sacroiliac joint motion palpation may be accomplished in the prone position with the examiner's first digit placed on the first sacral tubercle as a base reference and the thumb on the superior medial aspect of the PSIS, immediately lateral to the sacroiliac joint (Fig. 5.99). This is adapted from the recommended standing position for SI joint motion palpation in the older child and adult, with the same motion of hip abduction and

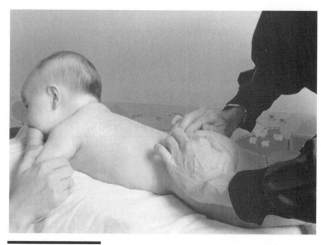

Figure 5.95.   Lumbo-sacral examination. The neonate is nursing for security and comfort.

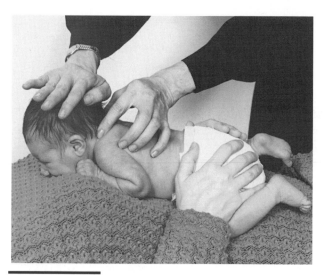

Figure 5.93.   Palpation of the cervical spine with the fingers and thumb.

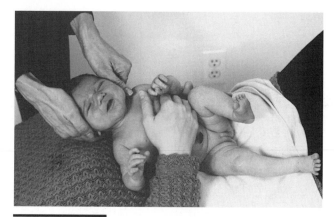

Figure 5.96.   Motion palpation of the cervical spine.

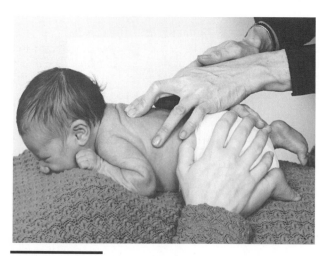

Figure 5.94.   Thoracic spine static palpation.

flexion being instituted as the motion is evaluated within the joint. Any degree of fixation or aberrant movement should be recorded. Bilateral comparison is an integral component of this exam. It is within normal limits for the sacroiliac joint motion of a newborn to be limited by as much 50–60% from the weight-bearing expectation due to immature development of the articular structures and soft tissue function. These pelvic joints do not complete their biomechanical development until the weight bearing stresses introduced by walking create the "joint rhythm." This should be fully realized by approximately 12 to 18 months after the initiation of upright ambulation.

Cervical range of motion is best assessed by encouraging the baby to move her/his head by audibly drawing attention to the direction of the parent's or examiner's voice, or visually by using a brightly colored or black and white contrasting object, such as a small toy (Fig. 5.100). The ranges of flexion, extension, bilateral flexion, and bilateral rotation may be easily accomplished in this manner. Passive, gentle movement of the infant's head through full ranges of motion assists in determining the degrees of global cervical motion if the neonate is in a drowsy state (Brazelton's States 1, 2, or 3). Thoracic and lumbar ranges of motion may be observed with the patient lying in a prone or supine position. If in an awake and alert state, kicking of the legs and weak attempts to roll the trunk will often be noted. Additionally, testing of some of the infant reflexes will provide insight into spinal ranges of motion.

Spinal percussion can readily reveal any underlying spinal pathology. Light tapping with a reflex hammer directly over the spinous processes of each vertebrae may elicit a positive response that could be characterized by a sharp cry or inconsolable crying (Fig. 5.101). A positive response would dictate further investigation.

Orthopedic Examination

EXAMINATION OF THE HIPS

Although this examination is routinely performed in the birth room or neonatology unit, a comprehensive investigation is warranted by the chiropractor. Frequently, a cursory initial examination may not reveal the potential for problems of a

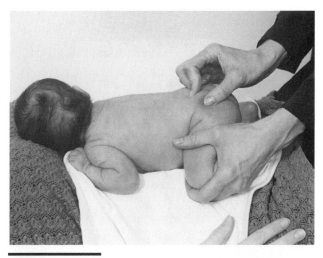

Figure 5.99.   Sacro-iliac joints: motion palpation.

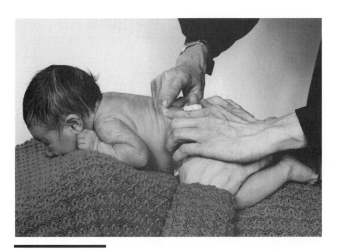

Figure 5.97.   Motion palpation of the thoraco-lumbar spine.

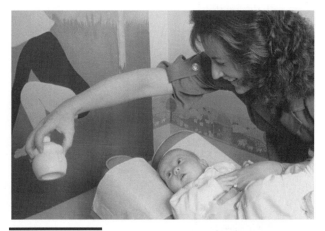

Figure 5.100.   Cervical range of motion examination. The neonate's gaze is directed towards the toy through all the ranges of motion.

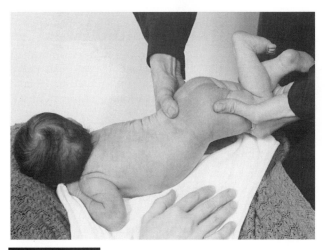

Figure 5.98.   Motion palpation of the first three sacral segments. Introduce flexion - extension as the thumb palpates the joint play and movement.

congenital or biomechanical nature. A further hip examination is recommended at 6 weeks of age, as it is recognized that a neonate presenting with normal hips at birth may subsequently dislocate at a later time. In assessment of the hip joints, a full range of circumduction must be attempted with concomitant observation and palpation of the involved structures, as well as the execution of salient orthopedic tests.

Congenital dislocation of the hip joint can occur in 1–19 per 1000 births (65). The left hip exhibits dislocation four times more commonly than the right. The etiology of this is normally in-utero constraint in which the left fetal hip is more adducted than the right. The polygenic factor is described as a familial recurrence of about 1 in 30 (65). The breech : vertex ratio of incident affected by presentation is 10:1 (65). Female to male ratio has been analyzed as 6:1, and there is some evidence of an elevated incidence with multiple congenital anomalies. Associated abnormalities that may proliferate the muscular dysfunction at the hip joint are congenital hypotonia, spina bifida, and arthrogryposis congenital multiplex.

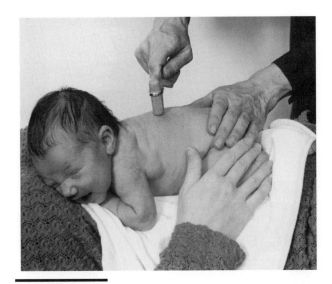

Figure 5.101.   Spinal percussion over each of the spinous processes with the use of a Taylor reflex hammer.

To adequately examine the hips, the neonate must be fully unclothed with the diaper removed. Observation and palpation for any obvious deformity, hemiatrophy, paralysis, edema, asymmetry, or coldness is essential (Fig. 5.102A, B, C). The defect associated with congenital dysplasia or dislocation of the hip may present in varying levels of severity. Subluxation of the hip is described when the femoral head and the acetabulum are in partial contact at birth. A total loss of contact between the femoral head and the acetabulum, with the femoral head usually displaced laterally and superiorly (because of muscular contracture), describes a frank dislocation of the hip. Reduced or absent development of the femur and acetabulum at birth connotes congenital hip dysplasia. Usually, the dysplasia progresses relentlessly as growth occurs unless the dislocation is corrected. Correction of the subluxation or dislocation in the early days or weeks of life will reverse the dysplasia with ensuing normal development of the hip joint structures. Signs of established dislocation may be manifest by unequal leg length and asymmetry of the thighs (Fig. 5.103A, B, C).

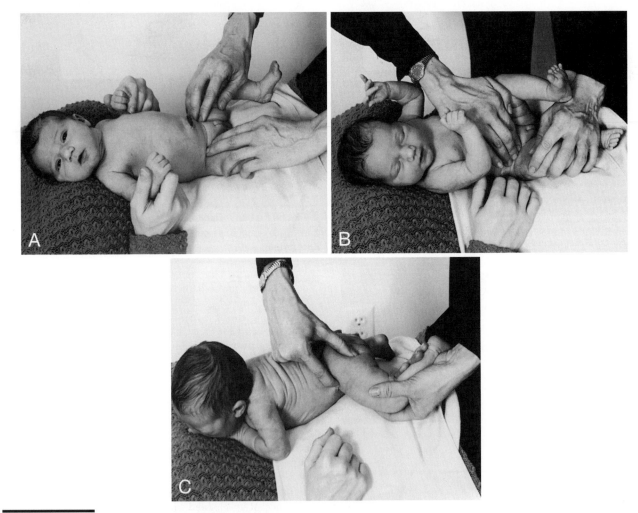

Figure 5.102.   A, Bilateral palpation of the hip joint around the acetabular rim; patient in the supine position. There should be comparison for symmetry. B, Palpation of the hip joints for evaluation of atrophy, edema, paralysis. Unilateral examination should be compared for symmetry in the supine position. C, Palpation of the hip joints in the prone position.

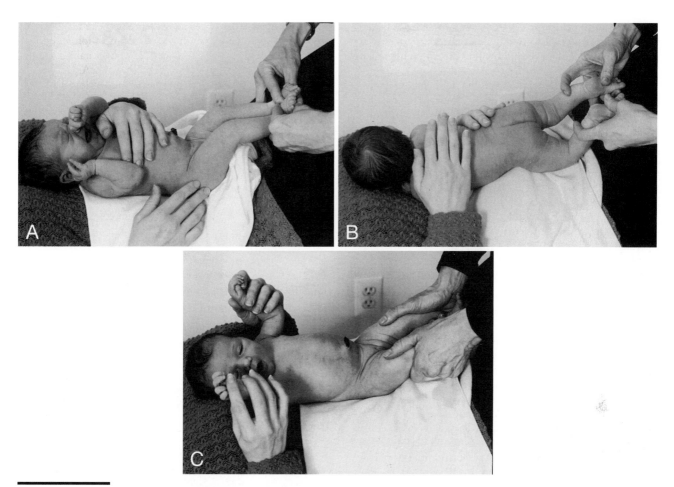

Figure 5.103.   A, Evaluation of leg length from the medial malleoli in the supine position. B, Evaluation of leg length in the prone position. There is increased resistance of the left leg as extension is attempted. C, Assessment of the supine infant for asymmetry of thigh development.

To establish the diagnosis of congenital hip dislocation, one must be able to demonstrate instability of the joint. This is achieved by proceeding with the Ortolani's reduction test and the Barlow's dislocation test. In Ortolani's test, the infant is placed comfortably in a supine position with the knees and hips flexed to 90 degrees or greater (Fig. 5.104). The joints are examined unilaterally, with the examiner's long finger being placed over the long axis and the greater trochanter of the femur and the thumb over the medial aspect of the upper thigh (Fig. 5.105). The thigh is slowly abducted and the examiner lifts the greater trochanter forward (Fig. 5.106). Any instability is perceived by a "slipping feeling" as the femoral head moves into the acetabulum. A sense of reduction may be discerned by concomitant palpation of a "clunk" with forward movement of the head of the femur.

Barlow's test is indicated in the hip joint, which presents with some degree of stability, but suspicion of hip dislocation prevails. This is performed in the opposite manner to Ortolani's test. The examiner's hand grasps the infant's thigh while stabilizing the opposite thigh with the other hand to introduce gentle downwards adduction of the hip joint (Fig. 5.107). For the hip to be dislocatable, adduction must be accompanied by

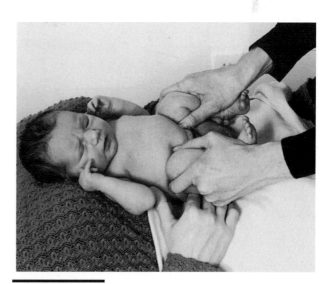

Figure 5.104.   Ortolani's test. The first step involves bilateral flexion of the thighs.

flexion and axial pressure. The dislocation may be palpated with a concomitant "clunk" as the femoral head moves over the posterior lip of the acetabulum (Fig. 5.108). This test is applicable until 4 to 5 months of age.

With normal movement of the hip joint and negative Ortolani's and Barlow's' test, the joint is considered to be stable. A "clicking" sound heard or palpated during the examination is considered to be normal in the absence of excessive movement of the femoral head. Clicking is usually the result of ligamentous laxity and is found in approximately 10% of neonates. If the femoral head remains within the joint and is able to be fully abducted, but Barlow's test creates posterior dislocation with adduction, the hip joint is termed a "dislocatable" joint. Complete dislocation of the hip joint is indicated by a positive Ortolani's test in which the hip cannot be abducted.

EXAMINATION OF THE LOWER EXTREMITIES

Asymmetry of the creases of the thighs and lower legs may indicate faulty orthopedic development (Fig. 5.109A, B). This should be observed from both anterior and posterior perspectives (Fig 5.109C). With mild asymmetry, the baby should be monitored on a continuous basis throughout the first year of life, when the normal mechanics of upright weight bearing and walking will introduce healthy stresses to promote symmetry.

Kernig's test performed on the neonate may not be the best indicator for meningeal irritation. Clinical features such as fever, irritability, cyanosis, high-pitched cry, and poor feeding are more significant; however, the test may be performed to ferret out pain or problems in the lower extremities or pelvis. This is evaluated with the infant in a supine position. The examiner gently lifts and flexes the hip and knee, then attempts to straighten the knee (Fig. 5.110). Resistance due to pain necessitates further investigation.

Measurement of thigh and calf circumferences is an excellent index of asymmetry suspicious of interrupted orthopedic development (Fig. 5.111A, B).

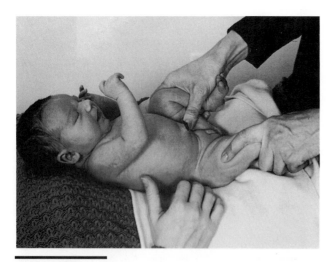

Figure 5.105.   Ortolani's test. Unilateral abduction of the thigh is performed to assess each hip joint separately.

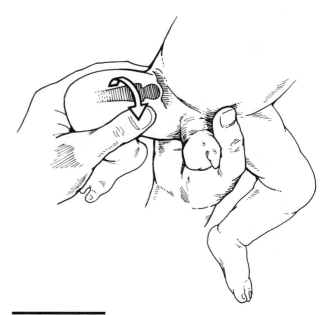

Figure 5.106.   Ortolani's test. Abduction of the hip in a flexed position will cause reduction of the hip if a dislocation is present.

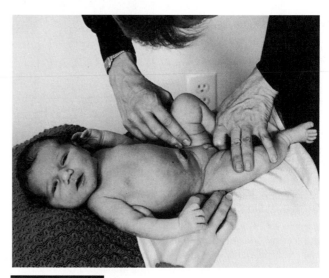

Figure 5.107.   Barlow's test. Unilateral flexion, adduction, downwards and axial pressure on the hip joint.

The feet should be examined for deformities. Mild postural aberrations may be observed; however, if the feet and ankle joints can be passively moved through the anticipated ranges of motion, continued monitoring is adequate. Abnormalities of the feet such as talipes equinovarus, talipes calcaneovalgus, and metatarsus varus are discussed in Chapter 14.

Birth Trauma

Injuries to the neonate may be sustained either during the labor or delivery process and, despite a decreasing incidence (65), birth injury remains a cause for concern to the obstetrician, the

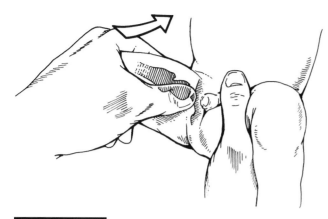

Figure 5.108. Barlow's Test. Flexion, adduction, and axial pressure of the femoral head produce a positive response of laxity or a palpable "clunk" in a positive test.

neonatal pediatrician, and the chiropractor. Birth injuries are second only to asphyxia and atelectasis as causes of neonatal mortality. Because of the attribution of birth injury to obstetric mismanagement, a high litigation rate has evolved, which has, in turn, created the practice of defensive obstetrics (66). A high caesarean rate has been cited as a likely consequence of this.

Modic (67) alleges that extreme flexion and rotation injuries are not uncommon in newborn infants and that acute hemorrhage or hemorrhagic necrosis may occur even in the absence of fracture. He further implicates flexion as the most conventional mechanism of injury at the craniovertebral junction. Towbin (68) describes the birth process as a potentially traumatic, crippling event for the fetus, even under optimal controlled conditions. He cites the primary etiology of injury during cephalic delivery as forceful, longitudinal traction, emphatically when combined with flexion and torsion of the vertebral axis. He comments that this traumatic mechanism is thought to be the most important cause of neonatal spinal injury (68–71).

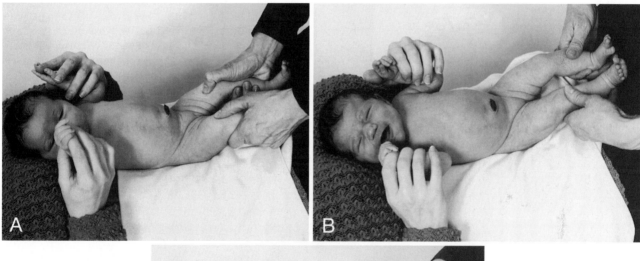

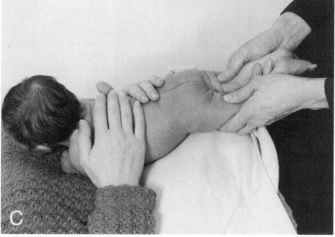

Figure 5.109. A, Assessment of symmetry of thigh creases in the supine position. Bilateral comparison. B, Assessment of symmetry of creases in the lower leg. Supine position; compare bilaterally. C, Assessment of symmetry of thigh creases in the prone position.

Towbin (68) reports that pathologic patterns of spinal injury at birth occurring as transectional spinal and brain stem lesions are observed with less frequency than with non-transectional lesions. He describes these nontransectional lesion patterns as inflicted upon the meninges, spinal nerve roots, or spinal cord. Meningeal lesions comprise permutations of dural laceration and hemorrhage, pia-arachnoidal congestion, and subarachnoid hemorrhage. Lesions altering the spinal nerve roots encompass perineural hemorrhage and laceration or avulsion of the spinal nerve root(s). Spinal cord lesions exhibit as laceration, edema and congestion, acute neuronal damage, focal hemorrhage or malacia and architectural distortion. Foderl (71) found, elucidated by Garde, that architectural

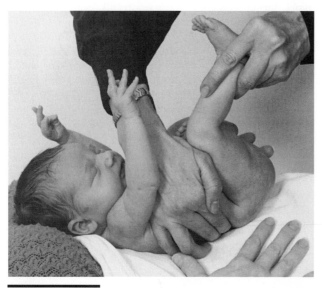

Figure 5.110.   Kernig's test.

distortion is evidenced as a buckling distortion created by reduction of the spinal cord canal seen with acute flexion of the spine. This was discovered to subject the spinal cord to direct compression injury.

Stolzenberg (72) in autopsy studies demonstrated latent fractures-dislocation of the vertebrae from the flexion mechanism of birth injury. Stanley et al (73) presented a radiologic review confirming fracture-dislocation of the cervical spine during delivery. They demonstrated that the consequent neuropathophysiology contrasted from tetraparesis with respiratory compromise and early death to minimal or transient deficits. This study additionally described anterior subluxation of the cervical spine as an integral etiology of airway compression.

Gorton and Marsden (74) suggest that spinal cord injury at birth occurs with greater incidence than previously considered. Yates (75) cites the significant frequency of vertebral artery damage encountered in the birth process as contributing to babies dying after delivery.

Vaginal delivery of the breech is incessantly implicated in birth trauma. Yet, an intensive study from the University of Manitoba (76) asserts the findings of a Canadian consensus panel in 1986, which concluded that planned vaginal birth should not only be permitted, but actually recommended for the large majority of breech fetuses; and that caesarean delivery was unjustified merely because the fetus was breech.

Birth injuries of the spinal cord resulting from breech extraction have been reported as early as 1870 by Parrot (77). Hyperextension of the fetal head is of major concern in breech presentation. Behrman has concluded that the etiology of this mechanism appears to originate from cervical extensor muscles spasm. Infantile paraplegia has been referenced by Ford (78) as being a rarely acknowledged outcome of breech delivery. Spinal cord and intracranial hemorrhage, and spinal cord lacerations are summarized by Pierson (79) as substantive

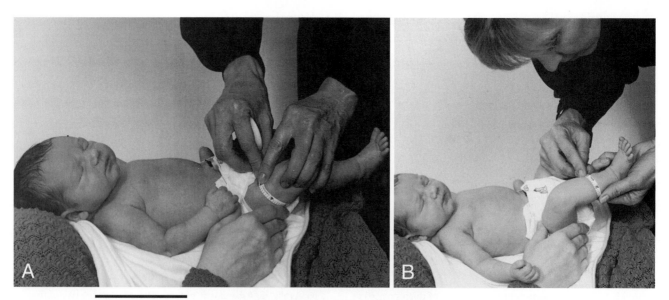

Figure 5.111.   A, Measurement of thigh circumference. This is compared bilaterally and recorded.
B, Measurement of calf circumference. This is compared bilaterally and recorded.

findings with breech delivery. He also described fractures of the vertebrae, typically a transverse separation of the upper epiphyseal plate of the sixth cervical vertebra. Pierson continues to implicate delivery trauma as one of the major causes in the ambiguous diagnosis of stillbirth in breech presentations. He concluded that birth injury and shock in breech deliveries cause greater fetal mortality and morbidity than asphyxia, that unnecessary haste in breech extractions often causes obstetrical complication leading to birth injuries, and that forced traction and suprapubic pressure could be avoided by obstetrically accommodating the long axis of the fetus to the axes of the maternal pelvis.

Further injuries incurred by vaginal breech delivery consist of hip dislocation, traumatic torticollis, and scoliosis. The typical skull deformation is visualized as a severely flattened vertex with an overhanging occiput.

Towbin (80) indicates that of all neonatal deaths, 10% have sustained a spinal cord injury. He stresses that respiratory depression in the neonate is the chief indication of such injury. This may lead to hypoxia and secondary damage to the cerebrum. Birth trauma affecting the brain stem and upper cervical spinal cord has been frequently summarized in the literature as being responsible for sudden infant death syndrome (SIDS). Banks et al (81) report that functional disturbances in the brainstem and cervical spinal cord areas related to the neurophysiology of respiration may contribute to the clinical findings associated with SIDS. They further assert that normal development of the respiratory control centers may be altered by genetic, biochemical, traumatic or biomechanical processes, which have been distressed by neonatal spinal constriction and compression as a result of birth trauma. They behold this as being contributory to SIDS.

It is also being stated in the obstetrical community that an increasing number of traumatic lesions are due to iatrogenic insult, sustained in the neonatal unit (82).

PREVALANCE OF BIRTH TRAUMA

Profound birth injury, repudiating asphyxia, occurs in 0.2 per 1000 live births (83) and is encountered more frequently in premature infants, and in breech presentations and deliveries. Comprehensive birth trauma is the eighth most common cause of neonatal mortality; in low birth-weight infants, it is the fourth most common cause of death.

The risk factors for injury sustained during the birth process are deliberated under the rubric of fetal and maternal factors, fetal malpresentation and malposition, cephalopelvic disproportion, prolonged and precipitate labor and obstetrician inexperience and incompetence.

Fetal factors encompass prematurity, intrauterine growth retardation, multiple pregnancy and fetal distress. The etiology of maternal determinants are summarily nulliparity, obesity, and short stature. Malpresentation and malposition are epitomized in breech presentations, brow, facial shoulder or compound presentations, occipitoposterior arrest, and deep transverse arrest. Cephalopelvic disproportion, while often regarded as a "catch-all" term to describe many labor difficulties, describes cases of macrosomia, macrocephaly,

contracted maternal pelvis, shoulder dystocia, severe cranial molding, and an unengaged fetal head.

OBSTETRICAL PROCEDURES IN BIRTH TRAUMA

Contemporary obstetrical procedures are predominant perpetrators of traumatic birth injury. Forceps delivery has long been imputed to be the etiological factor in myriad traumatic birth injuries. Shulman et al (84) report on transection of the spinal cord after mid-forceps rotation. They assert that in spinal cord transection in cephalic delivery, the lesion is most typically located in the upper cervical cord, most frequently resulting from rotational forces. Although mid or high forceps application contributes less to fetal morbidity than the abnormality of labor that required their use, depressed skull fracture and intracranial hemorrhage are distinct hazards.

Laisram (86) and Eastman (86) have revealed an increased frequency of cerebral palsy in correlation with the application of midforceps. There have been many controversial reports that there is a reciprocity between forceps usage and a reduction in the intelligence quotient (IQ) in the neonate. Friedman et al (87) described intelligence assessments at least up to 7 years of age, with the conclusion that those children who had been delivered by midforceps had lower mean IQs compared with children who were delivered by outlet forceps. High forceps operations describe the application of forceps before engagement of the presenting part. High pelvic delivery, either by forceps or vacuum extraction, may be associated with significant morbidity in both the mother and the fetus and "has no place in modern obstetrics" (88).

The vacuum extractor, obstetrically termed ventouse extraction, was re-introduced in the 1950s and is not without danger to the neonate. Although no long-term neurologic deficits have been documented resulting from this method of delivery, excessive occurrence of potentially dangerous complications such as cephalhematoma, intracranial hemorrhage, and skin abrasions have been amply documented. In one study, these complications ensued in 25 percent and 12 percent, respectively (89). The theoretical advantages of the vacuum extractor over forceps application comprises the aversion of insertion of the steel blades within the vagina and their positioning precisely over the fetal skull, as is required for safe forceps delivery; the ability to rotate the fetal skull without impinging on maternal soft tissues; and less intracranial pressure during traction. Use of the soft cup vacuum extractor is not associated with an increase in serious neonatal morbidity when compared with forceps, although frequency of cephalhematomas and retinal hemorrhage increases with the use of these implements. A common sequelae in the case room is initial application of vacuum extraction, which in many cases is not effective, followed by secondary deployment of forceps blades. The combined stresses of forced longitudinal traction, termed "tractoring" in obstetrical forceps usage, with critical axial rotation too often ensues in complex neonatal trauma.

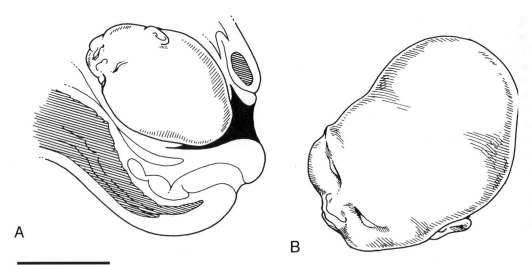

Figure 5.112.   A, The formation of a caput succedaneum as the fetus descends through the birth canal.
B, The formation of a caput succedaneum when the fetal head has been in a left position.

Caesarean section, while perceived by many maternity patients as non-traumatic to their unborn baby, in fact, presents significant etiology for not only fetal, but maternal well-being. Maternal morbidity is more frequent and likely to be more severe after caesarean section than after vaginal delivery (81). The reported antecedents for maternal morbidity from surgical delivery are hemorrhage, infection, and injury to the urinary tract.

Perinatal outcomes from caesarean section comprise depressed skull fractures, femur fractures, and fractures of other extremity bones. The fetus may be wounded during the incision into the uterus. Certainly, caesarean section is not a guarantee against fetal injury. Injury to the fetal spinal cord and brain can ensue where the skull of a preterm breech is entrapped in a small transverse uterine incision incorrectly judged to be adequate for delivery. There is some conjecture of respiratory distress being of higher incidence for a repeat caesarean section rather than for vaginal birth. Due to uterine contraction at incision or other circumstances, forceps may have to be applied to facilitate neonatal delivery. The trauma affiliated with forceps applications may pertain to this type of delivery.

The cited indications for surgical delivery are previous caesarean sections, breech presentations, failure to progress or dystocia, or fetal distress. Failure to progress in labor is the most common justification for caesarean section in the United States (90). Caesarean section is one of the most frequently performed surgical procedures in the US.

Not to be ignored are the potential implications for birth trauma perpetrated by manual delivery. A monumental amount of force can be executed by a pair of hands in the process of extricating the neonate. Similar injurious forces of longitudinal traction, axial rotation and extreme flexion or extension can be exercised, and perhaps augmented by using one's entire body weight as leverage. A frequent observation in case rooms is the placement of the physician's feet, thighs, or torso in such a manner as to effect increased force to extract the infant.

Due to the diversity of mechanisms of trauma during the birth process, the role of the chiropractic professional is becoming increasingly acknowledged as that of an integral member of the birth team. Observation of the biomechanism of the actual delivery of the neonate can further the clinical recognition of the vertebral subluxation complex incurred at birth. After the neonatal examination is performed immediately after delivery, the chiropractor can offer the opportunity for an initial cursory chiropractic examination to further confirm the neonate's neuromusculoskeletal well being. Should any clinical signs of spinal or related trauma be detected, a comprehensive examination should be recommended, in which the chiropractor performs an integrated and critical role. When a chiropractor cannot be present at the birth process, the infant should be referred for a routine chiropractic examination within a maximum of 48 hours after the birth process.

Birth trauma is evidenced by a number of clinical manifestations. The chiropractor should be aware of the signs and symptoms that herald the more routinely found neonatal conditions whose etiology is the birth or obstetrical process.

HEAD INJURIES

Caput succedaneum, although not obstetrically considered to be a traumatic injury, is a normal finding in the newborn. It is a localized, edematous thickening of the scalp formed by the effusion of serum. Pressure of the cervical ring causes obstruction of venous return, so that the part of the scalp that lies within the cervix becomes edematous (Fig. 5.112). The caput forms during labor and after the membranes have been ruptured. The caput is present at birth, begins to disappear immediately afterward, and usually disappears entirely after 24 to 36 hours. It is absent if the baby is stillborn, the contractions are poor, or the cervix is not applied closely to the head.

The location of the caput varies with the position of the head. In occiput anterior positions, the caput forms on the vertex, to the right of the sagittal suture in left occiput anterior and to the left in right occiput anterior positions. The size of the caput is an indication of the amount of pressure that has been exerted against the head. A large one suggests strong pressure from above and resistance from below. A small caput is present when the contractions are weak or the resistance feeble. The largest are found in contracted pelves after long, hard labor. In the presence of prolonged labor, a large caput suggests disproportion or occipitoposterior position, while a small one may indicate uterine inertia.

Cephalhematoma occurs in approximately one percent of newborn infants. This results from bleeding between the periosteum and the cranial bones, most often the parietal and less encountered the occipital bones. Its etiology is as a consequence of shearing or tearing of communicating veins during delivery. The extent of edema is limited by the underlying cranial bones, and it does not cross the suture lines. This is largely due to buffeting of the fetal skull against the maternal pelvis, which is seen principally in situations in which there is prolonged labor. It also commonly occurs during a forceps or ventouse (vacuum) extraction delivery. Subperiosteal bleeding is torpid and may not appear until the second day of life. Enlargement may occur during the first week and the swelling may persist for several weeks. The edge may be mistaken for a depressed fracture of the skull.

Concomitant complications of cephalhematoma may include an underlying linear skull fracture, neonatal jaundice due to resorption of the blood, calcification developing during resorption — not to be confused with a depressed skull fracture — or, infrequently, intracranial hemorrhage. When a cephalhematoma is observed, it requires immediate referral to a neonatologist or pediatrican. Differentiation of caput succedaneum and cephalhematoma is described in Table 5.8.

Subaponeurotic or subgaleal hemorrhage occurs rarely beneath the aponeurotic sheath uniting the two portions of the occipitofrontalis muscle of the scalp. This may be the consequence of trauma during delivery, particularly seen with ventouse extraction, or it may indicate the presence of a coagulation defect. These hemorrhages can spread over the scalp and may be fluctuant. Shock may result from the blood loss of a large subaponeurotic hemorrhage and transfusion may be recommended. This is seen particularly in black infants.

Skull fractures are prevalent as head injuries incurred during the birth process. Linear fractures usually require no specific treatment. Depressed fractures are most often affiliated with forceps application or head compression produced by the maternal sacral promontory. Large fractures may be associated with cerebral contusion, and neurosurgical consultation may be prudent. Depression of the skull may remain for many months post-natally.

Intracranial hemorrhages are frequently encountered as a result of head injuries in delivery trauma. This can also result from infections, coagulation disorders, circulatory disturbances, hypoxia, hypernatremia or erythroblastosis fetalis. It may also arise from a tentorium tear. The hemorrhage may manifest in either the subdural or subarachnoid layer, as well as being frequently encountered in the subependymal region. In the latter case, the hemorrhage may rupture into the ventricles or extend into the brain substance. Symptomatology and clinical signs appearing at birth and postpartum may comprise apnea, disturbed cardiac and respiratory function, a high-pitched shrill cry, opisthotonus, failure to breastfeed, muscular twitching, convulsions, and irritability and restlessness. A bulging fontanelle may be observed, as well as faulty temperature regulation. Opthalmoscopic examination may reveal abnormalities of the puplis and hemorrhage of the retina. The Moro reflex may be exaggerated initially or absent. Symptomatology may appear at birth, then disappear for a few days to return later. Immediate referral is indicated.

NERVE INJURIES

Neonates may present with a diversity of nerve injuries. These are most often a consequence of compression, stretching, axial rotation or twisting, hyperextension, hyperflexion or separation of neurologic tissue.

Pathologic classification of injuries to nerve tissues would include neuropraxia, characterized by nerve edema, axonotmesis involving complete peripheral degeneration with total recovery, and neurotomesis where complete division of all neurological structures transpires.

Facial nerve palsy may be due to either an upper or lower motor neuron lesion; however, clinical distinction is often difficult. Oblique application of the forceps blade can cause a pervasive injury to the lower motor neuron. The seventh cranial nerve may also be impaired by prolonged pressure on

---

Table 5.8. **Differentiation of Caput Succedaneum and Cephalhematoma**

Caput succedaneum	Cephalhematoma
Present at birth	May not appear for several hours
Soft, pits on pressure	Soft, does not pit
Diffuse swelling	Sharply circumscribed
Lies over and crosses the sutures	Limited to individual bones, does not cross suture lines
Movable on skull, seeks dependent portions	Fixed to original site
Is largest at birth and immediately begins to grow smaller, disappearing in a few hours	Appears after a few hours, grows larger for a time, and disappears only after weeks or months

the maternal sacral promontory. Upper motor neuron lesions are less frequent and due more to brain injury or nuclear agenesis, known as Moebius' syndrome.

The typical lesion of facial nerve palsy is clinically recognized by the inability to close the eye and lack of lower lip depression on crying, visualized on the affected side. This should be distinguished from asymmetrical crying facies in view of an absence of the depressor anguli oris muscle. In this condition, the eye is able to close normally; however, there is an inability of the mouth to move downward and outward on the affected side when the infant cries. Asymmetry customarily remains into adult life becoming less perceptible with time. It is a common familial trait. In the majority of cases, complete recovery transpires; however, permanent facial palsy can occur.

The etiology of brachial plexus injuries to the brachial plexus are most often the consequence of excessive lateral flexion, rotational or tractional forces applied on the neck during delivery. This results in brachial plexus palsy. These types of trauma are observed with manual or forceps delivery, with impacted shoulders or during vaginal delivery of the aftercoming head of a breech. In a study performed by Rubin (91), brachial plexus injury was encountered 17 times more frequently with breech than with cephalic deliveries.

There are three categories of brachial plexus injury (see also Chapter 12). The first is described as Erb's Palsy or upper brachial plexus palsy. This type is the most common type of obstetrical injury to the brachial plexus (92). Here, the fifth and sixth cervical nerve roots are injured. The clinical signs illustrate the arm being held in abduction with the elbow fully extended and the forearm pronated with the wrist fully flexed. This is also referred to as the "waiter's tip" position. Hernandez and Dias (93) contend that, although the majority of children with Erb's palsy will fully recover with minimal or no residual deformity, some children, because of muscle imbalance, develop persistent deformity of the shoulder consisting of internal rotation contractures, subluxation, or dislocation of the proximal humerus. The chiropractic role for reduction or correction of this neurologic injury is unequivocal. A significant population of chiropractors have received extensive training and clinical experience with extremities assessment and treatment. Often, infants afflicted with brachial plexus injury respond favorably and quickly to this approach and are offered indicative resolution where previously these cases have been suspended in dogmatic approaches.

The second form of brachial plexus injury involves the lower brachial plexus and is known as Klumpke's Paralysis, implicating a lesion to the seventh and eighth cervical and first thoracic nerve roots. The result is paralysis of the small muscles of the hand, with localized wrist drop and flaccid paralysis of the hand. Notably, the grasp reflex is absent.

Less frequently, total paralysis of the arm is encountered. All trunks of the brachial plexus are damaged in this lesion with resultant complete paralysis of the arm and concomitant flaccidity and sensory, trophic, and circulatory changes. Spinal cord injury is suspected when there is bilateral paralysis.

None of the three types of brachial plexus injury respond to active medical treatment. Passive movement of the joints can prevent contractures. Recovery of mild injuries usually occurs within a few days, although more severe lesions are not anticipated to recover spontaneously for 2 to 4 months. Gordon et al (94) conducted a study that displayed 85% recovery by 4 months of age, 92% recovery by 12 months, and 93% by 4 years of age (94).

Radial nerve injury results rarely from fracture of the humerus, experienced with difficulty in delivering the arm during breech or shoulder extraction. The deltoid region as an indicated site for intramuscular injection can result in radial nerve injury, largely due to the fact that the deltoid muscle of the newborn infant is so diminutive that correct localization of the needle point is difficult. It may also be illustrated after repeated brachial artery sampling of arterial blood.

Phrenic nerve palsy or damage to the cervical nerve roots C3, C4, and C5 is chiefly associated with brachial plexus palsy. This often causes severe respiratory distress because the neonate primarily breathes with the diaphragm rather than the intercostal muscles. Chest radiography displays the characteristic elevated hemidiaphragm or an immobile diaphragm. This is confirmed with ultrasound diagnostics.

Recurrent laryngeal nerve palsy is an infrequent outcome of birth trauma associated with excessive lateral traction of the cervical spine. This can cause congenital laryngeal stridor.

Spinal cord injury of the cervical region is infrequently confronted and associated with overstretching in difficult breech deliveries involving internal version and breech extraction. It can also occur in some cases of shoulder dystocia.

The mechanism of injury involves stretching of the cervical spinal cord from excessive traction techniques. This type of lesion may present with one of the following: a normal neonate at parturition, with later sequelae of respiratory depression, urinary retention and lower extremity paralysis; paraplegia from birth; a depressed health condition from birth including respiratory depression, shock, hypothermia, and infant death. Cervical spine radiography may illustrate a fracture or dislocation. A neurosurgical consultation may be required for pathologic differentiation and treatment. Pathology of hematomyelia or extradural hematomas are delineated through ultrasound and myelogram diagnostics of the cervical spinal cord. MRI also proves useful in this regard.

BONE AND JOINT INJURIES

A miscellany of bones and joints can be afflicted from birth trauma. Traumatic fractures of bone are often associated with the archetypal signs of fracture including edema, deformity, avoidance of movement and crepitus. Fractures of the upper limb bones are delineated by an asymmetrical Moro reflex or failure to spontaneously move one arm. The clavicle is the most frequently fractured bone during parturition. The incidence is reported to be 2.0–7.0 per 1000 live births. It is most frequently associated with shoulder dystocia, more so in the diabetic mother with a macrosomic infant or with a difficult breech or transverse delivery. A brief period of immobilization may be required. Chiropractic examination of the affected and adjacent areas can provide information regarding neurological tissue or associated joint damage. Brachial plexus injury should be ruled out.

When the humerus is implicated, the upper one-third of

the humeral shaft is most often fractured with concomitant considerable deformity. Radial nerve injury is sometimes associated. Immobilization is mandated in this circumstance, consisting of a plastic backslab or immobilization with a binder to the chest.

Femoral fracture may occur during breech extraction either vaginally or with caesarean section. The footling or double footling breech position is most at risk for this fracture. Immobilization with plaster, gallows traction or cutaneous traction and a Thomas splint is clinically indicated.

When multiple or other unusual fractures present at birth, osteogenesis imperfecta or non-traumatic injury should be speculated. Dislocations of joint and epiphyses separations are difficult to diagnose and require specialized orthopedic treatment.

SOFT TISSUE INJURIES

Soft tissue injuries are most commonly seen after forceps delivery, episiotomy, uterine incision at caesarean section, cephalopelvic disproportion, and fetal scalp electrode monitoring.

Erythema, lacerations, and abrasions are common; ecchymoses may be seen with traumatic deliveries, precipitate labor, preterm infants, poorly controlled deliveries, or abnormal presentations such as breech, brow, or facial.

Traumatic cyanosis, also labeled traumatic petechiae, occur over the head, neck, and upper chest after a difficult delivery. They eventuate frequently as a result of breech presentation and in infants born with the umbilical cord wrapped tightly around the neck. These petechiae may be related to a sudden increase in intrathoracic pressure during passage of the chest through the birth canal. These petechiae routinely fade within 2 to 3 days postnatally and do not require treatment, other than parental reassurance. Traumatic petechiae must be clearly distinguished from generalized petechiae associated with co-agulation disturbances.

Subcutaneous fat necrosis describes well-demarcated indurated areas in the skin resulting from applied pressure such as from forceps blades applied on the face. No medical treatment is required.

ORGAN INJURIES

Numerous visceral injuries can occur to the liver and spleen, adrenal glands, kidneys, and testicles during the birth process. Mechanical trauma can lead to a predominant injury termed parturitional crush injury of the liver. If suspected, referral to a neonatologist is essential.

An alarming number and scope of traumatic lesions are cited to be due to iatrogenic insults protracted in the neonatal intensive care unit. The etiology of these lesions is related to invasive procedures and technology necessary to salvage infants, primarily premature neonates of progressive lowered birth weight, and gestational age. Table 5.9 illustrates examples of iatrogenesis found in some neonates (95).

Doctors of chiropractic need an accurate and comprehensive evaluation of injuries incurred as a result of birth trauma and need to apply clinical treatment where indicated.

Table 5.9.   Examples of Iatrogenesis

Oxygen toxicity
    Retinopathy of prematurity
    Bronchopulmonary dysplasia
Hearing deficits
    Antibiotics
    Incubator noise
Cardiac failure from patent ductus arteriosus
Necrotizing enterocolitis
Rickets
Digit damage, nerve palsies, nasal deformities, oral deformities and bowel disturbance from catheters, tubes and needles
Premature thelarche
Postural deformities
    Scaphocephaly
    Narrow arched grooved palate
    External rotation of the hips and feet

BREASTFEEDING

All babies should receive breastmilk, as it is undoubtedly, as the advertisements suggest, nature's perfect food (see Chapter 11). The chiropractic professional plays an integral role in supporting the universal goal of all infants receiving breastmilk, ideally through the breasts of their mothers. A myriad of research indicates that breastmilk is superior nutrition for the infant (96–104).

The value of early and prolonged breastfeeding is inestimable. Human milk is perfectly formulated for infants' requirements with optimum levels of protein, vitamins, minerals, and essential nutrients compared with the milk of other species (97). Additionally, breastmilk is an exceptional method of conferring protection from infections during the time the baby's immune system is maturing. Breastfed infants have a significantly reduced incidence of colds, flus, and other infections, as well as less propensity for allergic manifestation. Montague (98) describes the reduction of learning disabilities in babies who have been breastfed. He further discusses their superior intellectual development, including higher IQ assessed in breastfed babies. Breast feeding promotes a healthy emotional bond between the mother and child.

Breastfeeding also prefers many health advantages on the mother. These include some protection against ovarian and premenopausal breast cancer and osteoporosis. The release of oxytocin while breast feeding facilitates uterine involution. Maternal weight loss is much more ensured with breast feeding during the first year of the infant's life. Lactation amenorrhea produces a contraceptive effect in mothers whose babies are exclusively breastfed due to the elevated prolactin levels and reduced nocturnal luteinizing hormone, although this should not be regarded as a foolproof method of contraception.

A current global concern is that the initiation rates of breastfeeding mothers wanting to breastfeed their babies through infancy into childhood are waning. The present world standard is that 85% of babies leaving the hospital are being breastfed (101). However, by 3 months of age, this percentage decreases dramatically to 50% or less of infants still being breastfed. Limited maternal leave for working mothers and work environments that do not facilitate breastfeeding or child care contribute to this problem. There is a distinct lack of education and commitment in the medical community to support continuous breastfeeding; this is compounded by the fact that a great majority of health care providers are inadequately informed. Further, our society suffers from the social stigma of living in a bottle-feeding culture. The international average age of weaning from breastfeeding is 4.2 years of age (102); however, in our culture, we shrink from the mainstream condemnation of babies being breastfed beyond 1 year of age. As chiropractors, we have a responsibility to participate in and support the movement toward a breastfeeding culture, so that our babies may reap the short and long-term benefits granted them by their natural birthrights. Availability of references on breastfeeding in the office is essential, as well as established referral to professional lactation consultants.

REFERENCES

1. Aimant J. X-ray pelvimetry of the pregnant adolescent. Obstet Gynecol 1976; 48-281.
2. Barge FH. Scoliosis. Identifiable causes, detection and correction, 2nd ed. Davenport, Iowa: Bawden Bros., Inc., 1986:76-78.
3. Bautch, Caruso, Nuzzi, Stady, Grilliot. The importance of a sacral base x-ray view in a complete lumbar study. Logan College of Chiropractic, 1982.
4. Kirkaldy-Willis WH. Managing low back pain. New York: Churchill Livingstone, 1983.
5. National Institute of Child Health and Human Development. National Registry for Amniocentesis Study Group. Midtrimester amniocentesis for prenatal diagnosis: safety and accuracy. JAMA 1976; 236:1471-6.
6. Simpson NE, Dallaire L, Miller JR, et al. Prenatal diagnosis of genetic disease in Canada: report of a collaborative study. Can Med Assoc J 1976; 115:739-48.
7. Hunter AG, Thompson D, Speevak M. Midtrimester genetic amniocentesis in eastern Ontario: a review from 1970 to 1985. J Med Genet 1987; 24:335-43.
8. Hess LW, Anderson RL, Golbus MS. Significance of opaque discolored amniotic fluid at second trimester amniocentesis. Obstet Gynecol 1986;67 (suppl):44-6.
9. Djalali M, Barbi G, Kennerknecht I, Terinde R. Introduction of early amniocentesis to routine prenatal diagnosis. Prenat Diag Aug 1992;12:8: 661-66.
10. Elajalde BR, de Elajalde MM, Aunca JM, Thelan D, Trujillo C. Prospective study of amniocentesis performed between 9 and 16 weeks gestation: its feasibility, risks, complications and use in early genetic prenatal diagnosis. Am J Med Genet 1990;35:188-96.
11. Evans MI, Drugan A, Koppitch FC, et al. Genetic diagnosis in the first trimester: the norm for the 1990s. Am J Obstet Gynecol 1989; 160:1332-6.
12. Rhoades GG, Jackson LG, Schlesselman SE, et al. The safety and efficacy of chorionic villus sampling for early prenatal diagnosis of cytogenetic abnormalities. N Engl J Med 1989;320:611-7.
13. Wilson RD, Kendrick V, Wittmann BK, McGillivray B. Spontaneous abortion and pregnancy outcome after normal first-trimester ultrasound examination. Obstet Gynecol 1985;67(Suppl):352-5.
14. Gilmore DH, McNay MB. Spontaneous fetal loss rate in early pregnancy. Lancet 1985;1:8420, 107.
15. Burton BK, Schulz CJ, Burd LI. Limb anomalies associated with chorionic villus sampling. Obstet Gynecol 1992;79:726-30.
16. Brambati B, Simoni G, Tavi M, Danesino C, Tului L, Privitera O, Stioui S, Tedeschi S, Primignani P. Transabdominal and transcervical chorionic villus sampling before 8 gestational weeks: efficiency, reliability and risks on 317 completed pregnancies. Prenat Diagn 1992; 12:787-99.
17. Holmes LB. Limb deficiency defects among 125,000 newborn infants. Am J Hum Genet 1992;51(Suppl):a18.
18. Eiben B, Hammans W, Goebel R. Fetal development after chorionic villus sampling. Lancet 1993;341:1037-38.
19. Report of NICHD Workshop on CVS and Limb and other Defects. J SOGC 1993:754-59.
20. Brewer T. Toxemia of pregnancy. Am J Obstet Gynecol 1964; 89:838.
21. Williams P. Nourishing your unborn child. New York: Avon,1974.
22. Baldwin R. Special delivery. Berkeley: Celestial Arts, 1986.
23. Schenker JG. Fetal alcohol syndrome: Current status of pathogenesis. Alcoholism: Clinical and Experimental Research 1990; 14:635.
24. Henry AK, Feldhausen J. Drugs, vitamins, minerals, pregnancy. Tucson, AZ: Fisher Books, 1989:40.
25. Compendium of Pharmaceutical Specialties. 13th ed. Ottawa: Canadian Pharmaceutical Association, 1995.
26. Butler NR, Goldstein H. Smoking in pregnancy and subsequent child development. Br Med J 1973:573-78.
27. Morris MB, Weinstein L. Caffeine and the fetus: Is trouble brewing? Am J Obstet Gynecol 1981; 140:607-11.
28. Scrisuphan W, Bracken MB. Caffeine consumption during pregnancy and association with late spontaneous abortion. Am J Obstet Gynecol 1986; 154:14-19.
29. Martin TR, Bracken MB. The association between low birth weight and caffeine consumption during pregnancy. Am J Epidemiol 1987;126, Nov 1987:813-18.
30. American Medical Association's Council on Scientific Affairs. Caffeine labelling. JAMA 1984; 252:803-06.
31. Diakow PRP, Gadsby TA, Gadsby JB, Gleddie JG, Leprich DJ, Scales AM. Back pain during pregnancy and labor. J Manipulative Physiol Ther 1991; 14:116-118.
32. Rungee JL. Low back pain during pregnancy. Orthopedics 1993;16:1339-44.
33. Abramson D, Roberts S, Wilson P. Relaxation of the pelvic joints in pregnancy. Surg Gynecol Obstet 1934;58:595-613.
34. MacLennan AH. Serum relaxin and pelvic pain of pregnancy. Lancet 1986; 2:235-236.
35. Mantero E, Crispini L. Static alterations of the pelvis, sacral, lumbar area due to pregnancy. Chiropractic treatment. In: Mazzarelli JP. ed. Chiropractic Interprofessional Research, Torino: Edizioni Minerva Medica,1982:59-68.
36. Fast A, Shapiro D, Ducommun EJ, Friedmann LW, Bouklas T, Floman Y. Low-back pain in pregnancy. Spine 1987;12(4)368-371.
37. Cunningham FG, MacDonald PC, Gant NF, Leveno KJ, Gilstrap LC. Williams Obstetrics. 19th ed.Appleton & Lange: Norwalk, CT, 1993:276.
38. Trillat P. Gynec et Obst 1926; 14:211.
39. Gibberd GF. The factors influencing the attitude of the foetus in utero. Section of Obstetrics and Gynaecology. Proc Royal Soc Med : 1223-1229.
40. Taylor HC. Breech presentation with hyperextension of the neck and intrauterine dislocation of cervical vertebrae. Am J Obstet Gynecol 1948; 56:381.
41. Aker PS, Cassidy JD. Torticollis in infants and children: a report of three cases. J Can Chiro Assoc 1990;34:13-19.
42. Hellstrom B, Sallmander U. Prevention of cord injury in hyperextension of the fetal head. JAMA 1968;202:1041-44.
43. Cunningham FC, MacDonald PC, Gant NF, Leveno KJ, Gilstrap LC. Williams Obstetrics, 19th ed. Appleton & Lange, 1993:504.
44. Burns JW. An unusual attitude of the child in utero. Clinical and laboratory notes. Lancet 1928;2:751-752.
45. Knowlton RW. A flying foetus. J Obstet Gynecol Br 1938; 45:834-835.
46. Kobak AJ. Deflection attitudes in transverse fetal presentations. Am J Obstet Gynecol, 1946; 51:582.
47. Fallon J. Textbook on Chiropractic & Pregnancy. Arlington, Va: ICA, 1994:112.
48. Anrig C. Chiropractic approaches to pregnancy and pediatric care. In: Plaugher G. ed. Textbook of clinical chiropractic: a specific biomechanical approach. Baltimore: Williams & Wilkins,1993:383-432.
49. Gimovsky ML, Schifrin BS. Breech management. J Perinat 1992; 12(2):143-151.
50. Goer H. Obstetric myths versus research realities.Westport, CT: Bergin & Garvey, 1995:107-111.
51. Simkin P, Whalley J, Keppler A. Pregnancy childbirth and the newborn. New York: Meadowbrook Press, 1991:178.
52. Lopes MA, Plaugher G, Walters P, Cremata E. Spinal Examination. In: Plaugher G, ed. Textbook of clinical chiropractic: a specific biomechanical approach. Baltimore: Williams & Wilkins, 1993;73-111.
53. Plaugher G, Doble RW, Lopes MA. Lower Cervical Spine. In: Plaugher G, ed. Textbook of Clinical Chiropractic A Specific Biomechanical Approach. Baltimore: Williams & Wilkins, 1993;295-301.
54. Plaugher G, Lopes MA. The knee-chest table: indications and contraindications. Chiropractic Technique 1990;2:163-167.
55. Dick-Read G. Childbirth Without Fear. 4th ed. New York, Harper & Row 1972:31-35.
56. Dick-Read G. Childbirth Without Fear. 4th ed. New York, Harper & Row, 1972:325-6.
57. Oxorn H. Human labor and birth. 4th ed.New York: Appleton-Century-Crofts, 1980:401.
58. Sinclair L, Young R. Mind body connection in the labour and birth process. Positive birthing and beyond workshop archives, 1995.
59. Cunningham FG, MacDonald PC, Gant NF, Leveno KJ, Gilstrap LC. Williams Obstetrics. 19th 4d. Norwalk, CT: Appleton & Lange, 1993: 378-379.

60. Friedman, EA. Use of labor pattern as a management guide. Hosp Top1968;46(8): 58-63.

61. Goer H. Obstetric myths versus research realities. Westport, CT: Bergin & Garvey, 1995:179-202.

62. Apgar V. A proposal for a new method of evaluation of the newborn infant. Curr Res Anest Analg 1953 32:260-274.

63. Lawrence R. Breastfeeding. 4th ed. St. Louis: Mosby, 1994.

64. Anderson RT. Angulation of the basiocciput in three cranial series. Current Anthropol 1983;24:226-228.

65. Hughes JG.4th ed. Synopsis of pediatrics. St Louis: Mosby, 1975:942.

66. Levene MI, Tudehope D. Essentials of neonatal medicine. 2nd ed. Oxford: Blackwell Scientific Publications, 1993:49,319.

67. Modic MT, Masaryk TJ, Ross JS. Magnetic resonance imaging of the spine. Chicago: Year Book Medical Publishers, 1989:217.

68. Towbin A. Latent spinal cord and brain stem injury in newborn infants. Devlop Med Child Neurol 1969;11:54-68.

69. Leventhal HR. Birth injuries of the spinal cord. J Pediat 1960;56:447-453.

70. Gordon N, Marsden B. Spinal cord injury at birth. Neuropadiatrie 1970; 2(1):112-118.

71. Foderl V. Die Halsmarquetschung. eine Unteract der geburtstraumatischen Schadigung des Zentralnervensystems. Arch Gyna 1931;143:598-603.

72. Stolzenberg F. Zerreissungen der intervertebralen Gelenkkapsein der Halswir-belsaule, eine typische Geburtsverletzung. Berl KlinWsehr 1911;48:1741-1743.

73. Stanley P, Duncan AW, Isaacson J, Isaacson AS. Radiology of fracture-dislocation of the cervical spine during delivery. AJR 1985; 145:621-625.

74. Gordon N, Marsden N. Spinal cord injury at birth. Neuropadiatrie 1970; 2(1):112-118.

75. Yates PO. Birth trauma to vertebral arteries. Arch Dis Child 1959; 34:436-441.

76. Pollock AN, Reed MH. Shoulder deformities from obstetrical brachial plexus paralysis. Skel Radiol 1989;18:295-297.

77. Parrot. Note sur an cas de rupture de la moelle, chez un nouveau-ne par suite de manoevres pendent l'accouchement. L'Union Med 1870; 11:137-141.

78. Ford FR. Breech delivery in its possible relations to injury of the spinal cord. Arch Neurol Psychiatr 1925; 14:742-750.

79. Pierson RN. Spinal and cranial injuries of the baby in breech deliveries. Surg Gynecol Obstet 1923; (Nov):802-815.

80. Towbin A. Latent spinal cord and brain stem injury in newborn infants. Develop Med Child Neurol 1969;11:54-68.

81. Banks BD, Beck RW, Columbus M, Gold PM, Kinsinger FS, Lalonde MA. Sudden infant death syndrome: A literature review with chiropractic implications. J Manip Physiol Ther 1987;10(5):236-251.

82. Levene, MI, Tudehope D. Essentials of Neonatal Medicine. 2nd ed. Victoria, Australia: Blackwell Scientific Publications, 1993:58.

83. Curran JS, Birth associated injury. Clin Perinatol 1981;8:111-130.

84. Shulman ST, Madden JD, Esterly JR, Shanklin DR. Transection of spinal cord. A rare obstetrical complication of cephalic delivery. Arch Dis Child 1971; 46:291-294.

85. Laisram N, Srivastava VK, Srivastava RK. Cerebral palsy—an etiological study. Indian J Pediatr 1992;59:723-728.

86. Eastman N, Hellman LM. Obstetrics, 12th ed. New York:Appleton, 1969.

87. Friedman EA. Disordered labor. Objective evaluation and management. J Fam Pract 1975;2:167.

88. Cunningham FG, MacDonald PC, Gant NF, Leveno KJ, Gilstrap LC. Williams obstetrics, 19th ed. Norwalk, CT: Appleton & Lange, 1993:556.

89. Gordon M, Rich H, Deutschberger J, Green M. The immediate and long term outcome of obstetric birth trauma. Am J Obstet Gynecol 1973;117:51-56.

90. Goer H. Obstetric myths versus research realities. Westport, CT: Bergin & Garvey, 1995:83-105.

91. Rubin A. Birth injuries: Incidence, mechanisms and end results. Obstet Gynecol 1964;23(2):218-221.

92. Hardy AE. Birth injuries of the brachial plexus incidence and prognosis. J Bone Joint Surg 1981;63-B(1):98-101.

93. Hernandez RJ, Dias L. CT evaluation of the shoulder in children with Erb's palsy. Pediatr Radiol 1988;18:333-336.

94. Gordon M, Rich M, Deutschberger J, Even M. The immediate and long term outcome of obstetric birth trauma, brachial plexus paralysis. Am J Obstet Gynecol 1973;92:122-130.

95. Levene MI, Tudehope D. Essentials of neonatal medicine, 2nd ed. Oxford: Blackwell Scientific Publications, 1993:57.

96. Simkin P, Whalley J, Keppler A. Pregnancy, childbirth and the newborn: the complete guide. Deephaven MN: Meadowbook Press, Simon & Schuster, 1991.

97. La Leche League International. The womanly art of breastfeeding, 3rd ed. Franklin Park, IL, 1981.

98. Montague A. Touching, 2nd ed. New York: Harper & Row, 1978:67.

99. Minchin M. Breastfeeding matters, 2nd ed. Armadale, Victoria, Australia: Allen & Unwin, 1989.

100. Lawrence RA. Breastfeeding: a guide for the medical profession, 4th ed. St. Louis, 1994:312.

101. Renfrew M, Fisher C, Arms S. Bestfeeding: getting breastfeeding right for you. Berkeley: Celestial Arts, 1990.

102. Martin J, White A. Infant feeding: 1985 Office of Population Censuses and Surveys. London: Her Majesty's Stationery Office, 1988.

103. Nutrition Committee of the Canadian Paediatric Society and the Committee of Nutrition of the American Academy of Pediatrics. "Breast-Feeding: A Commentary in Celebration of the International Year of the Child." Pediatrics 1978; 62.

104. Garza C, Schanler RJ, Butte NF, Motil KJ. Special properties of human milk. Clin Perinatol 1987;14:11-32.

6 Exercise During Pregnancy

Debra W. Levinson and Judy A. Forrester

The recommendations for exercise in pregnancy have evolved with the recently increasing focus on fitness as an adjunct to health and well-being. Both benefits and risks have been hypothesized as resulting from exercise during pregnancy. The pregnant patient can stand to profit with appropriate consideration given to the stage of pregnancy, the pre-pregnant fitness quotient of the individual and the current health status of the mother and fetus. However, some adverse perinatal outcomes have been associated with exercise; specifically, the diversion of blood away from the splanchnic bed to the skeletal muscles could deprive the fetus of oxygen and nutrients leading to intrauterine growth retardation or fetal distress (1).

The 1985 guidelines for exercise during pregnancy developed by the American College of Obstetrics and Gynecology have been suggested as too stringent for well-conditioned, low risk, prenatal patients (2). Recent studies support the view that moderate fitness conditioning can augment maternal metabolic and cardiopulmonary capacities without altering fetal development or pregnancy outcome (3).

The initial hemodynamic change in pregnancy appears to be an increase in heart rate (4). This commences between 2 and 5 weeks and continues well into the third trimester. Elevation of stroke volume occurs slightly later than the heart rate and continues throughout the second trimester after an augmentation of venous return and a decrease of systemic vascular resistance and afterload. Myocardial contractility is likely to slightly increase.

Structural changes within the heart reflect the volume loading of pregnancy and include dilatation of the valve ring and increase in myocardial thickness. Plasma volume undergoes a 30 to 60 percent increase during pregnancy. There is also a 20 to 30 percent increase in red blood cell mass. The increase in blood volume occurs rapidly during the second trimester, and lessens near term. During exercise, plasma is filtered out from the capillary bed as a result of increased capillary pressure from working muscles (4). Maximal oxygen uptake and the work rate at the onset of blood lactate accumulation (OBLA) are not significantly altered during the course of a normal pregnancy (4).

Oxygen consumption can increase during pregnancy as the result of an increased number of red blood cells, an increasing tissue mass, and an increase in metabolic rate. Maternal and fetal oxygen consumption climaxes near term and is estimated to be 16 to 30 percent above nonpregnant values (5).

Regular recreational exercise increases the rate of growth in placental volume in the midtrimester of pregnancy, possibly due to an adaptive response to the intermittent stimulus of a reduction in regional blood flow (6). In addition, recreational exercise performed by well-conditioned women at or above a baseline conditioning level in mid and late pregnancy is normally associated with an increase in fetal heart rate (7). The indication of a diminished blood flow during exercise suggests the possibility of fetal oxygen supply being lowered and thus the fetal heart rate would be affected more by physical activity in late pregnancy (8). It has been stated that maternal exercise has no effect upon the birth weight, the newborn length, and the placental size, therefore, suggesting that physical activity in pregnancy seems to be neither beneficial nor detrimental to fetal growth (9).

Summarily, effects on the fetus by maternal exercise do not appear to contraindicate physical activity, provided due caution and consideration prevail.

Exercise and Pregnancy

The safety of the mother and infant is the primary concern in any exercise program. The goal of exercise both before and during pregnancy as well as during the postpartum period, should be to maintain the highest level of fitness consistent with maximum safety. The potential for maternal and fetal injury is significant because of the musculoskeletal and cardiovascular changes at this time. Therefore, any exercise recommendations should err on the conservative side.

With regard to the professional athlete who is physically well-trained, the approach may be to continue training under strict obstetrical observation to avoid a conflict between the patient's professional needs and the needs of the fetus. Although the athlete may wish to continue to train and compete, it may become extremely difficult for the professional or elite athlete to maintain a level of fitness that will allow her to continue beyond the 20th week of pregnancy (10). All professional athletes should plan to stop active competition between 16 and 20 weeks or earlier if they notice that they are experiencing difficulty (10). The female professional athlete who is under strict observation by her health care provider should expect to have the same pregnancy outcome as any other woman (10). The sole purpose of an exercise program during pregnancy is to maintain physical fitness and to prepare for labor and delivery, and not to challenge the limits of the fetus.

The growth and development of a new life requires the interaction of many of the body's systems. Exercise requires these complex interactions as well. In fact, pregnancy and exercise "share" certain body systems, including the metabolic system, the circulatory system, the respiratory system, and the musculoskeletal system (11). Because both exercise and pregnancy depend on common systems, they can interact with each other. For example, pregnancy changes the muscular and skeletal systems, which are also basic to the source for locomotion and balance of the individual. Exercise produces heat that can also disturb the developing fetus (11).

Planning Before Conception

Infant mortality rates decrease, not with better birth technology, but with pre-pregnancy planning, including proper exercise and nutrition. Equally important to eating well is giving the nutrients a chance to get where they are needed. Aerobic activity helps in this regard. When the heart and the circulatory system are stimulated into good performance, healthier organs, stronger connective tissue, and denser bones are built or maintained (12). Also, aerobic activity of the proper type, intensity, duration, and frequency, combined with a diet composed mostly of complex carbohydrates, is the best way to eliminate stored toxins (13).

Guidelines for Prenatal Exercise

The following guidelines are based on the unique physical and physiological conditions that exist during pregnancy. They will outline the general criteria for safety during the development of home exercise programs. This information was compiled from the American College of Obstetricians and Gynecologists Exercise during Pregnancy and the Postnatal Period (ACOG Home Exercise Programs) (12):

1. Regular exercise at least three times a week is preferable to intermittent activity. Competitive activities should be discouraged. However, in the case of a professional or elite athlete who is already accustomed to training at a high heart rate, it is probable that the pregnant athlete may be able to continue to exercise above the 140 heart rate limit recommended for the general pregnant population (10). Rare cardiovascular complications can also occur in athletes. As a result, warning signs include the appearance of palpitations and tachycardia during rest.

2. Vigorous exercise should not be performed in hot, humid weather or during a period of febrile illness.

3. Ballistic movements such as jerky, bouncy motions, should be avoided. Exercise should be done on a wooden floor or a tightly carpeted surface to reduce shock and provide a sure footing.

4. Deep flexion or extension of joints should be avoided because of connective tissue laxity. Activities that require jumping, jarring motions or rapid changes in direction should be avoided because of joint instability.

5. Vigorous exercise should be followed by a period of gradually declining activity that includes gentle stationary stretching. Because connective tissue laxity increases the risk of joint injury, stretches should not be taken to the point of maximum resistance.

6. The pregnant woman's heart rate should be measured at times of peak activity. Target heart rates and limits established in consultation with the health care provider should not be exceeded.

7. Care should be taken to gradually rise from the floor to avoid orthostatic hypertension. Some form of activity involving the legs should be continued for a brief period.

8. Liquids should be taken liberally before, during, and after exercise to prevent dehydration. If necessary, activity should be interrupted to replenish fluids.

9. Women who have led sedentary lifestyles should begin with physical activity of very low intensity and advance their activity levels very gradually.

10. Activity should be stopped and the health care provider consulted if any unusual symptoms appear.

As for the pregnant professional athlete, she can consider becoming pregnant while still being competitive. However, she should seek counselling immediately from a health care provider to learn the proper way of balancing the exercise regime with her pregnancy.

Some recommendations for athletes include having a dietary evaluation, a review of desired pregnancy dates, and counselling on potential limitations of pregnancy before conceiving.

In some cases concerning pregnant professional athletes, ovulation induction should be considered. Once pregnant, the professional athlete does not appear to face any problems specific to her professional status. Although few definitive studies exist, the available data indicates that professional athletes are at no greater risk (10).

The predominate maternal risks stem mostly from overuse injuries. Fetal risks are related to hyperthermia, dehydration, and premature labor. Intrauterine growth may occur with a higher frequency. After pregnancy, the athlete can return to competition as soon as they feel ready. Usually, the athlete can resume conditioning activities within 2–4 weeks of delivery (10).

In considering the average female pregnancy, seven guidelines should be followed:

1. The maternal heart rate should not exceed 140 beats per minute.

2. Exercise intensity should be low, well below the anaerobic threshold. An intensity of 50–60% maximal functional capacity (maximal oxygen consumption) will prevent excessive build up of exercise by-products and heat that could be delivered to the growing fetus.

Intensity can be guided by target heart rates, perceived exertion, and the talk test by being able to speak without the breath becoming too rapid.

3. Strenuous activities should not exceed 15 minutes in duration.

4. No exercise should be performed in the supine position after the fourth month of gestation is completed.

5. Exercises that employ the Valsalva maneuver should be avoided.

6. Caloric intake should be adequate to meet not only the extra energy needs of pregnancy, but also of the exercise performed.

7. Maternal core temperature should not exceed 38 degrees Celsius.

Contraindications or Cautions

The following recommendations are from the 1994 ACOG Guidelines. Women with the following signs or symptoms should not exercise at all:

1. Bleeding
2. Heart disease
3. History of 3+ spontaneous abortions or miscarriages
4. Incompetent cervix
5. Intrauterine growth retardation
6. Pregnancy-induced hypertension
7. Multiple babies (twins, triplets, etc.)
8. Placenta previa
9. Premature labor
10. Ruptured membranes

Women with the following signs and symptoms should only exercise with her caregiver's (health care provider's) permission:

1. Anemia/other blood disorder
2. Breech in the last trimester
3. Diabetes
4. Excessive obesity
5. Extremely sedentary
6. Extreme underweight
7. High blood pressure
8. History of bleeding during pregnancy
9. History of intrauterine growth retardation
10. History of precipitous labor
11. Irregular heart rhythms
12. Pulmonary disease
13. Thyroid disease
14. Vascular disease

Warning Signs and Symptoms

Exercise should stop immediately and the caregiver (health care provider) contacted if the patient experiences any of the following:

1. Back pain
2. Disoriented feeling
3. Extreme nausea
4. Marked swelling or fluid retention
5. Pubic pain
6. Sharp pain in abdomen or chest
7. Temperature is extremely hot, cold or clammy
8. Uterine contractions
9. Any vaginal bleeding
10. Decrease in fetal movement
11. Gush or fluid from vagina
12. Blurred vision
13. Dizziness
14. Fainting
15. Difficulty in walking
16. Shortness of breath
17. Pain or palpitations

Physiologic Changes During Pregnancy

The physiological changes during pregnancy require certain modifications to any general exercise program. Pregnancy increases maternal blood volume, heart rate, cardiac stroke volume and, consequently, cardiac output (14).

Normally, blood volume and associated cardiac output increase early in pregnancy (6 to 8 weeks of gestation) and reach a peak increase of 40 to 50 percent by the middle of the second trimester. Stroke volume and heart rate also increase early in pregnancy and peak by mid-pregnancy, with stroke volume increasing by as much as 30 percent and heart rate by 15 to 20 beats per minute. The total increase in body mass due to pregnancy to be served by this increased cardiac output is only 13 percent, with the majority of the increase occurring in late pregnancy (14).

Specific maternal cardiovascular alterations help accommodate fetal development. Cardiac output increases 30–50% during pregnancy, and the resting oxygen consumption rate increases by 30%. These cardiovascular factors can help facilitate exercise during pregnancy (15).

The increase in cardiac output creates a marked cardiovascular reserve in early pregnancy, when exercise is usually well tolerated. At this stage, some women report an improved exercise tolerance as compared with their pre-pregnancy level. In late pregnancy, however, cardiovascular reserve decreases as fetal needs increase.

The increase in blood volume is important because many complications of pregnancy, such as premature labor, hypertension, and in-utero fetal growth retardation, are associated with relative maternal hypovolemia or failure of plasma volume expansion. The condition "pregnancy anemia," usually seen in the second and third trimesters may be a true anemia in some women, but in most it reflects a plasma volume expansion that exceed the concurrent increase in red cell mass (14).

This process is similar to the pseudo-anemia that develops in long-distance athletes because of plasma volume expansion. The pseudo-anemia may be substantial evidence for encouraging women to start an exercise program before conception, thus improving cardiac reserve and possible preventing complications from hypovolemia (14).

During light to moderate intensity exercise, the mobilization and use of carbohydrates and fat suddenly increase at least sixfold and remain increased for a variable period of time post exercise (16, 17). New tissue growth may be inhibited due to the sudden release of energy.

In addition to the above cited changes, a pregnant woman experiences respiratory changes, weight gain, changes in energy levels and metabolism, and musculoskeletal changes such as an expanding uterus, which displaces the center of gravity anteriorly, resulting in progressive lumbar lordosis, which in turn, alters balance (14). The concern at this point is an increased susceptibility to injury. Increased lumbar lordosis adversely affects a woman's ability to exercise during pregnancy.

The impact of exercise can also cause membrane rupture, placental separation, premature labor, direct fetal injury, or umbilical cord entanglement (17). Because of these changes that occur during pregnancy, women may need to avoid or modify strenuous athletic activities and begin exercising conservatively.

Changes in the lumbar lordosis and the onset of anterior pelvic tilt affect a woman's posture and may make carrying extra weight difficult and painful. Extended periods of walking, even without extra loads, might become difficult, especially after the second trimester. Jogging and other weight-bearing activities can result in increased stress and micro shock of the joints (15).

During dynamic exercise, the blood flow in the splanchnic bed decreases in proportion to the increase in heart rate (18) and decreases in circulation to the uterus. The concern here is the lack of nutrients and oxygen available to the embryo or fetus. This could stimulate uterine contractions, causing preterm labor.

Some exercise positions during a dynamic workout may need to be modified. For example, exercise should not be performed in the supine position. When a pregnant woman lies on her back, the weight of the fetus may obstruct the flow of blood back to her heart and head. For this reason, exercise in the supine position has been contraindicated after the fourth month of pregnancy. Symptoms of obstructed blood flow include light-headedness or dizziness. If a pregnant woman should become light-headed in the supine position, she should be rolled on to her side until she feels better. Then she should slowly be assisted into an upright position (10).

Women who continue to exercise in a supine position after 4 months into their pregnancy, because they do not "feel" the symptoms of low blood flow to the head, should realize that the blood flow to the fetus may still decrease when in this position. Therefore, the fetus may experience negative effects even though the mother does not (10).

Body temperature and exercise intensity have a direct proportional relationship. During early pregnancy, the obvious concern is that exercise-induced hyperthermia will cause abortion or congenital abnormalities, particularly midline fusion defects of the central nervous system, heart, spine, and urogenital system (16).

Due to hormonal changes and the growing fetus, the body temperature of a pregnant woman usually starts one to two degrees higher than that of a non-pregnant woman (10). It is extremely important that pregnant exercisers take every precaution against overheating during exercise in a warm environment. Frequent elevation of the body temperature to over 102 degrees in the first trimester may increase the likelihood of neural tube defects in the fetus. Studies associating an increase in body temperature with neural tube defects have dealt with chronic heat exposure, not the heat generated by exercise. However, it is still wise for a pregnant exerciser to be conservative, because the heat generated during exercise can exacerbate chronic heat exposure (16).

The endocrine system's response to exercise is akin to that of stress. Abrupt hormonal changes take place. Blood levels of catecholamines increase briskly followed by increased secretion of glucagon, endorphin, prolactin and cortisol (16,17). The concern here is that this response will initiate uterine contractibility and impair other hormonally mediated adaptations to pregnancy (19–21).

Although some non-experimental reports have associated exercise during pregnancy with increased uterine contractions and prematurity and low birth weight, other well-conducted studies using objective measures do not support these claims.

In the later stages of pregnancy, dehydration from chronic heat exposure may precipitate premature labor. Temperature regulation also remains important during the postpartum period, especially if the mother is breast-feeding her infant. If a nursing mother becomes dehydrated from working in the heat, milk production will be difficult (19). Drinking plenty of fluids before, during, and after exercise is one of the best precautionary measures a mother can take.

Effects of Exercise on Existing Disease

This subject represents an area where a paucity of literature exists and where both potential risk and/or benefits of exercise during pregnancy can be great. In this regard, specific areas of interest include coexistent maternal cardiovascular, pulmonary and metabolic disease; the extremes of fetal growth; and several disease states unique to pregnancy. Because some of the research that has been done in this area involves animal models, the author has chosen only to cite the studies that have been conducted on human female subjects (22).

Cardiovascular Disease

The interaction between pre-existent cardiovascular disease and exercise during pregnancy has been examined in only a limited number of subjects with untreated rheumatic heart disease, which is rare today. These findings suggest that, with sufficient disease, the cardiac output response to exercise is reduced, which should induce increased splanchnic vasoconstriction to adequately supply the exercising muscle. Despite the increasing incidence of obstetrical patients with both surgically corrected and uncorrected congenital heart disease, there is virtually no data that directly addresses the issue of superimposing the cardiovascular stress of exercise on that of pregnancy (22).

There is no information dealing with the effects of physical activity in pregnancies complicated by pre-existing hypertension, lupus erythematosus, or peripheral vascular disease. The same is true for metabolic disease with the exception of diabetes mellitus. Likewise, the use of exercise to modulate fetal growth through its effects on placentatation and nutrient delivery has received scant attention.

Growth Abnormalities

The effect of exercise on fat mass and size at birth of the offspring of recreational athletes suggest that it may prove to be a useful therapeutic modality in women with a history of pregnancies complicated by either fetal growth restriction or fetal overgrowth (22).

Diabetes

Gestational diabetes occurs in 4–7% of the obstetric population. Insulin therapy and diet may not be the only or optimal treatment to attain euglycemia. The hormonal changes of pregnancy reduce peripheral insulin sensitivity and are further amplified in patients affected by gestational diabetes. Reduced insulin sensitivity can be reversed most efficiently with exercise. Exercise has been recognized for a long time as an adjunct or alternative therapeutic modality for type II diabetic patients (52). Pregnant diabetics have been denied this option in the past, primarily because of the potential fetal risks. Recent studies on fetal responses to exercise have removed some of the initial concerns (52).

Pilot exercise studies conducted in pregnant diabetics indicate that these patients' physiologic and metabolic responses are similar to healthy non-diabetics. No maternal or fetal adverse responses have been reported concerning pregnant diabetics engaging in mild to moderate physical activities. Nor have significant complications been reported in non-diabetic, physically active pregnant women (22).

To date, a few studies have tested several exercise prescription regimens for pregnant diabetics. These studies have assessed maternal and fetal safety and the efficacy of exercise prescription to improve carbohydrate tolerance and obviate insulin therapy (22). The prescribed exercise regimens include the following:

1. Artal: 20 minutes of bicycle ergometry (18 subjects) at 50% Vo2max after each meal (three times per day) for at least 5 days per week for 6 weeks before estimated date of confinement (EDC);
2. Jovanovic-Peterson: 2 minutes of arm ergometry (10 subjects) at less than 50% Vo2max (daily) for 6 weeks before EDC;
3. Bung: 45 minutes of bicycle ergometry (21 subjects) at 50% of Vo2max three to four times per week for at least 6 weeks before EDC.

All of these studies have demonstrated that exercise prescription is feasible in pregnant diabetics and may be used as an optional therapeutic approach even in previously sedentary gestational diabetics (22). The type, frequency, and intensity of exercise used in these studies were sufficient to attain and maintain euglycemia. Non–weight-bearing exercise appears to be particularly suited for these types of patients.

In the absence of either medical or obstetric complications, exercise prescription can be an optional or adjunct therapy for gestational diabetes. This concept has been endorsed by the second and third International Workshops on Gestational Diabetes (22).

Benefits of Exercise

The benefits of aerobic exercise for most non-pregnant individuals are familiar to most clinicians (15). Some benefits that might also be applicable to pregnant women include:

1. Reducing blood pressure
2. Decreasing other cardiovascular risks such as clot formation
3. Helping to maintain an ideal body weight
4. Managing stable diabetes

Exercise during pregnancy can also have a beneficial effect on the labor process and delivery. Pregnant women who exercise have shorter labor times, and faster, easier deliveries. Another benefit is the psychological "lift" perceived by those who exercise. Some studies show that women who exercised during pregnancy had higher self-esteem than those who did not. The cause and effect relationship between exercise and high self-esteem, however, has not been established. Studies also have demonstrated high self-esteem was associated with a decrease in the number of complaints of backaches, headaches, and fatigue in an exercising group of pregnant women compared with a non-exercising group of pregnant women. The exercise group also had less shortness of breath, probably because exercising women are more conditioned for difficult breathing (15).

If exercise continues after delivery, the benefits appear to continue. By promoting blood flow, exercise helps decrease varicosities, leg cramps, and peripheral edema.

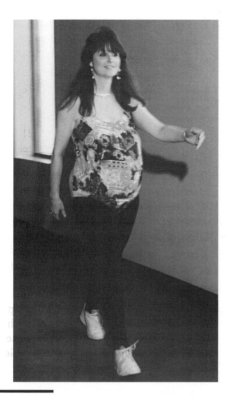

Figure 6.1. Walking is a supportive alternative to ballistic exercises.

Specific Recommendations for Exercise During Pregnancy

Jogging

It is recommended that women not start jogging during pregnancy. If jogging is initiated during pregnancy, it should be started at a low intensity and frequency, with monitoring for any of the symptoms listed previously (23).

Walking

Walking is a supportive alternative to jogging, cycling, and other intense exercises because it does not involve any ballistic (jerky, bouncy) movements, but also helps to condition the cardiovascular system (Fig. 6.1).

Cycling

Cycling can be started during pregnancy because it is not a weight-bearing activity. A stationary bicycle is safer than a standard bicycle, because of the changes in balance that can occur during pregnancy (Fig. 6.2).

Aerobics

The ACOG guidelines recommend that exercise in the supine position, as well as jerky, bouncing movements and deep flexion and extension, be avoided after 4 months gestation. Low impact aerobics may be easier for the pregnant woman to tolerate, especially in the third trimester (23) (Fig. 6.3).

Swimming

Swimming is considered by many to be the perfect aerobic exercise because it can be safely initiated during pregnancy. Swimming in excessively cold or hot water should be avoided.

Hydrotherapy

Immersion or hydrotherapy is one of the oldest forms of healing therapy. Its benefits have been touted since antiquity. Immersion, because of its diuretic and natriuretic effects, has even been proposed as therapy for patients with some forms of renal disease and patients with cirrhosis. The diuresis of immersion may have positive effects on the pregnant woman who is bothered by fluid retention. Water aerobics during pregnancy is a non–weight-bearing exercise that occurs in a "thermal-friendly" medium (10).

Weight Lifting

Lifting light weights for maintenance of strength can be cautiously continued throughout pregnancy provided proper breathing is performed and the Valsava maneuver is avoided, especially in those exercises that may strain the lower back (Fig 6.4) (e.g., dead lifts, bent-over rows and squats).

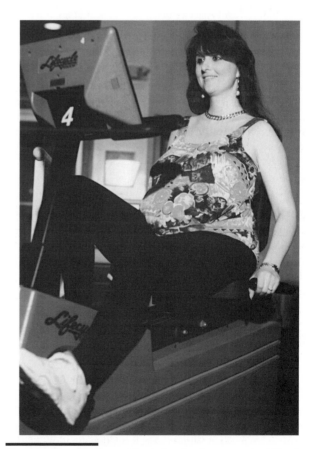

Figure 6.2. Stationary bicycle is safer than a standard bicycle.

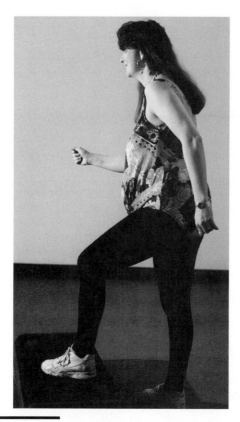

Figure 6.3. Low impact aerobics, such as stair steps, are considered more tolerable especially in the last trimester.

Contact Sports

Because of the potential for trauma to the abdomen, it is recommended that pregnant women avoid collision sports and some contact sports, especially football and field hockey. Basketball, volleyball, gymnastics, and horseback riding are also considered dangerous.

Racquet Sports

Racquetball, squash, and even tennis are thought to be fairly safe for pregnant women. However, as pregnancy progresses, the intensity of play should be reduced to prevent heat stress and injuries due to impaired coordination. Because these sports use unilateral movements, they could create imbalances in the musculoskeletal system.

Water Skiing

Water skiing should be avoided, because high speed falls cause forceful entry of water into the uterus via the vagina with subsequent miscarriage.

Scuba Diving

Experienced divers who are pregnant may continue making very conservative dives, not exceeding 1 atm in pressure (10 m [33 ft]). They should also limit the duration of the dive to 30 minutes or less. Deeper or longer dives and diving by inexperienced divers should be avoided because the compressed air environment can cause decompression sickness in the mother, as well as maternal acid base and nitrogen imbalances and intravascular air embolism in the fetus (53).

Downhill and Cross Country Skiing

Experienced downhill and cross-country skiers who are pregnant may continue to ski cautiously during pregnancy. Falling can be dangerous, and these sports should not be pursued by pregnant inexperienced skiers.

Ice Skating

Ice skating is more dangerous than snow skiing because falls on hard ice can cause more serious trauma. Skating should definitely not be engaged in by inexperienced skaters and should be pursued only with extreme caution by those with experience.

Yoga

Yoga has experienced popularity with pregnant women for two reasons. First is the relaxation effect that many women seek during their pregnancy. The second reason is the desire to maintain muscle tone and flexibility throughout gestation. Yoga should be accompanied by some form of aerobic exercise.

Relaxation

The skills of relaxation and good breathing help prepare a pregnant woman to cope with the challenge and discomforts associated with childbirth. Practicing relaxation and good breathing also has a positive effect on the fetus. Babies, both

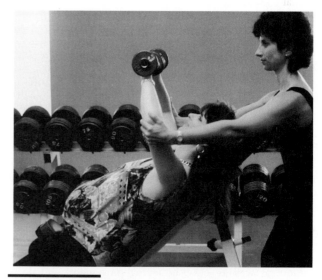

Figure 6.4. Lifting light weights for maintenance, as well as building strength, should be done cautiously.

before they are born as well as postpartum, thrive best in a calm and temperate environment; they need relaxed mothers.

Exercise Progression

The progression of physical activity is an important aspect of any exercise program. During pregnancy, the patient's energy levels tend to gradually fluctuate.

First Trimester

During the first trimester, physical fitness will decrease. Some women will perceive that the same amount of work will require more effort than before pregnancy and they will adjust their efforts accordingly. Other women, who try to continue pre-pregnancy activity levels, will need instruction on decreasing their efforts (10).

Second Trimester

In the second trimester, physical fitness will increase, although rarely to pre-pregnancy levels. A pregnant exerciser may be able to exert more effort during this trimester. If the exercise is comfortable for the pregnant participant and within the recommended guidelines, she should be allowed to continue. Remind her that she must not try to do the same amount of work she did before she was pregnant.

Third Trimester

As body weight increases in the third trimester, physical fitness will again decrease and the amount of work a pregnant exerciser does should be decreased as well. During this time, weight-bearing activities may become uncomfortable, and gradual transition to non–weight-bearing activities such as swimming and stationary cycling may become a reasonable alternative (10).

A progressive exercise program for pregnancy may move from traditional aerobics to low impact aerobics, then alternate low impact aerobics with a walking program, and finally shift to a total walking program. Most changes in exercise mode depend on the participant's comfort. Some women have been able to participate in regular dance-exercise classes and even lead classes until childbirth. Most women will need professional guidance for change.

Spinal Exercise

It is important to strengthen the muscles in the back during pregnancy. It can help to reduce lower back pain and increase flexibility. The benefits of good posture allow the back and neck to lengthen upward, so that the head is well balanced. The spine is then lengthened, allowing plenty of space to accommodate the baby.

As a chiropractor it is important to stress to the pregnant patient that good posture and maintaining a strong spine free from subluxation is vital to both the mother and the fetus' health (24,25).

Pre-Pregnancy Exercises

To choose a proper activity, it is important to remember that anything that moves the large muscle groups such as the arms and legs, simultaneously in a rhythmic manner will be sufficient in getting started. Some exercises may include walking, running, ballroom dancing or aerobic dance, rowing, cycling out in the open or on a stationary bike. A variety of these exercises increases the chances that all muscles will get worked and reduces the risk of imbalance or injury from overworking one particular muscle group (14).

Something as simple as a good brisk walk about three times a week for half an hour enhances the body's ability to handle toxins and improves calcium metabolism. A simple rule to remember which will help a woman preparing for pregnancy decide on the proper exercise duration for her fitness program, is that working the cardiovascular harder than normal for 15 minutes or more will strengthen it; anything shorter will still help, but is less effective (14). And finally, in terms of frequency, while the cardiovascular fitness will get stronger from an aerobic workout three times a week, if the aim is to burn more fat, five or six times a week is preferred. It should be noted that a woman's body needs a bit of fat, about 20 percent, to accept a pregnancy (14). Nature seems to want some insurance that the calories needed to complete the process are going to be there. Body fat can influence hormone levels (14).

If the woman is not used to exercising, start by doing movements against the resistance of gravity; do not use additional weight. Once this is achieved, some resistance such as small weights, can be added to the exercise program.

Remind the pregnant patient that all exercise programs should begin with a set of warm-up exercises for at least the first 5 minutes. The following exercises can be recommended to the pregnant patients. They are beneficial during pregnancy as well as safe and effective movements for postpartum exercise. All exercises should be done on both sides, left and right, to ensure equal balance in exercise strength. After completing an aerobic workout program, remember that a five minute cool down period is necessary, with light stretches and relaxation exercises, to bring the body temperature and heart rate back to normal. Cool down exercises also help to alleviate muscle stiffness after exercise.

Warm-ups and Cool-downs

The following maneuvers should be used as warm-ups and cool-down exercises.

Shoulder rolling: Instruct the pregnant patient to raise her shoulders up towards her ears, backwards and down (Fig 6.5).

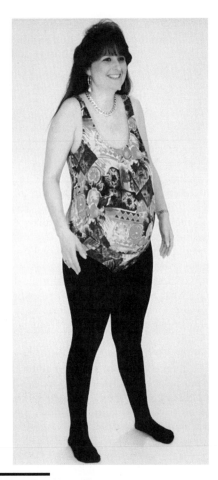

Figure 6.5.   Shoulder rolling.

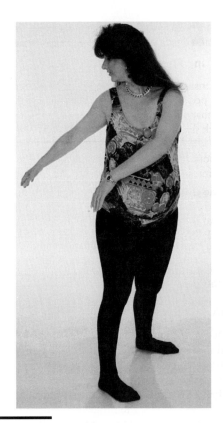

Figure 6.6.   Arm swinging.

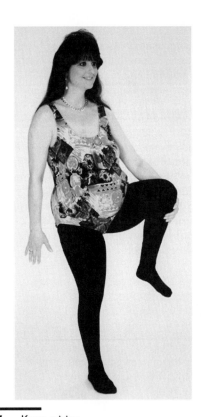

Figure 6.7.   Knee raising.

- Duration: Instruct her to continue rolling her shoulders in this backward circular motion six times.
- Benefits: The benefits of this exercise are to loosen the muscle in the shoulders and neck.

Arm swinging: Instruct the patient to begin by swinging her arms from side to side, keeping the arms at shoulder height and swinging gently and easily (Fig 6.6).

- Duration: Instruct her to continue this exercise six times on each side.
- Benefits: This exercise releases any stiffness in the shoulders, increases blood circulation, and stretches the upper back muscles.

Knee raising: Instruct the patient to bring her right knee up towards her chest and tell her to hold it for two seconds then have her do the left side (Fig 6.7).

- Duration: This should be repeated four times on each side for 2-second intervals.
- Benefits: The benefits of this exercise are that it loosens the knee and pelvic joints, and gives abdominal organs a gentle massage.

Neck Relaxing Exercises

Flexion/Extension: Instruct the patient to sit in a comfortable cross-legged position. Instruct her to relax her head forward and to hold that position for 10 seconds. Then have her relax her head back slowly and hold for 10 seconds (Figs. 6.8, 6.9).

- Duration: Instruct her to repeat this exercise three times in each direction for 10 second intervals.
- Rotation: Instruct her to bring her head back into the center looking straight ahead, then direct her to turn as far to the right side as possible and hold for 10 seconds. Now, have the patient turn to the left side and hold for 10 seconds (Fig 6.10).
- Duration: Repeating this three times in both directions for 10-second intervals.

LATERAL FLEXION

Finally, instruct the patient to bring her head back to the center and her shoulders down and relax looking straight ahead. Instruct her to drop her head toward her right shoulder for 10 seconds and then to do the same thing with the left shoulder (Fig 6.11).

- Duration: Instruct her to repeat the exercise three times in each direction.
- Benefits: The benefit of this exercise is that it relieves tension in the neck and upper back.

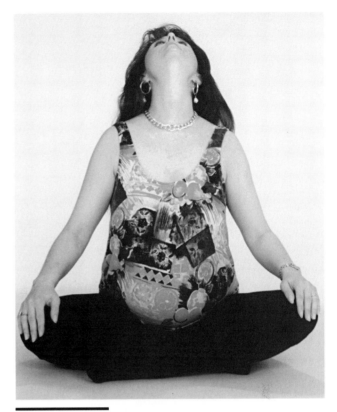

Figure 6.9.   Cervical flexion/extension.

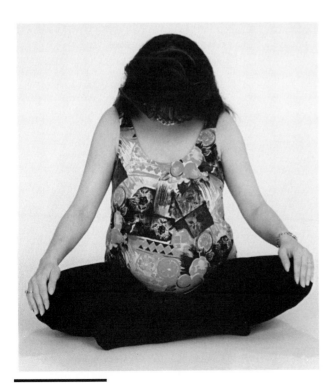

Figure 6.8.   Neck relaxing exercises.

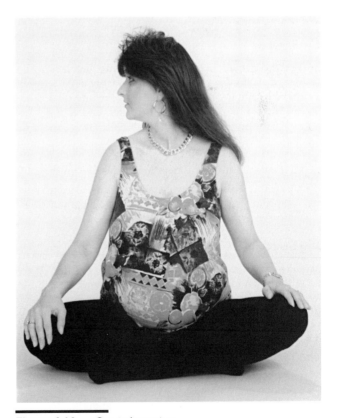

Figure 6.10.   Cervical rotation.

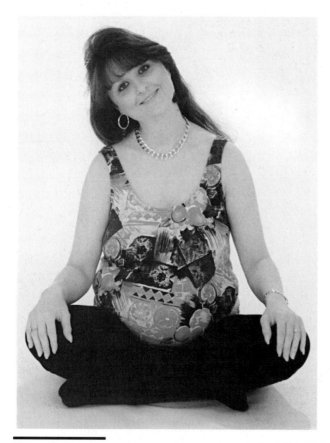

Figure 6.11.   Cervical lateral flexion.

Cat Stretch

Instruct the patient to come forward onto her hands and knees with a flat back. Have her round her back upward towards the ceiling while her head flexes looking toward her knees (Fig 6.12). As the patient relaxes into a flat back position have her extend her head looking toward the ceiling (Fig. 6.13).

- Duration: Have the patient repeat this five times.
- Benefits: This stretches all anterior muscles from knee joints to facial muscles. It also stretches all posterior muscles from hamstring to the neck extensors.

Dog Stretch

Have the patient leave her hands remaining on the floor. Have her push her buttocks up towards the ceiling and heels to the floor. She should repeat two times looking towards her knees (Fig 6.14).

- Duration: Have her hold the stretch for 15 seconds.
- Benefits: This removes fatigue and brings back lost energy. It relieves pain and stiffness in heels, strengthens the ankles, tones the legs, eradicates stiffness in region of shoulder blades and arthritis of shoulder joints is relieved.

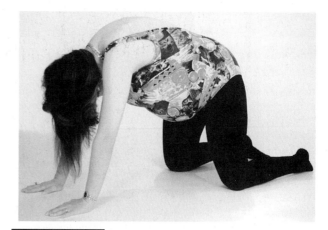

Figure 6.12.   Cat stretch: rounded back position.

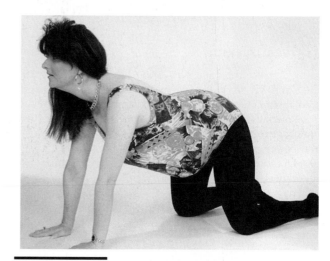

Figure 6.13.   Cat stretch: flat back position.

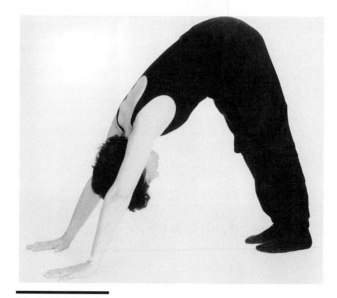

Figure 6.14.   Dog stretch: beyond the first trimester, a pregnant woman should avoid any position that places her head below her heart.

Lumbopelvic and Lower Limb Exercises

Butterfly

Have her bring the soles of her feet together to allow the knees to relax out to the sides (Fig. 6.15). Gently bringing the knees up and down like the wings of a butterfly. Have her relax her knees and come forward as far as she can, attempting to touch her feet with her head. Have her come up slowly and breathe (Fig 6.16).

- Duration: Have her repeat this exercise three times slowly.
- Benefits: This exercise is helpful in alleviating stiffness in legs and tones the spine. It stretches the sacro-illiac joints as well as the ilio-femoral ligaments.

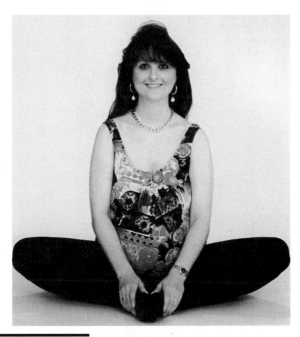

Figure 6.15. Butterfly: the soles of her feet are together allowing the knees to relax out to the sides.

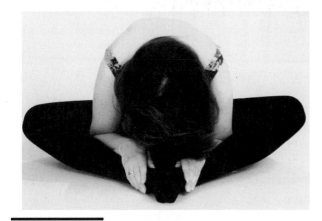

Figure 6.16. Butterfly: forward bend.

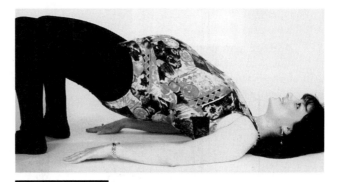

Figure 6.17. Bridge.

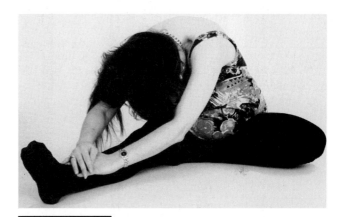

Figure 6.18. Alternate leg stretch.

Bridge

Have the patient lying on her back with the knees bent, heels next to buttocks and her hands on the floor next to her sides, palms facing down. Have her begin by slowly raising up her pelvis, lifting her buttocks off the floor as well as her lumbar and thoracic spine. Then have her slowly lower down, first the mid back, then lower back and then buttocks to the floor and relax (Fig. 6.17).

- Duration: Have her hold the pelvis up for 10 seconds and then release slowly. Have her repeat this exercise three times.
- Benefits: This exercise is helpful in eliminating or minimizing pregnancy backache, relieves neck strain, tones and tightens the thighs.

Alternate Leg Stretch

Have the patient spread her legs hip distance apart in front. Then tell the patient to bend her right leg and place the sole of the foot on the inside of the left thigh. Have the patient facing towards the right leg, then tell her to take her arms and stretch them up along side their ears and relax forward bringing the head as close as possible to the right knee, without bouncing or straining themselves. Slowly have them come up and repeat the stretch to their left side (Fig. 6.18).

- Duration: Repeat the exercise two more times on each side.
- Benefits: This exercise stretches the muscles and the connective tissues in the hamstrings and lower back. It increases the blood circulation in the abdominal organs, and gives a gentle stretch to the knee tendons and muscles.

Squat

Have the patient stand and then squat down with her feet flat on the floor, palms together in front of the chest and elbows pressing against her knees. Instruct her to hold the stretch for 20 seconds while breathing normally. Have her sit back on the buttocks and relax her legs (Fig. 6.19).

- Duration: Have her repeat the exercise one time. Have her work up to holding the exercise for 1 minute.
- Benefits: The benefit here is that it increases flexibility in the knee joints and relieves lower back pressure. It also relaxes the pelvic floor muscles.

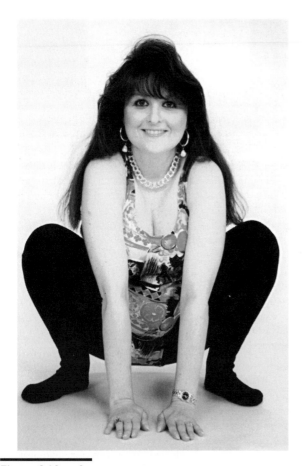

Figure 6.19. Squat.

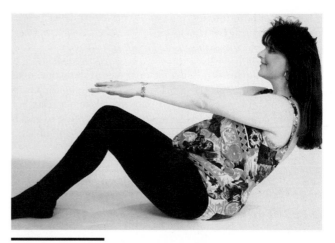

Figure 6.20. Pregnancy sit ups: rolling back one vertebra at a time.

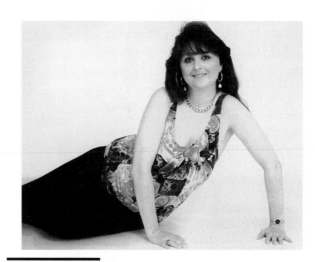

Figure 6.21. Pregnancy sit ups: rolling over onto the left side, to sit up and repeat the exercises.

Abdominal Exercises

Pregnancy Sit-ups

In a seated position, have her bend her knees with her arms extended in front of her over her knees. Have her slowly roll back one vertebra at a time until the shoulders recline, then tell her to sit up and repeat the sit up exercise three times (Figs. 6.20, 6.21).

- Duration: Have the patient work up to 10 repetitions.
- Benefits: This exercise strengthens the abdominal muscles and strengthens the anterior neck muscles.

Alternate Leg Raise

Have the patient stretch her legs out in front on the floor. Instruct the patient to put her hands underneath her pelvis, palms facing down. Have her slowly raise one leg up towards her head, without forcing or straining herself. Instruct her to inhale while raising her leg, hold for 20 seconds, then lower her leg slowly while exhaling. Instruct her to repeat on the opposite leg. If lower back discomfort or pain exists have her bend the opposite leg bringing her foot on the floor towards her pelvis (Fig 6.22).

- Duration: Have her repeat the exercise three times on each side. Hold for 20 seconds while breathing normally.
- Benefits: This exercise stretches the hamstring muscles while strengthening the abdominal muscles.

Pelvic Floor Exercises

Exercises for the Birth Canal or Pelvic Floor

The pelvic floor is the layer of muscles which form a sling across the base of the pelvis and support the bladder, uterus and rectum. The sphincter muscles surround the passages to the anus, vagina and urethra. Pregnancy and childbirth increases the strain on these muscles.

To become familiar with these muscles, tell the patient to do the following exercises:

1. While urinating, stop urine flow midstream.
2. Void a little more and then contract again.
3. Once they have accomplished steps 1 and 2, interrupt the flow several times during each urination.
4. Once they know how to contract these muscles, then tell them to try it when they are not urinating, several times a day.
5. Contracting the sphincter muscles along with the pelvic floor muscles, then release them slowly from front to back.

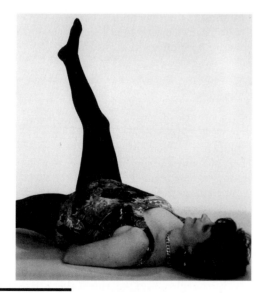

Figure 6.22.   Alternate leg raise.

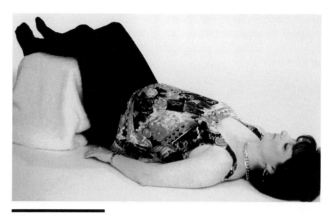

Figure 6.23.   Position 1: relaxation.

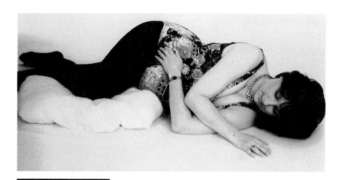

Figure 6.24.   Position 2: relaxation.

Relaxation Positions

The relaxation exercises help to deeply relax the muscles and the nervous system, releasing stored tension, and anxieties while restoring a state of peace. Just 20 minutes of complete relaxation is equal to 2 hours of sleep. It is a useful energizer for the pregnant patient. It prepares pregnant women for relaxation periods between contractions and helps to keep their blood pressure within normal range.

Position 1

If the patient is having any low back discomfort or varicose veins, tell her to arrange a few pillows comfortably under the legs to elevate them approximately one and a half feet off the ground, when resting at home. Instruct the patient to lie back and relax. Demonstrate to the patient that the small of the back should be resting flat on the floor (Fig. 6.23). This position helps varicosity.

Position 2

Instruct the patient to lie only on the left side, which allows proper circulation for the baby. Have her prop one pillow under the head and the second one between her knees. Instruct the patient to bend the right leg slightly, so that it comes forward. The spine should be parallel with the ground (Fig 6.24). Instruct the patient to lie in a comfortable position, close the eyes and relax. Have the patient imagine taking a journey through the body from the feet to the head, constantly breathing and feeling totally relaxed. Tell the patient to think of each part of the body, each muscle, bone, and joint and relax them gradually all the way up to their facial features, by wrinkling and relaxing their face, mouth and eye brows to release tension.

Benefits: This exercise aids pregnant patients with insomnia.

Pelvic Tilt

From a chiropractic perspective, maintenance of the pelvic tilt throughout pregnancy is imperative to ensure appropriate biomechanics, as well as provide a healthy uterine environment for the fetus (Fig 6.25). The third trimester patient can be taught to perform this in a supported squat. She should be encouraged to keep her feet as flat on the ground as possible, then gently flex her knees outward. Once they are comfortably abducted, she then "scoops" the pelvis forward and maintains this position for 5–10 seconds.

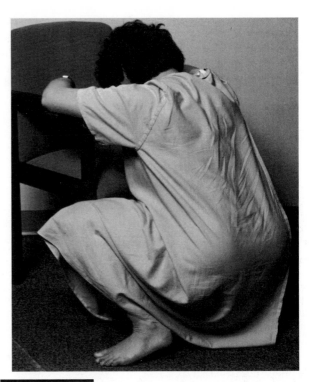

Figure 6.26.   Pelvic tilt: supported squatting position.

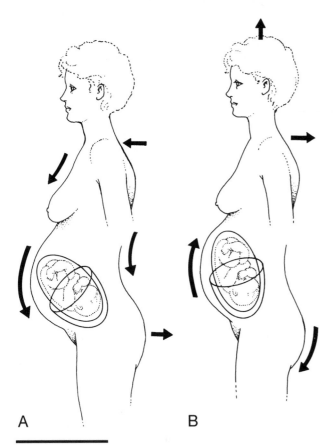

A   B

Figure 6.25.   Pelvic tilt. During pregnancy, maintaining a pelvic tilt improves not only postural and biomechanical considerations, but supports the fetus in a more comfortable position. This imposes less stress on the uterine muscle and ligaments, and potentially reduces the possibility for in-utero constraint. A, Compromised, faulty posture with no pelvic tilt. B, Erect posture with full pelvic tilt well-maintained.

Full relaxation should occur in between 4 or 5 of these movements (Fig 6.26). The "all fours" position is valuable for promoting pelvic tilt in the later stage of pregnancy. The elbows should be supported comfortably on a chair and the knees positioned slightly posterior under the hips (Fig 6.27A). The patient should then ease herself backwards, stretching out of her arms and moving the pelvis backwards above the knees as far as the distended uterus will allow (Fig 6.27B). At no time should the back be allowed to extend downwards. This can be repeated in a gentle rocking motion with slow, sustained stretches for three to four repetitions. This is also an excellent position to facilitate the fetal head being maintained in the occiput anterior position.

Precautions

Although certain exercises have precautions, many women will have no problem performing these and other exercises all the way through the gestational period. The patient should consult her midwife and/or health care provider before beginning any exercise regimen.

Give your pregnant patients the following advice in guiding them toward a safe and effective exercise plan:

1. Instruct them to discuss their intention to do these exercises with their obstetrician, midwife or primary health care provider.
2. If an exercise hurts, have the patient check to see if they are doing it correctly. If discomfort persists, tell them to

omit that exercise from the regimen. They can always try it again in a few days; the baby may change position by that time and may allow the woman to continue the exercise as normal.

3. In using the exercises to speed your recovery, don't practice those exercises in which the buttocks are higher than the shoulders, until all postpartum bleeding has ceased to avoid air rushing into the still open blood vessels at the placental site. Eliminate the exercise in which the head is below the heart, after the first trimester, to avoid dizziness.

Exercise During the Postpartum Period

The physiological changes of pregnancy remain until 6–12 weeks after birth. Hormones will not return to normal levels in nursing mothers until they stop breast-feeding. Many of the guidelines for exercise during pregnancy still apply to the postpartum period (10).

All exercise modes for physical fitness, including aerobic activities can be resumed after pregnancy. Few women are able

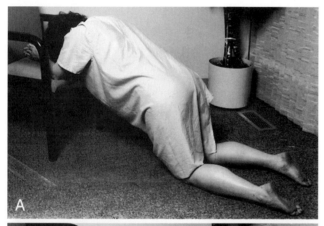

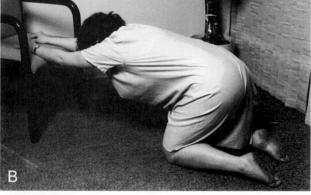

Figure 6.27. A, Pelvic tilt: "all fours" position. Relaxing with flat back (never arched or extended downward). Weight of the hips should be slightly forward over the knees. B, Pelvic tilt: "all fours" position. Movement backwards with weight backwards over the knees. Pelvic tilt is introduced and maintained while in this position.

to resume activity within a week after delivery; more women begin to exercise again around the sixth week. However, each woman should consult with her doctor to determine the best time to resume exercise.

Most women resume their exercise program by walking for 6 to 8 weeks and gradually switch to the mode of exercise they prefer. Those women who resume dance exercise early in the postpartum period may report the sensation of the uterus falling. The uterus is not actually falling, of course, and the sensation should disappear once the muscles regain their former tone.

Abdominal exercises are still important to firm up the muscles of the stomach. Continuing lower back exercises will help control low back pain, and additional instruction in lifting and carrying should help prevent lower back problems and fatigue. Abdominal and lower back exercises used in non-pregnancy patients can be safely incorporated into the postpartum exercise program (10).

Exercise frequency, duration, and intensity will depend on the fitness and goals of the new mother. To maintain fitness, a postpartum exerciser will probably have to work out 2 to 3 times per week for 20 to 30 minutes. To improve fitness, she may have to increase the frequency to three to four times per week and the duration to 30 minutes. If she also wants to lose excess fat gained during pregnancy, her exercise program should emphasize long duration, low intensity exercise four to five times per week. Because exercise intensity during pregnancy was low, any increase in intensity should be made gradually and as comfort indicates (10).

Summary

There are inherent benefits to exercise: it maintains muscle tone, strength, and endurance; protects against back pain; and is felt to have a positive effect on energy level, mood and self-image. These benefits can be appreciated during pregnancy and the postpartum period, if precautions are taken in consideration of the woman's special needs during these times. An individualized, closely monitored exercise program can help promote fitness and at the same time, ensure the safety of women during pregnancy and the postpartum period (26).

Women who exercised before pregnancy and continued to do so during pregnancy tended to weigh less, gain less weight, and deliver smaller babies than women who were mostly sedentary; all women, regardless of initial level of physical activity, decrease their activity as pregnancy progresses; physically active women appear to tolerate the demands of labor better; and exercise can be used as an alternative and safe therapeutic approach for gestational diabetes.

Pregnancy should not be a state of confinement, and cardiovascular and muscular fitness can be reasonably maintained with proper guidance. It is beneficial to encourage the expectant mother to condition herself before the onset of the greatest physical challenge she and her fetus will experience during the course of the pregnancy—labor and delivery (22).

REFERENCES

1. Schick-Boschetto B, Rose NC. Exercise in Pregnancy. Obstet Gynecol Surv 1991; 47(1):10-13.
2. Hunter S, Robson SC. Adaptation of the maternal heart in pregnancy. Br Heart J 1992;68(6):540-543.
3. Wolfe LA, Mottola MF. Aerobic exercise in pregnancy: an update. Can J Appl Physiol 1993;18(2):119-47.
4. Pernoll ML, Metcalfe J, Schlenker TL, Welch JE, Matsumoto JA. Oxygen consumption at rest and during exercise in pregnancy. Resp Physiol 1975;25: 285-293.
5. Hatch MC, Xiao-Ou Shu, McLean DE, Levin B, Begg M, Reuss L, Susser M. Maternal exercise during pregnancy, physical fitness, and fetal growth. Am J Epidemiol 1993;137,10:1105-14.
6. Clapp JF, Rizk KH. Effect of recreational exercise on midtrimester placental growth. Am J Obstet Gynecol 1992; 167(6):1518-21.
7. Clapp JF, Little KD, Capeless EL. Fetal heart rate response to sustained recreational exercise. Am J Obstet Gynecol 1993; 1993;168(1):198-205.
8. Revelli A, Durando A, Massobrio M. Exercise and pregnancy: A review of maternal and fetal effects. Obstet Gynecol Surv 1992; 47(6):355-367.
9. Grisso JA, Main DM, Chiu G, Synder ES, Holmes JH. Effects of physical activity and life-style factors on uterine contraction frequency. Am J Perinatol 1992;9(5/6): 4889-492.
10. Mittelmark RA, Wallace JP, Wiswell RA, Drinkwater BL. Exercise in pregnancy, 2nd ed. Baltimore: Williams & Wilkins, 1991: 231-246, 313-319.
11. Wallace JP, Rabin J. Lactic acid accumulation in mother's milk during maximal exercise. Med Sci Sports Exerc 1986; 18:547.
12. American College of Obstetricians and Gynecologists. Exercise During Pregnancy and Postpartum Period, Number 189, February, 1994.
13. DeLyser F. Jane Fonda's new pregnancy workout and total birth program. New York: Simon and Schuster, 1989:38-39.
14. Paisley JE, Mellion MB. Exercise during pregnancy. Am Fam Physician 1988; 38:143-144.
15. Jarski RW, Trippett DL. The risks and benefits of exercise during pregnancy. J Family Practice 1990; 30:185-189.
16. Clapp J. A clinical approach to exercise during pregnancy. Clin Sports Med 1994;13,2:443-55.
17. Artal R, Platt LD, Sperling M, et al. Exercise in pregnancy, I. Maternal cardiovascular and metabolic responses in normal pregnancy. Am J Obstet Gynecol 1981; 140: 123.
18. Cooper KA, Henyor SW, Boyce S, et al. Fetal heart rate and maternal cardiovascular and cathecholamine responses to dynamic exercise. Aust NZ J Obstet Gynecol 1987; 27:220.
19. Gorski J. Exercise during pregnancy: maternal and fetal responses. A brief review. Med Sci Sports Exerc 1985;17: 407-16.
20. Hytten F, Chamberlain G. Clinical physiology in obstetrics, ed 3. London: Blackwell Scientific, 1991.
21. Metcalfe J, Steck MK, Barron DH. Maternal physiology during gestation. In: Knobil E, Neil J. (eds). The physiology of reproduction, New York: Raven Press, 1988: 1995-2021.
22. Clapp JF, Rokey R, Treadway JL, Carpenter MW, Artal RM, Warrnes C. Exercise in pregnancy. Med Sci Sports Exerc 24, 6; S296-7.
23. Hall DC, Kaufmann DA. Effects of aerobic and strength conditioning on pregnancy outcomes. Am J Obstet Gynecol 1987; 157:1199-203.
24. Moore PR. Chiropractic care for the pregnant patient. Dig Chiro Econ 1983; May/June:60-61.
25. Penna M. Pregnancy and chiropractic care. ACA J Chiro 1989; Nov:31-33.
26. ACOG: Pregnancy, work and disability (Technical Bulletin, No. 58). Washington DC, ACOG, 1980.

Clinical and Radiological Assessments

7 History and Physical Assessment

Monika A. Buerger

The purpose of this chapter is to provide the doctor of chiropractic with the basic procedures necessary to evaluate the infant, toddler, preadolescent, and adolescent patient. The reader is referred to other sources for additional physical examination information not covered in this chapter (1,2). The focus of this chapter is on the case history and physical examination of the skin, head and neck, thoracic cavity, and abdomen. In this text, general orthopedics is presented in Chapter 14, the neurological examination in Chapters 5 and 13, and the spinal examination in Chapter 9. The chiropractor should also be able to determine the extent of injury/illness, the type of treatment necessary, the amount/length of treatment necessary, and appropriate referral, if required.

The "chiropractic" portion of the pediatric evaluation may be performed before or after the general physical examination. In many instances, while performing the physical examination, portions of the spinal evaluation can also be incorporated. It is important for chiropractors to keep in mind their knowledge of the spine and nervous system and how it may or may not relate to any findings during the history or physical examination of a particular patient.

It is important for the physician to establish a relationship with various professionals in their community specializing in the field of pediatrics. Such relationships can be crucial to encourage co-management of the pediatric patient. A network of professionals should include, but are not limited to pediatricians, dentists, orthopedists, neurologists, ophthalmologists, optometrists, psychologists, nutri-

tionists, physical therapists, speech therapists, audiologists, internists, dermatologists, and allergy specialists. A working relationship with a diagnostic imaging center and laboratory familiar in dealing with the pediatric patient is also important.

General Considerations

Physical assessment of the pediatric patient includes a complete and detailed history, comprehensive physical examination, and complete chiropractic evaluation. Before beginning any procedures, an authorization to treat a minor must be signed by the parent or legal guardian of the child.

A systematic approach to the evaluation of a patient may be remembered by using the acronym HIPPI RON LT. The order of evaluation is history, inspection, palpation, percussion, instrumentation, range of motion, orthopedic evaluation, neurologic evaluation, laboratory testing (special tests), and treatment. The doctor of chiropractic must also include a complete spinal evaluation before determining the appropriate course of treatment.

History

The history is a way of collecting comprehensive data that will depict the child's health and development from conception to the present time as well as help anticipate any future health concerns. History taking is an important step in establishing trust and confidence with any patient; it is especially important in dealing with the pediatric patient. The parents or caretakers need to know that their child is in competent and safe hands. A thorough history will also give the doctor information on how best to educate the parents or caretakers on a "wellness" or "dis-ease" lifestyle. Pediatrics is a unique area among the medical community because the emphasis of care is placed on disease prevention and parental guidance to a healthy lifestyle. This approach has always been a primary focus of the chiropractic profession and must be considered a part of the care received from the doctor of chiropractic. When discussing healthy lifestyle choices with the parents, regular chiropractic check-ups should be considered as a part of disease prevention.

It is recommended that the entire history be taken before beginning the physical assessment portion of the evaluation. When obtaining the history of the adolescent patient, there may be portions of the history where the child may feel more comfortable answering the questions in the absence of their parents. For example: the psycho-social portion of the history dealing with recreational, sexual, and social issues.

The following is a history outline recommended for the chiropractic pediatric patient:

1. Identifying data (ID). Name, nickname, sex, date of birth, birthplace, first and last name of each parent, day and work phone number of each parent, home address of child and each parent.
2. Source of history (SH). Record the source of given history information (e.g., patient, father, mother, other medical reports).
3. Chief complaint (CC). Depending on the child's age, attempt to record the chief complaint in their own words. It should be made clear in the records if the chief complaint is a concern of the child, parent, or a third party (e.g., teacher, daycare provider, grandparent).

HISTORY OF PRESENT ILLNESS (HPI)

The current injury/illness should be recorded in a chronological fashion from the onset of signs/symptoms to the present. The nature and timing in which the injury/illness began, the location, the severity, in comparison to the current presentation, and any previous treatment, should all be carefully recorded. Symptoms should be described in terms of onset, timing, location, quality, quantity, severity, duration, associated manifestations, and factors that influence the symptoms (e.g., what makes it better, what makes it worse). When taking the history, one must remember that children may not know the meaning of specific terms often used to obtain information. For example: the child may not know what pain or tenderness means, but they will understand "hurt." They may not be able to describe where the "hurt" is, but they are able to point. They may not understand intensity, but will understand "not very much" or "a lot." Therefore, it is helpful to have the child point to what "hurts"; then use words or examples that the child will understand to retrieve more detailed information.

With children, it is often wise to find out if there is a secondary gain to their injury/illness (e.g., not having to attend school or not having to do chores).

PAST MEDICAL HISTORY (PMH)

BIRTH HISTORY

The birth history is important for the doctor of chiropractic to determine the amount of trauma the spine or cranium may have sustained during the birth process. The parent or caregiver should be educated on the traumatic effects the birthing process may have on the child's spine and nervous system. Birthing trauma can lead to vertebral subluxations in the newborn and go undetected, leading to various neuropathophysiologic effects. The cause of trauma in most instances is due to a forceful tractioning of the spine while in a hyperextended position. Longitudinal traction with rotation and flexion, or excessive lateral bending, also can cause injury (3).

PRENATAL

Establish what the mother's health status was before and during the pregnancy. What was the mother's age? What was the mother's gravida status and para status. Were there any prior miscarriages? If so, how many and how long ago? Were any drugs (prescription or otherwise) used before or during the pregnancy (this includes alcohol). How much weight was gained during the pregnancy? Were there any complications with the pregnancy? Were there any parental concerns regarding the pregnancy, delivery, or care of that particular child? What was the term of the child (full term or premature)?

NATAL

Ask the duration and extent of difficulty of both labor and delivery. Was labor spontaneous or induced? Was the delivery "natural" or was it caesarean? If it was caesarean, what was the reason? Were forceps, vacuum extraction (suction cup) or other devices used? Did the mother require any type of analgesic drug? What was the position of the child at birth (e.g., vertex, transverse, breech). Was the child born in a hospital, home, or birthing center? Excessive tractional forces during vaginal delivery, breech births, caesarean births, use of forceps or vacuum extractors all can result in trauma to the cranium, cervical and thoracic spine.

NEONATAL

What was the child's Apgar scores? Was there any need for resuscitation efforts? Were there any particular problems with feeding, respiration, cyanosis, jaundice, anemia, convulsions, congenital anomalies or infections? What was the mother's health status postpartum?

FEEDING/NUTRITIONAL HISTORY

INFANCY

Was the child solely breastfed, breastfed along with supplemental feeding, or solely supplementally fed? If some type of supplemental feeding took place, what did it consist of? What was the frequency and duration of feedings? Were there any difficulties associated with the feedings (e.g., spitting-up, not latching, not wanting to eat from the right or left breast, colic, or diarrhea)? Sometimes, due to irritation caused by an upper cervical vertebral subluxation, one will find that the child will not want to latch-on or feed when his head is turned toward one particular side. There is also the possibility that the infant is unable to turn his head to one particular side because of joint restriction due to a vertebral subluxation (e.g., with an ASRP atlas, the child may not be able to turn their head far enough to the left to comfortably nurse at the right breast).

EARLY CHILDHOOD

At what age did the child begin to eat solid foods? How were foods introduced, one at a time or many at one time? Did there seem to be any allergic reactions to certain foods? If so, which foods were they and what type or reaction occurred?

CHILDHOOD, PRE-ADOLESCENT, AND ADOLESCENT

What are the child's current and past eating habits? Is she eating large quantities of fast foods (See Chapter 17)? Is she eating foods with good nutritional content? Is there evidence of any eating disorders such as anorexia nervosa or bulimia. If an overeating or undereating disorder is suspected, a 14-day food intake diary may be helpful to make a proper assessment.

CHILDHOOD ILLNESSES AND EXPOSURES

CHILDHOOD ILLNESSES

Does the child have a history of chickenpox, mumps, measles, rubella, rubeola, rheumatic fever, or whooping cough? At what age did they experience the illness? Were there any complications due to the illness? What was the extent of the illness and what type of treatment was rendered? Other illnesses that should be inquired about in the history include: chronic ear aches/infections, asthma, chronic colds/flu, or headaches. These may be indicative of a compromised immune system due to vertebral subluxation or other factors.

RECENT EXPOSURES

Were there any recent exposures to contagious childhood illnesses that should be noted? What was the nature of the exposure and have there been any signs or symptoms of the disease?

TRAVEL/PETS

Has there been any recent or past travel to other countries or other locations? Has there been any exposure to animals?

OPERATIONS/INJURIES/HOSPITALIZATIONS

Record the dates/ages of each incident. If there is a history of past injuries, what were the circumstances surrounding them? What medical procedures were performed and by who were they performed? Was a blood transfusion necessary? Was therapy or chiropractic care necessary? Are there any current repercussions arising from the incident? Are the medical records available for your review if necessary?

ALLERGIES

Does the child have a history of allergies to any medications or foods? Have they shown any signs of eczema, urticaria, or hypersensitivity to insect bites or pollens? As with any patient suffering from allergies, children should be checked for vertebral subluxations. Specific areas that should be examined are: C6–T3 for thyroid involvement and T7–T12 for adrenal involvement (4). The lower lumbar spine (L4–L5) and the second sacral segment should also be examined for subluxation. Nutritional support with antioxidant vitamin supplements is also recommended. For those suffering from pollen allergies, eating honey made from local bee pollen may help build up an immunity to local pollens.

SPECIAL TESTING OR SCREENING PROCEDURES

Record the date/age and results of any special tests or screening procedures performed on that specific child, for example: blood tests for hematocrit levels, blood lead levels, or sickle cell anemia. Were any vision, hearing, urinalysis or tuberculin tests performed? Was there any testing for genetic or high-risk disorders?

VACCINATIONS

Record the ages/dates of any vaccinations. Were there any reactions; if so, to what extent? If vaccines have not yet been administered, is the intention that they will be in the future? The doctor of chiropractic should have knowledge regarding the potential risks/benefits in relation to immunizations (see Chapter 3). The chiropractor should be able to offer the parent literature on various vaccines and the risks associated with them as well as educate them on why vaccines may or may not be necessary for their children. Rather than advising the parent(s) to vaccinate or not to vaccinate, the chiropractic doctor should focus on educating the parent(s) on the subject and allowing the parent(s) to make the decision they feel is most appropriate for their child.

GROWTH AND DEVELOPMENT

The developmental history is especially important for the infant and toddler ages for detecting and/or treating any abnormalities of physical growth, psychomotor development, intellectual retardation, or behavioral disorders.

PHYSICAL GROWTH

What is the child's current weight and height? Has there been any period of rapid weight gain or weight loss? Has there been a progressive growth and maturity pattern, and has the child shown normal tooth eruption and loss patterns? If the child is being treated regularly in your office, it is advisable to obtain an updated physical growth history at various ages. The recommended ages are: 1, 2, 5, 10, and 16.

DEVELOPMENTAL MILESTONES

These are specific tasks and/or accomplishments achieved by the majority of normal children by a certain predictable age. Examples are: lifts chin at 6–8 weeks, rolls over at 3–5 months, sits without support at 6–8 months. (Table 7.1). Record ages/dates when major milestones were attained.

PSYCHO-SOCIAL DEVELOPMENT

This area deals with information regarding the child's lifestyle, behavior, environment, emotional, and cognitive functioning. Questions should be reflective of the patient's age. The adolescent patient may be more comfortable in the absence of their parents and may be more likely to answer your questions truthfully. The following are some areas to touch on in relation to psycho-social development:

1. Sleep patterns: amount, frequency of naps, nightmares, sleep walking.

2. Toileting: age toilet training was introduced, age that bowel and bladder control were attained, occurrence of accidents or enuresis. If enuresis is reported, evaluation of the fifth lumbar, second and third sacral segments, and the T11 to L2 spinal segments should be checked for vertebral subluxations. The most common vertebral levels associated with enuresis are the second and third sacral segments. The upper cervical spine should also be evaluated for vertebral subluxations in a child with enuresis (3).

3. Speech: record any stuttering, lisping, or hesitation of speech patterns. Verbally interact with the child to obtain some sense of their vocabulary (e.g., number of words in their vocabulary, clarity of words, understanding of words).

4. Discipline: What is the child's temperament (behavioral style) and how does the parent/caretaker respond to it. Does the discipline style used appear to be successful? Does the child demonstrate negativism, withdrawal from others, temper tantrums, or aggressive behavior? Children suffering from "attention deficit hyperactivity disorder" (ADHD) may tend to demonstrate aggressive behavior. They show little thought or regret for any of their actions, even if they involve injury to others. These children are easily distractible and impulsive and are often unpopular with their peers. Any child with hyperactive tendencies should be checked for vertebral subluxations. Special attention should be paid to the upper cervical region (i.e., occiput to C3) (3).

5. Schooling: Does/did the child attend day care or pre-school? At what age did the child begin kindergarten? What is the current child and parent satisfaction with the schooling? Are there any specific academic achievements or concerns regarding schooling? Is there a history of an attendance problem?

6. Recreational: Is the child involved in any recreational activities? If so, was it the child's choice to participate or the parents' decision? If the child participates in sports do they participate in team sports or individual sports?

7. Sexuality: Is the child comfortable with his/her sexual orientation? What is their relationship with members of the opposite sex? Do they have any questions regarding conception, pregnancy, contraception, or sexually transmitted diseases? Is their relationship with their parent(s) one that permits discussion of sexual concerns?

8. Personality: What is the child's degree of independence/autonomy? What is their relationship with parents, siblings, peers, and teachers? What is their self-image? What do they feel their major assets are?

FAMILY HISTORY (FH)

Obtain a family history of parents, siblings, and grandparents. Is there a family history of any medical conditions such as heart disease, high blood pressure, diabetes, stroke, kidney disease, tuberculosis, cancer, AIDS, arthritis, anemia, headaches, mental illness, alcohol, or drug abuse? If so, what type of treatment was given? Is there a history of any infant or childhood deaths or congenital anomalies? Are the parents living or deceased? If living, what are their ages? If deceased, was there a known cause of death? If the child is adopted, ask the adoptive parents if there is any known family medical history.

REVIEW OF SYSTEMS (ROS)

The review of systems is designed as a "safety net" to assess any problems/concerns that may not have surfaced during the other portion of the patient history. Ask a few general questions in each system. If there is a system (area) of concern, more detailed questions should be asked in order to rule-in or rule-out any possible dysfunction/disorder:

1. General: weight changes, energy level, sleep patterns, growth patterns, fever, fatigue.

2. Skin: birthmarks, rashes, pallor, sweating, itching, bleeding, swelling, dryness, color changes, lumps, changes in hair or nails.

3. Head: headaches, head injuries, dizziness.

4. Eyes: vision disorders, pain, redness, excessive tearing, glasses.

5. Ears: hearing disorders, infections, dizziness, ringing in ears, discharge.

6. Nose and sinuses: frequent colds, nasal stuffiness, hay fever, nosebleeds, drainage, discharge, sinus troubles.

7. Mouth and throat: dental or gum problems, sore throats, speech problems, hoarseness, sore/enlarged tongue, last dental examination.

8. Lymphatics: enlarged and/or painful lymph nodes.

Table 7.1.   **Developmental Milestones**

1-2 months

Observational activities

Holds head up

Raises head prone 45 degrees

Turns head and eyes to sound

Acknowledges faces

Follows objects through visual fields

Drops objects (toys)

Is alert in response to voices

Activities reported by parents

Smiles responsively and spontaneously

Recognizes parents

Language Capabilities

Engages in vocalization (coos)

3-5 months

Observational activities

Smiles, laughs, gurgles

Holds head high and raises body with hands while in a prone position

Reaches for and brings objects to mouth

Makes "raspberry" sound

Sits with support (head steady)

Holds rattle briefly

Follows objects 180 degrees

Activities reported by parents

Anticipates food on sight

Rolls from front to back

Turns from back to side

Excited upon recognizing familiar people

Language capabilities

Squeals

Babbles, initial vowels

Gutteral sounds ("ah," "go")

Consonants: m, p, b

Vowels: o, u

6-8 months

Observational activities

Imitates "bye-bye"

Reaches

Sits alone for a short time

Some weight bearing

Passes object from hand to hand in midline

First scoops up a pellet then grasps it using thumb opposition

Activities reported by parents

Rolls front to back and back to front

Is indifferent to the word "no"

Language capabilities

Babbles/Imitates speech sounds

Syllables: da, ba, ka

9-11 months

Observational activities

Sits alone

Pulls to stand

Stands alone

Creeps

Imitates pat-a-cake and peek-a-boo

Uses thumb and index finger to pick up pellet

Activities reported by parents

Feeds self finger foods

Walks supported by furniture

Follows one-step verbal commands (e.g., "Come here", "Give it to me")

Language capabilities

MaMa/DaDa nonspecifically

Approximates names: baba/bottle

12 months

Observational activities

Walks with support or independently

Pincer grasp

Gives toys upon request

Brings two blocks together; tries to build tower

Releases objects into cup after demonstration

Activities reported by parents

Points to desired objects

Looks for hidden objects

Language capabilities

MaMa/DaDa specific

Jargon begins (own language)

2-3 words understandable

18 months

Observational activities

Throws ball

Climbs/descends stairs with aid

Turns pages

Uses a spoon

Identifies body parts

Table 7.1. *(continued)* **Developmental Milestones**

Seats self in chairs

Scribbles spontaneously

Builds tower of 3-4 blocks

Activities reported by parents

Feeds self

Carries and hugs doll

Understands a 2-step command

Language capabilities

Says 4 to 20 words

Consonants: t, d, w, h, n

2-word phrases understandable

24 months

Observational activities

Kicks ball

Holds cup securely

Points to named objects or pictures

Jumps off floor with both feet

Stands on one foot alone

Builds tower of 6-7 blocks

Climbs/descends stairs unaided

Turns pages of a book singly

Activities reported by parents

Verbalizes toilet needs

Mimics domestic activities

Pulls on simple garments

Language capabilities

3-word phrases understandable

Use of pronouns: mine, me, you, I

Vowels uttered correctly

Approximately 270 words

30 months

Observational activities

Refers to self as I

Copies a crude circle

Walks backwards

Begins to hop on one leg

Holds crayon in fist

Activities reported by parents

Helps put things away

Language capabilities

Carries on a conversation

Uses prepositions

36 months

Observational activities

Shares playthings

Copies a circle

Holds crayon with fingers

Imitates a vertical line

Builds a tower using 9-10 blocks

Gives first and last name

Activities reported by parents

Dresses with supervision

Rides tricycle using pedals

While looking at picture book able to answer "what is . . . doing"?

Language capabilities

Some degree of hesitancy and uncertainty common

Intelligible 4-word phrases

Approximately 900 words

3-4 years

Observational activities

Walks on heels

Climbs/descends stairs with alternating feet

Responds to command to place objects in, on, or under table

Draws a circle when asked to draw a person (man, boy, girl)

Knows own sex

Finger opposition

Begins to button and unbutton

General knowledge: Full name, age, address (2 out of 3)

Activities reported by parents

Takes off shoes and jacket

Feeds self at mealtime

Language capabilities

Intelligible 5-word phrases

Approximately 1540 words

Answers questions using plurals, personal pronoun, and verbs: ("What do you want to do that is fun?")

4-5 years

Observational activities

May stand on one leg for at least 10 seconds

Runs and turns without losing balance

Tiptoes

Tells a simple story

Table 7.1.   *(continued)* **Developmental Milestones**

Knows the days of the week ("What day comes after Monday?")

Draws a person (Head, 2 appendages, and possibly 2 eyes. No torso.)

Counts to 4 by rote

Begins understanding rules (right and wrong)

Cuts and pastes

Gives appropriate answers to: "What must you do if you are sleepy? Hungry? Cold?" Etc.

Activities reported by parents

Dressing and undressing without supervision

Buttons clothes and laces shoes but does not tie

Self-care with toilet needs (May need help wiping)

Plays outside for at least 30 minutes

Language capabilities

Intelligible 4-word phrases

Approximately 1540 words

Uses plurals, personal pronouns, and verbs

5–6 years

Observational activity

Skips

Catches a ball

Copies a + that is already drawn

Tells own age

Knows right and left

Draws a recognizable person with at least 8 details

Understands the concept of 10 (Is able to count out 10 objects)

Describes favorite television program or video in some detail

Activities reported by parents

Goes to school unattended or meets school bus

Helps with simple chores at home (Taking out the garbage)

Good motor capability but little aware of dangers

Language capabilities

Intelligible 6–7 word sentences

Approximately 2560 words

6–7 years

Observational activities

Copies a triangle

Knows morning, afternoon, night

Draws a person with 12 details

Uses a pencil for printing name

Reads several one-syllable printed words (dog, cat, boy, my, see)

Language capabilities

Intelligible 5-word phrases

Approximately 1540 words

7–8 years

Observational activities

Hops twice on each foot

Finger opposition (5 seconds)

Copies a diamond shape

Counts by 2s and 5s

Ties shoes

Knows what day of the week it is

Draws a person with 16 details

Adds and subtracts one-digit numbers

Language capabilities

Adult proficiency

No evidence of sound substitution (e.g., fr for thr)

8–9 years

Observational activities

Defines words more appropriately by use ("What is an apple?" "A fruit.")

Answers appropriately to questions such as: "What should you do if a playmate hits you without meaning to do so?" "What should you do if you break something that doesn't belong to you?"

Is learning to borrow and carry in addition and subtraction

9–10 years

Observational activities

Walks heel to toe with eyes closed

Knows the day, month, and year

Recites the months in order (Fifteen seconds, one error)

Learning simple multiplication

10–12 years

Observational activities

Jump and clap three times

Draws vertical lines

Multiplication and simple division

Tanner staging of pubertal development

14 years

Observational activity

Tanner staging of pubertal development

16 years

Observational activity

Tanner staging of pubertal development

Modified from Behrman R.E, Kliegman R, eds. Nelson essentials of pediatrics. Philadelphia: W.B. Saunders Co., 1990:80-82.

9. Neck: pain, lumps/masses, thyroid problems, wryneck (torticollis), "swollen glands."

10. Breasts: pain, discharge, masses, asymmetry, self-examinations.

11. Respiratory: cough, sputum (color, quantity), difficulty breathing, wheeze, frequent colds, exercise intolerance, hemoptysis, tuberculin test, bronchitis, asthma, history of chest x-rays.

12. Cardiovascular: heart murmur, heart abnormalities, high blood pressure, rheumatic fever, dyspnea, chest pain, palpitations, edema, cyanosis.

13. Gastrointestinal: abdominal pain, nausea, vomiting, diarrhea, constipation, colic, food intolerance, vomiting of blood, excessive belching or passing of gas, jaundice, bloody or tarry stools, hepatitis, liver or gall bladder problems.

14. Urinary: pain, frequency, infections, enuresis, blood in urine.

15. Genito-reproductive: male: age of onset of puberty, hernias, undescended testicle, testicular pain or swelling, discharge from or sores on penis, sexually transmitted diseases, sexual activity, sexual concerns; female: age at menarche, regularity, frequency and duration of periods, dysmenorrhea, last menstrual period, excessive abdominal and/or back pain or bleeding associated with menstrual cycles, sexually transmitted diseases, sexual activity, pregnancies, sexual concerns, vaginal abnormalities, ovarian cysts, discharge, itching.

16. Musculoskeletal: pain or swelling in joints, joint stiffness, arthritis, pain in muscles or bones, congenital abnormalities, sports injuries, scoliosis, gait abnormalities, back or neck pain. Inconsistencies in the history in this area are especially important in detecting suspected child abuse or maltreatment (see Chapter 2).

17. Neurological: fainting, blackouts, seizures, paralysis, local weakness, numbness, tingling, memory, personality changes, abnormal movements or vocalizations, difficulties with handwriting, balance/coordination, CNS infections, delayed development, school functioning.

18. Psychiatric: nervousness, tension, mood, memory, behavior, depression, hallucinations.

19. Endocrine: thyroid problems, heat/cold intolerance, excessive sweating, diabetes, excessive hunger, thirst, or urination.

20. Hematologic: anemia, bruising, bleeding, past transfusions.

Physical Examination

The physical examination of the pediatric or adolescent patient should be performed in a head-to-toe fashion, similar to the examination of the adult patient. For the uncooperative or difficult patient, such as the hyperactive child, you may need to alter the order of your examination process to encourage patient compliance. The "IPPI RON" portion of the examination may be done in two fashions. The first is by performing inspection of the entire body, then palpation of the entire body, then percussion of the entire body. The second and usually most effective way, is by performing the entire "IPPI" sequence on one specific area (e.g., head, chest, abdomen) starting at the head and working downwards. This approach is followed by all range of motion, orthopedic and neurologic tests, as well as the special cranial and spinal evaluations. It is important that you not force the child to do something that may be frightening or uncomfortable.

When examining the infant, toddler, or school-aged child, it is advisable to have the parent(s) or caregiver of the child in the examination room with you. This will help make the child feel more secure; patient confidentiality is usually not an issue at this young of an age. With the adolescent patient, it may be more appropriate not to have the parent(s) or caregiver in the room during the physical examination. This may allow the adolescent to feel that they can be more candid in discussing any of their particular concerns. It is important that you tell both the parent and the adolescent that any discussion between the doctor and patient will remain confidential. However, any possible health concerns must be brought to the attention of the parent if the child is not of legal age. The doctor should verify confidentiality laws in their particular state that pertain to this issue (see Chapter 18). To avoid any possible legal issues, male practitioners examining female patients may want to have a female assistant accompany him during the examination.

The Skin

Visual examination of the skin should be done with proper lighting. Starting from head to toe, pay close attention to any cuts, bruises, burns, or distinctive pattern marks (e.g., hand prints, cigarette size burns, curling iron burns) which may indicate some form of intentional injury. If there is a history of a recent automobile accident, look for any possible bruising from seat belts or cuts from broken glass. Identify any birthmarks or lesions present and record them. Use descriptive terms in regard to size, color, shape, number, location, distribution pattern, and type (e.g., macule, papule, pustule). The doctor may want to use a magnifying glass to better visualize smaller lesions.

Obtain a history of when the lesions first occurred, and determine if there have been any secondary changes, or if itching is associated with the lesions. A Polaroid picture may be helpful to track any changes that may occur over time. Yellowness of the skin can occur from the ingestion of carrots and other foods containing carotene; if the sclarae of the eyes also appear yellowish in color, jaundice is likely. Intense yellowness of the skin may be due to the presence of increased amounts of indirect bilirubin; while yellow-green may indicate the presence of increased direct bilirubin.

Cyanosis of the skin may be due to lead poisoning, cardiac dysfunction, or respiratory dysfunction. If there is a metallic gray blue quality to the cyanotic appearance, suspect methemoglobinemia.

Examination of the skin should go beyond visualization and

include palpation. Check the tone and texture of the skin feeling for any raised lesions, edema, or muscle spasticity. To check for hydration, take a fold of loose skin around the abdomen and roll it between your thumb and forefinger. If the child is well hydrated, it will return to normal immediately upon release.

A number of skin conditions may affect the pediatric and adolescent patient. Some conditions will present themselves the same in various age groups, while others are more prevalent at certain ages. Lesions due to drug reactions, as well as to an allergic or contact dermatitis should always be kept in mind. No single drug produces an invariably typical pattern; however, the main offenders tend to be the barbiturates, anticonvulsants, and antibiotics. This following section will list a few of the more common skin conditions seen in the pediatric and adolescent patient.

INFANTS

MILIA

These lesions present as multiple white pinheadsized papules over the chin, forehead, nose and cheeks. They are present in up to 40% of newborns (5) and will disappear over the course of several weeks.

VASCULAR LESIONS (HEMANGIOMAS)

Capillary hemangioma (i.e., strawberry hemangioma) are irregularly shaped red areas frequently found over the occiput, upper eyelids, forehead, and upper lip. Oftentimes they are not present at birth, but appear within the first few months of life as marked vascular growths raised above the skin. These hemangiomas grow rapidly for approximately 1 year, plateau, and then begin to involute. Fifty percent resolve spontaneously by age five, 70% by age seven, 90% by age nine, and the rest by adolescence (5). Usually, no intervention is necessary unless there is an obstruction of a vital area (e.g., airway or visual obstruction).

PORT WINE STAINS

Port wine stains are flat hemangiomas present at birth that do not involute with age. They appear unilaterally on the side of the face or an extremity. If the port wine stain affects an extremity, there may be local overgrowth of soft tissue and bone in that area. When a port wine stain involves the first branch of the fifth cranial nerve (i.e., trigeminal), it can be associated with a vascular malformation of the ipsilateral meninges and cerebral cortex (e.g., Sturge-Weber syndrome). Seizures, mental retardation, hemiplegia, and glaucoma are also associated with Sturge-Weber syndrome.

INFLAMMATORY DERMATOSES

Infantile Atopic Dermatitis (Eczema). Eczema consists of red, itchy papules and plaques associated with oozing and crust formation. The lesions are located on the cheeks, forehead, scalp, trunk, or extremities. They typically appear after 2 months of age and are primarily on the extensor surfaces initially. After infancy, involvement of the flexural creases (e.g., antecubital, popliteal, neck) predominates. The infantile form may last 2 to 3 years. Seventy percent of affected children have first degree relatives exhibiting some form of allergic disease; 30–50% of children will go on to develop allergic rhinits or asthma (6). In some infants and children, IgE antibody to one or more foods can be demonstrated. Foods implicated most frequently in atopic dermatitis include egg white, milk, legumes (including peanut butter), wheat, and corn. Certain foods, especially citrus fruits and tomatoes, may induce facial erythema in children with atopic dermatitis. Special attention should be paid to the sympathetic nervous system for vertebral subluxations, especially levels T9–T12 for suprarenal function (4).

SCALING DERMATOSES

Psoriasis. These lesions are red, well-demarcated plaques with a silvery scale, which have a predisposition for the extensor surfaces of the extremities, scalp, and buttocks. Guttate (droplike) psoriasis is a common form in children that often follows an episode of streptococcal pharyngitis by the second or third week. Sunlight or artificial ultraviolet light may prove beneficial in these cases.

Seborrheic Dermatitis. In seborrheic dermatitis, red scaling eruption occurs predominantly on the scalp, eyebrows, eyelashes, perinasal, presternal, and postauricular areas. The folds of the neck and groin may also be affected. In infants, the scalp can be affected with a greasy, yellow colored, scaly rash called cradle cap. Most cases remit spontaneously.

Diaper Dermatitis. These lesions are diffuse and scaly erythema with papular, vesicular, and pustular lesions confined to the lower abdominal, perineal, and gluteal regions. In severe cases, ulcerations may be seen. The usual cause is moisture from wet diapers.

TODDLERS

CAFE-AU-LAIT SPOTS

These spots are irregular or well-circumscribed macules varying from dark brown to chestnut or yellowish in color. The most common locations are the lower lumbar region, buttocks, back of the neck, shoulders, chest, and oral mucosa. Solitary cafe-au-lait spots may be seen in normal individuals; however, the occurrence of 4 or more is uncommon. Neurofibromatosis may be suspected if greater than 6 smooth well-defined lesions at least 1.5 cm or larger are present (7).

URTICARIA (HIVES)

Urticaria consists of multiple (occasionally single) macular lesions, consisting of localized edema (wheal) with surrounding erythema. Pruritus is frequently intense. Most commonly, acute urticaria (lasting less than 6 weeks) is caused by a hypersensitivity reaction to food, drugs, insect bites, infections, contact allergens, or inhaled substances. Chronic urticaria (lasting more than 6 weeks) can be a sign of an underlying disorder, such as occult infection hepatitis B, or connective tissue disease.

IMPETIGO

Traditional Impetigo. These erosions are covered by honey-colored crusts. They spread easily and are contagious. They usually are not painful, but may be itchy. Staphylcocci and group A streptococci are the causative agents in these cases.

Bullous Impetigo. These erosions are covered by honey-colored crust with a border filled of clear fluid. Staphylococcus aureus is the causative agent in these cases.

VARICELLA (CHICKENPOX)

Mild systemic symptoms such as fever, malaise, or rash may be the predecessor to red macules that rapidly become tiny vesicles on a red base (6). They form pustules, crust, and then form scabs. Lesions erupt in crops and usually stop forming after 5–7 days. They typically begin centrally and spread peripherally involving the trunk, face, scalp, extremities, nose, mouth, ears, and intestines. The incubation period for chickenpox ranges from 10–20 days, most typically being between 14–16 days.

HAND, FOOT, AND MOUTH DISEASE (COXSACKIE)

Children younger than age 10 are most commonly affected (5). Mild fever, anorexia, and soreness of the throat and mouth may be present 2–3 days before the outbreak of lesions. Red macules, which progress to vesiculation and ulceration appear on the soft palate, tongue, pharynx, and gingiva. At the same time, a maculopapular rash develops containing clear, watery fluid. The limbs, hands, and feet are the usual sites of the skin lesions although the buttocks may also be affected. The lesions will last for 3–4 days and regress spontaneously. Coxsackie is highly contagious with an incubation period of approximately 2-6 days. It is often seen in settings where there are large groups of children (e.g., daycare centers, pre-school, elementary school). The peak season for Coxsackie is late summer through early fall.

SCHOOL-AGE, PREADOLESCENT AND ADOLESCENT

SCABIES

These lesions are pruritic papules, vesicles, pustules, and linear burrows appearing in the webs of the fingers, axillae, wrists, waist, nipples, and genitals. In infants, the palms, soles, head, and neck may also be affected. Scabies is contagious and appears approximately 4 to 6 weeks after the initial contact. Often times complaints of intense itching, especially at night, accompany these lesions.

SCARLET FEVER

This disorder presents as a diffuse erythema characteristically appearing 24–48 hours after the onset of phyrangitis. Upon palpation, the lesions have the texture of coarse sandpaper. The rash first appears in the axillae, groin, and neck; however, within 24 hours the rash becomes generalized. Creases of the fingers, groin, and the antecubital fossae may appear with an accentuation of erythema (Pastia lines). A circumoral pallor around the lips and a rash on the tongue gives the appearance of a "strawberry tongue."

SEBORRHEIC DERMATITIS

These are red scaling eruptions. In adolescents, it commonly appears as flaking of the scalp, eyebrows, postauricular areas, or flexural areas. Antiseborrheic shampoos may be helpful to clear flaking of the scalp. Topical steroid ointments can be applied to areas of the skin that are affected.

PSORIASIS

These lesions present as red, well-demarcated plaques with a silvery scale. In the school aged, pre-adolescent, and adolescent child, psoriasis is commonly seen on the scalp, knees, elbows or other sites of repeated traumas. Psoriasis is often chronic with periods of exacerbations and remissions.

PITYRIASIS ROSEA

This disorder frequently begins as a single, pink, oval lesion, which may be scaly. Five to seven days later, crops of lesions appear commonly on the trunk. It is a benign, self-limiting disorder of unknown etiology. The rash may be preceded by a prodrome of headache and malaise.

TINEA CORPORIS (RINGWORM)

This skin disorder has dull red, ring-shaped lesions with a raised border of scaly papules, vesicles, or pustules. The lesions may appear on any body surface.

ACNE

The onset of adolescent acne is between ages 8 and 10 in 40% of the children. The early lesions are usually limited to the face and are primarily closed comedones (whiteheads) (5).

The Head/Hair

The doctor should visually inspect the head for any asymmetries, bumps, bruises, or cuts. Palpate the head for any prominences or edema (see Chapters 2, 10).

INFANT

In the infant, palpate the suture lines and fontanelles for any abnormalities. The sutures can be felt as slightly depressed ridges, and the fontanelles as soft concavities. The anterior fontanelle is the largest (4-6 cm) and normally closes between 4 and 26 months; the posterior fontanelle (1-2 cm) normally closes by 2 months of age (8). The head may be percussed using the index or middle finger. Percussion over the sutures before fusion will create a "cracked-pot" sound. The anterior fontanelle should be examined with the infant in an upright position to eliminate the effects of gravity. Check for the presence of any bulging or depressed areas. Bulging of the anterior fontanelle may indicate increased intracranial pressure found in infectious and neoplastic diseases of the central nervous system or with obstruction of the ventricular circulation. Depression of the anterior fontanelle is found with decreased intracranial pressure and may be a sign of dehydration in the infant.

The circumference of the head should be measured regularly during the first 2 years of life. Using a soft plastic centimeter tape, measure over the occipital, parietal, and frontal prominences so as to obtain the greatest circumference. Head growth rate reflects the rate of brain growth; if there is doubt as to whether growth rate is normal, there are reference tables in various pediatric text books on normal values (see Chapter 14). Half of ultimate brain growth is completed by 9 months of age and 75% is completed by age 2 (8).

The shape of the infant's head should be examined for any possible abnormalities or asymmetries. The shape may be altered by premature fusion of the cranial sutures (craniosynostosis). Another alteration in shape, flattening of the occiput, may be seen within the first months of life if the infant spends a lot of time in the supine position. The flattening will disappear as the baby becomes more active and spends less time in the supine position.

TODDLER

Observe any asymmetries or abnormalities of the head. Palpate for any bumps or points of tenderness; the child may squirm in an attempt to "get away" when tender areas are palpated. Children at this age tend to acquire injuries of the head via falls while learning how to walk and run. Palpate the anterior fontanelle for closure. If it is still open, then measure its size. Examine the hair and eyebrows for texture, quantity, and patterning. Abnormalities in hair may be associated with systemic disease or abnormality. For example, dry, coarse, brittle hair may be associated with congenital hypothyroidism.

SCHOOL-AGE, PREADOLESCENT AND ADOLESCENT

Observe any asymmetries or abnormalities of the head. Palpate the entire head for any bumps or points of tenderness; children of this age tend to be more active in sports leading to traumas. Examine the hair and eyebrows for texture, quantity, and patterning. Alopecia (hair loss) may be present and the cause should be determined. Cited below are some of the most common disorders associated with hair loss in the school age, pre-adolescent, and adolescent patient.

ALOPECIA AREATA

This disorder presents as well-circumscribed areas of complete or almost complete hair loss. The scalp is smooth with no signs of inflammation. Hair loss usually begins suddenly and total loss of scalp and body hair may develop.

TINEA CAPITIS

This is a fungal infection of the scalp. It is most common in the pre-pubertal patient and is characterized by a patch of short broken-off hairs. The patches of hair loss may be scaly or they may be marked with inflammation, bogginess, and pustules called "kerion."

TRICHOTILLOMANIA

This disorder is defined as irregular areas of hair loss of varying lengths. The scalp is generally normal. It is a self-inflicting disorder (pulling one's own hair) that may result from habitual behavior in normal individuals; it is also found in children who have significant underlying psychiatric illness (9).

TRACTION ALOPECIA

This is chronic, recurrent tension on hair from ponytails or braided hair styles.

MYOTONIC DYSTROPHY

Myotonic dystrophy is frontal baldness usually developing during childhood. Muscle myotonia, weakness, and an immobile facies are early clues.

The Face

The majority of the facial examination will be through visual inspection. It should begin by observing the child during the taking of the history, paying attention to the overall alertness and expressions of the child. Does the child appear happy, sad, lethargic or expressionless? Is the face pale or puffy appearing? Inspect the face for any asymmetries which may be a clue for a 7th cranial nerve palsy. Trauma during the birthing process may result in facial paralysis; not uncommonly, it is the result of pressure on the peripheral portion of the nerve during forceps delivery, by the maternal sacral promontory, or occasionally by bone fragments in skull fractures.

Congenital hypothyroidism may present itself by puffy eyelids, a depressed nasal bridge, poor muscle tone, widely spaced eyes, and an enlarged tongue. The child may appear lethargic, the skin will be dry and cool, and the neck is thick and short. The infant patient may show signs of hypothyroidism as early as the first week of life presenting with a hoarse quality to their cry, low food intake and intense, prolonged jaundice. Upper respiratory tract allergies will present with classic signs such as dark shadows under the eyes; called allergic shiners, horizontal skin creases under the lower lids; called Dennie's lines, and a horizontal crease just above the tip of the nose; called a nasal pleat (from wiping the nose in an upward fashion). The child will often times present with an open mouth because of the inability to breath through the nose due to nasal congestion.

The Eyes

For the chiropractor, it will be important to do a general assessment of the eyes in the pediatric patient. The chiropractor should be able to screen for any abnormalities that may require a referral to a pediatric ophthalmologist or optometrist for a more complete evaluation. Because examination of the eyes is not the specialty of the chiropractor, the general ophthalmoscopic examination should be left to other health professionals specializing in this particular field. However, visual inspection of the eyes should be done checking for size, shape, spacing, and symmetry. Slanting eyes that are widely spaced are common in many chromosomal abnormalities (e.g., Down's Syndrome).

In cases in which there is a history of recent trauma or neurologic dysfunction is suspected, one should check pupillary size, equality, accommodation, and light reaction.

EYELIDS

Ptosis, drooping of one or both upper eyelids, may be congenital or acquired in nature. Congenital ptosis is commonly due to extraocular muscle abnormalities or central nervous system abnormalities while acquired ptosis is more commonly associated with inflammatory type diseases or injury to the oculomotor nerve supplying the levator palpebrae superioris muscle.

Acute or chronic blepharitis, inflammation of the eyelids, is common in children and is often associated with seborrhea or staphylococcal infections. Frequent rubbing or itching of the eyes, due to allergies, may contribute to staphylococcal contamination. In blepharitis, the lid margins are red with hard, brittle, yellowish scales present. Complications may include lid ulceration, abscess formation, chronic conjunctivitis, and keratitis.

Hordeolum(stye) and chalazion are inflammatory masses of the eyelids. A hordeolum is a staphylococcal infection around the hair follicle of the eyelashes or of the gland of Zeis. It produces a painful, tender, mass on the lid margin, which looks like a boil. Drainage of exudate occurs spontaneously; however, application of moist, warm compresses may accelerate the process.

A chalazion is a painless, beady nodule of the eyelid. It may point externally or internally and occasionally may become inflamed. Chalazions may subside with no intervention; however, surgical drainage is often required.

Viral diseases are also common causes of eyelid infections in children, one of the most common being primary herpes simplex. It is characterized by small vesicles, often unilateral, and associated with conjunctivitis.

Tumors of the eyelids are most commonly the result of a hemangioma. Hemangiomas grow rapidly during the first year of life and then begin to involute spontaneously (see earlier section). Visual obstruction may be of concern depending on location and size.

CONJUNCTIVA

Conjunctivitis is common in the pediatric patient. It may be bacterial, viral, or allergic in nature and is rarely serious except in the newborn.

Bacterial conjunctivitis may be classified as hyperacute, acute, or chronic. Hyperacute bacterial conjunctivitis has a rapid onset and involves both the lid and the cornea. It has a purulent discharge, marked edema, pain, tenderness, accompanied with regional lymphadenopathy. Neisseria gonorrhoeae and Neisseria meningitis are the causative agents.

Acute bacterial conjunctivitis has a mucopurulent discharge. It is associated with tearing, irritation, and the eyelids sticking together on wakening. Staphylococcus, pneumococcus, or hemophilus are the causative agents.

Chronic bacterial conjunctivitis may have varying symptoms such as the sensation of a foreign body in the eye, red eyes, or a mucopurulent discharge of the eyelids upon waking. The causative agents are here are Proteus, Staphylococcus aureus, or Moraxella.

Allergic conjunctivitis is the result of a hypersensitive reaction to foods, pollens, dust, fungus, or other airborne irritants. Redness, itching, burning, tearing, sensitivity to light, the feeling of "sand" in the eyes, or a mucopurulent discharge are all symptoms of allergic conjunctivitis.

Subconjunctival hemorrhages are bright red patches in the exposed part of the bulbar conjunctiva. They are not uncommon in children and are the result of a secondary infection, trauma, bleeding disorder, or a sudden increase in venous pressure (e.g., coughing or sneezing). Reddish discoloration of the eyes may also be due to elevated hemoglobin and hematocrit which causes engorgement of the conjunctival blood vessels. This is often seen in patients with heart defects.

EVALUATION OF VISION

INFANT

By the age of 2–4 weeks, the infant will begin fixating on objects and by 5–6 weeks, visual tracking can be observed in the normal infant. At about 3 months of age, the infant's eyes will begin converging and the baby will begin to reach for objects. Visual acuity is obtained when an object is focused onto the fovea centralis and the fovea has the ability to fixate on it. It is poor at birth (approximately 20/400), but increases rapidly during the first 6 months to 20/40. To assess visual acuity, conduct a central fixation test. Using your thumb to cover one eye at a time; let the uncovered eye fixate on a small brightly colored object at a distance of 1 ft. By 6 months of age, the infant should be able to fixate and follow the object.

If considerable deviation of the eyes is evident by simple inspection, the likely diagnosis is strabismus. Strabismus is classified as either paralytic or nonparalytic. Paralytic strabismus is associated with central nervous system disease or anatomical maldevelopements of the ocular muscles and may have a sudden onset. If only slight deviation is present, one can test for strabismus by either the corneal light reflection test or the cover-up test (Fig. 7.1). Children with a persistent head tilt or face turn may have strabismus with little eye deviation. Infants often demonstrate signs of strabismus because of undeveloped eye muscles. This can be considered normal up to 6 months of age. If deviation of the eyes persists after 6 months of age, referral to an ophthalmologist is recommended. Children with epicanthal folds may demonstrate pseudostrabismus (the appearance of strabismus without the dysfunction).

TODDLER

The aforementioned examinations for strabismus should be applied to the toddler patient. If eye deviations are not corrected, they may lead to amblyopia exanopsia (suppression amblyopia). This condition is one in which visual images have

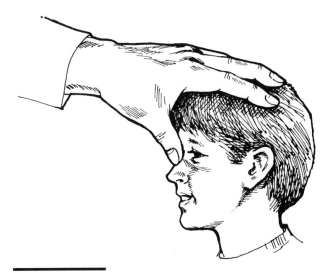

Figure 7.1. The doctor's hand should be placed on the top of the child's head with the thumb placed in front of one eye while the other eye is observed for movement. The thumb is then removed and both eyes are observed for movement. If one or both eyes move, a strabismus could be present. The test is repeated on the opposite eye. Modified from Hoekelman RA. The pediatric physical examination. In: Bates B, ed. A guide to physical examination, 2nd. ed. Philadelphia: J.B. Lippincott Co., 1979:393.

been suppressed in the deviated eye and macular vision never develops; the result is reduction of visual acuity.

Visual acuity in the young toddler is tested very subjectively; observe if the child reaches or follows objects when placed in front of them. Also, ask the parents if they have noticed any abnormal behavior when playing or observing the child at home. By age 3–4, most children will cooperate with a formal visual screening using the Snellen tumbling "E" chart. Place the chart eye level at a distance of 20 feet. Have the child keep both eyes open while occluding one eye at a time. The child should be able to tell which way the open legs of the "E" are pointing (you may have them use their hand and point their finger-tips to the direction of the open legs). By age 5, the child should be able to read the 20/40 line. A two-line visual difference between the eyes should be considered for referral to a pediatric ophthalmologist.

Pre-adolescent/Adolescent

The same procedures used for the infant and toddler ages can be applied to the pre-adolescent and adolescent ages. By age 7, the child should have a visual acuity of 20/20 using the Snellen eye chart. Myopia (nearsightedness) and colorblindness are commonly diagnosed during the adolescent years.

The Ears

Begin by visually inspecting the position of the ears. A low position (below the level of the eyes) or small deformed auricles may be an indication of a brain defect or congenital kidney abnormality, especially renal agenesis.

Inspection of the auricle and periauricular tissues can be done by checking for the four D's: discharge, discoloration, deformity, and displacement. Discharge from the ear canal can be the result of primary otitis externa or chronic untreated otitis media. The discharge may be thick and white in appearance; it may accompany a bright pink or red canal. To differentiate between otitis externa and otitis media, pull on the pinna of the ear; if this elicits pain, otitis externa is the likely diagnosis. Prolonged moisture in the ear canal promotes bacterial and fungal growth which predisposes the child to otitis externa. An equal mixture of rubbing alcohol and white vinegar used as a rinse in the ears will help keep the ears dry and keep bacteria from growing. If the discharge is accompanied with perforation of the tympanic membrane, otitis media should be suspected. The presence of foreign bodies in the ear is common with children. If left in the ear for a period of time, an inflammatory response may develop, which in turn may produce a foul-smelling purulent discharge.

Discoloration in the form of eccymosis over the mastoid area is called "Battles sign." It is associated with trauma and should be considered an emergency. Erythemic discolorations of the pinna and/or mastoid area are often associated with displacement conditions which will be in the following section.

Deformity of the ears may develop from intrauterine positioning or could be the result of hereditary factors. The deformities are of minor concern unless gross deformities are present. Gross deformities of the external ear are often associated with anomalies of the middle and inner ear structures. These anomalies may create hearing disabilities; therefore, these children should be referred for further evaluation and diagnosis.

Displacement of the pinna away from the skull is a distressing sign associated with mastoiditis. Additional signs of mastoiditis include erythema and tenderness over the mastoid area, erythema of the pinna, fever, and purulent discharge. Other conditions associated with displacement of the pinna are parotitis, primary cellulitis, contact dermatitis, and edema secondary to insect bites.

AUDITORY EXAMINATION

Infants/Toddlers

Auditory screening for infants and toddlers is rather crude. Oftentimes, while taking the child's history from the parents, subjective complaints are the first indicator that an auditory deficit may exist. For the toddler ages, the parent may complain that the child does not listen to commands or that they do not repeat familiar words often spoken to them. If the child has begun forming words, evaluate the clarity of the words along with the tone in which they speak; unusually loud speech may accompany a child with a hearing deficit. Remember to evaluate the clarity of the words based on the child's age. Get a clear picture from the parent on time spent working with the child building a vocabulary (e.g., Does the child attend daycare or is there a stay-at-home parent who spends time working with the child?). Children of these age groups can be tested by making a loud startling nose (e.g., clapping your hands behind their head or slamming a door) to see if there is a blink or startled response. A deaf child will not blink in response to a loud startling noise. Due to the invasive nature of the otoscopic evaluation, this should be left until the end of the complete examination for the infant and toddler ages.

PREADOLESCENT/ADOLESCENT

Auditory screening for the pre-adolescent and adolescent ages is also very subjective. Ask the children if they sit towards the front or the back of classes at school and if they have any difficulty in hearing teachers. You may want to question them on their grades to rule out any learning disorders related to a hearing deficit. As you speak with a child, listen to the enunciation of words, the tone in which the child speaks, and his or her ability to listen to instructions. These are all crude ways in which defective hearing may first be suspected. If any suspicion is raised, referral for more sophisticated diagnostic testing should be done. Otoscopic evaluation may be done at this time or at the end of the complete examination.

OTOSCOPIC EVALUATION

The otoscopic evaluation can be performed by having the child in the supine position with his or her head turned to the opposite side of the ear to be examined or with the child seated and the head slightly tilted to the opposite side being examined (for the apprehensive child, you may want to have the child sit on the parent's lap) (Fig. 7.2).

Before examining the older toddler or a younger school-aged child, you may ease his/her anxiety by showing the light of the otoscope and playing a "hide and seek" game. Tell the

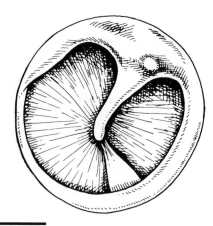

Figure 7.3.   Structures of the ear drum. Modified from Bates B. A guide to physical examination, 2nd. ed. Philadelphia: J. B. Lippincott Co., 1979:59.

child that you will be putting the light in his or her ears so that you can see if anything is hiding in them (e.g., Barney, monsters, trains, etc.). Explain that the child must sit very still so that you don't scare whatever may be inside the ears. Begin by putting the otoscope only partway in the ear (very gently) and take it out quickly, gaining more of the child's confidence. Do this in both ears first, unless there is a suspicion of an infection. If this is the case, the "good ear" should be examined first, followed by the ear with the complaint.

The canal should appear pink and flesh colored, while the tympanic membrane will appear pearly grey and semi-transparent in color. Structures of the ear drum are shown in Figure 7.3. Cerumen (wax) may be present and have a orange, yellow, or brown color. Because the younger child tends to be more active, you should hold the otoscope in an inverted position with your hand lightly rested on the child's head. Therefore, if the child moves suddenly, it will be easier to control the depth of penetration of the otoscope. This reduces the potential for injury or pain to the child. To best visualize the auditory canal of the infant patient, the pinna should be pulled inferior and posterior. For the older child, you may pull the auricle superior and posterior as in the adult patient.

The Nose

Check the nose for any drainage or foreign bodies. As with ears, younger children often enjoy putting foreign objects into various orifices of the body and they often get stuck there. A green, foul smelling , purulent discharge from only one side of the nose is common with a foreign object being left in the nose. Allergic rhinitis and congestion are common with children. Often times, the overuse of nasal sprays causes nasal mucosa irritation and upon inspection, you will find a red, flaky mucosa. Epistaxis may accompany the intrusion of foreign bodies or irritation of the nasal mucosa. To visualize the anterior portion of the nose, push up on the tip of the nose (be sure you have appropriate lighting in the examining room). To see deeper into the nostrils, use a large speculum attached to the otoscope.

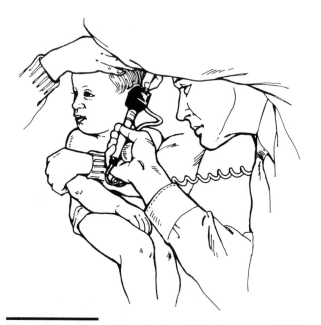

Figure 7.2.   Otoscopic evaluation of the infant patient. Modified from Algranati PS. The pediatric patient: an approach to history and physical examination. Baltimore: Williams & Wilkins, 1992:79.

The Throat/Mouth

Because of the smallness of the oral cavity in the infant, the activity level of the toddler, and the fear of gagging on the tongue depressor in the older child, examination of the mouth and throat in the pediatric patient can be quite a challenge. For the infant and toddler ages, if you have the child in the supine position with his or her neck hyperextended, it will often result in the child opening his or her mouth spontaneously. This will make it easier to insert the tongue depressor and hopefully avoid a struggle. With the older child, ask the child to open his or her mouth and pant like a puppy dog or say "ha ha"; this will help lower the posterior portion of the tongue for better visualization of pharyngeal structures. The size and appearance of the tonsils should be noted. In children, the tonsils are relatively large; they will appear even larger when they protrude out of their fossa as the tongue is protruded (when the child says "ha ha") or when the gag reflex is elicited. The adenoids are not normally visible unless they are extremely enlarged. Examination of the throat should include palpation of the anterior throat. Feel for any enlarged, fixed or hardened lymph nodes. If the child squirms or winces on palpation of the lymph nodes, you may presume that it is tender. These are all signs of possible infection; a referral for further diagnostic tests may be appropriate.

Lymph nodes in a healthy child should be soft, mobile, and non-tender. Inspect the throat, from an anterior view as well as a lateral view, in the vicinity of the thyroid gland looking for any enlargement or asymmetry. After inspection, palpate the thyroid for enlargement. Standing behind the child as he or she remain seated, bring your hands around the front of their neck and gently palpate the isthmus and lateral lobes for size, texture, and symmetry. The size of the lateral lobes should approximate the size of the terminal phalanx of the child's thumb. As you are palpating, ask the child to swallow, this will help in evaluating size and/or the possibilities of any nodules that may be present.

ACUTE PHARYNGITIS AND TONSILLITIS

Over 90% of cases of sore throat and fever in children are due to viral infections. Treatment for viral pharyngitis should be strictly symptomatic and antibiotics are contraindicated (5). Common signs of viral pharyngitis are fever, throat ulcers, vesicles, runny nose, and cough. Approximately 10% of sore throat and fever cases in children are of streptococcal derivation. These cases present with common symptoms of cervical adenitis, petechiae, a swollen red uvula, and tonsillar exudate. The only way the definitive cause of pharyngitis can be determined is through a throat culture or a rapid identification test. Unfortunately, oftentimes antibiotics are prescribed without such a test being performed and the causative agent is viral in nature. Viral infections do not respond to antibiotic therapy; however, the prescribed antibiotics may act to further weaken the immune system and strip the body of its natural flora, thus creating an opportunity for further, and more resistant infections to develop.

Recurrent pharyngitis may be brought on by mouth breathing, postnasal drip, or "school evasion problems."

ACUTE STOMATITIS

Recurrent Aphthous Stomatitis (Canker Sore). These are painful ulcerations lasting approximately 1–2 weeks. They are found on the inside of the lips and throughout the mouth. They are often recurrent throughout a person's life and are often misdiagnosed as herpes simplex. An allergic response or a decreased autoimmune response is normally the cause. The pain associated with the ulcers can be diminished be avoiding foods with salt or acid; switching from a bottle to a cup in infants is also helpful. Measures that can be harmful are: smallpox vaccine, systemic antibiotics, chemical cautery, and lactobacillus containing agents.

Herpes Simplex. This disorder presents with multiple ulcers on the tongue, inner lips, bucal mucosa, and gingiva, lasting 7–10 days, often associated with fever and tender cervical nodes. The child may experience difficulty swallowing, which may interfere with eating or drinking. Treatment should be focused on symptomatic relief as described for recurrent stomatitis. Topical corticosteriods should be avoided as they may result in a spread of the infection.

Thrush. These are white curd-like plaques located mainly on the buccal mucosa. The causative agent is Candida albicans and normally is not invasive unless there is an abrasion of the mouth. Common symptoms are soreness of the mouth and refusal to eat; diaper rash may be associated. Thrush often resembles left-over milk but is easily differentiated by scraping the plaques. Milk will easily be wiped away, while thrush does not scrape away and will sometimes cause bleeding. The use of antibiotics may contribute to thrush.

The Heart

The examination of the heart in the pediatric patient is much the same as that of the adult. Heart sounds are louder because of the thinness of the chest wall. They will also be higher pitched and of shorter duration than those of the adult. The point of maximum impulse (PMI) is at the fourth intercostal space until about age 7, after which it drops to the fifth intercostal space. It will be to the left of the midclavicular line until age 4, at the midclavicular line between ages 4–6, and to the right of it at age 7 (8). A thorough history and physical examination will provide important clues to the possibility of heart disease in the pediatric patient, such as a history of a first-degree relative with heart disease. A history of excessive perspiration and difficulties in feeding are two of the most common complaints of early congestive heart failure.

INSPECTION

Begin by inspecting the precordium for any abnormal pulsations (this is best done by using tangential lighting). Next, visually inspect the skin, lips, nails, and mucous membranes for any appearance of cyanosis. This should be done in proper (preferably natural) lighting, since fluorescent lights may cause a false appearing cyanotic tinge. A cyanotic difference between the upper and lower extremities occurs as a result of pulmonary vascular disease and a patent ductus. This will also lead to clubbing of the toes but not the fingers. In early clubbing of the nails, the angle between the nail and nail base straightens and the nail base will have a spongy feel upon palpation. The normal angle between the nail and nail base is approximately 160 degrees and the nail base is firm upon palpation. Signs of early clubbing, especially of the thumb nails, may appear as early as 3 months of age. In late clubbing, the base of the nail becomes visibly swollen. Clubbing of nails may also be indicative of hypoxia and chronic bacterial endocarditis.

PALPATION

Begin by palpating the precordium and PMI for any thrills or heaves (thrills are said to feel like cat's purrs). The ball of the hand should be used for this procedure as it is generally more sensitive in detecting thrills or heaves; the pads of the fingers are more sensitive for analyzing pulses. Next, palpate all pulses for strength and regularity. A diminished femoral pulse should raise suspicion of coarctation of the aorta. In young children, the femoral pulse may be the easiest to evaluate heart rate. The average heart rate by age is provided in Table 7.2.

PERCUSSION

Percuss the heart borders for size. The heart in the pediatric patient will seem to percuss larger because of its horizontal positioning; this is not to be confused with cardiomegaly. Percussion is best performed by placing a hyperextended middle finger of one hand firmly on the child's chest. Using the middle finger of the opposite hand (the plexor), tap over the nail portion of the hand placed on the chest. Tap with the tip of the plexor finger, not the pad of the finger. Strike one or two times in each location, keeping your technique uniform in all areas examined.

INSTRUMENTATION

AUSCULTATION

As with the otoscope, allow the child to become familiar with the stethoscope before beginning auscultation. Warm-ing the stethoscope before placing it on the child's chest or back is also helpful. Auscultation of the heart can be difficult, especially with the active or apprehensive child. Therefore, it is important to have the parent(s) assistance. The examination room should be quiet while performing the auscultation portion of the exam. The ideal situation for auscultation of the infant patient is while it is asleep. They will also tend to be quieter while eating or sucking on a pacifier. Both the infant and toddler may do better with the parent holding the infant in a cradled position. The older child may be distracted if given a toy to hold or something to stare at.

Using both the bell and the diaphragm, listen to each heart sound paying close attention to the heart rate, rhythm, and intensity. In order, listen to the following areas:

1. Aortic area (second right intercostal space close to sternum)
2. Pulmonic area (second left intercostal space close to sternum)
3. Erb's point (third left intercostal space close to sternum). Murmurs of aortic and pulmonic origin may often be heard here.
4. Tricuspid area (fifth left intercostal space close to sternum)
5. Mitral (apical) area (fifth left intercostal space just medial to the midclavicular line). To remember the name and order of each area to be auscultated, one may think of the acronym "A PET Monkey."

S1 is loudest over the apex, and S2 is loudest at the upper left sternal border. The splitting of S2 along with the normal widening upon inspiration should be noted. A normal S3 may be heard at the apex or lower left sternal border. Differential diagnosis of abnormal heart sounds will not be discussed as it goes beyond the scope of this text.

BLOOD PRESSURE

The width of the blood pressure cuff in the pediatric patient should be one-half to two-thirds the width of the extremity. A cuff that is too narrow will elevate the blood pressure reading. Oftentimes in early childhood, heart sounds are not audible due to a deeply placed or narrow brachial artery. In such cases, one can use palpation of the radial artery at the wrist to determine the child's systolic blood pressure (diastolic pressure can not be determined by palpation of the radial pulse). The point at which the radial pulse is first felt is approximately 10 m Hg lower than that of the systolic pressure determined using auscultation of the brachial artery. Average blood pressures by age are depicted in Table 7.3.

SPECIAL TESTS

Special tests to rule out heart abnormalities could include radiographic, laboratory, and electrocardiograph studies. The chiropractor should refer to a pediatric cardiologist if heart abnormalities are suspected.

Table 7.2.   **Average Heart Rate of Infants and Children at Rest**

Age	Average Heart Rate
Birth	140
1–6 months	130
6–12 months	115
1–2 years	110
2–6 years	103
6–10 years	95
10–14 years	85
14–18 years	82

Modified from Lowrey GH. Growth and development of children, 8th ed. Chicago: Year-Book, 1986:246.

Table 7.3. Normal Values for Blood Pressure

| Age (yr) | Percentile (syst/dias) (mm Hg) | |
	50%	95%
2	96/60	112/78
6	98/64	116/80
9	106/68	126/84
12	114/74	136/88

The neonate range is: systolic: 40-80 mm/Hg; Diastolic: 20-55 mm/Hg. Modified from Silverman BK. Practical information. In: Flesher GR, Ludwig S, eds. Textbook of pediatric emergency medicine, 3rd. ed. Baltimore: Williams & Wilkins, 1993:1735.

RHEUMATIC FEVER

Acute rheumatic fever (ARF) is related to group A, beta streptococcus infection. The typical presentation is 2–6 weeks after a streptococcal infection such as pharyngitis. The presence of a new heart murmur of mitral or aortic insufficiency upon auscultation is strong evidence of carditis. Visual examination of the skin in a patient with acute rheumatic fever may reveal an erythemic rash non-specific to rheumatic fever. It is found on the inner aspects of the arms, thighs, and on the trunk. It is non-pruritic with wavy margins. It may be transitory and may be brought out by heat or a warm bath.

In chronic rheumatic heart disease, subcutaneous nodules that are firm, nontender, and movable are found over bony prominences of large joints and external surfaces of the elbows, knuckles, knees, ankles, scalp, and along the spine. They may be difficult to see but may be felt upon palpation. These nodules are often associated with severe carditis.

BACTERIAL ENDOCARDITIS

Bacterial endocarditis is not common in the pediatric patient. It is most often associated with a history of rheumatic heart disease, or preceding dental, urinary, or intestinal procedures. Classical skin lesions with bacterial endocarditis include splinter hemorrhages of the nails, conjunctival hemorrhages, and Janeway lesions (small, painless nodules). A spiking fever and enlarged spleen are also common signs.

The Lungs and Thorax

As with the entire physical assessment, a complete and careful history are important beginnings of the lung and thorax examination. Assessing the rate, ease, depth, rhythm, and symmetry of respiration is important in ruling out respiratory dysfunction and/or pulmonary disease.

Infants and young toddlers are prone to diaphragmatic breathing; therefore, respiratory rates for these age groups are more easily obtained by observing abdominal excursions. Placement of the stethoscope under the child's nose or auscultation of the chest may also be useful to determine the respiratory rate of a child in this age group. For the older child, observation or palpation of the thoracic cage may be used to determine the respiratory rate. The range of normal respiratory rates for infants and children are listed in Table 7.4.

An increase in respiratory rate (100 + per minute) is seen in children with bronchial asthma or diseases that cause lower respiratory tract obstruction. The respiratory rate of premature as well as full-term newborns may alternate between periods of rapid breathing and periods of apnea. Apnea of 20 seconds or greater duration may indicate a risk for sudden infant death syndrome (SIDS).

INSPECTION

The younger child's clothing should be removed from the waist up. With the pre-adolescent and adolescent female, it is best to have them wear a body suit, bathing suit, or patient gown (especially for the male chiropractor). Begin by checking the thoracic index (the ratio of the transverse diameter to the anteroposterior diameter) of the chest. In infancy, the ratio is approximately equal because of a more rounded thorax. At 1 year of age, the ratio is 1.25, at age 6, it is 1.35 without much change thereafter. Check the sternum for pectus excavatum or carinatum; the xiphoid process can often be seen protruding anteriorly beneath the skin of the infant and young toddler because of the thin musculature of the chest.

With the child in a quiet and relaxed manner, observe respiratory pattern, rate, and depth. Watch for symmetry of chest movements upon inspiration and expiration. In the pre-adolescent and the adolescent patient, check for rib cage height asymmetry. This may be an early indication of possible scoliosis.

PALPATION

Palpation of the thorax is helpful in assessing the following:

1. Reported areas of tenderness
2. Observed areas of abnormalities
3. Respiratory excursions
4. Vocal or tactile fremitus

Table 7.4. Average Respiratory Rates for Normal Infants and Children

Age	Respirations per Minute
Newborn	30–75
6–12 months	22–31
1–2 years	17–23
2–4 years	16–25
4–10 years	13–23
10–14 years	13–19
15+	same as adult

Modified from Cloutier MM. Pulmonary diseases. In: Dworkin PH. Pediatrics. Baltimore: John Wiley & Sons, In., 1987:266.

Begin by palpating any areas of reported tenderness. If no areas are reported as being tender, begin palpating at the level of the clavicles working downward. When palpating the posterior thorax of the infant, have the parent either hold or lie the child on the parent's chest. For the older toddler, pre-adolescent, and adolescent patient, have the child seated with hands folded in front (tell him to give himself a big hug). To palpate the anterior thorax, have the child in a supine position. Be careful not to tickle the child while palpating.

Respiratory excursions should be checked in the older toddler, pre-adolescent, and adolescent patient. To check the anterior thorax, place your thumbs along the anterior costal margin while wrapping the rest of your hands laterally around the rib cage. For the posterior thorax, place your thumbs parallel to the tenth rib. Tell the child to take a deep breath. As the thorax expands, look for symmetrical movement of your thumbs and feel for the range and symmetry of respiratory movement (Fig. 7.4A, B).

Using the ball of one of your hands, palpate for fremitus. Fremitus refers to palpable vibrations transmitted through the bronchopulmonary system to the chest wall when a person speaks. In the infant patient, this can be checked when the baby cries. For the older patient, have them repeat the words "ninety-nine" or "one" while palpating over the lung fields. Fremitus will be decreased or absent when there is bronchial obstruction, fluid in the pleural space, or the patient's voice is decreased. An increase in fremitus will be noticed over the larger bronchi and over consolidated lungs (Fig. 7.5A, B).

PERCUSSION

Percussion is used to determine if the lung fields are air-filled, fluid-filled, or solid. Normal air-filled lungs should have a resonance sound when percussed. In the infant, the normal lung fields will be hyperresonant throughout. A dull or flat sounding lung field may be indicative of fluid filled lungs or pleural space or a solid mass in the lung or pleural space. An example of a "dull" sound can be found when percussing over the heart or liver. While percussion over the thigh will resemble a "flat" lung sound.

Percussion of the lung fields in the infant can be done using only one finger to tap the thoracic wall or the finger–on–finger method described for percussion of the heart. The finger–on–finger method is the preferred method for the older toddler, pre-adolescent, and adolescent patient.

INSTRUMENTATION

Auscultation

Because the infant's chest is so small, the bell or a small diaphragm stethoscope should be used to allow for maximum localization of findings. It is advisable to warm the stethoscope before placing it on the child's chest. Apprehensive children may be calmed if they are allowed to touch and/or listen through the stethoscope before auscultation begins.

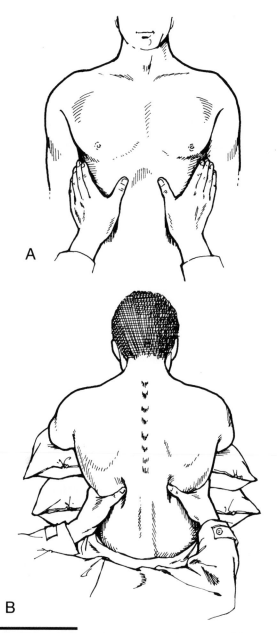

A

B

Figure 7.4. A, Assessing respiratory excursion of the anterior chest. Modified from Bates B. A guide to physical examination, 2nd ed. Philadelphia: J.B. Lippincott Co., 1979:129. B, Assessing respiratory excursion of the posterior chest. Modified from Bates B. A guide to physical examination, 2nd ed. Philadelphia: J.B. Lippincott Co., 1979:121.

As is the case with heart sounds, respiratory sounds in the pediatric patient will be louder than the adult patient because of the thinness of the chest wall. There are three kinds of normal breath sounds:

1. Vesicular
2. Bronchovesicular
3. Bronchial or tubular

Vesicular breath sounds are low pitched, soft sounds heard over most of the lung fields. Bronchovesicular breath sounds are of medium pitch and medium intensity. They are heard below the clavicles and between the scapulae, especially on the right side. Bronchial or tubular breath sounds are high pitched, loud sounds heard over the trachea. Abnormal breath sounds include wheezes, rales, rhon-chi, or friction rubs. Wheezes or rhonchi may be heard with asthma or bronchitis. Audible wheezes are more common with infants and young toddlers because of small lumen of the bronchial tree. Wheezing may occur with only slight swelling of the mucous membrane or a small production of mucous.

In the older toddler, pre-adolescent and adolescent patient, listen for spoken and whispered voice sounds. Ask the child to say "ninety-nine" or "eee" while auscultating; the sounds should be muffled. Next, have the child whisper "ninety-nine," one should hear the words only faintly while ascultating.

ASTHMA

Asthma is the most common chronic lung disorder in children. Between 80–90% of those affected will have their first episode by 4–5 years of age (6). Asthma is defined as spasms or swelling of the bronchial tubes and their mucous membranes. The disease is intermittent and is characterized by recurrent episodes of coughing, wheezing, tightness of the chest, and dyspnea. Severity and recurrence of episodes is greatly influenced by mental or physical fatigue, exposure to various fumes, endocrine changes at various stages in life, stress, and by various emotional situations.

Several classifications of asthma may be the probable cause for the attack. Exercise-induced asthma (EIA) occurs in up to 95% of asthmatic children; cold dry air is often the stimulus. Allergic or extrinsic asthma occurs before 2 years of age and is often associated with foods, pollens, dusts, and animals. Children with allergic asthma will often suffer from eczema as well. Nonallergic or intrinsic asthma is often associated with temperature changes, cold air, odors, smoke, viral infections and menses (6).

For the chiropractor, it is helpful to classify asthma as either "wet" or "dry." Asthmatics suffering from excessive production of thick, tenacious mucous will present with a "wet" sound during respiration. They often have trouble sleeping and can get air into their airways but have trouble with expiration. Vertebral levels associated with the parasympathetic nervous system should be checked for subluxations (occiput to C5, the sacrum and ilia) (10). In the pediatric patient, retrolisthesis of the unfused second sacral tubercle is a common finding in asthmatic patients. Having the child inhale steam may be helpful in loosening up the mucous, making it easier for the child to expel it from the air passages.

Children suffering from "dry" asthma present with a dry, hoarse cough during the attacks. Dry asthma is most often associated with the sympathetic nervous system. As stated previously, changes in endocrine function and menses are known triggers for asthma. The sympathetic nervous system is associated with these functions, therefore, vertebral levels associated with sympathetic functions should be checked for subluxations. Particular attention should be paid to the C6–T3 levels for thyroid function and the T7–T12 levels for suprarenal function. It is helpful, although not easy, to have the parent take the child off of milk, sugar, and chocolate products. Supplementation with vitamins A, C, E, and B Complex is also helpful (4).

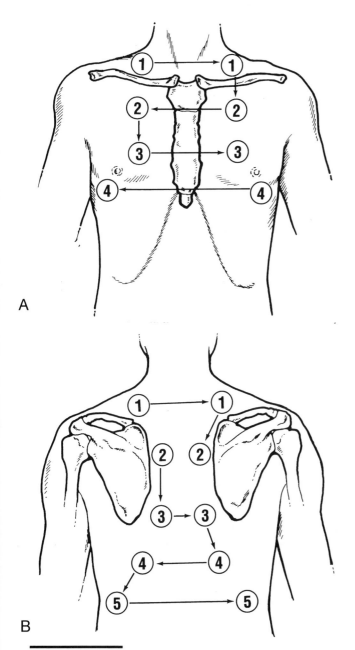

Figure 7.5. A, Palpation for fremitis over the anterior lung fields. Modified from Bates B. A guide to physical examination, 2nd ed. Philadelphia: J.B. Lippincott Co., 1979:130. B, Palpation for fremitis over the posterior lung fields. Modified from Bates B. A guide to physical examination, 2nd ed. Philadelphia: J.B. Lippincott Co., 1979:122.

CROUP

Croup is one of the most common infectious upper airway obstructions in children (AKA: acute infectious laryngotracheobronchitis). It is usually viral in nature and most often affects children in the fall and winter months. Viral croup results in inflammation and edema of the subglottic space, thus, causing the airway obstruction. It is characterized by a hoarse voice, inspiratory stridor and a deep brassy cough sounding like a "barking seal." Respiratory distress may develop slowly or acutely. Labored breathing and marked suprasternal, intercostal, and subcostal retractions are present upon examination. The majority of children are not seriously ill, although airway obstruction may become severe. In severe cases, the need for an artificial airway may become necessary. The child should be checked for vertebral subluxations paying close attention to the upper cervical area (occiput to C2) and the thoracic spine (T2–T7) (4).

The Abdomen

The order for examination of the abdomen is changed slightly in that palpation is done last. Therefore, the order is: inspection, percussion, auscultation, light palpation, and deep palpation. If there is a complaint of a tender area, that area should be palpated last. Ask the older child if he or she must use the restroom before beginning the abdominal examination; a full bladder can be quite uncomfortable. If possible, have the child in the supine position for the entire abdominal exam. This may be difficult with the toddler patient, therefore, you may have to perform the examination with the child sitting or standing. The examination will not be as accurate, but it will be superior to not performing the procedures at all. With the older child, it is helpful to place a pillow under the knees to help relax the abdominal muscles. For examination of the infant and toddler, relaxation of the abdominal muscles can be obtained by holding the knees in a flexed position with one hand while palpating with the second hand. Have the child's arms down at his or her sides, not above the head. With the arms above the head, the abdominal muscles become stretched and tight, making palpation difficult.

INSPECTION

The abdomen in the infant will be protuberant due to the poorly developed abdominal muscles. This "pot belly" appearance is commonly seen in children up until adolescence. It is most apparent when the child is sitting and dramatically decreases when he or she is supine.

The child should already be unclothed (waist up) from the lung and thorax portion of the physical examination. For the pre-adolescent and adolescent female, it is easiest to have her wear a gown or shirt that can be "rolled" up to expose the abdomen. From the right side of the patient, inspect for rashes, scars, lesions, or discoloration. Silver striae discoloration is indicative of stretching, while purple-pink striae is indicative of Cushing's syndrome.

An abdominal venous pattern is often noticeable until puberty. Observe the overall contour and symmetry of the abdomen. An infant with a concave abdomen should immediately be checked for a diaphragmatic hernia with possible displacement of abdominal organs into the thoracic cavity. An asymmetric bulging abdominal wall may be indicative of an enlarged organ and/or abdominal mass. A bottle of sugar water or milk should be fed to the infant patient. If pyloric stenosis is present, peristaltic waves will be seen going from left to right across the abdomen. These waves will become more intense and frequent with further feedings.

Inspect the umbilicus for shape, signs of inflammation or hernia. In the infant, the umbilical stump dries up and falls off within 1 to 2 weeks. Some serous fluid or blood may continue to ooze from the site for several days after. By approximately 1 month of age, the cord site will be covered with new skin. Infants are prone to umbilical hernias, ventral hernias, and diastasis (recti midline vertical outpouching of the abdomen). They are considered normal variants and usually disappear by early childhood. These variants are usually not observable until 2 to 3 weeks of age and are easily detected when the child cries.

INSTRUMENTATION

AUSCULTATION

Auscultation of the abdomen should be done before palpation and percussion since the latter may alter the frequency and quality of bowel sounds. Listen to all four quadrants noting the frequency and quality of bowel sounds. Abdominal sounds may include gurgles, clicks, or growls. The frequency of sounds has been estimated anywhere from 5 to 34 times per minute. An increase in frequency or pitch of bowel sounds may be associated with intestinal obstruction or diarrhea. Decreased or absent sounds may be associated with paralytic ileus or peritonitis. To determine if bowel sounds are in fact absent, listen for at least 2 minutes in the area just inferior and to the right of the umbilicus.

PERCUSSION

Percussion of the abdomen in the pediatric patient is the same as in the adult patient. It is useful for general assessment of the liver (and sometimes the spleen) size and for the assessment of air in the stomach and/or bowels. Because children are prone to swallowing air while feeding or crying, one may expect to find a great amount of air within the stomach and intestinal lumen of the pediatric patient. Percuss the abdomen in all four quadrants listening for dullness or tympany. Tympany will usually be more prevalent. Dullness in the suprapubic area is due to a distended bladder. The liver, when percussed, will also be dull. Percussion of liver borders should begin below the umbilicus (in an area of tympany, not dullness) and the examiner works upwards in the right midclavicular line. Identify and mark the lower border of the liver when the first sound of dullness is heard. To identify the upper border of the liver, begin in the area of lung resonance and percuss downwards in the midclavicular line. The first sound of dullness will represent the upper border of the liver. In a small child, the liver may falsely appear as being enlarged because of the smallness of the child's overall chest and abdominal cavity in proportion to the liver size.

The spleen can be percussed as a small oval area of dullness near the left tenth rib, just posterior to the midaxillary line. Splenic dullness can often be obscured by gastric or colonic air tympany. Percuss the lower left anterior rib cage for gastric air bubble tympany of the stomach.

LIGHT PALPATION

Begin palpation of the abdomen with light, gentle pressure. This will help relax and reassure children that you are not going to hurt them. Palpation should be done on an unclothed abdomen with the pads of the fingertips and with the fingers together. If the child is apprehensive or ticklish, have the child place his or her hands on top of yours and ask that the child do the pushing. Children often enjoy participating in the examination; in addition, their participation will help distract them so that the abdominal muscles will be relaxed.

Using light dipping motions, feel all quadrants of the abdomen. Indentify any palpable organs or masses. Note any areas of tenderness, rigidity, or increased resistance. If the abdominal muscles are not relaxed, encountering voluntary resistance is not uncommon. Make sure the abdominal muscles are relaxed before going on to deep palpation. Any areas that produced tenderness or are suspect for pathology should be palpated last during deep palpation.

DEEP PALPATION

Deep palpation is mostly used to identify organs and masses. Using the palmar surfaces of the fingers, palpate all four quadrants. If any masses are detected, note their size, location, shape, consistency, tenderness, pulsations, and mobility (e.g., does the mass move with respiration or with applied pressure?). To differentiate between a mass of the abdominal wall and a mass within the abdominal cavity, have the patient tighten his or her abdominal muscles by raising his or her head and shoulders up off the examination table. If the mass is in the abdominal wall, it will remain palpable, whereas an intra-abdominal mass will be obscured by muscular tension. The most common "mass" found in the pediatric patient is that of fecal matter in the colon. It will often palpate as hard round balls in the left lower quadrant and will be freely mobile. Occasionally you may be able to outline a sausage-shaped mass filling the entire descending colon. Check tender areas for rebound tenderness that may be suggestive of peritoneal inflammation. Rebound tenderness is performed by pressing slowly but firmly into the abdominal cavity and then quickly withdrawing the hands.

The Liver. The liver can be palpated by standing on the right side of the patient. Place your left hand underneath the patient at approximately the level of the eleventh and twelfth rib. The liver can be felt more easily if there is slight anterior pressure applied with the left hand. The right hand is placed just lateral to the rectus muscle below the lower border of liver dullness with the fingers pointing cephalad. Press in and up, feeling for the edge of the liver (approximately 1–2 cm below the right costal margin). In children, the edge of the liver is more often palpable than not. A normal liver edge will present as a firm, sharp, regular ridge with a smooth surface. Having the child take a deep breath with his or her stomach (not with the chest)

may help make the liver more palpable. If palpable, trace the liver edge medially and laterally by repeating the procedure.

The Spleen. To palpate the spleen, remain on the right side of the patient. Reach your left arm across the patient's chest and "hook" your fingers around the left posterior aspect of his or her rib cage. Support and press forward the left side of his or her rib cage. Place your right hand low enough to be sure that you are below a possibly enlarged spleen. Be careful not to have your hand too close to the costal margin; this will not allow for sufficient mobility to reach up and under the rib cage. Have the patient take a deep breath as you press in and up toward the spleen. Try to feel the edge or tip of the spleen as it comes down to meet your fingertips. This procedure can be repeated with the patient on his or her side with the hips and knees flexed. In this position, gravity helps to bring the spleen forward and to the right into a palpable position. A slightly enlarged spleen may be palpable in the older infant and older child. However, a normal spleen is often difficult to palpate, especially in the older child.

The Kidneys. To palpate both kidneys, remain on the patient's right side placing your left hand underneath the patient between the rib cage and iliac crest on the side being examined. Place your right hand below the costal margin on the side being examined. Because the kidneys lie deep in the posterior aspect of the abdominal cavity, palpation of the kidneys is deeper than that of the liver. As the patient takes a deep breath, try to feel the inferior portion of the kidney come down between your fingers. Another method is the kidney "entrapment" test. The hand placement is the same as before. At the peak of inspiration, press your fingers together quickly (more pressure should be applied with the superior hand than the inferior hand), have the patient breathe out, and then stop breathing briefly. Slowly release the pressure of your hands feeling for the kidney to slip between your fingers back into its normal position. The kidney "punch" test is performed with the patient in the seated position and is often done during examination of the back. Place the palm of your left hand flat on the patient's back over area of the kidneys. Using the ulnar surface of your right fist, strike your left hand. The patient should notice a jar or thud, but no pain.

APPENDICITIS

Appendicitis is the most common cause of acute abdominal pain in older children and adolescents. Clinical signs and symptoms include a 1–2 day history of periumbilical crampy or dull pain followed by nausea and anorexia with or without vomiting. The abdominal pain remains fairly constant and is localized in the lower right quadrant at McBurney's point. A positive rebound test is common in this area. If the appendix ruptures, the abdominal pain may subside and is usually followed by high fever, abdominal wall muscle rigidity due to voluntary guarding, and involuntary muscle spasms. Atypical presentations are common with young children and may include normal white blood cell counts and fever at 100–102 degrees. Urinalysis may show mild pyuria and occasionally proteinuria.

Table 7.5.   **Distinguishing Characteristics of Abdominal Pain in Children**

Disease	Onset	Location	Referral	Quality	Comments
Irritable bowel syndrome	Recurrent	Periumbilical	None	Dull, crampy, intermittent, duration 2 hr	Family stress, school phobia, onset about 5 yr old
Esophageal reflux	Recurrent, 1 hr after meal	Substernal	Chest	Burning	Sour taste in mouth, Sandifer syndrome
Duodenal ulcer	Recurrent, between meals, at night	Epigastric	Back	Severe burning, gnawing	Relieved by food, milk, antacids
Pancreatitis	Acute	Epigastric, left upper quadrant	Back	Constant, sharp, boring	Nausea, emesis, tenderness
Intestinal obstruction	Acute or gradual	Periumbilical—lower abdomen	Back	Alternating cramping (colic) and painless periods	Distention, obstipation, emesis, increased bowel sounds
Appendicitis	Acute	Epigastric, localized to right lower quadrant	Back; pelvis if retrocecal	Sharp, steady	Nausea, emesis, local tenderness, fever
Meckel diverticulum	Recurrent	Periumbilical—lower abdomen	None	Sharp	Hematochezia
Inflammatory bowel disease	Recurrent	Lower abdomen	Back	Dull cramping, tenesmus	Fever, weight loss, hematochezia
Invagination of bowel	Acute	Periumbilical—lower abdomen	None	Cramping, with painless periods	Hematochezia, guarded position with knees pulled up
Lactose intolerance	Recurrent with milk products	Lower abdomen	None	Cramping	Distention, bloating, diarrhea
Urolithiasis	Acute, sudden	Back	Groin	Sharp, intermittent, cramping	Hematuria
Urinary tract infection	Acute, sudden	Back	Bladder	Dull to sharp	Fever, costochondral tenderness, dysuria, urinary frequency

Modified from Andreoli TE, Carpenter CCJ, Plum F, Smith LH. Cecili's essentials of medicine. Philadelphia: J.B. Lippincott Co., 1986:261.

Additional examination procedures to assess possible appendicitis include:

1. Rovsing's sign: press deep into the left side of the lower abdominal quadrant. Pain felt in the right lower quadrant may accompany appendicitis.
2. Abdominal pin prick: lightly and evenly touch the patient's skin with a pinpoint, testing in lines down both sides of the abdomen. Hyperesthesia of the right lower quadrant may accompany appendicitis.
3. Positive hip flexion or hip extension tests: with the patient's legs bent and feet resting on the examination table, place your hand over the patient's knee and have him or her flex the leg against your hand. Next, have the patient turn on the left side and extend the right leg at the hip. Pain on either maneuver constitutes a positive psoas sign, suggesting irritation of the psoas muscle by an inflamed appendix.
4. Obturator test: With the patient's knee flexed, flex the patient's right thigh at the hip and rotate the leg

internally. Pain in the right hypogastric area constitutes a positive obturator sign suggesting irritation of the obturator muscle by an inflamed appendix.

The differential diagnoses of suspected appendicitis or general abdominal pain should include pancreatitis, urinary tract infection, intestinal obstruction, and lactose intolerance. In the pre-adolescent and adolescent female, reproductive organ involvement should be ruled out (e.g. ovarian cysts, salpingitis, tubal pregnancy). Table 7.5 presents the distinguishing characteristics of abdominal pain in children. Patients with a suspected diagnosis of acute appendicitis should be referred to an emergency room.

URINARY TRACT INFECTIONS (UTI)

The pain associated with a urinary tract infection is acute and sudden. The pain is dull to sharp in nature and is located in the lower back area with possible referred pain to the bladder. The signs and symptoms associated with a UTI are fever, urinary frequency, dysuria, and costochondral tenderness. The spine should also be evaluated for vertebral subluxations paying particular attention to the lower thoracic (T9–T12) and the upper lumbar levels (L1–L2) (4). The use of unsweetened cranberry juice to cause the urine to become more acidic and create an unpleasant environment for bacterial growth may also be helpful. Increasing the water intake beyond the recommended eight glasses daily is recommended. Patients unresponsive to conservative measures should be referred for possible antibiotic therapy. UTIs are sometimes associated with streptococcal infections.

DYSMENORRHEA

Dysmenorrhea is the most common gynecologic complaint of adolescent females, with an incidence of about 60% (5). Dysmenorrhea can be divided into primary and secondary dymenorrhea; the determining factor being any underlying pelvic disease.

PRIMARY DYSMENORRHEA

Primary dysmenorrhea is that disorder in which no organic pelvic disease is detectable. It can be divided into two categories: primary spasmodic dysmenorrhea and psychogenic dysmenorrhea. Primary spasmodic dysmenorrhea accounts for 80% of cases of adolescent dysmenorrhea and most often affects women under 25 years of age (5). The pain associated with this type of dysmenorrhea begins once the menstrual cycle becomes ovulatory, which is 6–18 months post menarche. It is thought to be from excessive amounts of prostaglandins that causes uterine contractions, hypoxia, and ischemia. Prostaglandins also sensitize pain receptors and lower the pain threshold. Symptoms associated with spasmodic dysmenorrhea are lower abdominal cramps that may refer into the low back and thighs, nausea, vomiting, diarrhea, and urinary frequency. Symptoms most often start with the onset of flow or just before and last 1–2 days.

Psychogenic dysmenorrhea normally begins at menarche.

The pain may last for the duration of flow and is associated with anticipation of menses. School and/or work avoidance should be ruled out as possible secondary gains.

SECONDARY DYSMENORRHEA

Secondary dysmenorrhea is due to an underlying pelvic pathology. The most common cause of secondary dysmenorrhea in the adolescent patient is infection or endometriosis. Pelvic cramping of recent onset, excessive bleeding, vaginal discharge, or intermenstrual spotting are indicators of infection. The use of intrauterine devices are common causes of pelvic infections. Pain due to endometriosis usually begins more than 2 years after menarche. In cases of primary or secondary dymenorrhea, the spine should be checked for vertebral subluxations paying special attention to vertebral levels T12–L5 and the pelvis. Hypothyroidism may be associated with premenstrual syndrome; therefore, the cervicothoracic junction (C6–T3) should also be examined for vertebral subluxations (10).

COLIC

Colic is described as unexplained extreme fussiness, not related to eating, that occurs within the first 3 months of life. It typically begins at about 2–3 weeks of age and gradually declines by the third month. It is more common in the late afternoon and evening hours. Common characteristics of colic include sudden onset of intense crying for no known reason, stomach bloating, and drawing of the legs upward towards the chest. There is no known cause of colic. It has been speculated that immaturity of the central nervous system in infants, gastrointestinal intolerance to milk, or family distress may somehow be associated with colic. The infant should be checked for vertebral subluxations paying special attention to the upper cervical spine (occiput to C2) and the mid-thoracic spine (T4 to T9) (3).

REFERENCES

1. Flesher GR, Ludwig S, eds. Textbook of pediatric emergency medicine, 3rd ed. Baltimore: Williams & Wilkins, 1993.
2. Rudolph AM, Hoffman JIE, Rudolph CD. Rudolph's pediatrics, 20th ed. Stamford, CT: Appleton & Lange, 1996.
3. Anrig Howe C. Chiropractic approaches to pregnancy and pediatric care. In: Plaugher G, ed. Textbook of clinical chiropractic: a specific biomechanical approach. Baltimore: Williams & Wilkins, 1993:383-432.
4. Carr E, Donahue J. The notes: Gonstead seminar notes. Mt. Horeb, WI: Gonstead Seminar of Chiropractic (no copyright date).
5. Hathaway WE, Hay WW, Groothuis JR, Paisley JW. Current pediatric diagnosis and treatment. 11th ed. Norwalk, CT: Appleton & Lange, 1993.
6. Behrman RE, Kliegman R, eds. Nelson essentials of pediatrics. Philadelphia: W.B. Saunders Co., 1990.
7. Yochum TR, Rowe LJ. Essentials of skeletal radiology. Baltimore: Williams & Wilkins, 1987:888.
8. Bates B. A guide to physical examination, 2nd ed. Philadelphia: J. B. Lippincott Co., 1979
9. Algranati PS. The pediatric patient: an approach to history and physical examination. Baltimore: Williams & Wilkins, 1992.
10. Plaugher G, Lopes MA, Konlande JE, Doble RW, Cremata EE. Spinal management for the patient with a visceral concomitant. In: Plaugher G, ed. Textbook of clinical chiropractic: a specific biomechanical approach. Baltimore: Williams & Wilkins, 1993:356-382.

8 Diagnostic Imaging

Christopher Kent, Gregory Plaugher, David Borges,
Karen M. Borges, David M. Steiner, and David L. Cichy

Diagnostic imaging represents an integral component of chiropractic practice. This is evidenced by the widespread presence of plain film x-ray equipment in chiropractic offices and the increasing utilization of more advanced imaging such as MRI, CT, and bone scans.

This chapter will present the more salient clinical issues surrounding the application of plain film and advanced imaging in a chiropractic pediatric practice. The focus of this chapter is on plain film radiography and roentgenometric analysis of the spine although basic information on computerized axial tomography (CT) and magnetic resonance imaging (MRI) is also presented. The role of diagnostic imaging in the analysis of spinal development, congenital variants, fracture, neoplasm, infection, and epiphyseal disorders is also discussed.

Although diagnostic imaging can be used for all regions of the human body, we have specifically limited the discussion in this chapter to the spinal column and pelvis. Specific radiologic manifestations of disorders affecting the appendicular skeleton are discussed elsewhere in this text. There are other more complete works available to the chiropractor for the general study of plain film radiography (1–4), and these should be accessed by the reader.

Plain Film Radiography

Plain film radiography is the mainstay of imaging in most chiropractic practices. Approximately 80% of the private practices in the United States have x-ray facilities (5). A 1993 survey of U.S. chiropractors by the National Board of Chiropractic Examiners found that the use of x-ray examination to determine the presence of pathology, fracture, dislocations or other significant findings was rated the highest in importance of the 45 cited activities that chiropractors performed. According to the survey, chiropractors also use x-ray examination with high frequency to either update the x-ray examination and/or perform new x-rays on a patient whose condition has changed and/or who has a new condition (6).

Plain film radiography remains the primary imaging modality in the case of neuromusculoskeletal injuries and should direct the clinician to any further diagnostic investigations, such as CT or MRI (7). Radiographic examination in clinical practice is essential for a variety of reasons. Chiropractors have realized the value of being able to image the spinal column to rule out the presence of diseases such as neoplasm (e.g., pathologic fracture) and spine infections, that would necessarily alter how an adjustive intervention would be applied, if at all. During adjustments, substantial forces are applied to the vertebral column (8–11). Should bone weakening diseases be present, then the applied forces should be altered accordingly so as not to cause harm to the patient. Plain film radiography has been used to rule out (to the extent possible) these pathologic processes.

Since many patients who present for chiropractic evaluation have syndromes relating to joint pathology, it is important to evaluate the integrity of these structures in order to obtain a more accurate diagnosis (12). Chiropractors share this diagnostic imperative with orthopedists, neurologists and rheumatologists.

The ability of plain film to image the intersegmental and global posture of the spinal column and end-range mobility has been thought to be of clinical importance in terms of the application of a specific adjustment or rehabilitative exercise (13–21). There is still much needed research to perform to thoroughly assess the clinical utility of plain film radiography in practice (15, 22–24).

Vertebral Subluxation Complex

The vertebral subluxation complex (VSC) has a number of components (26–30). These spinal changes associated with the VSC include kinesiologic, myologic, neurologic and histologic factors.

Hildebrandt (19) has reviewed the clinical basis for chiropractic spinography. Chiropractic spinography can be defined as a roentgenological diagnostic procedure that uses postural (weight-bearing) x-rays for the principal purpose of evaluating the spinal column and pelvis for evidence of clinically significant biomechanical irregularities (19). The use of x-ray examination in the chiropractic profession dates back to 1910, when B.J. Palmer used the device initially as a research tool to evaluate the accuracy of spinal palpation. In later years, the x-ray was used as a common diagnostic procedure for the detection of abnormal spinal biomechanics (25).

Global postural spinal problems can be examined through external postural analysis and global range of motion assessed through goniometry (26–31). However, global assessments are limited since they primarily evaluate the extrinsic spinal musculature. The intersegmental biomechanical effects on the ligamentous elements, fixation dysfunction, normal motion and instability, in fact all intersegmental phenomena, can be more accurately assessed with plain film techniques (32). No alternative and less invasive procedures are currently available to the practicing chiropractor for accurately assessing the intersegmental kinesiologic components of the subluxation complex.

Clinical research and observation suggests spinal biomechanical compromise can occur in utero (constraint positions) or as a result of birth trauma (21,33). Multiple microtraumatic episodes and macro traumas can occur in the child throughout spinal development. During the formative years, shear stress deformities, changes in the instantaneous axis of rotation and altered intersegmental biomechanics create the environment for abnormal vertebral cartilaginous and osseous remodeling resulting in permanent structural deformity (34).

Radiographs should not be used independently to rule out the presence of a joint abnormality (i.e., subluxation) requiring an adjustment. As with most diagnostic tests, plain film is great for the interpretation of some things and completely unnecessary for others. To evaluate the multiple component nature of the subluxation, tests should be weighed differently when evaluating particular patients, spinal regions, or injury scenarios. The clinical and/or symptomatic picture should always be correlated with radiologic findings since the subluxation is a multivariate complex. The practitioner should first find the location (i.e., segmental level) of the joint abnormality on the patient and not on the radiograph. Factors that are proposed to be weighed heavily in the clinical examination are the presence of edema, tenderness, and joint fixation.

PREVENTION OF DEFORMITY AND INJURY

Chiropractic care may be more effective if it prevents the vertebral subluxation complex from causing the development of permanent osseous or soft tissue asymmetry (12). The pediatric spine is particularly vulnerable as the cartilage of the fetus makes its transition to bone in the adult. In some families of patients, there may be genetic predilection for the development of certain spinal problems.

To the extent possible, applying preventive adjustments to motion segments that may not yet be symptomatic could have the potential for minimizing abnormal cartilage and bone formation during the growth of the child. This logic applies as well to the promotion of certain exercise levels or postural practices and the limiting of others.

Some spinal anomalies can best be detected through plain film. Low cost combined with minimal risks, when used judiciously, makes plain film examination the imaging modality of choice in most circumstances. The presence of a small cervical central canal, measured from the lateral cervical radiograph, should alert the attending clinician and athlete that certain sports, in which the potential for neck trauma is high, must be avoided (35).

LIGAMENTOUS INJURIES

The onset of disc degeneration in the early stages often corresponds with the onset of symptoms (36), although some individuals will experience no symptoms. In these patients, early signs of spinal degeneration such as retrolisthesis or disc dehydration can only be determined through objective analytical procedures, such as plain film radiography or magnetic resonance imaging (MRI) combined with palpatory signs of inflammation such as edema or tenderness.

In low back disorders, the first pathological changes occur in the annulus. These early changes take the form of small circumferential separations between the annular lamellae. Evidence of lamellar separation has been reported as early as 8 years of age (36). In the vast majority of disc injuries, healing occurs in the form of granulation tissue and vascularization. The new blood supply comes from the outer annulus and the end-plate (36,37).

Recent advances in imaging technology have allowed better visualization of ligamentous structures, such as the intervertebral disc. Paajanen et al. (38) used MRI to study disc degeneration in young, low-back pain patients. The average age of the patients was 20 years. Fifty-seven percent of those suffering from low-back pain had one or more abnormal lumbar discs. A control group of pain-free individuals was also analyzed with MRI. Approximately 35% of these individuals showed signs of degeneration. End-plate changes, detected radiographically, were associated with disc degeneration. Therefore, damaged end-plates are likely one etiological and/or associated factor in the development of disc degeneration. Many of the MRI detected abnormal joints had no marked radiographic changes. Early degenerative disc disease may exist long before there is loss of disc height or other obvious radiographic findings of degenerative joint disease (39).

Paajanen et al. (38) did not evaluate subtle postural changes with plain film radiography, nor movement abnormalities. Because disc degeneration begins at an early age, it is important for the chiropractor to direct adjustments into the motion segment that do not cause further stress to the annular fibers. The avoidance of long axis rotational forces is one method for reducing the chance for disc injury with an adjustment (40).

Incorporating alignment and movement considerations during the delivery of an adjustment will less likely result in ligamentous injury to the spine. Ligamentous damage could result from a misdirected thrust by moving the joint further into the direction of ligamentous sprain (i.e., into the direction of hypermobility), or potentially cause a separation of the endplate at its attachment to the disc.

LOW BACK PROBLEMS

Olsen et al. (41) assessed the prevalence of low back pain in a cohort of 1242 adolescents (11–17 yr). Approximately 30% of the adolescents had low back pain. One third of the individuals with low back pain reported restricted activity and 7.3% sought medical attention. Based on the results of the investigation, the authors suggested that low back pain is a serious public health problem. If one third of the adolescent population is experiencing symptomatic back problems, others may have underlying subclinical pathology (i.e., subluxation with only mild sprain). Low back pain is a frequent reason for adult patients to seek chiropractic care, and "spinal manipulation" has received endorsement as an efficacious treatment from two independent reviews (42,43).

Plain film radiography is a highly efficient means for detecting subtle alignment changes in the spine, thought to be of importance to chiropractors in directing treatment in patients. In addition, tropism, transitional segments, lumbar scoliosis and leg length inequality are all structural entities that are readily identifiable with plain film which can alter both the direction and site of a high velocity low amplitude thrust and other treatments (e.g. heel lift). The presence of these structural changes in the low back also impacts the clinical diagnosis and prognosis of the patient. Although the findings that are typically seen on plain film radiographs of patients with low back pain are not necessarily relevant to a practitioner of internal medicine or a physical therapist since they will do little to direct the approach to treatment, these findings do have direct applicability to the adjustment/management issues facing the chiropractor (6,15,44).

CLINICAL EXAMINATION

Spinal trauma will usually result in signs of inflammation, especially over the posterior aspect of the spinous processes where ligamentous sprain injury due to hyperflexion moves the supraspinous ligament through the greatest arc of motion. The presence of the signs of inflammation may warrant radiographic examination. Signs of inflammation include palpable spinal tenderness (45), edema or erythema. Palpable tenderness is relatively reproducible in interexaminer reliability experiments (45,46).

When physical abnormalities such as skin temperature asymmetries (47–49), the red response (50), or skin texture abnormalities suggestive of autonomic disturbances or denervation supersensitivity (51,52) exist, then radiographs are usually indicated for the assessment of other components of the subluxation such as alignment and movement changes (15). These palpatory and instrument findings, indicative of inflammation or subclinical neuropathology, should guide the clinician towards further investigation (e.g., plain film), to address the need, if any, for the application of a specific adjustment.

ASYMPTOMATIC SUBLUXATION

The chiropractic paradigm incorporates the idea that abnormal spinal function, such as reduced movement (20,53–55) or alignment abnormalities (56,57), are significant and warrant chiropractic intervention (i.e., adjustment). The argument that early chiropractic intervention should be used, regardless if a patient has symptoms, lends support for the use of objective means of assessment, such as plain film radiography. Exacting analysis and treatment could theoretically avert more serious problems later or alleviate currently silent nerve pathology, thus influencing the general health of the patient. Long-term prospective investigations will need to be performed to address the salient issues surrounding the asymptomatic spinal subluxation and its putative effect on general health outcome measures (e.g., the quality and quantity of life).

KINESIOPATHOLOGY

Kinesiopathologic factors associated with spinal trauma include intersegmental postural and movement abnormalities as well as global assessments of spinal function and posture. Abnormal patterns of movement, compensatory hypermobility due to fixation dysfunction, and spinal and pelvic misalignments (i.e., positional dyskinesia) are entities that should be scrutinized carefully when evaluating the spinal column for signs of trauma or functional disturbances.

FIXATION DYSFUNCTION

If movement irregularities, such as reduction in global range of motion or intersegmental abnormalities such as fixation dysfunction or hard end-feel are present, then radiographic assessments are usually indicated because there is likely to be adjustive intervention for these dysfunctions (15). The information derived from the radiograph is likely to be useful in the delivery of care (i.e., ruling out contraindications, identifying anomalies, and determining patterns of thrust consistent with improved biomechanics). Limited information is available on the use of various radiographic findings as outcome measurements. Bronfort and Jochumsen (32) report on a series of patients with low back pain in whom functional radiographic examinations of the low back were obtained. An analysis of a subset of the cohort of adults who had low back pain and received spinal adjustments demonstrated improvements in intersegmental motion after treatment.

POSITIONAL DYSKINESIA

Upper Cervical Spine. Biedermann (20), a manual medicine practitioner, studied biomechanical problems (i.e., subluxation) of the upper cervical spine in newborns. Approximately 135 babies who were available for follow-up were reviewed in the report. The babies were referred to the author because of asymmetrical posture, and the case histories included the following disturbances:

1. Tilt posture of the head or torticollis
2. Head tilt in flexion
3. Uniform sleeping patterns; the child cries if the mother tries to change its position
4. Fixation of the sacroiliac joints
5. Extreme sensitivity of the neck to palpation
6. Loss of appetite

The symptoms described by the patients' parents could be due to a variety of pathologic conditions. Biedermann states that if motor asymmetries, sleeping alterations, or facial scoliosis are present, then the suboccipital articulations should be evaluated for blockages (i.e., fixation dysfunction). He also advocates the use of plain film radiographs for determining malalignment of the suboccipital region and for determining the appropriate vector of force during the adjustment. In addition, the radiograph is used for the detection of malformations. Biedermann states that basing treatment on information not taken from the radiograph is why his colleagues probably do not have as favorable results. A high proportion of the newborns in this study experienced prolonged labor times during delivery when compared with normal babies. Most patients only required 1–3 adjustments before remission of symptoms occurred. However, no long-term follow-up of these patients was reported. These findings parallel the clinical observations of many practicing chiropractors and indicate that chiropractic care for newborns is promising. Further research on suboccipital subluxation, including prospective controlled studies, should be undertaken to control for the natural history of these disorders.

Lumbar Retrolisthesis. Plaugher et al. (56), in a retrospective consecutive case analysis of pretreatment and comparative radiographs from 49 adult outpatients attending a chiropractic clinic, found that retrolisthesis of the L5 or L4 vertebra reduced about 34% after an average of eight adjustments directed at the level of displacement. No statistically significant change was detected in a retrospective control group. The doctor whose records were scrutinized usually performed comparative evaluations just before the tenth visit and the patients usually continued care on an individual basis after this comparative analysis. Twenty-five patients who entered the clinic between January 1, 1986 and March 1, 1986 had their records added to another 25 patients who entered the clinic between April 1, 1986 and June 1, 1986. Because of poor quality radiographs in one case, a total of forty-nine patients were analyzed. There were 31 females (63%) and 18 males (37%). The mean age was 44 yr (SD = 20 yr). The most common complaint at entrance was low back pain, occurring in 79% of the population. Fifty-three percent of the patients had mid-back or neck symptoms. Sixty-four percent of the patients had referred pain to either shoulder, or upper and/or lower extremity. Forty-seven percent of the patients had viscerosomatic or somatovisceral symptoms. Patient complaints included, headache, constipation, dysmenorrhea, shortness of breath, and nervousness.

Sacral Base and Lumbar Lordosis Angles. In the aforementioned study (56), measurements were also made of the sacral base angle and the lumbar lordosis angle in the adult patients. No statistically significant changes were observed pre- and post-treatment. The length of time between analyses was about 1 month, and occurred before the tenth office visit. The use of these radiologic parameters as outcome measurements in short-term trials (i.e., less than 1 month) of chiropractic adjustments is questionable.

Banks (57) has shown that reduction of the hyperextension component of the lower lumbar motion segments is readily attainable in adults with side posture manipulation. A statistically significant decrease in the average disc angle at the involved level was detected in his sample of 13 patients with clinical diagnoses of facet syndrome (i.e., hyperextension of the lower lumbar and lumbosacral disc spaces with concomitant facet jamming).

Cervical Lordosis. Plaugher et al. (56) observed no significant change in the cervical lordosis after examination of the initial and comparative radiographs. The average number of cervical and upper thoracic adjustments delivered between the initial and comparative radiographs was 6.5. All patients who reported for care were analyzed, regardless of the level of adjustment.

These findings contrast with the results of Leach (58) who showed significant post-treatment improvement in the cervical lordosis, in the magnitude of 2–5°. Because Leach's study did not evaluate the reliability and examiner measurement error of his analysis, these results can be questioned.

Giesen et al. (59) evaluated radiographic findings in children with hyperactivity disorder as part of a small scale time-series study in seven patients. A moderate level of correlation was found between pretreatment radiographic findings and baseline skin conductance levels. In four of the seven subjects, the number of positive x-ray findings reduced after specific adjustive treatment.

A case report has been presented by Thornton (60) of a 13-year-old patient with a cervical kyphosis. Three specific adjustments to the atlas subluxation was followed by a complete return of the normal cervical lordosis.

Harrison et al. (61), in a preliminary study of adult patients, evaluated the efficacy of cervical extension-compression traction in the restoration of the cervical lordosis. Treatment was approximately 3 to 4 months. Their pilot study demonstrated a positive effect of this treatment on the lordosis. The addition of supine-positioned diversified spinal manipulation including lateral flexion and rotational forces combined with prone drop-table adjustments, did not enhance the effect demonstrated with extension-compression traction treatment alone. The results of this study should provide the impetus for a large-scale, controlled clinical trial. Research should also focus on the type and duration of treatment that is most effective in restoring the cervical lordosis. Comparison clinical trials of different techniques should be a high priority for the chiropractic profession.

Coronal Plane Spinal Posture. Grostic and DeBoer (62), using a retrospective design, compared atlas laterality ($\pm\theta Z$) after specific adjustments. The data, from a sample of 523 case files, tended to show a reduction is this type of displacement after chiropractic care. Plaugher et al. (56) detected no changes in the posture of the shoulder girdle (42 patients) or scoliosis magnitude (18 patients) in their retrospective consecutive case analysis. These patients were primarily adults with scoliosis. Each patient received an average of eight adjustments between examinations. Although there are several case studies describing the role of chiropractic care in the patient with scoliosis (see Chapter 14), more formal prospective trials are needed to adequately address the plethora of issues facing the attending clinician, especially in the case of mild (i.e., <20°) curvatures.

Transverse Plane Posture. Grostic and DeBoer (62), in a retrospective study of case files, found that Y-axis rotational subluxation of the atlas reduced after specific adjustments.

Leg Length Inequality. In the pediatric patient, the clinical assessment of leg length is irrelevant for a newborn, someone who is nonambulatory, or in an active toddler who never stops moving. Most of the clinical application of leg length inequality evaluation pertains to the juvenile or adolescent.

Should leg length inequality be detected below the level of palpatory findings of injury, then radiographic assessment of the more caudad areas is often indicated (15). This is due to the fact that pelvic unleveling can cause compensational changes (i.e., scoliosis) in the spine above. Plain film usage must always answer the question of whether the information obtained is to be of clinical benefit. The findings from the radiographic examination are likely to alter the therapeutic course by providing alignment information.

The issue of whether the leg lengths should be equal at a certain stage in a child's life, considering the fact that leg length growth may be far from even, deserves discussion. Asymmetrical growth that evens out later should be balanced with the appropriate clinical goal of avoiding asymmetrical loading on the endplates during skeletal maturation, resulting in slight wedging of the vertebrae (i.e., Heuter-Volkmann Law) (34). If orthotic inserts are prescribed, then follow-up low-exposure radiographic investigation with the appliances worn needs to be performed to assess periodic and final leg length. All appliances, from heel lifts to orthotic inserts must be continually posturally evaluated (iliac crest height) at each chiropractic visit during a child's growth (63). An appliance, if incorrectly applied, can cause permanent vertebral deformation through bone remodeling and asymmetrical epiphyseal plate growth (34). The high prevalence of leg length inequality in adults (64–66) should alert the clinician to the potential for this type of asymmetry in children.

Primum Non Nocere

After trauma, the need to be specific is even more crucial when an adjustment is administered because of the patient's acute pain. Sometimes patients, with minimal history of trauma (e.g., uncomfortable sleeping position), will present with a painful alteration of movement or posture (67). Most practitioners with experience find that patients such as these as well as individuals with severe disc injury can be managed chiropractically, where indicated. The subject of adjusting patients with acute spinal fractures and dislocations is also discussed in this text (see Chapter 19). The chiropractor needs to impart the same importance of radiographic findings in the acute patient, as in the case of the chronic or asymptomatic individual undergoing chiropractic care. Having thorough examination procedures is the best method for minimizing misdiagnosis and therefore the misapplication of technique/care.

Disorders such as neoplasm, fracture, or severe anomaly (e.g., agenesis of the dens, occipitalization, etc.) can be readily detected radiographically. Their identification could potentially avert a serious complication should an adjustment be applied with too much force, in an inappropriate direction, or at a contraindicated segmental level. Spinal abnormalities occur in significant number in referral practices (68).

Reasonable caution must be exercised when using specific contact, high-velocity low-amplitude adjustments (55). Greater practitioner attention needs to be given to the potential for causing injury if forces are inappropriately applied to a spine. A treatment considered of such putative benefit cannot be considered with the same rationale as having no potential for harm, no matter what the applied technique. It is the authors' opinion that directing one's attention to biomechanical parameters, derived from plain film radiographs, when applying a biomechanical treatment such as an adjustment, will likely result in the most favorable outcome for the patient and the least chance for further injury (15).

No discussion of "above all do no harm" can be made without mentioning the risks of ionizing radiation. Here the doctor has the responsibility to ensure that the risk is made as low as reasonably possible by using x-rays judiciously, with the greatest attention to decreasing exposure through high speed (e.g., 1200 RSV) systems, shielding, filtration, and the minimizing of retake examinations.

Nature of X-ray Examination

When radiographing any patient, especially a young child, certain clinical questions must be answered before the exposure. "Will the information obtained be of clinical benefit? Is this benefit greater than the risk of the future effects of ionizing radiation?" and "Will the information gained change the treatment plan?" These questions can only be answered by the treating doctor of chiropractic, on a case by case basis, with the necessary clinical documentation demonstrating the need for such exposure (69).

The U.S. Bureau of Radiological Health emphasizes the importance of clinical judgment in selecting radiographic procedures. The Bureau also recognizes the right of the attending doctor to make benefit vs. risk determinations in selecting radiographic procedures. A Bureau publication states, in part: In almost every medical situation, when the physician feels there is reasonable expectation of obtaining useful information from roentgenological examination that would affect the care of the individual, potential radiation hazard is not a primary consideration.

The physician should retain complete freedom of judgment in the selection of roentgenologic procedures, and (the physician) should conform to good technical practices (1).

In selecting any type of examination, a given procedure should be considered "necessary" under the following circumstances:

1. The outcome of the test will be used in determining the nature of the treatment administered.
2. The test itself is reliable.
3. More cost effective procedures that are equally reliable or more reliable are not available.

Indications

For examination of the skeleton, there is no modality to match the time and cost effectiveness of the plain film radiograph (70,71). Plain film studies remain the primary diagnostic evaluation (6,7) and should direct the doctor's approach to further diagnostic testing.

A past or present history of trauma (72), including a difficult birth, is the most frequent indication for skeletal radiographic evaluation (73). In addition, congenital, neoplastic, and infectious conditions may warrant radiographic studies. The authors propose the following indications for pediatric radiologic examination, acknowledging the fact that any examination or treatment should only be directed at the discretion of the attending doctor who will need to address the individual clinical scenario and the patient risks and benefits associated with any examination or treatment proposed:

1. History of trauma with clinical signs suggestive of fracture, dislocation, or subluxation

2. Clinical suspicion of infection or neoplasm

3. Clinical evidence of a congenital or developmental anomaly (e.g., Down's syndrome), which could alter the nature of the chiropractic care rendered, or which may itself require treatment

4. When clinical findings are equivocal, and the suspected condition can be detected or ruled out by plain film radiography

5. When other examination procedures do not disclose the complete nature of the condition, and the patient is not responding favorably to care

6. To characterize the biomechanical component of the vertebral subluxation complex when such characterization would likely alter the chiropractic care (i.e., the directions and locations of adjustive intervention) and less hazardous or more accurate alternative examinations are not available

7. To evaluate patient response to chiropractic care when such evaluation would likely alter the nature of the care being rendered, and less hazardous or more accurate alternative examinations are not available

Contraindications

All clinical examination results are reviewed by the attending chiropractor. The doctor responsible for the care of the patient must then make a judgment based on the patient's clinical needs. Contraindications for plain film examination include instances when no possible change in the doctor's treatment procedures can be anticipated from the results of the examination. The age of the patient, as well as the doctor's ability to image the spine appropriately (i.e., positioning difficulties) will vary substantially from patient to patient, stressing the need for astute clinical judgment in deciding whether a radiograph is needed, and if so, what views are most important and have the most favorable diagnostic yield with as little risk imparted to the patient.

For patients in whom x-ray exposure would be very harmful (e.g., leukemia), radiography is usually not the initial imaging modality of choice. Axiomatic contraindications for x-ray examination include for financial gain or as a habitual practice with no regard for the clinical circumstances of the patient (23).

Comparative Examination Indications

Rowe et al. (12) have outlined ten indications for comparative plain film radiographic examination. Some indications are necessarily more applicable to different pediatric populations (e.g., adolescent vs. neonate). Indications for comparative examination are listed:

1. When clinical evaluation procedures (e.g., pain questionnaires, motion palpation findings, instrumentation findings) do not correlate with the information from the most recent radiographic examination.

2. If the patient was initially x-rayed in an acute or antalgic position, since changes in tonicity of the paraspinal musculature would alter the postural configuration of the spinal column.

3. If the patient's clinical symptomatology does not improve within a 4- to 6-week period. There may be instances in which comparative radiographs would be required before these time periods. The major determining factor would be if physical findings do not correlate with the initial radiographs. A second chiropractic opinion is often helpful, if the attending physician is contemplating a comparative examination.

4. If there has been the introduction of a foot orthotic (e.g., heel lift) and the physician needs to determine the postural adaptation to the device.

5. There is an alteration in the orthopedic or neurologic findings unexplainable without a radiograph. In many instances, additional diagnostic tests, such as electronic thermography or electromyography, may be more appropriate for gaining the necessary information critical to case management.

6. There has been a traumatic insult since the initial radiograph.

7. To monitor a potentially progressive scoliosis.

8. To follow a pathological process such as degenerative joint disease, fracture healing, or post-traumatic ligamentous rupture, laxity or creep.

9. If initial radiographs were not performed in an upright weight-bearing position or with the patient improperly positioned.

10. To monitor response to treatment in terms of biomechanical parameters if the information derived from the radiograph is likely to alter case management.

Comparative Examination Contraindications

Rowe et al. (12) have also proposed four situations in which comparative radiologic examination is contraindicated.

1. When there is any possibility of pregnancy (unless not performing the procedure would place the mother at risk)

2. In the absence of objective clinical findings indicating the need for comparative examination

3. When no possible change in treatment procedures would be anticipated from the examination

4. When appropriate filtration, shielding, and high speed screen/film (e.g., 1200 RSV) are not being used

Ionizing Radiation

Unfortunately, the various sorts of useful information derived from radiographs must be weighed against the harmful effects of ionizing radiation. There are potential negative biological effects of human exposure to ionizing radiation. Exposure effects are cumulative. The use of ionizing radiation in examining any patient, including children and adolescents, should be based on clinical need.

Growing concern for the hazards of ionizing radiation and the availability of alternative imaging techniques may cause our reliance on plain film to change. The best course to take is to minimize exposure by using the latest technology for patient protection. According to a recent National Research Council report, low doses of x-radiation pose a human cancer risk three to four times higher than previously reported. The report also noted that some fetuses exposed to radiation face a higher than expected risk of mental retardation (74). Radiation protection is particularly important when x-raying infants, children, adolescents, and adults in their reproductive years. The effects of radiation in individuals with high rates of cellular division (i.e., children) are greater. The physician should always adhere to the principle of "as high as reasonably achievable" with regard to diagnostic yield, and "as low as reasonably achievable," with regard to radiation exposure. Retake examinations should be minimized.

HOW MUCH RADIATION?

With modern technology, the amount of radiation that patients receive has been substantially reduced (75–77). Some sacrifice in film quality might be observed with the very high speed systems currently available (e.g., 1200 RSV) (78). This potential reduction in the clinical utility of high speed systems, however, has not been subjected to scientific verification. A 400–800 screen/film speed (79) coupled with a high frequency generator, high kilovoltage factors, shielding over the breasts, gonads, and eyes, and Niobi-X filtration (12), produces dosages that are much less than technology could provide only a decade ago.

A report by Kalmar et al. (80) states that using higher kilovoltage, 1200 high-speed screen systems, leaded compensation filters and shielding of sensitive structures, demonstrated an immediate dose reduction of approximately 75%, continuing to 95% before image quality became unreliable. They concluded that using readily available radiation reduction equipment, satisfactory image quality can still be obtained.

One Rad is equivalent to 1000 mRad. An AP full spine x-ray exposed at 88 inches (224 cm) with a 1200 speed system for an averaged size adult (77 kg) results in approximately 65 mRAD of exposure (81). It is not known how harmful this quantity of radiation is to adults or children because no long-term studies currently exist.

GENETIC EFFECTS

Radiation-induced genetic effects have not been observed to date in humans. The largest source of material for genetic studies involves the survivors of Hiroshima and Nagasaki, but the 77,000 births that occurred among the survivors showed no evidence of genetic effects (82).

PREGNANCY

There is evidence that 1000 mRad of exposure to a fetus in the first trimester of gestation will result in an increase in the prevalence of carcinoma by 0.6 deaths per 1000 (82). The occurrence of cancer death from natural causes is approximately 1.4 per 1000. From 1000 mRAD of exposure during pregnancy, the occurrence of mental retardation and small head size increases. A pregnant female should usually not be exposed to radiation unless the trunk and pelvis can be adequately shielded, or if not performing the examination would jeopardize the health of the mother (12, 83).

CANCER

Little information exists on the effects of radiation from diagnostic x-rays on the incidence of cancer in the general population. Evans et al. (84) determined that radiation-induced leukemia represented approximately 1% of all cases. Less than 1% of all cases of breast cancer are due to the effects of diagnostic radiography (85). Evans et al. (84) concluded that x-rays for diagnostic purposes have only a small influence on the occurrence of leukemia and breast cancer.

Thyroid neoplasms can result from exposure to high levels of diagnostic x-rays. Pillay et al. (86) report on two patients who received between 90 and 525 rads of total exposure after an initial diagnosis of congestive cardiac failure at age three. Radiographic procedures also included catheterization. Both children were diagnosed with thyroid cancer at age 14.

Chromosomal abnormalities associated with ionizing radiation have been reported, but usually involve frequent repetition or extremely high radiation levels not typically encountered in diagnostic radiography (12, 87–89).

RISK ASSESSMENT

The scientific controversy surrounding the determination of the magnitude of the health risk from low level radiation should not divert public attention from the fact that even conservative estimates place risks from radiation well within the range of risks from other perils that are considered acceptable. One approach to risk education is through the presentation of quantified risk estimates, such as one in a million chance of dying or a decrease in life expectancy as a result of exposure to a variety of hazards. The carcinogenic risk of radiation exposure is 100–200 deaths per million people exposed per Rad per year. The exposure to a typical patient should be far less than 1 Rad (see How Much Radiation?) (90, 91).

There is no conclusive evidence to show any shortening of the life span even in radiologists who are exposed to much more radiation than would be received by a patient, as the result of diagnostic use of roentgen rays (92).

The use of ultra-high speed cassette/film and longwave length filters will likely reduce the risks associated with ionizing radiation exposure further. But as with most controversial areas in health care, much research will be needed before more accurate assessments of risks and benefits can be made for low levels of diagnostic radiation.

GENERAL CONSIDERATIONS

Several inherent pitfalls are involved in imaging pediatric spines. Patient motion is an ever present problem. Even when short exposure times are used to limit the effects of motion on the finished radiograph, a true postural study may be difficult to obtain. Immobilization of an uncooperative patient can yield a film that is useful diagnostically, but may not accurately depict postural pathomechanics. If an unclear or improperly exposed film is likely to result from a particular examination (i.e., due to patient positioning difficulties), then that view should be omitted rather than exposing the child to unnecessary radiation. Radiographic procedures for children and adults should include every safety precaution to ensure the lowest possible exposure to ionizing radiation. Biological effects from exposure to ionizing radiation are both tissue and dosage dependent. The breast, eyes, and gonads are extremely sensitive to radiation and can be selectively shielded for many radiographic examinations. Taking appropriate safety measures (i.e., shielding), including the use of long film focal distances can significantly reduce the entrance skin exposure to the patient (93). The information that follows should be used as a summary guide for clinicians and technologists who perform x-ray examination so that the appropriate technical precautions are taken to minimize radiation exposure.

All doctors need to determine their clinical and diagnostic needs and then maximize the available equipment to minimize the radiation exposure to both the patient and the technician. As with any piece of equipment, regular calibration checks of the generator by an x-ray physicist is recommended (94). During this check, re-alignment of the central ray to the cassette will minimize abnormal projection magnification.

Potential trade-offs should be considered when attempting changes in radiographic technique. Two representative examples are presented:

1. Decreased exposure times are attainable with an increased processor chemistry temperature. However, the chemistry will oxidize more rapidly at higher temperatures and will require greater maintenance for consistent films.

2. The KVP can be increased resulting in a greater proportion of high energy photons and less exposure time (resulting in a lower entrance skin dose). The high KVP technique will then result in graying (loss of contrast) of the image, which can decrease diagnostic quality (94–96).

FILM-SCREEN SPEEDS

Although an 800–1200 film screen speed combination suffices for most radiologic assessments, especially in the case of a pediatric patient, there are situations when the need for detail may outweigh the benefit of reduced patient exposure (12). This can occur when there is a potential spinal or extremity fracture in which the use of lower speed screens may be more appropriate for issue of high detail. A careful history and physical examination will dictate which screen/film speed is most appropriate. The chiropractor can more effectively care for the individual patient by matching the appropriate system to the specific clinical presentation by having available one high speed system of 800–1200 for spinography, and one slower speed system, of 200–400, for more detailed evaluations (12).

Presently the fastest screen/cassette/film on the market was introduced by Kodak as a 1200 speed system comprising Lanex Fast screen with Kodak PDH-1 film. It substantially decreases radiation exposure while producing a diagnostic quality image.

In the darkroom, some of the high speed films (e.g., 1200) are very sensitive to many light spectrums. The technologist should adhere to the recommended safety light provided by the manufacturer of the film. One can test a sheet of unexposed film by holding it up in the safety light. If the film develops clear, then the safety light spectrum is within the tolerance of the film.

Although not yet in widespread use, cassette intensifying screens with a 1200 screen-film combination speed are recommended for spinographic evaluation of pediatric patients to reduce entrance skin exposure (ESE). Comparative radiographs and x-rays used to assess spinal motion should also have a minimum 1200 screen/film speed.

FILM SIZES

Depending on the child's size, a smaller film size can be substituted for the standard 14 × 36 in., for full spine radiographs. The technician should measure from the occiput to the lower sacrum to include all sacral segments. Allowing for slight magnification of the image, if the measurement is less than 17 inches, then a 14 × 17 in. film size can be used. Strict collimation should be used, excluding the skull and femurs from exposure.

For sectional radiography or bending films, the smaller film sizes (e.g., 8 × 10, 10 × 12, or 14 × 17) are more appropriate.

If the entire spine needs to be imaged, then full spine views are preferable to sectional studies due to the necessary overlap and double exposure in two regions of the spine (12). Comparative dosimetric evaluations between full spine and sectional radiography have shown lower exposure levels with full spine (97). Phillips (98) has reported on the comparative diagnostic utility of full spine versus sectional radiographs. In a survey of Diplomates of the American Chiropractic Board of Radiology, it was judged that although adult full spine x-rays are inferior in the quality of diagnostic detail compared with sectionals, the diagnostic information/yield obtained from both procedures was essentially the same.

POSITIONING

X-ray positioning demands can be challenging for a child. They may need to hold a stance or opposition that might be painful. Thoroughness during positioning is essential for radiographs obtained for the purpose of imaging spinal biomechanics. Positioning instructions should be carefully explained to the child and adapted so that the child can reduce motion artifacts and the need for unnecessary repeat radiographs. If a child cannot stand still (e.g., cerebral palsy patient or infant), parental assistance may be necessary. Lead shielding (e.g., apron, gloves) can be provided to the assisting parent. The assistance of an outside radiological facility may be necessary in some unusual circumstances.

COLLIMATION

The smallest possible collimation of the x-ray beam is preferred during the exposure. In addition to protecting the patient and the technician from excessive dosage, collimation also increases the quality of the radiograph by reducing the amount of scatter radiation thus improving contrast and detail. Ideally the exposed radiograph should have two edges that reveal the collimator (99). It is not appropriate for the entire skull and three-fourths of the femurs as well as the lateral aspects of the trunk and arms to be exposed in a full spine radiograph.

SHIELDING

Shielding for the reproductive organs, thyroid gland, and bone marrow protection should be provided (100–102). Because children undergo more rapid cellular division than adults, they are more susceptible to the mutagenic effects of ionizing radiation. Also, cellular compaction in most glands is greater than in the adult, causing a potentially greater proportion of risk per square inch of surface area exposed to ionizing radiation. Lead contact shields can be placed directly on the patient, especially in front of the eyes and gonads.

Breast tissue is very sensitive to radiation and must be shielded from the x-ray beam. This can be accomplished through collimator mounted or contact shielding (12) without compromise to spinal and pelvic evaluations.

The thyroid gland should be shielded whenever possible due to its high radiosensitivity (86). Systems that offer partial shielding of this gland are currently available (102) (Fig. 8.1A,B).

GRIDS

Grids reduce the amount of secondary exposure and improve the film quality. They are coordinated with the x-ray unit, depending on the highest KVP usually used. Because a high kilovoltage technique (e.g., 100–110 KVP) is recommended for most spinal column assessments due to the decreased entrance skin dose, a higher grid ratio of 10:1 to 12:1 is preferred (12, 103).

Grids minimize scatter radiation by allowing most useful electrons to pass through perpendicular to the cassette, thereby

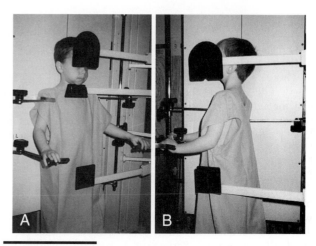

Figure 8.1. Bolin x-ray shielding.

increasing film clarity. Most grids are rated by the ratio of the depth of the grids to the width and the number of lines per inch.

GRID FOCUS

A problem seen in some clinics can be the lack of coordination between the radiographic grid focus distance and tube distance. This distance should be known and strictly adhered to for optimum radiographs. It is the doctor's responsibility to check this equipment requirement. Some technicians may not be aware of this important consideration during the initial equipment set-up, especially if unusual (but appropriate) distances are used during radiography (i.e., > 84 inches for full spines) (90).

FILTRATION

Prepatient filtration is integral to producing good quality radiographs. Due to variances in size and density of various regions of the spine and pelvis, prepatient filtration can modulate the x-ray beam, thereby creating more uniform penetration. This is especially important when full spine evaluations are being made.

Prepatient filtration systems that accommodate for tissue density and thickness have been used in the chiropractic profession and have improved diagnostic quality while at the same time reducing ESE (104). Because no shielding contacts the patient, this filtration is hygienically positive. Additionally, the radiation is attenuated at the collimator. When properly used, pre-patient filtration focuses on the body part of study and selectively minimizes radiation exposure.

BUCKY STAND SHIELDING

Bucky stand shielding is another quality barrier for scatter radiation reduction. Lead sheeting placed behind the bucky as close as possible to the cassette will minimize post-entry rebound scatter radiation. This is a relatively inexpensive safeguard.

LONG WAVELENGTH FILTRATION

Long wavelength filtration such as Niobi-X is currently available (12). The element niobium is used to reduce the low energy, long wavelength radiation. At short film focal distances (FFD), this type of filtration can substantially reduce exposure.

In the clinical arena, Niobi-X radiation filters significantly reduce the ESE. Field testing using the Kodak Lanex/PDH-1 film with the Niobi-X filter revealed an approximate 50% reduction of millirems (mR) compared with exposure without the Niobi-X filter. This Lanex/PDH-1 film with the NIOBI-X filtration combination equates to an approximately 90% reduction of mR in the AP cervical spine study with a patient who has 10 cm body part thickness when compared with the average of the Nationwide Evaluation of X-ray Trends tabulated by the Bureau of Radiological Health Jan 1, 1981 to December 31, 1981 (80, 105, 106).

FILM FOCAL DISTANCE

The shorter the film focal distance, the more magnification of the patient on the radiograph. Shorter FFDs also result in more marked apparent distortions of patients when they have been improperly positioned for the exposure. As the distance between the tube and patient is increased, there is less angulation, or angle of inclination, between the focal spot and the object (12). A longer FFD also results in less patient exposure and is therefore recommended (107).

HIGH FREQUENCY GENERATORS

Ultra high frequency generators decrease exposure time, and lower overall patient dose, as well as increase technical accuracy and consistency of imaging. These generators produce a higher quality image with greater image contrast detail (12, 108).

AUTOMATIC TIMERS

Automatic exposure timers have experienced a recent resurgence in popularity due to increased electronic technology. Each cassette houses a sensor that detects the pre-set radiation exposure required for an optimum exposure. Once the pre-set radiation has been sensed, a signal is sent back to the radiographic controller, which is attached to the generator and the exposure is stopped. The timer allows an optimum KVP and MA setting for body density and thickness, and the time is automatically stopped by the sensor. This equipment is most helpful for doctors who are meticulous about patient placement. The sensor must be located behind the object desired. Any deviation of the desired body part from the sensor will result in a substandard radiograph (94).

SPLIT SCREENS

Non-homogeneous speed intensifying screens (i.e., split screens) for full spine radiographs can also compensate for regional variation in size, but result in more radiation exposure to the patient. Their use is outdated due to the advances made in prepatient filtration (12). It is recommended that doctors currently using this technology switch to homogenous high speed screen/film systems (e.g., 1200 speed).

PROCESSING

Film processing chemistry must be carefully maintained. A properly performing circulation pump will keep the chemicals at the same concentration throughout the tank.

PATIENT POSITIONING AND EQUIPMENT ALIGNMENT

The x-ray beam must be perpendicular to the bucky and the patient. If the beam is not centralized, this will result in postural distortion of the area under examination. In addition, measurements of the pelvis, including the femoral heads are affected from this offcentering. The pelvis is especially susceptible to rotational (y axis) malpositioning (109). A foot positioning grid should be used to reliably position the patient on a level surface (110, 111) (Fig. 8.2).

The patient should always be positioned in the upright posture whenever possible. Recumbence tends to lessen the effects of gravity on the spine, minimizing displacements of the motion segments (12, 112, 113).

For the toddler through adolescent, the patient's heels are placed parallel to the bucky at one of three grid lines. The heels should be kept equidistant from the midline of the foot positioning grid and approximately four to eight inches apart. The patient should be instructed to maintain their natural foot flare and to keep the knees in a locked position. A potential problem with foot placement markers is the tendency for patients to stand with their feet to match the marks thus altering natural foot flare.

Immobilization straps attached to the bucky are available for stabilizing those patients who have tremor or sway while standing. These straps should be used only to stabilize and not to distort the patient's normal gravitational standing posture.

When attempting x-ray examination of the pediatric patient, the doctor should explain carefully the procedures that are being performed. More time is needed for these examinations, especially in the case of the infant or toddler. An informed and cooperative child will minimize the potential for re-take examinations.

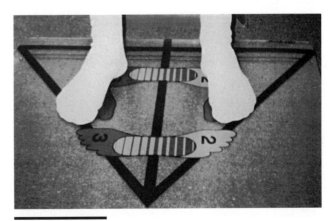

Figure 8.2.   Foot positioning grid.

Normal Developmental Anatomy of the Spine

Accurate interpretation of pediatric radiographs is dependent on an understanding of the appearance of ossification centers at various stages of development and a thorough knowledge of normal radiographic anatomy. Many normal findings can mimic injury and lead to an incorrect diagnosis (114, 115).

The earliest evidence of the developing axial skeleton is the notochord. Along each side of the notochord are paired somites composed of mesodermal tissue. The anteromedial aspect of each somite is termed the sclerotome. Each sclerotome can further be subdivided into a cephalad portion and a caudad portion. The upper portion of one sclerotome and the lower portion of another give rise to the vertebral body.

The central portion of each sclerotome gives rise to an intervertebral disc. The residual notochord forms the nucleus pulposus of the disc.

At puberty, five secondary ossification centers appear in a typical vertebra. There is one at the tip of each transverse process, one on the superior and inferior aspects of the vertebral body, and one at the tip of the spinous process.

In cervical vertebrae where bifid spinous processes occur, there are two separate ossification centers at the distal aspect of each spinous process. The atlas, axis, and C7 are atypical cervical vertebrae, and follow different patterns. The atlas usually has three ossification centers. There is one ossification center for each lateral mass present in fetal life, and a third center in the anterior arch, which appears at about 1 year of age. The axis develops from five primary and two secondary ossification centers. This configuration is to permit development of the dens, which is thought to be the "lost" vertebral body of the atlas. The primary centers include two in the neural arch, one in the vertebral body, and two in the dens. The first of the two secondary centers occurs at the base of the dens, and corresponds to the "would be" intervertebral disc. The other secondary center is on the inferior aspect of the vertebral body. C7 has two separate ossification centers in the costal processes, which if they fail to unite may result in the development of cervical ribs (116, 117). Each lumbar vertebra has two additional secondary ossification centers for the mamillary processes.

The sacrum develops from five segments, which normally fuse into a single mass by the 25th year. The coccyx is formed from four centers (118).

Congenital Variants

NON-SEGMENTATION

A lack of segmentation of the primitive sclerotome results in a "block vertebra" (Figs. 8.3–8.5). In the cervical spine, this occurs most frequently at the C5/C6 and C2/C3 levels. Non-segmented vertebrae appear structurally as one, and function as one. Failure of the non-segmented vertebrae to contribute to the composite motion of the region affected may lead to hypermobility and degenerative changes at other segmental levels, often above the site of non-segmentation.

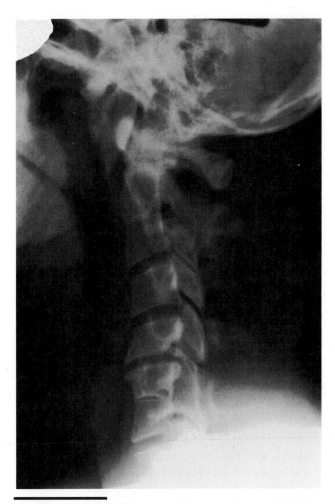

Figure 8.3.   Non-segmentation (block vertebrae) of C2-C3 and C6-C7.

When non-segmentation occurs at the occipital-atlantal articulation, the term "occipitalization" is applied (Fig. 8.6). Although non-segmentation by itself rarely produces neurologic compromise, brain stem or cord compression have been reported in cases of upper cervical fusion (119–121).

MacGibbon and Farfan (122) studied various common anatomical variants demonstrable on plain films of the lumbar spine. Six hundred forty-two subjects were studied. The investigators reported that two main types of anatomic spinal variations are identified in the majority of individuals. The presence of L4–L5 injury and degeneration is likely to be associated with the following anatomical factors:

1. A high intercrestal line passing through the upper half of L4

2. Long transverse process on L5

3. Rudimentary rib

4. Transitional vertebra (Fig. 8.7)

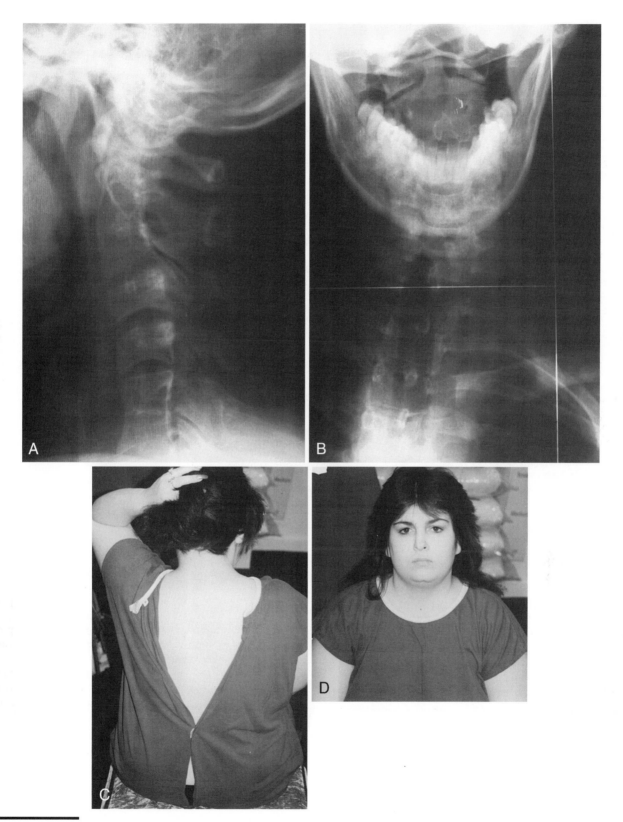

Figure 8.4.   A, Non-segmentation of C2-C3 and C6-C7. B, AP view of patient in Figure 8.4A. Notice the lack of coronal plane symmetry of the block vertebrae. C, Posterior view of patient in Figure 8.4A and B. Notice the short neck. D, Anterior view of patient in Figure 8.4A-C. A moderate head tilt is evident.

L5–S1 degeneration was associated with the following:

1. An intercrestal line passing through the body of L5
2. Short transverse processes on L5
3. No rudimentary rib
4. No transitional vertebra

DOWN'S SYNDROME

Other variations may also occur in the upper cervical spine. In children, the atlanto–dental interspace should not exceed 5 mm (1). An increase may be due to congenital absence of the transverse ligament as seen in Down's syndrome. Although previously considered of little clinical significance, increased participation by such children in athletic activity (e.g., special Olympics) requires careful assessment of the upper cervical spine. Radiologic studies, including flexion/extension views, are advocated for such children at about 2 1/2 to 3 years of age to assess possible atlantoaxial subluxation (123–126). Juvenile rheumatoid arthritis or traumatic rupture of the transverse ligament may also result in an increased atlanto–dental interspace (127,128).

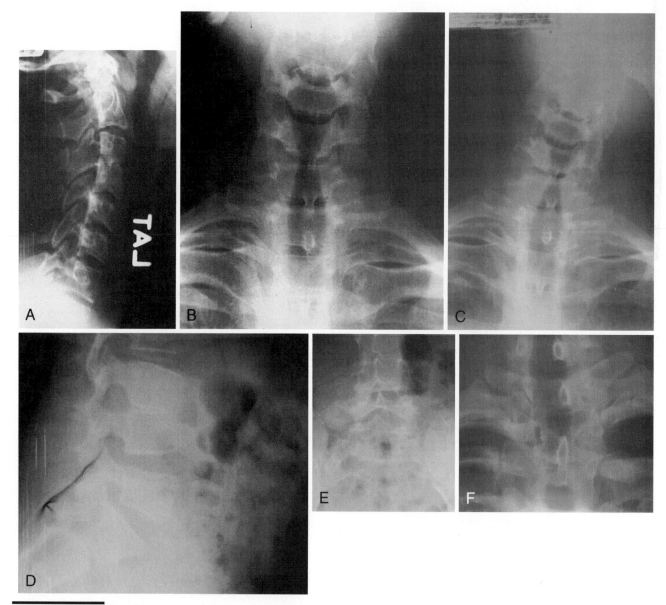

Figure 8.5. A, Lateral view of congenital block vertebrae of C3-C4. B, AP view of patient in Figure 8.5A. There is a wedge malformation at the C3-C4 level leading to cervical scoliosis and head tilt. C, Right lateral bending radiograph of the patient de-picted in Figure 8.5A-B. The wedge shape of C3-C4 is more no-ticeable in this radiograph. D, Lateral view of non-segmenta-tion of L3-L4. E, AP view of non-segmentation of L3-L4. F, AP view of non-segmentation at T2-T3.

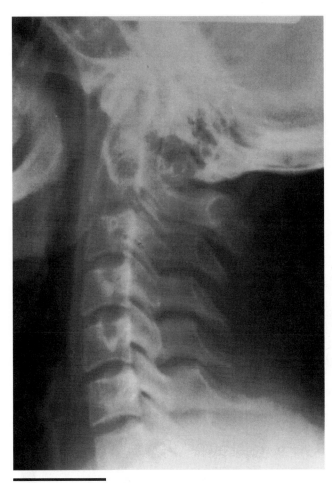

Figure 8.6.   Occipitalization.

ODONTOID PROCESS VARIATIONS

Variations also occur in the development of the odontoid process. The tip of the dens develops from an ossification center, which appears at age 2 and unites at 10 to 12 years. If such union does not occur, a terminal ossicle remains. If the dens remains ununited at its base, the condition is termed os odontoideum (Fig. 8.8A–D). Instability and cord compression may result (129). Hypoplasia or congenital absence of the dens may also occur, resulting in an unstable articulation (130). Unstable os odontoideum, although rare, should be considered in the differential diagnosis of a child complaining of neck pain with decreased mobility. The diagnosis will be confirmed by stress radiographs taken in the extremes of flexion and extension (131).

KLIPPEL-FEIL SYNDROME

This condition is characterized by multiple block vertebrae of the cervical spine. The patient may present with a short neck, low hairline, and genitourinary anomalies. The condition predisposes the spine to injury and possible cord damage (132) (see Nonsegmentation).

SPRENGEL'S DEFORMITY

Congenital non-descent of the scapula can often be detected clinically. Radiographs will demonstrate an omovertebral bone in 30–40% of cases (133).

CERVICAL RIBS

Ribs may arise from a lower cervical segment (Fig. 8.9). These ribs may cause neurovascular compression (scalenus anticus syndrome) later in life, but are usually only contributing factors. In children, they are usually asymptomatic (134).

BUTTERFLY VERTEBRA

A sagittal cleft in a vertebral body may occur, usually in the thoracic or lumbar spine. Most are asymptomatic and clinically insignificant (135).

HEMIVERTEBRA

Failure of the lateral half of a vertebral body to develop produces a lateral hemivertebra. The inevitable consequence is a scoliosis. Rarely, a dorsal or ventral hemivertebra oc-

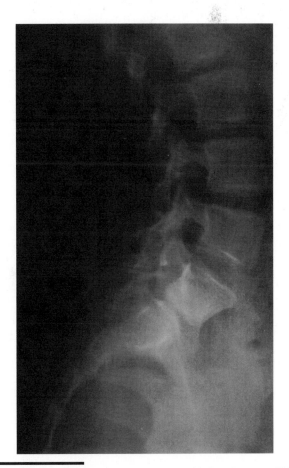

Figure 8.7.   Transitional segment of L5-S1. Sacralization of L5 in a 6-year-old female.

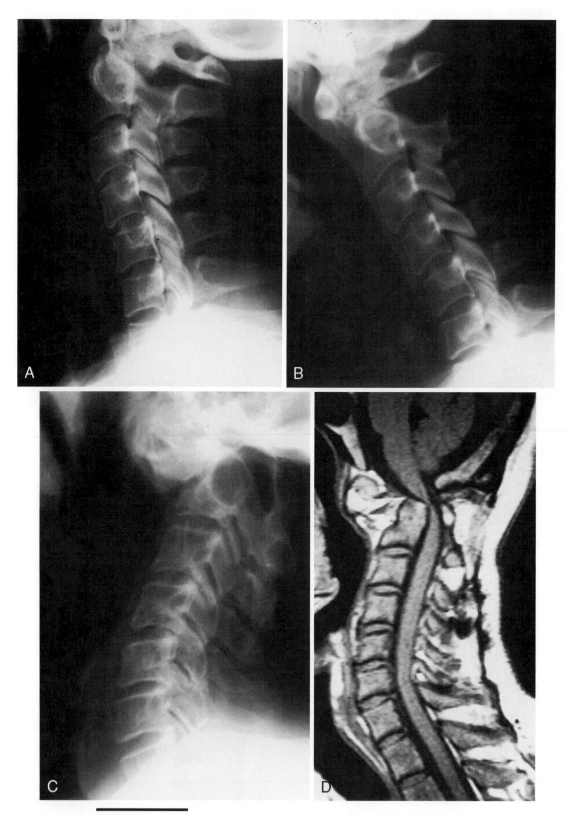

Figure 8.8.   A, Neutral lateral radiograph of os odontoideum. B, Flexion view of os odontoideum. Compare the spinolaminar line to that in Figure 8.8A. C, Os odontoideum. D, MRI of patient in C.

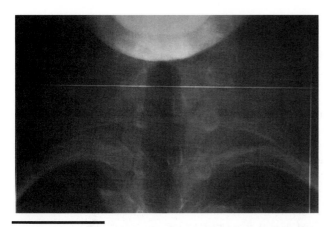

Figure 8.9.   Cervical ribs. This patient has a superior end-plate burst fracture of C7 (see Chapter 19) leading to the widening interpedicular distance at that level.

curs, which may cause an alteration of lordotic and kyphotic curves (136).

SPINA BIFIDA OCCULTA

Spina bifida occulta is a failure of fusion of the posterior elements of a spinal segment without meningeal protrusion. It is often seen at the L5–S1 levels and is usually of little clinical significance (Fig. 8.10A–E). It does not increase susceptibility to athletic injury (124). Spina bifida is a serious condition in which there is protrusion of the spinal membranes, with or without cord tissue, through absent posterior vertebral arches.

FACET TROPISM

Asymmetry of the facets at the L5/S1 level may produce asymmetrical biomechanics and joint dysfunction (137) (Fig. 8.11). Their identification provides a more complete analysis for the purposes of motion palpation or motion x-ray interpretation.

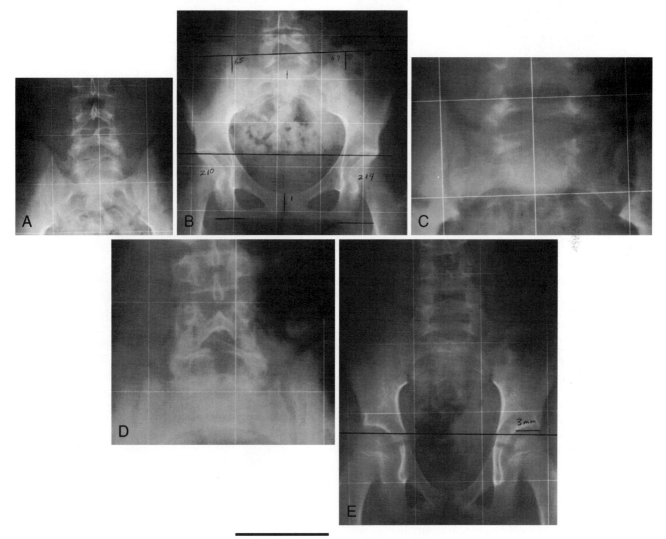

Figure 8.10.   A-E, Spina bifida occulta.

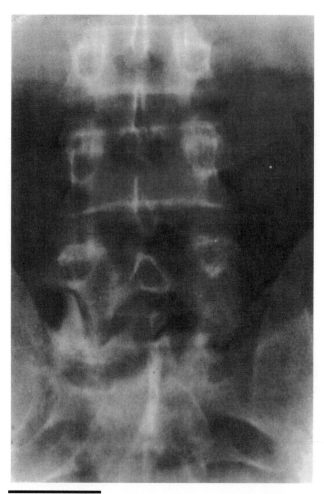

Figure 8.11.   Facet tropism at L5-S1.

SLIPPED CAPITAL FEMORAL EPIPHYSIS

This condition is usually seen in children older than 10 years. It may be associated with a specific traumatic episode or may appear gradually. A limp with hip pain is the characteristic clinical presentation. Males are more commonly affected than females. Overweight children are also more likely suffer from this condition. Radiologically, a widening of the growth plate is seen initially. An abnormal relationship between the femoral neck and femoral head may be appreciated. This condition can also cause an aseptic necrosis of the femoral head with resultant deformity. AP and frog leg views are recommended in the assessment of slipped capital femoral epiphysis (1).

Post Natal Abnormalities

"PSEUDO" SUBLUXATION

The concept of a "pseudo subluxation" has been presented by many different authors throughout the years. The differentiating factor in pseudo subluxation vs. subluxation is that in the former, the spinolaminar line is preserved and not in the latter. Physicians and radiologists learned early on, the problems in mislabeling certain injuries that could have resulted in unnecessary surgical operations, these findings have more relevance to the practitioner using nonoperative methods (e.g., chiropractor). Some recent publications present radiographs diagnosed as pseudo subluxation. However, other biomechanical abnormalities are clearly of clinical use to chiropractors.

Since most patients are x-rayed because they have suffered a trauma to the spine or have pain, the labeling of a pseudosubluxation may be a result of poor interpretive skills (142). Labeling something as normal when a clinical scenario is present does a disservice to the patient. The

KNIFE CLASP DEFORMITY

Spina bifida occulta in association with an elongated L5 spinous process may result in painful and limited extension (138) (Fig. 8.12).

TRANSITIONAL VERTEBRAE

Lumbarization of S1 or sacralization of L5 may occur (see Nonsegmentation). Tini et al. (139) examined 4000 radiographs and concluded that persons with transitional vertebrae did not exhibit any more backaches than controls. Abnormal mechanics produced by the condition, however, may lead to premature disc degeneration at other levels (140).

CONGENITAL HIP DYSPLASIA

Deformities of the acetabulum and dislocation of the femur from an anomalous acetabulum characterize this condition. Radiologic manifestations of congenital hip dysplasia were described by Putti (141). Putti's triad consists of a small or absent proximal femoral epiphysis, lateral displacement of the femur, and increased angulation of the acetabular roof.

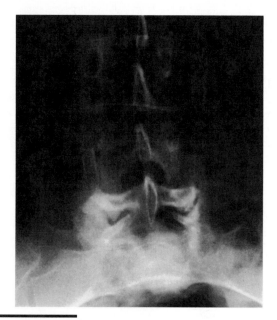

Figure 8.12.   Knife-clasp deformity.

scenario of perhaps overdiagnosing spinal biomechanical abnormalities in children stems from the observation that many asymptomatic individuals exhibit similarly minimal findings. Radiographs should always be correlated with the presenting clinical picture. A "normal" radiograph, in the presence of a symptomatic patient should not be weighed very heavily in resolving the lack of agreement between the two examinations. If the patient is asymptomatic, some of these findings may have less clinical relevance to the patient. Their potential effects on future spinal growth, deformity, or neurologic health should be carefully outlined to the patient or guardian.

SPINAL CORD INJURY WITHOUT RADIOGRAPHIC ABNORMALITY (SCIWORA)

Some patients with spinal cord injury will have "normal" or near normal radiographs. This is due to the potential lengthening of the spinal column without a commensurate increase in the elasticity of the spinal cord. In cadaver studies it was determined that the canal can stretch up to 2 inches due to the elasticity of spine ligaments. The spinal cord can only stretch about a 1/4 inch before injury or rupture occurs (143). This mismatching of elasticity accounts for, in part, neural injury seen in normal radiographic vertebral anatomy. Mechanisms for SCIWORA include simple anatomical differences as well as transient subluxation, reversible disc protrusion, vasospasm, and vascular occlusion. Dickman and Rekate (143) have provided a list of the most possible mechanisms for SCIWORA (Table 8.1).

STRUCTURAL AND FUNCTIONAL VARIATION

In addition to structural variation, functional variation in the pediatric spine warrants careful consideration by the chiropractor. Sullivan et al. (144) examined lateral cervical radiographs on 100 normal children and discovered that in 20% of cases, C2 appeared subluxated anteriorly on C3. This phenomenon is usually observed in children younger than 9 years of age, and is due to the more horizontal facet orientation in the younger child. It is particularly pronounced in flexion (145). The preservation of the spinolaminar line differentiates true subluxation from pseudo subluxation (146). Whether these "normal" findings represent early changes predisposing to subluxation degeneration has not been explored. Following subjects with these purportedly "normal" "pseudo subluxations" throughout life and comparing the incidence of degenerative changes in the spine with controls is suggested as an area for additional research.

ATLANTO-OCCIPITAL HYPERMOBILITY AND SUDDEN INFANT DEATH SYNDROME

A triple blind study of sudden infant death syndrome (SIDS) and non-SIDS infants was undertaken by Schneier and Burns (147). Analysis of radiographs of 53 infant cadavers revealed that in all cases in which the atlas inverted into the foramen magnum, SIDS was listed as the cause of death. However, not all SIDS infants exhibited atlas

Table 8.1.   Mechanisms of SCIWORA

Direct spinal cord traction
1. Longitudinal spinal cord traction
2. Root traction/avulsion

Direct spinal cord compression
1. Transient compression
    a. Ligamentous bulging
    b. Reversible disc protrusion
    c. Transient subluxation of vertebrae
2. Persistent compression
    a. Occult fracture with spinal cord compression
    b. Spinal epidural hematoma
    c. Persistent disc herniation
    d. Occult subluxation/instability

Indirect spinal cord injury
1. Transmission of externally applied kinetic energy to spinal cord (spinal cord concussion)

Vascular/ischemic injury
1. Vascular occlusion, dissection, spinal cord infarction
2. Vasospasm
3. Hypotension, impaired spinal cord perfusion

Reprinted with permission from Dickman CA, Rekate HL. Spinal trauma. In: Eichelberger MR, ed. Pediatric Trauma, St. Louis: Mosby Year Book, 1993:368.

inversion. Atlas inversion is the condition in which the atlas posterior arch is positioned within the foramen magnum (Fig. 8.13A, B). These investigators also reported that measurements made on neutral, flexion, and extension radiographs suggested that a correlation may exist between atlanto-occipital hypermobility and SIDS. Some cases of atlas inversion may represent occipital subluxation into hyperextension (i.e., -θX, antero-superior condyle) with compensatory hyperflexion at the atlanto-axial level (Fig. 8.13C).

ADJUSTING CONSIDERATIONS FOR DEVELOPMENTAL VARIANTS

Hadley (4) lists five causes of neurologic compromise in cases of cervical spine anomalies and notes that symptoms often do not appear until the second or third decade of life:

1. Constriction of the foramen with resultant pressure on nervous structures
2. Adhesions
3. Ischemia from interference with blood supply

4. Interference with the dynamics of the cerebrospinal fluid between the ventricles and subarachnoid spaces causing hydrocephalus

5. Increased pressure within the cerebellar fossa from basilar impression or invagination

Forceful adjustments, particularly those employing rotation of the head, should be avoided. This does not mean that patients with spinal anomalies should be categorically denied the potential benefits of chiropractic care. If the decision is made to apply gentle adjusting procedures, the response of the patient should be carefully monitored. If an adverse reaction occurs, an alternative procedure or no procedure at all should be considered.

The authors suggest that the chiropractor consider the following when selecting adjustment techniques for patients demonstrating nonsegmentation:

1. Nonsegmentation without neurologic compromise. A simple block vertebra in the absence of neurologic compromise does not contraindicate traditional adjusting techniques. The two nonsegmented vertebrae are considered as one unit. Pathomechanically, nonsegmentation at one vertebral level may lead to compensatory hypermobility and degeneration at other vertebral levels (4). The increase in hypermobility would usually contraindicate an adjustment at that specific spinal level; and

2. Nonsegmentation with neurologic compromise. Great care should be exercised in both evaluating and treating patients with evidence of neurologic compromise. Neurologic symptoms that appear to be related to position or motion can indicate instability. Adjustments and patient postures would be contraindicated at a neurologically unstable motion segment. Magnetic resonance imaging permits exquisite visualization of soft tissue structures and is the initial study of choice in patients presenting with neurologic symptoms.

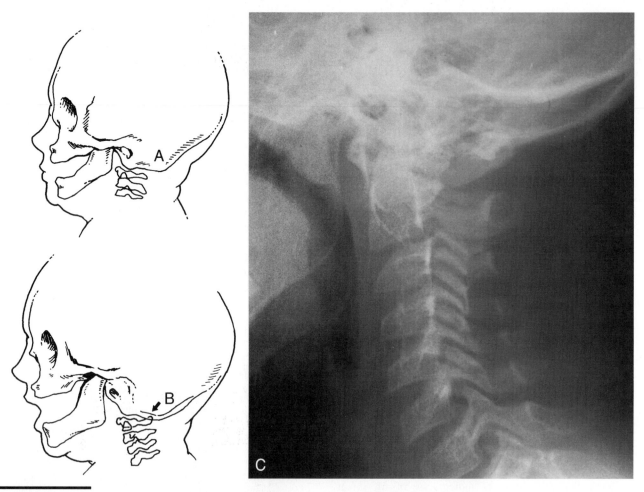

Figure 8.13. A, Normal lateral. B, Atlas inversion or -θX of the occiput on atlas (AS condyle). C, Atlas inversion or AS condyle (-θX). The "V" sign is present at the atlanto-dental inter- space indicating stretch or sprain of the superior fibers of the transverse ligament.

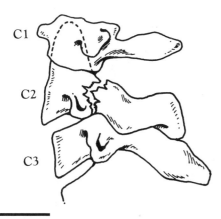

Figure 8.14.   Hangman's fracture of C2.

PEDIATRIC SPINE FRACTURES

Children younger than age 16 account for 7% or less of injuries to the spine (148, 149). Although pediatric spine injuries are relatively uncommon, their prompt recognition and proper management are essential in chiropractic practice. See Chapter 19 for further information on the management of adolescent patients with acute spinal fractures and dislocations.

Motor vehicle (including motorcycle) accidents account for more than 50% of the injuries, with team sports, diving injuries, and physical abuse accounting for most of the remainder. The most common areas of injury are the cervical spine and the thoracolumbar junction (152). In cases of spinal trauma, plain AP and lateral radiographs should be taken of the entire cervical, thoracic, and lumbar spine. This is due to the high occurrence of contiguous and non-contiguous injuries (153, 155). If an abnormality is detected on plain films, computed tomography (CT) may be useful in characterizing bony abnormalities (152, 156). In cases of neurologic involvement, magnetic resonance (MR) imaging is the technique of choice (157–159).

Denis et al. (160) reported that 50% of deaths due to pediatric spine injuries were associated with injuries to the occipito-atlanto complex. According to Henrys et al. (161), upper cervical injuries are more common in children and adolescents. The Powers ratio (162) can be used to assess such injuries on plain radiographs. This ratio is between the distances of the basion to the posterior arch of the atlas and the distance from the anterior arch of the atlas to the opisthion. Powers ratio should be equal to or less than 1 in the normal cervical spine.

UPPER CERVICAL FRACTURES

Jefferson fractures are rare in children. Two cases, ages 7 and 12 years, have been reported in the literature (153). The most frequently encountered fracture of the axis is the dens fracture (163, 164), although five cases of bilateral pedicle (hangman) fractures in children were reported by Pizzutillo et al. (165) (Fig. 8.14). Jefferson fractures are usually not neurologically unstable (166). Many have been treated with entirely conservative methods.

LOWER CERVICAL FRACTURES

Lower cervical spine fractures are seen more frequently in adolescents than young children (153). Most are associated with flexion-compression injuries in collision sports (167). Motor vehicle accidents are another important cause of these injuries (see Chapter 4).

THORACO-LUMBAR FRACTURES

A variety of fractures may present in the pediatric thoracic and lumbar spine. The most common vertebral fracture seen in children younger than 10 years of age is the compression fracture (152). The cause is a compressive flexion force. Schmorl's nodes occur from excessive compression loading (Fig. 8.15). Seatbelt injuries can result in a compressive distractive force leading to the Chance fracture (see Chapter 19). Fracture through the bone as well as soft tissue damage may result, although the ligaments are usually spared (168).

SPINE INJURY FROM PHYSICAL ABUSE

Gunshot injuries (Fig. 8.16) and child abuse (see Chapter 2) are other causes of spine fractures (160). Avulsion fractures of the spinous processes in the cervical spine and compression fractures in the thoracic and lumbar region may occur as a consequence of violent shaking (169,170).

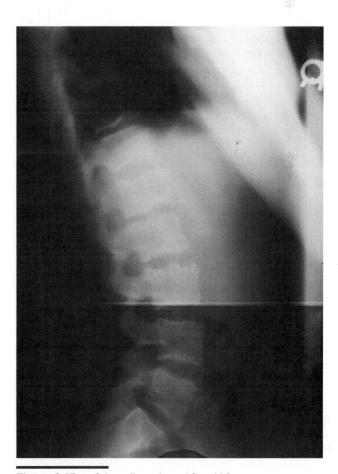

Figure 8.15.   Schmorl's nodes at L3 and L2.

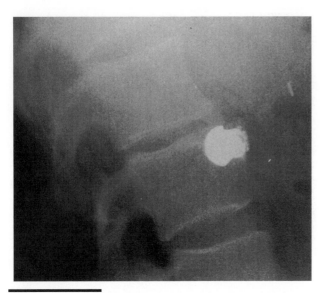

Figure 8.16. Gunshot wound at the L2 vertebra. The L2 vertebra was adjusted +Z several years post injury.

Radkowski (171) has presented seven specific points that the astute clinician should consider regarding suspected child abuse and the interpretation of plain film radiographs:

1. The radiographic manifestations of the abused or battered child combined with the clinical findings are usually so specific that there is little doubt regarding the appropriate diagnosis.

2. Most of the conditions considered in the differential diagnosis may be readily identified by a careful interpretation of the clinical history, physical, and laboratory data.

3. Children with pre-existing disease may also be abused and/or neglected.

4. Innocent trauma to bone may cause lesions that simulate battering.

5. Although the radiographic findings may be classical for abuse-related trauma, careful attention should be given to the overall bone mineralization and architecture to rule out predisposing disease.

6. A conclusion should be drawn from adequate studies. An effort should be made to resolve apparent discrepancies in radiologic findings by different imaging modalities.

7. Thorough knowledge of the medical, social, and dietary history of the child is essential in a complete evaluation of someone suspected of being abused (171).

PEDIATRIC SPINE NEOPLASMS

Spine tumors in children are relatively uncommon when compared with adults. In Western Populations, children younger than age 15 account for only 1 in 200 of all cancers (172). Because patients with signs of neurologic impairment that may or may not be due to a mechanical lesion may be brought to the attention of chiropractors, it is important to carefully differentially diagnose a mechanical lesion from a malignant cord tumor. Cancer is more common in younger children. Half the cumulative risk occurs within the first 6 years of life (172). About one-third of all childhood cancers are leukemias and of these, 80% are acute lymphoblastic leukemia. Between one quarter and one fifth of childhood cancers are brain or spinal cord tumors. Of these, one-third are astrocytomas (172).

Although it has been estimated that 80% of adults will seek professional care at some time for back pain, only 2% of children and adolescents presenting at an orthopedic clinic reported back pain (173). Others (174) have reported that the most frequent reason for a visit to a chiropractor by a child was for respiratory and ENT (e.g., otitis media) conditions. It is unknown how often patients with neoplasm first present to chiropractors. Spine tumors in children may be primary benign tumors, primary malignant tumors, or metastatic tumors.

PRIMARY BENIGN TUMORS

Osteochondroma. This tumor is simply an exostosis. It is the most common benign tumor of bone, although only 2% occur in the spine. Seventy-five percent of osteochondromas occur below age 20, and males are more frequently affected than females (175). Spinal osteochondromas rarely cause symptoms (176). Osteochondromas arise from metaphyseal sites in other bones, with 50% being found in the shoulder and knee. Radiographic findings in extraspinal lesions include a pedunculated mass presenting with a "coat hanger" or "cauliflower" appearance. This finding is characteristic in the knee, hip, and ankle.

Osteoid Osteoma. About 1% of spine tumors are osteoid osteomas, seen more frequently in males than females, and usually appearing between the ages of 10 and 25 years. The posterior elements are involved more frequently than the vertebral body. The lumbar spine is more frequently affected than the cervical or thoracic region. Common extraspinal sites include the femur and tibia. Radiologically, osteoid osteoma presents with a lucent nidus surrounded by reactive sclerosis (Fig. 8.17). Localized pain, worse at night and relieved by aspirin, is characteristic of the disease (177). Osteoid osteoma is one of the most frequent causes of a painful scoliosis (178).

Osteoblastoma. Approximately 40% of these lesions occur in the spine (179). Most patients are younger than 30 years of age, and the posterior elements are involved more frequently than the vertebral bodies. Radiologically, an expansive lesion with a thin, clearly defined rim is characteristic (180). Like osteoid osteoma, pain is usually the presenting symptom. Unlike osteoid osteoma, however, the pain is not worse at night (181).

Aneurysmal Bone Cyst. Although these tumors account for only 1% of primary bone tumors, 11 to 22% occur in the spine. The lesion is usually painful. Neurologic deficit may result from the expansile nature of the tumor (182, 183) (Fig. 8.18). Most aneurysmal bone cysts are found in the 5- to 20-year-old age group, and females account for about 60% of cases (184). Extraspinal sites most commonly affected are the femur and tibia. A "blown out" appearance is characteristic. According to Yochum and Rowe (1), the aneurysmal bone cyst is the only benign bone tumor known to cross the epiphyseal plate.

Eosinophilic Granuloma. This lesion occurs in the second or third decade of life and may not be a true neoplasm. The clinical presentation is often that of an adolescent with back pain. Vertebra plana often occurs, but neurologic deficit is rare. In the absence of neurologic deficit, the condition is self limiting, and reconstitution of height is the rule. This condition was previously reported as Calve's disease, incorrectly believed to be a form of juvenile ischemic necrosis (1, 185).

Simple Unicameral Bone Cyst. Simple bone cysts are very rare in the spine. Two cases have been reported in the literature (186, 187). Most unicameral bone cysts occur in the humerus or femur. These cysts are most prevalent in the 2- to 20-year-old age group, and males are affected more frequently than females. These lesions are characterized radiologically by a geographic lucency. The lesion is asymptomatic unless a pathological fracture occurs, which is common. A "fallen

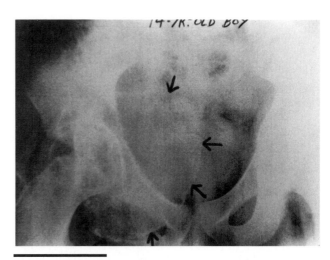

Figure 8.18.   Aneurysmal bone cyst.

fragment" of cortex freely floating within the cyst is considered pathognomonic, but does not occur in all cases (188).

PRIMARY AND METASTATIC TUMORS

Astrocytoma. Astrocytomas were formerly graded on a scale of 1 through 4, with a grade 1 being benign and a grade 4 denoting malignancy. This system has been supplanted by the terms astrocytoma, anaplastic astrocytoma, and glioblastoma.

Shafrir and Kaufman (189) presented a case report of a 4-month-old boy who had torticollis since birth. The chiropractor did not take radiographs of the patient. Roentgenograms obtained after presentation as a tetraplegic following a chiropractic adjustment demonstrated widening of the pedicle widths, indicative of a space-occupying lesion. An infant presenting with a persistent congenital torticollis should undergo radiographic examination for a potential skeletal anomaly (i.e., Klippel-Feil) or a widened interpedicular distance suggestive of spinal cord tumor.

Multiple Myeloma. The most common primary malignant tumor in bone, multiple myeloma, usually occurs in patients older than age 50, but rarely is seen in young patients. Multiple lytic lesions and altered serum proteins are characteristic (173). The vertebrae, ribs, pelvis, and skull are the sites most frequently affected.

Ewing's Sarcoma. This tumor rarely involves the spine, but when it does, localized pain is usually present. The 5–20-year-old age group is most affected. Metastasis can occur. This is an aggressive and potentially fatal tumor (1, 173). Long bones frequently affected include the femur, tibia, and pelvis. An "onion skin" periosteal reaction in long bones is classical, accompanied by underlying intramedullary destruction (188).

Malignant Lymphoma. Osseous lesions are seen in about 15% of persons with lymphoma. An "ivory vertebra" appearance in a patient with Hodgkin's disease is characteristic (188). This

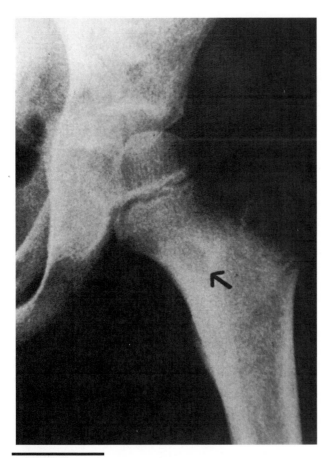

Figure 8.17.   Osteoid osteoma.

condition may be seen in young adults. Metastasis can occur. Lymphoma is a potentially fatal tumor (190).

Osteosarcoma. Primary involvement of the spine is rare, and spinal osteosarcoma is usually due to metastasis. Less than 2% originate in the spine. The condition is most commonly seen in the second decade of life. Spinal involvement may be difficult to treat. The condition is potentially fatal (191, 192). Osteosarcoma typically affects the 10- to 25-year-old age group and is more common in males. Most cases involve the knee, particularly the distal femur. A "sunray" periosteal reaction with Codman's triangles is often present. Osseous lesions may be sclerotic, lytic, or mixed (1, 188).

Chondrosarcoma, fibrosarcoma, and chordoma rarely occur in children or adolescents. Metastasis to the spine in children is most frequently from neuroblastoma and leukemia (173). Neuroblastomas are tumors of infancy and childhood. The peak incidence is at 2 to 3 years, and are uncommon after 7 to 8 years. Neuroblastomas arise in sympathetic nervous tissue, most frequently in the abdomen. An adrenal gland is often involved. The presenting finding is usually an abdominal mass (193). When metastasis to the spine occurs, destruction of a pedicle may be the earliest radiographic sign. Larger lesions may be lytic, mixed, or sclerotic (173).

PEDIATRIC SPINE INFECTIONS

Infections in the pediatric and adolescent spine are uncommon in the United States. When infections do occur, the route is usually hematogenous. There are four main categories of pediatric spinal infections (194, 195).

DISCITIS

This condition usually follows a benign course. Low grade fever, irritability, back rigidity, muscle spasm, and tenderness may present clinically. Treatment consists primarily of immobilization and rest. Antibiotics are sometimes used, although this treatment is controversial (196). Radiographically, the condition demonstrates collapse of the affected disc, narrowing of the disc space, and marginal destruction with sclerosis of the end plates (Fig. 8.19). Usually the condition is localized to one site (193). Computerized tomographic (CT) scans may be helpful in the differential diagnosis of discitis especially in early and atypical clinical presentations or in the case of a nonspecific plain film examination (197).

NON-TUBERCULOSIS VERTEBRAL OSTEOMYELITIS

This rare condition is far more serious than disc space infection. Toxemia may be evident. High fever can occur, and the child will appear very ill. Back pain may be present. Staphylococcus aureus is the most common bacteria isolated (195). The radiographic appearance of osteomyelitis includes osteolysis with severe deformity, not the isolated endplate involvement that characterizes discitis (198). In the patient with osteomyelitis, the radiographic examination can yield a range of findings including a normal radiograph or subtle soft-tissue swelling to frank bone changes (199). Radionucle-

ide bone scans may be helpful in the differential diagnosis of the child that presents with bone pain, joint tenderness, soft-tissue swelling and erythema, fever, and bacteremia (199).

TUBERCULOSIS OF THE PEDIATRIC SPINE

The age of onset of this condition is usually between 2 and 5 years of age. The most common site is the thoracic and lumbar vertebral bodies. A reversal of the height:width ratio of the vertebral bodies may occur. The radiographic changes can appear worse than the clinical condition of the patient. Advanced bony destruction may be evident. An "ivory vertebra" may be seen, as well as an associated abscess. The condition can lead to neurologic involvement and skeletal deformity. The disease is associated with poor sanitation and housing conditions. Most pediatric cases in the United States are in immigrant children (195).

SPINAL EPIDURAL ABSCESS

These are among the most serious infections of the spine and may lead to paraplegia and death. The patients often present with pain, high fevers, and appear very ill. Unlike osteomyelitis, however, plain film radiographs often appear normal. Magnetic resonance imaging is the technique of choice in such cases (200, 201) (Fig. 8.20).

JUVENILE RHEUMATOID ARTHRITIS

Juvenile rheumatoid arthritis (JRA) is an important chronic disease affecting the joints of children. It is important to remember that articular disease is only one manifestation of rheumatoid disease. When the arthritis is associated with splenomegaly, lymphadenopathy, and pericarditis, the condition is termed Still's disease. The disease usually begins at 3 to 5 years of age with pain, swelling, and stiffness in the

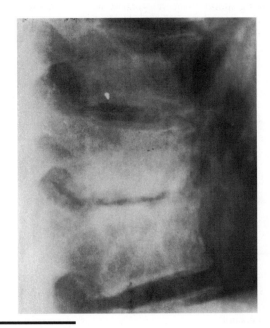

Figure 8.19. Discitis.

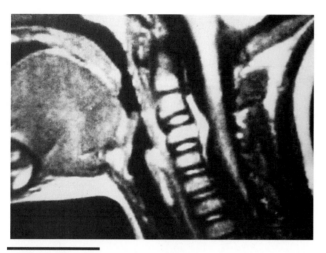

Figure 8.20.   Spinal epidural abscess.

knee. The joints of the hands, hips, and cervical spine are likely to become involved. Radiographic signs of peripheral involvement include soft tissue swelling, osteoporosis, periostitis, marginal erosion, and joint space narrowing (193). Cervical spine involvement is characterized by an increase in the atlanto-dental interval, odontoid erosion, subluxation, apophyseal joint erosions, disc narrowing, and generalized osteopenia (1).

ANKYLOSING SPONDYLITIS

Ankylosing spondylitis is a condition that begins in late adolescence or early adulthood. Most cases affect males. Clinically, low back pain is the usual presenting symptom. As the condition progresses, stiffness will also develop as a byproduct of ligamentous ossification. Decreased chest excursion may also occur. Radiologically, the first evidence of ankylosing spondylitis is irregularity in the sacro-iliac joints. Erosion followed by bony ridging is characteristic. In the vertebrae, ossification of the spinal ligaments leads to a "bamboo spine" appearance. Earlier signs include "squaring" of the vertebral bodies, vertebral body corner erosions, and reactive sclerosis in response to inflammation. The HLA B27 antigen is almost universally present, although most cases do not have the rheumatoid factor. In addition to the skeleton, cardiopulmonary, ocular, gastrointestinal, and genitourinary manifestations of ankylosing spondylitis have been reported (1,188).

SCLERODERMA

Progressive systemic sclerosis, known as scleroderma, is a connective tissue disorder or unknown etiology. Adult and child manifestations of the disease can differ, especially in the hands. In a radiologic survey of 12 children with this disease by Shanks et al. (202), no osteolysis or erosions of the hands was evident although two children did have flexion deformities. Soft tissue atrophy was seen in three-fourths of the patients' hand radiographs. Tuft resorption was detected in two-thirds of patients and generalized osteopenia was present in all but two patients.

SCOLIOSIS

Scoliosis may be due to muscular imbalance, structural asymmetry, decompensation of adaptational curves, or be idiopathic in nature (203). Adolescent idiopathic scoliosis is, in part, a hereditary condition (204). Recent investigators have reported abnormal proprioceptive function believed to be due to a posterior column abnormality. Abnormal vibratory sensation in both upper and lower extremities suggests that the lesion is located in the cervical spinal cord (205).

SCHEUERMANN'S DISEASE

This condition is sometimes known as juvenile kyphosis or Scheuermann's kyphosis. The etiology is controversial, but is believed to be due to an abnormality of the cartilaginous endplate. This results in anterior Schmorl's node formation (206, 207) (Fig. 8.21). The 13-17 age group is most frequently affected (208). Bradford (209) has proposed that the following criteria are most accurate for determining the presence of Scheuermann's kyphosis:

1. Hyperkyphosis greater than 40°
2. Wedging of 5° or more at one more vertebrae
3. Apparent loss of disc space height
4. Endplate irregularities

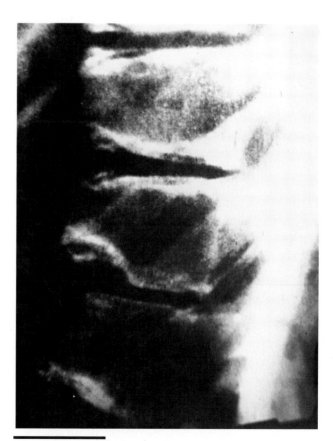

Figure 8.21.   Scheuermann's kyphosis (disease).

LEGG-CALVE-PERTHES DISEASE

The condition was originally described by Legg of Boston, Calve of France, and Perthes of Germany in 1910 (210–212). Legg-Calve-Perthes disease is an avascular necrosis affecting the capital femoral epiphysis. Males are affected more than females. The condition is usually unilateral. Weight bearing may lead to deformity. Crutches can reduce weight bearing. The disease is self-limiting. Legg-Calve-Perthes disease affects one in 820 boys and one in 4500 girls (213). The condition is most common in children between 4 and 7 years of age. The disease occasionally affects older children and adolescents (214). Early appearance of the disease is associated with a more favorable prognosis than late onset (215). The condition is rare in blacks and persons of Chinese descent (216, 217). A family history is present in about 6% of cases (218). The disease is associated with urban areas and occurs with greater frequency in families of lower socioeconomic status (217). Bilateral involvement is present in about 10% of cases and should suggest the possibility of hypothyroidism (219). The etiology is controversial, although the pathology is osteonecrosis (220,221). Necrosis is observed in both the marrow and trabeculae. Healing is associated with revascularization of the necrotic portion of the femoral head (219). The time required for the entire process varies from 2 to 8 years. Four stages describe the progress and resolution of the disease:

1. Avascular stage
2. Revascularization
3. Repair
4. Deformity (220)

Toby et al. (222) have proposed that MRI be used to further evaluate avascular necrosis of the hip. They point out that areas of necrosis and the articular cartilage are easily identified with MRI. MRI also provides information concerning the shape of the femoral heads in Legg-Calve-Perthes disease that is of comparable quality to that obtained from arthrography although the former is not an invasive test, and general anesthesia is not needed. MRI is also superior to a pin-holed collimated bone scan in the precise identification of avascular areas and the percentage of femoral head involvement. Revascularization in Legg-Calve-Perthes disease is easily detected with MRI, which may provide important information for the potential discontinuation of treatment (e.g., bracing, crutches) (222).

OTHER EPIPHYSEAL DISORDERS

Numerous eponymic disorders of developing epiphyseal centers have been described. Some are believed to be due to trauma or overuse (e.g., Sever's disease of the os calcis and Osgood-Schlatter's disease of the tibial tubercle). Others are thought to be due to osteonecrosis.

Sever's Disease

Heel pain with an associated irregularity in the calcaneal apophysis is the classical presentation of Sever's disease.

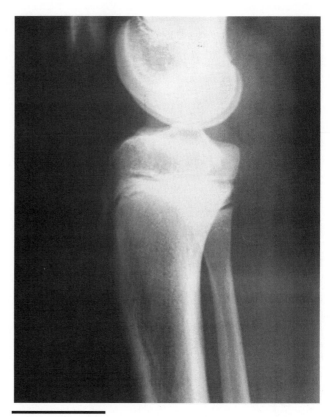

Figure 8.22.   Osgood-Schlatter's disease.

Yochum and Rowe (1), however, consider a fragmented, sclerotic, irregular calcaneal apophysis to be a normal finding and encourages eliminating the concept of Sever's disease.

Osgood-Schlatter's Disease

This condition is now considered an avulsion injury rather than a form of aseptic necrosis. It most frequently occurs in children 10 to 15 years of age and affects more males than females. The clinical presentation includes local pain, tenderness, and swelling over the tibial tubercle. Radiographically, there is avulsion and fragmentation of the tibial tubercle with soft tissue swelling (193) (Fig. 8.22).

SPONDYLOLYSIS AND SPONDYLOLISTHESIS

The incidence of spondylolysis is 4–6% (223). Most cases occur during the adolescent growth spurt. Spondylolysis is a stress fracture in most instances; although, sudden macrotrauma in hyperextension can produce an acute lesion (224) (see Chapter 19). Anterior displacement of the involved vertebral body may lead to pathomechanical changes although the association of the condition with back pain varies (Fig. 8.23).

RICKETS

Rickets (meaning to twist) is a disease rarely seen today. It is due to a deficiency of vitamin D or an abnormality of vitamin D metabolism. Radiologically, changes are best seen in the distal radius and around the metaphyseal end of the involved bone,

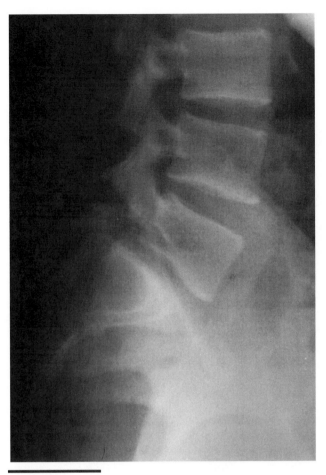

Figure 8.23. Spondylolysis and spondylolisthesis of L5.

and fraying of the metaphyseal margins (188) (Fig. 8.24A, B). In addition to disturbances in growth, other symptoms can include, tetany, listlessness, and generalized muscular weakness. Fractures occur frequently (225).

SCURVY RICKETS

Scurvy is caused by a deficiency of vitamin C and is found almost exclusively in infants fed on pasteurized or boiled milk preparations (2). Radiologically, there is widening of the metaphyses with accentuation of the adjacent metaphyseal plate, which has a lucency underlying it. The epiphysis may present a "ring sign" lucency under its subchondral margins (188).

LEAD POISONING

Lead poisoning can occur with or without symptoms. Radiographs demonstrate opaque transverse lines in the metaphyses of long bones. These lines may persist into adulthood. Lead poisoning occurs in children who eat old paint containing lead or inhale lead in dust particles, although other sources must also be considered. Transverse lines in newborn infants may be the result of drugs given during pregnancy (193).

Systematic Approach to Radiographic Interpretation

The use of a systematic approach to radiographic interpretation should assist the doctor in developing good film reading habits that will eventually become second nature. In the following section of this chapter, the reader is presented first with each individual skeletal radiograph (e.g., lateral cervical, AP full spine) and a protocol to its interpretation. For each view,

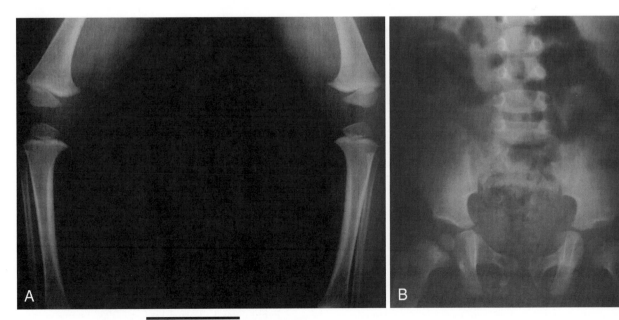

Figure 8.24. A, Rickets. B, Rickets. AP pelvic view of the same patient as in A. Notice the asymmetry of the obturator foraminae.

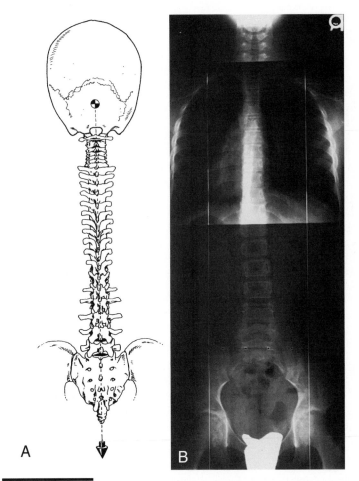

Figure 8.25.   A, Schematic of normal coronal plane posture of the spine.
B, Radiograph of near normal coronal plane posture of the spine.

a general "checklist" for interpretation is presented. Following each checklist is a table of common abnormalities that may be evident on the radiograph. These lists are not "all inclusive." Roentgenometric analysis (i.e., spinography) of spinal biomechanics is presented for each radiographic view. Spinography is used to evaluate the global postural and intersegmental static positions of the spinal column and pelvis. In the case of radiographs of the spine taken at the extremes of movement (e.g., lateral bending, flexion), spinographic procedures are presented to assist in the interpretation of vertebral motion. The chiropractor is encouraged to develop specific and thorough examination procedures consistent with the needs of the individual patient and the adjustive techniques employed by the doctor (226, 227).

ROENTGENOMETRICS/SPINOGRAPHY

Roentgenometrics involves the measurement of anatomical structures from radiographs. These measurements can be quantitatively based (i.e., mm or degrees) or assessed in a more qualitative manner. For example, an assessment of lateral bending of the lumbar spine may simply compare the relative efficiency of a motion segment to laterally flex to the right side

when compared with the left. Chiropractic spinography can be defined as a roentgenological diagnostic procedure that uses postural (weight-bearing) x-rays for the principal purpose of evaluating the spinal column and pelvis for evidence of clinically significant biomechanical irregularities (19).

STATIC ASSUMPTIONS

Certain assumptions of normal need to be made when analyzing the static upright posture of the spinal column, not the least of which is the assumption that the spinal column is at its highest efficiency when the individual is standing erect on both feet and that the spine is relatively straight when viewed in the coronal plane. The presence of structural anomalies (e.g., hemivertebra) decreases the validity of certain static assumptions in addressing the supposed optimal spinal position. These anomalies will also have direct impact on "normal" functioning of the motion segment.

For the sagittal plane, an assumption is made that there should be a balanced interplay between the lumbar lordosis, thoracic kyphosis and cervical lordosis (228). Some authors (229) have maintained that the spinal curves that are evident in the sagittal plane can be quantitatively evaluated and that deviation from this model represents abnormal spinal posture. The assumptions made for the spinographic analyses presented here are:

1. When an individual is x-rayed in the coronal plane while in the standing position with approximately equal weight on both feet, the spine is at its optimum if it does not deviate laterally and is relatively straight (Fig. 8.25A, B)

2. When an individual is x-rayed in the sagittal plane, there should be a lordotic configuration of the lumbar lordosis with the apex of the curve at L3. The thoracic kyphosis should have its apex at T6–T7 and the cervical lordosis should have its apex at C4–C5. In addition there should be a relative balance of the magnitude of curve in each spinal region. A vertically drawn gravitational line should demonstrate that each spinal curve's apex is furthest from the gravitational line (Fig. 8.26A–C). Harrison et al. have presented a model for the normal cervical lordosis (229).

DYNAMIC ASSUMPTIONS

As is the case when analyzing static upright posture, certain basic assumptions need to made when analyzing the movement of the spine at its extremes of bending. As is the case for the static upright posture, vertebral development is assumed to be symmetrical, and there will be minimal osseous malformation as this will have an effect on the function of the spine accordingly.

For movements such as lateral bending, there is an assumption that the quantity of movement both globally and on the intersegmental level will be relatively symmetrical in patients without dysfunction. There is also an assumption that coupled movements of the spine are relatively predictable (54, 230).

In the analysis of spinal position at the extremes of lateral bending, an assumption is made that the spine is most normal when the quantity of movement at each spinal level is approximately the same as that at adjacent levels and that there are gradual increases and reductions in spinal movement as one moves from one spinal region to another. There should not be abrupt changes in the quantity of movement such that one

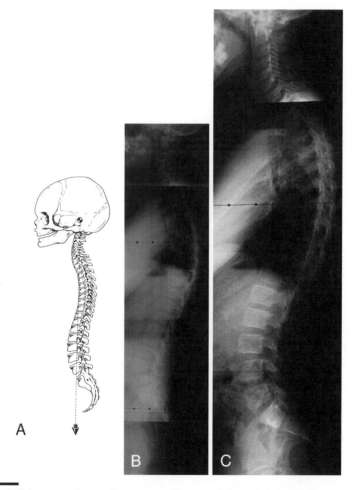

Figure 8.26.   A, Schematic of normal posture in the sagittal plane. B, Relatively normal sagittal curves. C. Relatively normal sagittal plane posture. Hyperflexion of C1 on C2 is present.

motion segment exhibits minimal movement while its neighbor demonstrates substantial motion.

Gracovetsky and Farfan have proposed a model for the mechanism of the lumbar spine during lifting and locomotion (231).

NOMENCLATURE

The International Listing System. The right-handed orthogonal coordinate system (RHOCS) is used in the biomechanics community and in some chiropractic circles for communication of the kinematic aspects of the spinal column (232, 233). Vertebral position and movement can be accurately and unambiguously described with this listing system for all six degrees of freedom of the motion segment (i.e., translation and rotation along or about the three cardinal axes (Fig. 8.27)). Since the RHOCS has been proposed as an international standard for defining body parts, it is referred to as the "international system" (234). This system should be the primary method of communication for the various configurations and movements of the motion segment and should be adopted by the chiropractic profession (234). Continuation of multiple, sometimes arbitrary, listing systems leads to confusion in the student and among practitioners especially when referral of a patient is required. The use of different points of reference when using the various (often conflicting) systems has not been helpful especially in state licensure standardization or instruction.

Instructors of technique should come to some consensus on this issue of nomenclature. Basic chiropractic technique research such as force parameters and patterns of motion should be communicated to the biomechanics community at large using the RHOCS or International system (232–234).

The X axis runs from the center of the motion segment straight left (+X) or right (-X) (Fig. 8.28). The Z axis runs from the posterior (-Z), to the anterior (+Z) through the X axis, while the Y axis, which is also referred to as the longitudinal axis, runs in a caudal (-Y) cephalad (+Y) direction. Rotation clockwise (+θ), or counterclockwise (-θ), is determined by looking from the negative pole of the axis towards the positive end and noting the direction of rotation. Rotation can also be determined by using the right-hand rule. By pointing the right thumb in the direction of the positive pole of the axis under scrutiny, the fingers will then curl in the direction of positive rotation (+θ). Translation is movement along the axis and can be in a positive or negative direction. Figure 8.29 demonstrates rotation around the X-axis. Flexion motion equates with +θX and extension is -θX. Lateral flexion is described as rotational movement around the Z-axis (Fig. 8.30). Figure 8.30 depicts the Y-axis. The reader is reminded that interpretation of rotation around the Y-axis must be done by looking from the negative pole of the axis towards its positive end. Spinous rotation to the right is the same as clockwise rotation around the Y-axis (i.e., +θY). External or lateral movement of the right PSIS is denoted also as +θY (Fig. 8.31).

By convention, the listing of movement or position of the motion segment is with respect to the vertebra below (232–234). This is in contrast to many "upper cervical" listing schemes that list the atlas with respect to the occiput. For these scenarios, the occiput would be listed with respect to the atlas.

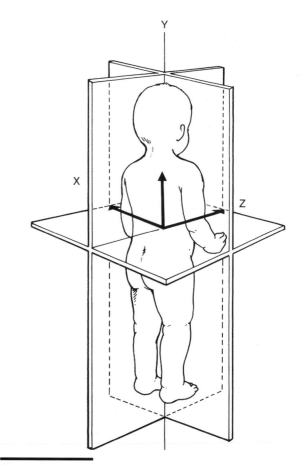

Figure 8.27.   The three (X-Y-Z) cardinal axes/planes of the body.

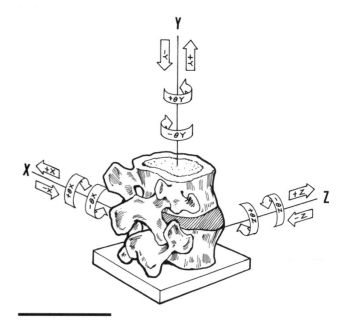

Figure 8.28.   The international listing system at the motion segment level.

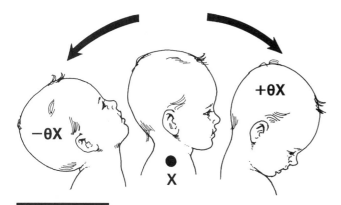

Figure 8.29.   Sagittal plane rotation around the X axis.

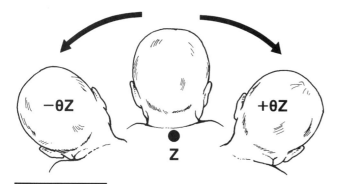

Figure 8.30.   Coronal plane rotation around the Z axis.

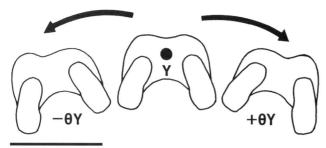

Figure 8.31.   Transverse plane rotation around the Y axis.

A necessary exception in terms of segmental contact and point of reference occurs at the lumbosacral junction. In some instances, in which there is failure of extension motion (S1–L5) and the posterior disc space remains open during this movement, it is often preferred to use an S1 tubercle contact to create an extension movement at the motion segment. The term base posterior sacrum (S1 -θX) is used to describe this type of dysfunction (Fig. 8.32). Because the contact point is the sacrum for the adjustment, this segment is listed. The dysfunction exists at the L5–S1 motion segment so the sacrum is listed with respect to L5. The sacral base is moved from a posterior to anterior direction during the adjustment, creating an extension moment at L5–S1. The base posterior sacrum is primarily listed as such due to the posterior to anterior

direction of correction. An individual listing of the sacrum can have varying degrees of ± θ X and retrolisthesis depending on the architectural characteristics of the articulations. Anomalies such as sagittally oriented facets at L5–S1 may allow larger degrees of posterior translation than in coronally oriented facet planes.

Palmer-Gonstead-Firth. The Palmer-Gonstead-Firth (PGF) listing system of vertebral misalignments are abbreviations for descriptions of motion segment alignment characteristics (234). The listing describes the positional state of a vertebra relative to its subjacent foundation. Table 8.2 has been included, which shows what each letter of a listing represents. This has been combined with the right-handed orthogonal coordinate or international system. The letters used in the PGF and International listing systems and their meaning are presented. Generally, the first letter of the listing denotes translation along the Z axis, the second letter is for rotation of the vertebrae around the Y axis. The third letter is for listing any lateral flexion positional dyskinesia. If there is a lateral flexion malposition of the vertebra, this is listed with the PGF system in relation to the direction of spinous rotation (i.e., right or

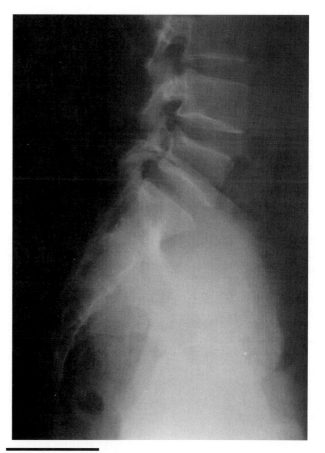

Figure 8.32.   Base posterior sacrum. -θX movement of S1 in relation to L5 or ±θX rotation of L5 in relation to S1. Correction is made by using S1 as the segmental contact point for the posterior to anterior adjustment.

Table 8.2.   **PGF Listings Transformed into the International Listing System**

AS (Anterior-superior)	$+\theta X$
PI (Posterior-inferior)	$-\theta X$
A (Anterior)	$+Z$
P (Posterior)	$-Z$
L (Left)	$-\theta Y$
R (Right)	$+\theta Y$
RS (Right-superior)	$-\theta Z$
LS (Left-superior)	$+\theta Z$

The PGF listings use the spinous process as the reference point for C2 through L5.

Table 8.3.   **Examples of Multidimensional PGF and International Listings**

Direction	PGF	International
Anterior	A	$+Z$
Posterior	P	$-Z$
Right (spinous)	R	$+\theta Y$
Left (spinous)	L	$-\theta Y$

left). If the spinous has rotated toward the open or superior side of the wedge (opposite the direction of lateral flexion), this is noted as an "S." If the spinous has rotated toward the closed or inferior side of the wedge, this is listed with an "I." Two examples are presented which also have the component of posteriority/retrolisthesis/-Z listed with them (Table 8.3). The International system lists lateral flexion positional dyskinesia as a rotation, around the Z axis (clockwise $(+\theta)$ or counterclockwise $(-\theta)$).

Listings for the pelvic ring are somewhat more complex. Some assumptions must be made regarding the axes of rotation for the pelvic bones to meaningfully describe their positional states. The forces that injure the joint can arise from a variety of different loads. Both acute as well as chronic injury can lead to joint deformity. The presence of swelling, pain and restriction of motion should lead the examiner in attempting to determine the precise mechanisms of injury. The adjustment is directed at moving the sacroiliac joint towards alignment and at the same time improving the mobility of the fixated joint.

In most cases the best and safest method for the adjustment is to move the joint three-dimensionally towards center, always the opposite direction that produced the ligamentous sprain of the joint (235). Adjustment options must be numerous due to the tremendous varieties of injury patterns that can present in the pediatric spine. Because children can have a variety of different acceleration/deceleration, blunt injuries and falls, the clinician needs to have a variety of different adjustment techniques. Adjustments are described later in this text.

A blow to the ASIS can cause the joint to gap at the front or posterior aspect of the sacroiliac joint. The joint can also become sprained at its caudad or cephalad pole. Multiple combinations of the above injury locations are possible, depending on the exact force mechanisms of the trauma.

ILIUM POSITIONAL DYSKINESIA

Internal or external rotational misalignment (positional dyskinesia) of the ilium (the PSIS acts as the moving landmark) with respect to the sacrum is essentially a rotation around the Y axis (see Fig. 8.31). The ilium is listed with respect to the sacrum (S2 serves as the stationary landmark).

External ilium movement (PSIS moving away from midline) is listed with an "Ex" and internal movement with an "In". The international system denotes internal and external ilium rotations relative to the sacrum as movements around the Y axis. An Ex ilium on the right would be a clockwise rotation around the Y axis and would be listed as $+\theta Y$. An In ilium on the left side would also be a clockwise rotation and would be listed as $+\theta Y$. It therefore becomes important to list the side of the sacroiliac involvement/fixation when determining which side of the misaligned pelvis should be adjusted. One side is fixated and the other is in compensation (i.e., normal or hypermobile motion). The compensatory SI joint can often be more tender than the joint that exhibits fixation dysfunction. Occasionally bilateral fixation occurs.

Antero-superior motion of the PSIS relative to the sacrum ipsilaterally is listed as "AS" and postero-inferior motion as "PI". This type of movement is essentially an oblique rotation around the X axis. In the International System an AS would be listed as $+\theta X$ and a PI as $-\theta X$. If there are large amounts of translations posteriorward ($-Z$) or anteriorward ($+Z$) then this too can be listed.

Sacrum. Rotation of the sacrum relative to the ilium at the sacroiliac joints in the PGF system is listed as a posterior rotation on either the right or left side (e.g., P-R or P-L). There is no listing for anterior sacrum rotation in this system since the ilium would be adjusted from posterior to anterior in these instances. A P-R sacrum is essentially a counterclockwise rotation around the Y axis and would be listed as $-\theta Y$. A P-L sacrum would be listed as $+\theta Y$.

C2–L5. Hyperextension of the vertebral body is commonly listed as inferior or "inf". This movement is a rotation around the X axis and would be listed as $-\theta X$ in the international system. Contact points for adjusting the vertebrae are abbreviated and follow the main listing:

m = mamillary process, sp = spinous process, t = transverse process, la = lamina

National System. The National system uses the vertebral body as the point of reference for rotational and lateral flexion listings (Table 8.4). So, LP becomes left (body) posterior instead of spinous process to the right (R) as in the PGF system.

Houston Conference or Medicare Listings. Medicare or Houston conference listings use anatomical descriptors of body positions. These listings are transformed into the international system in Table 8.5.

Listings for Fixation Dysfunction. Movements of the motion segment are easily listed with the International system (Table 8.6). Fixation dysfunction can be represented with a descending arrow just preceding the listing of the particular movement. If motion is increased in a particular direction, then the arrow preceding the listing can be oriented upward. If the movement of the joint is the same as when last examined, a "no change" could be listed with a horizontal arrow or by "no △."

Houston Conference Motion Restriction Listings. The Houston conference also resulted in listings for describing fixation dysfunction of the motion segment. The term "restriction" is used to describe the direction of movement lacking at the motion segment.

AP Pelvis and Lumbar

The AP pelvis and lumbar radiograph can usually be obtained from a sectional single exposure view of the pediatric patient on a 14 × 17 film. Analysis of these spinal regions can also be accomplished from an AP full spine radiograph. Figure 8.33

Table 8.4. National Listings Transformed into the International Listing System

F	Flexion malposition	$+\theta X$
E	Extension malposition	$-\theta X$
RLF	Right lateral flexion malposition	$+\theta Z$
LR	Left rotational malposition	$+\theta Y$
A	Anterolisthesis (spondylolisthesis)	$+Z$
R	Retrolisthesis	$-Z$
L	Laterolisthesis (right or left)	$\pm X$

Table 8.5. Houston Conference or Medicare Listings Transformed into the International Listing System

Flexion $= +\theta X$

Extension $= -\theta X$

Anterior translation $= +Z$

Posterior translation $= -Z$

Right lateral bending $= +\theta Z$

Left lateral bending $= -\theta Z$

Right translation $= -X$

Left translation $= +X$

Right rotation (spinous left) $= -\theta Y$

Left rotation (spinous right) $= +\theta Y$

Caudal translation (e.g., compression) $= -Y$

Cephalad translation (e.g., traction) $= +Y$

Table 8.6. Body Part Movements Described with the International Listing System

Extension restriction $\downarrow -\theta X$

Right rotational restriction $\downarrow -\theta Y$

Left rotational restriction $\downarrow +\theta Y$

Flexion restriction $\downarrow +\theta X$

Right lateral flexion restriction $\downarrow +\theta Z$

Left lateral flexion restriction $\downarrow -\theta Z$

Table 8.7. AP Pelvis Checklist

Procedure

1. Check pedicles
2. Check endplates
3. Check density of bodies
4. Check facet facings
5. Check pelvic brim and hip joints
6. Check spinous processes
7. Check transverse processes
8. Check SI joints
9. Check soft tissues
10. Check for abnormal gas patterns

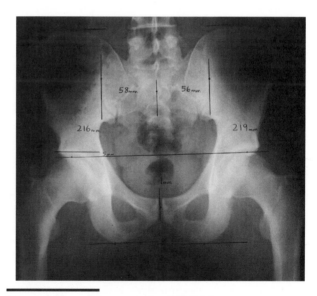

Figure 8.33. Anteroposterior (AP) Pelvis.

depicts an AP pelvic radiograph. This sectional study was collimated to a full spine but shielded to L3 and exposed only a 14x17 section of the pelvis to reproduce the distortion characteristics of a full spine x-ray with the central ray at the xiphoid process. The radiograph was exposed using a 1200 screen/film combination. Table 8.7 lists the protocol for general interpretation of the AP pelvis. Table 8.8 lists the findings that can be detected on an AP pelvic radiograph.

AP Pelvis Roentgenometrics. The Gonstead pelvic marking system (219) is based on the assumption that sacroiliac joint disrelationships and femur head unleveling can be measured on a standard antero-posterior full spine or antero-posterior pelvic radiograph. The diagnosis of leg length inequality through measurement of unleveling of the femur heads is relatively common (64, 65). In contrast, the use of pelvic marking techniques to assess sacroiliac joint disrelationships is more rare. A study by Plaugher and Hendricks looked at the Gonstead pelvic marking system (110) to determine the extent of agreement of ratings between two different examiners using identical methodologies. They found excellent levels of reliability for evaluating static configurations of the human pelvis with radiographs. Further, there appears to be good time-course (i.e., 45 min and 18 days) stability for patient positioning when evaluating these structural parameters (111).

Table 8.8.	**Conditions that Demonstrate Findings on the AP Lumbar Pelvic Radiograph**

Metastatic carcinoma

Spina bifida

Knife clasp deformity

Spondylolisthesis

Transitional segment

SI joint pathology

Ankylosing spondylitis

Subluxation

Dislocation

Fracture

Facet tropism

Legg-Calve-Perthes disease

Congenital hip dysplasia

Slipped capital femoral epiphysis

Adynamic ileus

Table 8.9.	**Checklist for the AP Thoracic Radiograph**

Procedure

1. Check pedicles for osteolytic activity

2. Check vertebral endplates

3. Check density of vertebral bodies

4. Check spinous process

5. Check ribs

6. Check clavicles

7. Check soft tissues

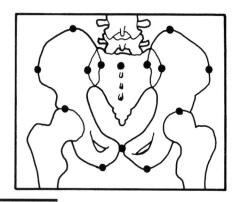

Figure 8.34. Reference points (dots) placed.

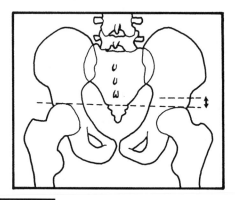

Figure 8.35. Femur head line.

Marking Procedure. Very small dots (i.e., less than .5 mm in diameter) are drawn at the top (cephalad portion) of both femur heads with a soft x-ray pencil (Fig. 8.34). Two dots are also placed at the tops of both ilia, at like anatomic locations, equidistant from either the lateral or medial margins of the iliac crests. Dots are drawn at the most inferior margins of both ischia, again, at like anatomic locations.

At the right and left lateral borders of the sacrum, medial to the radiolucent line that lies between the posterior aspect of the sacroiliac joint on the iliac bone and the lateral border of the sacrum, two additional dots are placed (see Fig. 8.34). The points selected, in addition to being at equal heights in the cephalo-caudal direction, should also reflect similar contours of the right and left sacroiliac joints.

A dot is placed at the center of the S2 tubercle. If there is incomplete ossification in this area, then a point is selected that bisects the distance between the right and left "pedicle" opacities on the sacrum. S2 and S3 tubercles are alternative locations for the center sacral point.

A dot is placed that bisects the pubic symphysis about midway between the cephalad and caudal portions of the pubic bone (see Fig. 8.34).

Next a parallel ruler is used to scribe a line that connects the femur head points (Fig. 8.35), termed the femur head line (FHL). In this analytical procedure, all other lines that are drawn on structures of the pelvis are either perpendicular or parallel to the FHL. These additional lines will pass through the remaining dots that are placed on the radiograph and should be about three inches in length (Fig. 8.36).

The parallel rule is used for the placement of the additional lines. The ruler should always be grasped near its center with pressure exerted equally around the mid point of the device. The operator should be careful to not allow the hand to "drag" along the radiograph, thus preventing symmetrical pressure to be applied to the instrument. Some practice in rolling the ruler in a straight direction is usually necessary before using it for clinical analyses. Radiographic illuminators placed in a slanted position seem to ease the use of the instrument.

The parallel is rolled cephalad from the FHL until it reaches the first dot placed at the top of one of the iliac crests. A 3-inch line is scribed through this point. The rule is then rolled further cephalad until the point on the other innominate is reached and another three inch line is drawn. The parallel is then rotated 180 degrees and rolled in a similar manner towards the caudal portions of the two innominate bones. In a similar manner as the tops of the iliac crests, two three inch lines, parallel to the FHL, are scribed through the ischia points.

The parallel rule is then placed perpendicular to the FHL and rolled horizontal to mark the two lateral borders of the sacrum. The parallel should be stopped at the S2 tubercle point and a three inch line drawn. With the parallel at the S2 point, another three inch line is drawn at the caudal portion of the parallel near the pubic symphysis. This line will bisect the dot placed in the center of the pubic symphysis only if no misalignment of this structure exists. In most individuals the line will usually be placed to the right or left of the center of the pubic symphysis.

With the parallel in its upright position with the leading edge oriented cephalad, the side portion of the rule is placed at the edge of the radiograph. The parallel is then rolled caudad until the edge of the rule comes in contact with the superior border of either or both femur head(s). If there is discrepancy in the height of both femur heads, then a 3-inch line is scribed above the more caudad femur head thereby facilitating the assessment of any right/left femur head height difference.

All measurements should be rounded to the nearest .5 millimeter. Mensuration begins with an assessment of femur head height. If a discrepancy in femur head height is present,

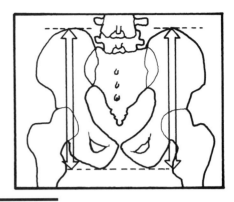

Figure 8.37. Measurement of the long axes of the innominates.

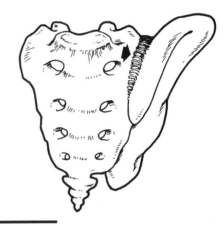

Figure 8.38. Upper SI joint sprain that is associated with the "PI" ilium subluxation.

then this is quantified in mm and termed the measured deficiency (MD) on the side of the more caudal femur head (See Leg Length Inequality).

The long axis lengths of the two innominates are measured next (Fig. 8.37). The longer of the two innominates is considered to have rotated in a posterior inferior direction ($-\theta X$) and is categorized as a PI. Posterior-inferior displacement of the innominate (PSIS as the reference point) is believed to be associated with sprain of the SI joint at its superior margin (Fig. 8.38). The shorter innominate is listed as an AS (anterior superior) and consists, in part, of a positive rotation around the X axis that causes a sprain at the inferior margin of the SI joint (13) (Fig. 8.39). The difference between the right and left innominate lengths, in mm, is denoted as a subscript to the listing. This measurement reflects only right/left differences, the magnitude of that difference is affected by not only sprain movement of one articulation, but also contralateral sacroiliac motion at the extreme of its physiologic range or beyond, if laxity is present. The measurement is also affected by radiographic magnification; about 24% at an FFD of 72 inches. Magnification could be considered an asset in the instance where examiner error in marking is a smaller component of the magnified innominate measurement. However,

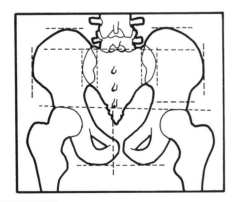

Figure 8.36. Roentgenometric lines placed.

the downside is that any improper patient positioning artifacts would be increased in the case of magnification due to shorter FFDs.

The type of sprain at the articulation is wholly dependent on the direction and magnitude of the major injuring vector (MIV). More or less rotation (±θX) and translation (e.g., ±Z), coupled with individual anatomical variances results in an infinite variety of potential directions for subluxation and the adjustments, which should be directed opposite the major injuring vector.

Pelvic torsion around the X-axis has been studied by Drerup and Hierholzer (236, 237). Using a noninvasive procedure to identify external landmarks of the pelvis, they determined that femur head unleveling resulted in pelvic torsions around an oblique X-axis. Raising the leg one side with a foot lift, resulted in a posteriorward rotation (-θX) of the ipsilateral innominate. Cibulka et al. (238, 239), using a noninvasive inclinometer, found that pelvic torsion around the X-axis may be related to sacroiliac joint dysfunction and that reduction of the displacement could be obtained with manipulation.

Obturator Appearance of ±θX Displacements. The diagonal portion of the obturator foramen (Fig. 8.40) can be used to evaluate right/left differences in rotations about the X axis. The diagonal will be increased on the side of the PI (-θX) ilium and relatively decreased in length on the opposite AS side. The effect of ilium torsion on the appearance of the obturator foraminae can be easily demonstrated by using a flashlight to illuminate a model spine in front of a screen. The obturators have a characteristic right-triangle appearance when the central ray is directed above as in an AP full spine radiograph. On sectional films where the central ray is directed lower, this appearance is less noticeable, unless an increased sacral base angle is present in the patient.

Y-axis Rotation. Sacral positional dyskinesia around the Y axis is evaluated by measuring the distance from S2 to each lateral border of the sacrum (Fig. 8.41). Clockwise rotation around

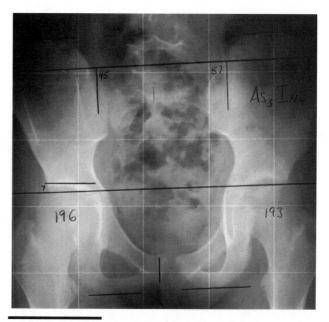

Figure 8.40.   Obturator foramen diagonal analysis for PI and AS ilium misalignments. The left obturator has an increased diagonal measurement (PI). The right obturator has a decreased diagonal measurement, associated with an AS ilium listing.

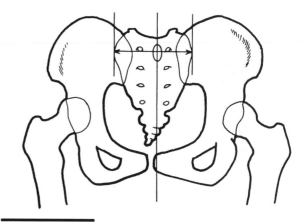

Figure 8.41.   Sacral rotation (Y-axis) measurement. There is an increased distance on the left side of the sacrum indicating posterior rotation on the same side (P-L, +θY).

the Y axis (posterior on the left side) will usually display a greater distance on the radiograph from S2 to the left lateral border of the sacrum (Figs. 8.42, 8.43). This positional dyskinesia is listed as P-L. Similarly, counterclockwise rotations are assumed to project as a greater distance from S2 to the right lateral border. This misalignment is listed as P-R. This type of displacement of a sprain at the upper and lower portions of the posterior portion of the SI ligaments. The lateral border of the sacrum is displaced posteriorward on one side. The opposite articulation is not necessarily sprained, although this probably occurs in rare instances; the MIV primarily affects one articulation.

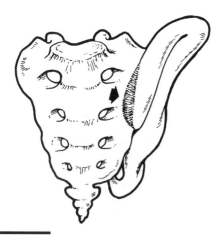

Figure 8.39.   Lower SI joint sprain that is associated with an "AS" ilium subluxation.

The lumbar spine will generally display Y axis rotational effects if a rotated sacrum is present below. The rotation is usually most prominent at the lower lumbar levels, gradually decreasing as one moves cephalad. As in the case presented in Figure 8.43, displacements of the ilia around the Y axis have been hypothesized to project as deviations of the symphysis pubis from the S2 tubercle (13) (Fig. 8.44A, B). If the symphysis displacement is clockwise (symphysis pubis deviated to the left or internal rotation of the PSIS on the left side), then the ilium is listed as In (internal) on the left or Ex on the right (Fig. 8.45). If the lateral borders of both iliac wings are visible on the radiograph, then a measurement of the distance from the lateral border of the crests to the medial border of the PSIS can be made (see Fig. 8.45).

Internal or medialward displacement of the PSIS is believed to result when trauma to the ventral aspect of the sacroiliac joint has occurred. Anatomical evidence of anterior SI joint disruption has been presented by Schwarzer et al. (240). They confirmed ventral tears in patients with suspected SI joint dysfunction. They also found that many of the patients with these types of injuries complained of groin pain. It is extremely important to remember that putative rotations around the Y axis (i.e., In and Ex displacements), can be obfuscated if malpositioning of the patient has occurred (241). Should malpositioning be a potential problem

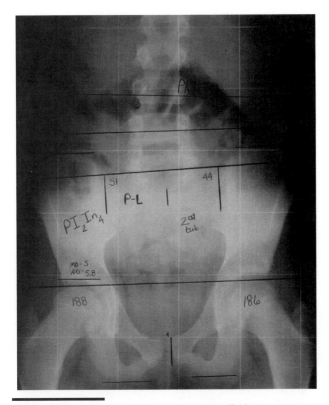

Figure 8.42.   Rotated sacrum subluxation (P-L).

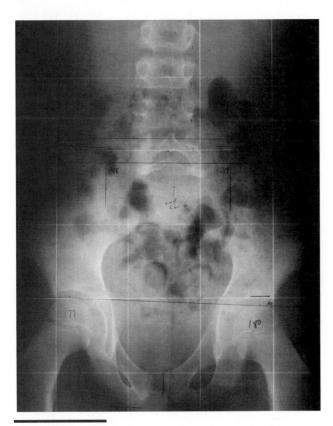

Figure 8.43.   Rotated sacrum subluxation. Notice the concomitant rotation of the lumbar spine.

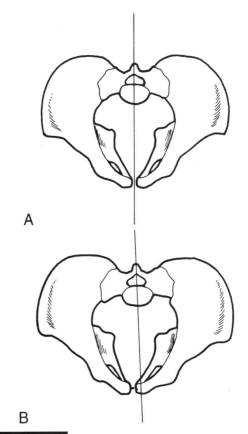

Figure 8.44.   A, Normal pelvis. B, Y-axis rotation of the innominates. Notice the deviation of the pubic symphysis with respect to the center sacral point.

Figure 8.45.   Displacement of the two ilia around the Y axis is evaluated by measuring the deviation of the pubic symphysis from the center sacral point. Sacral rotation is also pictured. The widths of the two iliac alae can also be measured to determine the presence of In/Ex ilium subluxation.

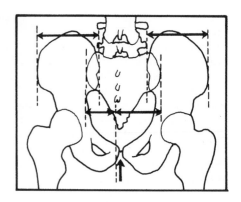

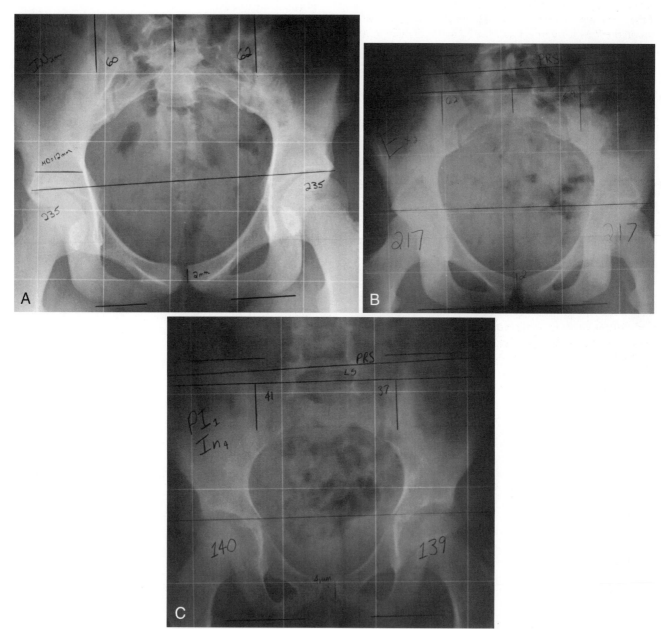

Figure 8.46.   A, The base of the obturator on the left has a decreased size with respect to the right side. B, "Ex" on the left and "In" on the right. Notice the differences in the widths of the obturator foraminae. C, The width of the obturator on the left is decreased indicating "In" subluxation on the left or "Ex" subluxation on the right.

because of poor quality control, there should be other confirmations of patient malpositioning, such as changes in the lumbar and sacral rotation and the width of the lesser trochanters, consistent with the particular direction of malpositioning. Radiographic findings of In/Ex need to be compared with static palpation findings of edema/tenderness and gluteal posture as well as the presence of any asymmetrical foot flare. Motion palpation is used to identify the side of fixation dysfunction. Bilateral fixations would be difficult to identify in bilateral motion palpation assessments. The patient's gait might be particularly altered in such instances.

Obturator Appearance of ±θY Displacements. The base portion of the obturator foramen is affected by rotations of the pelvis around the Y axis. Internal rotational (Y axis) misalignment of the PSIS makes the base measurement appear reduced when compared with the contralateral foramen (Fig. 8.46A–C).

Leg Length Inequality From Pelvic Subluxation. A leg length inequality may be demonstrated by a difference in the height of the right and left femur heads (Figs. 8.47, 8.48). A difference in leg length due to asymmetry of the femur or tibia or foot pronation, will cause the femur to be lowered on the side of the short leg. A discrepancy in femur head height may also result from projectional distortions of the femur head from patient malpositioning. Pelvic subluxation may also cause a change in the height of the femur head heights, either due to projectional distortion or biomechanical factors associated with certain sacroiliac subluxations (242). A PI (-θX) ilium causes the acetabulum to move in an anterior and superior direction. Heel contact is maintained in the standing upright position thus causing the acetabulum and femur head to be lowered on the side of subluxation (242). For an AS (+θX) ilium, even foot contact with the ground results in the opposite biomechanical effect; the femur head is raised on the side of AS subluxation (242). These theories are likely dependent on a variety of anatomical and physiological factors as well as the biomechanics of trauma. Well-designed biomechanical studies are needed to determine precisely what effects are occurring in most patients.

An anterior-superior, AS, and an internal, In, listed ilium, causes the acetabulum to move in a posterior and inferior direction. Heel contact forces the acetabulum to raise and hence appears on the AP film as a raised femoral head line.

With an Ex (Y axis) ilium misalignment, the acetabulum on the involved side is moved anteriorward. An In (Y axis) ilium misalignment causes the acetabulum to be moved in a posteriorward direction. The relative changes in position of the right and left femur heads results in projectional differences on the AP full spine radiograph. Because the central ray is positioned near the xiphoid process, there is a divergence of the x-rays at the periphery of the film. Because the more anterior femur head is intercepted by the x-rays first, it is projected lower than its more posteriorward positioned counterpart.

Walters (242) presents a ratio for determining the effects of pelvic misalignment on femur head height. This effect must be corrected for in the interpretation of leg length inequality prior

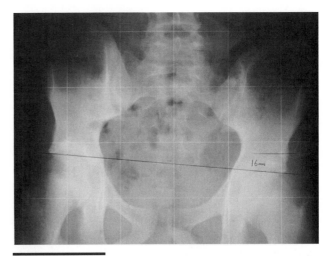

Figure 8.47.   16 mm measured deficiency on the right.

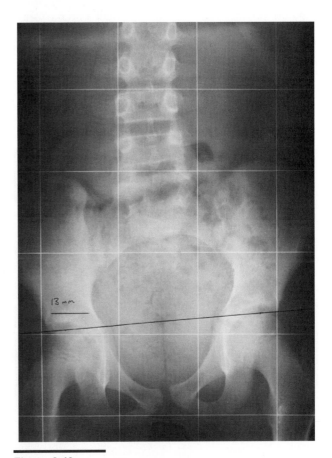

Figure 8.48.

to consideration of a heel lift or orthotic to correct a deficiency in length. For every 5 mm of ilium misalignment (derived from the subscript to the listing), this results in a 2-mm change in femur head height. The ratio is 1:0.4. The effect of ilium correction on the ipsilateral femoral head height projection on the AP film is as follows:

1. For every 5 mm of PI, or Ex correction, the femur head height will be raised 2 mm.

2. For every 5 mm of AS, or In correction, the femur head height will be raised 2 mm.

After correcting for the effect of pelvic misalignment on the femur head heights, this factor is subtracted or added to the measured deficiency, depending on the particular listing. The resulting measurement, the one used for prescribing a lift if indicated, is termed the actual deficiency or AD (Fig. 8.49). Pelvic misalignments are depicted in Figures 8.50 to 8.52. One side is listed for each figure. The side to be adjusted (the involved SI joint) is determined through motion palpation assessment of fixation dysfunction.

AP Lumbar Spine

Lateral Flexion (±θZ). The AP lumbar projection, either from a full spine or sectional radiograph, is placed on the illuminator with the patient's right side on the right portion of the viewbox. The radiograph should be oriented in a vertical direction with the vertical edge of the radiograph parallel to the edge of the illuminator.

For analysis of the L5–S1 motion segment small (i.e., less than 0.5 mm) dots are placed at the sacral notches (Fig. 8.53).

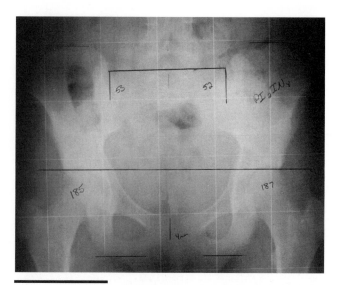

Figure 8.50.   PIIn subluxation on the right side.

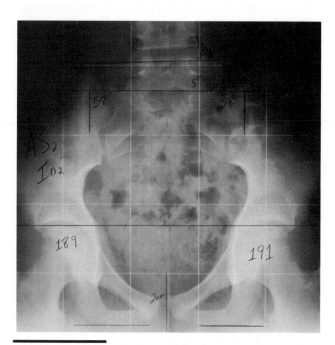

Figure 8.51.   ASIn subluxation on the left side.

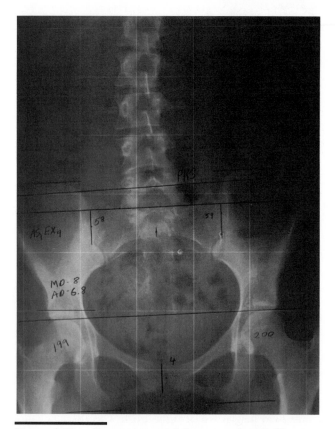

Figure 8.49.   8 mm measured deficiency on the left. The actual deficiency is 6.8 mm after correcting for the effects of the ilium subluxation on the left side.

A line should be scribed that intersects the sacral notch points and runs approximately the length of the parallel ruler. This is termed the sacral base line (SBL). Next, a line is scribed that represents the coronal plane (±θZ) posture of the fifth lumbar vertebra (see Fig. 8.53). The landmarks used to make this line can include the bottoms of both pedicles, the transverse process-body junctions, the endplates, or by simply using the parallel rule to obtain the "best fit" of all these structures. The examiner is concerned with determining if there is lateral flexion (±θZ) between the sacral base and L5 (i.e., wedging) (Fig. 8.54). The sacral base line and the FHL should be parallel if there are no sacral anomalies. If they are not, then there is probably malformation of the sacrum. Should malformation of the sacrum be present, then L5 wedging can be determined by comparing its posture to the FHL. A sacral base tilt-up radiograph (Fergusen projection) can be used to further evaluate the lumbosacral junction for an anomalous sacrum and any apparent wedging of the L5 disc space (243).

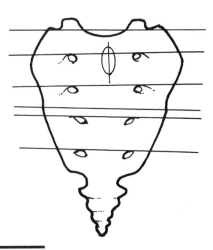

Figure 8.54.   To determine if an anomalous sacrum is affecting the coronal plane posture of the lumbosacral region, scribe lines parallel to the sacral foraminae. This schematic shows evidence of malformation.

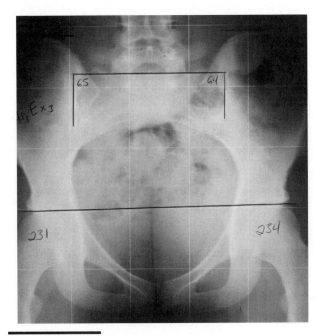

Figure 8.52.   ASEx subluxation on the left side.

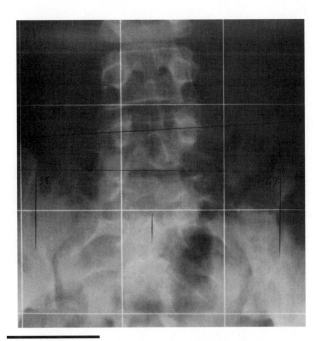

Figure 8.53.   Dots placed at the sacral notches with a horizontal line intersecting the two points. An endplate line is drawn at the superior portion of the vertebral body of L5. Lateral flexion to the left (-θZ) is present.

For L1 through L4, lines drawn parallel to the vertebral end plates are used to assess lateral flexion of the motion segment or the presence of asymmetrical, wedged-shaped vertebrae. These endplate lines are not markedly affected by rotational malpositioning of the patient (244). The vertebra under analysis is compared with its subjacent neighbor for the presence of wedging due to disc space asymmetry (Figs. 8.55–8.58).

Y Axis Rotation. To determine Y axis rotation of L5, the examiner should note the compensational position of the segments above (especially L4). If L4 is PL (-θY), then assume that L5 is PL as well unless an intersegmental torsional injury exists between L5 and L4. This will assure that the adjustment will not cause an increase in the compensation above.

Determination of axial rotation of motion segments from L4 through L1 can be suspected when the spinous process appears to be deviated laterally when compared to the subjacent vertebra. This deviation in the spinous process should be confirmed by inspecting the relative widths of the right and left pedicles since the spinous process is frequently anomalous. Again, the subjacent vertebra is used as the reference point. The pedicle on the side of body rotation will appear wide when compared to the pedicle on the side of spinous process deviation. As the pedicle narrows, there is a commensurate migration of the pedicle on the side of lumbar body rotation to move medially as the pedicle on the side of spinous rotation moves laterally (245, 246). It is unknown how often asymmetry of the spinous processes occurs in children. As an individual ages, the effects of asymmetrical muscular contraction will have demonstrable changes on the vertebral bony architecture. Van Schaik (247) has brought to light the observation that the oval shadow cast by the spinous processes on AP radiographs of the lumbar spine, is caused by its tip, rather than its base. Very large apparent deviations of the spinous process may not truly reflect vertebral rotation by necessity, therefore the clinician should use the analysis of pedicle shapes in order to confirm rotation.

If the patient is malpositioned in rotation for the radiograph, then multiple vertebral segments will demonstrate deviation of the spinous processes as well as the changes in pedicle dimensions; however, the practitioner must be astute at comparing the relative pedicle sizes and deviations of the spinous processes at two adjacent vertebral levels for any effect on intersegmental patterns. For all practical purposes the two vertebrae comprising one motion segment are equally distorted through patient malpositioning or off–centering of the central ray (248). Clinical findings associated with the rotation of the segment should be used as indicators of direction of injury. With regard to the vertebrae (C2–L5), the patient may

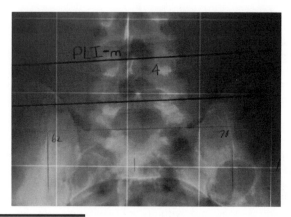

Figure 8.55. L4 PLI-m (-Z,-θY, -θZ). The contact point for the adjustment is the right mamillary process of L4.

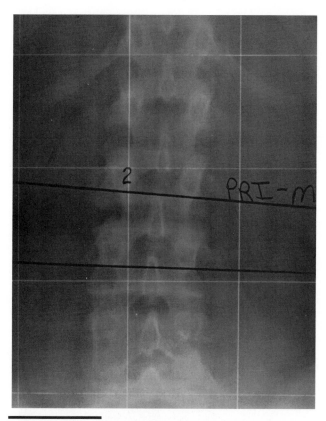

Figure 8.57. L2 PRI-m (-Z, +θY, +θZ). The contact point for the adjustment is the left mamillary process of L2.

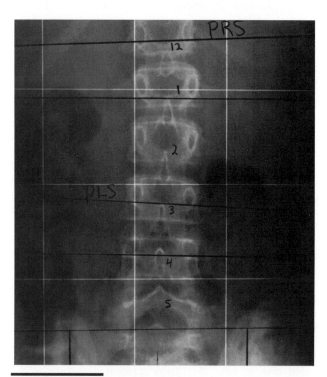

Figure 8.56. L3 PLS (-Z,-θY,+θZ). The contact point for the adjustment is the spinous process of L3.

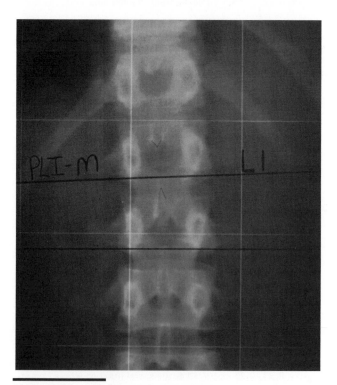

Figure 8.58. L1 PLI-m (-Z, -θY,-θZ). The contact point for the adjustment is the right mamillary process of L1.

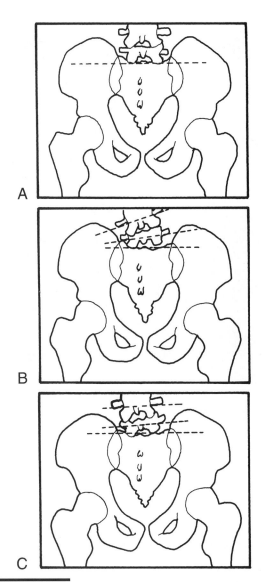

Figure 8.59. A, Sacral base line drawn. B, Lateral flexion of L5-S1 and L4-L5 is in the same direction (no special listing). C. Lateral flexion of L5-S1 and L4-L5 are in opposite direction (a special listing of L5 is present).

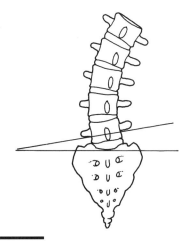

Figure 8.60. PRS-m (-Z,+θY, -θZ) of L5 (special listing). The left mamillary process of L5 is the contact point for the adjustment.

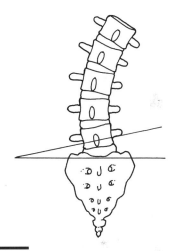

Figure 8.61. PLI-sp (-Z,-θY,-θZ) of L5 (special listing). The spinous process of L5 (approached from the left side) is the contact point for the adjustment.

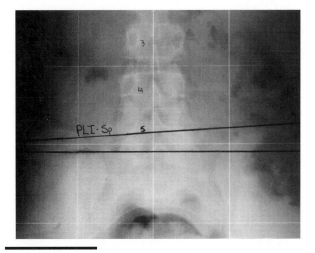

Figure 8.62. PLI-sp (-Z,-θY,-θZ) of L5.

describe more tenderness when the spinous process is pushed into the direction of deviation. This finding should not be weighed heavily in the acutely injured patient when marked soft tissue injury has occurred.

Contact points for PRI and PLI in the lumbar spine are the mamillary processes (e.g., PRI-m or PLI-m).

If the wedging at L4 is opposite of L5 (Fig. 8.59A–C), then there is a special listing of L5. Special listings include PRS–m (Fig. 8.60), PLS–m, PRI–sp and PLI–sp (Figs. 8.61, 8.62). Special listings occur only at L5 or L6, because of the doctor's ability to stabilize the sacrum during a side posture adjustment and are termed "special" because the contact point for the adjustment is on the closed side of the open wedge. The distraction on the closed wedge side is made possible through the stabilization procedure, difficult to obtain at other segments in the spine. This type of positioning in the case of a lateral scoliosis brings the patient's posture more in alignment during the adjustment. The convexity of the scoliosis is placed "up" in the side posture position. If no lateral flexion is present at a motion segment but a scoliosis in the region is present, then it is usually best to approach the adjustment from the convex side of the scoliosis (Figs. 8.63, 8.64).

AP LUMBAR, THORACIC AND CERVICAL SPINE: ANALYSIS OF POTENTIAL COMPENSATIONS AND SUBLUXATIONS

If the AP view of the lumbar spine is from a full spine radiograph, then the examiner can now determine the next true horizontal vertebra above L5 (compare with the grid lines or the edge of the film). Once the examiner has determined the

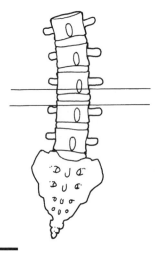

Figure 8.63.   PR (-Z,+θY) of L3. The adjustment is made with a spinous process contact from the right side.

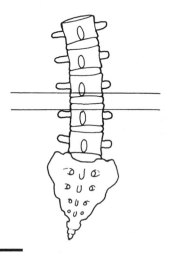

Figure 8.64.   PL-m (-Z,-θY) of L3. The adjustment is made with contact at the right mamillary process of L3.

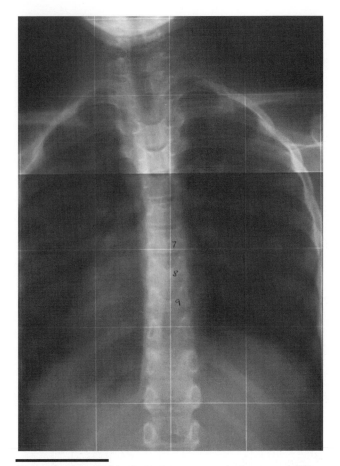

Figure 8.65.   T10 is the first segment to deviate away (-θZ) from true horizontal.

vertebra that is horizontal, the next vertebra to deviate away from horizontal is then marked (Fig. 8.65). Mark the wedging between the horizontal vertebra and the segment above. List this segment (Figs. 8.66–8.73). Determine rotation by observing the pedicle shadows and the deviation of the spinous. If ambiguous, look at the compensation immediately above. The compensation will usually magnify the direction of the subluxation. Using the direction of compensation as a guide to the direction of rotational malalignment of the subluxation will at the very least ensure that the adjustment will not increase the magnitude of the compensation. Make sure you compare rotation of the segment to the vertebra below. It is a relative assessment of rotation. Compare pedicle shadows closely. Continue this approach all the way up to C2, looking for the level vertebra, and the first segment which deviates away from horizontal. These are potential subluxations (249) but only represent misalignments in the coronal plane and so must be confirmed with motion analysis. Other freely movable segments are termed compensations.

AP THORACIC

Table 8.9 lists the protocol for the general interpretation of the AP thoracic. Table 8.10 lists the findings that may be visible on an AP thoracic view.

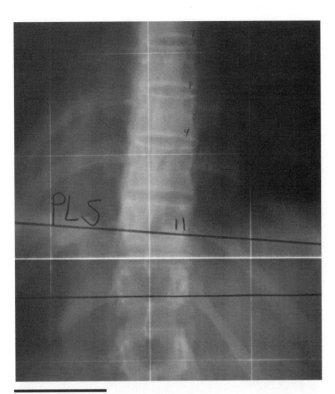

Figure 8.66.   PLS (-Z,-θY,+θZ) of T11.

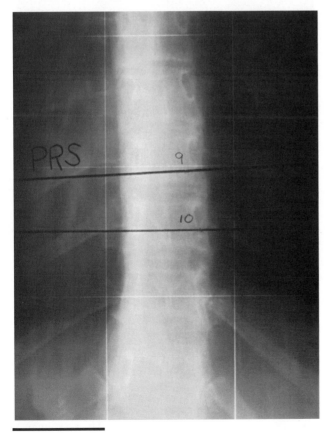

Figure 8.67.   PRS (-Z,+θY,-θZ) of T9.

LATERAL THORACIC

The lateral thoracic view can be scrutinized from the lateral full spine radiograph or as an isolated sectional study noting that identification of specific segments can be difficult on sectional views. Table 8.11 lists the protocol for the general interpretation of the lateral thoracic radiograph. Table 8.12 lists the findings that may be visible on a lateral thoracic view. Posterior displacement can sometimes be more easily detected by observing the anterior margins of the respective vertebral bodies. Hyperflexion of a disc space should be noted as a potential site of subluxation, confirmed by clinical findings of fixation dysfunction, edema, and tenderness.

AP OPEN MOUTH

The AP open mouth projection can be obtained from a well positioned AP full spine radiograph or from a sectional study of the area of interest. Table 8.13 lists the protocol for the general interpretation of the AP open mouth radiograph. Table 8.14 lists the findings that may be visible on an APOM.

ROENTGENOMETRICS FOR THE APOM

Mark the coronal plane posture of C2 by scribing a line along its endplate (Fig. 8.74). If difficult to see, then draw a line along the inferior aspects of both pedicles. Place dots at the junction of the transverse processes of C1 and the lateral masses. If difficult to see, then use the junctions between the posterior arch and the lateral masses. If also difficult to see, then place dots at the inferior medial corners of the lateral masses. Connect the dots. This line will represent wedging between C1 and C2. Place dots at the mastoid notches. Connect the dots. This line represents wedging between the occiput and C1 (Fig. 8.75). If difficult to see, then simply observe the tilt of the skull or the palatine plate.

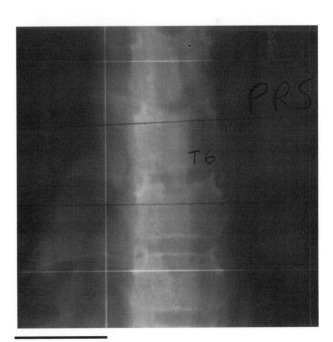

Figure 8.68.   PRS (-Z,+θY,-θZ) of T6.

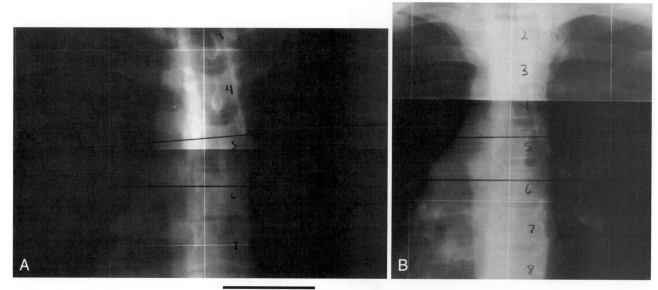

Figure 8.69.   A-B, PRS (-Z,+θY,-θZ) of T5.

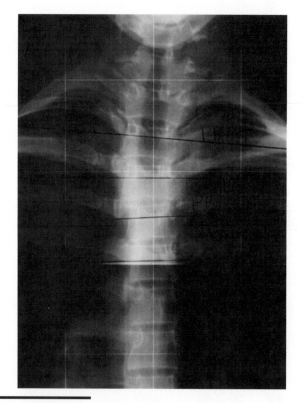

Figure 8.70.   PRS (-Z,+θY,-θZ) of T4 and PRI-t (-Z,+θY,+θZ) of T2.

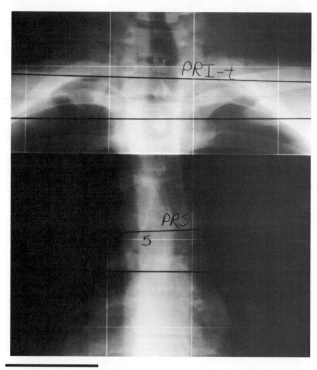

Figure 8.71.   PRS (-Z,+θY,-θZ) of T5 and PRI-t (-Z,+θY,+θZ) of T1.

Y-axis rotation is determined by observing for asymmetry of the lateral masses. Posterior rotation on one side is associated with a small lateral mass. Anterior rotation is associated with a wide lateral mass (Fig. 8.76). If one is attempting to determine Y-axis rotation of the occipital condyles in relation to C1 from the APOM, atlas rotation is noted. The rotation of the atlas (C1–C2) is usually opposite that of C0–C1. Three examples of upper cervical listings are depicted (Figs. 8.77–8.79).

AP Lower Cervical

The AP lower cervical projection can be obtained from an AP full spine radiograph or from a sectional study of the area of interest. Table 8.15 lists the protocol for the general interpretation of the AP lower cervical radiograph (APLC). Table 8.16 lists the findings that may be visible on an APLC.

Roentgenometrics for AP Lower Cervical

Endplate lines can be drawn just inside the endplate through the vertebral body. The lines should be extended laterally so that slight wedging can be identified. The inferior portion of the pedicles can also be used to draw the line representing the coronal plane posture of the segment. Usually lateral flexion is

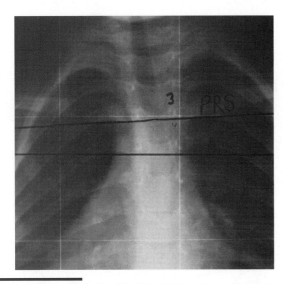

Figure 8.72. PRS (-Z,+θY,-θZ) of T4 in a 3-yr-old female.

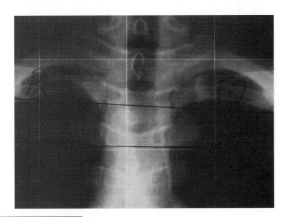

Figure 8.73. PLS (-Z,-θY,+θZ) of T2.

Table 8.10. **Conditions That Demonstrate Findings on the AP Thoracic Radiograph**

Metastatic carcinoma

Compression fracture

Spina bifida

Fractured ribs

Fractured clavicle

Table 8.11. **Checklist for the Lateral Thoracic Radiograph**

Procedure

1. Check pedicles
2. Check endplates
3. Check density of bodies
4. Check alignment of vertebral bodies
5. Draw George's line
6. Draw an anterior body line
7. Check disc spaces
8. Check soft tissues

Table 8.12. **Conditions that Demonstrate Findings on the Lateral Thoracic Radiograph**

Compression fracture

Metastatic carcinoma

Schmorl's node

Scheuermann's disease

Persistent notochord

Ankylosing spondylitis

Anterolisthesis

Retrolisthesis

of little magnitude in this region, unless an acute injury or upper thoracic scoliosis is present.

Y-axis rotation of the segment can be evaluated by observing for intersegmental deviations of the spinous process to either the right (+θY or left (-θY) (Figs. 8.80, 8.81). If the pedicles are visible, then rotation can be determined from these structures. The bifid spinous can be anomalous and give the appearance of rotation when there is little or none (Fig. 8.82).

CERVICAL OBLIQUES

The oblique cervical projection can be obtained from a sectional study of the area of interest with appropriate patient positioning. Table 8.17 lists the protocol for the general interpretation of the cervical oblique radiograph (APLC). Table 8.18 lists the findings that may be visible on a cervical oblique.

BASE POSTERIOR/VERTEX

The base posterior or vertex projection is used in various chiropractic technique systems to determine the presence of occipito-atlantal Y-axis rotation as well as to screen for other anomalies. Table 8.19 lists the protocol for the general interpretation of the vertex radiograph. Table 8.20 lists the findings that may be visible on the vertex view.

Table 8.13.   **Checklist for the APOM**

Procedure

1. Check dens for fracture, agenesis, and non-union. Beware of overlap of the incisors or posterior arch which could simulate fracture.
2. Check the atlas arches, particularly for fracture.
3. Note distance between dens and each lateral mass.
4. Check occciptoatlanto and atlantoaxial joints.
5. Check soft tissues.

Table 8.14.   **Conditions that Demonstrate Findings on the APOM Radiograph**

Ununited dens (os odontoideum or os terminale)

Dens fracture

Agenesis of dens

Occipitalization

Basilar invagination

Subluxation

Burst (Jefferson) fracture with displacement

Unilateral atlas arch fracture

Lateral listhesis

Non-union of posterior arch

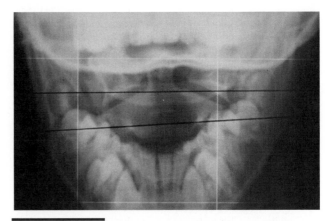

Figure 8.74. Roentgenometric lines for C1 and C2 are placed. $+\theta Z$ positioning of C1 with respect to C2 is present.

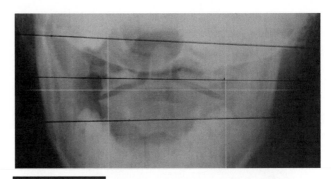

Figure 8.75. Roentgenometric lines for the occiput (C0), C1 and C2 placed. Lateral flexion ($+\theta Z$) of C1-C2 is present.

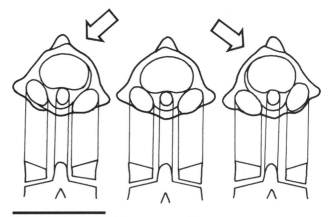

Figure 8.76. Normal is shown center. Notice the changes in the widths of the lateral masses on the right and left and the changes in the periodontoid spaces due to Y-axis rotation.

VERTEBRAL ARCH/PILLAR VIEW

Articular pillar views of the cervical spine are obtained in a P to A fashion with the patient's head rotated against the bucky. The tube is tilted 15° cephalad for the exposure. Table 8.21 lists the protocol for the general interpretation of the cervical pillar view. Table 8.22 lists the findings that may be visible on an articular pillar radiograph.

LATERAL LUMBAR/SACRUM

The lateral lumbar radiograph can be used to scrutinize not only the lumbar vertebrae but also changes visible on the lateral view of the sacrum. Table 8.23 lists the protocol for the general interpretation of the lateral lumbosacral. Table 8.24 lists the findings that may be visible on a lateral lumbosacral radiograph.

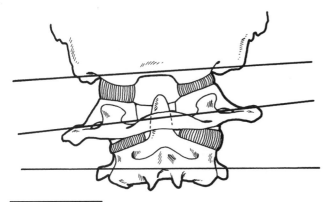

Figure 8.77. ASRA (+Z, -θX,-θZ,+θY) of C1. The first two letters of the listing are derived from the lateral radiograph (not shown).

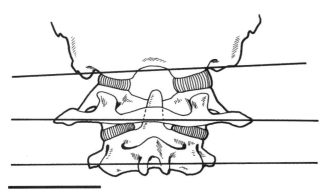

Figure 8.78. RS (-θZ) of C0.

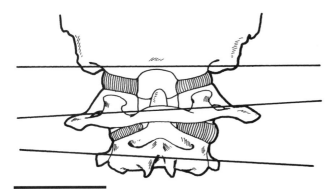

Figure 8.79. ASR (i.e., -θZ) of C1 and LS (+θZ) of C0.

Table 8.15.	**Checklist for the AP Lower Cervical Radiograph**

Procedure

1. Check tracheal shadow for deviation, which could indicate a soft tissue mass or swelling.
2. Check spinous processes for spina bifida, fracture (double spinous process sign), and rotation.
3. Check uncinate processes for fracture and degeneration.
4. Check laminae for fracture.
5. Check transverse processes for fracture.
6. Check pedicles for osteolytic activity and rotation.
7. Check vertebral endplates.
8. Check trabecular pattern.
9. Check for cervical ribs.

Table 8.16.	**Conditions that Demonstrate Findings on the AP Lower Cervical Radiograph**

Osteolytic metastatic carcinoma

Cervical ribs

Fractured transverse process

Fractured spinous process

Fractured uncinate process

Fractured lamina

Non-segmentation

Subluxation

Unilateral facet dislocation

Hemivertebra

Soft tissue mass

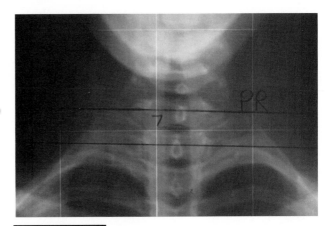

Figure 8.80. PR (-Z, +θY) of C7. The first letter of this listing is derived from the lateral radiograph (not shown).

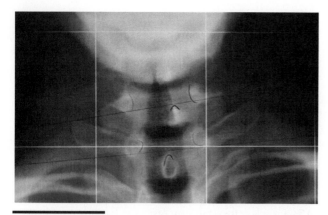

Figure 8.81. PRS (-Z,+θY,-θZ) of C7. Moderate lateral flexion (±θZ) is present at C7-T1 and T1-T2.

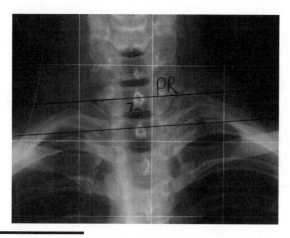

Figure 8.82. PR (-Z,+θY) of C7. Minimal Y-axis rotation of C7-T1 is present.

Table 8.17.   **Checklist for the Oblique Radiograph**

Procedure

1. Check foramina for alterations of size and shape.
2. Check pedicles for fracture or osteolytic activity.
3. Check joints for degeneration.

Table 8.18.   **Conditions that Demonstrate Findings on the Oblique Radiograph**

Uncinate process exostosis, causing foraminal encroachment

Foraminal enlargement due to a neurofibroma

Fractured pedicle

Degenerative changes in posterior joints

Subluxation

Dislocation

Table 8.19.   **Checklist for the Vertex Radiograph**

Procedure

1. Check atlas arches for fracture and non-union.
2. Check lateral masses for occipitalization.
3. Check dens for fracture and non-union.

Table 8.20.   **Conditions that Demonstrate Findings on the Vertex Radiograph**

Jefferson fracture

Unilateral arch fracture

Occipitalization

Dens fracture

Non-union of dens

Atlantoaxial rotatory fixation-subluxation

Table 8.21.   **Checklist for the Pillar View**

Procedure

1. Check the articular pillars for compression and burst fractures; compare left and right sides.
2. Check vertebral arches for fracture.

Table 8.22.   **Conditions that Demonstrate Findings on a Pillar View Radiograph (Lateral Lumbar)**

Compression fracture of articular pillar

Burst (comminuted) fracture of articular pillar

Vertebral arch fracture

ROENTGENOMETRICS

The rudimentary discs of the various sacral segments should be scrutinized for any widening at their posterior aspects. These displacements appear to be common in the pediatric population seen by chiropractors. Figures 8.83 and 8.84 demonstrate the posterior S3 subluxation. The segment is listed as posterior, in part, because the flexion malposition of S2–S3 (S2: +θX) is corrected by contacting the inferior motion segment (i.e., S3) and thrusting posterior to anterior causing extension to occur at S2–S3.

Posterior S2 subluxations appear to be the most common level of involvement. Segmental subluxations at S1–S2 are depicted in Figures 8.85 to 8.88. There are usually varying degrees of flexion between S1–S2 and retrolisthesis of S2 (with respect to S1). In addition to the identification of sacral subluxations, spondylolisthesis can be evaluated at the L5 level from the lateral radiograph (Fig. 8.89).

Table 8.23.	Checklist for the Lateral Lumbar Radiograph

Procedure

1. Check endplates.
2. Check density of bodies.
3. Check pedicles.
4. Check disc spaces.
5. Draw George's line.
6. Check soft tissues.
7. Check for sacral displacements.

Table 8.24.	Conditions that Demonstrate Findings on the Lateral Lumbar Radiograph

Retrolisthesis

Spondylolisthesis

Subluxation

Dislocation

Compression fracture

Burst fracture

Metastatic carcinoma

Schmorl's node

Avulsion fracture

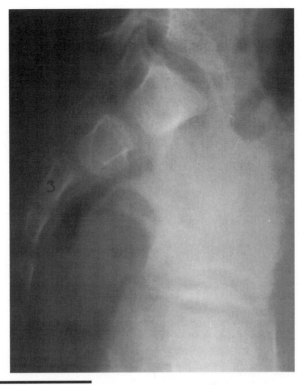

Figure 8.84. Posterior S3 (also S2) subluxation in a 10-yr-old female patient.

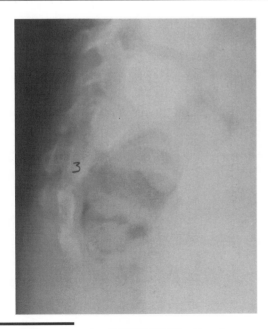

Figure 8.83. Posterior (+θX,S2-S3) S3 subluxation.

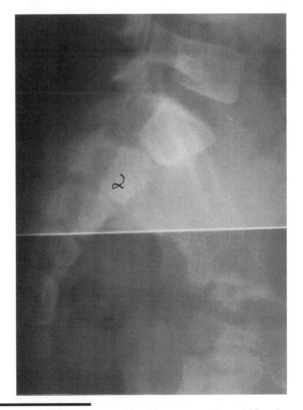

Figure 8.85. Posterior S2 subluxation in a 4-yr-old female patient.

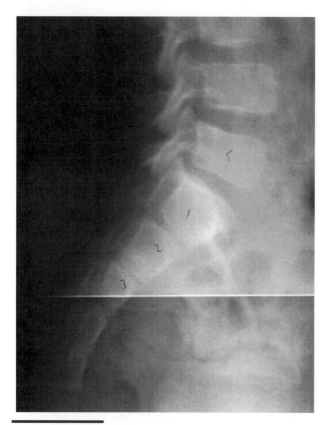

Figure 8.86. Posterior (+θX, S1-S2) S2 subluxation.

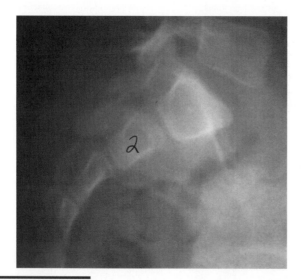

Figure 8.87. Posterior S2 subluxation. Hyperextension of L5-S1 is present.

will be two George's Lines present at each vertebra. The most anterior lines of the two vertebrae under inspection can be used to determine if any retrolisthesis is present. Patient malpositioning in rotation has little effect on these parameters, provided the appropriate vertebral points are used for comparison. Use the lateral radiograph to determine if L5 is

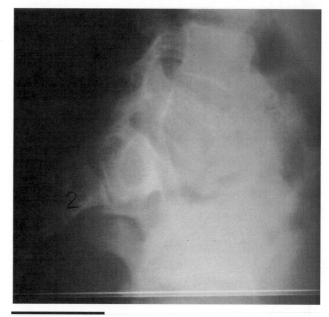

Figure 8.88. Posterior S2 subluxation in a 14-yr-old male patient.

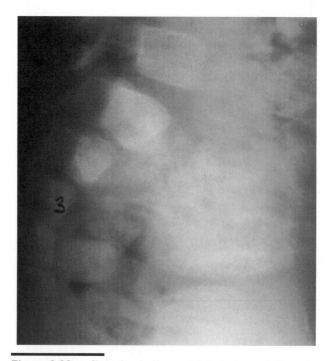

Figure 8.89. Slight (grade 1) spondylolisthesis of L5. Posterior S3 and S2 subluxations are also present.

Evaluation of retrolisthesis can be made radiographically with a high degree of reliability (56,250). While patient malpositioning may create an apparent retrolisthesis, this effect can be minimized by scrutinizing the appropriate George's Line. When rotation of the spine occurs about the Y-axis there

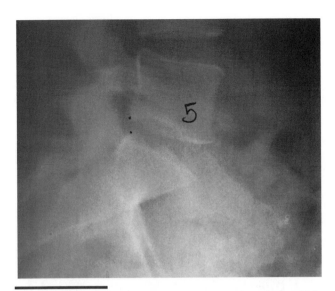

Figure 8.90. Dots placed for evaluating a retrolisthesis of L5.

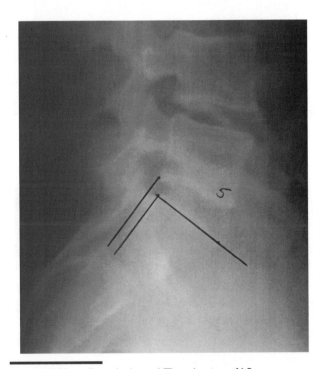

Figure 8.91. Retrolisthesis (-Z) evaluation of L5.

Figures 8.93 and 8.94. Figures 8.95 through 8.97 show varying degrees of hyperextension ($-\theta X$) (inferiority of the spinous process) concomitant with the retrolisthesis (-Z) displacement.

Figures 8.98 and 8.99 show a posterior L4 subluxation. L3 subluxations are depicted in Figure 8.100. Subluxation of L2 is shown in Figure 8.101.

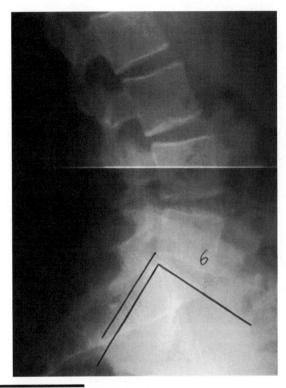

Figure 8.92. Retrolisthesis (posterior) L6.

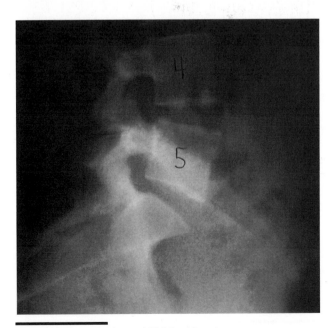

Figure 8.93. Posterior (-Z) L5 subluxation.

posterior (retrolisthesis). List L5 or L6 by placing a dot at the posterior-superior corner of S1 and at the posterior-inferior corner of L5 (Fig. 8.90). Next, a dot is placed at the anterior-superior corner of S1 (Fig. 8.91). An endplate line is drawn, ending at the posterior aspect of S1. The parallel ruler is used to construct a line descending at a right angle to the endplate line of S1. Finally, a line is drawn parallel to this line, descending from the posterior corner of L5. The amount of retrolisthesis is measured in millimeters. An L6 retrolisthesis is shown in Figure 8.92. Retrolisthesis of L5 is depicted in

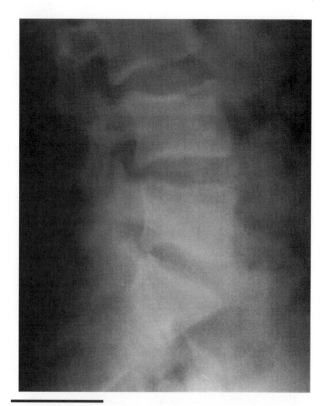

Figure 8.94. Posterior (-Z) L5 subluxation. End-plate depressions are present indicating compression injury.

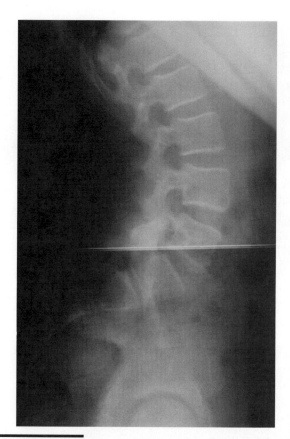

Figure 8.96. Postero-inferior (-Z,-θX) subluxation of L5. An increased sacral base angle and hyperlordosis is present.

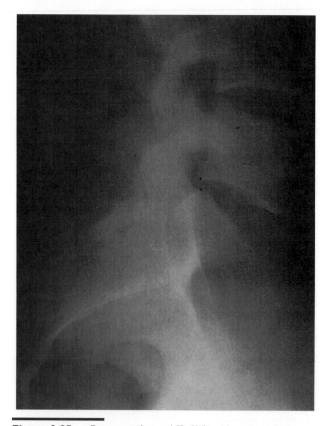

Figure 8.95. Postero-inferior (-Z,-θX) subluxation of L5.

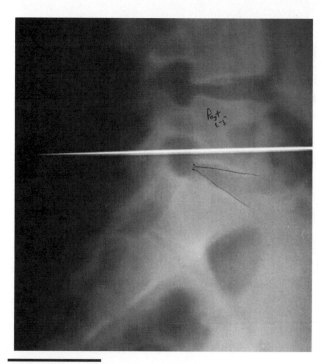

Figure 8.97. Postero-inferior (-Z,-θX) subluxation of L5. Hyperextension of the segment will tend to lessen the extent of the break in George's line.

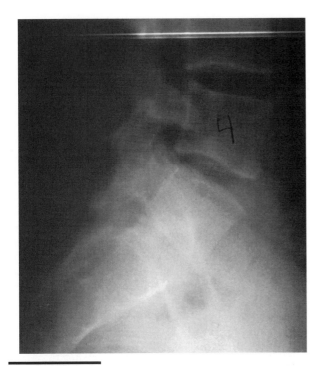

Figure 8.98.   Posterior L4 with sacralization of L5.

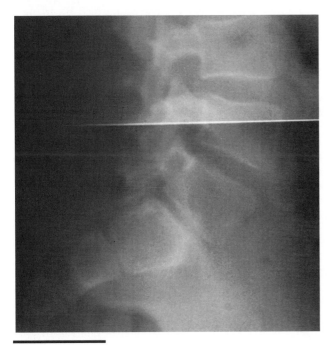

Figure 8.99.   Posterior L4 subluxation.

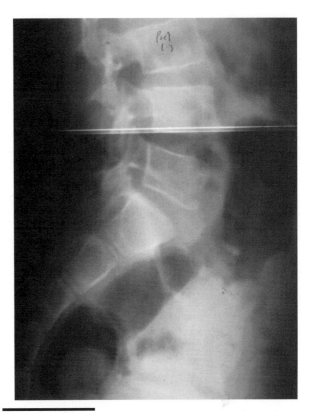

Figure 8.100.   Posterior L3 subluxation.

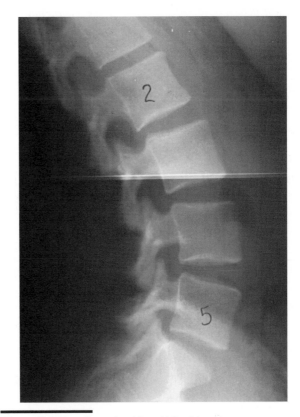

Figure 8.101.   Posterior L2 and L5 subluxations.

Instability (hypermobility) of the lumbar spine in the sagittal plane can also be detected radiographically. It is often the case that there may be retrolisthesis at both L5 and L4, but that during forward flexion the L4–L5 segment is moveable and persistent retrolisthesis remains at L5–S1. Although the L4–L5 motion segment is a frequent site of hypermobility, fixation dysfunction at this level can also occur.

If there is a spondylolisthesis, it is graded based on the method of Meyerding (see Chapter 19). In addition to retrolisthesis of the lumbar spine, other sagittal plane postural configurations can be detected. In one such instance, the lateral radiograph may demonstrate an abnormal shape of the normal wedge-like configuration of the L5–S1 disc (see Fig. 8.32). The space will either be parallel or widened at the posterior aspect of the joint space. Motion palpation findings may reveal a blockage to extension movement at L5–S1 (31). The radiograph can be used to detect the fixation dysfunction (12). There will usually be marked edema and tenderness at the L5–S1 level. If there is a base posterior (disc parallel or open in the back), then note this. Finally, the sacral base angle should be marked and measured.

LUMBAR OBLIQUES

Lumbar oblique radiographs can be used to further evaluate equivocal findings evident on standard AP and lateral views of the lumbar spine. Table 8.25 lists the protocol for the general interpretation of the lumbar oblique. Table 8.26 lists the findings that may be visible on a lumbar oblique radiograph.

LATERAL CERVICAL

The lateral cervical radiograph can be obtained as a sectional study or from a lateral full spine radiograph. Adequate visualization of the cervicothoracic junction should be made, if this is an area of clinical interest. Table 8.27 lists the protocol for the general interpretation of the lateral cervical radiograph. Table 8.28 lists the findings that may be visible on a lateral cervical.

Table 8.25. **Checklist for the Lumbar Oblique Radiograph**

Procedure

1. Check pars.
2. Check pedicles.
3. Check articular surfaces.

Table 8.26. **Conditions that Demonstrate Findings on the Oblique Lumbar Radiograph**

Spondylolysis

Subluxation

Dislocation

Metastatic carcinoma

Facet joint arthropathy

ROENTGENOMETRICS OF THE LATERAL CERVICAL RADIOGRAPH

Upper Cervical C0-C1. Draw the odontoid line (OL) and the odontoid perpendicular line (OPL) (Fig. 8.102). Place a dot at the anterior tubercle of C1 and in the posterior arch at the back. Connect these dots. Wedging greater than 5° may indicate AS displacement (+Z,-θX) (Fig. 8.103A, B). Hyperflexion of C1 is signified as AI (+Z,+θ X) (Fig. 8.104A, B). The remainder of any atlas listing is derived from the AP radiograph. Y axis rotation of atlas is determined by observing the sizes of the lateral masses. The mass which is anteriorly rotated is wider.

The atlantodental interval should be checked for possible anteriorward translation of the atlas. The shape of the predens space (i.e., ADI) should also be scrutinized. With hyperextension of the atlas on axis, there may be a widening of the caudad portion of the ADI. With flexion injury, partial transverse ligament sprain, and AI displacement, the predens space takes on a "V" shape (251) (Fig. 8.105). The ADI should increase with flexion (Fig. 8.106). Young patients (e.g. < 5 yr) have shown a slight increase in the ADI with flexion. However, the displacement should not be greater than 5 mm (Fig. 8.107).

Observe the space between the posterior arch of atlas and the posterior aspect of the occiput (Fig. 8.108). If closed down, then this signifies an AS condyle (confirmed by taking a radiograph in flexion to see if it opens up) (Fig. 8.109A, B). If the space diverges at the posterior (Fig. 8.110), then the patient may have a PS condyle (confirmed by taking a radiograph in extension).

Lateral Cervical (C2–C7). Mark the cervical spine (C2–C7). Draw lines that represent the wedging between each cervical segment. The lines are drawn through the vertebral bodies but represent disc wedging (Figs. 8.111, 8.112). These lines should be relatively perpendicular to George's line. In a lordosis, the lines converge at the posterior. The line that converges the most at the posterior should be listed. This is a potential subluxation. When the segment is hyperextended, it is listed as "inferior" (i.e., spinous process inferior) (e.g., PRS-inf or PLI-la-inf). For listing contact points, a lamina or spinous process abbreviation follows the listing. The following are examples: PRI-la, PLI-la, PR-sp, PL-sp.

Flexion–subluxation injury to the cervical presents as a posterior widening of the spinous processes, evident on the neutral projection or exacerbated with a stress film in flexion (252). These radiologic changes can often be subtle and require careful scrutiny to avoid overlooking an injury. The clinical picture should always be considered when interpreting the radiographic findings. The physical signs associated with flexion injuries of the cervical spine range from pain and muscle spasm to complete tetraplegia (252).

The anterior to posterior cervical curve can be present in a variety of configurations (Fig. 8.113). Its magnitude can be quantified by measuring the angles of each individual segment (Fig. 8.114).

Table 8.27.   Checklist for the LateralCervical Radiograph

Procedure

1. Check the posterior arch of atlas for fracture, non-union, occipitalization, or basilar invagination.

2. Check the ADI (atlanto-dental interval) for enlargement. A measurement exceeding 3 mm in an adult or 5 mm in a child may indicate a damaged transverse ligament, a congenital anomaly, or an inflammatory process.

3. Check for agenesis, fracture, or non-union of the dens.

4. Draw the following lines (visualize or mark the film).

    A. Anterior body line

    B. George's line

    C. Spinolaminar junction line

5. This will divide the cervical spine into three columns:

    A. Anterior column. Check the vertebral bodies for evidence of fracture, dislocation, alterations of trabeculae, and alterations of density.

    B. Middle column. The distance between George's line and the spinolaminar line roughly defines the sagittal diameter of the spinal canal. A measurement under 12 mm (at an FFD of 72 in.) may indicate stenosis. An unexplained increase of this measurement at a given segmental level may indicate fracture. When checking the middle column, the chiropractor should also look for abnormalities of the posterior joints.

    C. Posterior column. Check the spinous processes for evidence of fracture. Determine any abnormalities which may be present, and determine the cause. Sesamoid bones in the ligamentum nuchae are common, and should not be misinterpreted as fractures.

6. Check the intervertebral disc spaces and vertebral endplates.

7. Check the retropharyngeal space, which is measured from the anterior portion of the C-2 body to the posterior border of the pharynx. This measurement should not exceed 7 mm. The retrotracheal space is measured from the anterior aspect of the C-6 body and the posterior border of the trachea. This measurement should not exceed 22 mm. An increase in either of these measurements indicates prevertebral hemorrhage or soft tissue swelling.

Table 8.28.   Conditions That Demonstrate Findings on the Lateral Cervical Radiograph

Ponticus posticus	Burst fracture
Non-union of posterior arch	Non-segmentation
Fracture of posterior arch	Cervical kyphosis
Fracture of dens	Metastatic carcinoma
Non-union of dens	Laminectomy
Agenesis of dens	Osteoporosis
Down's syndrome	Subluxation
Rheumatoid arthritis	Dislocation
Ankylosing spondylitis	Anterolisthesis
Spinous process fracture	Retrolisthesis
Compression fracture	

Anterior carriage of the head can be quantified by measuring in millimeters the distance from the posterior-superior aspect of C2, to a line ascending vertically from the posterior-inferior margin of C7 (Fig. 8.115).

Quantifying the degree of cervical curve can serve as one objective outcome measurement for treatment (Fig. 8.116A, B). Several examples of configurations of the cervical, as well as segmental subluxations, are shown in Figures 8.117 through 8.128.

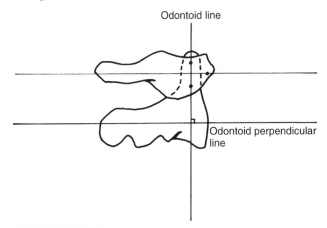

Figure 8.102.   C1-C2 roentgenometric analysis. The odontoid line (OL) is constructed by placing dots at the apex and the base of the dens.

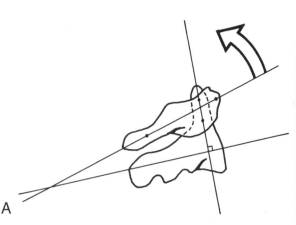

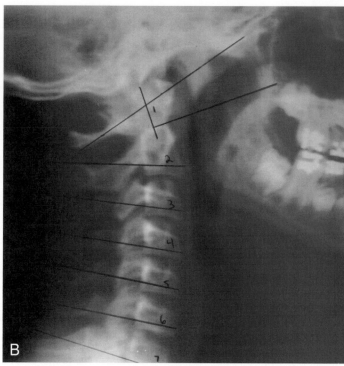

Figure 8.103. A, Antero-superior (AS) (+Z,-θX) movement of the anterior tubercle is detected by noting a greater than 5° angulation between the anterior to posterior atlas plane line and the odontoid perpendicular line (OPL). Confirmation of a motion restriction at this level is made with a radiograph taken in flexion. B, AS (-θX) of C1.

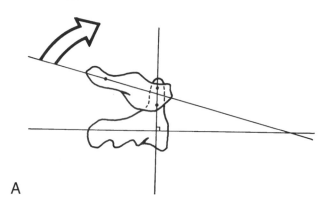

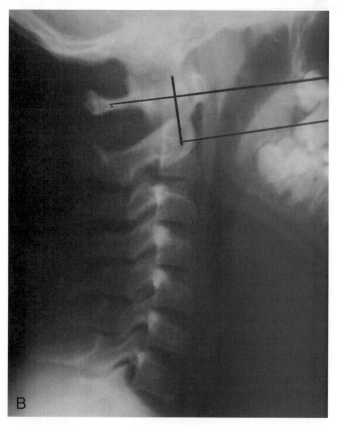

Figure 8.104. A, Antero-inferior (anterior tubercle) atlas listing. B, Antero-inferior (+θX) subluxation of C1.

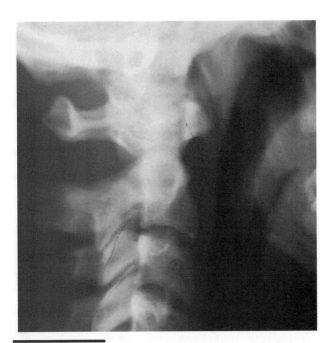

Figure 8.105. "V" sign at the ADI in the 20-yr-old male patient.

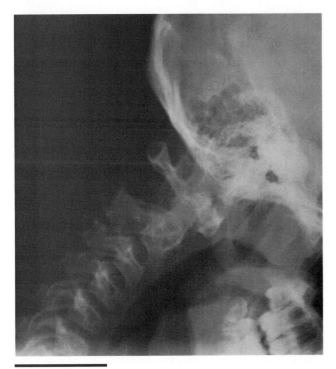

Figure 8.106. Increased ADI with flexion.

Yousefzadeh et al. (253) have investigated the normal sagittal diameter of the pediatric cervical spine from lateral radiographs. They note that gradual widening of the lower canal and even ballooning of the mid canal are often detected in normal children, 10 years old or younger. Occasionally adolescents up to 18 years of age may show these normal

variations from the funnel shape of the cervical spinal canal. For this reason the diagnosis of cervical cord tumors from lateral radiographs is not valid. In adults, however, canal widening is considered more clinically significant (253).

BENDING OR STRESS RADIOGRAPHS

Lumbar Lateral Bending. Lateral bending radiographs of the lumbar spine are obtained with an 8x10 film size and either a

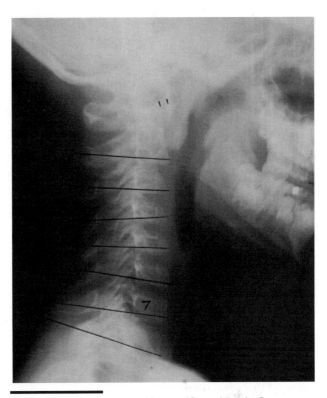

Figure 8.107. Increased ADI in a 13-yr-old male. Postero-inferior (-Z,-θX) subluxation of C7 is also present.

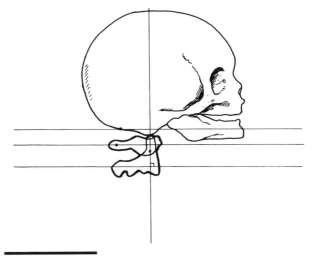

Figure 8.108. Normal occipito-atlantal spacing.

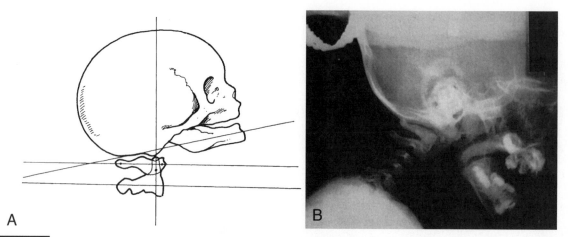

Figure 8.109. A, AS condyle (-θX) subluxation. B, AS (-θX) condyle subluxation during passive flexion. Notice the lack of separation of the occiput from the posterior arch of the atlas.

Reproduced with permission from Plaugher G, ed. Textbook of clinical chiropractic: a specific biomechanical approach. Baltimore: Williams & Wilkins, 1993:402.

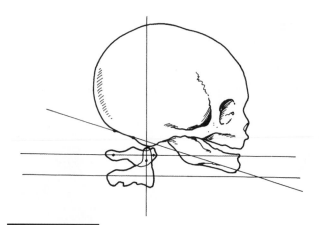

Figure 8.110. PS condyle (+θX) subluxation.

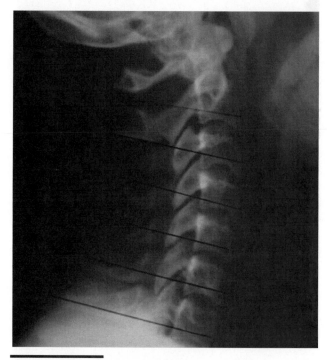

Figure 8.111. Endplate lines placed at C2-C7. This patient is hypolordotic in the lower cervical spine.

straight AP exposure or with a cephalad tilt of the beam to compensate for the lumbar lordosis and to allow better visualization of the lumbosacral junction (254). Endplate lines are drawn at each vertebral level and compared intersegmentally. Normal lateral flexion involves ipsilateral side-bending of the motion segment to the side the patient bends. This motion is usually accompanied by a coupling motion of the spinous process towards the side of tilt (i.e., +θZ with +θY). A second coupled motion, not visible on AP lumbar lateral bending views, consists of either flexion in the case of a spine beginning in extension, or an extension coupling, if the spine was prepositioned in flexion (255). Analysis of coupled axial rotation should be performed at the intersegmental level, taking into account motion at the sacroiliac joint, and by making a comparison of the pedicle shadows, segment to segment.

Grice (256) has presented four general categories of movement that are detectable on AP lumbar lateral bending radiographs. Type one is considered normal motion with ipsilateral movement of the spinous process towards the side of

bend (Fig. 8.129). In Type 2, normal lateral flexion is present but the spinous moves to the convex side of bend (Fig. 8.130). Grice (256) considers this finding to represent the first stage of abnormal biomechanics. He theorizes that this pattern of movement is due to the multifidi, sacrospinalis or psoas muscles becoming the prime movers, due to either hyperactivity, or as a result of weakness of quadratus lumborum.

In Type 3 motion, normal coupled movement of the spinous process is present, but there is failure of the motion segment to laterally flex towards the direction of side-bending

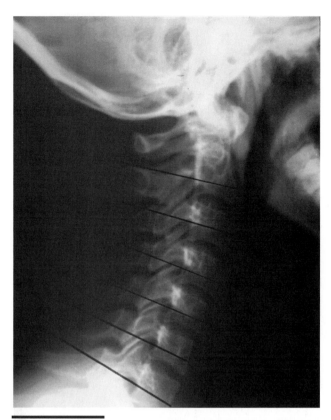

Figure 8.112.   Endplate lines placed at C2-C7. This patient is hypolordotic at the C5-C6 level.

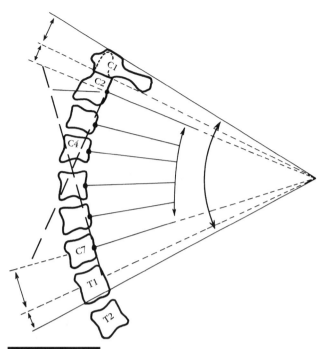

Figure 8.114.   Roentgenometric analysis for absolute and relative rotation angles of the cervical spine in the sagittal plane. The Ruth Jackson physiologic stress lines are shown forming an absolute rotation angle for the lordosis. Relative rotation angles are the degree of flexion-extension ($\pm\theta X$) at individual motion segments. For quantifying in degrees the magnitude of the cervical lordosis, the individual segmental angulations (relative rotation angles) are summed. Modified from Harrison DD, Jackson BL, Troyanovich S. The efficacy of cervical extension-compression traction combined with diversified manipulation and drop table adjustments in the rehabilitation of cervical lordosis: a pilot study. J Manipulative Physiol Ther 1994; 17:458.

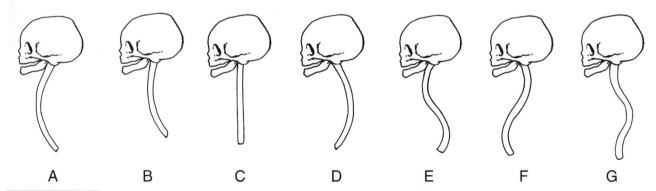

Figure 8.113.   A-G, Various configurations of the cervical curve. A, Lordosis. B, Hypolordosis. C, Straight (military posture). D, Kyphotic. E, Kyphotic (lower) and lordotic (upper). F, lordotic (lower) and kyphotic (upper). G, Lordotic (lower), kyphotic (mid), and lordotic (upper). Modified from Harrison DD, Jackson BL, Troyanovich S. The efficacy of cervical extension-compression traction combined with diversified manipulation and drop table adjustments in the rehabilitation of cervical lordosis: a pilot study. J Manipulative Physiol Ther 1994; 17:459.

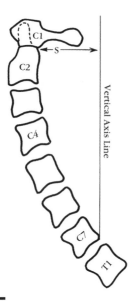

Figure 8.115. Roentgenometric analysis of anterior translation of the head and upper cervical spine. Modified from Harrison DD, Jackson BL, Troyanovich S. The efficacy of cervical extension-compression traction combined with diversified manipulation and drop table adjustments in the rehabilitation of cervical lordosis: a pilot study. J Manipulative Physiol Ther 1994; 17:459.

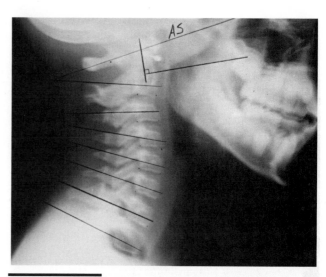

Figure 8.117. Cervical lordosis from C3-C7. C3 is positioned postero-inferior (-Z,-θX) and C2 is positioned antero-superior (+Z,+θX). The atlas anterior tubercle is slightly positioned antero-superior (i.e., -θX), likely in compensation for the flexion deformity below.

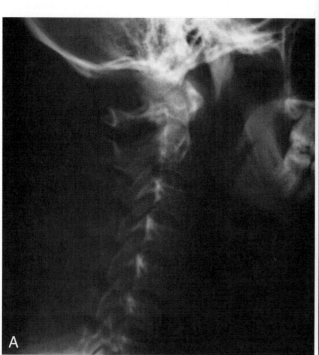

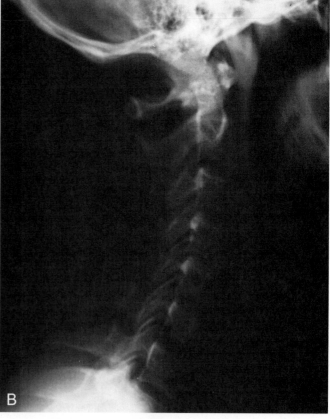

Figure 8.116. A, Pretreatment radiograph. The patient is slightly kyphotic at the C4-C5 level. B, Post-treatment (after specific adjustments) radiograph. The curve is now in a more lordotic configuration.

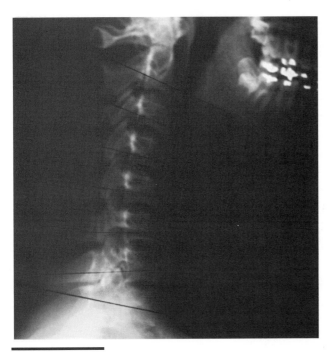

Figure 8.118. Postero-inferior (-θX,-Z) C7. Kyphotic cervical curve.

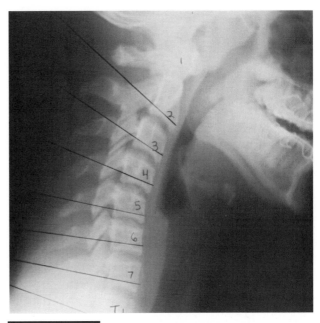

Figure 8.120. Postero-inferior (-θX,-Z) C7. Kyphotic cervical curve.

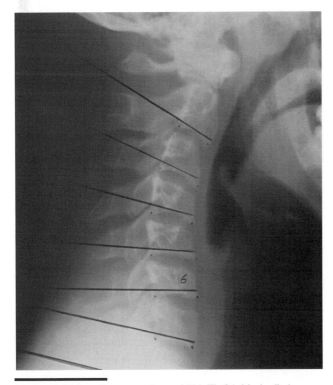

Figure 8.119. Postero-inferior (-θX,-Z) C6. Markedly kyphotic cervical curve.

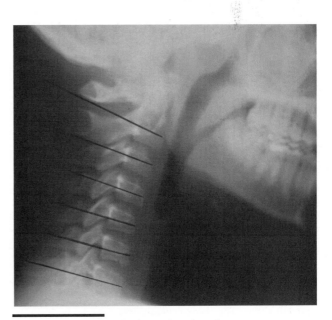

Figure 8.121. Straight (i.e., military) neck posture.

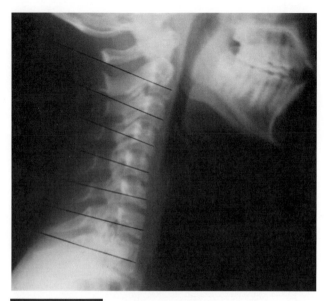

Figure 8.122.   A lordotic-kyphotic-lordotic cervical curve C1-T1. Notice the hyperextension at the C1-C2 level.

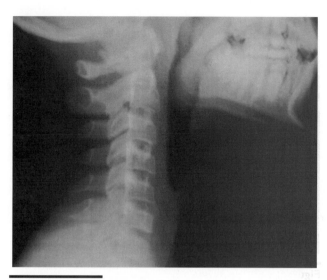

Figure 8.125.   Antero-superior (-θX) positioning of C1. The curve is mildly kyphotic at C3-C4.

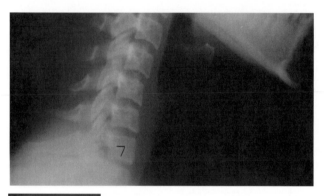

Figure 8.123.   Postero-inferior (-θX,-Z) C7. Notice the small interspinous space between C7-T1. Compare to C6-C7.

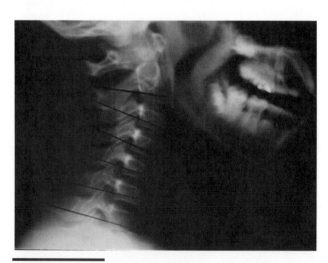

Figure 8.124.   The child's cervical curve is in a kyphotic (lower) and lordotic (upper) posture.

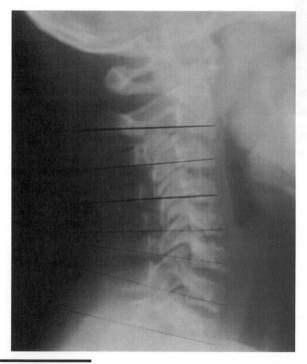

Figure 8.126.   Anterior (+Z) translation of C1 is present ("V" sign). The cervical curve is lordotic (lower) and kyphotic (upper).

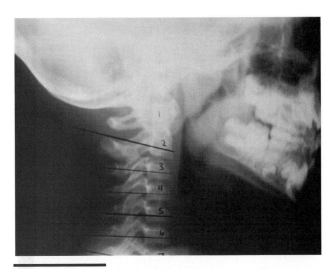

Figure 8.127. Anterior (+Z) translation of C2 is present in this patient with no cervical lordosis.

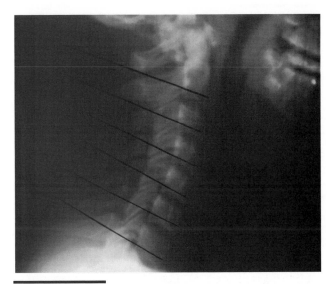

Figure 8.128. Decreased lordosis at C5-C7 with hyperextension (-θX) of C1.

(Fig. 8.131). Hyperactivity of the quadratus lumborum, internal derangement of the disc, or contractures of the iliolumbar ligaments or intertranversarii muscles could all potentially cause Type 3 motion.

In Type four motion, there is failure of the motion segment to laterally bend or have normal Y-axis rotational coupled motion (Fig. 8.132). Grice (256) theorizes that this type of motion dysfunction is due to ligamentous injury or internal disc derangement. Marked multifidi involvement or combined multifidi-intertransversarii spasm may also be causative factors (256).

Analysis of lumbar intervertebral motion is considered important in the etiology, diagnosis and treatment of many spinal pathologies (257). Figures 8.133 through 8.136 demonstrate several potential findings in the case of a disc lesion or

other musculo–ligamentous dysfunction affecting the motion segment (254). Lateral bending radiographs of the lumbar spine of two patients are shown in Figures 8.137 to 8.139.

Flexion–Extension Stress Radiographs of the Lumbar Spine. Various investigators have provided measurement systems for

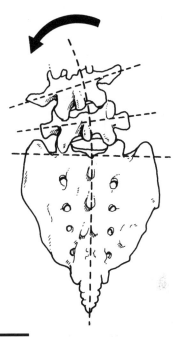

Figure 8.129. Type 1. Normal motion at L4-L5. Side bending is associated with spinous rotation (Y-axis) towards the ipsilateral side of bend.

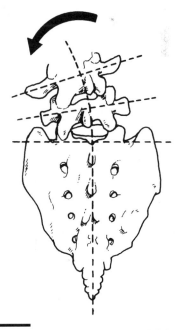

Figure 8.130. Type 2. Normal motion at L5. Lack of normal coupled motion at L4 during the main motion of side bending.

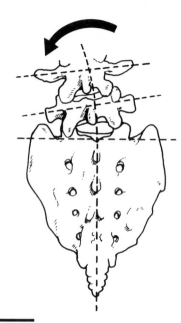

Figure 8.131.   Type 3. Normal motion at L5. Lack of side bending at L4. Spinous rotation towards the concave side of bend is still present.

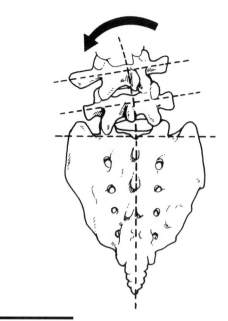

Figure 8.132.   Type 4. Normal motion at L5. No lateral flexion or coupled Y-axis rotation during side bending at L4.

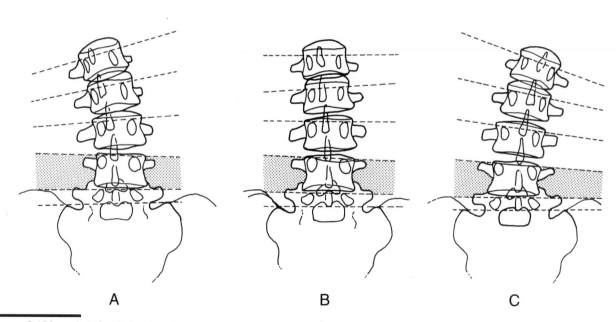

A   B   C

Figure 8.133.   A, Left side bending showing no lateral flexion at L4-L5 due to disc herniation at L4-L5. B, Standing neutral posture. C, Right side bending. Modified from Weitz EM. The lateral bending sign. Spine 1981; 6:391.

analyzing translational (Z-axis) and rotational (X-axis) movements on lateral lumbar radiographs. Movements of the cervical spine during flexion and extension can also be analyzed for the presence of hypermobility and hypomobility. In pediatric patients who have substantial ligamentous injury, radiological signs of instability or hypermobility may be present. Lumbar spine instability in the adult has been studied

by Dupuis (258); however, investigation of the natural history for this disorder is not available in the pediatric population. Because progressive instability of the lumbar spine is basically a chronic disease, effects may not be seen until late adolescence. Acute instability, capable of causing neurological injury with normal movements of the patient, is a complex discussion and is beyond the scope of this chapter.

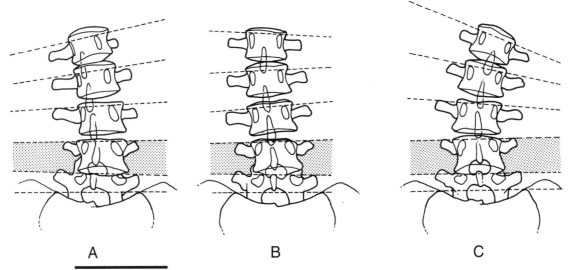

Figure 8.134. A, Left side bending. B, Standing neutral posture. C, Right side bending. Modified from Weitz EM. The lateral bending sign. Spine 1981; 6:392.

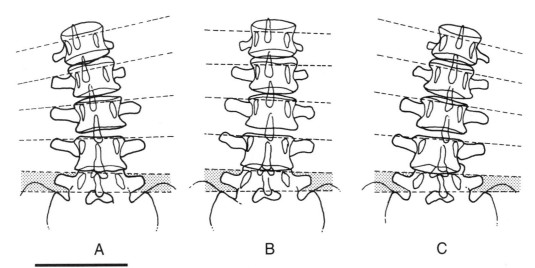

Figure 8.135. A, Left side bending. B, Standing neutral posture. C, Right side bending. Modified from Weitz EM. The lateral bending sign. Spine 1981; 6:392.

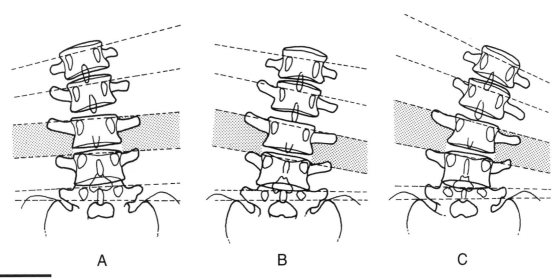

Figure 8.136. A, Left side bending. There is lateral disc herniation at L3-L4. B, Standing upright neutral posture. C, Right side bending. There is also a midline disc herniation at L4-L5 but this does not restrict lateral flexion at that level. Modified from Weitz EM. The lateral bending sign. Spine 1981; 6:394.

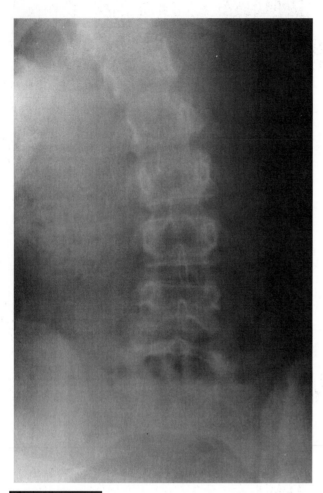

Figure 8.137. Left side bending in a 9-year-old female patient with back pain. There is decreased left lateral flexion (-θZ) and normal coupled rotation (-θY) at L5.

Lateral Bending Stress Radiographs of the Thoracic Spine. The thoracic spine can be analyzed in lateral flexion for the presence of fixation dysfunction and/or abnormal coupling patterns. The normal coupled motion of Y-axis rotation results in the spinous process moving towards the contralateral side of bend (259) (Fig. 8.140A–D). As lateral flexion of the spine moves to the more caudad thoracic motion segments, there is very little coupled motion. Y-axis rotation is very limited at the lower thoracic levels and the coupling patterns of Y-axis rotation likely approaches zero at T12 and then moves to an opposite pattern in the upper and lower lumbar spine. When analysis is made of thoracic motion lateral flexion, the lumbar spine should not be laterally flexed with the lower thoracic elements. Three cases of lateral bending dysfunction of the thoracic spine are presented in Figures 8.141 to 8.143.

Flexion–Extension Radiographs of the Cervical Spine. Acute unstable injuries of the cervical spine can be detected radiographically, although radiological signs of vertebral displacement may not be present for spinal cord injuries to have occurred (see SCIWORA). In the case of stress radiographs of

the cervical spine in an acutely injured patient, only active flexion should be obtained, and then, only after careful scrutiny of the lateral radiograph for signs of fracture, dislocation, or marked subluxation. The reader is cautioned that passive movements of the head towards flexion in the presence of a transverse ligament rupture could cause serious neurological injury or prove fatal for the patient. Stress movements of the cervical spine may provide the clinician with important information regarding fixation dysfunction or signs of hypermobility at the motion segment.

Lateral Bending of the Cervical Spine. Lateral bending and coupled motions of Y-axis rotation can be analyzed from lateral bending radiographs of the cervical spine. As with the lumbar spine, four patterns of movements are typically encountered. In Type 1 or normal motion the vertebral bodies tilt towards the ipsilateral side of bend with Y-axis coupled motion that results in the spinous process moving towards the convex side of lateral bend (Fig. 8.144).

Type 2 motion involves only an abnormal coupling pattern of the spinous process moving towards the side of tilt. Normal lateral flexion remains (Fig. 8.145).

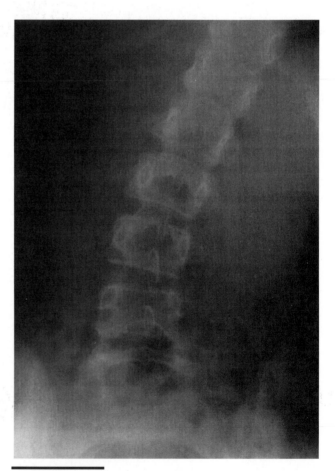

Figure 8.138. Same patient as in Figure 8.156. Right side bending. There appears to be increased right lateral flexion (+θZ) at the L4-L5 level.

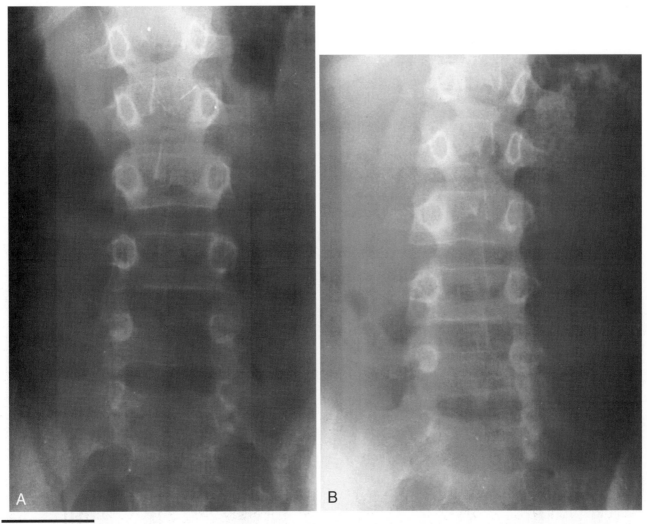

Figure 8.139. A, Left side bending in an 11-year-old male with back pain. There is decreased lateral flexion (-θZ) at L4-L5 and

L5-S1. B, Same patient as in Figure 8.158A. Right side bending. There is decreased right lateral flexion (+θZ) at L5-S1.

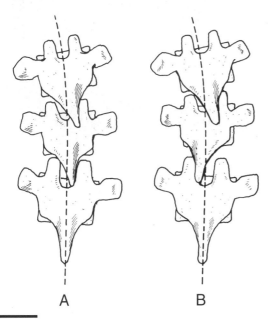
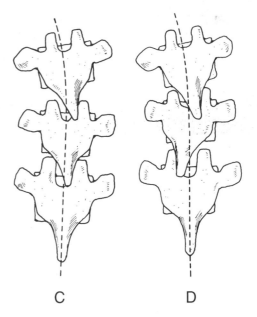

Figure 8.140. A, Normal motion (Type 1). With lateral flexion as the first direction of movement, there is coupled rotation of the spinous process to the convex side of bend. B, Absent

coupled motion. C, Absent lateral flexion but coupled Y-axis rotation motion is present. D, Absent lateral flexion and coupled Y-axis rotation.

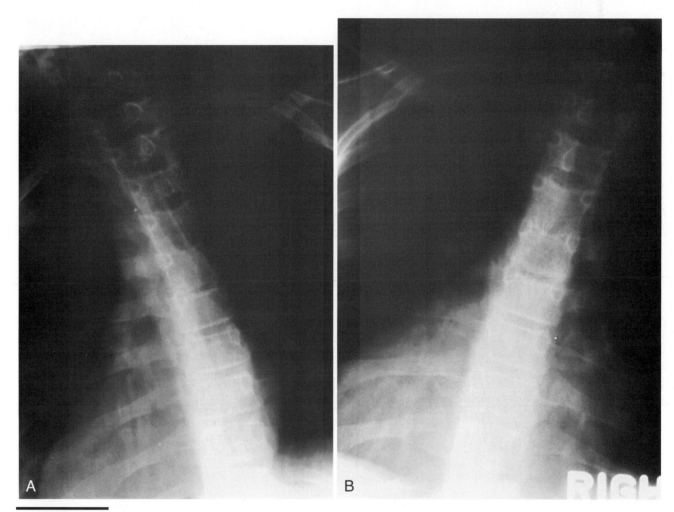

Figure 8.141. A, 10-year-old male. Left side bending. Relatively normal motion is present, The patient is likely bending the upper portion of the lumbar spine with the thoracic spine.

B, Right side bending. Decreased right lateral flexion (+θZ) motion is present at T2-T3, T4-T5 and T6-T7.

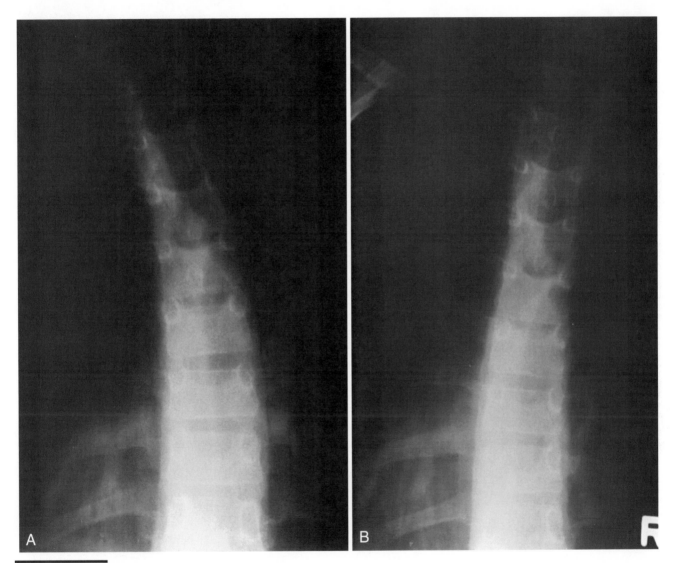

Figure 8.142.   A, Eleven year old male. Left side bending. There is decreased left lateral flexion (-θZ) at T4-T5. B, Right side bending. There is decreased right lateral flexion (+θZ) at T5-T6, T6-T7 and T9-T10.

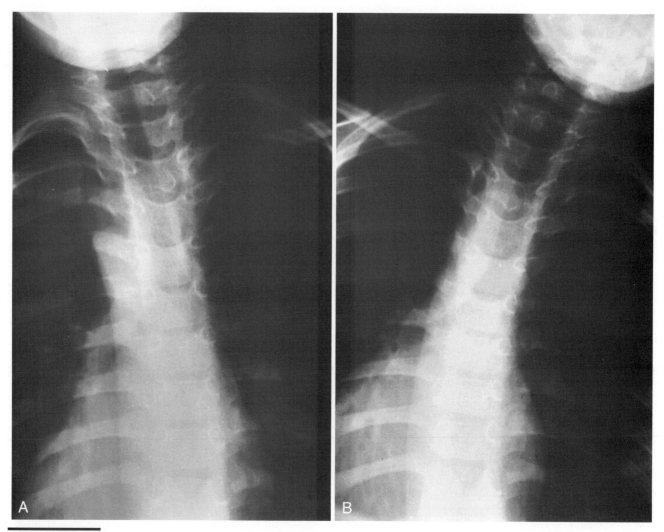

Figure 8.143.   A, Six year old male. Left side bending. There is decreased left lateral flexion (-θZ) at T8-T9-T10. B, Right side bending. There is decreased right lateral flexion (+θZ) at T4-T5.

Decreased coupled spinous rotation to the convexity (-θY) is also present at T4.

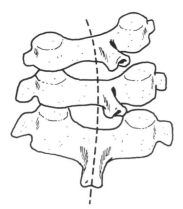

Figure 8.144.   Type 1. Normal lateral flexion and coupled Y-axis rotation.

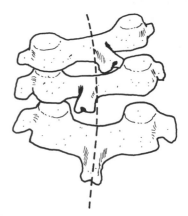

Figure 8.145.   Type 2. Normal lateral flexion. Middle segment does not have normal coupled motion.

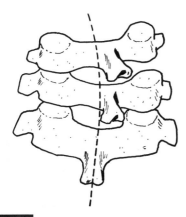

Figure 8.146. Type 3. Absent lateral flexion but coupled rotation remains at the middle segment.

Type 3 motion displays normal coupled movement of the spinous process, but there is restriction in the range of lateral flexion (Fig. 8.146).

Type 4 motion is ascribed to a motion segment that is not exhibiting lateral flexion or proper coupling motion (Fig. 8.147). Figures 8.148A, B and 8.149A,B depict two patients with lateral bending dysfunction of the lower cervical and upper thoracic spine.

Clinical Radiologic Case Studies

The following brief radiologic case studies are from one chiropractor's outpatient clinic. The practitioner used the exam findings of tenderness and edema, skin temperature asymmetries detected through a bilateral thermocouple device, and fixation dysfunction determined through intersegmental range of motion palpation, as well as symptomatology to determine the motion segment(s) involved. The radiograph was then used to determine the primary segment involved and the listing for adjustive correction.

Most illustrations are from sectional radiographs with a 1200 screen/film speed. The technique for the specific contact, short lever arm adjustments provided was Gonstead (260). All thrusts were of high velocity and short amplitude. For further examination/adjustment information please consult Chapter 9.

S1, S2, AND S3 SUBLUXATION

This 5-year-old Latino male patient has an alteration in gait and posture of the lower extremities. He walks with his feet turned inward (i.e., pigeon toed). There is an apparent retrolisthesis of S3 in relation to S2 (Fig. 8.150). These same findings are present between S2 and S1. There is a grade 1 spondylolisthesis of L5 (see Chapter 19). Separation of the pars interarticularis is demonstrable on the lateral projection. Oblique radiographs were not taken because they have low diagnostic/therapeutic yield. The AP radiograph was unremarkable.

CLINICAL COURSE

The patient was adjusted two times at S3, one time at S2 and three times at S1 in the side posture position over a one month period. Adjustments were initiated at S3 because of the posterior widening of the rudimentary disc space between S3 and S2 and the fact that S3–S2 serves as a foundation motion segment to S2–S1. After a therapeutic trial the doctor determined the primary or major subluxation in this patient was the L5–S1 motion segment. The contact point was the SI tubercle and this segment was translated forward (+Z) coupled with a slight flexion (+θX) movement. The patient's feet position returned to a straight position.

C1, C7, S2, AND S3 SUBLUXATION

This 8-year-old white male has had severe sinus symptoms and chronic ear infections for five years. He has near constant bronchial congestion. The child has had tympanostomy tubes placed in both ear drums. Medical recommendations included surgery for the sinus condition which prompted the referral of the child for chiropractic evaluation. Both the sinus problems and the ear infections were controlled through chiropractic adjustments at motion segments exhibiting signs of subluxation. The lateral lumbar radiograph demonstrates a posterior widening of the rudimentary disc between S1 and S2 and between S2 and S3 (Fig. 8.151). The lateral cervical radiograph discloses a reduction in the cervical lordosis with slight extension of the C1–C2 motion segment (Fig. 8.152). C7 is displaced posteriorly (-Z) and is extended (-θX).

CLINICAL COURSE

The patient was adjusted at C1 in the seated position. The side posture position was used to adjust the sacral segments. Over a 2-week period, three adjustments were administered at C1, two adjustments at S3 and two adjustments at S2. The upper cervical and sacral adjustments are thought to primarily affect the parasympathetic divisions of the autonomic nervous system (261,262) and are more related to disorders such as otitis media, nocturnal enuresis and certain types of asthma (33). After 2 weeks of care the otitis media in this patient resolved. The

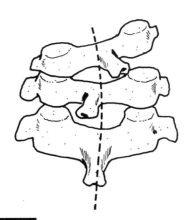

Figure 8.147. Type 4. Absent lateral flexion and coupled rotation at the middle segment.

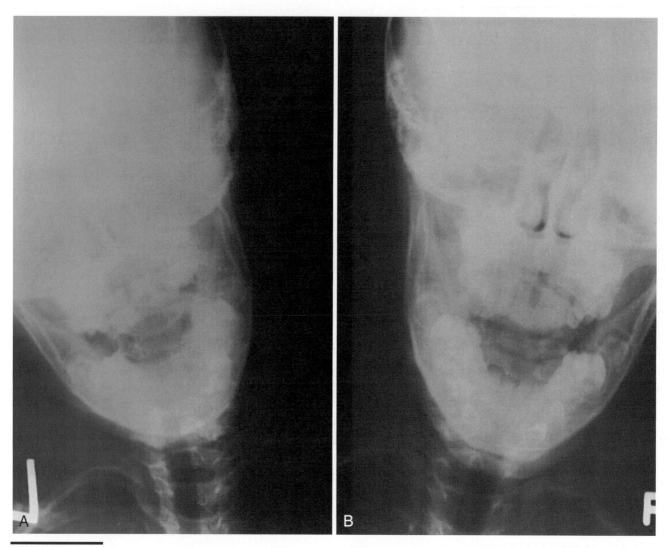

Figure 8.148.   A, 6-year-old male. Left side bending. More lateral flexion of the upper cervical spine is evident when compared to the radiograph of right side bending (see Fig. 8.148B).

Decreased left lateral flexion (-θZ) is present at T2-T3. B, Right side bending. There is decreased right lateral flexion (+θZ) at the upper cervical region (C0-C1-C2) and at T1-T2.

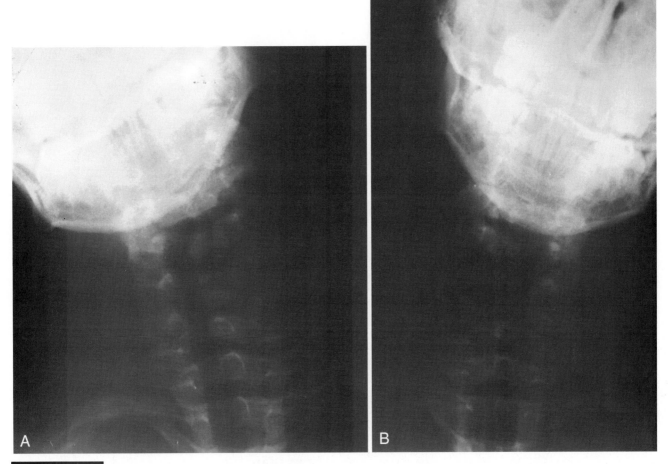

Figure 8.149. A, 11-year-old male. Left side bending. There is decreased left lateral flexion (-θZ) and coupled rotation (+θY) at C7-T1. B, Right side bending. There is decreased right lat-

eral flexion (+θZ) and coupled rotation (-θY) at T1. Decreased right lateral flexion (+θZ) is also present at C7.

patient was then adjusted on 14 occasions over a two and a half month period at C7 in the seated position. The patient began to notice improvement in his sinus congestion after the third adjustment to C7. The patient returns on an as needed basis, usually when his sinuses become congested. There has been no recurrent otitis media.

L3 AND L5 SUBLUXATION

This 15-year-old white female presented for chiropractic evaluation with complaints of dysmenorrhea, low back pain and right leg pain. The lateral lumbar radiograph demonstrates a slight retrolisthesis at L5 and L3 (Fig. 8.153). The AP lumbopelvic view discloses a left lateral flexion malposition (-θZ) at L3 with concomitant left spinous rotation (-θY) (Fig. 8.154). Left spinous rotation throughout the lower lumbar spine is consistent with the rotated sacrum subluxation P-R (-θY). The obturator foraminae are asymmetrical. The right obturator has an increased diagonal and base when compared to the left side. These findings are consistent with a PIEx (-θX,+ θY) ilium misalignment on the right and an ASIn (+θX, +θY) ilium misalignment on the left. The right lesser trochanter appears to be slightly larger than the left. This could

be due to (-θY) malpositioning of the patient or external rotation of the right femur. However, the pelvic misalignments listed are the opposite displacements that would result from -θY malpositioning.

CLINICAL COURSE

The patient was initially adjusted at L5 over the course of six visits. Then, she was adjusted three times at L3 over a 1-month period. All adjustments were performed in the side posture position. Although both segments were subluxated initially, adjustments were begun at L5 only because this was considered the foundational subluxation and was more related to the low back and leg pain. It is likely that a change in the lower lumbar position will have a greater effect on the overall posture of the spine, than a more cephalad motion segment.

After the first adjustment, the low back pain completely resolved. The leg pain was absent by the sixth visit. Adjustments were begun at L3 during the patient's menstrual cycle. No cramping occurred during this cycle.

The patient moved out of state and was lost to follow-up. The right sacroiliac joint exhibited fixation dysfunction which was not addressed during the 4 weeks she was under care. Had

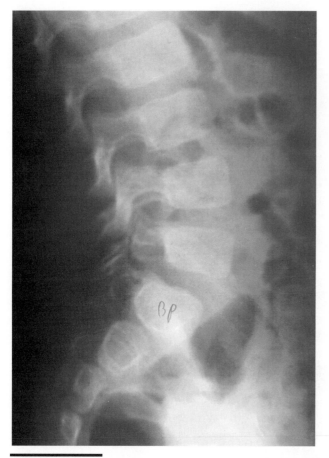

Figure 8.150.

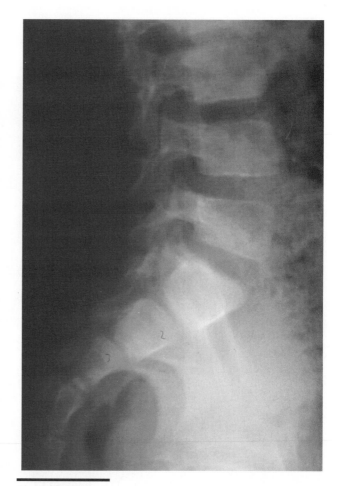

Figure 8.151.

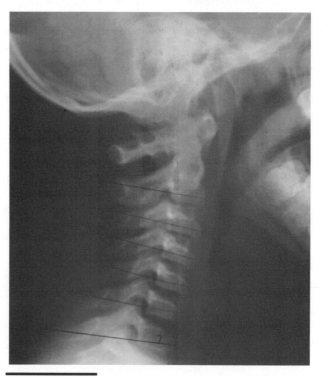

Figure 8.152.

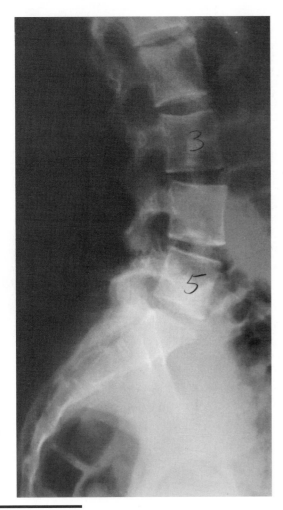

Figure 8.153.

she resumed care, then adjustments to the sacrum misalignment (P-R, -θY) would likely have been performed. This subluxation would be adjusted to decrease the overall Y axis rotation of the lower lumbar spine and to provide more stability (e.g., more symmetrical loading) for the L5–S1 and L3–L4 motion segments.

C5, C7, AND S2 SUBLUXATION

This 11-yr-old white female presented with complaints of low back pain, nocturnal enuresis and a bilateral inward foot flare. The lateral lumbar radiograph demonstrates a posterior S2 subluxation (Fig. 8.155). There are also multiple endplate invaginations in the lumbar spine, consistent with a history of compressive loading. The patient related falling off her bicycle onto her buttocks on several occasions. She also recalled falling from a tree on one occasion onto her buttocks.

On the AP lumbopelvic radiograph there is a measured deficiency of 5 mm on the left (Fig. 8.156). A slight rotation of the sacrum is present (△ to "P₂-R"). There is a slight rotation of the lumbar spine (-θY) that is more marked at the upper lumbar levels.

The lateral cervical radiograph demonstrates a kyphotic cervical spine with a "V" sign present at the atlanto-dental-interval (Fig. 8.157). The atlas is listed as AI (+θX) and there is extension (-θX) present at C5, C6 and C7.

CLINICAL COURSE

The patient was adjusted at S2 on eight visits over 3 months. The patient related an improvement in the nocturnal enuresis after two adjustments at the S2 level. After three months the nocturnal enuresis and low back pain had resolved. She was adjusted at C7 four times, then at C5 for eleven visits over a three month period. The cervical adjustments were performed in the seated position and the sacral adjustments were done in the side posture position.

C5 AND C6 SUBLUXATION

This 12-year-old white male presented for chiropractic evaluation with asthmatic symptoms, allergies and sinusitis. The lateral cervical radiograph demonstrates a reduction in the cervical lordosis (Fig. 8.158). Notice the endplate lines at C5 and C6 that disclose hyperextension (-θX) malposition of C5 and to a lesser extent at C6. Antero-posterior full spine radiographs were unremarkable.

CLINICAL COURSE

The patient was adjusted at C6 in the seated position. The patient received two adjustments over a one week period. C5 was to be adjusted but the patient discontinued care. The

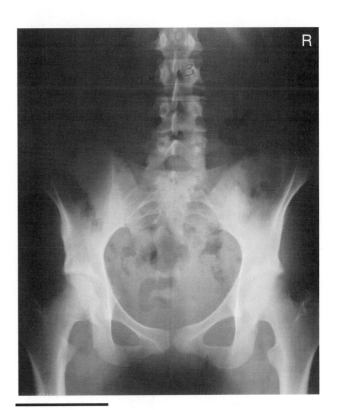

Figure 8.154.

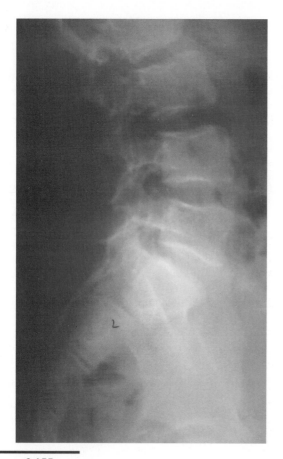

Figure 8.155.

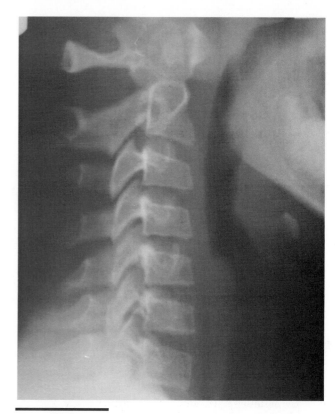

Figure 8.157.

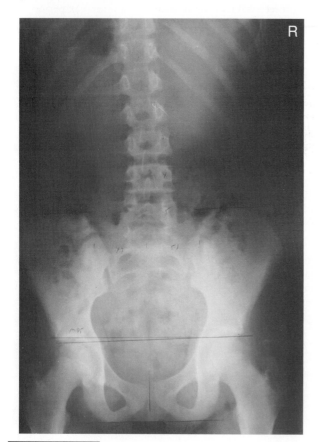

Figure 8.156.

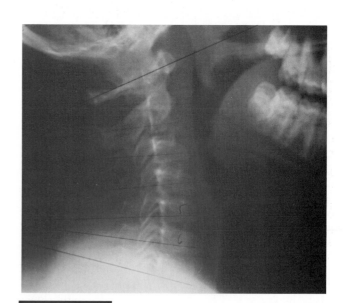

Figure 8.158.

patient's father had wanted the patient to receive chiropractic care but the patient's mother did not, indicating that he only needed medical care for his problems.

C3 SUBLUXATION

In 1993 this 6-year-old Latino female presented for chiropractic evaluation with a complaint of severe eye allergies (i.e., chronic vernal conjunctivitis) that she has had for three years duration. The lateral cervical radiograph demonstrates a retrolisthesis (-Z) and hyperextension (-θX) misalignment at C3 (Fig. 8.159). There is also a reduction in the cervical lordosis. The APOM was unremarkable.

The patient has a pine cone-like texture growth under her right upper eyelid, causing a corneal abrasion. Symptoms include severe pain and reduced vision. Any irritant causes a stabbing eye pain with swelling and irritation to her right eye for three days following a stimulus. Her past history for this problem included visits to 14 different medical doctors including various pediatricians, ophthalmologists and other eye specialists, allergists, homeopathic doctors, and emergency room physicians. Eye surgery had been performed in 1992. The patient had been prescribed eye drops, corticosteroids, antihistamines, antibiotics, antibacterial drops, and allergy injections for eight months. This patient's subluxation could have resulted from any number of several significant traumas that the child had encountered during her young life prior to the onset of the eye symptoms. Her past history included an incident where she dove head first from a high-chair on to the kitchen floor, resulting in a minor concussion. The patient had fallen down a staircase and

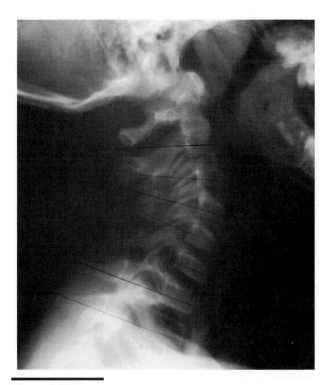

Figure 8.159.

impacted onto a railing that resulted in seven stitches from a forehead laceration. She had also fallen from a jungle gym at school and hit her mouth on the bottom bar. This mechanism of injury alone could have easily produced a hyperextension subluxation of C3. She sustained a cut to the gums that required six stitches. During one six month period the patient had experienced six black eyes ranging from injuries such as diving from a table into a room to tripping over her feet and hitting her head on a nearby chair.

CLINICAL COURSE

The patient was adjusted at C3 in the seated position. She received twelve adjustments over the course of one month in the summer of 1993 and returned to her home in Spain until the following summer in 1994, when she received three adjustments. The patient related that her symptoms were resolved up to the spring of 1994, when they had subsequently returned, but with decreased severity. The patient desired being treated on more than one occasion but intercontinental travel prevented this. At the time of this writing (early 1995), the patient's symptomatology was not totally resolved but the severity had been reduced. The frequency and duration of pain had been reduced since initiating chiropractic care. At the beginning of care the child appeared very sad and withdrawn. Following treatments this behavior changed to that of a more normal 6-year-old girl who was feeling healthy.

C1 AND C6 SUBLUXATION

This 17-year-old white male presented for chiropractic evaluation with a complaint of deafness in the right ear since the age of 4. The patient had suffered marked head and neck trauma at the age of 3. He has additional complaints of neck pain, headaches, allergies and sinusitis.

The lateral cervical radiograph demonstrates a kyphotic posture of the cervical spine (Fig. 8.160). The endplate lines disclose hyperextension (-θX) at C6. Notice the increase in disc space height at the anterior aspect of this motion segment.

The APOM demonstrates a lateral flexion malposition of C1-C2 (Fig. 8.161). There is a slight increase in the width of the right lateral mass consistent with anterior rotation (+θY) on that side. The atlas is listed as ASRA (+Z,- θX, -θZ,+ θY). Additional radiographs of the full spine were unremarkable.

CLINICAL COURSE

The patient was adjusted at C6 in the seated position. The patient received eleven adjustments over a 6-week period. Following the first adjustment, the patient noticed a decrease in neck pain. At 6 weeks, there was a complete resolution of the neck pain, headaches and sinus problems. No appreciable change in the deafness was noticed while under care. The patient moved out of state and was lost to further follow-up.

C4 AND S2 SUBLUXATION

This 6-year-old white female presented for chiropractic evaluation with complaints of leg cramps and headaches. The lateral cervical radiograph demonstrates slight hyperextension (-θX) and retrolisthesis (-Z) at C4 as evidenced by the convergence

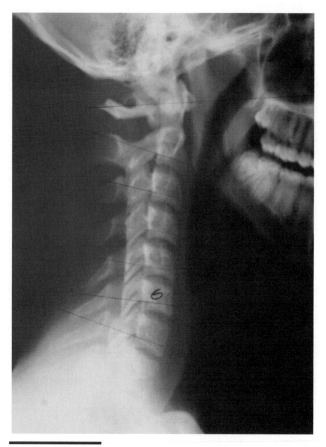

Figure 8.160.

of the endplate lines (Fig. 8.162). These findings are present to a lesser extent at C3 and also at C2.

The lateral lumbar radiograph discloses a posterior S2 subluxation (Fig. 8.163). There is widening of the posterior aspect of the rudimentary disc between S1 and S2. The patient was malpositioned slightly for this exposure creating the double George's line appearance throughout the lumbar spine.

CLINICAL COURSE

The patient was adjusted at C4 in the seated position. She received eight adjustments over a one month period with a complete resolution of symptomatology. Her headaches improved after the first adjustment but did not completely resolve until the eighth visit. Adjustments to S2 were performed in the side posture position. A total of five adjustments to S2 were provided. After the third S2 adjustment, the leg cramps had resolved. The patient received an additional two adjustments at S2 while asymptomatic because of persistent edema at S2 and hypomobility during extension of the lumbar spine. The patient maintains an active lifestyle, (e.g., roller skating, falls, etc.) and returns for care on an as needed basis.

C6, L3 AND ILIUM SUBLUXATION

This 17-year-old white female presented for chiropractic evaluation with a primary compliant of dysmenorrhea (e.g.,

painful cramping). She has secondary complaints of headaches and sinusitis. The lateral cervical radiograph demonstrates a kyphotic posture of the cervical spine (Fig. 8.164). Notice the severe hyperextension (-θX) malposition of C6 with concomitant retrolisthesis (-Z).

The AP cervical radiograph discloses a slight upper thoracic scoliosis that is somewhat compensated for in the mid cervical spine (Fig. 8.165). C6 is listed as a PRS.

The lateral lumbar radiograph shows a retrolisthesis (-Z) at L3 (Fig. 8.166). There is also a healed and fused subluxation between S4 and S5

The AP lumbopelvic radiograph demonstrates a right convex lumbar scoliosis consistent with a measured deficiency of 9 mm and an actual deficiency of 11 mm on the right (Fig. 8.167). The right ilium lists as PI3In7 and the left ilium as AS3Ex7. The third lumbar is listed as PLI-m (−Z, −θY, −θZ).

CLINICAL COURSE

The patient was adjusted at C6 in the seated position. She received thirteen adjustments over a two month period with a complete resolution of the headaches and sinus symptoms. The patient was also adjusted thirteen times at L3, initially in the side posture position, but later with greater ease at the knee-chest table. The patient's flexible lumbar spine was more easily accommodated for the adjustment in the knee-chest position. The menstrual cramps were improved during the course of treatment but the patient found the care to be too time consuming (she was a first year college student). There was no further follow-up of this patient.

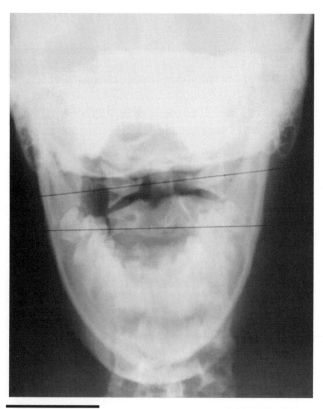

Figure 8.161.

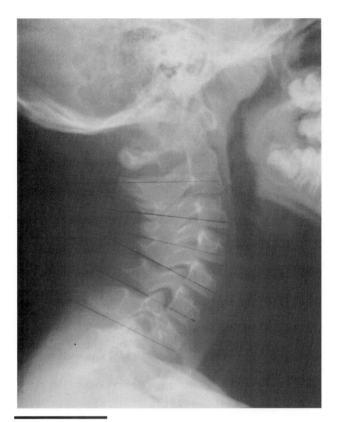

Figure 8.162.

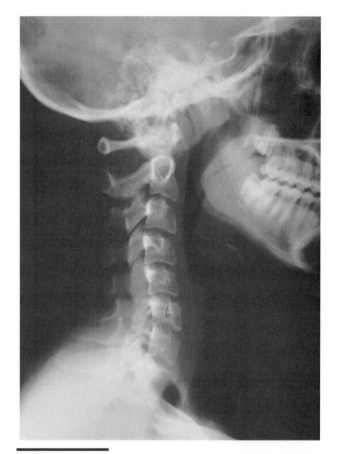

Figure 8.164.

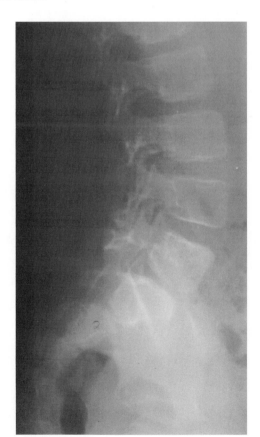

Figure 8.163.

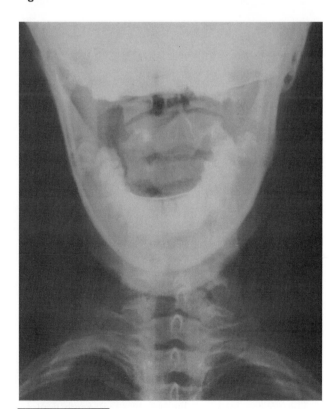

Figure 8.165.

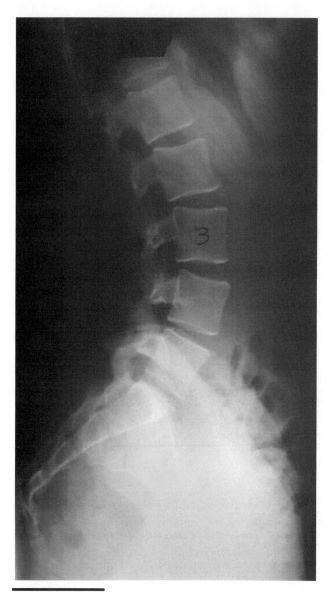

Figure 8.166.

C2, S2, AND ILIUM SUBLUXATION

This 9-year-old white male presented for chiropractic evaluation with complaints of neck pain and severe bilateral toe-in foot flare, which the patient has had since birth. The history included multiple episodes of otitis media with myringotomy at the age of 4. The patient has no current ear problems. The lateral cervical radiograph demonstrates a hypolordosis with a slight retrolisthesis (−Z) and hyperextension (−θX) malposition at C2 (Fig. 8.168).

The pre-treatment lateral lumbar radiograph demonstrates an accentuated lumbar lordosis with a posterior S2 misalignment (Fig. 8.169) (compare to Fig. 8.171).

The pre-treatment AP lumbopelvic radiograph demonstrates a mild left convex thoracolumbar scoliosis (Fig. 8.170).

CLINICAL COURSE

The patient was adjusted at C2 in the seated position on twenty-six occasions over a twelve month period. After these adjustments, there was complete resolution to the neck pain. After the third adjustment, the patient related an improvement in neck pain which was usually constant. The patient had also developed a pattern of self manipulation of the cervical spine prior to initiating care in an attempt to reduce the neck pain. The patient followed through with the lengthy course of care in order to achieve a complete reduction in symptomatology and the related clinical subluxation findings.

The patient was adjusted 20 times in the side posture position at S2. The left ilium was adjusted as an Ex (−θY) on 12 visits with the involved side towards the side posture table.

The bilateral toe-in foot flare improved but did not completely resolve. It appeared to be worsened following certain sporting activities. This postural finding was of 9 years duration. The patient had tried reversing shoes, braces and ankle-leg casts. All procedures had failed and the patient was subsequently referred for chiropractic evaluation.

The post-treatment lateral lumbar radiograph demonstrates a slight decrease in the lumbar lordosis and a slight reduction in the posterior S2 subluxation (Fig. 8.171).

The post-treatment or comparative AP lumbopelvic radiograph (Fig. 8.172) discloses a reduction in the thoracolumbar scoliosis.

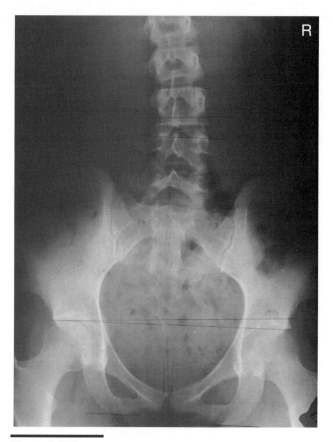

Figure 8.167.

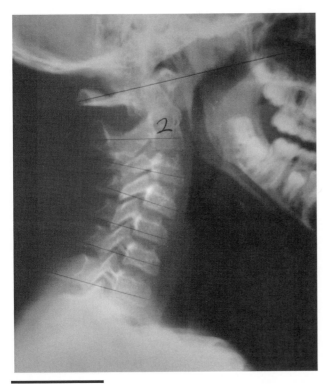

Figure 8.168.

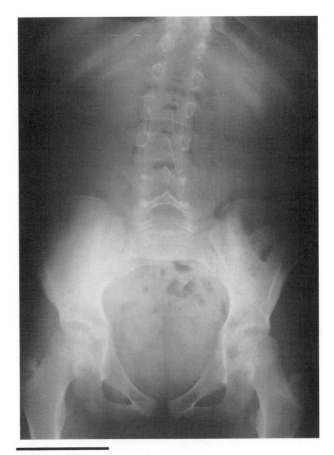

Figure 8.170.

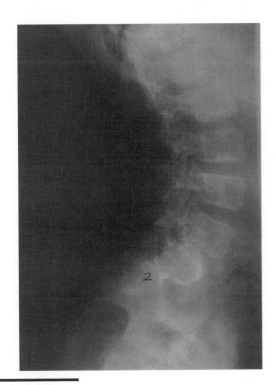

Figure 8.169.

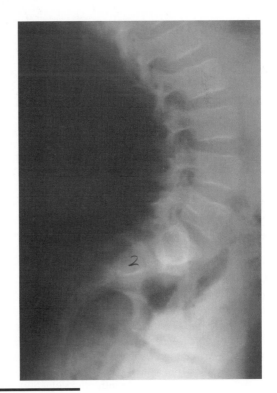

Figure 8.171.

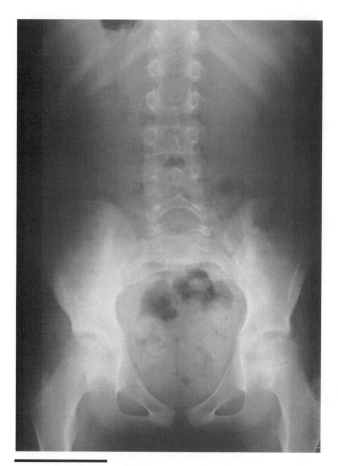

Figure 8.172.

C5 SUBLUXATION

This is a 4-year-old white male with scoliosis and sinus congestion. The lateral cervical radiograph discloses a hyper-extension ($-\theta X$) subluxation at C5 (Fig. 8.173). There is also an increase in the atlanto dental interval. The AP cervical view of this patient shows that the cervical spine is not compensating for the lateral deviation in the thoracic spine (Fig. 8.174). The AP thoracic radiograph discloses the moderate thoracolumbar scoliosis and the AP lumbopelvic view discloses a lateral flexion malposition at L3, perhaps contributing to the lateral deviation above (Fig. 8.175). L3 is listed as PLS ($-Z$, $-\theta Y$, $+\theta Z$).

The lateral lumbar radiograph demonstrates a posterior S2 subluxation with a widening of the posterior aspect of the rudimentary disc space between S1 and S2 (Fig. 8.176).

CLINICAL COURSE

The patient was adjusted at C5 in the seated position on 20 occasions over a two and a half year period. The sinus congestion resolved after ten adjustments although if the child gets a cold, then the sinuses are troublesome. One to two adjustments usually makes the patient asymptomatic again. The patient returns on an as needed basis only and other segments of the spine are adjusted when indicated. Follow-up (approx. 4 yr) full spine radiographs indicate a reduction in the scoliosis on the AP view (Fig. 8.177). The lateral view demonstrates a persistent S2 subluxation (Fig. 8.178).

C1 AND S2 SUBLUXATION

This is a 6-year-old black female patient with a history that includes frequent colds, headaches and sore throats. The patient also has a medialward deviation of both knees. The lateral cervical radiograph demonstrates a hypolordosis of the cervical spine with a slight increase in the ADI (Fig. 8.179). There is incomplete ossification of the posterior arch of atlas.

The AP cervical view demonstrates a lateral flexion mal-position at C1 (Fig. 8.180). The atlas is listed as ASRA ($+Z$, $-\theta X$, $-\theta Z$, $+\theta Y$). The AP radiographs of the full-spine in two exposures of the same patient demonstrate a slight scoliosis or convexity of the thoracic spine (Fig. 8.181). A close-up of the AP and lateral radiographs demonstrates spina bifida occulta at L1 and T12 (Fig. 8.182). The lateral of the lumbar spine demonstrates congenital absence of the spinous process at L1 and T12 and a S2–S1 misalignment (Fig. 8.183).

CLINICAL COURSE

The patient was adjusted at C1 in the seated position. She received 14 adjustments over a 6-month period. During this time, 10 adjustments were administered to S2 with the patient in the side posture position. There was a complete resolution of her symptomatology.

C3 SUBLUXATION

This 10-year-old white male presented for chiropractic evaluation with a complaint of neck pain. The patient actively participates in football and soccer. The pretreatment lateral

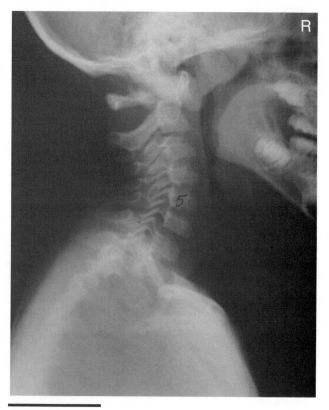

Figure 8.173.

(+θY) ilium was also adjusted twice during this time with the involved side towards the table. The patient's foot flare returned to normal after chiropractic care. The patient did not return for additional care or follow-up because of the time involved and distance to the chiropractor's clinic.

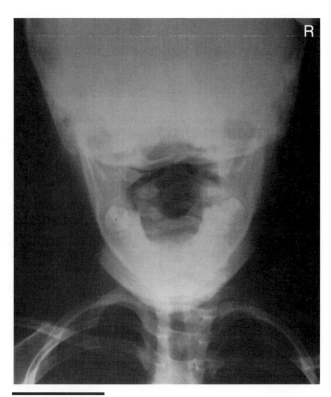

Figure 8.174.

cervical radiograph discloses a retrolisthesis of C3 with concomitant hyperextension of the vertebra (Fig. 8.184).

The patient was adjusted at C3 in the seated position. The patient received 22 adjustments over a 7-month period. There was complete resolution of his symptomatology. The post-treatment lateral cervical radiograph demonstrates a reduction in the C3 -Z misalignment (Fig. 8.185).

C2 AND ILIUM SUBLUXATION

This patient is a 4-year-old white female who had previously been diagnosed with a learning disability. The patient has a bilateral toe-in foot posture that is more pronounced on the right side. The lateral cervical radiograph demonstrates a slight posterior displacement of C2 (Fig. 8.186).

The AP cervical radiograph discloses a left head tilt that appears to be in compensation for a mild thoracic scoliosis below (Fig. 8.187). The AP lumbopelvic radiograph demonstrates a widening at the base of the right obturator foramen (Fig. 8.188). A right Ex ilium subluxation will create the foregoing obturator appearance and is consistent with the patient's right toe-in foot posture. The lateral lumbar radiograph of the same patient demonstrates a slight reduction in the lumbar lordosis at the upper lumbar levels (Fig. 8.189). The L4–L5 motion segment is the most anterior. There is a posterior S3 subluxation.

CLINICAL COURSE

The patient was adjusted at C2 in the seated position. She received two adjustments over a 2-month period. The Ex

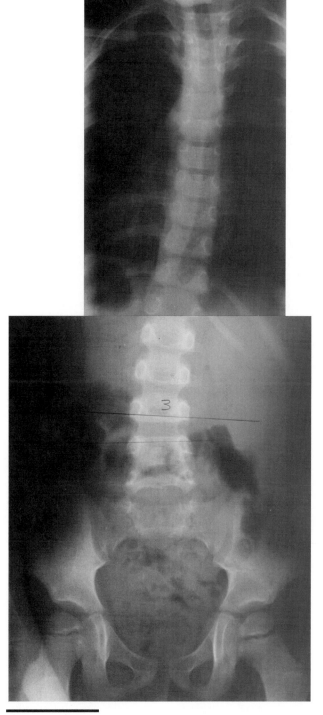

Figure 8.175.

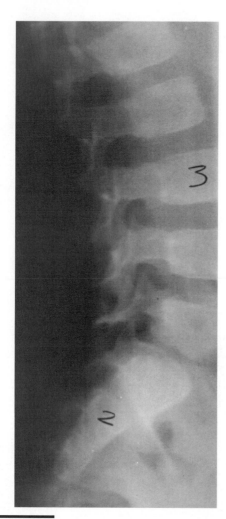

Figure 8.176.

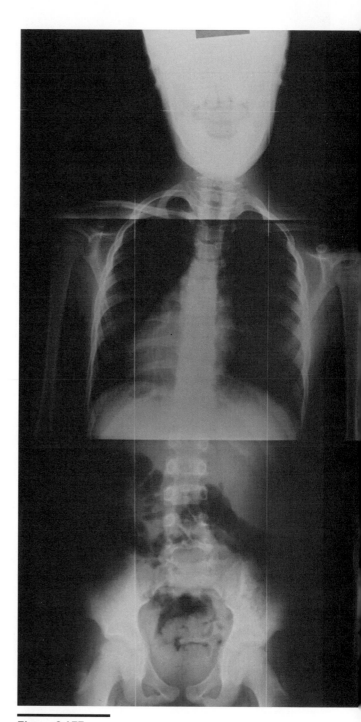

Figure 8.177.

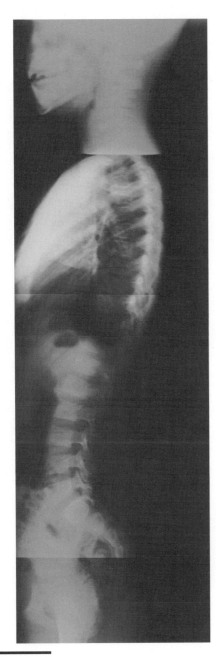

Figure 8.178.

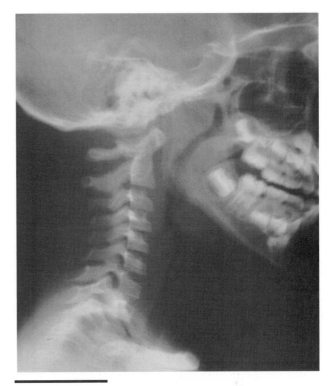

Figure 8.179.

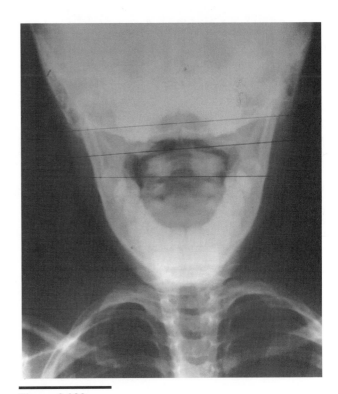

Figure 8.180.

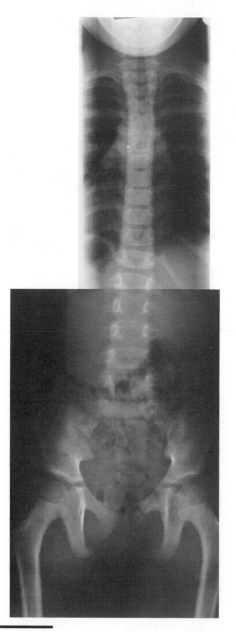

Figure 8.181.

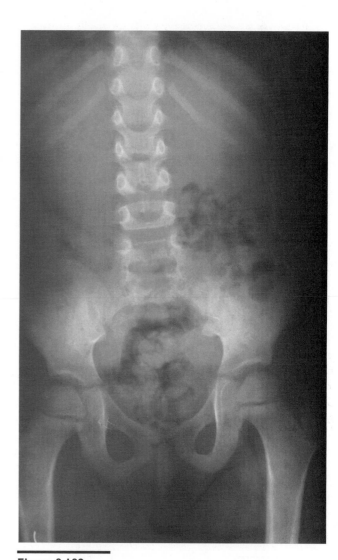

Figure 8.182.

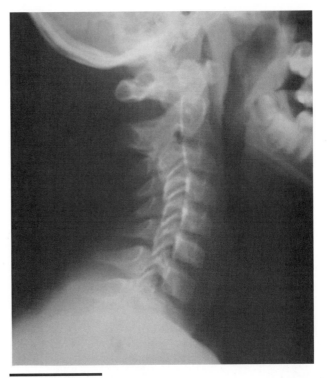

Figure 8.184.

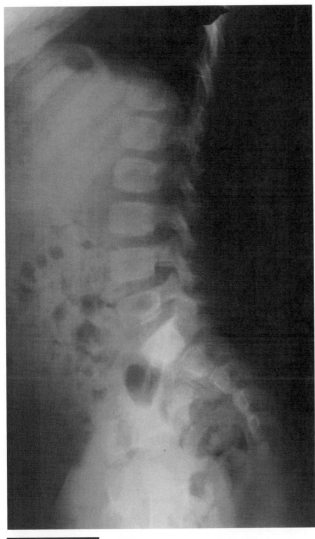

Figure 8.183.

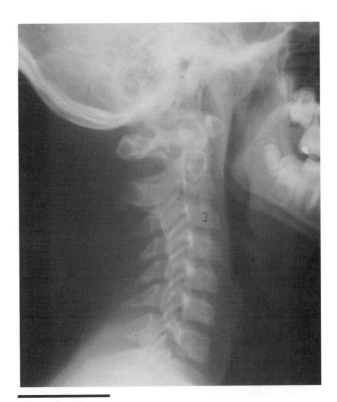

Figure 8.185.

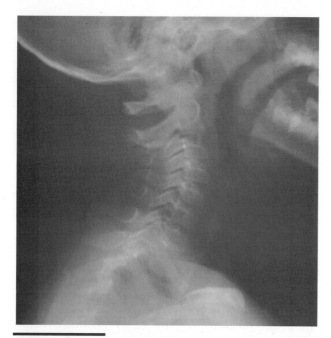

Figure 8.186.

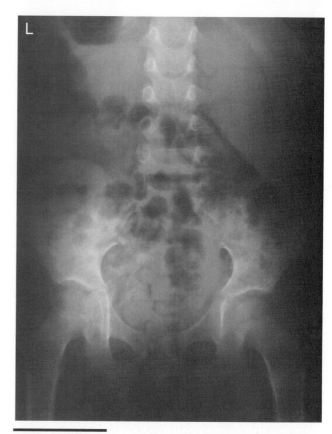

Figure 8.188.

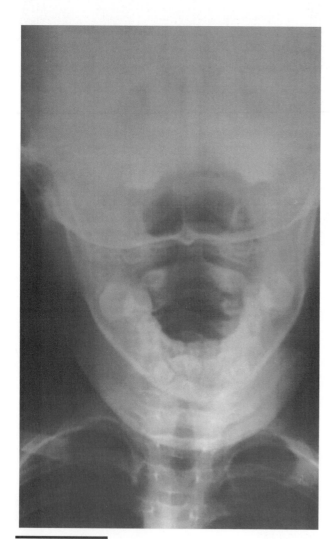

Figure 8.187.

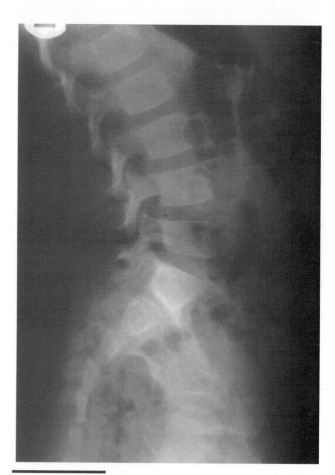

Figure 8.189.

S2 SUBLUXATION

This patient is a 5-year-old overweight Latino male. The primary history includes nocturnal enuresis. The lateral lumbar radiograph demonstrates a posterior S2 misalignment (Fig. 8.190).

The AP lumbopelvic radiograph discloses a left leg measured deficiency of 10 mm (Fig. 8.191). There is an AS1In3 ilium subluxation on the left. Both SI joints were found to be freely movable when motion palpated and were therefore not adjusted.

CLINICAL COURSE

The patient was adjusted at S2 in the prone position on the hi-lo table as well as in side posture. The patient received 30 adjustments over a 4-year period. After three adjustments the patient noticed a decrease in the frequency of the nocturnal enuresis. This case is particularly complicated by the fact that the patient participates in football, soccer, karate and judo. When the patient has fallen on his buttocks or suffers other type of trauma to the low back, he becomes symptomatic again. There has not been a total resolution of the nocturnal enuresis.

C5, C6, L2, AND SACRUM SUBLUXATION

This 13-year-old black male patient has complaints of severe allergies and migrainous headaches. The lateral cervical radio-

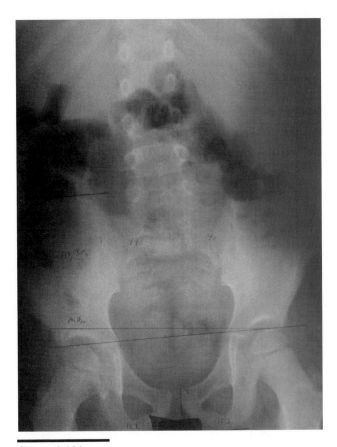

Figure 8.191.

graph demonstrates a kyphotic posture (Fig. 8.192). There is a hyperextension ($-\theta X$) subluxation at C5 and to a lesser extent at C6.

The AP cervical radiograph discloses slight right spinous rotation of the upper cervical spine, especially at C2 (Fig. 8.193). This appears to be compensatory for a very mild upper thoracic scoliosis. The AP lumbopelvic radiograph of the same patient demonstrates a mild right convex lumbar scoliosis (Fig. 8.194). There is asymmetry in the appearance of the obturator foraminae. The right obturator has findings of a decreased base and diagonal measurement. This is consistent with an ASIn ilium subluxation. The left obturator has findings (increased base width and increased diagonal measurement) consistent with a PIEx ilium subluxation. The lateral lumbar radiograph was unremarkable.

CLINICAL COURSE

The patient was adjusted at C6 in the seated position. He received six adjustments to this segment over two and a half years. After C6 was first adjusted, the chiropractor eventually moved up to C5, also adjusting this segment in the seated position. Thirty adjustments were administered to C5 over the two and one half year period. After the first adjustment the headaches resolved completely. After ten adjustments the patient began to notice a positive change in his allergies with less drainage of the sinuses. The patient also had a right sacroiliac joint fixation. The sacrum was adjusted as P-R ($-\theta Y$)

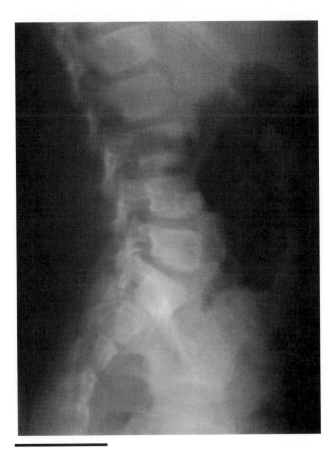

Figure 8.190.

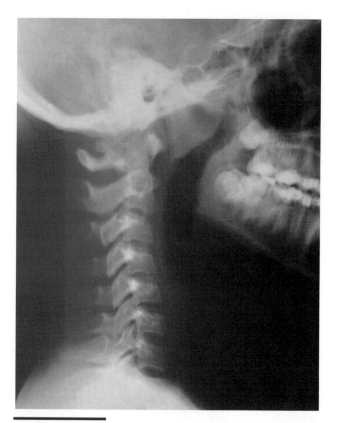

Figure 8.192.

in the side posture position. Ten adjustments were administered to the right SI joint over the two and one half year period. The patient was also adjusted at L2 on three occasions in the side posture position. There was a complete resolution of the patient's symptomatology.

C6 SUBLUXATION

This 12-year-old black female suffered neck trauma and presented for chiropractic evaluation with a complaint of headaches. The lateral cervical radiograph demonstrates a kyphotic cervical curve (Fig. 8.195). The AP radiograph of the cervical spine was unremarkable.

CLINICAL COURSE

The patient was adjusted at C6 in the seated position. The patient received 22 adjustments over a 10-month period. By the fourth adjustment, the patient noticed a diminution in her symptoms and by the fifteenth adjustment she was asymptomatic.

C3 SUBLUXATION

This 2-year-old white male was evaluated because of a history of recurrent otitis media with effusion. The lateral cervical radiograph demonstrates slight hyperextension of the upper cervical segments C2-C5 (Fig. 8.196). Notice the break in the spinolaminar line at C3 with respect to C4. An APOM radiograph was not obtained due to difficulties in patient positioning.

CLINICAL COURSE

The patient was adjusted at C3 (+Z, +θX) in the seated position. He received six adjustments over a 4-week period and had a complete resolution of symptomatology. The patient cooperated easily and fully during the adjustment procedure and appeared to enjoy the process.

C4 SUBLUXATION

This 8-year-old white female presented for chiropractic evaluation with a complaint of headaches. The lateral cervical radiograph discloses a slight hyperextension subluxation at C4 as evidenced by the convergence of the endplate lines at the posterior (Fig. 8.197). Notice the closeness of the C4 and C5 spinous processes. The atlas has an anterior-inferior (+θX) malposition. The APOM was unremarkable.

CLINICAL COURSE

The patient was adjusted at C4 in the seated position. The patient received three adjustments over a 1-week period. She responded favorably to care but the patient did not return for additional care or follow-up because she moved out of state.

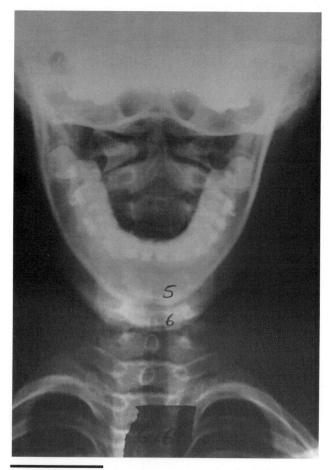

Figure 8.193.

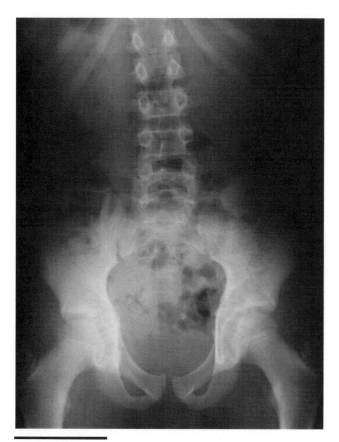

Figure 8.194.

C5 SUBLUXATION

This 13-year-old Latino male patient presented for chiropractic evaluation with complaints of sinus congestion and headaches. The lateral cervical radiograph demonstrates a cervical hypolordosis (Fig. 8.198). When compared with the surrounding motion segments, there is slight convergence of the endplate line towards the posterior at C5 on C6.

CLINICAL COURSE

The patient was adjusted at C5 in the seated position. He received twenty-five adjustments over a twelve month period with a complete resolution of symptomatology. The patient was asymptomatic after the twelfth adjustment but continued care to reduce the clinical signs of subluxation (e.g., edema, hypomobility, etc.).

C3 AND C4 SUBLUXATION

This patient is a 5-year-old Latino male. He has a history of recurrent ear and upper respiratory infections. The lateral cervical radiograph demonstrates a retrolisthesis at C3 and C4 (Fig. 8.199). Notice the break in both the spinolaminar and George's line at these two segments. The patient was malpositioned for the exposure. This is evidenced by the overlap of the jaw over the cervical spine. Y axis rotation of atlas is also visualized. An APOM was not obtained because of positioning problems.

CLINICAL COURSE

The patient was adjusted (+Z, +θX) at C4 and C3 in the seated position. He first received three adjustments at C4 and then seven at C3 over a 3-month period. At that time there was no symptomatology. The doctor began with the adjustments at the C4 segment to have a potentially greater effect on the

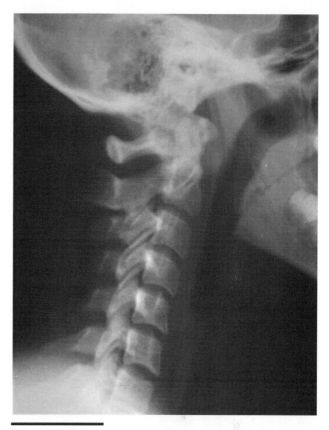

Figure 8.195.

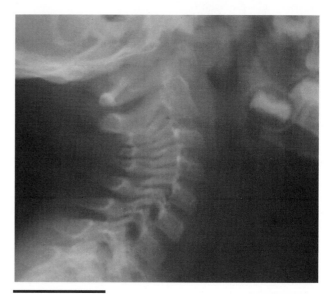

Figure 8.196.

segments above by changing the foundation. After this was done, C3 was considered the major subluxation in this patient. Improvement in symptoms was noticed after the first adjustment. By the sixth visit all symptomatology was resolved.

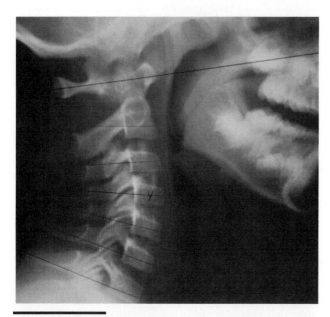

Figure 8.197.

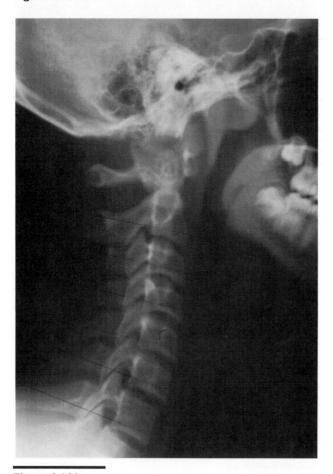

Figure 8.198.

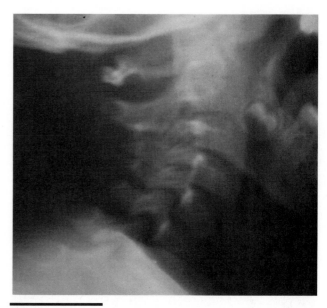

Figure 8.199.

C2 AND C3 SUBLUXATION

This patient is a 5-year-old Latino male. His twin is depicted in Figure 8.199. As does his brother, this twin also has a history of recurrent ear and upper respiratory infections. The lateral cervical radiograph discloses slight hyperextension of the upper cervical spine at C1–C3 (Fig. 8.200). Although the lateral radiograph is well positioned, due to further positioning problems, an APOM was not obtained.

CLINICAL COURSE

The patient was adjusted (+Z, +θX) at C3 in the seated position. He received five adjustments over a 3-month period. The patient was also adjusted (+Z, +θX) at C2, again in the seated position. He received five adjustments over a three month period. After receiving the second adjustment the patient noticed some relief and by the ninth, the symptoms were totally resolved.

C3 AND S2 SUBLUXATION

This patient is a 7-year-old white male. He has a history of learning disabilities (i.e., dyslexia), attention deficit hyperactivity disorder (ADHD) (see Chapter 17), nocturnal enuresis, headaches, allergies, and wrist pain. The lateral cervical radiograph demonstrates a retrolisthesis (−Z) at C3 and hyperextension at C1 on C2 (Fig. 8.201).

The AP cervical radiograph demonstrates an upper thoracic convexity (Fig. 8.202). There is also a right head tilt. The lateral lumbar radiograph of the same patient demonstrates a posterior S2 subluxation (Fig. 8.203). Notice the posterior widening of the rudimentary disc between S1 and S2.

CLINICAL COURSE

The patient was adjusted (+Z, +θX) at C3 in the seated position. He received twenty adjustments over a one and a half year period. The atlas was adjusted in the seated position on twelve different occasions during this time period. S2 was adjusted while in the side posture position during twenty-five visits for the year and a half of care. By the fifth adjustment, there was resolution of the nocturnal enuresis. The S2 segment was adjusted on subsequent occasions because of the high activity level of the patient and the various falls he underwent. After the fifteenth adjustment there was resolution of the

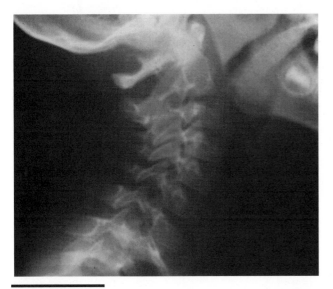

Figure 8.200.

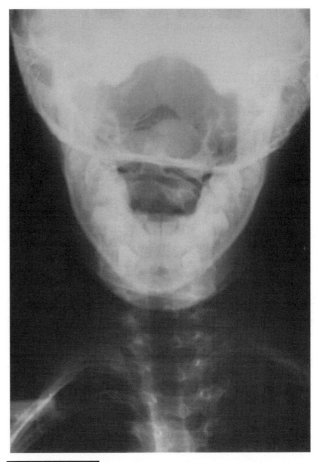

Figure 8.202.

headaches and wrist pain. The patient's learning disabilities, dyslexia, and ADHD were related by the patient and his family to be 90% improved. The child's grades in school improved. At the initiation of chiropractic care, the child was one year behind in school. After a year and a half of care he was at the normal grade level. After chiropractic care for one and a half years, the patient moved and was lost to any further follow-up.

S2 SUBLUXATION

This 9-year-old Latino male presented for chiropractic evaluation with a complaint of hyperactivity, for as long as the child could remember. The lateral lumbar radiograph demonstrates a posterior S2 subluxation (Fig. 8.204). Notice the posterior widening of the rudimentary disc between S1 and S2.

CLINICAL COURSE

The patient was adjusted at S2 in the side posture position. After 10 adjustments over a 2-month period, there was a resolution in the symptomatology.

ILIUM SUBLUXATION

This 5-year-old oriental female presented for chiropractic evaluation with a toe-in foot posture on the right side. She had leg pain, was constipated, and had a history of recurrent bladder

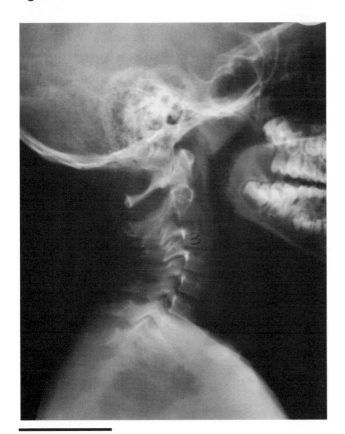

Figure 8.201.

infections. She had experienced these symptoms for approximately one and a half years.

The AP lumbopelvic radiograph demonstrates a right leg length deficiency of 6 mm (Fig. 8.205). The actual deficiency is only 3 mm due to the effect of the PIEx (−θX, +θY) ilium on the same side. The Ex (+θY) ilium finding is consistent with the patient's foot flare.

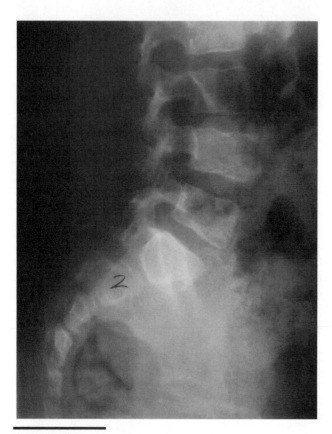

Figure 8.203.

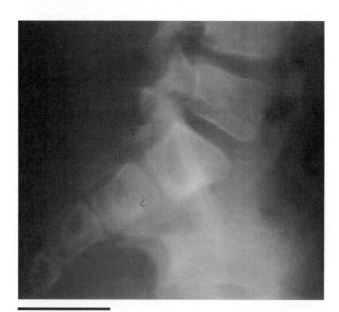

Figure 8.204.

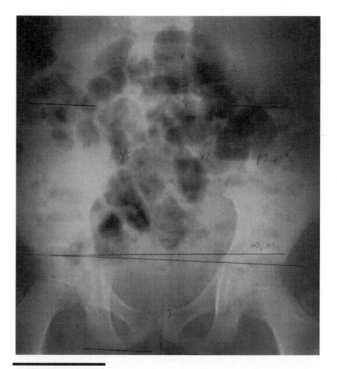

Figure 8.205.

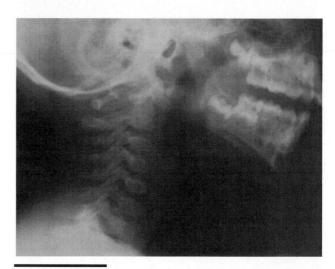

Figure 8.206.

CLINICAL COURSE

The patient was never adjusted. After the initial examination, the patient did not return for care. There was no follow-up on this patient.

OCCIPITAL CONDYLE AND CI SUBLUXATION

This is a 2-year-old Indian female patient. The patient had learning disabilities. At 2 years of age, she was unable to walk or talk. The lateral cervical radiograph demonstrates a hypolordotic cervical spine (Fig. 8.206). There is hyperextension of the upper cervical spine. The decrease in the joint space between the occiput and the posterior arch of atlas is a sign of an AS (−θX) condyle subluxation. There is also hyperextension present at C1–C2.

CLINICAL COURSE

The patient was first adjusted at C1 and later at C0 (i.e., occiput) in the seated position. Eight adjustments were delivered to the atlas and 12 adjustments were administered to the occiput over a 10-month period. The atlas only was adjusted initially for the first month. Skin temperature findings were present at the upper cervical level and both C0–C1 and C1–C2 motion segments exhibited fixation dysfunction on palpation. After both motion segments were freely movable, then adjustments were administered alternately on subsequent visits, depending on which joint was more fixated. After each adjustment, the patient would attempt to utter words that were uninterpretable. By the twelfth adjustment the patient was able to walk slowly with the aid of her mother by her side. There was no further follow-up on this patient. It was observed that at each visit, the child was difficult to deal with or adjust. She always appeared very nervous and in distress. Touching the child on the shoulder or touching her head would cause her to burst out with severe yelling and screaming rampages. Due to positioning problems, an APOM radiograph was not obtained.

C1 AND C3 SUBLUXATION

This is a 5-year-old white male patient. He has recurrent ear infections. A medical doctor had recommended myringotomy with insertion of tympanostomy tubes but the parents declined the surgery for their son. The lateral cervical radiograph discloses a hypolordosis (Fig. 8.207). There is a retrolisthesis present at C3 and the atlas is in a hyperextended position.

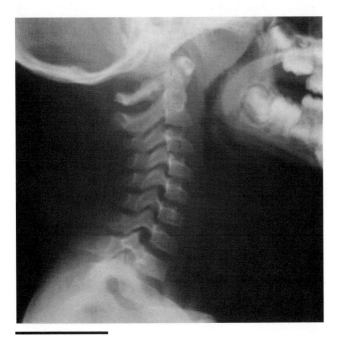

Figure 8.207.

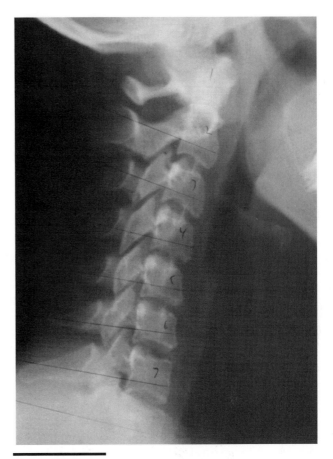

Figure 8.208.

CLINICAL COURSE

The patient was adjusted at C3 in the seated position. He received seven adjustments over the course of 4 months. The patient was also adjusted on three occasions at C1, also in the seated position. There was a complete resolution of symptomatology. At 2 years follow-up, the patient has had no signs or symptoms of any problems with his ears.

C7 AND T2 SUBLUXATION

This is a 17-year-old Indian female patient. She has a complaint of severe daily headaches. The lateral cervical radiograph demonstrates a kyphotic cervical spine (Fig. 8.208). There is a hyperextension (−θX) malposition at C7 as evidenced by the converging endplate lines at the posterior. The atlas is also in an extended position.

CLINICAL COURSE

The patient was adjusted posterior to anterior at T2 in the seated position. She received six adjustments over a two and a half year period. Over the same time period, the patient received 34 adjustments at C7. After 6 months of care there was resolution of the headache symptomatology. Physical work and stress would sometimes periodically provoke a headache. The patient returned on as needed basis whenever a headache recurred.

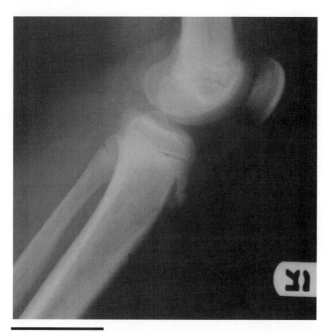

Figure 8.209.

OSGOOD SCHLATTER'S DISEASE

This is a very athletic 9-year-old black female patient. She has a complaint of right knee pain. The lateral knee radiograph demonstrates Osgood-Schlatter's disease (Fig. 8.209).

CLINICAL COURSE

The patient was instructed to apply cryotherapy to the knee as well as to tape it and use a brace to restrict movement. She was provided crutches and advised to avoid weight-bearing for 4 weeks. During the 4 weeks, she returned to the clinic on six occasions to have the avulsed bone adjusted (i.e., tapped upon) to approximate the fragment to the host bone. After 4 weeks of treatment there was a complete resolution of symptoms. The patient was advised to wear a light knee brace support for several additional months.

C2 AND L5 SUBLUXATION

This is a 16-year-old white female patient. She has complaints of migraine headaches (1x to 2x/month), tension headaches, neck pain and dizziness several times each month and low back pain which is daily upon arising in the morning. The low back pain is also aggravated with prolonged sitting. She has had these symptoms for approximately 4 years. Since beginning menstruating, the patient has experienced dysmenorrhea with every menstrual cycle.

The lateral cervical radiograph demonstrates a slightly hypolordotic lower cervical spine and a slight retrolisthesis (-Z) and hyperextension (−θX) at C2 (Fig. 8.210).

The APOM radiograph of the same patient demonstrates a left lateral flexion malposition (−θZ) at C2 with concomitant right spinous rotation (+θY) (Fig. 8.211A). C2 is listed as PRS

(−Z, +θY, −θZ). The patient's lateral lumbar radiograph demonstrates a retrolisthesis at L5 (Fig. 8.211B). Notice the break in George's line between L5 and S1.

CLINICAL COURSE

The patient was adjusted at C2 in the seated position. The patient received 25 adjustments to this segment over a one and a half year period. There was complete resolution of the headaches. She was also adjusted at L5 on 22 occasions over the same period of time in the side posture position. The dysmenorrhea was improved with less duration and severity of symptoms. The low-back pain returned if the patient sat for excessive periods of time. The patient returned for care on an as needed basis.

C3 SUBLUXATION

This 4-year-old Latino female patient has a history of recurrent otitis media. The lateral cervical radiograph demonstrates a reduction in the cervical lordosis in the lower cervical region (Fig. 8.212). There is a retrolisthesis (-Z) present at C3. A flexion malposition at C6 and C7 is present and T1 is in a relatively extended position when compared to the above spinal levels. Due to positioning difficulties, an APOM radiograph was not obtained.

CLINICAL COURSE

The patient was adjusted at C3 in the seated position. She received six adjustments over a 5-week period with complete

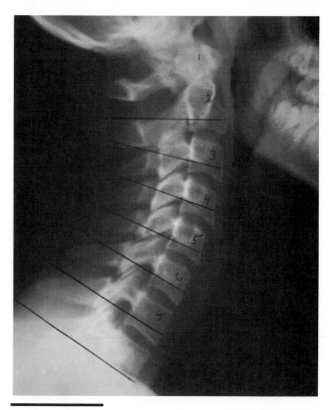

Figure 8.210.

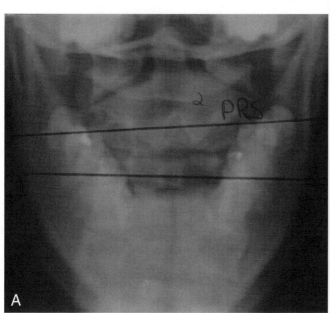

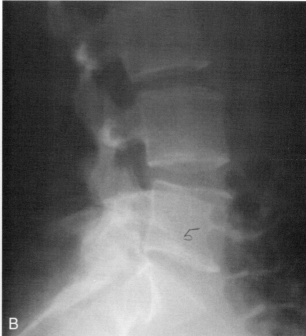

Figure 8.211A,B.

resolution of symptoms. Due to a hearing deficit, the patient's pediatrician had recommended myringotomy with placement of tympanostomy tubes. These procedures were not performed.

S2 AND ILIUM SUBLUXATION

This is a 4-year-old black male patient. His left foot flares inward, a postural problem that had been noticed by the child's parents since he began walking. The lateral lumbosacral radiograph discloses a slightly posterior S2 subluxation (Fig. 8.213) with a similar slight posterior widening of the posterior portion of the rudimentary disc at S2–S3. The AP lumbopelvic radiograph demonstrates a large anatomical leg length deficiency on the left side (Fig. 8.214). This appears to cause a left convex lumbar scoliosis above. There is an AS1Ex2 (+θX, −θY) ilium listing on the left side. The left foot flare is consistent with an Ex (−θY) ilium listing on the same side.

Clinical Course

The patient was adjusted at S2 in the side posture position. The patient received two adjustments over the course of 3 weeks. During this time period the patient also was adjusted at the left ilium (ASEx, +θX, −θY) with the involved side down in the side posture position. After the fifth visit there was a resolution of the foot posture abnormality.

C5 AND S2 SUBLUXATION

This is a 8-year-old Latino female patient. She has complaints of leg pain and headaches. The lateral cervical radiograph demonstrates a cervical hypolordosis (Fig. 8.215) with a

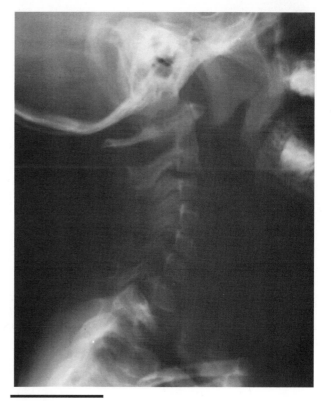

Figure 8.212.

kyphosis at C2–C3. The endplate lines demonstrate a hyperextension (−θX) malposition at C5.

The lateral lumbosacral radiograph of the same patient demonstrates a posterior S2 subluxation (Fig. 8.216). Notice

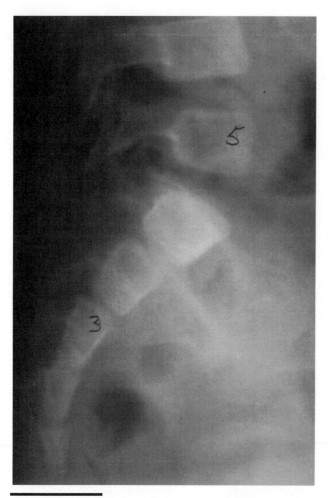

Figure 8.213.

the widening at the posterior aspect of the rudimentary disc between S1 and S2.

CLINICAL COURSE

The patient was adjusted at C5 in the seated position. She received 15 adjustments over a 5-month period. During the same period, the patient received 12 adjustments at S2 in the side posture position. The patient returns for care on an as needed basis. The patient's headaches still recur but are not as severe. Although more periodic care was recommended to the patient, this advice was not heeded. There was complete resolution of the leg pain.

C1 AND C2 SUBLUXATION

This 9-year-old Latino male patient has a history of severe asthma. Prior to receiving chiropractic care he been taking various medications for the control of his asthma. The APOM demonstrates a lateral flexion (+θZ) malposition at C1 (Fig. 8.217). The atlas listing is A-LP (+Z, +θZ, −θY). The "A" component of the listing was derived from the lateral cervical radiograph shown in Figure 8.218.

On the lateral exposure the ADI is slightly increased but within normal limits (Fig. 8.218). Additional radiographs of the full spine were obtained but were unremarkable.

CLINICAL COURSE

The patient was adjusted at C2 and C1 in the seated position. Fifteen adjustments were delivered to C2 and 25 adjustments to C1. The patient showed improvement by the fifth adjustment. After 5 months, there was complete resolution of symptomatology. The patient is seen on a maintenance basis. After being checked on each visit, the patient may or may not receive an adjustment. Since he has been under care, the patient has not used any medications.

L5 AND S2 SUBLUXATION

This is a 7-year-old white female patient presented with a complaint of nocturnal enuresis. The lateral lumbar radiograph demonstrates a retrolisthesis of (-Z) of L5 (Fig. 8.219). There are nuclear invaginations present at the vertebral endplates of all lumbar levels, a sign of compression trauma.

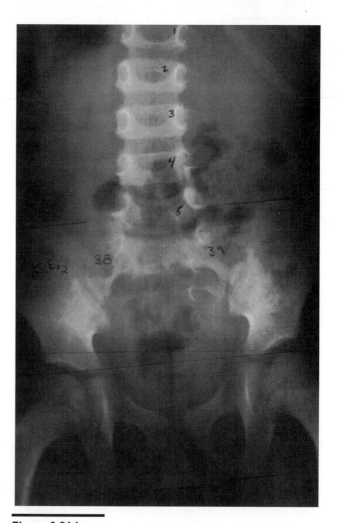

Figure 8.214.

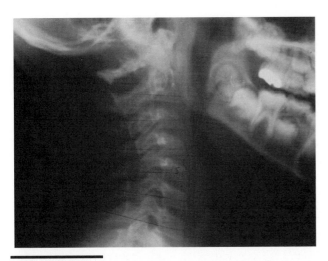

Figure 8.215.

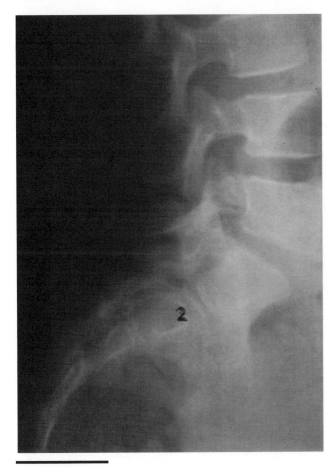

Figure 8.216.

right side. The ilia were not adjusted because the sacroiliac joints were found to be freely movable.

CLINICAL COURSE

The patient was adjusted in the side posture position on one occasion at S2 and on three visits at L5 over the course of 2 weeks. There was a complete resolution of symptomatology. The patient was lost to further follow-up because she moved out of state.

C1 SUBLUXATION

This is a 4-year-old black male patient with nocturnal enuresis. The APOM demonstrates a right lateral flexion malposition of the atlas (Fig. 8.221). The atlas listing is AILP (+Z, +θX, +θZ, +θY). The lateral cervical radiograph demonstrates an antero-

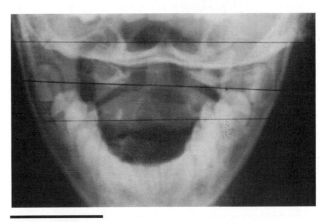

Figure 8.217.

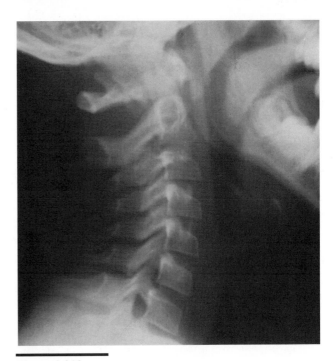

Figure 8.218.

On the AP lumbopelvic radiograph there is a slight left spinous process deviation (−θY) of L5 when compared to the S1 tubercle (Fig. 8.220). The obturator appearance demonstrates a narrow base on the left, consistent with an In (+θY) ilium listing on the left and an Ex (+θY) ilium listing on the

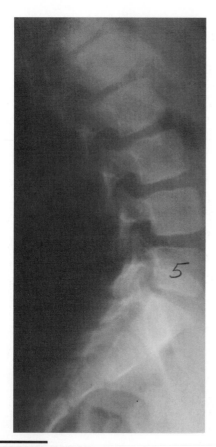

Figure 8.219.

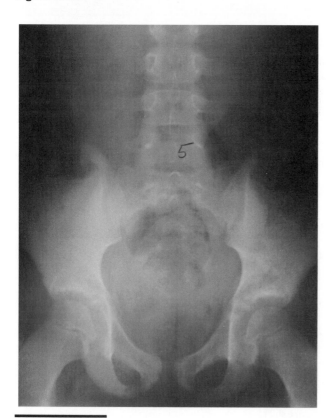

Figure 8.220.

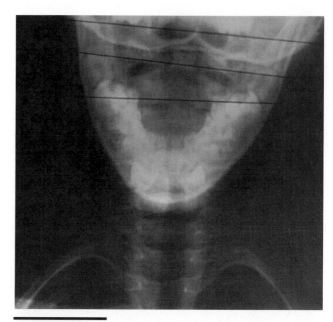

Figure 8.221.

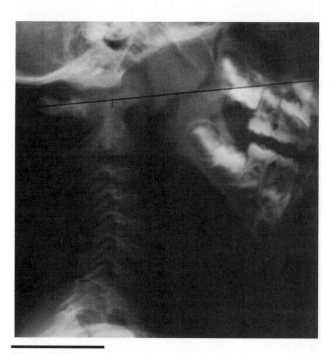

Figure 8.222.

inferior (+Z, +θX) position of the atlas (Fig. 8.222). A decreased cervical lordosis is also present. Radiographs of the lumbar spine were unremarkable.

CLINICAL COURSE

The patient was adjusted at C1 in the seated position. He received four adjustments over a 4-week period. The patient did not return for any additional care and no follow-up on this patient was obtained.

C6 SUBLUXATION WITH UPPER CERVICAL ANOMALY

This is a 12-year-old black male patient who has a history of recurrent otitis media and headaches. The lateral cervical radiograph demonstrates a decreased cervical lordosis (Fig. 8.223). There is a hyperextension ($-\theta X$) malposition at C6. Notice the close proximity of the C6 and C7 spinous processes. The APOM demonstrates an anomalous atlas-axis articulation on the right side (Fig. 8.224).

CLINICAL COURSE

The patient was adjusted at C6 in the seated position. He received 14 adjustments over a 10-week period and had a complete resolution of symptoms. The patient began to show improvement after the second adjustment and was asymptomatic by the fourteenth.

C2 SUBLUXATION

This is a 3-year-old white male patient. He has recurrent bouts with otitis media on a monthly basis. A medical doctor's suggestion that antibiotics be taken on a "daily maintenance basis" prompted the chiropractic referral. The lateral cervical radiograph demonstrates a decreased cervical lordosis (Fig. 8.225). Lateral flexion of the upper neck has caused the atlas ring to be visualized. Due to patient positioning problems an APOM radiograph was not obtained.

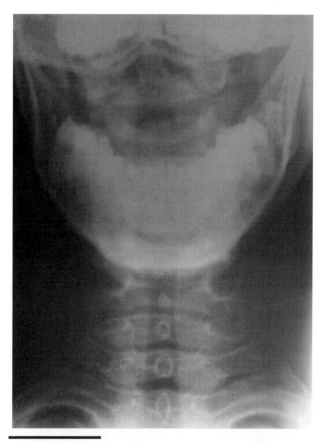

Figure 8.224.

CLINICAL COURSE

The patient was adjusted ($+Z$, $+\theta X$) at C2 in the seated position. He received 30 adjustments over a two and a half year period and had a complete resolution of symptomatology. The patient had noticed improvement after the first few adjustments but several months of care were needed before the patient became completely asymptomatic. He was at this time a very active child and falls or plays hard often. After the child suffers a fall he may develop an ear infection. Adjustment at the subluxation appears to resolve the complaint after one or two adjustments to C2. The patient no longer takes any medications for the otitis media.

S2 SUBLUXATION

This is a 10-year-old black male patient with a complaint of chronic diarrhea of 1 year duration. The lateral lumbar radiograph discloses a posterior S2 subluxation (Fig. 8.226). Notice the marked posterior widening of the joint space between S1 and S2. The AP lumbopelvic radiograph was unremarkable.

CLINICAL COURSE

The patient was adjusted at S2 in the side posture position. He received eight adjustments over a 5-week period. There was complete resolution of symptoms. Improvement in the diarrhea was noted by the third adjustment and was resolved by the eighth.

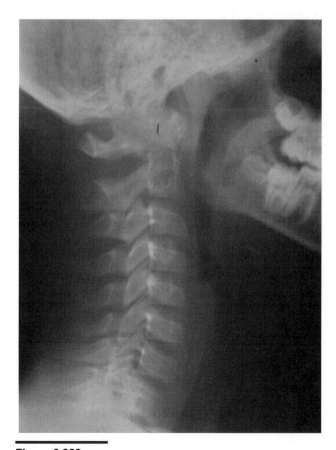

Figure 8.223.

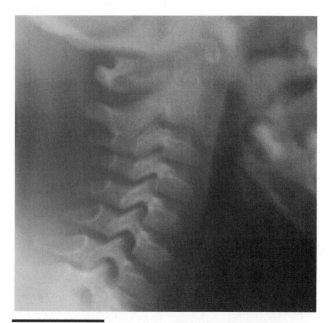

Figure 8.225.

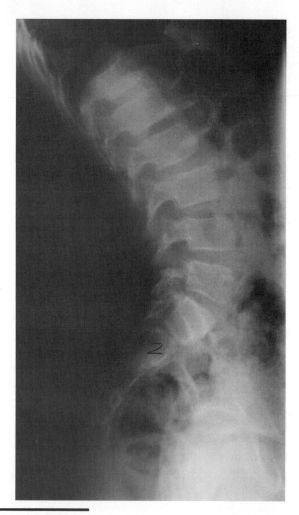

Figure 8.226.

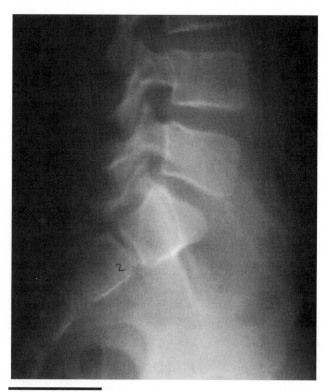

Figure 8.227.

S2 SUBLUXATION

This is an 11-year-old white male patient with a complaint of low back pain when sitting. The lateral lumbar radiograph demonstrates a posterior S2 subluxation (Fig. 8.227). Notice the widening of the joint space at its posterior aspect between S1 and S2.

CLINICAL COURSE

The patient was adjusted at S2 in the side posture position. He was administered 12 adjustments over a 2-month period. There was complete resolution of symptomatology. Improvement in the low back pain was noticed after the first adjustment to S2. The AP lumbopelvic radiograph was unremarkable.

S2 AND ILIUM SUBLUXATION

This is a 10-year-old white male patient with a complaint of nocturnal enuresis. The lateral lumbar radiograph demonstrates a posterior S2 subluxation and a slight retrolisthesis of L5 (Fig. 8.228). The AP lumbopelvic radiograph discloses a measured deficiency of 4 mm on the left that causes a very slight left convex lumbar scoliosis (Fig. 8.229). An Ex1 (−θY) ilium on the left is noted. There is a more demonstrable change at the obturator. The left obturator base is wider than the left, indicative of a left Ex (−θY) ilium or a right In (−θY) listing.

CLINICAL COURSE

The patient was adjusted at S2 in the side posture position. He received three adjustments over a 2-week period. During this time, the patient also received one adjustment to the left ilium (Ex, −θY) also in the side posture position. The patient's enuresis persisted and there was no improvement in symptomatology. There was no further follow-up on this patient because he moved out of state.

C7 SUBLUXATION

This is a 17-year-old white male patient. He participates in martial arts and wrestling and has complaints of "allergies," sinusitis, headaches, shoulder pain, and knee pain. The lateral cervical radiograph demonstrates a kyphotic posture (Fig. 8.230). An anterolisthesis is present at C6. The APOM radiograph was unremarkable.

There is an increase in the glenohumeral joint space on the right side, indicative of an antero-inferior subluxation of the humerus (Fig. 8.231).

CLINICAL COURSE

The patient was adjusted (+Z, +θX) at C7 in the seated position. The patient received 13 adjustments over a 2-year period. Although the patient's problems are related to the sporting activities, he does not follow a structured chiropractic care plan and only returns on as needed basis. The patient is

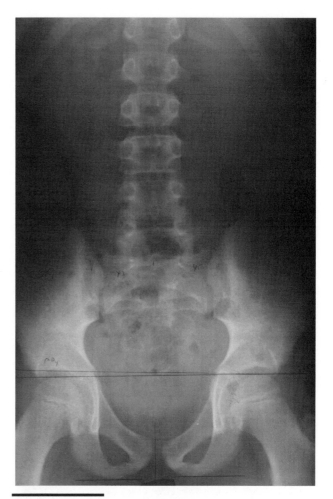

Figure 8.229.

usually in marked pain but becomes much improved after the treatment. The patient's anterior-inferior shoulder (i.e., humerus) has been adjusted on five occasions. The patient's right knee has also been adjusted (radiograph not pictured) and he has received three adjustments to this joint.

C3 SUBLUXATION

This is a 7-year-old male patient who presented for chiropractic evaluation with a diagnosis of ADD. A pediatrician's suggestion for the child to begin Ritalin medication prompted a chiropractic referral The child also has a "lazy" left eye that turns medialward. The past history included multiple episodes of otitis media. The lateral cervical radiograph demonstrates a retrolisthesis (-Z) and hyperextension position (-θX) of C3 (Fig. 8.232).

CLINICAL COURSE

The patient received fifteen adjustments at C3 in the seated position over the course of ten weeks. The lazy left eye was normalized after the first adjustment. The patient's ADD has appeared to improve while under care. At the time of this writing, the patient was entering his eleventh week of care.

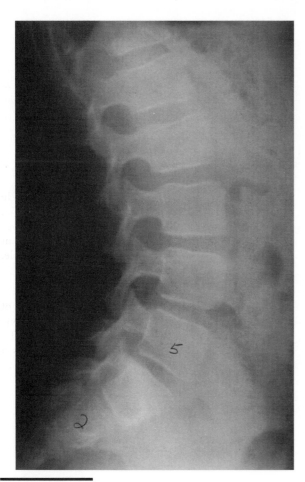

Figure 8.228.

Additional radiographs of other regions of the spine were unremarkable.

ILIUM SUBLUXATION

This patient is a 21-month-old black female. The patient has a stiff left hip upon rising in the morning. The hip also becomes stiff after sitting for too long a period of time. The left foot flares outward. The patient has experienced these symptoms for about 12 months. The AP lumbopelvic radiograph demon-

strates a left ASIn (+θX, +θY) ilium misalignment (Fig. 8.233). Notice the asymmetrical appearance of the obturator foraminae. The left obturator has a reduced base and diagonal, consistent with a left AsIn (+θX, +θY) misalignment.

CLINICAL COURSE

The patient was adjusted as a left ASIn (+θX, +θY) ilium in the side posture position on her mother's lap. The involved side was placed up. She received 14 adjustments over a 3-month period. There was a complete resolution of the leg and hip stiffness. The improvement in these symptoms was very gradual over the course of care. The post treatment (approx. 3 months) radiograph demonstrates a reduction in the ilium misalignment (Fig. 8.234). Notice the symmetrical appearance of the obturator foraminae compared with the pretreatment radiograph.

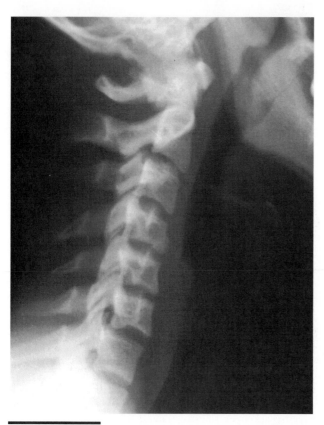

Figure 8.230.

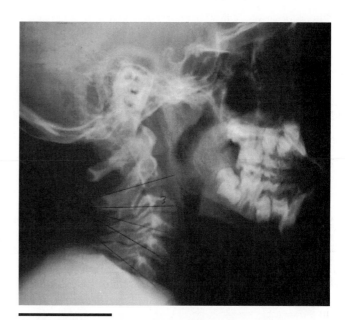

Figure 8.232.

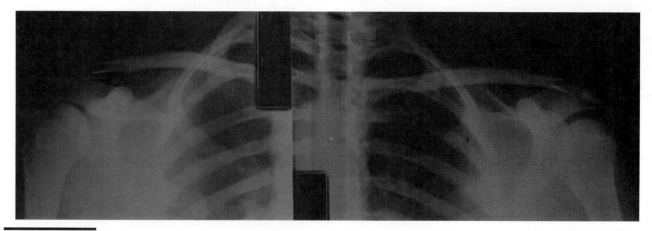

Figure 8.231.

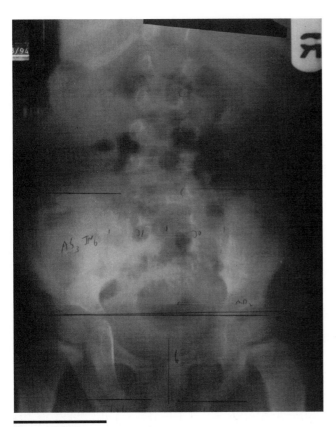

Figure 8.233.

Computed Tomography

Contemporary technologies, such as computed tomography and magnetic resonance imaging, are useful in identifying pathoanatomical changes of the axial skeleton. Their application in situations where clinical and/or radiological findings of spinal dysfunction are equivocal is especially relevant. More importantly, however, CT and MRI provide information about the integrity of the spinal column (e.g., fracture) and spinal cord (e.g., tumor), that is simply unavailable with conventional radiography and clinical examination tools.

Computed tomography or CT scanning is an imaging technique which produces cross sectional (axial) images of body structures using x-radiation. The technique was developed in Great Britain in the early 1970s (263). Sagittal, coronal, and oblique images can also be produced by computer reconstruction. Sensitive electronic detectors record the radiation passing through the body part under examination. The output of the detector array is fed to a computer. The computer produces an image on a cathode ray tube.

The image may be recorded on photographic film. A CT examination of the spine begins by producing a digital locator film. The locator is similar in appearance to a lateral radiograph. Two protocols are commonly employed in spine imaging. The first is the angulated gantry protocol. In this procedure, axial images are acquired parallel to the disc being examined. This procedure provides optimal visualization of

the relationship of the disc margin to the thecal sac and nerve roots. The chief disadvantages of the angulated gantry procedure are that there are gaps in the coverage of the spine, and that reformatting in other planes is impossible or suboptimal.

The alternative technique is to take parallel contiguous axial scans with no gantry angulation through the entire anatomical region. This technique permits reformatting in other planes and eliminates the gaps produced by the angulated gantry technique. However, since more slices are produced, more time is required, and there is a greater radiation burden. Some CT software may permit reformatting the data collected in this manner to produce axial images through the plane line of the discs, thus realizing the advantages of both protocols.

Since CT is an x-ray based procedure, it shares many advantages and disadvantages of radiographic imaging. The technique involves exposure to ionizing radiation. Scatter can cause artifact. The beam hardening effects of bone can result in suboptimal visualization of soft tissue structures. CT is not able to provide the degree of differentiation of soft tissue structures possible with magnetic resonance imaging. However, the ability of CT to image cortical bone and calcified lesions assures its place in the imaging armamentarium, particularly for cases involving trauma or bony abnormalities.

Imaging of the Vertebral Subluxation Complex

Many clinicians consider degenerative disease of the spine to be an affliction affecting middle aged and older patients. In

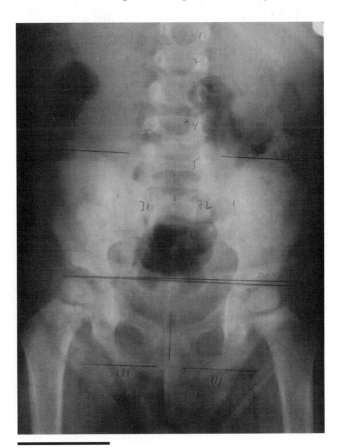

Figure 8.234.

actuality, the roots of spinal degenerative disease may be patho-mechanical changes which occur in childhood. Disc degeneration typically begins in males after the first decade of life, and in females after the second decade. By age 40, 80% of male discs and 65% of female discs exhibit moderate degeneration. The most common cause of disc degeneration is believed to be mechanical (264). Torsional stress, sometimes complicated by poor disc nutrition and vascular changes in the capillary networks of the vertebral endplates has been proposed as a major etiologic component in degenerative disc disease (265–267).

The importance of correcting early childhood vertebral subluxations cannot be overemphasized. Histologically, the cartilaginous vertebral end plate is composed of hyaline cartilage attached to the bone by a thin layer of calcified cartilage. Degenerative change demonstrates microfractures at the bone-cartilage interface. Focal necrosis, fissuring, and tears of the annulus fibrosus are seen as the degenerative process progresses. Large clefts develop in the discs which may produce the vacuum phenomenon seen on plain radiographs and CT scans. As the disc space decreases, new bone formation is seen around the periphery of the discs. Anterior disc herniation leads to spondylosis deformans, producing osteophytes (268–271). Manifestations of subluxation degeneration which may be demonstrated infolding of the ligamentum flava, osteophytosis, and bony sclerosis. An important advantage of CT imaging in the analysis of lumbar subluxation is the ability to visualize the thecal sac, the nerve roots, and intervertebral disc tissue.

Functional CT is very useful in the evaluation of rotary subluxation of the upper cervical spine (Fig. 8.235). This condition is often associated with torticollis in children. The etiology is usually traumatic. Axial images are acquired in the neutral position and with rotation. The space between the odontoid process and each lateral mass can be measured (272–275). White and Panjabi (276) have described three types of rotatory subluxation:

Type I. Unilateral anterior atlantoaxial subluxation.

Type II. Posterior atlantoaxial subluxation.

Type III. Associated anterior and posterior subluxation.

Other Applications

Computed tomography may be employed to assess developmental variants in the spine, as well as fractures, dislocations, neoplasms, inflammatory lesions, and infections. Osseous anomalies which can be appreciated on CT images include butterfly vertebra, limbus vertebra, os odontoideum, cleft vertebra, congenital absence of pedicle, Schmorl's nodes, and Cupid's bow. CT is also capable of demonstrating neural developmental variants such as conjoined nerve roots and cystic nerve root sleeve dilation (277–285).

Extraspinal applications include imaging of the head, particularly following trauma, and imaging of the viscera (286,287).

Magnetic Resonance Imaging

Magnetic resonance imaging produces high resolution images of the living human body without exposure to ionizing radiation. The principal disadvantages of the procedure are the relatively high expense and limited availability (288). MR imaging is particularly useful if a soft tissue lesion is suspected. Pediatric conditions reported in the literature successfully imaged with MR include: adolescent disc herniation (289), space occupying lesions of the CNS (290), herpes simplex encephalitis (290), disc disease (291), spinal tumors (292), tethered cord (292), post-traumatic lesions (293), metabolic disorders (293), and congenital malformations (293).

Technology

The body part under examination is placed within a powerful magnetic field. The magnetic field may be produced by permanent magnets or superconductive electromagnets cooled with liquid helium and liquid nitrogen. Most clinical MR imaging employs hydrogen as the element of interest, although other elements, such as sodium, potassium, and

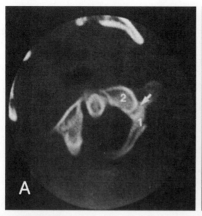 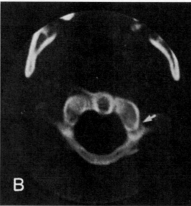 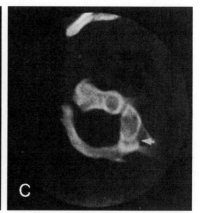

Figure 8.235. Atlanto-axial rotary subluxation. Axial C1-C2-level 10-mm thickness 30/3000 head rotation to the right (A). Neutral (B). Left rotation shows a fixed rotation (rotary subluxation) of C1 on C2 such that the C2 and C1 lateral mass rela- tionships are unchanged with a change in head-body position. Reproduced with permission from Grossman CB. Magnetic resonance imaging and computed tomography of the head and spine. Baltimore: Williams & Wilkins, 1990:425.

fluorine, may also be imaged. Because much of the human body is composed of water and fat, hydrogen imaging permits exquisite visualization of soft tissue structures.

Hydrogen protons can be represented as tiny spinning magnets with north and south poles. When placed in a steady, powerful magnetic field, they align in the direction of the magnetic poles and "wobble" or precess at a specific frequency. The scanner then introduces a powerful radio wave timed to this frequency called the Larmor resonance frequency. This frequency is determined by the strength of the magnetic field and the element being imaged. This pulse of radio frequency energy temporarily knocks the protons out of alignment. After the RF pulse is turned off, the protons snap back into position, emitting a weak radio wave. This signal is received by a coil and processed by a computer. Images of the body part being examined are displayed on a cathode ray tube. Most MR systems can produce axial, sagittal, and coronal images. Some equipment is capable of producing oblique images.

MR imaging is unique in that it does not employ ionizing radiation and has no known adverse effects. The images produced offer very good resolution. In chiropractic practice MR imaging may be useful in the detection and evaluation of vertebral subluxations, disc lesions, neoplasms, brain, cord, and nerve lesions.

IMAGING TECHNIQUES

The radiologist performing an MR study must specify several parameters:

1. Plane: axial, coronal, sagittal, or oblique;
2. Slice thickness: Thinner slices produce better detail, but require longer imaging times;
3. Matrix size: The number of pixels (picture elements) also affects picture detail. The greater the number of pixels, the better the detail. Again, better resolution results in longer imaging times;
4. Signal averages: The more signal averages, the better the detail, but the longer the imaging time;
5. Pulse sequences: There are three pulse sequences used in clinical MR imaging. These are spin-echo, gradient echo, and inversion recovery. The most widely used is the spin echo sequence;
6. Image weighting: Pulse duration determines the "weighting" of the image. T1 weighted images use shorter pulses, while T2 weighted images use longer pulses. Spin echo sequences involve two parameters, TE (echo time) and TR (repetition time).

From a clinical standpoint, these factors determine the relative brightness of different tissues. Tightly bound hydrogen, such as the hydroxyapatite found in calcific structures, produces little or no signal. However, the hydrogen in water and fat will produce high signal intensity if appropriate parameters are employed. Depending on the parameters selected, the MR image will emphasize either structures with high concentrations of fat or structures with high concentrations of water. Of particular interest to chiropractors are the following sequences:

Table 8.29. Relative Signal (Brightness) of Different Tissues on a T1 Weighted Spin Echo Sequence

White	Gray	Black
Fat	Bone marrow	Air
	Brain	
	Abdominal viscera	
	Muscle	
	Body fluids	
	Cortical bone	

1. T1 weighted spin echo. T1 weighted images are sometimes called "fat images." Structures containing fat appear bright. In the spine, the vertebral bodies contain marrow fat. In the absence of pathology, vertebral bodies will appear bright on T1 weighted images. In pathologies where the marrow fat is replaced, changes in signal intensity will cause the vertebral bodies to appear brighter or darker. T1 weighted images employ relatively short pulses, and do not take nearly as long to produce as T2 weighted images;
2. T2 weighted spin echo. T2 weighted images are often termed "water images." Water rich structures, such as the nucleus pulposus and CSF appear light. Fat-containing structures appear dark. T2 weighted images require much longer imaging times than T1 weighted images. T2 weighted images are useful in evaluating disc desiccation. These sequences also help identify edematous lesions, and provide dramatic differentiation of disc, CSF, and cord;
3. Gradient echo/partial flip angle imaging. Different manufacturers apply different terms to this technique, which produces a "pseudomyelographic" effect. The image is similar in appearance to a T2 weighted image. Partial flip angle images require much less time to produce than T2 weighted images.

Table 8.29 summarizes the relative signal (brightness) of different tissues on a T1 weighted spin echo sequence.

MR IMAGES

Edema may occur secondary to infection, infarction, tumor, trauma, or demyelinization. On T1 weighted images, edema appears dark. On T2 weighted images, edema has an intense signal and appears white (295, 296).

Tumors involving fluid filled cysts behave similar to edematous tissues, while tumors involving calcification may be difficult to detect using present MR techniques. Calcified tumors are better imaged using CT techniques. It is difficult to reliably differentiate benign from malignant tumors with current MR techniques. Metastatic bone disease results in decreased signal on T1 weighted images. This is due to replacement of the marrow with tumor cells. T2 weighted images may demonstrate increased signal intensity (297–300).

Table 8.30.   Checklist—Cervical Spine MRI

Sagittal images

1. Check the craniocervical junction, paying particular attention to Chiari malformation, pannus formation, cranial settling, etc.

2. Check the pituitary.

3. Examine the brain stem, cerebellum, and any other brain tissue visible on the films.

4. Check the spinal cord, looking for contour changes and intrinsic pathology.

5. Examine the CSF signal on the "myelo" images, checking primarily for contour changes. Be sure to evaluate the 4th ventricle and related intracranial structures, which are usually visible on c-spine spines.

6. Evaluate the intervertebral foramina on the parasagittal images for patency or stenosis.

7. Check the vertebral bodies. Determine any changes in the marrow signal on both the T1 and T2 weighted images.

8. Check the intervertebral discs, noting any evidence of thinning, desiccation, bulging, or herniation.

9. Scan the posterior aspects of the vertebral bodies, drawing a mental "George's line." Check for uplifting of the epidural venous plexus and fat which may be caused by a disc bulge, herniation, or posterior osteophyte. Determine if the disc is contained or not contained.

10. Scan the anterior aspects of the vertebral bodies looking for spondylotic changes.

11. Examine the soft tissues anterior to the vertebral bodies.

12. Check the spinous processes.

13. Examine the soft tissues posterior to the vertebral bodies.

Axial images

1. Check any abnormalities noted on the sagittal images.

2. Check the craniocervical junction.

3. Evaluate the marrow signal in each vertebral body.

4. Evaluate the disc signal at each motion segment.

5. If a disc bulge or herniation is present, determine the following:

    a. Is it symmetrical (bulge) or focal (herniation)?

    b. If focal, note the direction (central, lateral, far lateral) and degree of herniation in mm.

    c. Is there pressure on the cord or thecal sac?

    d. Are the intervertebral foramina patent?

    e. If an osteophyte is also present, or if it is not possible to differentiate disc from osteophyte, this should be noted.

6. Check for osteophytes, including anterior spondylotic changes, posterior osteophytes, and exostoses from the uncinate processes.

7. Check the spinal canal, including cord and CSF signals. Note any evidence of stenosis.

8. Check the emerging nerve roots and intervertebral foraminae.

9. Examine the posterior joints.

10. Check the major vessels, including carotid arteries, jugular veins, and vertebral arteries where visible.

11. Check the paraspinal muscles for symmetry, ability to discern layers, and hemorrhage.

12. Examine the spinous processes, articular pillars, and laminae.

13. Check the soft tissues anterior to the spine, including laryngeal and thyroid areas.

Blood that is flowing rapidly appears dark because of turbulence and high velocity. Slowly flowing blood often appears bright (301). Inflammatory diseases of the spinal cord, such as multiple sclerosis and transverse myelitis, will demonstrate intense (bright) signals on T2 weighted images when acute. Multiple sclerosis more frequently produces subtle changes in cord intensity. T1 weighted images of the spinal cord demonstrate changes in cord contour, while T2 weighted images demonstrate increased signal (brightness) where water content is high, such as CSF. Discitis and osteomyelitis may be evaluated using a combination of T1 and T2 weighted images (302–304).

Intervertebral disc disease demonstrates low signal intensity (brightness) due to desiccation and degeneration. Herniations may also cause changes in cord contour, nerve root compression, and edema (305).

Contraindications to MR Imaging

The two absolute contraindications to MR imaging are cardiac pacemakers and ferrous cerebral aneurysm clips. Claustrophobic and uncooperative patients are poor candidates for MR imaging. Unlike CT scans, where patient motion will degrade the image only on the slice(s) where the motion occurred, movement during an MR scan degrades all the slices in that scan. The effects of strong magnetic fields on biological systems, particularly during pregnancy, have not been fully explored. Although no adverse effects have been reported following MR imaging, its use in pregnancy should be restricted to those cases where it is deemed absolutely necessary and there is no less hazardous alternative. Ferromagnetic foreign bodies, implanted electrical stimulator wires, and metal prosthetic heart valves also are relative contraindications to MR studies (294–297).

CLINICAL MR APPLICATIONS

Magnetic resonance imaging has been used as an adjunct in the diagnosis of a wide variety of conditions affecting the spine and contiguous structures. Myelopathy (306), cervical spondylosis (306), cervical disc disease (307), epidural fibrosis (308), hypertrophy of the ligamentum flava (309), canal stenosis (309), facet degeneration (309), disc herniation (308,310-314), infection (315), arachnoiditis (316), Chiari malformation (317), syringomyelia (318), cord impingement (319), multiple myeloma (320), neurofibromatosis (321), cord compression (322), vertebral hemangioma (323) and metastatic malignancies (324) are examples of conditions which can be detected on MR images. Extraspinal lesions which can be appreciated on MRI include osseous pathologies involving marrow replacement, soft tissue tumors, soft tissue manifestations of trauma, and some occult fractures (325). MR imaging of the extremities, therefore, may be valuable in the assessment of selected pediatric cases.

A SYSTEMATIC APPROACH TO THE ASSESSMENT OF SPINAL MRI IMAGES

Some chiropractors may have limited experience in the interpretation of MR images. The following checklist for the

Table 8.31.   Examples of Possible Findings from MR Images

Disc bulge

Herniated nucleus pulposus

Degenerative disc disease

Degenerative joint disease

Syrinx

Tumor

Chiari malformation

Rheumatoid arthritis

Congenital/developmental variants

Fracture

Dislocation

Metastasis

Infection

Hemorrhage

cervical spine (Table 8.30) may be helpful to doctors as an aid in the interpretation of MRI reports (326). The authors strongly suggest that the attending doctor view the films, and locate any abnormalities mentioned in the report. In some cases, the radiological report may fail to describe certain clinically relevant information or the images can be misinterpreted. The conditions presented in Table 8.31 are examples of possible findings that can be visible on MR images. The list is only illustrative and not all inclusive and the clinician is encouraged to expand the list.

Table 8.32 presents a checklist protocol for analysis of MR images of the lumbar spine. Table 8.33 is an abbreviated list of possible abnormalities that are detectable with MRI. These conditions are examples, and the list is only illustrative and not all inclusive. The clinician is encouraged to expand the list.

Comparison of CT and MR Imaging

Generally, CT is superior in imaging bone, or pathologies associated with calcification. MR is superior for evaluating soft tissue structures, particularly the brain and spinal cord. Since CT involves the use of x-radiation, metallic implants may produce scatter artifact. Because of the beam hardening effects of bone, MR is the technique of choice for imaging posterior fossa structures. Mirvis et al. (327) believe that CT is superior to MR for demonstrating fractures. In suspected disc lesions, there is controversy. CT has a distinguished track record in imaging herniated discs, particularly in the lumbar spine. However, improvements in MR technology have resulted in a growing number of clinicians favoring MR for the evaluation of disc lesions.

Table 8.32.   **Lumbar Spine—Checklist for the MR Image**

Sagittal images

1. Check the vertebral bodies. Determine any changes in the marrow signal on both the T1 and T2 weighted images.

2. Check the intervertebral discs, noting any evidence of thinning, desiccation, bulging, or herniation.

3. Scan the posterior aspects of the vertebral bodies, drawing a mental "George's line." Check for uplifting of the epidural venous plexus and fat which may be caused by a disc bulge, herniation, or posterior osteophyte. Determine if the disc is contained or not contained.

4. Scan the anterior aspects of the vertebral bodies looking for spondylotic changes.

5. Examine the soft tissues anterior to the vertebral bodies, particularly the abdominal aorta.

6. Check the spinal cord, looking for contour changes and intrinsic pathology. Examine for evidence of arachnoiditis.

7. Examine the CSF signal on the "myelo" images, checking primarily for contour changes.

8. Evaluate the intervertebral foramina on the parasagittal images for patency or stenosis.

9. Check the spinous processes.

10. Check for a tethered cord, spina bifida, and lipoma.

Axial images

1. Check any abnormalities noted on the sagittal images.

2. Evaluate the marrow signal in each vertebral body.

3. Evaluate the disc signal at each motion segment.

4. If a disc bulge or herniation is present, determine the following:

    a. Is it symmetrical (bulge) or focal (herniation)?

    b. If focal, note the direction (central, lateral, far lateral) and degree of herniation in mm.

    c. Is there pressure on the thecal sac?

    d. Are the intervertebral foraminae patent?

    e. If an osteophyte is also present, or if it is not possible to differentiate disc from osteophyte, this should be noted.

5. Check for osteophytes, including anterior spondylotic changes and posterior osteophytes.

6. Check the spinal canal, including cord and CSF signals. Note any evidence of stenosis, congenital or acquired. Look for clumped nerve roots and meningeal thickening suggestive of arachnoiditis. Examine for diastomyelia, conjoined nerve roots, etc.

7. Check the emerging nerve roots and intervertebral foraminae.

8. Examine the posterior joints. Check for asymmetry (tropism) and degenerative changes.

9. Check the kidneys.

10. Check the psoas muscles.

11. Examine the abdominal aorta and any other major vessels visible on the image.

12. Check the paraspinal muscles for symmetry, ability to discern layers, and hemorrhage.

13. Examine the spinous processes, and check for spina bifida, meningomyelocele, etc.

Table 8.33. **Abbreviated List of Possible Abnormalities That Can Be Detected with MRI**

Disc bulge

Herniated nucleus pulposus

Degenerative disc disease

Degenerative joint disease

Fracture

Dislocation

Tumor

Congenital/developmental variants:

    a. Spina bifida

    b. Diastomyelia

    c. Tethered cord

    d. Spinal stenosis

    e. Other types of dysraphism

Arachnoiditis

Metastasis

Infection

Hemorrhage (295)

Selection of Imaging Techniques in Pediatric Back Pain

Subluxation, Pain and Dysfunction

In adults with low back pain, two representative studies (328,329) have failed to demonstrate a correlation between neutral position and lateral bending x-ray findings, and the patients' symptoms. The lack of correlation primarily stems from the observation that many asymptomatic individuals have "abnormal" radiographs. Similar studies testing correlation, if any, with plain film radiography have yet to be performed. Low back pain has a relatively high prevalence among adolescents (41,330). The relevance of low back pain to the decision making process resulting in the ordering of radiographs would likely be different if a practitioner (e.g. internist) used varying analytical protocols and different treatment procedures (331,332).

The medical doctor usually treats all minor degenerative changes and biomechanical irregularities of the spine in similar fashion (e.g. medications, rest, exercises). The chiropractor, in contrast, uses these often subtle radiological changes to alter how forces are applied to the spinal column during a specific contact, short lever arm adjustment (15). Chiropractors have not primarily used radiographs to identify the source of pain, per se, but rather to determine biomechanical factors that would aid in the delivery of adjustments.

Pain may or may not be a good indicator of where the doctor should adjust the patient. Hypermobile motion seg-

ments can cause more pain than their hypomobile counter parts. Therefore, using subjective criteria alone for the determination of the segmental level (i.e. the point of therapeusis) at which to radiograph or adjust is somewhat problematic. However, the general region of pain, and certainly known referral patterns, will often point to the correct area for examination.

Pain can be an important outcome measure for the effectiveness of various treatments although it is not the only parameter chiropractors should consider as an outcome measure. The chiropractor can more appropriately care for the health of individuals if the focus is on both objective (e.g., x-ray, palpation) and subjective (e.g., pain) parameters.

Although using the radiograph to identify an abnormality or to render a diagnosis is possible, the radiograph of the spine has historically been used to determine the direction of thrust (or line of drive) and to confirm the diagnostic impression that has been worked out clinically. Following the initial history and physical examination, signs of subluxation may be identified. The methods used during this clinical assessment may include static and motion palpation, postural analysis, and noninvasive instrumentation such as goniometer, skin temperature devices and other tools to assess the multifaceted nature of the lesion.

In the case of a pediatric or young adult patient, overt symptoms are usually minimal shortly following an injury. But residual joint disability due to ligamentous trauma and subsequent scarring of the motion segment may develop a chronic or permanent pattern of movement, if motion is not introduced to a fixated segment through an adjustment.

Back pain is a relatively uncommon complaint in children compared to adults, although adolescents have a high prevalence for the disorder. Such complaints warrant a thorough investigation. Although the primary responsibility of the chiropractor is to locate and correct vertebral subluxations, it is also imperative that the chiropractor be familiar with conditions which may contraindicate certain adjusting techniques, or conditions where interdisciplinary management is indicated. Although it is estimated that 80% of the adult population will suffer from back pain, complaints of back pain are relatively uncommon in the younger pediatric age groups (e.g. toddler, juvenile). Proper epidemiologic studies need to be performed in order to determine the true prevalence and incidence of this disorder.

Vertebral subluxations have been implicated as significant etiologic factors in a variety of conditions (333-336). Subluxation can also be associated with congenital or developmental variation (337). Many vertebral subluxations are asymptomatic, or produce symptoms quite distant from the anatomical site of involvement. Spinal subluxations are also associated with local tenderness (338). Thus, it is important for the chiropractor to recognize the far reaching consequences of vertebral subluxation in the developing spine. The use of plain film spinography to characterize subluxations is indicated if the information to be gained cannot be obtained through clinical examination (339).

In many cases of pediatric back pain, subtle clinical signs and symptoms may be due to major pathology (340) (Fig. 8.236). The chiropractor should be alert to this possibility, and carefully evaluate the case. A thorough history, physical examination, and appropriate imaging studies are imperative. The selection of appropriate imaging techniques, including plain radiographs, CT, and MRI studies is discussed in the next section.

History and Examination

The onset, character, and progression of pain should be considered. Pain which occurs suddenly following trauma suggests subluxation, strain/sprain, dislocation, or fracture. Children are relatively active, and thus suffer muscle strain less frequently than adults. Overuse syndrome may result in athletes as a consequence of repeated unrepaired microtrauma. This may be due to improper conditioning or improper technique. In such cases, the pain will usually resolve following 2-3 minutes of limited activities. It is useful to ask if the pain is constant, or if it is aggravated by activity (341). Back pain which progresses, if accompanied by signs and symptoms of systemic illness, or if associated with neurological signs requires careful investigation. Altered gait, muscular weakness, or foot drop suggest the possibility of a progressive neurological process. Bowel or bladder dysfunction may indicate intraspinal pathology.

Fever, malaise, irritability, and an elevated ESR can indicate an infectious process such as discitis, meningitis, or osteomyelitis. Rheumatic disorders, as well as hematologic disorders such as sickle cell anemia and acute leukemias may result in back pain (342). See Chapters 7 and 9 for the discussion of examination procedures.

Neoplasm

Primary osseous tumors are uncommon, although back pain with an accompanying scoliosis should alert the chiropractor to this possibility. The most common primary pediatric vertebral osseous tumors are osteoid osteoma (Fig. 8.237), osteoblastoma (benign), aneurysmal bone cyst (Fig. 8.238), Ewing's sarcoma, and eosinophilic granuloma. Primary lymphoma occurs less commonly (343,344).

Spinal cord tumors are usually slow growing. As such, symptoms are often insidious. Weakness is the most common presenting complaint, although 25-30% also report having a dull ache confined to a few spinal levels, or nerve root pain. Astrocytomas and ependymomas are the most frequently encountered pediatric intramedullary tumors. Pain or other symptoms may be aggravated by Valsalva maneuvers (345,346).

Infection

Discitis refers to an inflammatory condition affecting the intervertebral disc. It is generally thought to be infectious, although cultures of biopsy specimens are positive in only about 25% of cases. The organism most frequently isolated is Staphylococcus aureus. Epidemiologically, discitis occurs most frequently in children under 10 (median age is 6 years). Symptoms include non-radiating back pain, malaise, anorexia, and irritability.

Vertebral osteomyelitis often presents a similar clinical picture, but affects children over 10 years of age. A coexisting infectious focus is often found at a distant anatomical site. Plain radiographs are usually negative early in the disease. As the condition progresses, the disc space appears violated. Bone scans may be helpful in determining the extent of involvement, but provides very little anatomical information. Magnetic resonance imaging, although more expensive, provides better characterization of the lesions. Pediatric spine infections are classically treated with antibiotics, however some medical authorities suggest that childhood discitis is a self limiting condition with a benign course, and that neither biopsy nor antibiotics are necessary (347,348).

Mechanical and/or traumatic
  Vertebral subluxation
  Muscle strain
  Overuse syndrome
  Scheuermann's disease
  Herniated nucleus pulposus
  Spondylolisthesis
  Scoliosis
  Fracture
  Dislocation
Infectious
  Discitis
  Osteomyelitis

Neoplastic Osseous
  Osteoid osteoma
  Benign osteoblastoma
  Aneurysmal bone cyst
  Ewing's sarcoma
  Eosinophilic granuloma

Spinal cord and extramedullary
  Astrocytoma
  Ependyoma
  Lipoma
  Neurofibroma (rare in children)
  Meningioma (rare in children)

Rheumatic
  Ankylosing spondylitis
  Psoriatic arthritis
  Reiter's syndrome
  Enteric arthritis (associated with
    enteritis or colitis)

Hematologic
  Leukemia
  Sickle cell anemia

Figure 8.236.   Various potential causes of pediatric back pain.

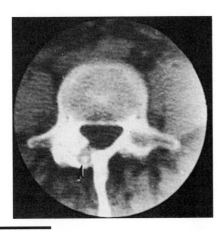

Figure 8.237. Osteoid osteoma. A central nidus is present in this case. Reproduced with permission from Grossman CB. Magnetic resonance imaging and computed tomography of the head and spine. Baltimore: Williams & Wilkins, 1990:435.

Scheuermann's Disease

The etiology of this condition has been the subject of much debate. Scheuermann proposed that the condition represented a form of avascular necrosis (349). It is now thought to be a spondylodystrophy caused by cumulative trauma. This process is believed to result in traumatic growth arrest and vertebral endplate fractures. It is felt that there is heightened vulnerability to the condition during the adolescent growth spurt. Clinically, the patient presents with a rigid kyphotic thoracic spine and dull, not radiating pain. The pain is aggravated by activity and relieved by rest or positional changes. Individuals with Scheuermann's disease are twice as likely to develop back pain as the general population (350).

Spondylolisthesis

Spondylolysis refers to a defect in the pars interarticularis. It is currently thought to be a stress fracture resulting from cumulative trauma (351,352). Children and adolescents who participate in gymnastics and contact sports are more likely to develop the condition. Spondylolisthesis is an anterior slipping of one vertebral segment over another, and is often associated with bilateral spondylolysis. The most common anatomical site is fifth lumbar. Patients with spondylolisthesis frequently present with low back pain which is aggravated by activity, especially hyperextension motions, and relieved by rest (353). There may be an associated step defect in some patients, a prominent L5 spinous process or increased sacral base angle. In young patients, with a small anterolisthesis, these findings may not be evident on physical examination (See Chapter 15).

Disc Herniation

Although disc herniations are rare in infants and children, the prevalence of disc lesions in adolescents is increasing (354).

There is often a history of trauma, and herniation of the nucleus pulposus is more likely to occur in athletes than the general adolescent population. Two thirds of adolescents with disc herniations present with back pain, and one third have sciatica as their chief complaint. Back stiffness, hamstring tightness, and an associated gait disturbance should alert the chiropractor to the possibility of HNP. Clinical examination will reveal a marked decrease in straight leg raising. Vertebral endplate fractures and avulsion fractures may also be present (355).

Scoliosis

Although scoliosis may have profound effects in the affected patient, the condition is usually without pain. When suspected clinically, spinographic x-ray examination is indicated to evaluate the condition. Follow-up spinographs should be taken to assess response to chiropractic care and to monitor the correction or progression of the scoliosis. In addition, spinographs are valuable in determining spinal listings, and characterizing the disc block subluxation (356) (See Chapter 14). A painful scoliosis may be due to muscle spasm or may herald a serious pathology (357). Pathologies which present with a painful scoliosis include osteoid osteoma, benign osteoblastoma, pyogenic infection, eosinophilic granuloma, and aneurysmal bone cyst (354,355).

SELECTION OF IMAGING TECHNIQUES IN BACK PAIN

According to King (340) every pediatric patient who presents with back pain should have AP and lateral radiographs taken of the affected area. Other authorities recommend AP and lateral radiographs be taken of the entire spine in cases of trauma (358-360). The rationale is the high incidence of contiguous and non-contiguous injuries. From a chiropractic perspective, full spine radiographs permit the characterization of primary and compensatory changes (12).

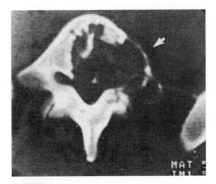

Figure 8.238. Aneurysmal bone cyst. Reproduced with permission from Grossman CB. Magnetic resonance imaging and computed tomography of the head and spine. Baltimore: Williams & Wilkins, 1990:436.

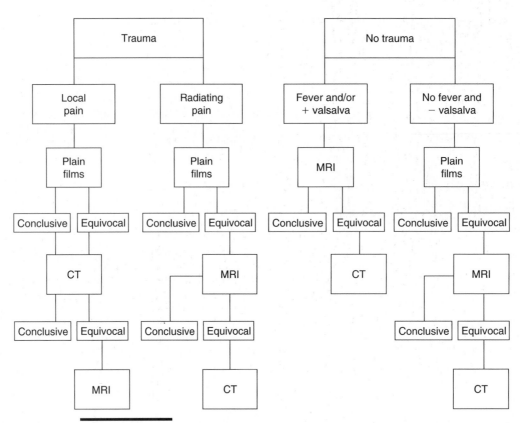

Figure 8.239. Imaging flow-chart for the pediatric patient with back pain.

The plain film spinograph is usually the initial imaging study of choice in evaluating the pediatric spine. Plain films are inexpensive and readily available, and with good technique, the radiation burden is low. In cases of pediatric back pain, however, plain films alone may not be adequate. If plain films fail to disclose the cause of the condition, CT or MRI studies may be appropriate.

In cases where visualization of bone is desired, such as suspected fractures and osseous neoplasms, CT examination generally follows plain film radiography. CT provides direct, high resolution imaging in the axial plane. For many conditions, it offers superior sensitivity compared to plain films. CT, however, is more expensive than plain film radiography. It also involves exposure to ionizing radiation.

Magnetic resonance imaging (MRI) is the technique of choice for soft tissue imaging. In cases of suspected spinal cord tumors, other extraosseous neoplasms, demyelinating disease, syrinx, Chiari malformation, or infection, MRI is indicated.

MRI is also useful in the evaluation of disc lesions. MRI has the ability to image directly in multiple planes. Although more expensive than CT, its superior sensitivity in soft tissue imaging, as well as freedom from exposure to ionizing radiation makes MRI an attractive technique for pediatric imaging. Some children may find it difficult to remain still while undergoing MRI examination. Also, the noise produced by some imagers may be frightening to the child. The availability of a virtually silent, open MRI imager (ACCESS,

by Toshiba America MRI) makes pediatric MRI without sedation practical. A parent may accompany the child in the magnet room, providing comfort and security. This system is of particular interest to chiropractors who are reluctant to have their patients sedated.

Plain film radiography remains the imaging technique of choice for most cases of pediatric back pain (361). The limitations of plain film studies must be borne in mind when the possibility of infection, neoplasm, or demyelinating disease is suggested by the history and clinical findings. In such cases, magnetic resonance imaging may be the initial imaging technique of choice. In all cases, individual clinical need must determine which imaging techniques are selected, and under what circumstances. Figure 8.239 displays an algorithmic approach to imaging decisions in the pediatric patient with back pain.

REFERENCES

1. Yochum TR, Rowe LJ. Essentials of skeletal radiology, 2nd ed. Baltimore: Williams & Wilkins, 1995.
2. Reed MH, ed. Pediatric skeletal radiology. Baltimore: Williams & Wilkins, 1992.
3. Swischuk LE. Differential diagnosis in pediatric radiology. Baltimore: Williams & Wilkins, 1984.
4. Hadley LA. Anatomico-roentgenographic studies of the spine. Springfield: Charles C. Thomas, 1964.
5. Statistics on chiropractic offices and equipment. J Am Chiro Assoc 1987; 24:56-61.
6. Job analysis of chiropractic. National Board of Chiropractic Examiners. Greeley, CO, 1993:73; Appendix E:11.

7. Clark CR, Igram CM, El-Khoury GY, Ehara S. Radiographic evaluation of cervical spine injuries. Spine 1988; 13:742-747.
8. Kawchuk GN, Herzog W, Hasler EM. Forces generated during spinal manipulative therapy: a pilot study. J Manipulative Physiol Ther 1992; 15:275-278.
9. Wood J, Adams A. Forces used in selected adjustments of the low back: a preliminary study. Res Forum 1984; 1:16-23.
10. Herzog W, Conway PJ, Kawchuk GN, Zhang Y, Hasler EM. Forces exerted during spinal manipulative therapy. Spine 1993; 18:1206-1212.
11. Conway PJW, Herzog W, Zhang Y, Hasler EM, Ladly K. Forces required to cause cavitation during spinal manipulation of the thoracic spine. Clin Biomech 1993; 8:210-214.
12. Rowe SH, Ray SG, Jakubowski AM, Picardi RJ. Plain film radiography in chiropractic. In: Plaugher G, ed. Textbook of clinical chiropractic: a specific biomechanical approach. Baltimore: Williams & Wilkins, 1993:112-149.
13. Herbst RW. Gonstead chiropractic science and art. Mt. Horeb, WI: Sci-Chi Publications 1968.
14. Cremata EE, Plaugher G, Cow WA. Technique system application: the Gonstead approach. Chiropractic Technique 1991; 3:19-25.
15. Plaugher G. The role of plain film radiography in chiropractic clinical practice. Chiro J Aust 1992; 22:153-161.
16. Plaugher G, ed. Textbook of clinical chiropractic: a specific biomechanical approach. Baltimore: Williams & Wilkins, 1993.
17. Palmer BJ. The subluxation specific-the adjustment specific. Davenport, IA: Palmer School of Chiropractic, 1934.
18. Faucret B, Mao Wm Nakagawa T, Spurgin D, Tran T. Determination of bony subluxations by clincial, neurolgical and chiropractic procedures. J Manipulative Physiol Ther 1980; 3:165-176.
19. Hildebrandt RW. Chiropractic spinography and postural roentgenology-part 2: clinical basis. J Manipulative Physiol Ther 1981; 4:191-201.
20. Speiser RM, Aragona RJ, Heffernan JP. The application of therapeutic exercises based upon lateral flexion roentgenography to restore biomechanical function in the lumbar spine. Chiro Res J 1990; 1(4):7-16.
21. Biedermann H. Kinematic imbalances due to suboccipital strain in newborns. J Manual Med 1992; 6:151-156.
22. Haldeman S, Chapman-Smith D, Peterson D, eds. Guidelines for chiropractic quality assurance and practice parameters. Gaithersburg, MD: Aspen Publishing Company, 1992.
23. Phillips RB. Plain film radiology in chiropractic. J Manipulative Physiol Ther 1992; 15:47-50.
24. Taylor JAM. Full spine radiography: a review. J Manipulative Physiol Ther 1993; 16:460-473.
25. Hildebrandt RW. Chiropractic spinography and postural roentgenology-part 1: history of development. J Manipulative Physiol Ther 1980; 3:87-92.
26. Lantz CA. The vertebral subluxation complex. Part 1. An introduction to the model and the kinesiological component. Chiro Res J 1989; 1(3):23-36.
27. Nansel D, Cremata E, Carlson J, Szlazak M. Effect of unilateral spinal adjustments on goniometrically-assessed cervical lateral-flexion end-range asymmetries in otherwise asymptomatic subjects. J Manipulative Physiol Ther 1989; 12:419-27.
28. Dishman R. Review of the literature supporting a scientific basis for the chiropractic subluxation complex. J Manipulative Physiol Ther 1985; 8:163-174.
29. Gatterman MI. Foundations of chiropractic: subluxation. St. Louis: Mosby-Yearbook, 1995.
30. Pettibon BR. Pettibon method for cervical x-ray analysis and instrument adjusting. Tacoma, WA: (self-published), 1968.
31. Lopes MA, Plaugher G, Cremata EE, Walters PJ. Spinal examination. In: Plaugher G, ed. Textbook of clinical chiropractic: a specific biomechanical approach. Baltimore: Williams & Wilkins, 1993:73-111.
32. Bronfort G, Jochumsen OH. The functional radiographic examination of patients with low back pain: a study of different forms and variations. J Manipulative Physiol Ther 1984; 7:89-97.
33. Anrig CA. Chiropractic approaches to pregnancy and pediatric care. In: Plaugher G, ed. Textbook of clinical chiropractic: a specific biomechanical approach. Baltimore: Williams & Wilkins, 1993:383-432.
34. White AA, Panjabi MM. Clinical biomechanics of the spine, 2nd ed. Philadelphia: J.B. Lippincott, Co., 1990:132.
35. Scher AT. Spinal cord injuries in rugby players. J S Afr Sports Med 1988; 3(2):12-13.
36. Farfan HF. Mechanical disorders of the low back. Philadelphia: Lea & Febiger, 1973.
37. Moore RJ, Vernon-Roberts B, Fraser RD. Changes in endplate vascularity after an outer annulus tear in sheep. Spine 1992;17:874-878.
38. Paajanen H, Erkintalo M, Kuusela T, Dahlstrom S, Kormano M. Magnetic resonance study of disc degeneration in young low-back pain patients. Spine 1989; 14:982-985.
39. Schiebler ML, Camerino VJ, Fallon MD, et al. In vivo and ex vivo magnetic resonance imaging evaluation of early disc degeneration with histopathologic correlation. Spine 1991;16:635-640.
40. Slosberg M. Side posture manipulation for lumbar intervertebral disk herniation reconsidered. J Manipulative Physiol Ther 19994; 17:258-262.
41. Olsen TL, Anderson RL, Dearwater MS. The epidemiology of low back pain in an adolescent population. Am J Publ Health 1992; 82:606-608.
42. Shekelle PG, Adams AH, Chassin MR, et al. The appropriateness of spinal manipulation for low-back pain. Rand R-4025/1-CCR/FCER, Santa Monica, CA. 1991.
43. Manga P, Angus D, Papadopoulos C, Swan W. The effectiveness and cost-effectiveness of chiropractic management of low-back pain. Ontario: Kenilworth Publishing, 1993.
44. Klemp DD. Letter to the editor. J Manipulative Physiol Ther 1992; 15:331.
45. Keating JC, Bergmann TF, Jacobs GE, Finer BA, Larson K. Interexaminer reliability of eight evaluative dimensions of lumbar segmental abnormality. J Manipulative Physiol Ther 1990; 13:463-470.
46. Boline PD, Haas M, Meyer JJ, et al. Interexaminer reliability of eight evaluative dimensions of lumbar segmental abnormality: Part II. J Manipulative Physiol Ther 1993; 16:363-374.
47. Plaugher G. Skin temperature assessment for neuromusculoskeletal abnormalities of the spinal column. J Manipulative Physiol Ther 1992; 15:365-381.
48. Plaugher G, Lopes MA, Melch PE, Cremata EE. The inter- and intraexaminer reliability of a paraspinal skin temperature differential instrument. J Manipulative Physiol Ther 1991; 14:361-367.
49. Ebrall PS, Iggo A, Hobson P, Farrant G. Preliminary report: the thermal characteristics of spinal levels identified as having differential temperature by contact thermocouple measurement (Nervo Scope). Chiro J Australia 1994; 24:139-146.
50. Wright HM, Korr IM, Thomas PE. Local and regional variations in cutaneous vasomotor tone of the human trunk. Neural Transmission 1960; 22:34-52.
51. Gunn CC, Milbrandt WE. Early and subtle signs in low-back sprain. Spine 1978; 3:267-81.
52. Gunn CC, Milbrandt WE. Tenderness at motor points-a diagnostic and prognostic aid for low back injury. J Bone Joint Surg 1976; 58A:815-825.
53. Rahlman J. The mechanism of intervertebral joint fixation. J Manipulative Physiol Ther 1987; 10:177-187.
54. Carrick FR. Treatment of pathomechanics of the lumbar spine by manipulation. J Manipulative Physiol Ther 1981; 4:173-178.
55. Carrick FR. Cervical radiculopathy: the diagnosis and treatment of pathomechanics in the cervical spine. J Manipulative Physiol Ther 1983; 6:129-37.
56. Plaugher G, Cremata EE, Phillips RB. A retrospective consecutive case analysis of pretreatment and comparative static radiological parameters following chiropractic adjustments. J Manipulative Physiol Ther 1990; 13:498-506.
57. Banks SD. Lumbar facet syndrome: spinographic assessment of treatment by spinal manipulative therapy. J Manipulative Physiol Ther 1983; 6:175-180.
58. Leach RA. An evaluation of the effect of chiropractic manipulative therapy on hypolordosis of the cervical spine. J Manipulative Physiol Ther 1983; 6:17-23.
59. Giesen JM, Center DB, Leach RA. An evaluation of chiropractic manipulation as a treatment of hyperactivity in children. J Manipulative Physiol Ther 1989; 12:353-363.
60. Thornton RE. Cervical kyphosis. J Clinical Chiropractic 1971; Archives Ed. 1:192-193.
61. Harrison DD, Jackson BL, Troyanovich S, et al. The efficacy of cervical extension-compression traction combined with diversified manipulation and drop table adjustments in the rehabilitation of cervical lordosis: a pilot study. J Manipulative Physiol Ther 1994; 17:454-464.
62. Grostic JD, DeBoer KF. Roentgenographic measurement of atlas laterality and rotation: a retrospective pre- and post-manipulation study. J Manipulative Physiol Ther 1982; 5:63-71.
63. Aspegren DD, Cox JM, Trier KK. Short leg correction: a clinical trial of radiographic vs. non-radiographic procedures. J Manipulative Physiol Ther 1987; 10:232-238.
64. Friberg O. The statics of postural tilt scoliosis; a radiographic study on 288 consecutive chronic LBP patients. Clin Biomech 1987; 2:211-219.
65. Giles LGF, Taylor JR. Lumbar spine structural changes associated with leg length inequality. Spine 1982; 7:159-162.
66. Lawrence D, Pugh J, Tasharski C, Heinze W. Evaluation of a radiographic method determining short leg mensuration. ACA J Chiro 1984; 21(6):57-59.
67. Plaugher G. Lumbar spine. In: Plaugher, ed. Textbook of clinical chiropractic: a specific biomechanical approach. Baltimore: Williams & Wilkins, 1993.
68. Rowe ML. Low back pain in industry, a position paper. J Occup Med 1969; 11:161-169.
69. Fickel TE. Organ - specific dosimetry in spinal radiography: an analysis of genetic and somatic effects. J Manipulative Physiol Ther 1988; 11: 3-9.
70. Morrissy RT. Clinical and radiologic evaluation of spinal disease. In: Bradford DS, Hensinger RM, eds. The pediatric spine. New York: Thieme, Inc., 1985:31.
71. Yochum T, Rowe L. Essentials of skeletal radiology. Baltimore: Williams & Wilkins, 1987.
72. Davis D, Bohlman H, Walker AE, Fisher R, Robinson R. The pathological findings in fatal craniospinal injuries. J Neurosurg 1971; 34:603-613
73. Eiken M. Roentgen diagnosis of bones. Chicago: Year Book Medical Publishers, 1975.
74. Ellett W: Biological effects of ionizing radiation (BEIR V). National Research Council. Washington, DC, 1990.
75. Drummond D, Ranallo F, Lonstein J, Brooks HL, Cameron J. Radiation hazards in scoliosis management. Spine 1983; 8:741-748.
76. Hellstrom G, Irstam L, Nachemson A. Reduction of radiation dose in radiologic examination of patients with scoliosis. Spine 1983; 8:28-30.

77. Nash CL, Gregg EC, Brown RH, Pillai K. Risks of exposure to x-rays in patients undergoing long-term treatment for scoliosis. J Bone Joint Surg 1979; 61A: 371-374.

78. Eastman Kodak Company. Rochester, NY 14650.

79. Du Pont Co. Burbank, CA, 91505.

80. Kalmar JA, Jones JP, Merritt CR. Low dose radiography of scoliosis in children: a comparison of methods. Spine 1994; 19:818-823.

81. State of California. Department of Health Services. Radiation Inspection Findings and Acknowledgment. Bachman Chiropractic Office, Fremont, CA, 1991.

82. U.S. Nuclear Regulatory Commission. Regulatory Guide. Office of Nuclear Regulatory Research. Regulatory Guide 8.13; December, 1987.

83. Mossman KL, Hill LT. Radiation risks in pregnancy. Obstet Gynecol 1982; 60:237-242.

84. Evans JS, Wennberg JE, McNeil BJ. The influence of diagnostic radiography on the incidence of breast cancer and leukemia. N Engl J Med 1986; 315:810-5.

85. Boice JD, Land CE, Shore RE, Norman JE, Tokunaga M. Risk of breast cancer following low-dose radiation exposure. Radiology 1979; 131:589-597.

86. Pillay R, Graham-Pole J, Miraldi F, et al. Diagnostic x-irradiation as a possible etiologic agent in thyroid neoplasms of childhood. J Pediatrics 1982; 101:566-568.

87. Nordenson I, Beckman G, Beckman L, Lemperg R. Chromosomal aberrations in children exposed to diagnostic x-rays. Hereditas 1980; 93:177-179.

88. Wall BF, Rae S, Darby SC, Kendall GM. A reappraisal of the genetic consequences of diagnostic radiology in Great Britain. Br J Radiol 1981; 54: 719-730.

89. Howe J, Yochum TR. X-ray, pregnancy and therapeutic abortion: a current perspective. ACA J Chiro 1985; 19(4):76-90

90. Twibble DA. Estimation of health risk from low-level radiation. Postgrad Radiol 1984; 4:383-401.

91. Sinclair WK. Effects of low-level radiation and comparative risk. Radiology 1981; 138:1-9.

92. Juhl JH. Paul and Juhl's essentials of roentgen interpretation, 4th ed. New York: Harper & Rowe, 1981.

93. Boal TJ, Wikinson LE, Walker RJ, Costantin SA, Einsiedel PF. Patient doses from x-ray units owned by chiropractors in Victoria. Chiro J Australia 1994; 24:91-98.

94. Department of Health Services: Radiologic Health Section. Syllabus on Diagnostic X-ray Radiation Protection for Certified X-ray Supervisors and Operators, January 1982.

95. Shrimpton PC, Jones DG, Wall BF. The influence of tube filtration and potential on patient dose during x-ray examinations. Phys Med Biol 1988; 33:1205-1212.

96. Reuter, Conway, McCrohan, Sueiman. Average radiation exposure values for three diagnostic radiographic examinations. Radiology 177(3):341-346.

97. Hardman LA, Henderson DJ. Comparative dosimetric evaluation of current techniques in chiropractic full-spine and sectional radiography. J Manipulative Physiol Ther 1981; 25:141-145.

98. Phillips RB. An evaluation of chiropractic x-rays by the diplomate members of the American Chiropractic Board of Roentgenology. ACA J Chiro 1980; 14:S80-S88.

99. HEW Publication: a practitioner's guide to the diagnostic x-ray equipment standard. J Manipulative Physiol Ther 1978; 1:260-264.

100. Gyll C. Gonadal protection for the paediatric patient. Radiography 1988; 54(613):9-10.

101. Kuntz F. A simple method of protecting the breasts during upright lateral radiography for spine deformities. Radiolc Technol Volume 55/Number 1 532-535.

102. Bolin DE. 1803 Lansing Ave. N.E., Salem, OR 97303.

103. Hildebrandt RW. Chiropractic spinography. 2nd. ed. Baltimore: Williams & Wilkins, 1985.

104. Buehler MT, Hrejsa AF. Application of lead-acrylic compensating filters in chiropractic full spine radiography: a technical report. J Manipulative Physiol Ther 1985; 8:175-180.

105. Kohn ML, Gooch AW, Keller WS. Filters for radiation reduction: a comparison. Radiology Volume 167 Number 1 256-257.

106. Aragona R, et al. A.S.B.E. Fellowship Commission on X-ray Safety, Patient consumer protection and standards of care in spinal and dental diagnostic roentgenography and academy recommendations to develop equitable chiropractic practice standards of care guidelines (data available on request). The American Academy of Applied Spinal Biomechanical Engineering, 1992:1-120.

107. Sherman R. Teleradiography: extending the focus film distance. J Can Chiro Assoc 1986; 30:143-144.

108. Yochum TR. Evolution to revolution. Amer Chiro 1990; (Sept):25-28.

109. Schram SB, Hosek RS, Silverman HL. Spinographic positioning errors in Gonstead pelvic x-ray analysis. J Manipulative Physiol Ther 1981; 4:179-181.

110. Plaugher G, Hendricks AH. The inter- and intraexaminer reliability of the Gonstead pelvic marking system. J Manipulative Physiol Ther 1991; 14:503-508.

111. Plaugher G, Hendricks AH, Doble RW, et al. The reliability of patient positioning for evaluating static radiological parameters of the human pelvis. J Manipulative Physiol Ther 1993; 16:517-522.

112. Denslow JS, Chace JA, Gutensohn OR, Kumm MG. Methods in taking and interpreting weight-bearing x-ray films. J Am Osteopath Assoc 1955; 54:663-670.

113. Lowe RW, Hayes TD, Kaye J, Bagg RJ, Luekens CA. Standing roentgenograms in spondylolisthesis. Clin Orthop 1976; 117:80-84.

114. Reed MH. Pediatric skeletal radiology. Baltimore: Williams & Wilkins, 1992.

115. Keats T. An atlas of simulated fractures. In: Felson B, ed. Roentgenology of fractures and dislocations. New York: Grune & Stratton, 1978:19.

116. Foreman S, Croft A. Whiplash Injuries. Baltimore: Williams & Wilkins, 1988.

117. Bullough P, Boachie-Adjei O. Atlas of spinal diseases. Philadelphia: J.B. Lippincott, 1988.

118. Goss CM (ed). Gray's Anatomy. Philadelphia: Lea & Febiger, 1966.

119. Lovell W, Winter R. Pediatric orthopedics. Philadelphia: J.B. Lippincott, 1978.

70. National Council on Radiation Protection, Report No. 17,33, 34. NCRP Publications, Washington D.C., 20008.

120. Wiesel S, Rothman R. Occipitoatlantal hypermobility. Spine 1979; 4:187-191.

121. Dunsker S, Brown O, Thompson N. Craniovertebral anomalies. Clin Neurosurg 1980; 27:430-439.

122. MacGibbon B, Farfan HF. A radiologic survey of various configurations of the lumbar spine. Spine 1979; 4:258-266.

123. Pueschel SM, Scola FH, Pezzullo JC. A longitudinal study of atlanto-dens relationships in asymptomatic individuals with Down syndrome. Pediatrics 1992; 89:1194-1198.

124. Letts M, MacDonald P. Sports injuries to the pediatric spine. Spine: State of the Art Reviews 1990; 4(1):49.

125. Pennecot G, Leonard P, Peyrot S, et al. Traumatic ligamentous instability of the cervical spine in children. J Ped Orthop 1984; 4:339-345.

126. Kopits S, Perovic M, McKusick P. Congenital atlantoaxial dislocations in various forms of dwarfism. J Bone Joint Surg 1972; 54A:1349.

127. Martell W, Holt J, Cassidy J. Roentgenologic manifestations of juvenile rheumatoid arthritis. AJR 1962; 88:400.

128. Nathan F, Bickel W: Spontaneous axial subluxation in a child as the first sign of juvenile rheumatoid arthritis. J Bone Joint Surg 1968; 50A:1675-1678.

129. Minderhound J, Braakman R, Pennig L. Os odontoideum: clinical, radiographic, and therapeutic aspects. J Neurol Sci 1961; 8:521.

130. McRae D. The significance of abnormalities of the cervical spine. AJR 1960; 84:3.

131. Lefebvre S, Vallee D, Cassidy JD, Dzus AK. Unstable os odontoideum in young children. J Can Chiro Assoc 1993; 37:141-144.

132. Hensinger R, Lang J, McEwan G. Klippel-Feil syndrome: A constellation of associated anomalies. J Bone Joint Surg 1974; 56:1246-1253.

133. Jenkinson S. Undescended scapula with associated omovertebral bone: Sprengel's deformity. J LA State Med Soc 1977; 129:13-14.

134. Lord J, Rosati L. Thoracic outlet syndromes. Clinical Symposia 1971; 23:1-32.

135. Schmorl G, Junghans H. The Human Spine in Health and Disease. New York: Grune and Stratton, 1971.

136. Murray R, Jacobson H. The radiology of skeletal disorders. New York: Churchill Livingstone, 1977.

137. Farfan H, Sullivan J. The relationship of facet orientation to intervertebral disc failure. Can J Surg 1967; 10:179-185.

138. Starr W. Spina bifida occulta and enlargement of the fifth lumbar spinous process. Clin Orthop 1971; 81:71.

139. Tini P, Wieser C, Zinn W. The transitional vertebra of the lumbosacral spine: Its radiological classification, incidence, prevalence, and clinical significance. Rheumatol Rehabil 1977; 16:180-185.

140. Castellvi A, Goldstein L, Chan D. Lumbosacral transitional vertebrae and their relationship with lumbar extradural defects. Spine 1984; 9:493-495.

141. Putti V. Early treatment of congenital dislocation of the hip. J Bone Joint Surg 1929; 11(A):798.

142. Wakeley CJ, Cassar-Pullicino VN, McCall IW. Case of the month: not so pseudo. Br J Radiol 1991; 64:375-376.

143. Dickman CA, Rekate HL. Spinal trauma. In: Eichelberger MR, ed. Pediatric trauma. St. Louis: Mosby Year Book, 1993:362-377.

144. Sullivan C, Brewer A, Harris L. Hypermobility of the cervical spine in children: A pitfall in the diagnosis of clinical dislocation. Am J Surg 1958; 95:636.

145. Papavasiliou V. Traumatic subluxation of the cervical spine during childhood. Orthop Clin North Am 1978; 9:945.

146. Fielding J, Hensinger R. Fractures of the cervical spine. In: Rockwood C, Wilkins K, King K (eds) Children's fractures. Philadelphia: J.B. Lippincott, 1984.

147. Schneier M, Burns RE. Atlanto-occipital hypermobility in sudden infant death syndrome. J Chiropractic Res Clin Invest 1991; 7(2):33.

148. Bohlman H. Acute fractures and dislocations of the cervical spine: an analysis of three hundred hospitalized patients and review of the literature. J Bone Joint Surg 1979; A1:1119-42.

149. Henrys P, Lyne E, Lifton C, Salciccioli G. Clinical review of cervical spine injuries in children. Clin Orthop 1977; 129:172-6.

152. Mann D. Spine fractures in children and adolescents. Spine: State of the Art Reviews 1990; 4(1):25.

153. Evans D, Bethem D. Cervical spine injuries in children. J Pediatr Orthop 1989; 9:563-8.

154. Hubbard D. Injuries of the spine in children and adolescents. Clin Orthop 1974; 100:56-65.

155. Kewalramani L, Tori J. Spinal cord trauma in children: neurologic patterns, radiologic features, and pathomechanics of injury. Spine 1980; 5:11.

156. McAfee P, Yuan H, Frederickson B, Lubicky J. The value of computed tomography in thoracolumbar fractures. J Bone Joint Surg 1983; 65A:461-473.

157. Bale J, Bell W, Dunn V, et al. Magnetic resonance imaging of the spine in children. Arch Neurol 1986; 43:1253-6.

158. Fitz C. Diagnostic imaging of children with spinal disorders. Pediatr Clin North Am 1985; 32:1537-58.
159. Duthoy M, Lund G: MR imaging of the spine in children. Eur J Radiol 1988; 8(3):188.
160. Denis F, Winter R, Lonstein J. Pediatric spinal injuries. Proceedings of 22nd Annual Meeting of Scoliosis Research Society. September 15-19, 1987. Vancouver, BC, Canada.
161. Henrys P, Lyne E, Lifton C, Salciccioli G. Clinical review of cervical spine injuries in children. Clin Orthop 1977; 129:172-176.
162. Powers B, Miller M, Kramer R, et al. Traumatic anterior atlanto-occipital dislocation. Neurosurgery 1979; 4:12-17.
163. Martinez S, Morgan C, Gehwiler J, et al. Unusual fractures and dislocations of the axis vertebra. Skeletal Radiol 1979; 3:206.
164. Sherk H, Nicholson J, Chung S. Fractures of the odontoid process in young children. J Bone Joint Surg 1978; 60A:921-924.
165. Pizzutillo P, Rocha E, D'Astous J, et al. Bilateral fracture of the pedicle of the second cervical vertebra in the young child. J Bone Joint Surg 1986; 68A:892-896.
166. Rowe DJ. Chiropractic management of spinal fractures and dislocations. In: Plaugher G, ed. Textbook of clinical chiropractic: a specific biomechanical approach. Baltimore: Williams & Wilkins, 1993:326-355.
167. Kewalramani L, Krauss J. Cervical spine injuries resulting from collision sports. Paraplegia 1981; 19:303-312.
168. Chance G. Note on a type of flexion fracture of the spine. Br J Radiol 1948; 21:452.
169. Kleinman P, Zito J. Avulsion of the spinous process caused by infant abuse. Radiology 1984; 151:389-391.
170. Cullen J. Spinal lesions in battered babies. J Bone Joint Surg 1975; 57B:364-366.
171. Radkowski MA. The battered child syndrome: pitfalls in radiological diagnosis. Pediatr Ann 1983; 12:894-903.
172. Stiller CA. Malignancies. In: Pless IB. The epidemiology of childhood disorders. New York: Oxford university Press, 1994:439-472.
173. Galasko C. Tumors of the spine. Spine: State of the Art Reviews 1990; 4(1):101.
174. Spigelblatt L, Laine-Ammara G, Pless IB, Guyver A. The use of alternative medicine by children. Pediatrics 1994; 811-814.
175. Harsha WA. The natural history of osteocartilagenous exostoses (osteochondroma) Am Surg 1954; 20:65.
176. Novick G, Pavlov H, Bullough P. Osteochondroma of the cervical spine: case reports. Skeletal Radiol 1982; 8:13-15.
177. Pettine K, Klassen R. Osteoid osteoma and osteoblastoma of the spine. J Bone Joint Surg 1986; 68A:354-361.
178. Mehta M, Murray O. Scoliosis provoked by painful vertebral lesions. Skeletal Radiol 1977; 1:223.
179. DeSouza Dias L, Frost H. Osteoblastoma of the spine: a review and report of eight new cases. Clin Orthop 1973; 141-151.
180. Marsh BW, Bonfiglio M, Brady LP, et al. Benign osteoblastoma: range of manifestations. J Bone Joint Surg 1975; 57A:1-9.
181. Janin Y, Epstein J, Carris R, Kahn A. Osteoid osteoma and osteoblastoma of the spine. Neurosurgery 1981; 8:31-38.
182. Capanna R, Albisinni U, Picci P. Aneurysmal bone cysts of the cervical spine. J Bone Joint Surg 1985; 67A:527-531.
183. Hay M, Paterson D, Taylor T. Aneurysmal bone cysts of the spine. J Bone Joint Surg 1978; 60B:406-411.
184. Tillman BP, Dahlin DC, Lipscomb PR, et al. Aneurysmal bone cyst: an analysis of ninety-five cases. Mayo Clin Proc 1968; 43:478-495.
185. Makley J, Carter J. Eosinophilic granuloma of bone. Clin Orthop 1986; 204:37.
186. Dawson EG, Mirra JM, Yuhl ET, Lasser L. Solitary bone cyst of the cervical spine. Clin Orthop 1976; 119:141-143.
187. Wu KK, Guise ER. Unicameral bone cyst of the spine: a case report. J Bone Joint Surg 1982; 63A:324-326.
188. Griffiths HJ. Basic Bone Radiology. Norwalk, CT: Appleton-Century-Crofts, 1981.
189. Shafrir Y, Kaufman BA. Quadriplegia after chiropractic manipulation in an infant with congenital torticollis caused by a spinal cord astrocytoma. J Pediatr 1992; 120:266-269.
190. Reimer R, Chabner B, Young R. Lymphoma presenting in bone. Ann Intern Med 1977; 87:50-55.
191. Fielding J, Fietti V, Hughes J, Gabrielian J. Primary osteogenic sarcoma in the cervical spine. J Bone Joint Surg 1976; 58A:892-894.
192. Friedlander G, Southwick W. Tumors of the spine. In: Rothman R, Simeone F, eds. The spine, 2nd ed. Philadelphia: W.B. Saunders, 1982.
193. Silverman FN, Kuhn JP. Essentials of Caffey's pediatric x-ray diagnosis. St. Louis: Mosby Year Book, 1990.
194. Dich V, Nelson J, Haltalin K. Osteomyelitis in infants and children. A review of 163 cases. Am J Dis Child 1975; 129:1273-1278.
195. Apel D, Tolo V: Infections of the spine in childhood and adolescence. Spine: State of the Art Reviews 1990; 4(1):85.
196. Boston H Jr, Bianco A Jr, Rhodes K. Disc space infections in children. Orthop Clin North Am 1975; 6:953-964.
197. Sartoris DJ, Moskowitz PS, Kaufman RA, Ziprkowski MN, Berger PE. Childhood diskitis: computed tomographic findings. Radiology 1983; 149:701-707.
198. White JI, Gardner VO, Takeda H. Back pain in the pediatric patient: assessment and differential diagnosis. Spine: State of the Art Reviews 1990; 4(1):1.
199. Gilday DL, Paul DJ, Paterson J. Diagnosis of osteomyelitis in children by combined blood pool and bone imaging. Radiology 1975; 117:331-335.
214. Schoenecker P. Legg-Calve-Perthes disease. Orthop Rev 1986; 15: 561.
200. Fisher E, Green C Jr, Winston K. Spinal epidural abscess in children. Neurosurgery 1981; 9:257.
201. Angtuaco E, McConnell J, Chadduck W, Flanigan S. MR imaging of spinal epidural sepsis. Am J Roentgenol 1987; 149:1249-1253.
202. Shanks MJ, Blane CE, Adler DD, Sullivan DB. Radiographic findings of scleroderma in childhood. AJR 1983; 141:657-660.
203. Kent C. ICA Medicare manual. International Chiropractors Association. Davenport, IA, 1973.
204. Bunnell WP. The natural history of idiopathic scoliosis. Clin Orthop 1988; 229:20-25.
205. Green N: Adolescent idiopathic scoliosis. Spine: State of the Art Review Series 1990; 4:211.
206. Ippolito E, Ponseti I. Juvenile kyphosis: histological and histochemical studies. J Bone Joint Surg 1981; 63A:175-182.
207. Resnick D, Niwayama G. Intravertebral disk herniations: cartilaginous (Schmorl's) nodes. Radiology 1978; 126:57-65.
208. Alexander C. Scheuermann's disease. A traumatic spondylodystrophy? Skeletal Radiol 1977; 1:209.
209. Bradford D. Juvenile kyphosis. Clin Orthop 1977; 128:45.
210. Legg A. An obscure affection of the hip joint. Boston Med Surg J 1910; 162:202.
211. Calve J. Sur une forme particuliere de pseudo-coxalgie greffee sur des deformations characteristiques de l'extremitie superieure du femur. Rev Chir 1910; 30:54.
212. Perthes G. Uber arthritis deformans juvenilis. Dtsch Z Chir 1910; 107:111.
213. Wyngaarden J, Smith L. Cecil textbook of medicine. 16th ed. Philadelphia: W. B. Saunders, 1982:1349.
214. Schoenecker P. Legg-Calves-Perthes disease. Orthop Rev 1986; 15:561-574.
215. Clarke T, Finegan T, Fisher R, Bunch W, Grossling H. Legg-Calve-Perthes disease in children less than four years old. J Bone Joint Surg 1978; 60A:166-168.
216. Sutro C, Pomeranz M. Perthes disease. Arch Surg 1937; 34:360.
217. Baker D, Hall A. The epidemiology of Perthes disease. Clin Orthop 1986; 209:89-94.
218. Edgren W. Coxa plana: A clinical and radiological investigation with particular reference to the importance of the metaphyseal changes for the final shape of the proximal part of the femur. Acta Orthop Scand Suppl 1965; 84:1.
219. Resnick D, Niwayama G. Diagnosis of bone and joint disorders. Philadelphia: W. B. Saunders, 1988.
220. Ferguson A Jr. The pathology of Legg-Perthes disease and its comparison with aseptic necrosis. Clin Orthop 1975; 106:7-18.
221. Dolman C, Bell H. The pathology of Legg-Calve-Perthes disease. A case report. J Bone Joint Surg 1973; 55A:184-188.
222. Toby EB, Koman LA, Bechtold RE. Magnetic resonance imaging of pediatric hip disease. J Pediatric Orthopedics 1985; 5:665-671.
223. White J, Gardner V, Takeda H. Back pain in the pediatric patient: assessment and differential diagnosis. Spine: State of the Art Review Series 1990; 4(1):1.
224. Wiltse L, Widell E, Jackson D. Fatigue fracture, the basic lesion in isthmic spondylolisthesis. J Bone Joint Surg 1975; 57:17-22.
225. Stedman's medical dictionary, 25th ed, illustrated. Baltimore: Williams & Wilkins, 1990:1364.
226. Kent C. Protocols for the analysis of plain skeletal radiographs. Dig Chiro Econ 1988; 31(3):70.
227. Kent C. A systematic approach to the evaluation of cervical spine radiographs. International Review of Chiropractic 1989; 45(5):23.
228. Voutsinas SA, MacEwen GE. Sagittal profiles of the spine. Clin Orthop 1986; 210:235-242.
229. Harrison DD, Janik TJ, Troyanovich SJ, Holland B. Comparisons of lordotic cervical spine curvatures to a theoretical ideal model of the static sagittal cervical spine. Spine 1996; 21:667-675.
230. Frymoyer JW, Frymoyer WW, Wilder DG, Pope MH. The mechanical and kinematic analysis of the lumbar spine in normal living human subjects in vivo. J Biomech 1979; 12:165-172.
231. Gracovetsky S, Farfan H. The optimum spine. Spine 1986; 11:543.
232. Panjabi MM, White AA, Brand RA. A note on defining body parts configurations. J Biomech 1974; 7:385-87.
233. White AA, Panjabi MM, Brand RA. A system for defining position and motion of the human body parts. Med Biol Eng 1975; 13:261-65.
234. Gerow G. Osseous configurations of the axial skeleton: specific application to spatial relationships of vertebrae. J Manipulative Physiol Ther 1984; 7:33-38.
235. Lopes MA, Plaugher G. Vertebral subluxation complex. In: Plaugher G, ed. Textbook of clinical chiropractic: a specific biomechanical approach. Baltimore: Williams & Wilkins, 1993:52-72.
236. Drerup B, Hierholzer E. Automatic localization of anatomical landmarks on the back surface and construction of a body-fixed coordinate system. J Biomech 1987; 20:961-970.
237. Drerup B, Hierholzer E. Movement of the human pelvis and displacement of related anatomical landmarks on the body surface. J Biomech 1987; 20:971-977.
238. Cibulka MT, Rose SJ, Delitto A, Sinacore DR. Hamstring muscle strain treated by mobilizing the sacroiliac joint. Phys Ther 1986; 66:1220-1223.

239. Cibulka MT, Delitto A, Koldehoff RM. Changes in innominate tilt after manipulation of the sacroiliac joint in patients with low back pain. Phys Ther 1988; 68:1359-1363.
240. Schwarzer AC, Aprill CN, Bogduk N. The sacroiliac joint in chronic low back pain. Spine 1995; 20:31-37.
241. Schram SB, Hosek RS, Silverman HL. Spinographic positioning errors in Gonstead pelvic x-ray analysis. J Manipulative Physiol Ther 1981; 4:179-181.
242. Walters PJ. Pelvis. In: Plaugher G, ed. Textbook of clinical chiropractic: a specific biomechanical approach. Baltimore: Williams & Wilkins, 1993:150-189.
243. Tilley P. Cephalic angle film for sacral base visualization. J Am Osteopath Assoc 1968; 67:1153-1157.
244. Zengel F, Davis BP. Biomechanical analysis by chiropractic radiography: Part 3. Lack of projectional distortion on Gonstead vertebral endplate lines. J Manipulative Physiol Ther 1988; 11:469-473.
245. Gunzberg R, Gunzberg J, Wagner J, Fraser RD. Radiological interpretation of lumbar vertebral rotation. Spine 1991; 16:660-664.
246. Russel GG, Raso VJ, Hill D, McIvor J. A comparison of four computerized methods for measuring vertebral rotation. Spine 1990; 15:24-27.
247. Van Schiak JPJ, Verbiest H, Van Schaik FDJ. Isolated spinous process deviation: a pitfall in the interpretation of AP radiographs of the lumbar spine. Spine 1989; 14:970-976.
248. Zengel F, Davis BP. Biomechanical analysis by chiropractic radiography: Part 2. Effects of x-ray projectional distortion on apparent vertebral rotation. J Manipulative Physiol Ther 1988; 11:380-389.
249. Herbst RW. Gonstead chiropractic science and art. Mt. Horeb, WI: Sci-Chi Publications 1968.
250. Shaffer WO, Spratt KF, Weinstein J, Lehmann TR, Goel V. The consistency and accuracy of roentgenograms for measuring sagittal translation in the lumbar vertebral motion segment. Spine 1990; 15:741-750.
251. Bohrer SP, Klein A, Martin W. "V" shaped predens space. Skeletal Radiol 1985; 14:111-116.
252. Webb JK, Broughton RBK, McSweeney T, Park WM. Hidden flexion injury of the cervical spine. J Bone Joint Surg 1976; 58B:324-327.
253. Yousefzadeh DK, El-Khoury GY, Smith WL. Normal sagittal diameter and variation in the pediatric cervical spine. Radiology 1982; 144:319-325.
254. Weitz EM. The lateral bending sign. Spine 1981; 6:388-397.
255. Panjabi MM, Yamamoto I, Oxland T. How does posture affect coupling in the lumbar spine? Spine 1989; 14:1002.
256. Grice AS. Radiographic, biomechanical and clinical factors in lumbar lateral flexion: Part 1. J Manipulative Physiol Ther 1979; 2:26-34.
257. Stokes IAF, Wilder DG, Frymoyer JW, Pope MH. Assessment of patients with low-back pain by biplanar radiographic measurement of intervertebral motion. Spine 1981; 6:233-240.
258. Dupuis PR, Yong-Hing K, Cassidy JD, Kirkaldy-Willis WH. Radiologic diagnosis of degenerative lumbar spinal instability. Spine 1985; 10:262-276.
259. Plaugher G, Lopes MA. Clinical anatomy and biomechanics of the spine. In: Plaugher G, ed. Textbook of clinical chiropractic: a specific biomechanical approach. Baltimore: Williams & Wilkins, 1993:12-51.
260. Plaugher G. Advances in the Gonstead technique. In: Lawrence DJ, et al. eds. Advances in Chiropractic, Mosby-Yearbook, 1995.
261. Plaugher G, Lopes MA, Konlande JE, Doble RW, Cremata EE. Spinal management for the patient with a visceral concomitant. In: Plaugher G, ed. Textbook of clinical chiropractic: a specific biomechanical approach. Baltimore: Williams & Wilkins, 1993:356-382.
262. Harris W, Wagnon RJ. The effects of chiropractic adjustments on distal skin temperature. J Manipulative Physiol Ther 1987; 10:57-60.
263. Housenfield G: Computerized transverse axial scanning (tomography). Br J Radiol 1973; 46:10.
264. Miller J, Schmatz B, Schultz A. Lumbar disc degeneration: correlation with age, sex, and spine level in 600 autopsy specimens. Spine 1988; 13:173-178.
265. Farfan H, Cossette JW, Robertson GH, Wells RV, Kraus H. The effects of torsion on the lumbar intervertebral joints: the role of torsion in the production of disc degeneration. J Bone Joint Surg 1970; 52A:468-497.
266. Holm S. Nutrition of the intervertebral disc: solute transport and metabolism. Gothenburg, Sweden. University of Goteborg, doctoral dissertation. 1980.
267. Svensson H, Vedin A, Wilhelmsson C, Andersson GB: Low back pain in relation to other diseases and cardiovascular risk factors. Spine 1983; 8:277-285.
268. Lyons G, Eisenstein S, Sweet M. Biochemical changes in intervertebral disc degeneration. Biochim Biophys Acta 1981; 673:443-453.
269. Bernick S, Cailliet R. Vertebral end plate changes with aging of human vertebrae. Spine 1982; 7:97-102.
270. Milgram J. Osteoarthritic changes at the severely degenerated disc in humans. Spine 1982; 7:498-505.
271. Kirkaldy-Willis W, et al. Pathology and pathogenesis of lumbar spondylosis and stenosis. Spine 1978; 3:319-328.
272. Dietemann JL, Doyon D, Aubin ML, Manelfe C. Cervico-occipital junction: normal and pathological aspects. In Manelfe C: Imaging of the Spine and Spinal Cord. Raven Press. New York, NY, 1992.
273. Kowalski HM, Cohen WA, Cooper P, Wisoff JH. Pitfalls in the CT diagnosis of atlantoaxial rotary subluxation. AJR 1987; 149:595-600.
274. Fielding JW, Stillwell WT, Chynn KY, Spyropoulos EC. Use of computed tomography for the diagnosis of atlanto-axial rotatory fixation. A case report. J Bone Joint Surg 1978; 60A:1102-1104.
275. Ono K, Yonenobu K, Fuji T, Okada K. Atlantoaxial rotatory fixation. Radiographic study of its mechanism. Spine 1985; 10: 602-608.
276. White AA, Panjabi MM. The clinical biomechanics of the occipitoatlantoaxial complex. Orthop Clin North Am 1978; 9:867-878.
277. Kricun R, Kricun ME. Computed tomography. In: Kricun ME. Imaging modalities in spinal disorders. Philadelphia: W.B. Saunders Co, 1988.
278. O'Riordain DS, O'Connell PR, Kirwan WO. Hereditary sacral agenesis with presacral mass and anorectal stenosis. Br J Surg 1991; 78:536-538.
279. Shapiro J, Herring J. Congenital vertebral displacement. J Bone Joint Surg 1993; 75A:656-662.
280. Hoeffel JC, Bernhard C, Regent D. CT appearance of aneurysmal bone cyst of the spine in childhood. J Bone Joint Surg 1993; 75A:656.
281. Fredericks BJ, de Campo JF, Sephton R, McCredie DA. Computed tomographic assessment of vertebral bone mineral in childhood. Skeletal Radiol 1990; 19:99-102.
282. Wiener MD, Martinez S, Forsberg DA: Congenital absence of a cervical spine pedicle: clinical and radiologic findings. AJR 1990; 155:1037-1041.
283. Ulmer JL, Elster AD, Ginsberg LE, Williams DW 3d: Klippel-Feil syndrome. CT and MR of acquired and congenital abnormalities of the cervical spine and cord. J Comput Assist Tomogr 1993; 17: 215-224.
284. Sener RN, Ripeckyj GT, Otto PM, Rauch RA, Jinkins JR. Recognition of abnormalities on computed scout images in CT examinations of the head and spine. Neuroradiology 1993; 35:229-231.
285. Sarwar M. Imaging of the pediatric spine and its contents. J Child Neurol 1990; 5:3-18.
286. Schnitzlein HN, Hartley EW, Murtagh FR, Grundy L, Fargher JT. Computed tomography of the head and spine. Baltimore: Urban & Schwarzburg, 1983.
287. Webb WR, Brant WE, Helms CA. Fundamentals of body CT. Philadelphia: W.B. Saunders Co., 1991.
288. Kent C, Gentempo P. Magnetic resonance imaging in chiropractic. Today's Chiropractic. Part I January/February 1989. Part II March/April 1989.
289. Gibson M et al. Magnetic resonance imaging of adolescent disc herniation. J Bone Joint Surg 1987; 69B:699.
290. Reither M. Indications for magnetic resonance tomography in diseases of the central nervous system in children. Padiatric und Padologie 1989; 24:123-135 (Published in German).
291. Currie C, Pendergrass H, Brun M. Magnetic resonance imaging of the spine. Am Fam Physician 1987; 36:155-160.
292. Bale J, Bell W, Dunn V et al. Magnetic resonance imaging of the spine in children. Arch Neurol 1986; 43:1253-1256.
293. Duthoy M, Lund G. MR imaging of the spine in children. Eur J Radiol 1988; 8:188-195.
294. Elster A. Magnetic resonance imaging: a reference guide and atlas. Philadelphia: J.B. Lippincott, 1986.
295. Moon KL Jr, Genant HK, Davis PL, et. al. Nuclear magnetic resonance imaging in orthopedics: principles and applications. J Orthop Res 1983; 1:104.
296. Beltran J, Noto AM, Herman LJ, Mosure JC, Burk JM, Christopforidis AJ. Joint effusions: MR imaging. Radiology 1986; 158:133-137.
297. Zimmer WD, Berquist TH, McLeod RA, et. al. Bone tumors: magnetic resonance imaging vs. computed tomography. Radiology 1985; 155:709-718.
298. Moon KK Jr, Genant HK, Helms CA, et. al. Musculoskeletal applications of nuclear magnetic resonance. Radiology 1983; 147:161-171.
299. Brady TJ, Gebhardt MC, Pykett IL, et al. NMR imaging of forearms in healthy volunteers and patients with giant cell tumor of bone. Radiology 1982; 144: 549-552.
300. Aisen AM, Martel W, Braunstein EM, et al. MRI and CT evaluation of primary bone and soft-tissue tumors. AJR 1986; 146:749-756.
301. Wong W. Practical MRI: a case study approach. Rockville, MD: Aspen Publishers, 1987.
302. Maravilla KR, Weinreb JC, Suss R, Nunnally RL. Magnetic resonance demonstration of multiple sclerosis plaques in the cervical cord. AJR 1985; 144: 381-385.
303. Maravilla KR, Weinreb JC, Suss R, Nunnally RL. Magnetic resonance demonstration of multiple sclerosis plaques in the cervical cord. AJR 1984; 5:685.
304. Modic MT, Weinstein MA, Pavlicek W, et al. Nuclear magnetic resonance imaging of the spine. Radiology 1983; 148:757-762.
305. Modic MT, Steinberg PM, Ross JS, Masaryk TJ, Carter JR. Degenerative disk disease: assessment of changes in vertebral body marrow with MR imaging. Radiology 1988; 166:193-199.
306. Wilberger J, Chedid M. Acute cervical spondylytic myelopathy. Neurosurgery 1988; 22:145-146.
307. Enzmann D, Rubin J. Cervical spine: MR imaging with a partial flip angle, gradient refocused pulse sequence. Radiology 1988; 166:467-472.
308. Bundschuh CV, Modic MT, Ross JS, Masaryk TJ, Bohlman H. Epidural fibrosis and recurrent disk herniation in the lumbar spine: MR imaging assessment. AJR 1988 150:923-932.
309. Grenier N, Kressel HY, Schiebler ML, Grossman RI, Dalinka MK. Normal and degenerative posterior spinal structures: MR imaging. Radiology 1987; 165: 517-525.

310. Ross JS, Perez-Reyes N, Masaryk TJ, Bohlman H, Modic MT. Thoracic disk herniation: MR assessment. Radiology 1987; 165:511-515.

311. Gibson MJ, Szypryt EP, Buckley JH, Worthington BS, Mulholland RC. Magnetic resonance imaging of adolescent disc herniation. J Bone Joint Surg 1987; 69B:699-703.

312. Hedberg MC, Drayer BP, Flom RA, Hodak JA, Bird CR. Gradient echo (GRASS) MR imaging in cervical radiculopathy. AJR 1988; 150:683-689.

313. Francavilla TL, Powers A, Dina T, Rizzoli HV. MR imaging of thoracic disk herniations. J Comput Assist Tomogr 1987; 11:1062-1065.

314. Alvarez O, Roque CT, Pampati M. Multilevel thoracic disk herniations: CT and MR studies. J Comput Assist Tomogr 1988; 12:649-652.

315. Karnaze MG, Gado MH, Sartor KJ, Hodges FJ, Hodges FJ. Comparison of MR and CT myelography in imaging the cervical and thoracic spine. AJR 1988; 150:397-403.

316. Ross JS, Masaryk TJ, Modic MT, et al. MR imaging of lumbar arachnoiditis. AJR 1987; 149:1025-1032.

317. Wolpert SM, Anderson M, Scott RM, Kwan ES, Runge VM. Chiari II malformation: MR imaging evaluation. AJR 1987; 149:1033-1042.

318. Woznica J, Bryc S. Diagnosis of syringomyelia by using the method of nuclear magnetic resonance. Neurol Neurochir Pol 1988; 22:43-48.

319. Shippel A, Robinson G. Radiological and magnetic resonance imaging of cervical spine instability: a case report. J Manipulative Physiol Ther 1987; 10:316-322.

320. Fruehwald FX, Tscholakoff D, Schwaighofer B, et al. Magnetic resonance imaging of the lower vertebral column in patients with multiple myeloma. Invest Radiol 1988; 23:193-199.

321. Lewis T, Kingsley D. Magnetic resonance imaging of multiple spinal neurofibromata-neurofibromatosis. Neuroradiology 1987; 29:562-564.

322. Takahashi M, Sakamoto Y, Miyawaki M, Bussaka H. Increased MR signal intensity secondary to chronic cervical cord compression. Neuroradiology 1987; 29:550.

323. Vieregge P, Schwachenwald R, Reusche E, Pressler M. Vertebral hemangioma with extradural spinal cord compression. Nervenarzt 1987; 58:705-710 (German and Russian).

324. Godersky JC, Smoker WR, Knutzon R. Use of magnetic resonance imaging in the evaluation of metastatic spinal disease. Neurosurgery 1987; 21:676-680.

325. Kent C, Gentempo P. Extremity MR imaging at 0.064T: applications in chiropractic practice. J Chiropractic Res Clin Invest 1991; 7(2):52.

326. Kent C, Gentempo P. A systematic approach to the evaluation of magnetic resonance images of the cervical and lumbar spine. Intl Rev Chiropractic 1993; 49(2):47.

327. Mirvis SE, Geisler FH, Jelinek JJ, Joslyn JN, Gellard F. Acute cervical spine trauma: evaluation with 1.5 T MR imaging. Radiology 1988; 166:807-816.

328. Phillips RB, Howe JW, Bustin G, et al. Stress x-rays and the low back pain patient. J Manipulative Physiol Ther 1990; 13:1127-33.

329. Haas M, Nyiendo J, Peterson C, et al. Lumbar motion trends and correlation with low back pain. Part I. A roentgenological evaluation of coupled lumbar motion in lateral bending. J Manipulative Physiol Ther 1992; 15:145-58.

330. Balague F, Dutoit G, Waldburger M. Low back pain in school children. Scan J Rehab Med 1988; 20:175-179.

331. Deyo RA, Diehl AK. Lumbar spine films in primary care: current use and effects of selective ordering criteria. J Gen Intern Med 1986; 1:20-25.

332. Deyo RA. Conservative therapy for low back pain. JAMA 1983; 250:1057-1062

333. Gutmann G. Blocked atlantal nerve syndrome in infants and small children. Intl Rev Chiropractic 46(4):37, 1990. (Reprinted from Manuelle Medizin Springer-Verlag, 1987).

334. Fysh P. Upper respiratory infections in children: a chiropractic approach to management. International Review of Chiropractic 1990; 46(3):29.

335. Klougart N, Nilsson N, Jacobsen J. Infantile colic treated by chiropractors: a prospective study of 316 cases. J Manipulative Physiol Ther 1989; 12:281-288.

336. Hart D, Libich E, Fischer S. Chiropractic adjustments of the cervicothoracic spine for the treatment of bronchitis with complications of atelectasis. Intl Rev Chiropractic 1991; 47(2):31.

337. McMullen M. Handicapped infants and chiropractic care: Down syndrome-Part I. Intl Rev Chiropractic 1990; 46(4):32.

338. Janse J, Houser R, Wells B. Chiropractic Principles and Technic, National College of Chiropractic. Chicago, IL. 1947.

339. Kent C. An overview of pediatric radiology in the chiropractic practice. Intl Rev Chiropractic 1990; 46(4):45.

340. King HA. Back pain in children. Pediatr Clin North Am 1984; 31:1083-1095.

341. Stanitski C. Management of sports injuries in children and adolescents. Orthop Clin North Am 1988; 19:689-698.

342. Forster A, Pothmann R, Winter K, Baumann-Rath CA. Magnetic resonance imaging in non-specific discitis. Pediatr Radiol 1987; 17:162-163.

343. Kozlowski K, Beluffi G, Masel J, et al. Primary vertebral tumors in children: report of 20 cases with brief review of the literature. Pediatr Radiol 1984; 14:129-139.

344. Azouz E, Kozlowski K, Marton D, et al. Osteoid osteoma and osteoblastoma of the spine in children. Pediatr Radiol 1986; 16:25-31.

345. Epstein F, Epstein N. Intramedullary tumors of the spinal cord. In: Shillito J, Matson D eds. Pediatric neurosurgery. New York: Grune and Stratton, 1982.

346. Barkovich A: Pediatric Neuroimaging. New York: Raven Press, 1990.

347. Boston H, Bianco Jr. A, Rhodes K. Disc space infections in children. Orthop Clin North Am 1975; 6:953-963.

348. Spiegel P, Kengla K, Isaacson A, et al. Intervertebral disc space inflammation in children. J Bone Joint Surg 1972; 54A:284-296.

349. Scheuermann H. The classic: kyphosis dorsalis juvenilis. Clin Orthop 1977; 128:5-7.

350. Alexander C. Scheuermann's disease: a traumatic spondylodystrophy. Skeletal Radiol 1:209, 1977.

351. Wiltse L, Widell E, Jackson O. Fatigue fracture: the basic lesion in isthmic spondylolisthesis. J Bone Joint Surg 1975; 57A:17-22.

352. Farfan H, Osteria V, Lamy C. The mechanical etiology of spondylolysis and spondylolisthesis. Clin Orthop 1976; 117:40-55.

353. Weir M, Smith D. Stress reaction of pars interarticularis leading to spondylolysis: a cause of adolescent low back pain. J Adolesc Health Care 1989; 10:573-577.

354. Afshani E, Kuhn J. Common causes of low back pain in children. Radiographics 1991; 11:269-291.

355. Bunnell W. Back pain in children. Orthop Clin North Am 1982; 13:587-604.

356. Barge F. Idiopathic scoliosis: identifiable causes—detection and correction. Bawden Bros., Davenport, IA. 1988.

357. Mehta M, Murray R. Scoliosis provoked by painful vertebral lesions. Skeletal Radiol 1:223, 1977.

358. Evans D, Bethem D. Cervical spine injuries in children. J Pediat Orthop 1989; 9:563-568.

359. Kewalramani L, Tori J. Spinal cord trauma in children: neurologic patterns, radiologic features, and pathomechanics of injury. Spine 1980; 5:11-18.

360. Hubbard D. Injuries of the spine in children and adolescents. Clin Orthop 1974; 100:56-65.

361. King H. Back pain in children. In: Weinstein SL, ed. The pediatric spine: principles and practice. New York: Raven Press Ltd., 1994:173-183.

PART IV

Clinical Techniques and "Dis–ease" Prevention

---

9 Spinal Examination and Specific Spinal and Pelvic Adjustments

Claudia A. Anrig

*T*he focus of this chapter is on the analysis and manual adjustive correction of subluxations affecting the spinal column and pelvis. It is the author's intent to provide as much detail as possible in the specific application of examination strategies as well as techniques which emphasize the return to normal motion segment and nervous system function.

Very little research exists on the efficacy of the various adjustive techniques described in this chapter. This is due in large part to the dearth of scientific information in general with respect to the various health professions (1), rather than any state of affairs unique to the chiropractic profession. In the interim however, patients must be treated because of the unique ethical contract between doctor and patient, regardless of the state of science. One is reminded that the individual patient presenting before a doctor was never in a clinical trial, and so it is extremely difficult to predict outcomes for this individual patient. The art of being a doctor is to apply methods which seem to have the best chance for optimizing function and hold the least possibility of attendant risk. The art in chiropractic includes an adjustment which moves the segment towards normal with the least trauma imparted to the associated soft tissue elements. All adjustments, especially those applied to the pediatric population require a high level of skill. Nonspecific introduction of forces into the delicate spine, due to an ignorance of biomechanics cannot be tolerated.

Insofar as many clinical applications are considered, the practitioner should base their approach on an understanding of normal biomechanics and the mechanisms of trauma coupled with a reasoned approach which attempts, to not only "do no harm," but which also moves the motion segment towards normal which is generally opposite the forces of injury. All of the adjustments presented in this chapter are extremely detailed in their presentation and should be based on the clinical circumstances of the individual patient. The fact that the pediatric spine can withstand many loads the child is subjected to throughout life should not lead to the naive assumption that a doctor can do no harm. Moreover, the application of adjustment techniques in the adult cannot be applied to the infant or toddler's spine. Size differences in the anatomic elements as well as the unique flexibility differences of the spinal column at different ages necessitates a specific approach.

The more salient adjustive procedures currently being used in the chiropractic profession are discussed. The treatise is not all–encompassing, but should serve as a basis from which the clinician can formulate a cogent analytical and adjustive plan. Certain techniques which do not move the motion segment three-dimensionally towards center, involve long lever-arm vectors, or otherwise compromise delicate neurological or vascular tissues (2), are specifically contraindicated and presented as such. The hope is that clinicians unfamiliar with adjustive care of children, or those who have been applying techniques in a nonspecific fashion to pediatric populations,

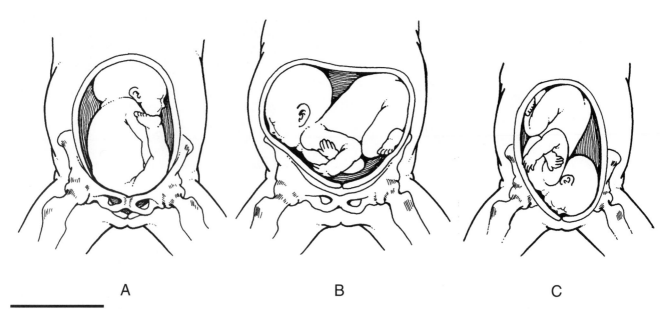

A   B   C

Figure 9.1.   A, Breech presentation. Notice the position of the legs. Modified from Graham JM. Smith's recognizable patterns of human deformation. 2nd. ed. Philadelphia: W.B. Saunders Co., 1988:86. B, Transverse lie presentation. Modified from Graham JM. Smith's recognizable patterns of human deformation. 2nd ed. Philadelphia: W.B. Saunders Co., 1988:95. C, Face presentation. Modified from Graham JM. Smith's recognizable patterns of human deformation. 2nd ed. Philadelphia: W.B. Saunders Co., 1988:96.

will begin to refocus their efforts toward the correction of the subluxation in as specific a manner as possible and with the least likelihood of doing harm. In this way, the application of chiropractic techniques can truly reach our youngest with the greatest potential for minimizing the deleterious neurological effects of spinal trauma.

Mechanism of Injury

A description of micro or macro trauma should be always considered as a part of the assessment process. The past and current history of the child may assist in understanding the cause of trauma to the pediatric spine and the vertebral subluxation complex (i.e., positional dyskinesia).

In-utero constraint (3–5) which includes breech, transverse lie, brow and facial presentations may be factors that lead to repetitive micro trauma to the spine (Fig. 9.1 A–C). The upper cervical region, specifically the occipital condyle should be suspected as a possible positional dyskinesia (i.e., AS or PS listing), as a result of in-utero constraint. Other complications to consider are the cervical and upper thoracic spine in an extended hyperlordotic presentation (e.g., facial, transverse) or the lumbosacral spine in a flexion position (i.e. breech).

The birth process is well documented as a potential source of trauma to the spine and spinal cord (4,6–10). The most common insult to the spine is forceful tractioning while the cervical spine is in hyperextension. Other forms of trauma are longitudinal traction with rotation and flexion or excessive lateral flexion (5). The use of any long lever device (e.g., vacuum extractor, forceps) as seen in Figures 9.2 and 9.3 or the

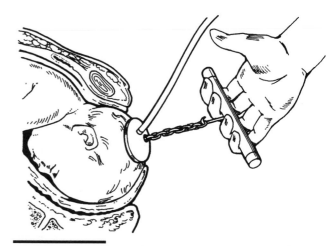

Figure 9.2.   Bird's modification of Malmstrom's vacuum extractor method. Modified from Pernoll ML, Benson RC. Current obstetric and gynecologic diagnosis and treatment. 6th ed. Norwalk: Appleton & Lange, 1987:496.

introduction of invasive techniques (e.g., caesarean, obstetrician hand dominance) should be documented as a possible neonate trauma.

The handling of newborns and infants may cause micro trauma to the spine. Diapering techniques (Fig. 9.4) lifting from the crib or car seat may place a strain on the spine with the undeveloped supporting muscles. Baby walkers (which are outlawed in some countries due to safety hazards) and jumpers

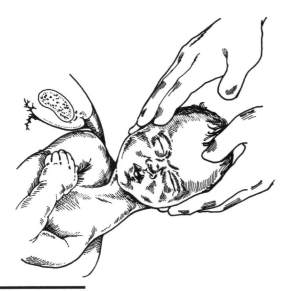

Figure 9.3. Delivery with upward traction applied to the head to deliver a posterior shoulder over the perineum. Modified from Wilson JR, Beecham CT, Forman I, Carrington ER, eds. Obstetrics and gynecology. St. Louis: CV Mosby, 1958:336.

place undue stress to the lower limbs and lumbopelvic region. An unsupported neck and upper thoracic spine while the caretaker is carrying the newborn may cause repetitive micro flexion and extension spinal trauma.

Falls are not uncommon with young children. A National Safety Council (11) noted that 47.5% infants were discovered to have fallen from a high place during their first year of life. The toddler is prone to repetitive compression forces on the buttocks when learning the skill of walking. The forward uncoordinated gait of the toddler often results in frontal skull strikes (e.g., into furniture). This mechanism of injury may result in extension or flexion trauma to the occiput, cervical and upper thoracic region.

The pre-schooler is no exception to falls (e.g., biking, playing, skating). Often sports activities are introduced into their lives (e.g., soccer, gymnastics) which brings asymmetrical forces into the developing spine.

Other spinal considerations for the child include sleep positions that are developed. Stomach sleeping habits are not suggested in the newborn/infant due to the possible link to SIDS (12). In addition this position is not recommended for any age, due to the biomechanical stress (e.g., rotation, favoritism to one side) at the cervical spine.

The school age child (5 to 18 yr) is prone to more traumas on the campus (7). This includes organized and unorganized sports. Playschool equipment (7,13) is a frequent site of trauma. Bicycles, skateboards, roller-skating, horseback riding, water slides, and diving (14,15) are a few common activities of the young. Hyperflexion and hyperextension of the neck, or compression of the buttocks or head can cause either spine or spinal cord injury (see Chapters 4 and 19).

Micro trauma may be seen in the form of postural insult due to behavioral habits. Poor sitting habits (e.g., slumping,

slouching) may contribute to stresses on the spine (Fig. 9.5). Schoolroom chairs in classrooms are often not ergonomically designed. Backpacks that are incorrectly carried on one shoulder or are too heavy, may be an asymmetrical strain on the spine (Fig. 9.6).

The leading cause of accidental death in children is vehicle related (7). Chapters 4 and 19 discuss in more detail the mechanisms of injury to the pediatric spine and nervous system.

Child abuse (see Chapter 2) is more common than one may suspect. Physical abuse often includes the forceful striking or shaking of the victim. Infants are not immune when violent shaking of the head occurs (14,16,17). Spinal cord trauma can result.

Management

Recording the history of the child can assist the practitioner in understanding not only the mechanism of injury, but the need for ongoing evaluation of the pediatric spine. The elimination of micro or macro trauma to the child is highly unlikely. Parents and children should be instructed and educated on how to diminish spinal injury.

The frequency of care should be individually assessed. The vertebral subluxation complex in its earliest stages may not manifest as a clinically symptomatic disorder (18). Objective findings, not necessarily a symptomatic picture alone, should be the criteria for its identification. The rendering of spinal adjustments in the young may be one of the most effective forms of contributing to the prevention of spinal dysfunction and other health disorders. Longitudinal studies should be conducted to determine the effectiveness of chiropractic care as part of a prevention program.

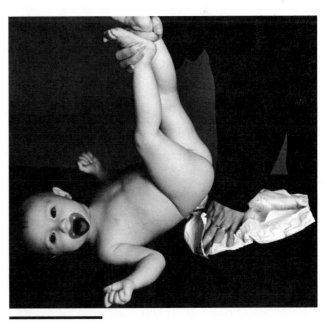

Figure 9.4. Certain diapering techniques may place unnecessary stress on the spine.

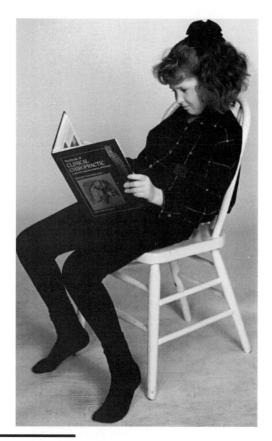

Figure 9.5.   Poor design and use of school chairs places repetitive stress on the developing spine.

During the consultation and after the clinical assessment of the patient, the doctor should thoroughly explain the objective findings. It is during this time that the doctor can inform the parents of three general phases of chiropractic care. Relief care which is the rendering of care until relief or stabilization of the condition is achieved. This varies from several weeks to several months. Visits are usually more frequent in the beginning and decrease as objective findings diminish. Reconstruction/rehabilitative care is the delivery of care to alter more permanently the biomechanical structure of the spine. This type of care would be required for example when a hypolordosis or kyphosis of the cervical spine or scoliosis is present. Frequency of visits varies depending on many factors; objective findings for biomechanical changes, age, lifestyle habits.

The third phase of care has been called by the following names; prevention or wellness. This program is the rendering of spinal adjustments when subluxations are present to allow the developing spine and its influence on the nervous system to have optimal function during the course of the child's developmental process. This program is similar to the preventive approach of dentistry. The evaluation of the spine will be generally more frequent than in dentistry due to the ongoing stresses and vulnerability of the spine. The frequency rate may

be greater if the child is going through a stage of increasing repetitive falls or stresses to the spine. The purpose of the visit is to evaluate the spine and to adjust if objective findings are present. It is negligent for the doctor to space out the visits when objective findings and the child's lifestyle warrants more frequent evaluation. At the other extreme, it is suspect to justify the necessity of high frequency/long term (i.e. daily visits for months) care by the practitioner.

An outline for evaluating the spine must be determined by many factors; age, environment, developmental stages, and activities. The purpose of a visit is to evaluate objectively for the necessity to adjust. If objective findings are not present, the doctor reschedules for the next visit. The neonate should be evaluated shortly after birth (within 48 hours). The newborn/infant should be examined on a regular schedule between 2 and 6 weeks unless a specific trauma results, in which case the child should be seen immediately. The more active toddler and pre-schooler may need an evaluation between 2 to 4 weeks due to their repetitive micro traumas.

For the less active pre-adolescent and adolescent patient, the frequency of care may vary from 2 to 6 weeks. The more active patient may require a closer evaluation visit frequency. This recommendation can vary for numerous reasons. If the patient is under care for a correction of a biomechanical disorder (i.e., scoliosis) or for an injury (e.g., auto, sports) the frequency and length of care will be increased.

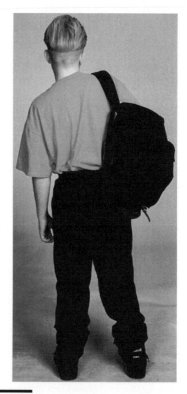

Figure 9.6.   Asymmetrical usage of the backpack places repetitive stress on the musculoskeletal system.

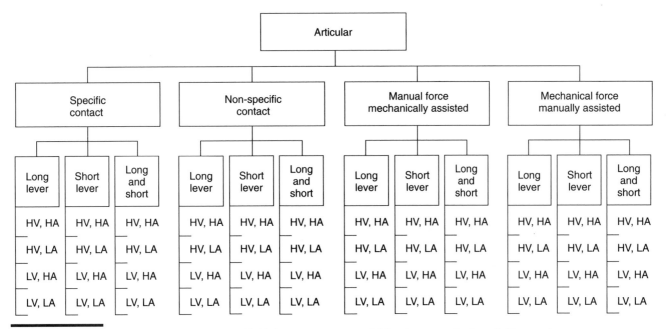

Figure 9.7. Articular procedure descriptions. H=High, L=Low, V=Velocity, A=Amplitude. Modified from Bartol KM. A model for the categorization of chiropractic treatment procedures. Chiropractic Technique 1991; 3:79.

Specific Contact, Short Lever-Arm Adjustive Techniques

The method of delivery that is emphasized is specific short lever arm adjustments (Fig. 9.7). The use of a listing system (see Chapter 8) allows for a systematic reference to the positional dyskinesia of the subluxated segment to be adjusted. The adjustment specifically directs a three-dimensional force away from the direction of misalignment. The advantage of specific adjusting allows for the protection of the supporting ligamentous elements. A short lever specific contact on the subluxated segment protects normal functional spinal units. The practitioner can protect the normal segments from introduction of unnecessary force during the adjustive thrust by the following considerations of preloading and end-range positions.

A specific adjusting approach includes patient management. Rather than randomly introducing multiple forces into spinal segments, the doctor limits the number of segments to be adjusted through a prior spinal evaluation. The rationale of limiting the segments to be adjusted allows for the practitioner to objectively assess the results.

Primum Non Nocere

"Above all, do no harm," should be the primary consideration of all health professionals. This principle should be applied for the examination as well as the adjustment. Acquiring knowledge of the relative positions of the vertebrae will prevent further joint insult. The adjustment should avoid introducing unnecessary forces into the neural elements, cartilage, disc and articular ligaments. No adjustment should ever be performed without evidence of a relative decrease in mobility at that articulation.

Hypomobility vs. Hypermobility

One major component of the vertebral subluxation complex is kinesiopathology. This begins with hypomobility of the vertebral segment. Commonly associated with hypomobility is the compensation of hypermobility within the same region of the spine (19). Symptoms related to the hypermobile region are not uncommon. Careful evaluation of the spine decreases the possibility of adjusting a hypermobile segment (12). Compensation in spinal regions has been brought forth by numerous individuals (e.g., Gonstead, Jirout, Gillet). Static and motion palpation can assist in detecting hypermobility with associated edema and tenderness. Introducing forces into a hypermobile or normally functioning joint is contraindicated.

Long Lever and Non-Specific Adjustments

Long lever contacts or general mobilization of a spinal region is not beneficial to the developing spine. The elastic properties of the spine and spinal cord dictates the elimination (or minimizing) of vectors that would introduce unnecessary and possibly harmful forces into the spine. Patient placement or the doctor's set-up should avoid the following forces and bending

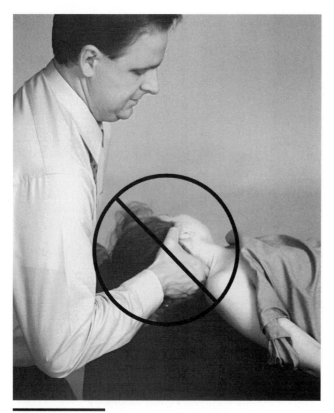

Figure 9.8. To pre-load the joint for the supine rotary break, it is necessary to position the cervical spine in extension, and Y-axis rotation.

moments; longitudinal traction, extension, rotation, flexion and lateral flexion.

Long lever techniques should not be performed on the pediatric spine. These adjusting procedures traditionally approach the spine with less specificity and the introduction of possibly harmful long lever forces. Examples of non-specific cervical techniques are supine or prone rotary breaks (Fig. 9.8), seated rotary break (Fig. 9.9) or hyper lateral flexion and rotation (Fig. 9.10). The thoracic spine receives unnecessary rotation with the upper thoracic thumb move (Fig. 9.11) or non specific mobilization as seen in the "anteriority" set-up (Fig. 9.12 A–C). The lumbar spine is susceptible to the introduction of rotation by poor upper torso stabilization (Fig. 9.13 A, B), excessive leaning or "kicking down" on the superior bent leg. Several general mobilization techniques which exist are the use of dangling or holding infants in the air either by their feet, under the axilla or hands wrapped around the thoracic spine and followed by a random snap, shake, or whip to the spine (Fig. 9.14).

Other contraindications to the adjustment are joint instability, destruction or fracture of the neural arch or segmental contact point (e.g., spinous process) and infection of the contact vertebra.

Patient and Doctor Placement

The patient should be placed in a neutral or near neutral position. Prone on a parent's lap, pelvic or hi-lo table, seated on a chair or side posture on the pelvic bench provide the neutral pre-patient setup. The doctor should stand in a position close to the patient and at an angle that allows for an optimal line of correction with the contact arm. The doctor should avoid placing the contact arm at an angle that would introduce a counter-productive force (e.g., rotation, lateral flexion).

Contact and Stabilization

The placement of the doctor's contact and stabilization hand is an important consideration. The anatomical size of the patient's segmental contact point (e.g., spinous, transverse, mamillary process) is part of the clinical assessment prior to the adjustment. Traditional contact hand positions (e.g., pisiform, thenar eminence, the length of the digit) may be too large and

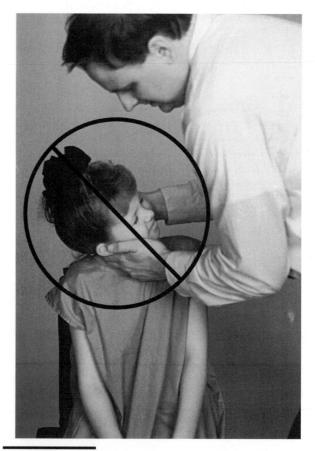

Figure 9.9. Long lever techniques are contraindicated for the pediatric spine.

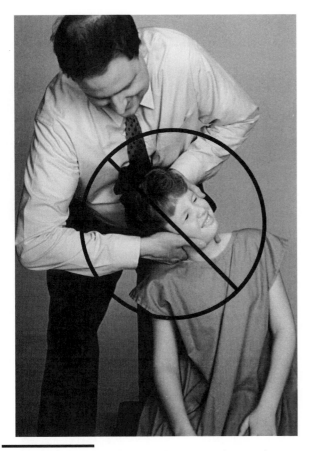

Figure 9.10. Lateral flexion with rotation places undue stress on the spinal elements.

contraindicated for the smaller pediatric spine. The possibility of overlapping several spinal segments or on to the ribs in the case of a thoracic contact, is likely with traditional contact hand set-ups (Fig. 9.15).

The distal end of a digit, specifically the fifth digit is ideal for the newborn, infant and toddler spine. The second digit is a choice for the larger contact processes. The pre-adolescent and adolescent may be contacted with a traditional hand set-up. The supporting hand is used to stabilize the spinal segments above and below the contact vertebra, or the crossed arms of the child in front of the chest in the side posture position.

Spinal Adjustment

Spinal adjustments are accomplished in two phases (21), the acceleration-deceleration process. The patient receives force during the adjustment from the mass of the doctor during deceleration after impact with the patient (22). The thrust or acceleration phase is the result of the doctor's mass and acceleration of the adjustive thrust which yields the force initiated by the doctor to reach the necessary impact velocity. In the deceleration phase, the doctor's mass is multiplied by the

deceleration which results in the actual adjustive force produced by the doctor-patient impact.

Other factors also contribute to the overall force the patient receives. The doctor's contact (e.g., pisiform, distal end digit) and the segmental contact point on the patient (e.g., mamillary, transverse process) contribute to the amount of force the patient receives. The presence of more soft tissue (e.g., infant brown fat) results in a greater dissipation of forces and a slower transference of energy (23,24) from the doctor to the patient. To minimize the force dampening effect, specific doctor and patient contact points are preferred.

Spine flexibility of the patient must also be considered. Tissue pull and pre-load tension are essential in the set-up procedure for the young spine. When performing a tissue pull (usually in the direction of the thrust), careful attention is paid to patient comfort. Pre-load tension is generally greater in the pediatric spine due to its flexibility. Pre-load is often greater than in a more rigid adult spine. The purpose of pre-loading is to prevent the need for extra force to reach the end range of motion of the segment. High acceleration thrusts will provide the force necessary to overcome the moment of inertia of the functional spinal unit. The deceleration phase is followed by a "hold" for 1-2 seconds (Figs. 9.16, 9.17) (25). The doctor should gradually release the contact after the "hold." The purpose of the "holding" after the adjustment is to affect the viscoelastic tissues with a more lengthy time component, thereby increasing the effectiveness of the adjustment on the elements. In preparing for the adjustment the doctor should interpret the "feel" of the patient's tolerances and adjustment requirements. Two patients may present with similar morphological characteristics, but require vastly different preloading, set-up time, relaxation, and force needed to accomplish the adjustment. The doctor's evaluation and clinical experience will allow for adaptability to individual patient needs.

The amount of force necessary to re-establish normal joint function varies with each patient. The patient's morphology

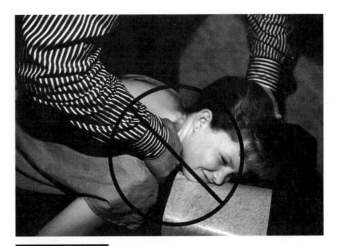

Figure 9.11. The diversified thumb move introduces unnecessary Y-axis rotation.

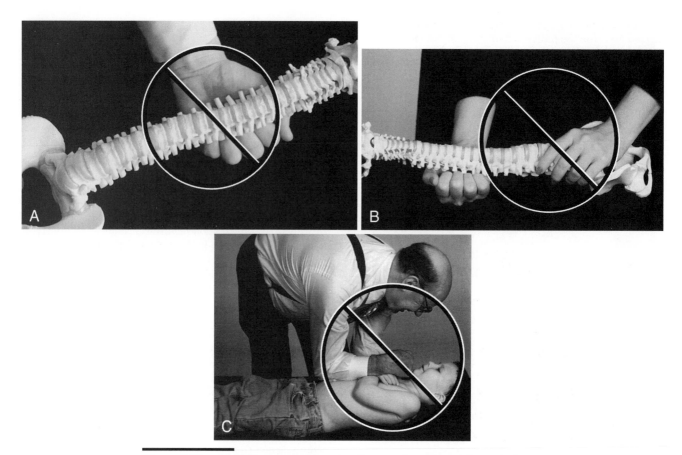

Figure 9.12.   A–C, The anterior thoracic adjustment is a non-specific manipulation for the developing spine. The doctor over contacts the spine and ribs.

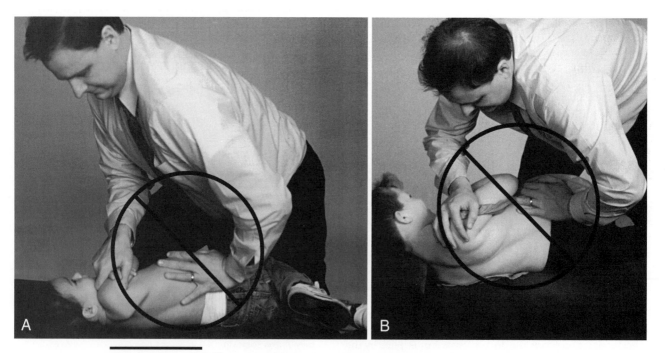

Figure 9.13.   A–B, Torso rotation introduces unnecessary forces into multiple spinal units.

and the doctor's adjustive skills are two important considerations. Studies on the peak force for the adjustment have been conducted for the adult spine (26-32). Although studies are lacking in children (and are warranted) some correlation may be drawn from the adult studies. Less force is necessary in the newborn/infant than the toddler, and less force for the toddler than the adolescent. The cervical spine requires more acceleration for the adjustment.

The audible cracking sound as a result of an adjustment is due to coaptation of articular gases in the synovial joints (33). After the coaptation of a joint, there is a refractory period (34). During the refractory period an increase of intra-articular movement is present. Introducing another force during this period may cause ligamentous strain.

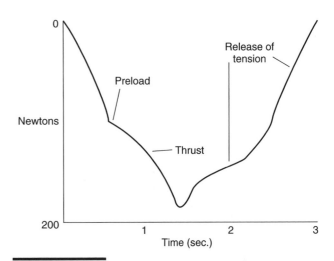

Figure 9.16. A qualitative graph of a set-hold type of adjustment thrust.

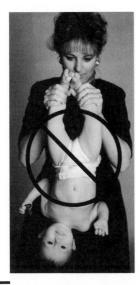

Figure 9.14. Dangling the infant by the ankles to perform a whipping movement of the spine is contraindicated.

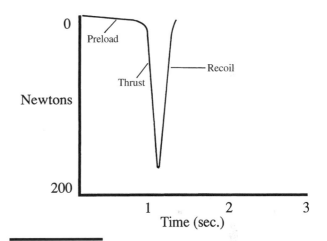

Figure 9.17. A qualitative graph of a toggle-recoil type of adjustment thrust.

Adjustments of the cervical and lumbar spine in the prone position may not necessarily result in cavitation of the joint, especially in the newborn/infant. The introduction of specific forces directed through the hypomobile joint (vertebral subluxation) is preferred over repeating random multiple forces (e.g. long lever) in the close proximity to the region of dysfunction.

Occipito-Atlantal (C0-C1)

Inspection

This examination procedure is somewhat limited in the evaluation process of C0-C1 and should be complemented by other assessments. In an upright position, inspect from

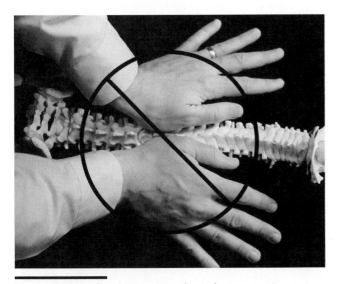

Figure 9.15. Overlapping several spinal segments may occur with a traditional hand contact.

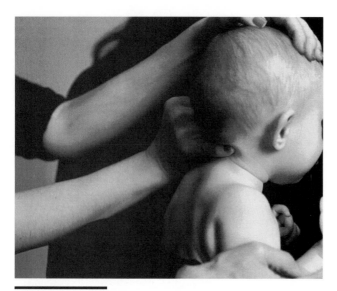

Figure 9.18.   The fifth digit is placed on the posterior-inferior aspect of the occiput.

the lateral view the position of the skull. The gaze of the patient should be in a horizontal plane to the floor. A skull in a superior head tilt may indicate an AS (-θX) condyle (anterior and superior). The PS (+θX) condyle (posterior and superior) will result in the head tilted inferior. The newborn, with under-developed cervical musculature, is difficult to inspect for postural abnormalities.

Static Palpation

Contact may be made by the fifth or second digit on the posterior-inferior aspect of the occiput (Fig. 9.18). Bogginess or edema may be detected if tissue injury is present. Posterior occiput rotation can palpate as soft tissue or muscle bulging.

Motion Palpation

The flexion or extension (-θX or +θX) range of motion is the primary motion to be evaluated. Contacting the condyle with the fingertips, slightly laterally flex the head to one side (Fig. 9.19). Once the articulation has been isolated, introduce a rocking motion consisting of flexion and extension. Repeat this procedure on the contralateral condyle. The PS condyle will manifest fixation during extension. The AS condyle will reveal joint restriction during flexion. To evaluate lateral flexion, slightly flex the head to the side approximately 5 degrees. Avoid creating unnecessary motion in the mid or lower cervical region. Normal lateral flexion will reveal a relaxation of the soft tissue components on the ipsilateral side of lateral flexion.

Instrumentation

The purpose of skin temperature analysis (e.g., Temp-o-scope, Nervoscope) is to obtain objective neurological evidence of a vertebral subluxation complex, and to monitor patient care. There is a probable connection between the nervous system

and intersegmental variations in skin temperature (35). Studies have been conducted to assess the reliability of the use of temperature differential instrumentation (36,37).

The Temp-o-scope (Fig. 9.20) and other similar instruments provide a qualitative assessment of thermal asymmetry. The instrument detects the temperature on both sides of the spine. The method for conducting the exam is dynamic scanning. A bilateral skin temperature difference is depicted as meter needle movement to one side or the other. The "reading" or "break" in temperature symmetry is considered significant if an abrupt "over and back" needle movement is seen over a one spinal segment distance. The amount of the temperature differential is thought to be directly proportional to the amount of neurophysiologic involvement due to the presence of VSC (20). The spinal subluxation in the acute stage often reveals a large variation in temperature. The temperature differential which reveals gradual diminishment is interpreted as improvement in the aberrant neurophysiology. Monitoring the intersegmental heat differential is one of several parameters of assessing and gauging patient progress in response to specific spinal adjusting. Table 9.1 lists the corresponding segmental level of temperature differentials.

The procedure of scanning small sections of the spinal column one after another is recommended for the paraspinal skin temperature instruments (36). To prevent air gaps forming

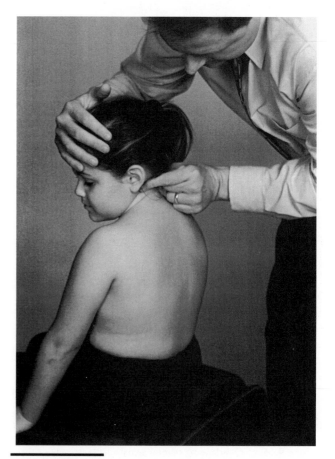

Figure 9.19.   Motion palpation of the occiput.

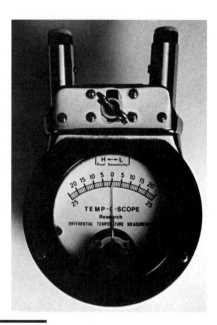

Figure 9.20. The Temp-o-Scope.

at the skin and thermocouple interface, the probes are maintained in perpendicular contact with the skin surface with sufficient pressure. The scanning glide is caudad to cephalad for T2-C0 and cephalad to caudad for T2 to S2 (S3 with the smaller patient). The nonamplified instrument should have a glide speed that does not exceed 0.5-1.0 cm/sec (20). To confirm a suspected temperature differential at a segmental level, the scan should be repeated several times. The accentuated differentials with a repeated scanning procedure are considered more significant than those that diminish. The validity of the procedure is decreased when the existence of moles or other lesions (e.g., blemishes, scar tissue, cysts) are in the path of the instrument glide. The glide and orientation of the instrumentation is modified for the presence of spinal curvature (i.e., scoliosis). Due to the rolling loose skin of the newborn/infant, any positive findings must be substantiated with other objective findings (e.g., tenderness or edema).

The existence of an intersegmental temperature differential does not, by itself, determine the presence of the vertebral subluxation complex. A spinal level with a neurophysiologic involvement is not considered as a subluxation when the presence of other subluxation parameters do not exist. Aberrant nervous system activity can occur at hypermobile functional spinal units (FSU). Hypermobility of the FSU can be a compensation for a restricted and subluxated FSU at another level, typically below the hypermobile segment (38).

C0-C1 TEMPERATURE SCANNING PROCEDURE

The neonate/infant is positioned across the lap or chest of the parent. The patient's head should be maintained in a neutral position during the scan. The toddler and older child is placed seated on the cervical chair to perform the procedure. In the upper cervical region the temperature differentials occur close together. The close proximity of C0-C2 makes it difficult to

determine the specific spinal level of the reading and must be confirmed with other objective findings. Suboccipital hair may also produce a spurious reading.

Radiographic Analysis

The lateral neutral posture of the occiput is analyzed in relationship to the atlas (see Chapter 8). The radiographic line that is drawn is called the foramen magnum line (FML). Due to the difficulty in identifying landmarks, assessing this region is performed by qualitative inspection. To create a maximal opening for the spinal canal, the foramen magnum line is fairly parallel to the AP atlas plane line. Deviation of the line in hyperflexion or hyperextension is considered abnormal. This assessment can be further substantiated with stress radiographic studies in flexion and extension and clinical assessments (Fig. 9.21).

On the lateral radiograph the FML is altered in relationship to the A-P atlas plane line. The FML will converge posterior on the AP atlas line with the AS condyle, reducing the space between the posterior arch of atlas and the foramen magnum. The PS condyle will appear as convergence of the two lines anteriorly, increasing the space between the posterior arch of atlas and the foramen magnum.

The AP radiograph (APOM) is used to determine if a RS ($-\theta Z$), LS ($+\theta Z$), or axial rotation (Y axis) exists. Lateral flexion positional dyskinesia (RS or LS) is determined by the transverse condyle line. The transverse condyle line (TCL) is scribed by like points on both sides of the condyles. The like points are the mastoid notches (on the temporal bones, the

Table 9.1. Corresponding Segmental Levels for Temperature Differentials[a]

C0-C2	The TDs occur very close together. A condyle or atlas subluxation may create a differential at any location between C2 and C0.
C2-T3	The TD should be inferior to the spinous process.
T4	The TD should be at the same level of the spinous process.
T5-T9	The TD should appear in the interspinous space above the spinous process of the involved vertebra.
T10-T12	The TD should be at the level of the spinous process.
L1-L5	The TD should appear at the level of the lower one fourth of the spinous process.
Sacroiliac and inferior	The TD should appear anywhere between the superior boundaries of the sacroiliac articulation.

[a]Modified from Herbst RW. Gonstead chiropractic science and art. Mt. Horeb, WI: Sci-Chi Publications, 1968:167–168.

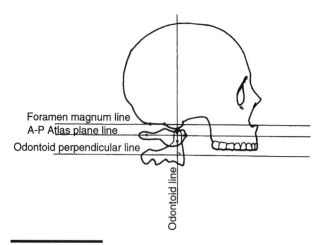

Foramen magnum line
A-P Atlas plane line
Odontoid perpendicular line

Odontoid line

Figure 9.21. Relatively normal alignment of C0-C1. Modified from Herbst RW. Gonstead chiropractic science and art. Mt. Horeb, WI: Sci-Chi Publications, 1968:133.

grooves of the mastoid process). Once the line has been drawn, it is compared to the atlas transverse plane line. It is considered normal when the two drawn lines are parallel in the coronal plane. A misalignment will manifest a divergence of the transverse condyle line from the atlas transverse plane line. A LS ($+\theta Z$) listing (divergence) will also appear as lateral flexion to the right side.

Condyle Y-axis rotation is analyzed also from the AP (APOM) radiograph. For a rotational subluxation to exist, it must also appear with a PS or AS and a LS or RS listing. If the condyle is in a rotational misalignment, the atlas will compensate with opposite rotation on the same side of misalignment. To list the condyle rotation, the atlas plane line is read for its axial compensation. The lateral mass of atlas will be smaller (posterior) if the condyle has rotated anteriorly. If the condyle has rotated posteriorly, the lateral mass of atlas will appear wider (anterior) to compensate for the axial rotation. The condyle rotation is listed as LP, LA, RP, or RA. The rotational misalignment should always be listed last (e.g., PSRSRP) (Table 9.2).

Table 9.2.   Occipital Condyle Listings

Gonstead Listing	International	Pattern of Thrust
PSRS	$+\theta X, -\theta Z$	Posterior to anterior, superior to inferior, right to left, through the C0-C1 joint plane line, with an inferiorward arcing motion toward the end of the thrust.
PSRSRA	$+\theta X, -\theta Z, +\theta Y$	Posterior to anterior, superior to inferior, right to left, through the C0-C1 joint plane line, the head is prepositioned in right rotation.
PSRSRP	$+\theta X, -\theta Z, -\theta Y$	Posterior to anterior, superior to inferior, right to left, through the C0-C1 joint plane line, the head is prepositioned in left rotation.
PSLS	$+\theta X, +\theta Z$	Posterior to anterior, superior to inferior, left to right, through the C0-C1 joint plane line, with an inferiorward arcing motion toward the end of the thrust.
PSLSLA	$+\theta X, +\theta Z, -\theta Y$	Posterior to anterior, superior to inferior, left to right, through the C0-C1 joint plane line, the head is rotated toward the side of contact.
PSLSLP	$+\theta X, +\theta Z, +\theta Y$	Posterior to anterior, superior to inferior, left to right, through the C0-C1 joint plane line, the head is prepositioned in right rotation.
AS	$-\theta X, +Z$	Anterior to posterior, superior to inferior, through the C0-C1 joint plane line.
ASRS	$-\theta X, -\theta Z$	Anterior to posterior, superior to inferior, right to left, through the C0-C1 joint plane line.
ASRSRA	$-\theta X, -\theta Z, +\theta Y$	Anterior to posterior, superior to inferior, right to left, through the C0-C1 joint plane line, the patient's head is prepositioned in right rotation.
ASRSRP	$-\theta X, -\theta Z, -\theta Y$	Anterior to posterior, superior to inferior, right to left, through the C0-C1 joint plane line, the patient's head is prepositioned in left rotation.

AS Condyle (-ΘX)

The AS condyle subluxation will reveal fixation and discomfort as the condyle is glided from anterior to posterior during motion palpation. Edema or bogginess is more difficult to assess. Lateral upright visual inspection will reveal a superior gaze to "the heavens." The more severe the AS condyle subluxation is, the greater likelihood of more severe neurological manifestations. A low APGAR score and depressed infant reflexes may be associated with this positional dyskinesia. The newborn or infant may be a slow developer or in more extreme cases can be high at risk (e.g., SIDS, sleep apnea). These patients have a tendency to be poor thrivers (e.g., low weight, poor appetite, weak cry). In the older infant, toddler, and pre-schooler, the parent may inform you that the child "head bangs" the crib or wall to fall asleep or when upset.

The AS condyle is not a common subluxation. It should be suspected if facial or brow trauma has occurred. In-utero constraint positions (e.g., brow or facial), obstetrical trauma, or a fall from a height (e.g., changing table, couch) are a few of the possible mechanisms of injury. An automobile accident with the child unrestrained or the toddler falling from a height and hitting the forehead, can also induce the AS condyle subluxation. An unusual injury history given by the parent or guardian that does not correlate with typical AS injuries should alert the doctor to the possibility of child abuse.

The AS condyle adjustment is performed supine on the newborn and infant. The sitting position set-up is usually performed once the cervical musculature is developed (e.g., toddler, pre-schooler). A condyle block (Fig. 9.22) is used in all AS condyle adjustments. Once the correct size of condyle block is selected, it is placed under the cervical spine supporting C1 to C7. The purpose of the condyle block is to stabilize the cervical spine when the thrust is performed.

SUPINE AS CONDYLE

The newborn or infant is placed supine on the pelvic bench. The crown of the head is placed close to the edge of the table. Depending on the arc of thrust necessary for correction, the doctor will squat or kneel directly superior to the infant's head. Once the condyle block is positioned, the parent can assist by gently holding the child in the supine position. The

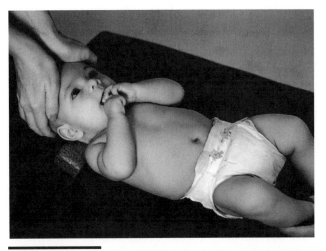

Figure 9.23.   The thenar eminences contact the glabella for the AS occiput.

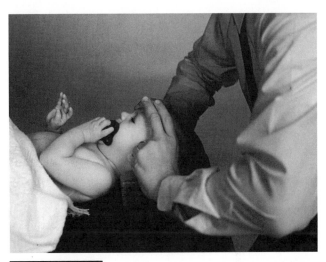

Figure 9.24.   Fingers on the glabella with the thumbs wrapped around the posterior occiput.

condyle subluxation without laterality or rotation will be corrected by contacting the glabella with both thenar eminences. The fingers will lightly wrap under the posterior occiput to create a slight lift (Fig. 9.23). A second hand set-up is the use of the second and third digit from both hands, contacting the glabella, with both thumbs wrapped under the posterior occiput to create a slight lift (Fig. 9.24) If condyle laterality exists, the doctor will position herself slightly to the same side of the listing. If the listing is LS the contact hand will be the left and vice versa. The contact will be the soft portion of the doctor's pisiform on the glabella (Fig. 9.25). The opposite hand will cup the posterior occiput and create a slight separation from the atlas. The thrust is an arcing anterior to posterior and slightly superior to inferior movement. Laterality (e.g., PSLS, PSRS) is corrected by the doctor's contact. To correct condyle rotation, the infant's

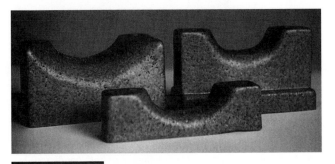

Figure 9.22.   The condyle block comes in a variety of sizes to accommodate the cervical spine.

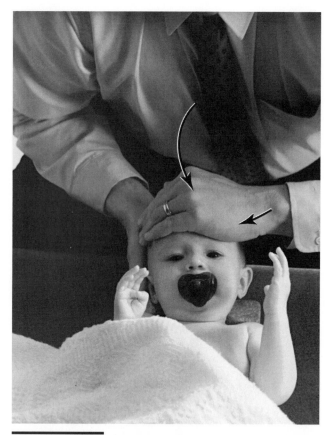

Figure 9.25. Single hand contact for an ASLS listing. The condyle block is used for all supine AS setups.

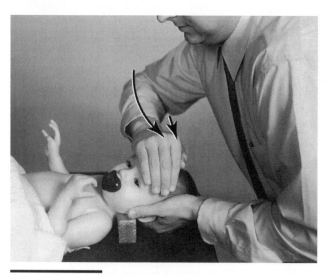

Figure 9.26. Slight head rotation of the infant's head away from the contact hand will correct the axial rotation in an ASRSRP listing.

head is pre-positioned with slight rotation prior to the thrust. For posteriority (e.g., PSLSLP, PSRSRP) the head is slightly rotated away from the contact hand (Fig. 9.26). The anterior listing of PSLSLA or PSRSRA is pre-positioned with slight

head rotation towards the side of the doctor's contact hand (Fig. 9.27).

Newborn/Infant

AS CONDYLE SUPINE DOUBLE THENAR ADJUSTMENT

Name of technique: Gonstead
Technique procedure: Supine AS condyle double thenar adjustment.
Example: AS ($-\theta$X, +Z) (Fig. 9.28).

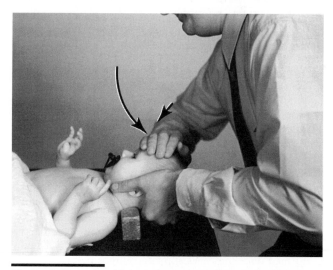

Figure 9.27. On the side of occiput laterality the doctor will squat or kneel behind the bench, contacting the glabella of the frontal bone on the side of laterality of the listing. The opposite hand will cup the posterior occiput and slightly lift to separate the occipito-atlantal joint. Head rotation towards the contact hand positions the infant for an ASRSRA listing.

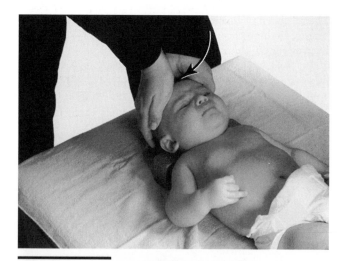

Figure 9.28. Supine AS condyle adjustment. Place both thenar eminences on the contact site. The fingers of both hands are wrapped around posterior to the occiput creating a slight lift. The doctor's elbows should stay close to the side of the body.

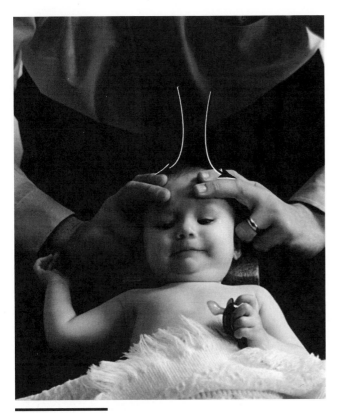

Figure 9.29. Supine AS condyle adjustment. Place the second and third digits of both hands on the contact site, the thumbs are wrapped around posteriorly to the occiput creating a slight lift. The doctor's elbows should stay close to the side of the body.

Contraindications: All other listings, hypermobility, normal functional spinal unit, instability, destruction of the cranium, fracture (pathologic or nonpathologic) of the frontal bone, infection of the contact bone or fracture of the ocular orbit.
Patient position: Supine at the distal end of the pelvic table. The condyle block is placed underneath the cervical spine to protect the C1–C7 region.
Contact site: The glabella.
Doctor's position: The doctor is kneeling or squatting cephalad to the patient.
Supportive assistance: The parent holds the upper and lower limbs to keep them from moving.
Pattern of thrust: Anterior to posterior, superior to inferior with an inferiorward arcing (scooping) movement across the lateral masses of C1.
Contraindication for the thrust: The newborn is unable to be maintained in a supine position.

AS CONDYLE SUPINE FINGER CONTACT ADJUSTMENT

Name of technique: Gonstead
Technique procedure: Supine AS condyle adjustment.
Example: AS (-θX, +Z) (Fig. 9.29).
Patient position: Supine at the distal end of the pelvic table.

The condyle block is placed underneath the cervical spine to protect the C1–C7 region.
Contact site: The glabella.
Doctor's position: The doctor is kneeling or squatting cephalad to the patient.
Pattern of thrust: Anterior to posterior, superior to inferior with an inferiorward arcing (scooping) movement across the lateral mass of C1.

ASRS CONDYLE SUPINE ADJUSTMENT

Name of technique: Gonstead
Technique procedure: Supine ASRS condyle adjustment.
Example: ASRS (-θX, -θZ) (Fig. 9.30).
Patient position: Supine at the distal end of the pelvic table. The condyle block is placed underneath the cervical spine to protect the C1–C7 region.
Contact site: The glabella.
Doctor's position: The doctor is kneeling or squatting cephalad and to the side of laterality.
Supportive assistance: The parent keeps the upper and lower limbs from moving.
Pattern of thrust: Anterior to posterior, superior to inferior, lateral to medial with an inferiorward arcing (scooping) movement across the lateral mass of C1.

SEATED AS CONDYLE

The younger child (e.g., toddler and preschooler) may be positioned on the cervical chair. To accommodate the height of the child, an elevation device (e.g., pelvic bench pillow, booster chair) may be used on the adjusting chair. The condyle block will be positioned behind C1–C7 and held there with the doctor's abdomen (Fig. 9.31). The stabilization strap or the parent's hand can also be placed on the child's abdomen and

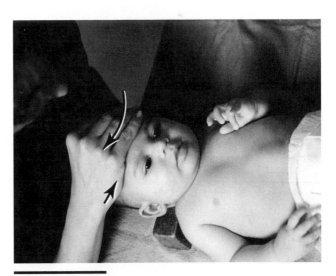

Figure 9.30. The doctor squats on the side of laterality, placing the right thenar eminence on the contact site for the ASRS listing. The stabilization hand is wrapped around the occiput creating a slight lift. The doctor's elbows should stay close to the side of the body.

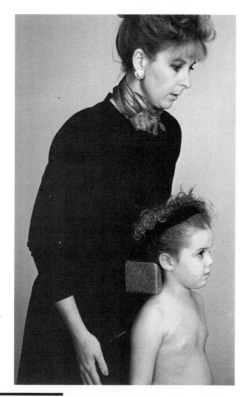

Figure 9.31. The condyle block is placed behind the patient's C1-C7 spine. The doctor's abdomen will hold the block.

chest to further stabilize the patient. For an AS listing, the flat palm of the doctor's hand will contact the center of the glabella and supra orbital margin. The opposite hand will overlap the contact hand for stabilization (Fig. 9.32). An alternative set-up is for the doctor to interlink the fingers (Fig. 9.33). Pre-tension at the joint is obtained with slight head flexion. Prior to the thrust, the doctor's elbows should be positioned close to the side of the body. This will provide for a smoother glide during the arc of the adjustment. Laterality is corrected by the doctor standing slightly towards the side of listing. The contact hand for a lateral misalignment (e.g., ASRS, ASLS) is the same hand as the side of listing. Condyle rotation (e.g., ASRSRP, ASLSLA) is corrected when the doctor pre-positions the head. For anteriority, the head is slightly rotated to the side of the contact hand (Fig. 9.34). Posteriority is corrected with slight head rotation away from the contact hand (Fig. 9.35).

Infant

AS CONDYLE SEATED ADJUSTMENT

Name of technique: Gonstead
Technique procedure: Seated AS condyle adjustment.
Example: AS ($-\theta X, +Z$) (Fig. 9.36).
Patient position: The infant is placed between the thighs of the doctor. The condyle block is placed underneath the cervical spine to protect the C1-C7 region.
Contact site: The glabella.
Doctor's position: The doctor applies thigh pressure to the patient and support to the condyle block with her abdomen.
Pattern of thrust: Anterior to posterior, superior to inferior,

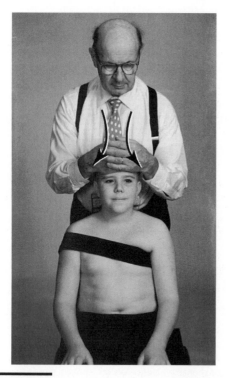

Figure 9.32. For the AS listing the flat palm of the doctor's hand contacts the center of the glabella, the opposite hand will overlap the contact hand.

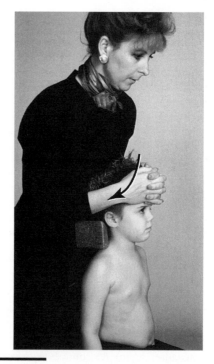

Figure 9.33. An alternative AS set-up is to interlink their fingers.

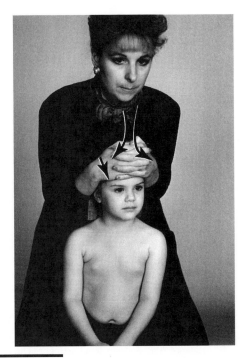

Figure 9.34.   For the ASLSLA listing the head is rotated to the side of hand contact.

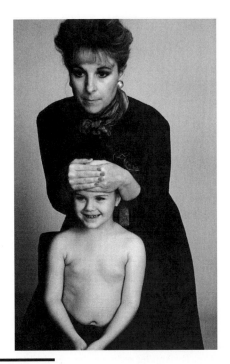

Figure 9.35.   The head is rotated away from the contact hand for the ASLSLP listing. The elbows are kept close to the side of the doctor.

with an inferiorward arcing (scooping) movement across the lateral masses of C1.

Toddler and Pre-Schooler

AS CONDYLE SEATED ADJUSTMENT

Name of technique: Gonstead
Technique procedure: Seated AS condyle adjustment.
Example: AS ($-\theta$X, +Z) (Fig. 9.37).
Patient position: The patient is seated on the cervical chair. The child may need to be raised on the chair (e.g., pelvic pillow, booster chair). The condyle block is placed behind the cervical spine to protect the C1–C7 region. The stabilization strap can be used.
Contact site: The glabella.
Doctor's position: The doctor stands behind the patient supporting the condyle block with her abdomen region.
Supportive assistance: The parent can support the upper chest from activity.
Pattern of thrust: Anterior to posterior, superior to inferior, with an inferiorward arcing (scooping) movement across the lateral masses of C1.
Contraindication for the thrust: The toddler or pre-schooler is unable to be maintained in a seated position.

ASLS CONDYLE SEATED ADJUSTMENT

Name of technique: Gonstead
Technique procedure: Seated ASLS condyle adjustment.
Example: ASLS ($-\theta$X, $+\theta$Z) (Fig. 9.38).
Patient position: The patient is seated on the cervical chair.

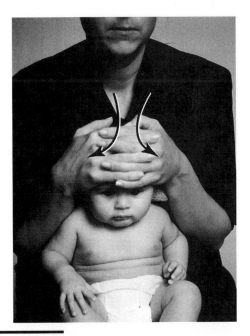

Figure 9.36.   The infant is placed between the thighs of the doctor. The doctor places either thenar eminence on the contact site for the AS listing. The stabilization hand is placed on top. A second alternative is interlocking the fingers. The doctor's elbows should stay close to the side of her body.

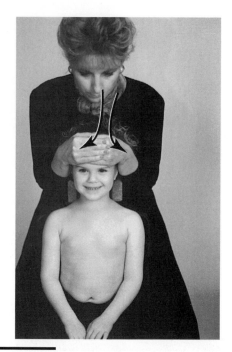

Figure 9.37.   The smaller child may be raised in the chair by a pelvic pillow for the AS setup. Either thenar eminence is placed on the contact site. The opposite (stabilization) hand is placed on top of the adjusting hand. A second option is interlocking the doctor's fingers of both hands and placing on the contact site. The doctor's elbows should stay close to the side of her body.

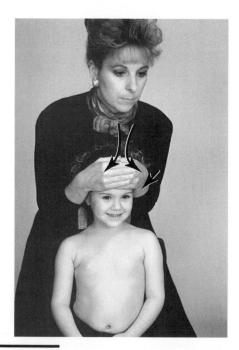

Figure 9.38.   Seated ASLS condyle adjustment. The left thenar eminence is placed on the contact site. The stabilization hand is placed on top of the adjusting hand. The doctor's elbows should stay close to the side of her body.

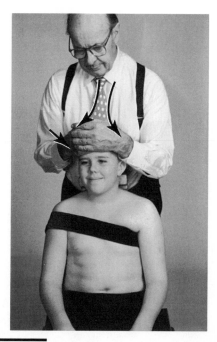

Figure 9.39.   Seated ASRSA condyle adjustment. The right thenar eminence is placed on the contact site. The stabilization hand is placed on top of the adjusting hand. The head is rotated slightly towards the doctor. The amount of rotation is in direct proportion to the amount of listing to be corrected. The doctor's elbows should stay close to the side of his body.

The condyle block is placed behind the cervical spine to protect the C1–C7 region. The stabilization strap may be used. Contact site: The glabella.

Doctor's position: The doctor stands behind the patient and slightly to the side of laterality. The doctor's abdomen supports the condyle block.

Pattern of thrust: Anterior to posterior, superior to inferior, lateral to medial, with an inferiorward arcing (scooping) movement across the lateral mass of C1.

Pre-adolescent and Adolescent

ASRSRA CONDYLE SEATED ADJUSTMENT

Name of technique: Gonstead

Technique procedure: Seated ASRSRA condyle adjustment. Example: ASRSRA ($-\theta X$, $-\theta Z$, $+\theta Y$) (Fig. 9.39).

Patient position: The patient is seated on the cervical chair. The condyle block is placed behind the cervical spine to protect the C1–C7 region. The stabilization strap may be used. Contact site: The glabella. Doctor's position: The doctor stands behind the patient and slightly to the side of laterality. The doctor's abdomen supports the condyle block. Pattern of thrust: Anterior to posterior, superior to inferior, lateral to medial, with an inferiorward arcing (scooping) movement across the lateral masses of C1.

PS (+ΘX) CONDYLE

The set-up for the newborn/infant is performed seated on the lap of the parent. The child will sit with the side of laterality away from the parent. The doctor can use one of two contact points for the adjustment. The distal end of the thumb or the thenar eminence (of the small handed doctor) will contact behind the infant's ear, and slightly above the mastoid process. The doctor's stabilization hand will contact the contralateral cervical musculature especially C1-C2. The fingers of the adjusting hand will wrap around the posterior aspect of the cervical spine. This method of stabilization will protect C1-C7 from receiving unnecessary motion during the thrust. Prior to the thrust, the parent should assist in stabilization by supporting the chest and back of the child. A second set-up is that the newborn/infant can be positioned between the legs of the doctor (Fig. 9.40). The chest or abdomen of the doctor will stabilize the child. Slight thigh pressure should be used by the doctor to prevent the child from shifting from the desired position.

The toddler, pre-schooler, or older child, should be seated on the cervical chair. Chest stabilization can be attained with the parent's hands or the stabilization strap. The doctor's thenar eminence will contact the supramastoid groove on the side of listing (Fig. 9.41). To eliminate interference from occipital hair, the doctor will first glide superior from the supramastoid groove and then slide down to set-up on the groove. The stabilization hand will contact the opposite mastoid and the fingers will wrap around the C1-C2 articulation.

Lateral flexion dyskinesia (e.g., PSLS, PSRS) will be corrected by contacting the mastoid on the side of laterality (Fig. 9.42). The pattern of thrust for a PSRS listing is: Posterior

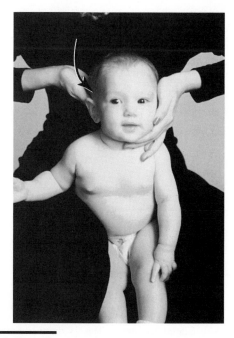

Figure 9.40.   The infant can be placed between the thighs of the doctor. The doctor stabilizes with the chest or abdomen, combined with a slight medial thigh pressure.

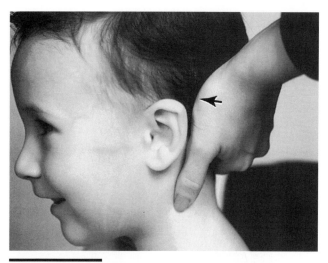

Figure 9.41.   The doctor's thenar eminence will contact the supramastoid groove on the side of listing.

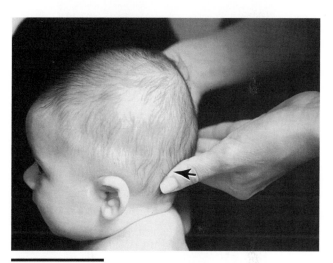

Figure 9.42.   Set up for a PSLS adjustment.

to anterior, superior to inferior, right to left, through the C0-C1 joint plane line, with an inferiorward arcing motion toward the end of the thrust. Condyle rotation is compensated for with pre-positioning of the patient. Anterior rotation (e.g., PSRSRA, PSLSLA) is corrected by slightly rotating the head towards the contact hand (Fig. 9.43). The posteriority listings of PSRSRP or PSLSLP are compensated by pre-positioning the child's head slightly away from the doctor's contact hand (Fig. 9.44).

Newborn and Infant

PSLS CONDYLE SEATED ADJUSTMENT

Name of technique: Gonstead
Technique procedure: Seated PSLS condyle adjustment.
Example: PSLS (+ΘX, +ΘZ) (Fig. 9.45) listing.
Contraindications: All other listings, hypermobility, normal

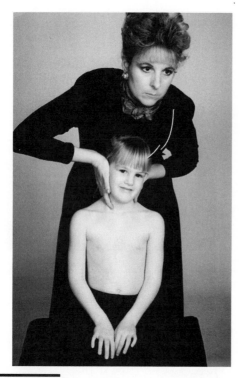

Figure 9.43. The head is rotated towards the doctor's contact hand for the PSLSLA listing.

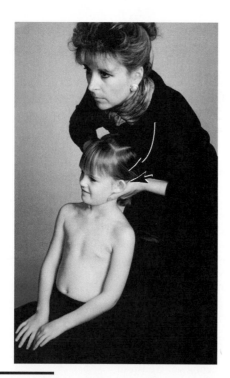

Figure 9.44. For the PSLSLP listing, the head is rotated away from the contact hand. The thrust is posterior to anterior, lateral to medial with an inferiorward arcing movement.

functional spinal unit, instability, destruction of the condyle, fracture (pathologic or nonpathologic) of the condyle bone, infection of the contact bone.

Patient position: The newborn/infant is placed on the lap of the parent. The involved side is facing the doctor.

Contact site: The left supramastoid groove.

Doctor's position: The doctor stands slightly to the side of laterality.

Supportive assistance: The parent supports the chest and back region.

Pattern of thrust: Posterior, superior to inferior, lateral to medial with an inferiorward arcing movement across the lateral masses of C1.

Contraindication for the thrust: The newborn is unable to be maintained in a seated position.

PSRS CONDYLE SEATED ADJUSTMENT

Name of technique: Gonstead

Technique procedure: Seated PSRS condyle adjustment.

Example: PSRS ($+\theta X$, $+\theta Z$) (Fig. 9.46) listing.

Patient position: The newborn/infant is placed on the lap of the parent, the involved side facing the doctor.

Contact site: The right supramastoid groove.

Doctor's position: The doctor stands slightly to the side of laterality.

Supportive assistance: The parent supports the chest and back region.

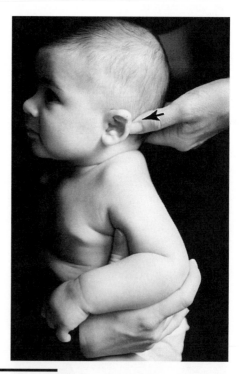

Figure 9.45. Seated PSLS setup. The left distal end of the adjusting thumb or the thenar eminence is placed on the contact site. The stabilization hand supports the cervical musculature on the opposite side.

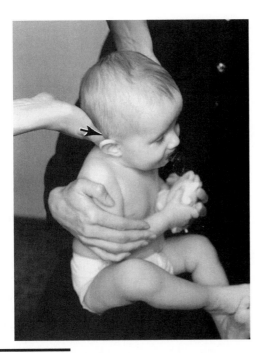

Figure 9.46. Seated PSRS listing. The right distal end of the adjusting thumb or the thenar eminence is placed on the contact site. The stabilization hand supports the cervical musculature on the opposite side.

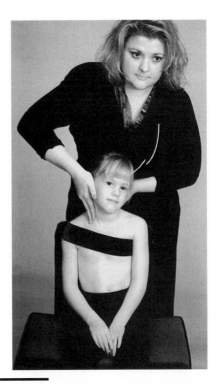

Figure 9.47. The PSLSLA condyle adjustment. The left thenar eminence is placed on the contact site. The stabilization hand is placed on the cervical musculature on the opposite side. The head is rotated towards the doctor. The amount of rotation is in direct proportion to the amount of listing to be corrected.

Pattern of thrust: Posterior to anterior, superior to inferior, lateral to medial with an inferiorward arcing movement across the lateral masses of C1.

Toddler and Pre-Schooler

PSLSLA CONDYLE SEATED ADJUSTMENT

Name of technique: Gonstead
Technique procedure: Seated PSLSLA condyle adjustment.
Example: PSLSLA ($+\theta X$, $+Z$, $-\theta Y$) (Fig. 9.47) listing.
Patient position: The patient is seated on the cervical chair. The child may need to be raised (e.g., pelvic pillow, booster chair). The stabilization strap can be used.
Contact site: The left supramastoid groove.
Doctor's position: The doctor stands behind the patient and slightly to the side of laterality.
Pattern of thrust: Posterior to anterior, superior to inferior, lateral to medial, with an inferiorward arcing movement across the lateral masses of C1.

Pre-Adolescent and Adolescent

PSRS CONDYLE SEATED ADJUSTMENT

Name of technique: Gonstead
Technique procedure: Seated PSRS condyle adjustment.
Example: PSRS ($+\theta X$, $-\theta Z$) (Fig. 9.48) listing.
Patient position: The patient is seated on the cervical chair. The stabilization strap may be used.
Contact site: The right supramastoid groove.

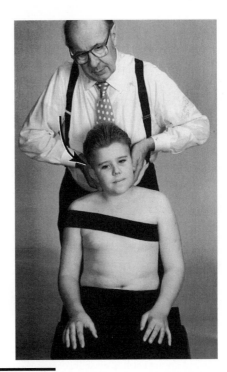

Figure 9.48. Seated PSRS condyle adjustment. The right thenar eminence is placed on the contact site. The stabilization hand is placed on the cervical musculature on the opposite side.

Doctor's position: The doctor stands behind the patient and slightly to the side of laterality.

Pattern of thrust: Posterior to anterior, superior to inferior, lateral to medial, with an inferiorward arcing movement across the lateral masses of C1.

PSRSRP CONDYLE SEATED ADJUSTMENT

Name of technique: Gonstead

Technique procedure: Seated PSRSRP condyle adjustment. Example: PSRSRP (+θX, –Z, +θY) (Fig. 9.49) listing.

Patient position: The patient is seated on the cervical chair. The stabilization strap may be used.

Contact site: The right supramastoid groove.

Doctor's position: The doctor stands behind the patient and slightly to the side of laterality.

Pattern of thrust: Posterior to anterior, superior to inferior, lateral to medial, with an inferiorward arcing movement across the lateral masses of C1.

Atlas (C1-C2)

The atlas subluxation is not as common in the pediatric spine as one might first suspect. Compensation in the upper cervical, particularly in the coronal plane, can result from a lower cervical subluxation. This is due to the righting reflex. Examination of the atlas should involve a multiparameter

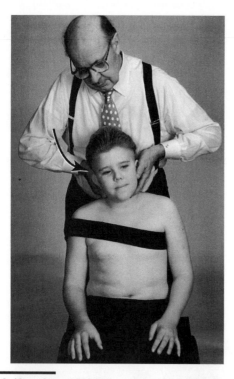

Figure 9.49. Seated PSRSRP condyle adjustment. The right thenar eminence is placed on the contact site. The stabilization hand is placed on the cervical musculature on the opposite side. The head is rotated away the doctor. The amount of rotation is in direct proportion to the amount of listing to be corrected.

approach. Relying on findings from the radiograph or static palpation alone is not sufficient to determine the need for an adjustment.

INSPECTION

With the patient in a seated position, the doctor may assess the atlas with inspection. If the atlas rotates posteriorly (e.g., ASLP, ASRP), the superficial muscle groups can bulge on the side of posteriority. The atlas that has rotated anteriorly (e.g., ASRA, ASLA), can present with a slight ipsilateral head tilt. To confirm lateral flexion malposition, request the patient to shut the eyes and then flex and extend the head for a few seconds. If lateral flexion fixation is present there may be a slight head tilt during the procedure or after resting in a neutral position.

STATIC PALPATION

Static palpation should be performed in the sitting position. The newborn or infant can be seated on the parent's lap and supported with the parent's hands on the chest and back of the child. The older child may independently be examined on a chair. The distal end of the fifth digit or the index digit is used to palpate the musculature. The static musculature examination is used to detect tissue edema or bogginess. The edema reaction at the tissues may be a response due to autonomic nervous system dysfunction or trauma to the region. If posterior rotation is present, a bulging or increased musculature will be palpated. The examiner should be aware that muscular asymmetry or skeletal malformation can influence the validity of these examination findings.

MOTION PALPATION

Motion palpation is conducted in the sitting position. As in static palpation, the parent may assist in the stabilization process of the smaller child or infant. The analysis of the atlas is to determine if fixation dysfunction is present in relationship to the axis (C2). The rotation and lateral flexion position of the atlas is ascertained with this procedure. The AS or AI component of the listing can be determined from the lateral radiograph.

To determine lateral flexion (±θZ) the doctor will need to contact bilaterally the transverse process of the atlas. The younger child can be contacted with the distal end of the fifth digit and thumb (Fig. 9.50 A,B). The larger child will be contacted with the second digit and thumb. The doctor should confirm the findings by reversing the palpation contact hand. This will reduce hand bias. With the doctor's stabilization hand on the crown of the head, laterally flex the head from side to side. Although the motion is not completely understood, it appears that the side contralateral to the fixation reveals the loss of motion. This appears as the lateral mass of C1 is raised on the contralateral side when C1 is laterally flexed onto C2 (39). The listing is confirmed with the APOM radiograph. The lettering assigned is "R" for right or "L" for left, following the AS (e.g., ASR, ASL) or AI (e.g., AIR, AIL).

The primary movement of the atlas-axis relationship is Y-axis rotation. Rotation (Y axis) can be determined very readily with motion palpation. First place the distal end of the

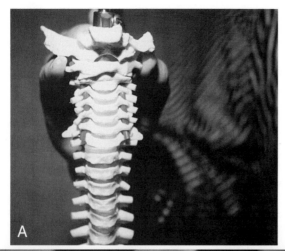

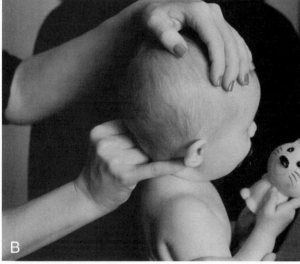

Figure 9.50. A–B, Depending on the size of the patient the fifth or second digit will contact one side of the atlas transverse process. The thumb contacts the opposite transverse process.

fifth or second digit at the anterior-lateral aspect of the transverse process of the atlas. Next slowly rotate the head from side to side. The side of rotational fixation will reveal restriction.

On the older child, the Dvorak's maneuver can assist in determining if an upper cervical (C1-C2) rotational fixation is present. Flex the child's head and rotate the spine from side to side (Fig. 9.51). The side of fixation will reveal restriction of motion. Once the side of laterality (± θZ) has been determined, rotation, if it exists, must be determined. A posteriorly rotated atlas will be confirmed when the doctor can demonstrate restriction of that movement. A left posterior atlas (e.g., ASLP) will reveal restricted range of motion when the doctor rotates the patient's head to the right. Likewise a clockwise (+θ) restriction of the atlas reveals right posteriority (e.g., ASRP). The left anterior atlas (e.g., ASLA) is determined when upon rotation the range of motion clockwise is re-

stricted. The ASRA listing is concluded when counterclockwise motion is diminished. The anterior "A" listing is often more difficult to determine.

INSTRUMENTATION

The newborn and infant are typically more difficult to assess with an instrument (e.g., Nervoscope, Temposcope) than the older pediatric patient. What is commonly referred to as "baby fat" or the brown fatty tissue present can interfere with the gliding procedure (Fig. 9.52). With the toddler, the doctor must be careful to take into account that the child may move during the procedure leading to an inaccurate reading. Stabilization is required to maintain the subject in a motionless neutral position (Fig. 9.53). The procedure for this examination is to glide the instrument from caudad to cephalad. Suboccipital hair is also another factor that may give a

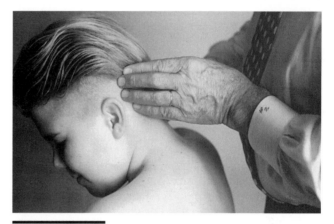

Figure 9.51. Dvorak's maneuver may reveal rotational fixation in the upper cervical (C1-C2) region.

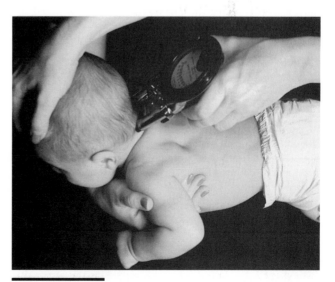

Figure 9.52. The infant's baby fat may interfere with the gliding procedure. The parent or doctor may have to assist with a superiorward skin pull.

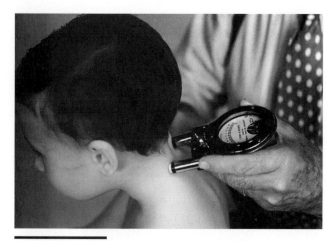

Figure 9.53. The doctor may stabilize the younger patient by bracing the shoulder or abdomen.

false positive finding. If a true positive finding does occur, the doctor must further determine through other examination methods if the reading reflects a C1 or C2 involvement, due to the proximity of the articulations.

RADIOGRAPHIC ANALYSIS

When analyzing the atlas, it is important to acknowledge the possible active involvement of adjacent segments in compensation. The primary biomechanical motion of the atlas is rotation around the odontoid process of the axis. Therefore the odontoid process is used as a reference point in the analysis of the atlas.

The lateral cervical radiograph is analyzed to determine the relationship between C1 and C2 (see Chapter 8). The odontoid will be divided with two dots. The first dot is placed at the base and center of the odontoid, the second dot at the center and superior aspect of the odontoid. Place a longitudinal line intersecting the two points. This line is called the odontoid line (OL). Through the mid-section of the body of the axis, draw a perpendicular line to the OL. This line is referred to as the odontoid perpendicular line (OPL).

To analyze the atlas, place one dot in the middle of the anterior tubercle, and the second dot at the middle junction of the posterior tubercle and the posterior arch. The drawn line between the two points is called the AP atlas plane line. Occasionally the lateral radiograph will reveal the atlas in a lateral flexion position. This will project a space between the posterior arch (rather than an overlap). In this case bisect the space that the lateral atlas tilt creates. If the AP line and the OPL are parallel, a normal atlas and axis relationship can be assumed. Slight atlas extension onto the axis can also be considered within normal limits.

To evaluate the coronal plane posture, an open mouth projection is analyzed. The axis line is drawn parallel at the superior aspect of the body of axis. This line is referred to as the "axis plane line (APL)." The APL represents the horizontal plane of atlas. To draw the line, choose two like points on the atlas. A reliable anatomical point is the transverse process-lateral mass junction. Often the superior border of the

transverse process is obstructed by overhanging of the occiput. If this is the case then the dot should be placed on the inferior transverse process where it intersects the lateral mass. The two dots are connected with a line. A normal atlas-axis relationship is present when the atlas plane line and the axis plane line appear parallel.

Anteriority (+Z)

The atlas may slightly slide anteriorward as it rotates around the X axis. The transverse ligament is responsible for the close relationship of the atlas to the axis. Rupture or severe stretching of the transverse ligament should be suspected if noticeable anterior slippage is viewed on the lateral radiograph. The contact point for the adjustment for the atlas is the antero-lateral portion of the transverse process.

Superiority/Inferiority ($\pm\theta$X)

The anterior tubercle can be referenced for the superiority or inferiority of the atlas on the lateral radiograph. Superiority or hyperextension positional dyskinesia is more common than inferiority/hyperflexion displacement. The superiority ($-\theta$X) misalignment is detected when the AP atlas plane line and the odontoid perpendicular line diverge anteriorly. Inferiority, which is rare, can be detected when the AP atlas plane line and the odontoid perpendicular line coverage anteriorly. The superior displacement is labeled "S" and follows the A listing. The inferior misalignment is given the letter of "I" and also follows the letter A. The listing of the atlas is AS or AI.

A second radiographic finding that can confirm the line analysis is to observe the space between the anterior portion of the dens and the posterior portion of the anterior tubercle of the atlas. When the AS listing is present this space will reveal an inverted "V," the AI listing will appear as a "V." It should be noted that the younger pediatric patient may show a marked space difference between the dens and tubercle. This increased atlas dens interspace (ADI) should not be interpreted as severe AS or AI misalignment. The normal ADI measurement of the pediatric spine is 1 to 5 mm. A greater measurement may be an indication of transverse ligament instability (i.e. tear or sprain) or ligament absence as seen in 25% of Down's patients (14,40).

Laterality $\pm\theta$Z ($\pm$X)

The atlas can rotate around the Z axis and move towards the convexity of lateral bend (termed laterality). The AP radiograph is used to establish laterality. On the side of laterality, the atlas transverse plane will appear with a superior lift of the atlas from the axis plane line. The two possible listings of laterality are ASR or ASL. The ASR listing would reflect the divergence of the two lines on the right side.

Rotation $\pm\theta$Y

The AP radiograph is used to determine the fourth letter of the atlas listing (Table 9.3), which is the Y-axis rotational component. The anatomical reference points to determine rotation are the lateral masses of atlas. Rotation is listed on the side of atlas laterality ($\pm\theta$Z). On the side of laterality, if the atlas rotates posterior, the lateral mass will appear smaller. Anterior rotation of the atlas appears as a larger width of the lateral mass on the side of laterality. The possible listings are ASRP, ASLP, ASRA and ASLA.

The indented concave surfaces of the lateral masses can be analyzed on the AP radiograph. Rotation can be analyzed by locating the radiolucency of the concave and indented upper medial surfaces of the lateral masses. The side of posterior rotation will manifest a narrower radiolucency and the anterior rotation, a wider appearance.

A third method of analyzing the radiograph for rotation is by comparing the occiput to atlas relationship. The transverse occiput line may descend on the side of atlas anteriority. This may appear as a convergence of the transverse occiput line towards the atlas plane line.

C1-C2 Adjustment

The atlas adjustment is adapted to the age and compatibility of the pediatric patient. The neonate and the infant should be adjusted in a side posture or seated position. For the side posture set-up, patient placement should be across the lap of the parent or on the pelvic table. In the case of patient placement on the pelvic table, the doctor should evaluate the space between the lateral cervical spine and the table. A space greater than one fourth of an inch should be reduced by the placement of a folded towel or supportive foam to prevent this space from causing an uncontrolled drop phenomenon during the thrust (acceleration) phase.

The neonate or infant should be placed with the atlas listing involved side up (e.g., ASR or ASL), the head and body in a neutral position, and the face towards the doctor. The practitioner should stand facing the patient. To eliminate anterior-lateral component of the listing (e.g., ASR or ASL) contact is made at the anterior-lateral aspect of the transverse process of the atlas. The contact is made by the distal end of the fifth or second digit (Fig. 9.54). The stabilization distal digit (e.g., fifth or second) contacts the nail bed of the contact digit. The doctor's forearms and stance should reflect the line of correction. To correct the posterior "P" component, the

Table 9.3. Atlas Listings

Gonstead Listing	International	Pattern of Thrust
ASR	(+Z), −θX, −θZ, (−X)	Right to left, through the C1-C2 joint plane line, inferiorward arcing motion toward the end of the thrust.
ASRA	(+Z), −θX, −θZ, −X, +θY	Right to left through the C1-C2 joint plane line, the head is rotated toward side of contact, an inferiorward arcing motion toward the end of thrust.
ASRP	(+Z), −θX, −θZ, (−X), −θY	Right to left, through the C1-C2 joint plane line, the patient's head is rotated away from the side of contact, an inferiorward arcing motion toward end of thrust.
ASL	(+Z), −θX, +θZ, (+X)	Left to right, through the C1-C2 joint plane line, an inferiorward arcing motion toward the end of the thrust.
ASLA	(+Z), −θX, +θZ, (+X), −θY	Left to right, through the C1-C2 joint plane line, the head is rotated toward the side of contact, an inferiorward arcing motion toward the end of the thrust.
AIR	(+Z), +θX, −θZ, (−X)	Right to left, through the C1-C2 joint plane line, a superiorward arcing motion toward the end of the thrust.
AIRA	(+Z), +θX, −θZ, −X, +θY	Right to left, through the C1-C2 joint plane line, the head is rotated toward the side of contact, a superiorward arcing motion toward the end of the thrust.
AIRP	(+Z), +θX, −θZ, (−X), −θY	Right to left, through the C1-C2 joint plane line, the head is rotated away from the side of contact, a superiorward arcing motion toward the end of the thrust.
AIL	(+Z), +θX, +θZ, (+X)	Left to right, through the C1-C2 joint plane line, a superiorward arcing motion toward the end of the thrust.
AILA	(+Z), +θX, +θZ, (+X), −θY	Left to right, through the C1-C2 joint plane line, the head is rotated towards the side of contact, a superiorward arcing motion toward the end of the thrust.
ASLP	(+Z), −θX, +θZ, (+X), +θY	Left to right, through C1-C2 joint plane line, the head is rotated away from the side of contact, an inferiorward arcing motion toward the end of the thrust.

doctor's stance should be slightly leaning forward towards the patient. For the anterior "A" listing, the doctor's stance should be slightly leaning away from the patient. The parent may assist by stabilizing the infant's head and body.

The sitting position is the ideal position for the infant or toddler. There are several possible sitting positions. The

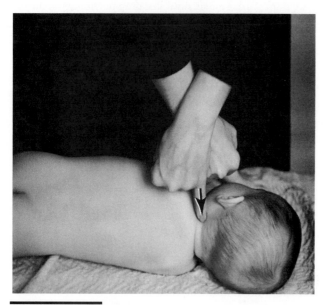

Figure 9.54. The atlas listing should be placed involved side-up for a side posture set-up.

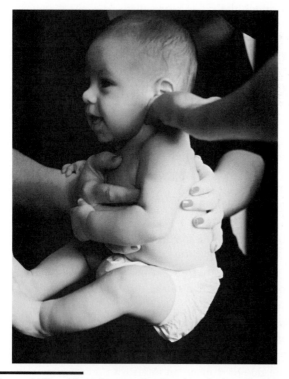

Figure 9.55. The infant may be placed on the lap of a parent for an atlas set-up. The parent will stabilize the infant.

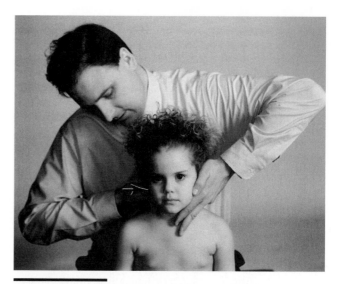

Figure 9.56. The taller doctor may place the toddler between the legs for an atlas set-up.

infant/toddler may be placed on the lap of an attending parent (Fig. 9.55). The parent should stabilize the child's chest and mid-thoracic spine. The side of laterality should be placed toward the doctor for set-up. A taller doctor may place the infant/toddler between their legs and apply slight thigh pressure for stabilization (Fig. 9.56). This procedure should only be chosen if the doctor can maintain their contact and stabilization arms in proper alignment.

The toddler or older child may sit independently in a cervical chair with a back support. The stabilization strap or the parent's hands are used to stabilize the chest. On the side of atlas laterality, the doctor will contact the anterior-lateral aspect of the transverse of atlas (e.g., ASR or ASL) with the distal portion of the thumb (Fig. 9.57). The rotational aspect of the listing (e.g., ASRP, ASRA, ASLP, ASRA) can be corrected by slightly rotating the head prior to the thrust. The posterior atlas (e.g., ASRP or ASLP) is corrected by turning the head away from the contact hand (Fig. 9.58). Anterior rotation (e.g., ASRA or ASLP) is corrected by rotating the head slightly towards the contact hand of the doctor. The opposite hand will be used to stabilize the opposite side of atlas laterality (Fig. 9.59). The stabilization hand will cup the ear and the fingers will point caudal to protect the C2-C3 articulation. The stabilization hand should not be used to create a counterforce. The thrust is given with a slight torque ($+\theta X$) to enhance the fluidity of the adjustment. A set and hold follows at the end of the adjustment.

Newborn and Infant

C1 ASL SEATED ADJUSTMENT

Name of technique: Gonstead
Name of technique procedure: Seated atlas adjustment.
Example: ASL ($+Z$, $-\theta X$, $+\theta Z$, $+X$) (Fig. 9.60) listing. AS

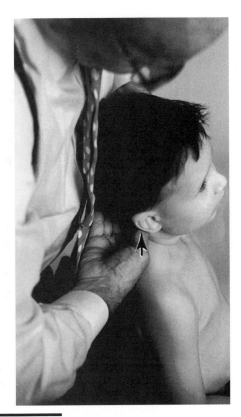

Figure 9.57. On the side of atlas laterality, the doctor will contact the antero-lateral aspect of the transverse process.

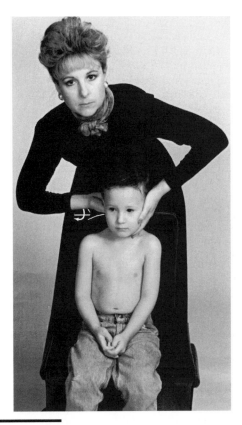

Figure 9.59. The head is rotated towards the side of the contact for the ASRA listing.

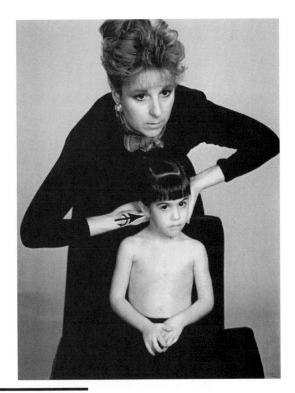

Figure 9.58. To eliminate the atlas posterior rotational listing, the head is rotated away from the contact site.

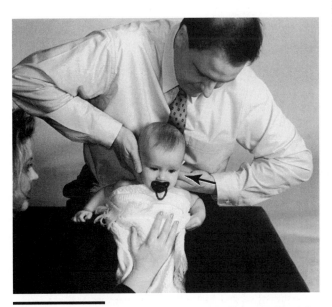

Figure 9.60. Seated ASL adjustment. The distal tip of the left thumb on the contact site. The stabilization hand is placed cupping the opposite ear and stabilizing the C2-C3 articulation and the lateral musculature.

(antero-superior, -θX), lateral flexion to the right (+θZ). Flexion and left lateral flexion fixation dysfunction.

Contraindications: All other listings, hypermobility, normal functional spinal unit, instability, pathologic fracture of the neural arch, infection of the neural arch or transverse process, destruction of the atlas, transverse ligament rupture.

Patient position: The newborn/infant is placed in between the thighs of the seated doctor. The doctor applies slight thigh pressure.

Contact site: Antero-lateral aspect of the transverse process of the atlas.

Supportive assistance: The parent should keep the torso from moving.

Pattern of thrust: Lateral to medial, inferiorward arc toward the end of the thrust.

Contraindication for the thrust: The newborn/infant is unable to be maintained in a seated position.

C1 ASL SIDE POSTURE ADJUSTMENT

Name of technique: Gonstead
Name of technique procedure: Side posture atlas adjustment.
Example: ASL (+Z, -θX, +θZ, +X) (Fig. 9.61) listing. AS (antero-superior, -θX), lateral flexion to the right (+θZ). Flexion and left lateral flexion fixation dysfunction.

Patient position: The newborn/infant is placed on its right side on the pelvic bench. The head piece of the hi-lo or knee-chest table or the lap of the parent may be used. A small rolled up towel or foam may need to be placed between the patient's lateral aspect of the cervical spine and table to reduce any air gap.

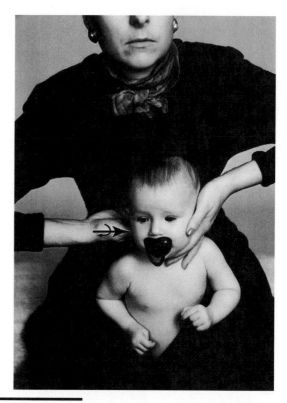

Figure 9.62. Seated ASRA adjustment. Distal tip of the right thumb to the contact site. The stabilization hand is placed cupping the opposite ear and stabilizing the C2-C3 articulation and the lateral musculature.

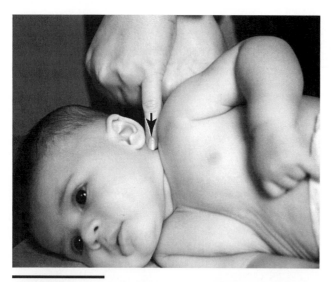

Figure 9.61. Setup for a lateral ASLS listing. The distal tip of the fifth or second digit, or thumb on the contact site. The stabilization hand will support the contact hand by placing the fifth or second digit, or thumb upon the nail bed of the contact hand.

Contact site: Antero-lateral aspect of the transverse process of the atlas.

Supportive assistance: The parent may need to stabilize the chest and/or lower limbs from activity.

Pattern of thrust: Lateral to medial, inferiorward arc toward the end of the thrust.

Contraindication for the thrust: The newborn/infant is unable to be maintained in a side posture position.

C1 ASRA SEATED ADJUSTMENT

Name of technique: Gonstead
Name of technique procedure: Seated atlas adjustment.
Example listing: ASRA (+Z), -θX, -θZ, -X,+θY (Fig. 9.62). AS (antero-superior, -θX), lateral flexion to the left. Flexion and left lateral flexion, and right axial rotation fixation dysfunction.

Patient position: The newborn/infant is placed in a seated position in the doctor's lap. The doctor applies slight thigh pressure.

Contact site: Antero-lateral aspect of the right transverse process of the atlas.

Pattern of thrust: Lateral to medial, inferiorward arc toward the end of the thrust.

Toddler and Pre-Schooler

C1 ASR SEATED ADJUSTMENT

Name of technique: Gonstead
Name of technique procedure: Seated atlas adjustment.
Example: ASR (+Z, -θX, -θZ, -X) (Fig. 9.63) listing. AS (antero-superior, -θX), lateral flexion to the right (+θZ). Flexion and right lateral flexion fixation dysfunction.
Patient position: The toddler/pre-schooler is placed on the cervical chair.
Doctor's position: The doctor stands behind and slightly to the side of laterality.
Contact site: Antero-lateral aspect of the right transverse process of the atlas.
Supportive assistance: The stabilization strap or the parent should keep the torso from movement.
Pattern of thrust: Lateral to medial, inferiorward arc toward the end of the thrust.

C1 ASRP SEATED ADJUSTMENT

Name of technique: Gonstead
Name of technique procedure: Seated atlas adjustment.
Example listings: ASRP (+Z, -θX, -θZ, -X, -θY) (Fig. 9.64). Antero-superior, lateral flexion to the left and right axial rotation.

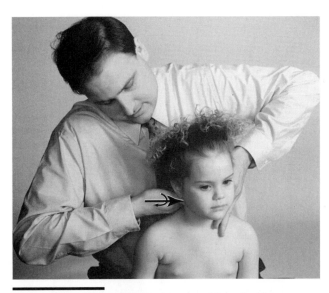

Figure 9.64. Seated ASRP adjustment. The taller doctor may place the patient between the thighs. Distal tip of the right thumb on the contact site. To correct the rotational component (-θY), the head is slightly rotated away from the side of contact. The amount of rotation is in proportion to the rotational component. The stabilization hand is placed cupping the opposite ear and stabilizing the C2-C3 articulation and the lateral musculature.

Patient position: The toddler/pre-schooler is seated between the thighs of the doctor.
Doctor's position: The doctor is seated on the pelvic bench or cervical chair.
Contact site: Antero-lateral aspect of the right transverse process of the atlas.
Supportive assistance: The stabilization strap may be used or a parent can stabilize the torso.
Pattern of thrust: Lateral to medial, inferiorward arc toward the end of the thrust.

Pre-adolescent and Adolescent

C1 ASL SEATED ADJUSTMENT

Name of technique: Gonstead
Name of technique procedure: Seated atlas adjustment.
Example listing: ASL (+Z, -θX, +θZ, +X) (Fig. 9.65). Antero-superior, lateral flexion to the right side.
Patient position: The patient is placed in a seated position on the cervical chair.
Contact site: Antero-lateral aspect of the left transverse process of the atlas.
Pattern of thrust: Lateral to medial, inferiorward arc toward the end of the thrust.

C1 AIL MODIFIED-TOGGLE ADJUSTMENT

Name of technique: Gonstead
Name of technique procedure: Modified toggle atlas adjustment for the AI listing.

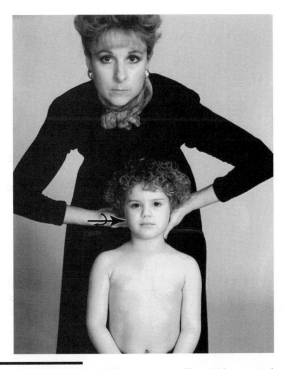

Figure 9.63. Seated ASR adjustment. The child may need to be raised on the chair by the pelvic pillow. The distal tip of the right thumb on the contact site. The stabilization hand is placed cupping the opposite ear and stabilizing the C2-C3 articulation and the lateral musculature.

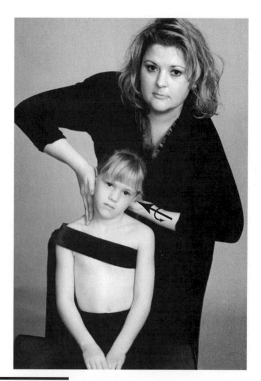

Figure 9.65.   Seated ASL adjustment. Distal tip of the left thumb on the contact site. The stabilization hand is placed cupping the opposite ear and stabilizing the C2-C3 articulation and the lateral musculature. Both arms should be opposed to each other when the set-up is completed.

Example listing: AIL (+Z, +θX, +θZ, +X) (Fig. 9.66). Antero-inferior, lateral flexion to the right. Extension and right lateral flexion fixation dysfunction.

Patient position: The patient is placed prone on the knee–chest or hi-lo table with the head rotated to the left side. To relax the paraspinal muscles, the arm of the involved side may be raised up over the head of the patient.

Doctor's stance: The doctor stands behind the patient.

Contact site: Antero-lateral aspect of the left transverse process of the atlas.

Pattern of thrust: Lateral to medial, superiorward arc toward the end of the thrust.

Lower Cervicals (C2-C7)

The cervical lordosis is formed by the wedge shape of the intervertebral discs (41,42). The magnitude of the lordosis is influenced by hyperplastic articular pillars (43), small facet angles (44) and short pedicles.

The cervical curve was previously thought to develop after birth at approximately 4-6 months of age, when the cervical spinal muscles are beginning to hold the head up. This however has been questioned. Bagnall et al. (45) suggests that at as early as nine and a half weeks (conceptual age), a well defined secondary curvature can be demonstrated.

Inspection

A hypolordotic or kyphotic cervical curve is the most frequent reaction to cervical trauma or as a compensation to a vertebral subluxation. If the vertebral subluxation is in an extension (posterior and inferior) position, the vertebrae above will compensate in a flexion posture. Further, the upper cervical region with hyperextension subluxations (e.g., AS occiput or AS atlas) can influence the mid-cervical spine with a corresponding postural kyphosis.

Rarely is hyperlordosis detected in the cervical spine. The thoracic spine can cause this type of postural reaction due to hyperkyphosis or compression fractures.

Motion Palpation

The zygapophyseal joints are part of a three joint complex. The two zygapophyseal joints contribute greatly to the overall stability of the region. It should be noted that the capsular ligaments are less taut in the cervical spine. This allows for increased range of motion.

The 45 degree angle (to the horizontal plane) of the zygapophyseal joints at C4 dictates the pattern of movement of the cervical vertebrae. At C7-T1 the facets are more vertical. There is a decreased +Z translation (anterior to posterior shear) motion at this level. In the lower cervical region the acuity of arc of movement is increased. The lower cervical arc is decreased with disc degeneration (46). This is seen more commonly in the mature adult spine. During flexion, the vertebrae will move anterior and superior. During extension the vertebrae will move posterior and inferior.

Coupling occurs with lateral flexion. At the segment level of C2-C3, for every 3 degrees of lateral flexion, there are 2

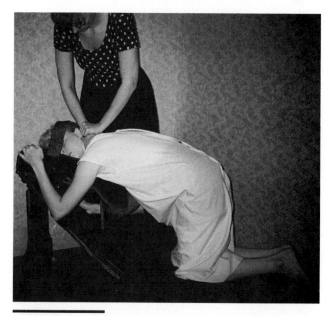

Figure 9.66.   The modified toggle set-up is used for the AIL listing. The knee-chest table is the suggested table. The soft portion of the cephalad (right) hand is placed on the contact site. The caudad (left) hand will wrap around the adjusting hand.

degrees of axial rotation (46). The coupling mechanism decreases as you descend to the lower cervicals. At C7-T1, there is 1 degree of axial rotation for every 7.5 degrees of lateral bending (46).

Dynamic Response

Vertebral injury (causing adhesion formation or edema) or long-term effects of impaired postural movements can result in fixation dysfunction. Dynamic reaction is seen with hypermobility in the region above the level of hypomobility (vertebral subluxation). The mid-cervical region will commonly respond with a hypermobile dynamic reaction. The midcervical region of the adult has the highest incidence of disc protrusion and degeneration in the cervical spine (47). Further, the mid-cervical spine is a common site for traction osteophytes. This architectural response is a sign of hypermobility and/or instability. It is contraindicated to adjust hypermobile segments. The region of hypermobility is commonly more tender or painful on palpation due to the postural compensation for the hypomobile segments below. Stress radiographs may assist in determining specifically the hypo and hypermobile segments of the pre-adolescent and adolescent patient.

There are two major types of motion palpation. They are "end play" and intersegmental range of motion. Current research suggests that "end feel" palpation is not reliable procedure (48). No intersegmental range of motion palpation studies have been performed. The reliability of motion palpation warrants further study within the chiropractic profession.

Intersegmental range of motion palpation is performed passively. Although the younger patient may inadvertently participate with this procedure, the examiner must be aware of this possibility and not hesitate to re-evaluate the region.

The position of the newborn and infant is typically prone on the parent's lap or against the chest of the parent. It is important that this position is stabilized in a neutral plane by the doctor and/or parent. Once the palpation position has been attained, the doctor then determines which of their distal digits will be used to palpate the lower to mid cervical region (C7-T1 to C2-C3).

The doctor should choose the distal digit which will be the most specific contact on the spinous process. Commonly, this will be the fifth digit (due to the smaller contact point) or the second digit for the toddler/pre-schooler spine (Fig. 9.67).

The contact will be made on the spinous process. With the opposite (stabilization) hand, the doctor contacts the crown of the infant's head. To introduce passive motion for intersegmental range of motion, the examiner will lightly flex and extend the skull in a rocking glide. The normal finding at the joint is a non-restrictive glide from posterior to anterior. If an extension positional dyskinesia ($-\theta X$ or posteriority and inferiority) is present, a restricted finding occurs when the spinous process does not complete the entire anterior ($+\theta X$, $+Z$) glide.

The posterior ($-Z$) listing is the most common in the newborn and infant. In the newborn/infant, through pre-adolescence, lateral flexion dyskinesia ($\pm\theta Z$) is generally not a major component of the listing. The superior or inferior

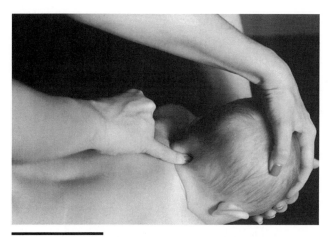

Figure 9.67.   The distal end of the fifth digit contacts the spinous process of the cervical vertebra. The opposite hand supports the crown of the head.

wedge is analyzed from the AP radiograph. Lateral flexion dyskinesia is more likely to be detected when the extension dyskinesia ($-Z$, $-\theta X$ or posteriority and inferiority) is not positionally corrected. The two most common patient groups to have lateral flexion dyskinesia are those younger children who may have a history of lateral cervical trauma or the adolescent without previous or properly performed spinal care.

To evaluate the pediatric spine for lateral flexion dyskinesia, the newborn/infant should be held in a sitting position by the parent. The parent should place one hand on the newborn or infant's chest and the other in the mid-thoracic spine. The older patient is seated. The doctor will place the smallest digit on one individual spinous process at a time (Fig. 9.68). Global motion palpation that attempts to scan two or more segments at a time is not encouraged (Fig. 9.69). The doctor will place the opposite hand on the crown of the head. From the neutral position, the doctor initiates the lateral bending of the cervical spine with the stabilization hand on the crown of the head. The motion begins in the neutral position and lateral bending is analyzed one side at a time. The soft tissue of the same or ipsilateral side of the bend will relax if there is no fixation of the segment. Generalized global scanning (e.g., left to right), although one form of analysis of the spine, should not be conducted as the primary or only assessment.

Assessing the coupling motion of spinous rotation PL and PR ($\pm\theta Y$) is more difficult. As lateral bending occurs, the spinous process should rotate to the contralateral side of lateral flexion. This axial rotation is greater in the upper cervical region and decreases to a smaller coupling movement in the lower cervical region.

The occurrence of spinous rotation is not as common in the young spine (e.g., newborn/infant, toddler/pre-schooler). Suspect this positional dyskinesia in rotational trauma to the spine or the long-standing vertebral subluxation that is compensating for lack of proper segmental function elsewhere in the spine. If the direction of spinous rotation and lateral flexion dyskinesia is questioned, it should be confirmed with lateral flexion stress radiographs and the anterior-posterior static view.

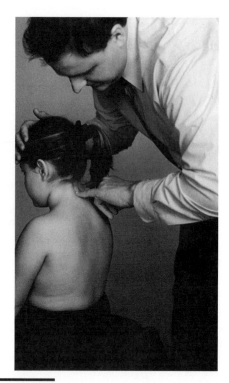

Figure 9.68.   The doctor initiates the lateral bending of the cervical spine with the stabilization hand. The motion begins in the neutral position and lateral bending is analyzed one side at a time.

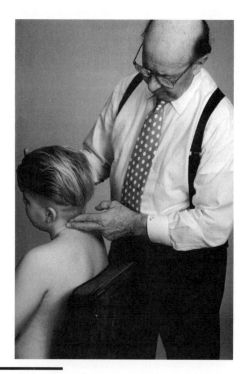

Figure 9.69.   Global scanning of cervical segments is not recommended.

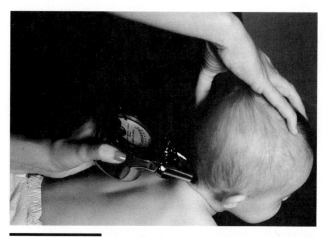

Figure 9.70.   Stabilizing the cervical spine is necessary to prevent infant movement during instrumentation scanning.

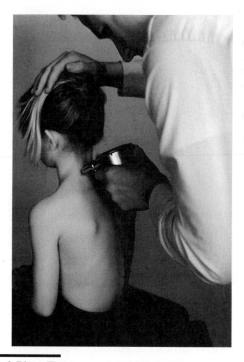

Figure 9.71.   The instrument is glided inferior to superior in the cervical spine.

Instrumentation

The newborn/infant is placed in the prone position (Fig. 9.70). The older child is assessed in a seated position (Fig. 9.71). The hand-held instrument is glided caudad to cephalad. The loose skin of the newborn/infant should be considered as a possible confounding variable. To stabilize the younger child, the doctor may need to hold the crown of the head.

Radiography

The neutral lateral cervical view is used to rule out any contraindications for the spinal adjustment. The lateral radio–

graph further provides analytical information on the position of the vertebral segment. Specifically hyperextended or flexed dyskinesia can be seen on this projection. Herbst (35) reveals that extension dyskinesia is highly correlated to segmental involvement. To confirm the finding, a flexion study would reveal little or no anterior to superior gliding. If the flexion study reveals appropriate $+\theta X$ motion in relationship with the segment below, this cephalad segment is not indicated for a spinal adjustment. An exception to this contraindication is if a lateral flexion study reveals decreased bending ($\pm\theta Z$) or rotation ($\pm\theta Y$).

The anterior-posterior radiograph (coronal plane) is used to determine rotational (e.g., PL, PR) and lateral flexion (e.g., PLS, PRS, PLI-la, PRI-la) components of the subluxation listing. See Chapter 8 for line analysis. If the AP static listing does not correlate with the intersegmental motion palpation findings, lateral bending radiographs may be warranted to accurately determine the nature of the subluxation.

In lateral stress radiographs, coupling action occurs with axial rotation (Y axis) and slight flexion (X axis) due to the angle of the facet joints. At the segments of C7-T1 the facets (coronal plane) are similar to the thoracic spine. At this vertebral segment only slight coupled axial rotation is present.

Lower Cervical Adjustment

The ages and compliance of the patient will determine the site for the cervical adjustment. The toddler may not be able to comply with the seated position, however the pre-schooler through adolescent should have no difficulty with the cervical chair position.

Biomechanical Considerations in Adjusting the Lower Cervical Spine

When the subluxation of the segment is in extension, it is imperative to contact the spinous process and "lift" the segment to a flexed position (or posterior and superior). This corrective motion is $+\theta X$ with $+Z$.

The neutral patient position seated in the cervical chair allows for the ideal set-up. In this position, the surrounding segments can be stabilized during the inferior to superior thrust. The recline of the chair is changeable; however the most upright position is recommended. The stabilization strap is suggested on the taller child to prevent forward motion during the thrust. For the left-sided contact (e.g., PL, PLS) the strap is placed over the right shoulder and the left shoulder for the right-sided contact. The smaller patient normally responds more easily to a parent stabilizing the child's torso with his/her hand(s).

In the set-up preparation by the doctor, the use of excessive lateral flexion to create a pre-load tension on the contact site should be avoided. Slight lateral flexion can assist in the pre-tension of the segment of the joint. Due to the flexibility of the pediatric spine, exaggeration of this position will introduce excessive coupling compensation and unnecessary spinous rotation. The set-up procedure for the chair adjustment is as follows:

1. Lower the patient's head into a flexed position. The doctor will create a tissue pull in the line of correction;

2. With the first digit (distal, lateral and palmar aspect), contact the inferior and lateral border of the spinous process or the medial aspect of the lamina (for lamina contacts);

3. The stabilization hand will assist in bringing the head into a neutral position and slightly posteriorward;

4. Slightly laterally flex (10-15 degrees) the head to the side of contact;

5. On the opposite side, place the stabilization hand on the cervical segments;

6. Following the line of correction, the contact hand and forearm will perform the thrust. The thrust is a very quick movement. The stabilization hand will not produce any force during the thrust; and

7. After the adjustment, the segment that has been contacted should be held for a moment. This will allow for the viscoelastic elements of the segment to respond.

8. To protect the vertebral arteries and the ligamentous elements of the joint, the doctor should avoid positioning or thrusting in the cervical spine with rotation or rotation with extension.

The pediatric patient should be seated in a neutral upright position. The legs should not be crossed and the hands should rest in a relaxed position on the lap. If the younger child is unable to touch his/her feet to the floor, they should be dangling in front of the chair.

The distal, lateral and palmar region of the doctor's first digit is the contact point for the adjustment. To increase stability for the first digit, the second to the fourth digit will be positioned behind as a back-up (Fig. 9.72A, B). To set up on a spinous process listing (e.g., P, PL, PR, PLS, PRS) the distal inferior aspect will be contacted. The doctor should further compensate his/her stance to correct spinous laterality. If the listing is PR the doctor will slightly stand to the right side of the patient. Tissue pull is performed to eliminate tissue slack and increase specificity of the adjustment. For the PR listing, the stabilization hand will tissue pull from right to left and inferior to superior. The inferior to superior tissue pull is important in the lower cervical region to assist in correcting the extension ($-\theta X$) component of the listing.

In the pre-adolescent and adolescent, the lamina listing may be present (e.g., PLI-la, PRI-la). This finding is confirmed on the AP radiograph. The contact point is the medial aspect of the lamina. To correct the lateral flexion component, the lamina is contacted on the opposite side of the listing (i.e., the left lamina is contacted for PRI-la). The tissue pull is the same procedure as for the spinous process contact. The inferiority of the listing is corrected when at the end of the thrust, a slight torque is introduced (i.e., clockwise for PLI-la and counter clockwise for PRI-la) by the doctor's contact hand. Prepositioning in lateral flexion likely has a greater influence on the lateral flexion fixation than the torque movement.

To stabilize the contact hand, the thumb of the thrusting hand contacts the ramus of the mandible. During the thrust, no

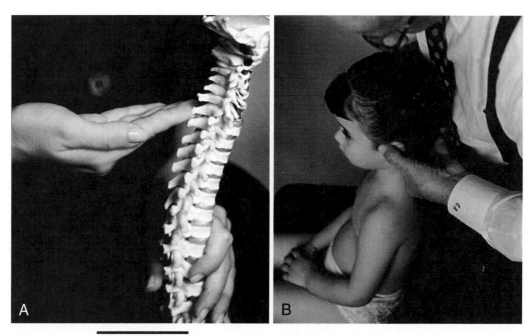

Figure 9.72. A–B, The first digit is supported by the second through the fourth digit as it contacts the spinous process or lamina listing.

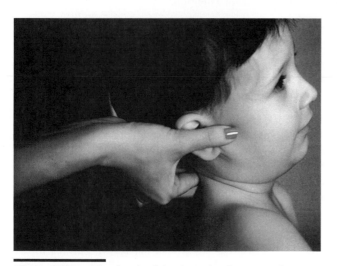

Figure 9.73. The thumb of the thrust hand contacts the ramus of the mandible. The contact should maintain an arch prior to and after the thrust.

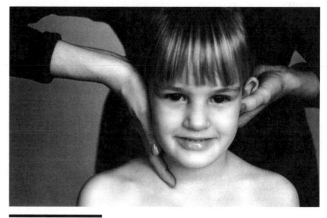

Figure 9.74. The palmar surface of the stabilization hand will contact the lateral cervical musculature.

pressure should be exerted from the thumb into the ramus. The thumb will move slightly forward (posterior to anterior) during the thrust. Prior, during and post thrust the contact hand should remain in the configuration of an arch (Fig. 9.73). The breaking of this hand posture increases the likelihood of introducing unnecessary rotation into the thrust.

On the opposite side of the thrusting hand, the palmar side of the stabilization hand will contact the cervical musculature (Fig. 9.74). The purpose of this contact is to stabilize the segments above and below the vertebra that will receive the thrust. The stabilization hand is not used to introduce any thrust or motion during the adjustment. To reinforce the vertebra that will be adjusted, the stabilization hand can

distribute slight inferiorward pressure to the segment below. This will create a foundation to set the vertebra upon.

With the taller adolescent, the posterior portion of the head can rest against the doctor's chest or abdomen for stabilization. The smaller patient should be elevated in the chair (e.g., by booster chair, pillow) to present the cervical spine for contact.

Considering the flexibility of the pediatric spine and specifically the component of elasticity, the following anatomical considerations, patient positions or thrust vectors should be avoided. Contraindications for cervical adjustments include:

1. Any other listing (i.e., set-up and thrust for a PR is performed as a PLI-La);
2. Normal FSU is present;
3. Infection of the contact vertebra;

4. Fracture or destruction of the neural arch or spinous process;

5. Long lever set-ups;

6. The doctor contacting broadly (overlapping segments) with the adjusting hand;

7. Bringing the segment to pre-tension with traction, extension, flexion, lateral flexion or rotation; and

8. Producing a thrust with unnecessary vectors as stated in item.

Table 9.4 presents different listings for the lower cervical spine (C2-C7).

Alternative Adjusting Procedures

The newborn, infant and toddler may not adapt well to the seated position so alternative positions are available. The newborn or infant can be placed in a prone position across the parent's lap. The patient may also be placed across the lap of the doctor. If the latter is chosen, the doctor must be careful to align the adjusting forearm for a posterior to anterior thrust and not to introduce any rotation. A side posture position can also be chosen as long as the newborn/infant can be maintained in a neutral position (Fig. 9.75). The doctor should stabilize the crown of the infant's head. Sitting the patient in an upright position can be accomplished with the assistance of the parent. The parent will seat the infant in an upright position on their lap, and support the chest and back with both hands (Fig. 9.76).

Table 9.4.   Examples of Adjustment Listings for the Lower Cervical Spine (C2–C7)

Gonstead	International
P (posteriority)	−Z
PL or PR	−Z, −θY or −Z, +θY
PLS or PRS	−Z, −θY, +θZ, or −Z, +θY, −θZ
PLI-Ia or PRI-Ia	−Z, −θY, −θZ or −Z, +θY, −θZ

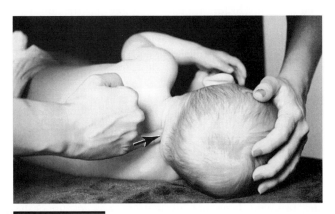

Figure 9.75.   Placed in the side posture position, the spinous process is contacted by the distal end of the fifth digit.

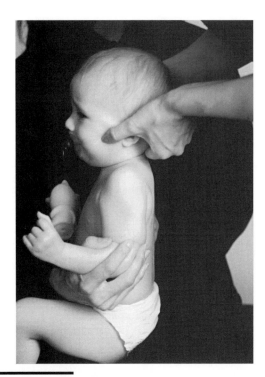

Figure 9.76.   The older infant may be placed on the parent's lap for a seated cervical set-up.

The doctor should carefully stabilize the opposite cervical musculature, to prevent the introduction of unnecessary forces to other segments.

The hi-lo or knee-chest table may also be an alternative for adjusting in a neutral position (Fig. 9.77A,B). If the two halves of the face pieces cannot be closed on the hi-lo table, rolling a small towel and placing it in the center may prevent the patient's smaller face from hitting the bottom of the head piece during the thrust. When using the knee-chest table, the stabilization strap or parent's hand may be used to stabilize the cranium. It should be noted that in the prone position, the cervical adjustment frequently does not create a pronounced audible.

Contact Digit and Stabilization

The parameters for choosing the contact digit are determined when the doctor evaluates the size of the involved vertebra and the suitable digit size that will specifically make the contact. A common error of the doctor is to choose the digit felt to have the most coordination to deliver a thrust. This often results in a digit too large (e.g., first digit of a large male hand on the spinous process of a newborn) to specifically contact the segment, leading to overlap on additional segments.

Particularly for the newborn, the traditional distal, palmar aspect of the second digit may not be specific enough. Depending on the size of the doctor's fingers, the fifth digit may substitute for the second digit in the seated cervical adjustment.

Depending on the position of the patient (i.e., prone or sitting) and the cervical muscular development, the doctor can stabilize the contact digit. If an older infant is prone on the lap of the parent, the doctor's contact is the distal end of the fifth

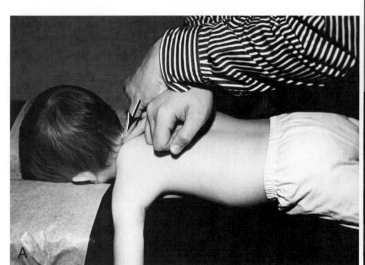
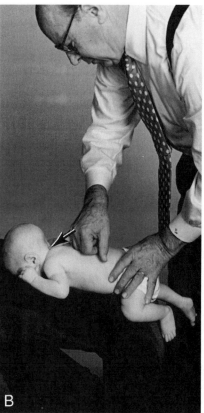

Figure 9.77. A, The hi-lo table may be used for cervical adjustments. B, The infant may be placed on the head piece of the knee chest table. The distal end of the fifth digit contacts the spinous process and the stabilization hand secures the infant's position.

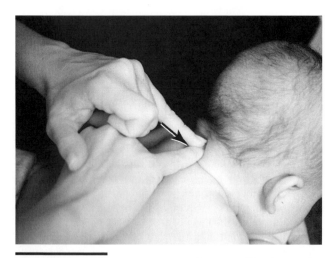

Figure 9.78. C2 posterior prone adjustment. The distal end of the fifth digit is placed on the contact site. To increase the depth of the thrust, the stabilization distal digit (e.g., fifth, second, thumb) will be placed on the adjusting nail bed. The doctor's forearms should follow the plane line of the joint.

digit. The use of the opposite hand for contact stabilization can only be used for the prone position. The second or fifth digit is placed on the contact nail bed. This stabilization procedure may be very helpful for those infants who manifest more developed cervical musculature.

Depending on the doctor's contact position (single digit or double digit), the doctor or parent may stabilize the newborn/infant during the prone set-up by placing a hand on the crown of the skull.

Prior to the thrust, the doctor must evaluate the position of their forearm. The forearm reflects the line of correction. The primary listing of the vertebral subluxation for particularly the newborn and infant is posteriority (-Z). The forearm placed in an incorrect position (lateral, too superior or inferior) should be properly aligned prior to the thrust.

Newborn and Infant

C2 POSTERIOR PRONE ADJUSTMENT

Name of Technique: Gonstead
Technique procedure: Prone cervical.
Example: Posterior (P, -Z) C2 listing (Fig. 9.78).
Contraindications: All other listings, normal functional spinal unit, instability, hypermobility, destruction or fracture of the spinous process or neural arch, and infection of the contact vertebra.

Patient position: The newborn/infant is placed prone across the lap of the parent, the knee–chest or hi–lo table. If spinous rotation exists (e.g., PL, PR) the side of laterality faces towards the doctor.

Doctor's position: The doctor stands inferior to the patient.

Contact site: The inferior lateral aspect of the spinous process.

Supportive assistance: The parent should keep the upper torso and lower limbs from movement.

Pattern of thrust: Posterior to anterior and inferior to superior with an arcing movement through the plane line of the intervertebral disc and facet articulations.

Contraindication for the thrust: The newborn/infant is unable to be stabilized in the prone position.

C3 POSTERIOR SEATED ADJUSTMENT

Name of technique: Gonstead.

Technique procedure: Seated cervical.

Example: Posterior (P, -Z) C3 listing (Fig. 9.79).

Patient position: The newborn/infant is placed seated on the lap of the parent. If spinous rotation exists (e.g., PL, PR) the side of laterality faces towards the doctor.

Doctor's position: The doctor stands behind the patient.

Contact site: The inferior lateral aspect of the spinous process.

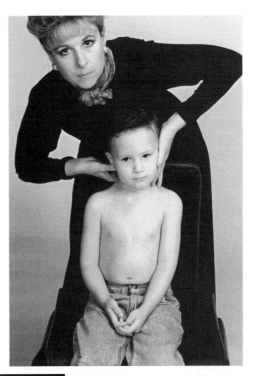

Figure 9.80. Seated C7 PR adjustment. The distal (and palmar) end of the right second digit is placed on the contact site. To increase adjusting hand stabilization, the third digit is placed next to the second digit. The contact hand thumb is placed on the ramus of the mandible. The contact thumb should not pull on the skin near the eye or be placed on the temporomandibular joint. The palmar surface of the stabilization hand is placed on the opposite lateral musculature of the cervical spine. The thenar eminence of the stabilization hand is below the ear and thumb along the angle of the jaw. The doctor's forearms should follow the plane line of the joint.

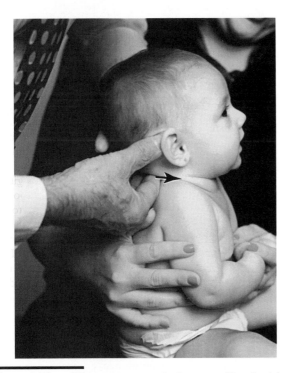

Figure 9.79. C3 posterior seated adjustment. The distal (and palmar) end of the right second digit is placed on the contact site. To increase adjusting hand stabilization, the third digit is placed next to the second digit. The palmar surface of the stabilization hand is placed on the opposite lateral musculature of the cervical spine. The thenar eminence of the stabilization hand is below the ear and thumb along the angle of the jaw. The doctor's forearms should follow the plane line of the joint.

Supportive assistance: The parent should stabilize the chest and back of the patient.

Pattern of thrust: Posterior to anterior and inferior to superior with an arcing movement through the plane of the intervertebral disc and facet articulations.

Contraindication to thrust: The newborn/infant is unable to be stabilized in the seated position. The doctor is unable to prevent the following vectors; excessive lateral flexion, extension or rotation during the thrust.

Toddler and Pre-Schooler

C7 PR SEATED ADJUSTMENT

Name of Technique: Gonstead

Technique procedure: Seated cervical chair.

Example: PR (-Z, +θY) C7 listing (Fig. 9.80).

Patient position: The toddler/pre-schooler is placed seated on the cervical chair. The child may need to be raised in the chair (e.g., by pelvic pillow, booster chair). The cervical strap can be used.

Doctor's position: The doctor stands behind and slightly to the side of laterality.

Contact site: The inferior right lateral aspect of the spinous process.

Pattern of thrust: Posterior to anterior and inferior to superior with an arcing movement through the plane of the intervertebral disc and facet articulations with a slight -θY rotation. The stabilization hand does not pull up during the thrust.

Contraindication for the thrust: The toddler/pre-schooler is unable to be stabilized in the seated position. The doctor is unable to prevent the following vectors: excessive lateral flexion, extension or rotation in the thrust phase.

C6 PR PRONE ADJUSTMENT

Name of Technique: Gonstead

Technique procedure: Prone hi-lo cervical.

Example: PR (-Z, +θY) C6 listing (Fig. 9.81).

Patient position: The toddler/pre-schooler is placed prone on the hi-lo table.

Doctor's position: The doctor stands on the right side and slightly inferior to the patient.

Contact site: The inferior right lateral aspect of the spinous process.

Pattern of thrust: Posterior to anterior and inferior to superior with an arcing movement through the plane of the intervertebral disc and facet articulations with a slight -θY rotation.

Pre-Adolescent and Adolescent

C5 PRS SEATED ADJUSTMENT

Name of Technique: Gonstead

Technique procedure: Seated cervical.

Example: PRS (-Z, +θY, -θZ) C5 listing (Fig. 9.82).

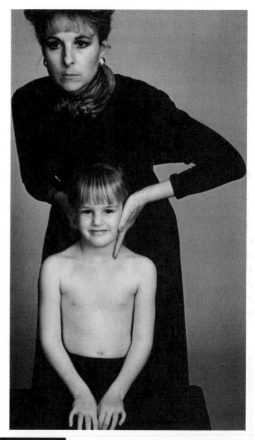

Figure 9.82. Seated C5 PRS adjustment. The distal (and palmar) end of the right second digit is placed on the contact site. To increase adjusting hand stabilization, the third digit is placed next to the second digit. The contact hand thumb is placed on the ramus of the mandible. The palmar surface of the stabilization hand is placed on the opposite lateral musculature of the cervical spine. The thenar eminence of the stabilization hand is below the ear and thumb along the angle of the jaw. The doctor's forearms should follow the plane line of the joint.

Patient position: The patient is seated on the cervical chair. The cervical strap may be used.

Doctor's position: The doctor stands behind and slightly to the side of laterality.

Contact site: The inferior right lateral aspect of the spinous process.

Set-up: The stabilization hand is placed on the top of the patient's head. The head should be slightly flexed to separate the spinous process. The contact digit is placed on the contact site. The head is brought up to a neutral position by the stabilization hand and then positioned on the contralateral musculature of the cervical spine. To relax the posterior musculature, the chin is raised slightly. The cervical spine is laterally flexed slightly (10 to 15 degrees) to the side of laterality. To preload the joint, apply a posterior to anterior (+Z) pressure with the contact digit. Head movement is restricted by the stabilization hand during the thrust. The stabilization hand does not pull up during the thrust.

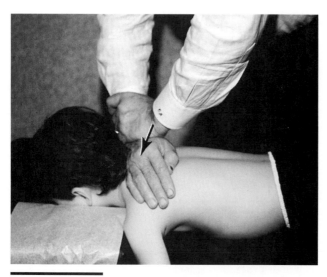

Figure 9.81. Prone C6 PR adjustment. The lateral border of the distal end of the right fifth metacarpal. To increase adjusting hand stabilization, the stabilization hand is placed on top of the adjusting hand with the fingers wrapped around the wrist.

Pattern of thrust: An arcing movement posterior to anterior and inferior to superior with a slight $-\theta Y$ rotation through the plane of the intervertebral disc and facet articulations. At the end of the thrust a slight counterclockwise torque is applied through the right center of mass of the segment that enhances right lateral flexion of the vertebra.

Contraindication for the thrust: The patient is unable to be stabilized in the seated position. The doctor is unable to prevent the following vectors: excessive lateral flexion, extension or rotation in the thrust phase.

C5 PRI-LA SEATED ADJUSTMENT

Name of Technique: Gonstead
Technique procedure: Seated cervical.
Example: PRI-la ($-Z$, $+\theta Y$, $+\theta Z$) C5 listing (Fig. 9.83).
Patient position: The patient is seated on the cervical chair. The cervical strap may be used.
Doctor's position: The doctor stands behind the patient and slightly to the opposite side of spinous process laterality.
Contact site: The medial portion of the left lamina.
Set-up: The stabilization hand is placed on the top of the

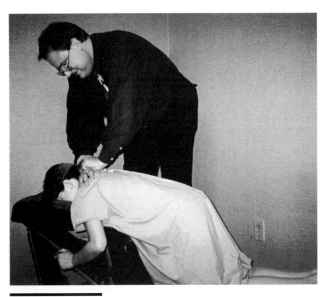

Figure 9.84.   C2 PR knee chest adjustment. The lateral aspect of the right fifth metacarpal is placed on the contact site. The stabilization hand is rested on top of the adjustment hand. The doctor's forearms should follow the plane line of the joint.

patient's head. The head should be slightly flexed to separate the spinous process. The contact digit is placed on the contact site. The head is brought up to a neutral position by the stabilization hand and then positioned on the contralateral musculature of the cervical spine. To relax the posterior musculature, the chin is raised slightly. The cervical spine is laterally flexed slightly (10 to 15 degrees) to the side of contact. To preload the joint, apply a posterior to anterior ($+Z$) pressure with the contact digit. Head movement is restricted by the stabilization hand during the thrust. The stabilization hand does not pull up during the thrust.

Pattern for the thrust: An arcing movement posterior to anterior and inferior to superior with a slight $+\theta Y$ rotation through the plane of the intervertebral disc and facet articulations. At the end of the thrust a slight counter clockwise torque is applied through the left center of mass of the segment that enhances left lateral flexion of the vertebra.

Contraindication for the thrust: The patient is unable to be stabilized in the seated position. The doctor is unable to prevent the following vectors: excessive lateral flexion, extension or rotation in the thrust phase.

C2 PR KNEE CHEST ADJUSTMENT

Name of technique: Gonstead
Technique procedure: Knee chest prone cervical.
Example: PR ($-Z$, $+\theta Y$) C2 listing (Fig. 9.84).
Patient position: The pre-adolescent or adolescent is positioned on the knee-chest table. The head strap is secured to stabilize the cervical region.
Doctor's position: The doctor stands inferior and to the side of spinous process laterality.
Contact site: The inferior lateral aspect of the spinous process.
Pattern of thrust: Posterior to anterior and inferior to superior

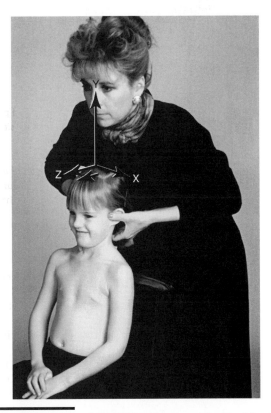

Figure 9.83.   Seated C5 PRI-la adjustment. The distal (and palmar) end of the left second digit is placed on the contact site. To increase adjusting hand stabilization, the third digit is placed next to the second digit. The contact hand thumb is placed on the ramus of the mandible. The palmar surface of the stabilization hand is placed on the opposite lateral musculature of the cervical spine. The thenar eminence of the stabilization hand is below the ear and thumb along the angle of the jaw.

with an arcing movement through the plane of the intervertebral disc and facet articulations. Contraindication for the thrust: The patient is unable to be stabilized in the knee chest position.

Thoracic Spine

The thoracic spine often manifests a compensation to a subluxation in a different spinal region. Full spinal analysis is necessary to eliminate the possibility of introducing a force into a compensatory area. The adjustment should only be performed at fixated segment(s). Lateral bending stress radiographs can assist in determining which segments are hypomobile compared to the hypermobile (compensatory) articulations.

Important considerations for thoracic analysis of the vertebral subluxation are the anatomical factors (e.g. facet planes, ribs, etc.) mechanism of injury and the extent of kyphosis. Often the thoracic spine is traumatized while the child is in a flexion position. If injury occurs in a flexed position, the damaged ligaments are unable to support the motion segment resulting in a flexion malposition (51). The spinal segment should be adjusted at the level of flexion trauma.

The thoracic spine is limited in its ability to compensate in a sagittal or extension plane. The adolescent spine can compensate creating a "dishing" effect, particularly at the T1-T6 region (49). The compensated dish region is usually painful, edematous and resilient to compressive palpation (+Z). The adjustment should occur at a segment caudal to the compensatory region.

Inspection

Observation of the thoracic spine should be done by examining the region unclothed. Inspect the shoulder height and scapular position (sagittal and coronal curvatures). Postural distortion may indicate vertebral subluxation, scoliosis, compensation reaction, congenital deformity or pathology. The kyphotic curve is observed to view the possible development of hyper or hypokyphosis.

Static Palpation

The newborn or infant should be palpated in the prone position. Across the lap of the parent or on the exam table, the doctor should palpate with the distal end of the fifth digit. Tenderness is typically elicited when upward pressure is applied to the inferior portion of the spinous process. The older pediatric patient can be seated (Fig. 9.85). Palpation for edema at the supraspinous, interspinous, or transverse region can be performed. The doctor should take note that often the lowest tender thoracic segment is often the hypomobile or subluxated segment.

The pediatric patient with years of long standing vertebral subluxation may have signs of compensation. The effects of long-standing compensation can be palpated as a tight or rope-like consistency of the associated musculature. Chronic subluxations in the older adolescent patient may demonstrate a hyperemia response when the doctor rubs over the area of involvement.

Motion Palpation

Patient placement is determined by the age and compliance of the patient to follow instructions. The newborn and infant should be placed in a prone position on the lap of the parent. The toddler can be seated on the lap of the parent. The pre-schooler, pre-adolescent and adolescent may be seated unassisted.

A light fingertip touch is placed on the spinous process. Motion palpation should be performed with a gentle glide with the younger patient and with a slight increase in pressure for the more developed spine. The use of too much pressure during the range of motion exam may invalidate any findings. The purpose of the examination is to detect fixation dysfunction. The detection of the hypomobile segment is considered the primary factor in determining the segment to be adjusted. The hypermobile segment is typically a compensatory response to a fixation dysfunction in a lower region. Other causes of hypermobility can be pathology or direct injury.

The age of the patient will determine which range of motion should be palpated. It should be noted that the doctor is not limited to the suggested palpation strategies presented. In the older child, lateral flexion (stress) radiographs will reveal or confirm findings (see Chapter 8).

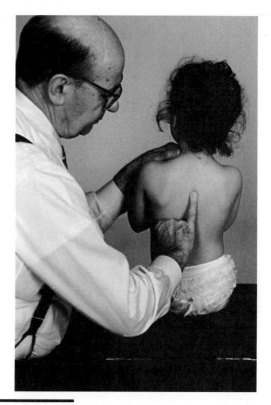

Figure 9.85. The static palpation examination is used to detect tenderness and edema at the interspinous and transverse process regions.

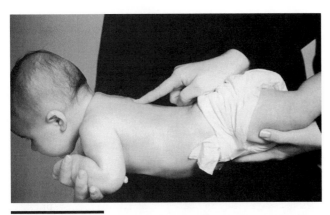

Figure 9.86.   The lower thoracic segments are palpated by raising and lowering the legs bilaterally.

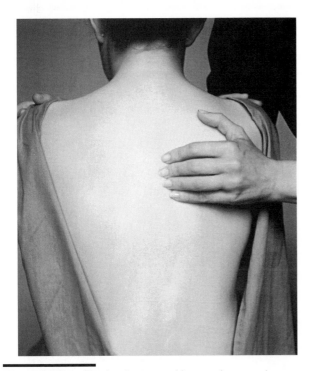

Figure 9.87.   One hand raises and lowers the arms that are crossed in front of the chest. The opposite hand will palpate the separation of the spinous process during flexion and approximation during extension.

The primary restricted dyskinesia pattern is the posterior to anterior (flexion and extension) movement. This examination should be performed on all age groups. The newborn/infant is examined in the prone position. The fifth digit, or second digit of the small-handed doctor, contacts the spinous process. The mid to upper thoracic region is palpated by lifting and lowering the chest of the newborn/infant. The lower thoracic region is palpated by raising and lowering the legs bilaterally (Fig. 9.86). The older patient is seated on a stool or cervical chair. The patient' arms are crossed in front of

the chest. The doctor passively raises and lowers the thoracic spine by contacting the arms at the crossed elbows in front. The other hand is used to examine separation of the spinous processes during flexion and approximation during extension (Fig. 9.87).

The older patient's examination should include lateral flexion (Fig. 9.88), rotation (Fig. 9.89), extension and rotation (Fig. 9.90) and extension and lateral flexion (Fig. 9.91). The lateral flexion analysis is performed by pushing the spinous process opposite the side of the passive lateral flexion. To evaluate rotation and coupled motions, the doctor should apply digital pressure on the spinous process on the younger child, and on the pre-adolescent and adolescent, the spinous or transverse process.

The upper thoracic region is more difficult to palpate. Two forms of palpating the upper thoracic region include extreme head and cervical extension (Fig. 9.92) or by crossing the arms in front of the child and raising and lowering the arms (Fig. 9.93).

Radiography

The full spine anteroposterior and lateral radiographs should be evaluated. The newborn, toddler and pre-schooler may not be radiographed due to difficulty in patient positioning. However, if trauma or other pathology is suspected a plain film radiograph is advised. To determine the size of film (i.e., 14x17 or 14x36) for a full spine evaluation, the doctor should

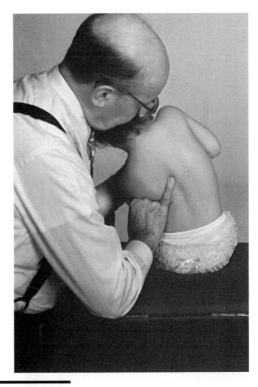

Figure 9.88.   The doctor's distal end of the digit contacts the spinous process. During passive lateral flexion the doctor pushes the spinous process in the opposite direction.

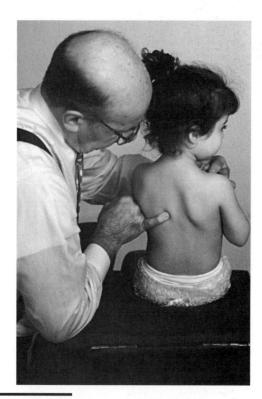

Figure 9.89. The doctor introduces rotation into the thoracic spine.

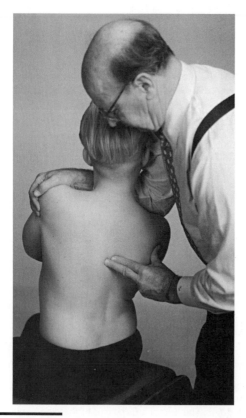

Figure 9.90. With the arms across the chest, the doctor introduces extension and rotation into the thoracic spine.

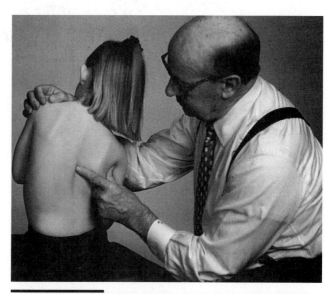

Figure 9.91. Extension and lateral flexion may be analyzed in the thoracic spine.

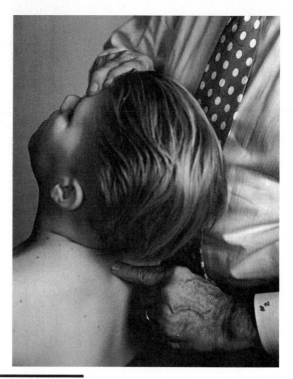

Figure 9.92. The upper thoracic region is palpated with extreme head and cervical extension.

measure the posterior aspect of the occiput to the sacrum/coccyx.

The anteroposterior view reveals the positional dyskinesia and can demonstrate scoliosis (see Chapter 15). The lateral projection will reveal the kyphotic curve. Thoracic line analysis is discussed in Chapter 8.

The lateral flexion thoracic view reveals information that can be very helpful in assessing the vertebral subluxation as it impacts the coupling reaction ($\pm\theta Z$ and $\pm\theta Y$). This evaluation may also be used to gauge progress in response to adjustive care and the management of thoracic scoliosis. Global thoracic lateral flexion studies may be further correlated with the AP static film to determine the listing of the segment. Therapeutic isometric maneuvers can be determined from the film analysis. The implementation of therapeutic exercises may be beneficial for spinal management and rehabilitation of scoliosis and other postural distortions.

Instrumentation

A paraspinal skin temperature instrument can be used for analysis of the thoracic spine. The newborn and infant should be placed in a prone position across the lap of the parent or on the exam table. The parent may assist the doctor by holding the legs and head in a neutral position (Fig. 9.94). The older patient can be seated. The younger child (i.e. toddler) may respond to

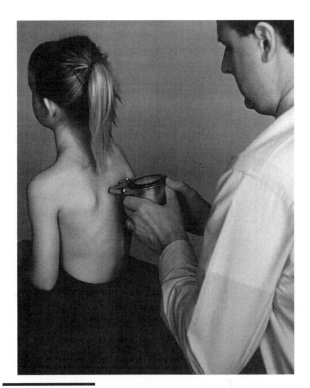

Figure 9.95. Skin temperature examination of the thoracic spine.

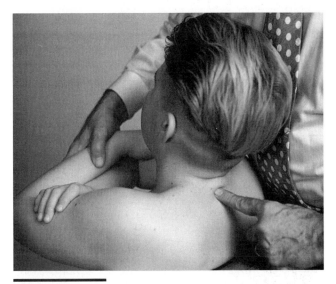

Figure 9.93. Crossing the arms in front of the patient, the doctor raises and lowers the arms to palpate the thoracic spine.

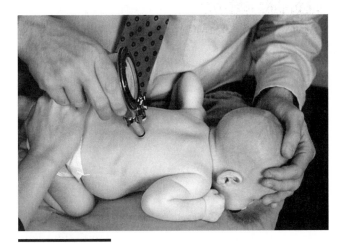

Figure 9.94. The infant is placed in the prone position and stabilized by a parent.

the glide of the instrument as ticklish and may have to be stabilized by the doctor's free hand on the abdomen or placed in a prone position. A smooth caudal glide with the handheld paraspinal skin temperature instrument (i.e., Temposcope, Nervoscope) is used to scan for temperature asymmetries. In one study, the Nervoscope was determined to have good inter- and intraexaminer reliability in the thoracic spine (36). Although this study was conducted on adult females, the clinical experience of the author suggests good reliability for the thoracic pediatric spine.

The "readings" in the thoracic region vary with the older weight bearing patient (Fig. 9.95). At the level of T1-T3, the temperature differentials (TD) will be detected inferior to the spinous process. The TD at T4 and at T10-12, are found at the level of the spinous process. The levels T5-T9 will reveal the TD in the interspinous space above the spinous process of the involved vertebra (35).

Thoracic Adjustment

The posterior (-Z) subluxation is the most common component of the listing for the younger pediatric spine. The contact point for posteriority is the spinous process. The newborn and infant can be placed across the lap of the parent or prone across the pelvic, knee-chest or hi-lo tables. Doctors should be aware of their stance prior to introducing a thrust. To set up for a posterior listing the doctor should stand caudal and centered to the patient. Standing to one side may inadvertently introduce an unnecessary vector (i.e., PL or PR) into the thrust. Due to the small anatomical size of the spinous process, the doctor should determine the appropriate digit to use for the contact. The neonate and infant should be contacted by the fifth digit on the spinous process with the other fifth digit on top of the nail bed (Fig. 9.96). For a deeper set in the infant and toddler, the doctor can replace the top digit with the second digit or thumb. The toddler's spinous process may be contacted with the second digit, with the stabilization digit (i.e., second digit or thumb depending on the depth necessary to produce an adjustment) on top of the nail bed of the contact digit. The larger-handed doctor can continue to use the fifth digit on fifth digit set-up (Fig. 9.97). The younger child (age 3 or 4) with a larger spinous process may be contacted with the thumb and the opposite thumb placed on top of the contact thumb nail bed (Fig. 9.98). The thrust for a posterior (–Z) listing is posterior to anterior (+Z). A less common listing is PL or PR. When a rotated spinous process exists, the doctor stands on the side of rotation. By assessing the patient with static and motion palpation and viewing the AP radiograph, the doctor can determine when it is appropriate to use the pisiform to contact the spinous or transverse process.

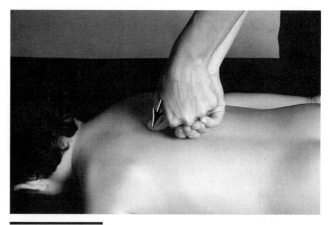

Figure 9.98.   The younger child with a larger spinous process may be contacted with a thumb on thumb set-up.

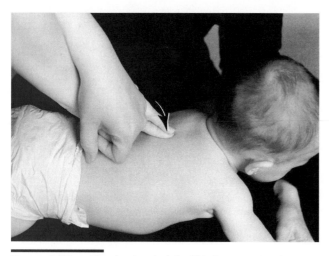

Figure 9.96.   The distal end of the fifth digit contacts the infant's thoracic spinous process.

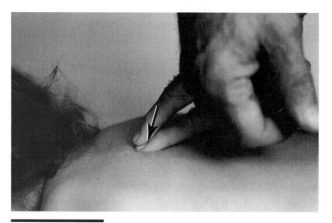

Figure 9.97.   The large-handed doctor may continue the use of the fifth digit on the thoracic contact site.

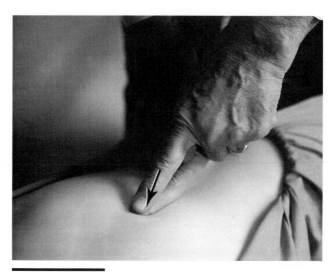

Figure 9.99.   The larger spinous process may be contacted with the distal end of the second digit.

Hi-lo Table

The hi-lo table can be used to deliver an adjustment to the toddler and older patient. The chest piece should be locked (unlike the adult table preparation of unlocking the chest piece) to prevent a rebound effect after the thrust phase. The single hand contact is the most common choice for the older pediatric spine. For the middle or lower thoracic adjustment, the contact hand is the cephalic or superior hand and the thrusting hand is the caudad or inferior hand. In the prone position, the upper thoracic region (T1–T3) should be contacted by the inferior hand.

For a listing of the spinous process, a specific contact must be made. The toddler or pre-schooler should be contacted by the distal end of the second digit, with the opposite second digit or thumb contacting the nail bed (Fig. 9.99). A doctor with a larger hand may choose to continue to use the fifth digit on the spinous process on the older child (Fig. 9.100) and place the opposite pisiform on the nail bed.

The larger spinous process can be contacted with the pisiform. For the posterior thoracic (–Z) listing, the doctor may stand to either side of the table. The doctor's stance and contact forearm should take into consideration the kyphotic curve and the plane line of the disc. The stance for T1–3 is slightly superior to the region with a 45 degree angle superior to inferior forearm. Standing neutral for a T4–T7 listing, the doctor's contact forearm is in a neutral plane. An inferior to superior 45 degree angle of the contact forearm will take into consideration the plane of correction for the lower thoracic (T8–T12) region. After pre-load tension has been created, the thrust must be delivered posterior to anterior (+Z) with no introduction of laterality. The AP radiograph determines the listing of spinous laterality ($\pm\theta Y$) and lateral flexion ($\pm\theta Z$). To correct the listing of PL or PR (–Z, $-\theta Y$ or –Z, $+\theta Y$), the doctor should stand on the side of spinous laterality. The doctor also stands on the side of spinous laterality to correct the listing of PLS or PRS (–Z, $-\theta Y$, $+\theta Z$ or –Z $+\theta Y$, $-\theta Z$). The spinous

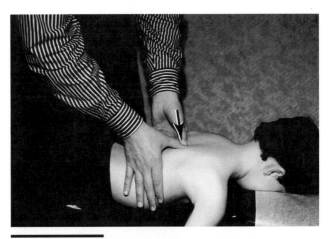

Figure 9.102.   Prone T9 posterior adjustment. The smaller patient is contacted with the distal end of a digit (e.g., fifth, second, thumb), and the larger patient with the soft portion of the pisiform. To increase the depth of the thrust, the digit (e.g., fifth, second, thumb) of the other hand is placed on the nail bed of the adjusting digit. The adjusting forearm must follow the joint plane line. For the pisiform contact, the stabilization hand rests on top of the adjusting hand.

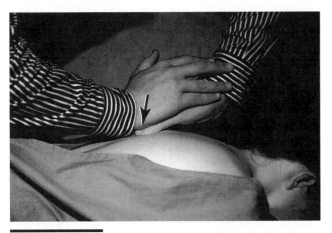

Figure 9.100.   The fifth digit-pisiform contact may be performed on the pelvic/slot bench or hi-lo tables.

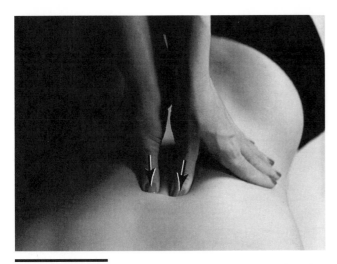

Figure 9.101.   The double thumb contact may be used on the transverse process contact.

process is contacted with the appropriate contact with the adjusting hand (i.e. pisiform, thumb with pisiform on nail bed). The pisiform contact will require the contact fingers to cross the spine.

The listing of PLI-t or PRI-t is also determined from the AP radiograph. The doctor will stand on the opposite side of the spinous rotation. The smaller transverse process should be contacted with a smaller contact point (i.e., fifth or second digit or thumb). Depending on the depth necessary to complete the thrust, the contact hand will rest on the nail bed with the fifth or second digit or pisiform. The larger transverse process is contacted with the pisiform. The hand and fingers do not cross the spine with this contact. Depending on the size of the transverse processes, the double thumb or double thenar contact can be chosen (Fig. 9.101). The doctor's thrust will only be initiated with one thumb or thenar. The PRI-t (–Z, $+\theta Y$, $-\theta Z$) is adjusted from posterior to anterior (+Z), with an inferiorward arcing motion ($+\theta Z$) at the end of the thrust phase.

T9 POSTERIOR PRONE ADJUSTMENT

Name of technique: Gonstead
Name of procedure: Prone Hi-lo adjustment.
Example: Posterior (–Z) T9 listing (Fig. 9.102).
Contraindications: All other listings, normal functional spinal unit, hypermobility, instability, destruction or fracture of the neural arch or spinous process, infection of the contact vertebra.
Patient position: The patient is placed prone on the hi-lo table. The hands rest on the hand plates.
Doctor's position: To either side of the table.
Contact site: The inferior portion of the spinous process.

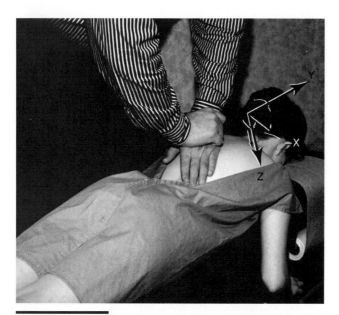

Figure 9.103. Prone T8 PLS adjustment. The soft portion of the left pisiform is placed on the contact site. The fingers cross the spine. The stabilization hand rests on top of the adjusting hand for the pisiform contact. The adjusting forearm must follow the joint plane line.

Tissue pull occurs with the stabilization hand from inferior to superior.
Pattern of thrust: Posterior to anterior and slightly inferior to superior.

T8 PLS PRONE ADJUSTMENT

Name of technique: Gonstead
Name of procedure: Prone hi-lo adjustment.
Example: PLS (-Z,-θY, +θZ) T8 listing (Fig. 9.103).
Patient position: The patient is placed prone on the hi-lo table. The hands rest on the hand plates.
Doctor's position: The doctor stands to the side of spinous laterality.
Contact site: The inferior left portion of the spinous process.
Tissue pull occurs with the stabilization hand from inferior to superior and lateral to medial.
Pattern of thrust: Posterior to anterior, lateral to medial with an inferiorward arcing motion towards the end of the thrust.

Knee Chest Table

The knee chest is another adjustment apparatus typically used for the older child (i.e. pre-adolescent, adolescent). The table receives its name from the position the patient will assume. The table should be prepared to the height of the patient (Fig. 9.104) allowing the spine to be level. The patient's face and chest are supported by the head and chest piece, and the lower thoracic and lumber spine is left unsupported. The knee-chest table allows for less restriction of the torso when a posterior to anterior adjustment is performed. This is not so when a normal flat table is used for the prone adjusting position. In the latter, the rib cage and torso provide increased stiffness to the

anteriorward thrust, thereby necessitating a proportional increase in the amount of force. Due to the flexibility of the developing spine and the unrestricted support to the region, the doctor must monitor the depth of the thrust. The magnitude of the thrust is decreased in the anteriorward direction during the adjustment. This is not so when a normal flat table is used for the prone adjusting position. Clinical experience reveals that the more flexible and shallow the sagittal curvatures are, the more easily the patient is adjusted in the knee-chest position (68). Conversely, the hyperkyphotic patient may be more easily adjusted on a typical flat or contoured table with support for the torso. Pre-load of the segment is established when the doctor translates the motion segment to a maximal +Z position. This +Z "tension" is achieved when the motion segment is preloaded at the end of the articulation's physiologic range of motion and before the paraphysiologic zone. The thoracic spine is translated anteriorly, similar to the lumbar spine, though less +Z translation is permissible due to the stiffness of the kyphosis during compression. Once the joint has been preloaded, a high velocity and short amplitude thrust is administrated. After the thrust phase, the doctor does not immediately release the contact, but rather, a "set and hold" for two seconds is performed.

T5 PLI-T KNEE CHEST ADJUSTMENT

Name of technique: Gonstead
Name of procedure: Knee-chest, pisiform contact.
Example: PLI-t (-Z, -θY, +θZ) T5 listing (Fig. 9.105).
Patient position: The patient is positioned on the knee-chest table with the thoracic spine slightly higher than the lumbar spine. The knees should be positioned so that the femurs can be perpendicular to the floor. The hands should rest on the hand plates.

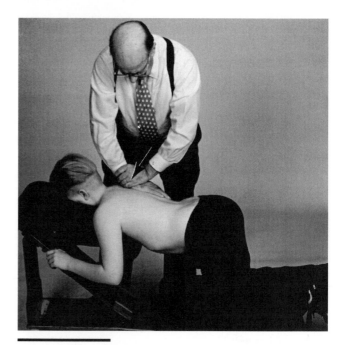

Figure 9.104. The knee chest table should be prepared to allow the spine to maintain a horizontal position.

Doctor's position: The doctor stands on the opposite side of spinous laterality and approximately center to the contact site. Contact site: The medial portion of the right transverse process. Tissue pull occurs with the stabilization hand from inferior to superior and medial to lateral.

Pattern of thrust: Posterior to anterior, with an inferiorward arcing motion toward the end of the thrust.

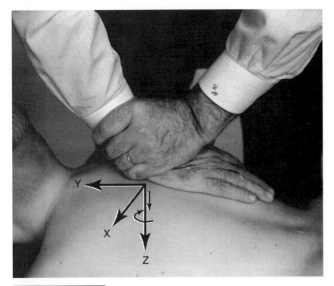

Figure 9.105.   T5 PLI-t knee chest adjustment. The soft portion of the right pisiform is placed on the contact site. The fingers do not cross the spine. The stabilization hand rests on top of the adjusting hand for the pisiform contact. The adjusting forearm must follow the joint plane line.

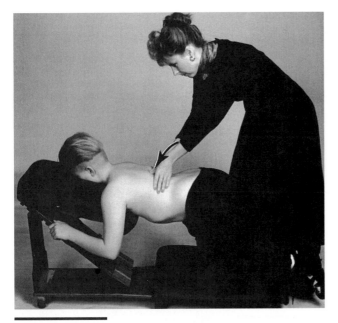

Figure 9.106.   T8 posterior knee chest adjustment. The thumbs (or second digits) are placed on the contact site. The adjusting forearm must follow the joint plane line.

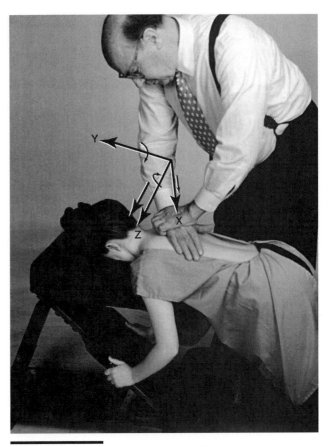

Figure 9.107.   T4 PRS knee chest adjustment. The soft portion of the right pisiform is placed on the contact site. The fingers cross the spine. The stabilization hand rests on top of the adjusting hand for the pisiform contact. The adjusting forearm must follow the joint plane line.

T8 POSTERIOR KNEE CHEST ADJUSTMENT

Name of technique: Gonstead

Name of procedure: Knee-chest, double thumb contact.

Example: P (−Z) T8 listing (Fig. 9.106).

Patient position: The patient is positioned on the knee-chest table with the thoracic spine slightly higher than the lumbar spine. The knees should be positioned so that the femurs can be perpendicular to the floor. The hands should rest on the hand rests.

Doctor's position: The doctor will stand inferior to contact site but may stand to either side of the table.

Contact site: The posterior, inferior portion of the spinous process.

Pattern of thrust: Posterior to anterior (+Z).

T4 PRS KNEE CHEST ADJUSTMENT

Name of technique: Gonstead

Name of procedure: Knee-chest, pisiform contact.

Example: PRS (−Z, +θY, +θZ) T4 listing (Fig. 9.107).

Patient position: The patient is positioned on the knee-chest table with the thoracic spine slightly higher than the lumbar

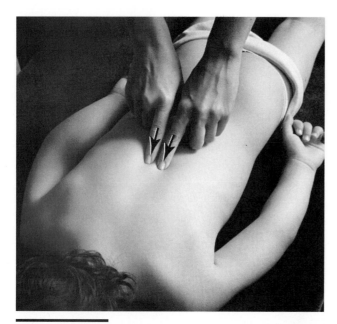

Figure 9.108. The smaller transverse process is contacted by the second digits.

spine. The knees should be positioned so that the femurs can be perpendicular to the floor.

Doctor's position: The doctor will stand on the side of spinous laterality and approximately center to the contact site.

Contact site: The inferior and right portion of the spinous process. Tissue pull occurs with the stabilization hand from inferior to superior and lateral to medial.

Pattern of thrust: Posterior to anterior, lateral to medial, with an inferiorward arcing motion towards the end of the thrust.

Pelvic Bench and Slot Table

The pelvic bench or slot table can substitute for the hi-lo table. The positioning, set-up and thrust is similar to that used with the hi-lo table. The mid and upper thoracic region is better suited for receiving the adjustment on the pelvic bench or slot table. Typically, the toddler and older child can be positioned for the adjustment on the pelvic and slot table. For a straight posterior listing accompanied by pronounced spinous process tenderness, a double transverse process contact can be made. Depending on the anatomical development of a segment, the doctor may contact the smaller transverse process with the second digits (Fig. 9.108). The larger transverse process of the pre-adolescent and adolescent may be contacted with the distal end of the thumb (Fig. 9.109). The older adolescent may be contacted with the following variations; double-thenar, double-pisiform, and pisiform-thenar.

The single hand contact is the most common choice for the developed pediatric spine. For the middle or lower thoracic adjustment, the contact hand is the cephalic or superior hand and the thrusting hand is the caudad or inferior hand. In the prone position, the upper thoracic region (T1–T3) should be contacted by the inferior hand.

Depending on the size of the transverse processes, the double thumb or double thenar contact can be chosen. The doctor's thrust will be through one thumb or thenar.

T8 POSTERIOR PRONE ADJUSTMENT

Name of technique: Gonstead
Name of procedure: Pelvic table, double thumb contact.
Example: P (–Z) T8 listing (Fig. 9.110).
Patient position: The patient is positioned prone on the pelvic or slot table. The arms are placed to the side of the patient.

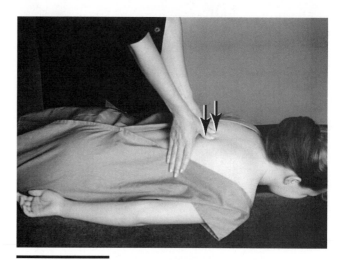

Figure 9.109. The larger transverse process may be contacted by the distal end of the thumbs.

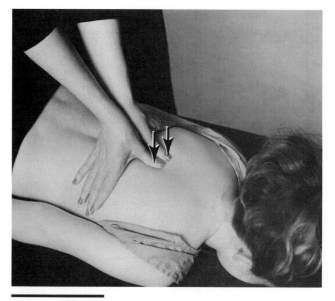

Figure 9.110. T8 posterior prone adjustment. The double thumb contact is placed on the transverse process of the T8 vertebra.

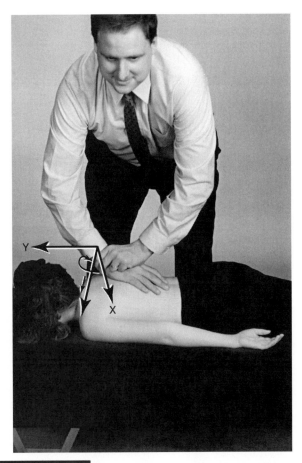

Figure 9.111. T6 prone adjustment. The soft portion of the right pisiform is placed on the contact site. The fingers do cross the spine. The stabilization hand rests on top of the adjusting hand for the pisiform contact. The adjusting forearm must follow the joint plane line.

Doctor's position: The doctor will stand inferior to the contact site and to either side of the table.

Contact site: The left and right portion of the transverse process.

Pattern of thrust: Posterior to anterior (+Z).

T6 PRS PRONE ADJUSTMENT

Name of technique: Gonstead

Name of procedure: Pelvic table, pisiform set-up.

Example: PRS (-Z, +θY, +θZ) T6 listing (Fig. 9.111).

Patient position: The patient is positioned prone on the pelvic or slot table. The arms are placed to the side of the patient.

Doctor's position: The doctor will stand inferior to the contact site and to the side of spinous laterality.

Contact site: The inferior and right portion of the spinous process. Tissue pull occurs with the stabilization hand from inferior to superior and lateral to medial.

Pattern of thrust: Posterior to anterior, lateral to medial with an inferiorward arcing motion toward the end of the thrust.

Cervical Chair

The upper thoracic region (T1-T4) may be adjusted in the cervical chair. This procedure is preferred for those children who can maintain a seated position. The doctor should stand behind the cervical chair, slightly to the side of spinous rotation PR or PL (-Z, +θY or -Z, -θY). For the listing of PRI-t or PLI-t (-Z, +θY, +θZ or -Z, -θY, -θZ) the doctor should favor the opposite side of spinous rotation to contact the transverse process. The contact point is the distal end of the second digit to the inferior aspect of the spinous or transverse process, depending on the listing. To provide stabilization, the middle finger should be placed adjacent to the index finger. The thumb of the contact hand should be placed on the ramus of the mandible (Fig. 9.112). This arch with the contact hand will decrease the possibility of introducing rotation or over contact of vertebral segments. The wrist of the doctor should be maintained in a neutral position. The palmar surface of the stabilization hand contacts the lateral surface of cervical spine. The thenar eminence will contact the sternocleidomastoid muscle and the thumb should be angled at a 45 degrees (anterior and inferior).

T1 PR SEATED ADJUSTMENT

Name of technique: Gonstead

Name of technique procedure: Cervical chair adjustment.

Example: PR (-Z, +θY) T1 listing (Fig. 9.113).

Patient position: Seated in the cervical chair. The stabilization strap or the parent's hands on the torso of the child may be used.

Doctor's position: Standing behind the patient, slightly to the right side.

Contact site: Inferior and right lateral aspect of the spinous process.

Pattern of thrust: Posterior to anterior (+Z), lateral to medial (-θY).

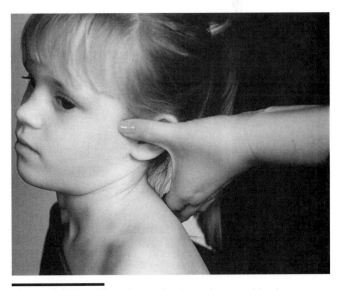

Figure 9.112. The adjusting hand arch is created by the second digit, the contact site, and the ramus of the mandible.

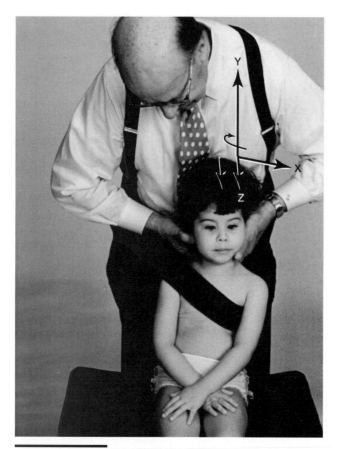

Figure 9.113. T1 PR seated adjustment. The distal end of the right second digit (palmar and lateral aspect) is placed on the contact point. The second digit is supported by the third digit. The right thumb is placed on the ramus of the mandible. An arch is formed by the thumb and contact digit. The stabilization hand (palmar) contacts the contralateral cervical musculature. A foundation for the adjustment is established by stabilizing the vertebra below and above the subluxation. Further stabilization may be provided by the head of the patient against the chest or abdomen of the doctor.

T3 PLI-T SEATED ADJUSTMENT

Name of technique: Gonstead
Name of technique procedure: Cervical chair adjustment.
Example: PLI-t (-Z, -θY, -θZ) T3 listing (Fig. 9.114).
Patient position: Seated in the cervical chair. The stabilization strap or the parent's hand on the chest of the child should be used.
Doctor's position: Standing behind the patient, slightly to the side opposite of spinous rotation.
Contact point: The right spinous lamina junction.
Pattern of thrust: Posterior to anterior (+Z) through the disc plane line, with an inferiorward (+θZ) arching motion towards the end of the thrust.

General Contraindications

General manipulation of the thoracic region is not indicated. The doctor must take great effort to not over-contact the involved region and unintentionally thrust into adjacent normal segments. Only with specific contacts can one expect a specific biomechanical change.

The osteopathic/chiropractic maneuver of manipulating the thoracic spine for the condition of "anteriority" is contraindicated with the pediatric spine. Depending on the size of the doctor's hand and the child's spine, several normal segments will receive a thrust with this maneuver.

Lumbar Spine

Inspection

Visual inspection of gait, postural analysis, static and dynamic intersegmental visualization, and observing global movement patterns provides important information as to the nature of the subluxation complex in the lumbar spine.

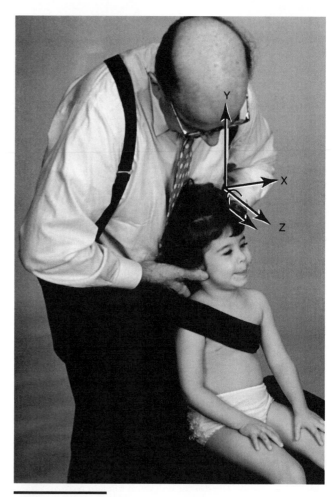

Figure 9.114. T3 PLI-t seated adjustment. The distal end of the right second digit (palmar and lateral aspect) is placed on the contact point. The second digit is supported by the third digit. The left thumb is placed on the ramus of the mandible. An arch is formed by the thumb and contact digit. The stabilization hand (palmar aspect) contacts the opposite cervical musculature.

Gait

The analysis of gait may reveal subtle signs of the subluxation complex manifested in the lumbo-pelvic region. A patient in pain may be observed to have guarded movement patterns with or without postural deviation. The lower limbs should be examined with radiographs if osseous involvement (e.g., Legg-Calve-Perthes, Osgood Schlatter's) is suspected.

Posture

Patient posture is a reflection of spinal architecture. Different postural states will have direct bearing on the function of the spine during movement (50). In the lumbar spine, the evaluation of posture can be influenced by the pelvic region and lower extremities.

The young toddler is often typified by a rounded and protuberant abdomen. This appearance varies with each child and disappears usually before the age of three. The protruding abdomen should not mislead the examiner in assuming the patient is hyperlordotic.

Due to the developmental stage of walking, this same age group is susceptible to repetitive falls onto the buttocks. This mechanism of injury can produce posteriority of the second or third sacral segment or a base posterior sacrum (see Chapter 8). A base posterior sacrum may induce a compensatory lumbar hyperlordosis.

Assessments of the sagittal plane may show a "lazy" or relaxed posture which can indicate lumbar hyperlordosis, or the "poker spine" associated with lumbar hypolordosis. Both disorders tend to cause compensatory changes in the thoracic and cervical region. Hyperlordosis of the lumbar spine is associated with a hyperkyphosis of the thoracic spine and anterior head translation. The straight lumbar spine is usually associated with a flattened thoracic spine and a kyphotic cervical curve.

The lumbopelvic region can be influenced by disorders of the lower limb. Genu recurvatum may lead to compensation above (e.g., lumbar hyperlordosis).

Static Palpation

The newborn or infant should be palpated in the prone position. The doctor should palpate with the distal end of the fifth digit. The older pediatric patient can be seated. Tenderness is typically elicited when upward pressure is applied to the inferior portion of the spinous process.

Motion Palpation

The neonate and infant are palpated in the prone position, across the lap of the parent or caretaker. The examiner should palpate with the fifth digit on the spinous process (Fig. 9.115). Posteriority of the segment is the most common subluxation in the lumbar region of this age group. The conditions of colic or constipation, which may cause a distended abdominal region, can complicate the palpatory assessment by causing a rigidity of the musculature of the lumbar and lower thoracic region. This rigidity can also occur in the crying infant. Soothing the infant or delaying the exam may be necessary in order to conduct a proper evaluation.

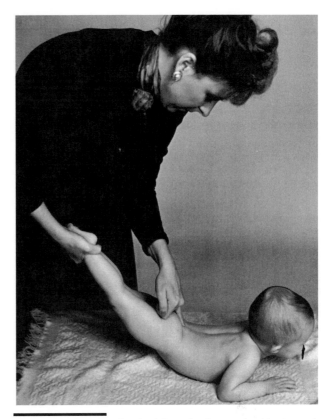

Figure 9.115.   Holding both legs, the doctor should raise and lower the legs palpating for restriction of posterior to anterior movement.

The toddler and older child may be palpated in a seated position. Selection of the correct digit to perform the exam will be necessary. The fifth or second digit is typically chosen to contact the spinous process. To perform a lateral flexion exam, the examiner should contact the inferior and lateral aspect of the spinous process. The practitioner introduces lateral flexion into the segment (Fig. 9.116). A normal lateral motion of the segment will cause relaxation of the ipsilateral soft tissues in the region to lateral and inferior spinous process. Coupling motion does occur. Lateral flexion produces a spinous rotation into the concavity of the lateral bend. Place the examining digit at the interspinous space and slightly to the side of the lateral bending. This movement is extremely difficult to palpate. Evaluation by lateral stress radiographs are recommended if the fixation dysfunction is difficult to determine.

Evaluate the extension movement in a seated position. During the extension motion, the spinous processes should move inferior (Fig. 9.117). The flexion motion is evaluated when the child is passively flexed forward (Fig. 9.118). The examiner should observe a separation of the spinous process. Due to the prominence of the spinous processes, the mid and upper lumbar segments are more easily palpated.

Instrumentation

The neonate can be examined in a prone position across the lap of the parent. The parent or doctor can hold the head and/or

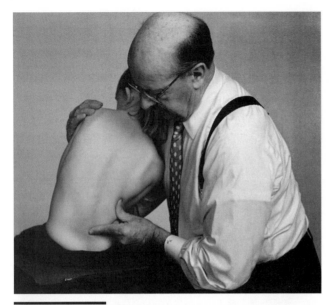

Figure 9.116. The inferior and lateral aspect of the spinous process is contacted by the doctor for the lateral flexion exam.

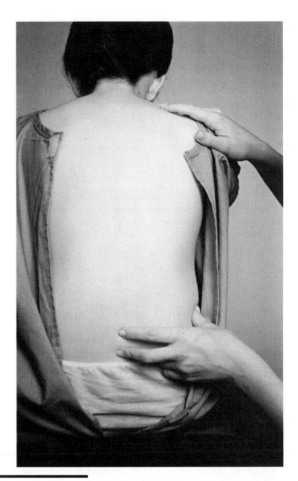

Figure 9.118. The flexion motion separates the spinous processes.

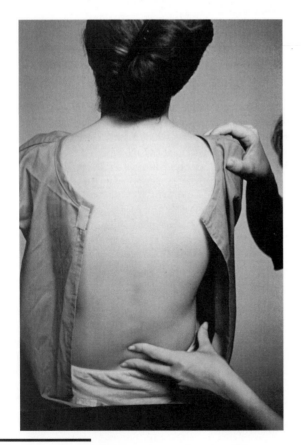

Figure 9.117. During extension motion, the spinous process should move anteroinferior.

pelvis of the subject in a neutral position. The probes of the instrument should be adapted to the child's spine, with perpendicular contact at the skin (Fig. 9.119). The glide is cephalad to caudad. The "reading" in the lumbar region (L1-L5) will be at the level of the lower one fourth of the spinous process. It should be noted that the reading does not indicate the level of subluxation. Due to loose skin, the glide of the instrument may cause a rolling effect of the skin. The reliability of the findings with this procedure when this occurs is questionable.

Lumbar Adjustment

PRONE POSITION

The neonate and infant are placed in the prone position. The preference is across the lap of a parent. Other prone positioning options are the hi-lo, knee-chest or pelvic tables. The neonate and infant should be carefully stabilized in a neutral position. The parent can assist in stabilizing the head and legs. To correct the most common positional dyskinesia, posteriority (–Z), the doctor is positioned inferior to the infant. The doctor should use the distal aspect of the fifth digit to contact the spinous process. The practitioner must constantly assess the size of their digits and the size of patient's spinous prior to rendering an adjustment.

When contacting the spinous process, the doctor will need to take more pre-load tension. If excessive "baby fat" (brown fat) exists, the doctor may have to perform a tissue pull (a cephalad skin pull) to eliminate heavy skin overlay. Once the skin is moved cephalad, the parent may assist in holding the skin.

For increasing the depth of the adjustment, the fifth digit can be contacted on the nail bed by the fifth, second digit or

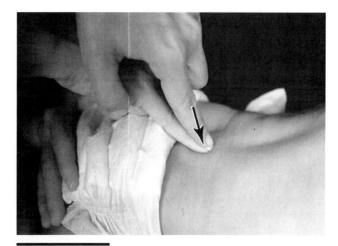

Figure 9.121. Second digit on the fifth contact.

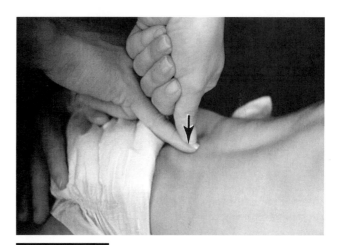

Figure 9.122. Thumb on the fifth digit.

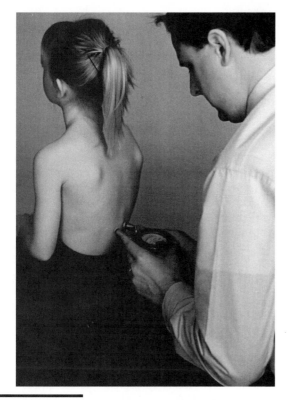

Figure 9.119. The instrumentation glide is from cephalad to caudad.

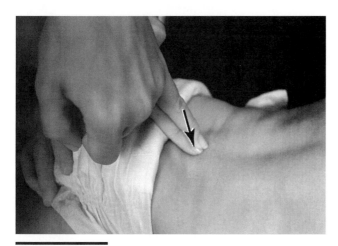

Figure 9.120. Double fifth digit contact.

thumb of the opposite hand (see Figs. 9.120 to 9.122). The forearm of the contact hand should be kept in a neutral position for the posterior listing. This will prevent the introduction of a lateral to medial movement. If a PL or PR (-Z, -θY or -Z, +θY) listing exists, the neonate or infant should be positioned in a prone position with the spinous rotation away from the parent.

Depending on the compliance and size of the toddler, a prone or side posture position may be chosen. The toddler in a prone position may be placed across the lap of the parent, on the pelvic or hi-lo tables, or across the chest portion of the knee chest table. The size of the toddler's spinous process and the doctor's finger will determine the necessary digit for the contact. For the prone position, the fifth digit, second digit, or thumb (of a small-handed practitioner) should contact the spinous process. To increase the depth of the thrust, the second digit, thumb or pisiform should contact the nail bed. The doctor should assess the set-up stance and forearm placement prior to the thrust.

SIDE POSTURE POSITION

The pelvic table is the table of choice for the side posture position to adjust the lumbar spine. The doctor should place the pillow to the end of table appropriate for the listing. The patient is requested to sit on the table so that the patient's head will ultimately rest on the pillow. The taller adolescent should be instructed to be seated in the center of the table. For the younger child it may be easier to reposition the pillow by the doctor than to reposition the patient. The inferior leg is positioned straight, and the older patient's inferior foot should hang over the edge of the table. The inferior foot position should allow for it to roll towards the doctor during the set-up and thrust. The superior leg should be bent, and the superior foot tucked behind the popliteal fossa of the inferior leg. The spine should be in a neutral position without any Y-axis torsion. The patient's shoulders should be positioned vertical, with the inferior shoulder pulled slightly caudal and the arms crossed in front of the chest. The doctor should stand in front of the lumbopelvic region and not leave this area during patient positioning.

The doctor will contact the segment to be adjusted with their cephalad hand. Contact should be made on the skin, taking a tissue pull in the direction of correction. The size of the spinous or mamillary process (which can be determined with the AP or lateral radiograph) will determine which contact hand point should be used. With the developed pre-adolescent and adolescent the pisiform can be chosen to contact the spinous or mamillary process. The smaller anatomical processes should be contacted with the second digit supported by the third digit on the contact nail bed (Fig. 9.123). This set-up is called a "finger push." This contact is not a pulling thrust (i.e. "pull move"). The pisiform and digit contact will both deliver a push type of thrust. The contact site may be brought to tension by rolling the patient slightly towards the

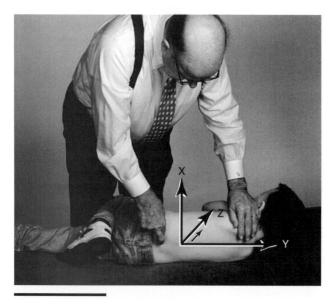

Figure 9.123. With the support of the third digit, the second digit contacts the spinous process. This set-up is called the finger push move.

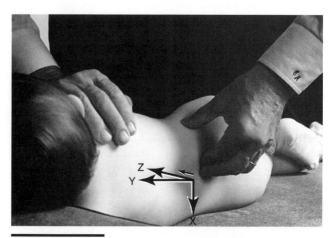

Figure 9.124. The finger push set-up is preferred for the smaller spinous process or mamillary process.

doctor at the level of the segmental contact point. The shoulder should be allowed to roll forward to eliminate or diminish thoracolumbar rotation. The larger pre-adolescent or adolescent (depending on height and weight of doctor) will require a body drop into the pelvis. This force should be directly opposite the contact hand or digit. It is not necessary to perform a body drop into the smaller child. In the set-up of the smaller patient, the parent may assist by stabilizing the legs. Parents should be instructed to stabilize the lower limbs and to prevent Y-axis rotation during the thrust. This assistance will allow the doctor to concentrate on stabilizing the upper body while performing the thrust without a pelvic drop. The doctor should be able to generate the required force through the contact shoulder and arm. Once the thrust has been completed, the segment should be held for 1-2 seconds.

Contraindications

Contraindications to adjusting in the side posture position include a doctor's inability to prevent thoracolumbar rotation, excessive body drop or multiple segmental contacts. The doctor should also not thrust if the patient lifts the inferior leg (reveals lack of relaxation) or arches the spine anteriorward while being rolled forward (a contraction of the erector spinae muscles). It should further be noted that in bone disorders such as Legg-Calve-Perthes or slipped femoral capital epiphysis the involved hip should be placed down or spinal correction conducted in a prone position.

The posterior listing (-Z) continues to be the common listing with the toddler. The lumbar adjustment for the toddler may be performed in a prone position (e.g., hi-lo, pelvic bench) or side posture position. The contact for a spinous or mamillary process should be with the finger(s) (Fig. 9.124). The listings of PL or PR (-Z, -θY, -Z, +θY) may be found in the young child (i.e., pre-schooler) who has been weight-bearing and has been a recipient of repeated micro or macro trauma. The spinous rotation to the left "L" (-θY) or right "R" (+θY) is determined from the AP radiograph. The patient should be adjusted with the involved rotation side up or in the prone position. The doctor should stand on the side of spinous rotation.

For the pre-schooler, pre-adolescent and adolescent, correction of the lumbar listing can be corrected with the side posture table. In the coronal plane, the vertebra may be tilted ($\pm\theta Z$). Years of repetitive activities, trauma, and asymmetrical weight bearing contributes to this listing component. The AP radiograph can be analyzed for the superior or inferiorly wedged listing. Superiority "S" ($\pm\theta Z$) is listed when the spinous process rotates ($\pm\theta Y$) towards the side of the superior wedge. When the spinous process rotates towards the inferior side of the wedge, the letter "I" is assigned. After listing the wedging, the spinous process "sp" or mamillary "m" contact points should be listed (e.g., PRI-sp, PLI-m).

Correction of Lateral Flexion Malposition and Lumbar Scoliosis

In the lumbar spine the wedging of the disc is corrected by pretensioning in side posture and thrusting from the opened side of the wedge towards the center. It is generally not recommended, to attempt to open the closed side by making a superiorward arcing motion during the thrust. This is due to the freely movable nature of the segment below. The one exception is the case of L5, since the sacrum and pelvis can remain relatively stable during an adjustment. If a lumbar scoliosis is present, then this supersedes the requirement for adjusting from the open towards the closed side of the wedge if the contact segment is L5 (35). The wedging of L4–L5 is used to determine if there is a special listing for L5. When there is wedging of L4, and is opposite the side of L5-S1 wedging then the L4 opened side is placed up in the side posture position. In this scenario, to decrease the lateral flexion component of the listing, the L5 segment is thrusted superiorly with a cephalad mild arcing motion towards the end of the thrust. If the AP radiograph, if no scoliosis or wedging is present at L4, then conventional or simple listings are used for L5.

Newborn and Infant

L5 POSTERIOR PRONE ADJUSTMENT

Name of technique: Gonstead
Name of technique procedure: Prone adjustment.
Example: Posterior L5 (-Z) listing (Fig. 9.125). Retrolisthesis

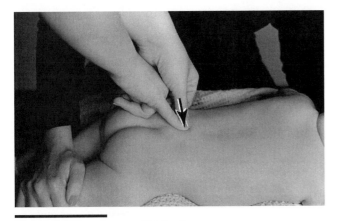

Figure 9.125.   A prone fifth lumbar setup.

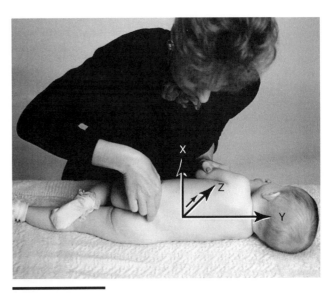

Figure 9.126.   L5 posterior side posture adjustment. The smaller spinous process is contacted by the second digit and supported by the third digit for a finger push. The stabilization hand contacts the anterolateral portion of the shoulder and axilla region with a slight cephalad distraction. Alternatively, the doctor can contact the crossed arms of the child to stabilize active arms.

of L5 with decreased anteriorward translation during flexion. Contraindications: All other listings, normal FSU, hypermobility, instability, destruction or fracture of the neural arch or spinous process, infection of the contact vertebra.
Patient position: Prone position across the lap of the parent.
Doctor's position: Standing behind the patient.
Contact site: Posterior, inferior border of the spinous process.
Adjusting and stabilization hand contact: The smaller spinous process is contacted by the distal end of the fifth digit. Depending on the depth necessary for the thrust, a stabilization digit (e.g., fifth, second, or thumb) will be placed of the nail bed of the adjusting digit.
Supportive assistance: The parent may stabilize the upper torso and lower limbs of the infant.
Pattern of thrust: A slight inferior to superior pattern followed with a marked posterior to anterior vector along the sacral base angle.
Contraindication for the thrust: The infant is unable to be maintained in a prone positioned.

L5 POSTERIOR SIDE POSTURE ADJUSTMENT

Name of technique: Gonstead
Name of technique procedure: Side posture, finger push adjustment.
Example: Posterior L5 (-Z) listing (Fig. 9.126). Retrolisthesis of L5 with decreased anteriorward translation during flexion.
Patient position: Right or left side posture position on the pelvic table. A small folded or rolled up towel may be required if the lateral cervical spine and the table shows a gap.
Doctor's position: Standing perpendicular to the smaller patient. As the height of the patient increases, the doctor will

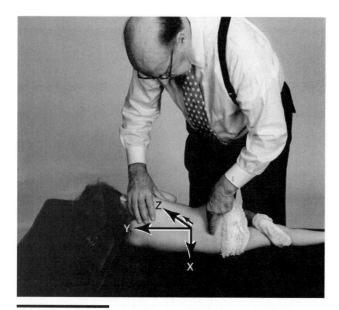

Figure 9.127.   The smaller spinous process is contacted by the second digit and supported by the third digit for a finger push. The larger spinous process may be contacted by a doctor with a smaller pisiform. The stabilization hand contacts the anterolateral portion of the shoulder and axilla region with a slight cephalad distraction. The finger push move allows for a specific setup for lumbar adjustment.

vary the degree of cephalad angle. The mature adolescent will have the same positioning as in an adult and the doctor will stand at a 45 degree angle facing cephalad.

Contact site: Posterior, inferior border of the spinous process.

Pattern of thrust: A slight inferior to superior pattern followed with a marked posterior to anterior vector along the sacral base angle. It is important to keep in mind that the sacral base angle is reduced when the patient lies in the side posture position. It is further reduced when the patient's thigh is flexed just prior to the thrust.

Contraindication for the thrust: The involved segment should not receive a thrust if the possibility exists of placing excessive y-axis rotation and/or flexion in the spine above the involved segment. This occurrence is more likely with the younger child who is either less cooperative and/or more flexible. Parent stabilization of the legs may assist the doctor to prevent unnecessary rotation.

Toddler and Pre-schooler

L5 POSTERIOR SIDE POSTURE ADJUSTMENT

Name of technique: Gonstead
Name of technique procedure: Side posture finger push adjustment.
Example: Posterior L5 (-Z) listing (Fig. 9.127). Retrolisthesis of L5 with decreased anteriorward translation during flexion.
Patient position: Right or left side posture position on the pelvic table.
Contact site: Posterior, inferior border of the spinous process.

Pre-adolescent and Adolescent

L5 POSTERIOR-INFERIOR SIDE POSTURE ADJUSTMENT

Name of technique: Gonstead
Name of technique procedure: Side posture adjustment.
Example: Posterior, inferior L5 (-Z, -θX) listing (Fig. 9.128). Retrolisthesis of L5 with decreased anteriorward translation and flexion during forward bending.
Patient position: Right or left side posture position on the pelvic bench.
Contact site: Posterior, inferior border of the spinous process.

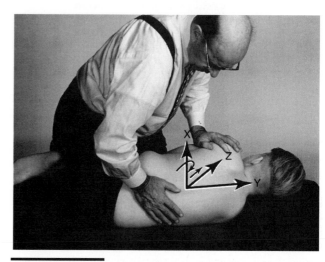

Figure 9.128.   Fifth lumbar Posterior, inferior (-Z,-θX) side posture adjustment. The larger spinous process is contacted by the pisiform, and the smaller spinous process is contacted by the second digit and supported by the third digit for a finger push.

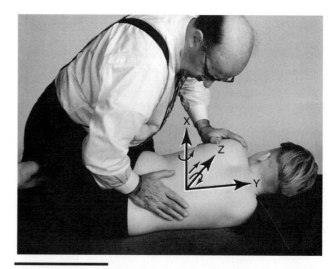

Figure 9.129.   PLS L5 side posture adjustment. The larger spinous process is contacted by the right pisiform, the smaller spinous process is contacted by the right second digit and supported by the third digit for a finger push.

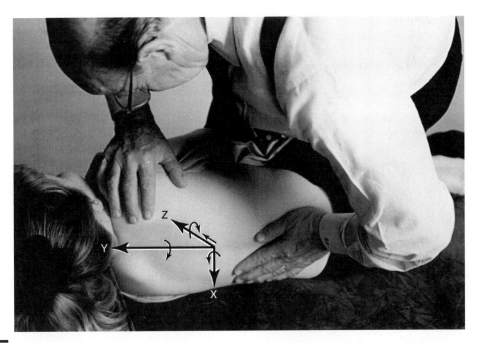

Figure 9.130.   PRS-inf L5 adjustment. The larger spinous process is contacted by the left pisiform, the smaller spinous process is contacted by the second digit and supported by the third digit for a finger push.

L5 PLS SIDE POSTURE ADJUSTMENT

Name of technique: Gonstead
Name of technique procedure: Side posture adjustment on the pelvic table.
Example: PLS (-Z, -θY, +θZ) L5 listing (Fig. 9.129). Retrolisthesis of L5 with decreased anteriorward translation and flexion during forward bending. Fixation dysfunction of right spinous rotation (+θY) and left lateral flexion (-θZ).
Patient position: Right side posture position on the pelvic table.
Contact site: Posterior, inferior, left lateral border of the spinous process. The tissue pull for the lateral flexion positional dyskinesia should be from superior to inferior.
Pattern of thrust: Posterior to anterior vector along the sacral base angle. It is important to keep in mind that the sacral base angle is reduced when the patient lies in the side posture position. It is further reduced when the patient's thigh is flexed prior to the thrust. Lateral to medial (+θY), with an inferiorward arcing motion (-θZ) toward the end of the thrust.

L5 PRS-INF SIDE POSTURE ADJUSTMENT

Name of technique: Gonstead
Name of technique procedure: Side posture adjustment.
Examples: PRS-inf (-Z, +θY, -θZ, -θX) L5 listing (Fig. 9.130). Retrolisthesis of L5 with decreased anteriorward translation and flexion during forward bending. Fixation dysfunction in left spinous rotation (-θY) and right lateral flexion (+θZ).
Patient position: Left side posture position on the pelvic table.
Contact site: Posterior, inferior, right lateral border of the spinous process. The tissue pull for the lateral flexion positional dyskinesia should be from superior to inferior.

Pattern of thrust: Slightly inferior to superior and posterior to anterior along the sacral base angle. It is important to keep in mind that the sacral base angle is reduced when the patient lies in the side posture position. It is further reduced when the patient's thigh is flexed prior to the thrust. Lateral to medial (-θY), with an inferiorward arcing motion (-θZ) toward the end of the thrust.

L5 PRS-M SIDE POSTURE ADJUSTMENT

Name of technique: Gonstead
Name of technique procedure: Side posture lumbar adjustment.
Example: PRS-m (-Z, +θY, -θZ) L5 listing (Fig. 9.131). Retrolisthesis of L5 with left lateral flexion positional dyskinesia and left body rotation. Left convex scoliosis with right lateral flexion of the L4–L5 motion segment necessitates using the left mamillary process as the contact point (special listing).
Patient position: Right side posture position on the pelvic table.
Contact site: Left mamillary process with the right pisiform. The fingers should be oriented along the axis of the spine.
Pattern of thrust: Posterior to anterior (+Z) with a superiorward arcing motion (+θZ) toward the end of the thrust.

L4 POSTERIOR ADJUSTMENT

Technique: Gonstead
Technique procedure: Side posture adjustment.
Examples: P (-Z) L4 listing (Fig. 9.132). Retrolisthesis (-Z) of L4. Fixation dysfunction of flexion.
Patient position: Side posture position on the pelvic table.

Contact site: Posterior, inferior border of the spinous process of L4.

Pattern of thrust: Posterior to anterior (+Z) through the L4–L5 disc plane with a slight inferior to superior vector of thrust.

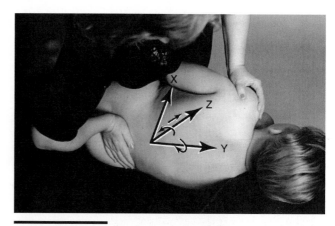

Figure 9.133. L3 PLS side posture adjustment. The larger spinous process is contacted by the right pisiform, the smaller spinous process is contacted by the right second digit and supported by the third digit for a finger push.

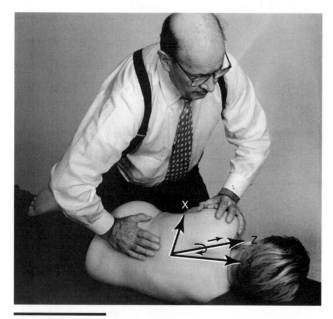

Figure 9.131. Contact is made on the left mamillary process by the right pisiform for the special L5 PRS-m listing. The stabilization hand contacts the anterolateral portion of the shoulder and axilla region with a slight cephalad distraction.

L3 PLS SIDE POSTURE ADJUSTMENT

Name of technique: Gonstead
Name of technique procedure: Side posture lumbar adjustment.

Example: PLS (-Z, -θY, +θZ) L3 listing (Fig. 9.133). Retrolisthesis of L3 with right body rotation and right lateral flexion positional dyskinesia.

Patient position: Right side posture position on the pelvic table.

Contact site: Posterior, inferior, left lateral border of the L3 spinous process.

Pattern of thrust: Posterior to anterior (+Z), lateral to medial (+θY) with an inferiorward arcing motion (-θZ) towards the end of the thrust.

L3 PLI-M SIDE POSTURE ADJUSTMENT

Name of technique: Gonstead
Name of technique procedure: Side posture adjustment with pisiform contact.

Example: PLI-m (-Z, -θY, -θZ) L3 listing (Fig. 9.134). Decreased anterior translation (+Z) motion of the segment, right lateral bending (+θZ) and left axial rotation (+θY). Retrolisthesis, lateral flexion malposition (-θZ) and left rotational (-θY) positional dyskinesia of L3.

Patient position: Left side posture position on the pelvic table.

Contact site: Right mamillary process with the left pisiform or digit of the doctor. The AP radiograph should be used to determine the location of the mamillary process in relation to nearby structures. The fingers do not cross the spine.

Pattern of thrust: Posterior to anterior (+Z) with an inferiorward arcing motion (+θZ) toward the end of the thrust.

L2 PRI-M SIDE POSTURE ADJUSTMENT

Name of technique: Gonstead
Name of technique procedure: Side posture adjustment with pisiform contact.

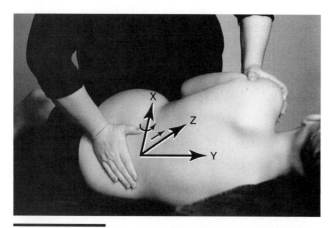

Figure 9.132. Fourth lumbar PL side posture adjustment. With the patient on their right side, the contact hand is placed so that the right pisiform is over L4, with the fingers pointing at approximately a 45 degree angle to the longitudinal axis of the spine. The patient is then rolled over towards the doctor with the pisiform contact thereby moving the L4-L5 articulation into the paraphysiological elastic zone. The patient's left shoulder is allowed to roll forward minimizing axial rotation of the spine. The doctor stabilizes the patient's pelvis onto the table.

Example: PRI-m (-Z, +θY, +θZ) L2 listing (Fig. 9.135). Decreased anterior translation (+Z) motion of the segment, left lateral bending (-θZ) and right axial rotation (-θY). Retrolisthesis, lateral flexion malposition (+θZ) and left rotational (+θY) positional dyskinesia of L2.

Patient position: Right side posture position on the pelvic table.

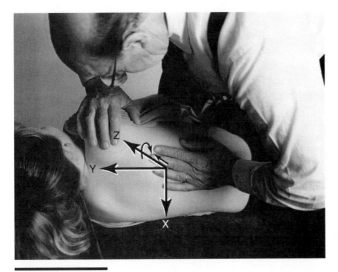

Figure 9.134. L3 PLI-m side posture adjustment. The patient is rolled over toward the doctor with the right pisiform contact, thereby moving the L3-L4 articulation from the neutral zone to the elastic zone (maximal preload or "tension"). The patient's shoulder is allowed to roll forward minimizing axial rotation of the spine. The doctor stabilizes the patient's pelvis into the table.

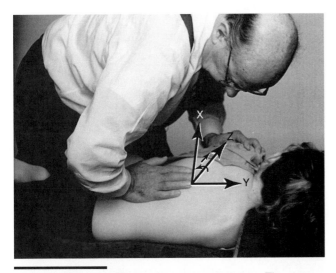

Figure 9.135. L2 PRI-m side posture adjustment. The patient is rolled over towards the doctor with the right pisiform contact, thereby moving the L2-L3 articulation from the neutral zone to the elastic zone. The patient's shoulder is allowed to roll forward minimizing axial rotation of the spine. The doctor stabilizes the patient's pelvis into the table.

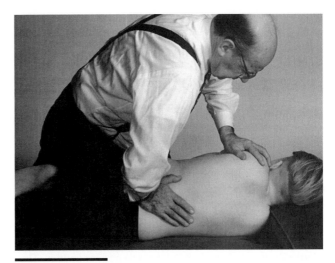

Figure 9.136. Base posterior side posture adjustment. With the patient on his right side the contact hand is placed so that the right pisiform is over S1, with the fingers pointing at approximately a 45 degree angle from the longitudinal axis of the spine. The patient is then rolled over towards the doctor with the pisiform contact thereby moving the S1-L5 articulation into the paraphysiological, elastic zone.

Contact site: Left mamillary process with the right pisiform or digit of the doctor. The fingers do not cross the spine.

Pattern of thrust: Posterior to anterior (+Z) (along the L2-L3 disc plane) with an inferiorward arcing motion (-θZ) toward the end of the thrust.

SACRAL BASE POSTERIOR SIDE POSTURE ADJUSTMENT

Name of technique: Gonstead
Name of technique procedure: Side posture adjustment for the base posterior (Fig. 9.136).
Example: Base posterior. Retrolisthesis (-Z) of sacral base and/or +θX positional dyskinesia of L5-S1. Decreased extension of the lumbosacral junction.
Patient position: On either the right or left side depending on the doctor's or patient's preference. If a lumbar scoliosis is present, then the convexity of the curve should be placed up.
Contact site: First sacral tubercle with a soft pisiform or digit contact.
Pattern of thrust: Posterior to anterior (+Z) through the lumbosacral articulation with a cephalad arcing motion (+θX) toward the end of the thrust.

L5 SPONDYLOLISTHESIS SIDE POSTURE ADJUSTMENT

Name of technique: Gonstead
Name of technique procedure: Side posture L5 adjustment (Fig. 9.137).
Example: L5 spondylolisthesis (Grade one or two) with decreased anterior translation of the sacral base during motion analysis. Grades 3 and 4 spondylolisthesis are usually adjusted in the prone position but can be performed in side posture provided adequate stabilization is made.

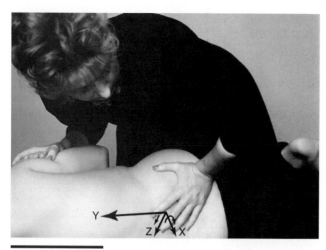

Figure 9.137.   L5 spondylolisthesis side posture position. The sacral tubercle is contacted by the pisiform, the smaller sacral tubercle is contacted by the second digit and supported by the third digit for a finger push.

Contraindications: All other listings, normal FSU, hypermobility, instability, destruction or fracture or infection of the sacrum.
Patient position: On either the right or left side depending on the doctor or patient preference. If a lumbar scoliosis is present, then the convexity of the curve should be placed up.
Contact site: Superior border of the S2 tubercle with a pisiform or finger push contact.
Pattern of thrust: Posterior to anterior (+Z) followed by an inferiorward arcing motion (-θX).

Knee Chest Table

As with the thoracic spine, the knee-chest table is more suitable for adjusting the lumbar spine of the older child (e.g., pre-adolescent, adolescent) than the toddler. The obese adolescent who is more difficult to position on the pelvic table may be an ideal candidate for this table. The face and chest are supported by a head or chest piece and the lower trunk is left unsupported (Fig. 9.138). The patient's knees rest on the base of the table. The chest piece or knee position can be adjusted so that the patient obtains a comfortable position with the spine relatively level from front to back. The segment being adjusted should be at the highest point on the spine, if possible.

General Indications

The knee-chest table provides a mechanical advantage to the doctor when adjusting the thoracic and lumbar regions. The knee-chest position lessens the amount of work by the doctor, which becomes critically important in the large or obese patient. In the typical side posture position for lumbar adjustments, the doctor must use coordination and strength to position the patient correctly and keeping them stable during and following the thrust. This table is also ideal with the smaller doctor who may have difficulty with the larger or obese adolescent or adult patient (51). The patient should be instructed to move as much as possible into the appropriate position.

The advantage of the knee-chest table for adjustments of the thoracic spine and lumbar spine for the larger patient is accomplished through the torso being allowed to move freely in an anteriorward direction during the thrust. This is not so when a normal flat table is used for the prone adjusting position for a thoracic or lumbar listing. In the latter, the rib cage and torso provide increased stiffness to the anteriorward thrust, thereby necessitating a proportional increase in the amount of force necessary. The magnitude of force is much less in nearly all knee-chest adjustments, compared to side posture. Since less force is needed to accomplish the adjustment, (from the lack of resistance offered by the unrestrained torso) the table is well equipped to handle those patients sensitive to high force techniques.

The table can be used for adjustments to all vertebral segments. The table is rarely used for adjustments to the sacroiliac articulations with the exception of the sacrum.

Adjustive Thrust

Since the mechanical advantage of the doctor is increased when the patient is in the knee-chest position, great care must be taken when the actual thrust is given (25). The patient should be completely relaxed and not supporting the chest with the upper extremities. The doctor guides the patient towards maximum +Z "tension," allowing the abdominal and pelvic area to protrude towards the knee-piece. The involved segment is then preloaded to tension. In this position, the bodies of the lumbar vertebrae are separated at the anterior, allowing for eased +Z translational movement of the segment.

Preload is applied to the spine by contacting the appropriate short lever arm (e.g., spinous, mamillary, transverse, or the cervical lamina) and translating the joint involved along the +Z axis to the limit of its physiological range. The transverse process of L5 can be used as a contact point if it is large enough with the adolescent spine. Care must be taken to translate the segment by taking into account the plane lines of the bodies of the vertebrae and the orientation of the articular facets. Directing the thrust through the spinal sagittal curves while minimizing vectors which create flexion or extension moments of the segment lessens the amount of longitudinal force encountered by the adjacent motion segments (25).

The maximal preloaded joint will receive a high velocity and short amplitude thrust. At the end of the thrust (i.e. at

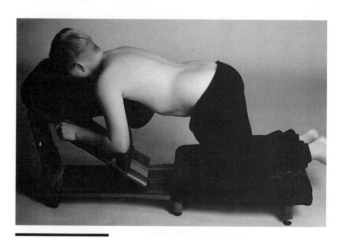

Figure 9.138.   Patient position on the knee-chest table.

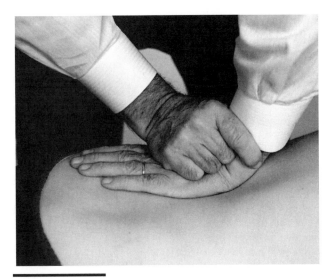

Figure 9.139.   The superior hand is used on the L2 listing.

maximum translation), the segment is held for one to two seconds, followed by a gradual "backing off" of the pressure. This allows for the viscoelastic tissues the time to adapt, providing an increase of adjustment effectiveness. The toggle-recoil thrust is contraindicated on the knee-chest table. This style of thrust to the flexible pediatric spine causes an unnecessary "whiplash" effect to the region. A lack of consideration to the specific type of thrusting action is perhaps the major misuse of the table (25). The thrust is given during maximal expiration, or between respirations, when the patient is completely relaxed.

Besides purely Z axis translatory movements, variation in contact points (e.g., spinous process, mamillary, transverse process) and the use of thrusting vectors which create motions in either the frontal (X-Y) or horizontal planes (X-Z) make the table useful for a variety of positional or dysfunctional configurations or movements of the segment (25).

Lumbar Adjustments

The chest support section should be positioned so that the patient's thoracic spine is level with, or slightly lower than, the lumbar spine (25). The knees are placed in a position such that the femurs are approximately five to ten degrees off vertical with the acute angle at the anterior. The doctor, facing the side of the patient, then places the most cephalad hand under the abdomen of the patient, instructing them to raise their abdominal area. This will cause the spinous processes to protrude, easing palpation. With the other hand, the doctor can then count to the appropriate segment they wish to contact for the adjustment. The spinous (preferred) or mamillary process is the short lever arm contact point. The transverse process of L5 can also be used for a contact point since it is much stronger at this level. The transverse processes of the other lumbar vertebrae should not be contacted since they have a propensity to be undeveloped, thin and weak. Fracture of a lumbar transverse process sometimes occurs (53). Evaluating the AP radiograph will determine the size of the mamillary process; the lateral radiograph reveals the size of the spinous process. Depending on the anatomical size of the contact point, the doctor must

determine what contact is made by the adjusting hand (e.g., soft pisiform, thumb, second or fifth digit).

The inferior hand is used for the contact point at the lower lumbar levels. Either hand can be used for L3 and the superior hand is used for the upper lumbar segments (Fig. 9.139). The doctor can stand behind the patient for double-thenar or the double-thumb contacts. The thrust is made with only one hand (Figs. 9.140, 9.141).

L5 POSTERIOR KNEE CHEST ADJUSTMENT

Name of technique: Gonstead
Name of technique procedure: Knee chest table adjustment.
Example: Posterior (–Z) L5 listing (Fig. 9.142). Retrolisthesis of L5 with decreased anteriorward translation during flexion.
Contraindications: All other listings, normal FSU, hypermobility, instability, destruction or fracture of the neural arch or spinous process, infection of the contact vertebra.
Patient position: Knee chest position.
Doctor's position: On either side of the patient facing perpendicular to the long axis of the spine.
Contact site: Posterior, inferior portion of the spinous process.

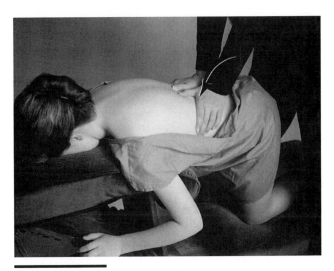

Figure 9.140.   The thrust is made with one hand.

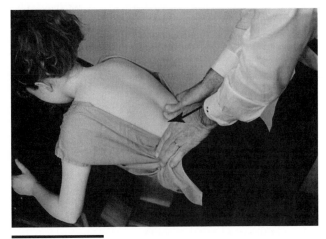

Figure 9.141.   The double thumb contact.

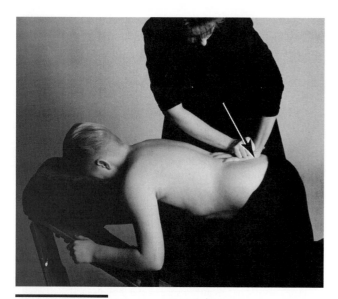

Figure 9.142. Fifth lumbar posterior adjustment.

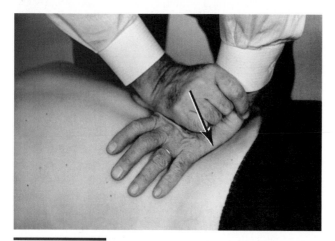

Figure 9.143. L5 PR-m adjustment. The right superior soft pisiform of the left adjusting hand is placed on the contact site. The support hand is placed over the contact hand.

Adjusting and support hand contact: The inferior soft pisiform contact. The support hand is placed over the contact hand. The supporting hand's pisiform can be placed over the pisiform of the contact hand.
Pattern of thrust: A slight flexion motion precedes the posterior to anterior thrust along the plane of the sacral base angle.
Contraindication to the thrust: The patient is unable to relax or cooperate to the position. The doctor is unable to specifically contact the smaller anatomical contact point with the adjusting hand.

L5 PR-m KNEE CHEST ADJUSTMENT

Name of technique: Gonstead
Name of technique procedure: Knee-chest table adjustment.
Example: PR-m L5 listing (Fig. 9.143). Retrolisthesis (-Z) of L5, right axial rotation (+θY).
Patient position: Knee chest position.
Doctor's position: On the opposite side of the mamillary

contact facing perpendicular to the long axis of the spine. The patient is stabilized with the doctor's knees.
Contact site: Left mamillary process.
Pattern of thrust: Posterior to anterior (+θZ) along the L2-L3 disc plane line, with an inferiorward arch motion (-θZ) toward the end of the thrust.

L4 PL KNEE CHEST ADJUSTMENT

Name of technique: Gonstead
Name of technique procedure: Knee-chest table adjustment.
Indications: PL L4 listing (Fig. 9.144). Retrolisthesis (-Z) of L4 and left spinous rotation (-θY).
Patient position: Knee chest position.
Doctor's position: On side of spinous rotation (i.e. left side) facing perpendicular to the long axis of the spine.
Contact site: Posterior, inferior lateral portion of the L4 spinous process.
Pattern of thrust: Posterior to anterior (+Z) thrust along the plane of the L4–L5 disc plane line with a slight lateral to medial (+θY) vector of thrust.

L3 PRS KNEE CHEST ADJUSTMENT

Name of technique: Gonstead
Name of technique procedure: Knee-chest table adjustment.
Example: PRS L3 listing (Fig. 9.145). Retrolisthesis (-Z) of L3 with right spinous rotation (+θY) and left lateral flexion (-θZ) positional dyskinesia.
Patient position: Knee chest position.
Doctor's position: On the right side of the patient facing perpendicular to the long axis of the spine.
Contact site: Posterior, right lateral portion of the spinous process.
Pattern of thrust: Posterior to anterior (+Z), lateral to medial (-θY) with an inferiorward arcing motion (+θZ) towards the end of the thrust.

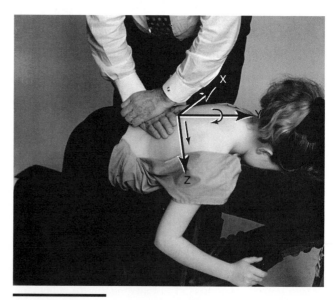

Figure 9.144. L4 PL adjustment. The inferior soft pisiform of the right adjusting hand is placed on the contact site. The support hand is placed over the contact hand.

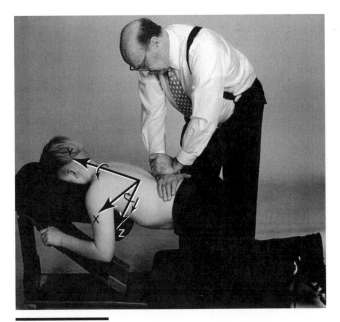

Figure 9.145. L3 PRS adjustment. The inferior or superior soft pisiform of the right adjusting hand is placed on the contact site. The support hand is placed over the contact hand.

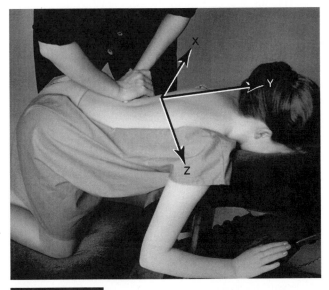

Figure 9.146. L2 PRI-m L2 adjustment. The thumb of the left adjusting hand is placed on the left mamillary process. The support pisiform is placed on the left thumb nail.

L2 PRI-M KNEE CHEST ADJUSTMENT

Name of technique: Gonstead
Name of technique procedure: Knee chest table adjustment.
Example: PRI-m L2 listing (Fig. 9.146). Retrolisthesis (-Z) of L2, right axial rotation (+θY) with left lateral flexion (-θZ).
Patient position: Knee chest position.
Doctor's position: On the opposite side of the mamillary

contact facing perpendicular to the long axis of the spine. The patient is stabilized with the doctor's knees.
Contact site: Left mamillary process.
Pattern of thrust: Posterior to anterior (+θZ) along the L2-L3 disc plane line, with an inferiorward arch motion (-θZ) toward the end of the thrust.

L1 POSTERIOR KNEE CHEST ADJUSTMENT

Name of technique: Gonstead
Name of technique procedure: Knee chest table adjustment.
Example: Posterior L1 listing (Fig. 9.147). Retrolisthesis (-Z) of L1.
Patient position: Knee chest position.
Doctor's position: Standing posterior to the patient.
Contact site: Right and left mamillary process.
Pattern of thrust: Posterior to anterior (+θZ) along the L1-L2 disc plane line, with an inferiorward arch motion (-θZ) toward the end of the thrust.

Pelvis

The pelvis is composed of two innominate bones, the sacrum, the coccyx and supporting tissues. The design of the pelvis allows for a transfer of the weight of standing to the lower limbs via the fifth lumbar. The pelvis allows for a variety of activities to be performed (e.g., standing, walking, sitting).

The sacroiliac joint is considered to be a true diarthrodial joint (67). The design of the innominate is auricular, fitting posterolateral to the cephalad half of the sacrum. The upper portion is vertical while the lower section is horizontal. The lower portion is close to the border of the sacrum, medial to the posterior superior iliac spine (54).

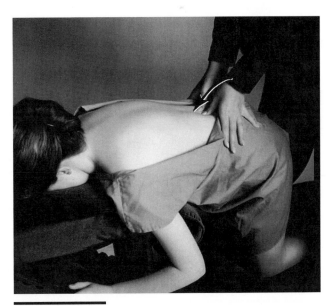

Figure 9.147. L1 Posterior double thumb adjustment. The right adjusting thumb is placed on the right mamillary process, the left adjusting thumb on the left mamillary process.

On the sacral surface the hyaline cartilage is three times as thick as the fibrocartilage found on the iliac surface (55). During the second fetal month the joint cavity is developed. The articular surfaces of the sacrum are first to develop grooves and ridges, followed by the ilium after puberty. The female articulation is built for mobility and parturition, while the male joints are built for strength and have extra ridges (extra and intra-articular tubercles) (56,57).

A sacroiliac subluxation is usually aggravated with prolonged standing and walking and is relieved with sitting. Disc problems in the lumbar spine will be aggravated with sitting.

Pain in the sacroiliac joint has been found in both increased and decreased mobility syndrome (58). One study (59) found that sacroiliac joint fixation was present in 28.1 percent of school age children 6-17 years of age. Lower back pain in the same study was present in 23.5 percent of the cases.

Pain from the sacroiliac joint may present as low back pain with pain and localized tenderness over the joint. This can extend further into the buttock, groin, genitalia, or trochanteric region (chiefly posterior, but also medial and anterior). Thigh pain, pain which may extend to the heel and lateral border of the foot, can also be attributed to a fixated sacroiliac joint (60-66).

The sacroiliac joint injury is often associated with a direct trauma to the pelvis with a twist at the time of impact or a lifting and twisting action. The pain is typically unilateral and reveals no neurological signs. The older patient may have more difficulty upon rising from a prolonged sitting position; pain

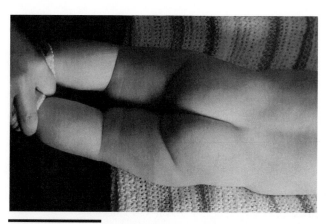

Figure 9.149.   The gluteal fold may be evaluated for the sign of an AS or PI ilium.

can be aggravated by walking. Commonly associated with this injury is stabbing pain with certain movements, specifically ipsilateral side bending when standing.

Postural Analysis

Postural analysis is conducted to determine abnormal postural and gravitational stresses on the spine. Of particular importance (in the coronal plane) is the relative levels of the posterior-superior iliac spines, the iliac crests, greater trochanters, gluteal folds and anterior-superior iliac spines. These observations provide initial indications of a level foundation, possible pelvic subluxations, and anatomical leg length inequality (LLI). The spine is examined for scoliosis and differentiation of functional or structural scoliosis is determined with Adam's test (Fig. 9.148). Foot pronation and the integrity of the longitudinal and transverse arch should be examined since these may contribute to LLI.

From the side observation is made of the spinal curves, particularly the degree of lumbar lordosis, pelvic tilt and abdominal muscle tone. Included in this examination is an analysis of gait. A shorter stride on one side may indicate a short leg or a fixation dysfunction at the sacroiliac joint. Foot pronation can be detected during the analysis of gait.

Inspection

From the posterior, the AS or PI ilium is visualized as asymmetric gluteal folds and iliac crest heights. An anatomical leg length inequality can also cause these findings. The newborn and infant (and occasionally the uncooperative toddler) are viewed in a prone position. The child (e.g., toddler, pre-schooler) capable of standing during the exam is viewed in the standing position. Although asymmetrical dimples (slightly inferior to the PSIS) may exist, there is also the possibility of either an AS or PI ilium. In the prone position the PI ilium will appear as a more marked gluteal fold and the AS ilium has a diminished fold (Fig. 9.149). While standing, the IN or EX ilium is evaluated by detecting asymmetry in the posterolateral iliac crests. The In ilium movement on the sacrum may cause a more flattened appearance of the soft tissue overlying the posterolateral portion of the ilium, whereas the

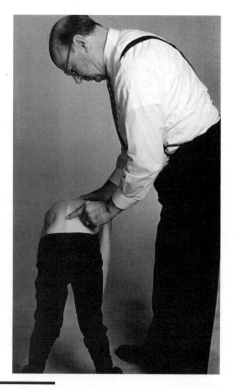

Figure 9.148.   The Adam's test evaluates for functional or structural scoliosis.

Ex ilium will demonstrate a more protuberant gluteus. In the prone position the undiapered infant with an In ilium may have a larger ilia width compared to the narrow ilia width of the Ex ilium.

A second way to detect the presence of the In or Ex ilium is by carefully lifting the infant under the axilla (Fig. 9.150). The In ilium will cause the foot on the same side of involvement to externally rotate. The Ex ilium will cause the foot on the involved side to be internally rotated. Foot flare can also be detected in the standing ambulatory child.

The base posterior sacrum may lead to compensation in the lower limbs with a "pigeon toe" or bilateral toe-in appearance. The rotated sacrum (e.g., P-L, P-R) may cause the ilium on the involved side to appear as an Ex ilium listing.

The lateral view should be examined for spinal curves, specifically the amount of lumbar lordosis and pelvic tilt. All postural evaluations of the pelvis should be confirmed by other examination findings (e.g. x-ray).

Gait

Gait analysis may reveal subtle signs of pelvic positional dyskinesia or fixation dysfunction. Since adaptive mechanisms often occur in a patient with a long-standing lesion, the gait abnormality may be obfuscated. Abnormal gait patterns are often more noticeable in the pediatric patient who has not had years of adaptation.

Lower limb positions and movement may be affected by both sacral or ilium subluxations. The fixated SI joint will often result in a decrease in the length of the stride ipsilateral. Uneven heel or sole wear of the shoe combined with an internal or external foot flare may be caused by an Ex or In ilium subluxation. Medial side heel wear of the shoe can also indicate the side of a functional or anatomical long leg; laterally worn heels may indicate the short leg side (67).

The sacral base posterior subluxation sacrum or in the unfused sacrum, a posterior second or third sacral segment (e.g., S2, -Z), may result in bilateral toe-in foot flare and/or a genu valgus waddling appearance during ambulation.

Severe occiput/atlas disrelationships can also influence a child's gait (20). An AS condyle (-θX restricted position of the occiput on the atlas) may be accompanied by bilateral outward toe flare. Toe walking may be caused by a PS occiput (+θX) or other upper cervical subluxation.

Static Palpation

The newborn or infant is placed in a prone position preferably across the lap of the parent. Depending on the size of the doctor's hand the small aspect of a digit (e.g., fifth, second,) is placed on either the superior or inferior medial margin of the PSIS. The practitioner will produce a light amount of pressure under the surface of contact moving along the entire length of the sacroiliac joint. Tenderness may cause the infant to react to the discomfort. Edema with the PI ilium is detected at the posterior superior area of the sacroiliac joint. The AS ilium edema is detected at the posterior inferior margin of the sacroiliac joint. The Ex ilium is associated with edema at the entire posterior region of the joint. The older child can be examined in either a seated or standing position.

Motion Palpation

The pelvis (sacroiliac joints) should be evaluated for fixation, dysfunction and compensatory hypermobility(19,62-64,68-70). There are numerous approaches to palpating this complex kinematic structure.

Newborn and Infant

The newborn/infant is placed prone across the lap of the parent or caretaker. If this is not possible, the prone position on the pelvic bench or the bottom section of the knee-chest is used. The doctor will place the small distal end of the palpating hand on the superior medial aspect of the PSIS. The leg of the involved side is raised and lowered several times (Fig. 9.151). If an AS ilium exists it may present with restriction and edema at the inferior margin. The PI ilium reveals fixation and edema at the superior portion of the sacroiliac articulation. The In and Ex ilium fixation is difficult to assess in the prone position.

The sacrum of the newborn/infant is evaluated in the prone position. The doctor should contact the involved sacral tubercle (e.g., S1, S2, S3) with the distal end of their digit. The doctor bilaterally raises and lowers the patient's legs creating an extension movement. If sacral posteriority exists, restriction of

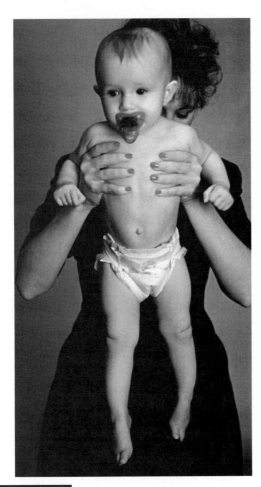

Figure 9.150.   The dangling legs of the infant may indicate an Ex or In ilium.

joint motion will be present. Sacral posteriority is the most common listing and is frequently overlooked in the newborn to pre-school age groups.

Sacral rotation (e.g., P-L, P-R) is extremely uncommon and difficult to detect in the newborn/infant. Mechanisms of injury that may warrant suspicion of this listing include in-utero constraint or the infant who has suffered a fall onto the pelvis.

Standing to either side, the doctor will contact the lateral aspect of the sacral ala with the distal end of the palpating digit. Careful consideration must be taken not to contact the PSIS or the sacral tubercle. While bilaterally raising and lowering the legs, the doctor moves the joint posterior to anterior (+Z) and slightly medial to lateral (±θY). If a rotated sacral tubercle exists the joint will generally present with both restriction and slight edema. Although rare, it has been noted by this author that severe sacral tubercle rotation (ex. P-L, -Z, -θY) can inhibit the infant's crawling development.

Toddler-Adolescent

PRONE SACRAL PUSH

The patient is placed prone on the pelvic or hi-lo table with the feet hanging off the edge. The chin must be maintained in a neutral position for those patients who are too short to reach

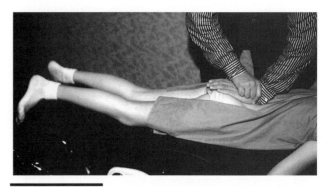

Figure 9.152. Normal sacroiliac motion occurs when the feet evenly externally rotate when posterior sacral pressure is applied.

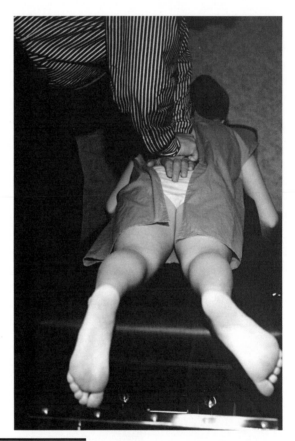

Figure 9.153. The right foot position reveals fixation on the ipsilateral side.

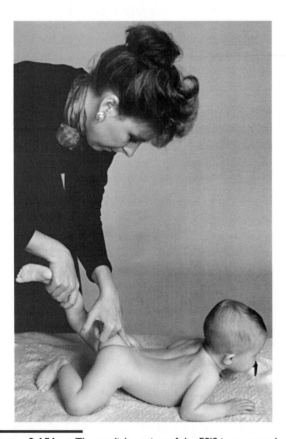

Figure 9.151. The medial portion of the PSIS is contacted by the palpating digit. The leg of the involved ilium is raised and lowered.

the face piece and dangle the feet off the table at the same time. The doctor will contact broadly the sacral tubercles (e.g., S2, S3) with the palpating hand. The smaller sacrum may be contacted with the thenar eminence or knife edge. The larger sacrum can be contacted by the pisiform. The doctor applies a firm posterior to anterior pressure. Normal sacroiliac motion occurs when the feet will evenly externally rotate when the posterior pressure is applied. When the pressure is released the feet should return to a neutral position. If there is a sacroiliac fixation, the foot on the fixated side will either move sideways or lift slightly during the posterior to anterior pressure (Figs. 9.152, 9.153).

SITTING LATERAL FLEXION

The doctor is squatted directly behind the seated patient. Contact each PSIS with the thumbs. Instruct the patient to actively side bend while not raising the buttocks from the seat (Fig. 9.154). The joint is considered to have normal motion when the PSIS stay level. An abnormal finding is when the fixated joint rides up on the contralateral side of bend.

A second version of the sitting lateral flexion of the sacroiliac articulation is evaluated by placing the tips of two digits just medial to the PSIS. Request the patient to bend from one side to the other. The examiner detects movement at the SI joint (Fig. 9.155). Palpation can be performed at both the superior and inferior margins of the joint. If a notable fixation is present, inspection may reveal that the contralateral buttock will raise when the spine is laterally flexed ipsilateral to the side of contact. The PSIS that raises more is likely the restricted articulation. Fixation at the SI joint will move the PSIS upward ipsilateral.

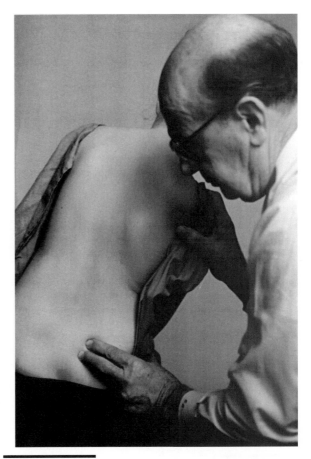

Figure 9.155. The use of two digits is a second version of the sitting lateral flexion examination.

SITTING ASSESSMENT OF AXIAL ROTATION

To palpate the sacroiliac joint, the doctor stands obliquely facing the ipsilateral side of contact. The doctor will place the contralateral third digit on the PSIS and the second digit on the sacrum. The ipsilateral hand is placed on the patient's opposite shoulder. The doctor initiates the rotation of the patient's slightly flexed trunk to the ipsilateral side. A normal movement should cause the sacroiliac joint and the fingers to separate. This examination is to be conducted bilaterally.

STANDING FLEXION

The patient is requested to stand with the doctor standing or kneeling (depending on the height of patient) behind the subject. To palpate the left SI joint movement, the doctor places the right third digit on the a tubercle (e.g., S2, S3) of the sacrum and the tip of the right index finger on the left PSIS. Instruct the patient to bend forward (Fig. 9.156). The normal joint motion during flexion will be a separation of the third and index finger. The test is repeated on the opposite side.

SITTING FLEXION

The seated patient is contacted by each of the doctor's thumbs on each PSIS. Request the patient to actively flex the trunk

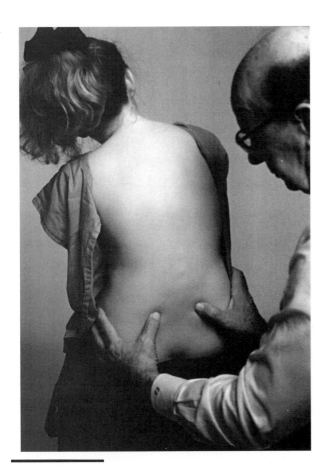

Figure 9.154. The sitting lateral flexion exam.

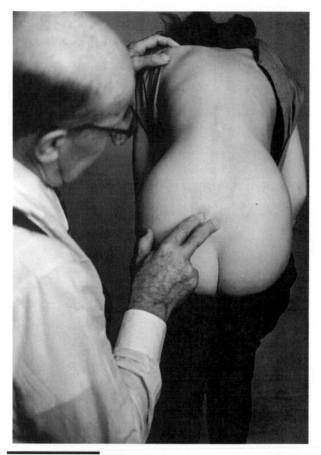

Figure 9.156. The normal joint motion for the Standing Flexion exam is separation of the digits while bending forward.

while not raising the buttocks from the chair (Fig. 9.157). During this motion both thumbs should remain level. If an ilium is fixated, the thumb over the PSIS on the fixated side will raise superiorly.

STANDING HIP FLEXION

The doctor stands (or kneels) behind the patient. Contacting one side of the PSIS with the ipsilateral thumb, the opposite thumb will contact the second sacral tubercle. The patient is instructed to lift the leg (ipsilateral of the PSIS contact) until it has achieved maximal hip flexion (Fig. 9.158). The motion findings are compared to the opposite side between the PSIS and S2. If a diminished downward movement is noted between the PSIS and S2, suspect possible fixation dysfunction. The younger child may need to be assisted by the parent standing anteriorly and stabilizing both shoulders.

Instrumentation

The hand held paraspinal temperature differential instruments (e.g. Nervoscope, Temposcope) can register temperature asymmetry in sacroiliac subluxation. The smaller patient may show a reading in the sacral area due to subluxation of an unfused sacral segment. With the older child a reading is more

likely to occur when the subluxation is in the acute, inflammatory condition. Chronic fixations may or may not register a temperature differential. To obtain a reading it is sometimes helpful to "tilt" the hand held instrument from side to side (i.e., $\pm\theta Z$ movement [Fig. 9.159]).

The newborn/infant is placed prone across the lap of the parent. The diaper will need to be lowered or removed. The older child (e.g., toddler, pre-schooler) can be seated. The doctor and/or parent may have to stabilize the ticklish child during the procedure.

Due to the nature of the positional dyskinesia, the PIEx subluxation may give a temperature differential at the upper sacroiliac joint. This region, specifically the Ex rotational component, is detectable due to the inflammation response to the fixation.

The base posterior sacrum will usually cause a temperature differential at the lumbosacral junction. However the fifth lumbar vertebra must be ruled out as the involved segment.

Pelvic Adjustments

The simple or compound ilium misalignment does not commonly occur in the newborn, infant or toddler, unless a marked trauma has been induced. This type of subluxation listing is difficult to assess due to the problems associated with effective patient positioning for the radiograph.

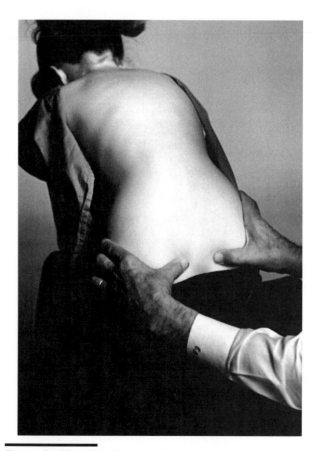

Figure 9.157. The Sitting Flexion procedure.

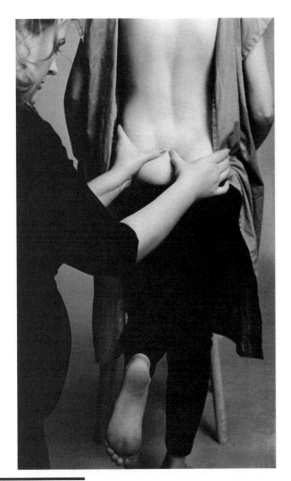

Figure 9.158. The patient raises the leg on the side of PSIS contact for the Standing Knee Bend exam.

PI ILIUM

The posterior inferior ilium (PI) occurs when the innominate PSIS rotates around an oblique X-axis and positions itself in a posterior and inferior position relative to the sacrum. Depending on the nature of the trauma, there will be more or less counter clockwise rotation around the X axis ($-\theta X$) and posterior translation along the Z-axis ($-Z$).

AP AND LATERAL RADIOGRAPH ANALYSIS

The vertical height of the innominate from the iliac crest to the ischial tuberosity is increased (see Chapter 8). On the AP radiograph, the size of the obturator foramen increases in its diagonal length. Further, the PI ilium causes the femoral head to appear lower, provided no leg length asymmetry exists. There may be an appearance of an increased sacral base angle or an increased lumbar lordosis.

CLINICAL FINDINGS

The gluteal fold will be more pronounced on the involved side of positional dyskinesia. During prone (newborn/infant) or standing static palpation, edema is detected at the posterior

superior region of the involved SI joint. To motion palpate the SI joint of the newborn/infant, the doctor raises and lowers the individual leg of the joint being palpated. The older child may be motion palpated as discussed earlier in this section. Static palpation will elicit tenderness and edema at the posterior superior portion of the PSIS. The PI ilium subluxation may cause an increased lumbar lordosis. A prone leg length check will likely reveal a short leg on the PI side, unless an anatomically increased leg length is present.

Newborn/Infant

PI ILIUM PRONE ADJUSTMENT

Name of technique: Gonstead
Name of technique procedure: Prone PI ilium push adjustment.
Indications: Right PI ($-Z$, $-\theta X$) subluxation (Fig. 9.160).
Contraindications: All other listings, hypermobility, instability, lytic metastasis in the region.
Patient position: The patient lies across the lap of the parent or caretaker. The involved side is towards the side of the doctor. The pelvic table may be used if the padding is comfortable.
Doctor's position: The doctor stands slightly inferior to the listing.
Contact site: The superior posterior aspect of the PSIS on the

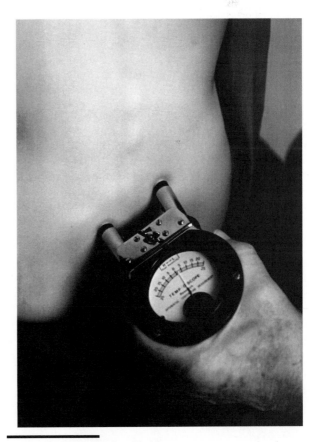

Figure 9.159. The hand held instrument may need to be tilted side to side to obtain a reading.

right ilium. The tissue pull is taken from superior to inferior by the stabilization (Lt.) hand.

Adjusting and stabilization hand contact: The following adjusting hand points may be used: digit on digit nail bed, thumb on thumb nail bed, pisiform on thumb nail bed.

Support assistance: The parent can stabilize the upper torso and lower limbs from movement.

Pattern of thrust: The doctor angles the adjusting elbow to allow the direction of thrust to be posterior to anterior (+Z) and inferior to superior (+θX) in the direction of the plane of movement of the sacroiliac joint.

Contraindication for the thrust: Inability of the newborn/infant to maintain the prone position.

PI ILIUM LEFT SIDE POSTURE ADJUSTMENT

Name of technique: Gonstead
Name of technique procedure: Side posture PI ilium push adjustment.

Indications: Left PI (-Z,-θX) subluxation (Fig. 9.161).

Contraindications: All other listings, hypermobility, instability, lytic metastasis in the region, inability to lie in the side posture position, congenital hip dislocation.

Patient position: The patient is placed in the side posture position on the pelvic bench. The PI listing is positioned involved side up.

Doctor's position: The doctor stands slightly inferior and oblique to the patient. The taller doctor may kneel at the side of the newborn/infant.

Contact site: The superior posterior aspect of the PSIS on the left ilium. Tissue pull is taken from inferior to superior by the stabilization (Lt.) hand. Depending on the doctor's hand size, a finger push (second digit supported by the third digit) or the pisiform of the caudad (Rt.) hand is applied to the posterior inferior border of the high side PSIS. The patient's high side knee is moved cephalad until the PSIS is felt to move back into the pisiform contact hand. The knee is then brought back slightly until the tension in the joint is felt to release.

Adjusting and stabilization hand contact: The caudal (Rt.) hand will deliver the adjustment. The following adjusting hand points may be used: soft pisiform, finger push and thumb. The newborn/infant's superior side knee is slightly bent and moved cephalad. The cephalad (Lt.) hand will stabilize the upper torso (holding the newborn/infant's crossed arms) perpendicular.

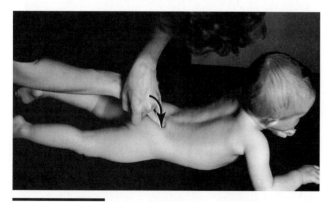

Figure 9.160.   The prone PI adjustment on an infant.

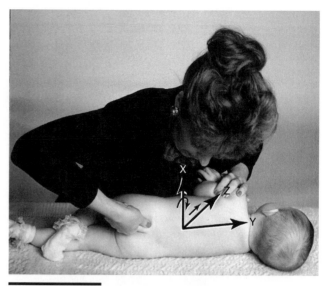

Figure 9.161.   Left PI ilium thumb push adjustment.

Supportive assistance: The bent and inferior straight leg can be stabilized by the parent. The parent is to assist in preventing lower body rotation.

Pattern of thrust: The doctor angles the adjusting forearm to allow the direction of thrust to be posterior to anterior (+Z) and inferior to superior (+θX) in the direction of the plane of movement of the sacroiliac joint.

Contraindication for the thrust: Inability of the newborn/infant to maintain a perpendicular position. The doctor is unable to minimize the introduction of rotation to the upper or lower body region.

Toddler and Pre-Schooler

PI ILIUM (RIGHT) PRONE ADJUSTMENT

Name of technique: Gonstead
Name of technique procedure: Prone PI ilium push adjustment.

Indications: Right PI (-Z, -θX) subluxation (Fig. 9.162).

Patient position: The patient lies prone on the pelvic or hi-lo table. Some toddlers may continue to cooperate across the lap of the parent or caretaker. The involved side is towards the side of the doctor.

Doctor's position: The doctor stands slightly inferior to the listing.

Contact site: The superior posterior aspect of the PSIS on the right ilium. Tissue pull is taken from inferior to superior by the stabilization (Rt.) hand.

Supportive assistance: The parent can stabilize the upper torso and lower limbs from movement.

Pattern of thrust: The doctor angles the adjusting arm to allow the direction of thrust to be posterior to anterior (+Z) and inferior to superior (+θX) in the direction of the plane of movement of the sacroiliac joint.

Contraindication for the thrust: Inability of the toddler or pre-schooler to stay in a prone position prior to engaging the thrust.

PI ILIUM (LEFT) PRONE ADJUSTMENT

Name of technique: Gonstead
Name of technique procedure: Prone PI ilium push adjustment.
Indications: Left PI (−Z, −θX) subluxation (Fig. 9.163).
Patient position: The patient lies prone on a pelvic or hi-lo

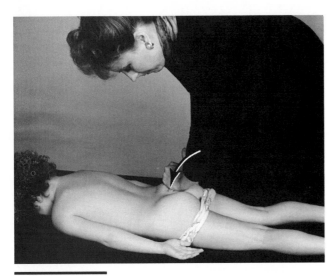

Figure 9.162.   Prone PI ilium thumb-pisiform adjustment on a toddler. The following adjusting hand points may be used; left pisiform on right thumb nail bed, left thumb on right thumb nail bed.

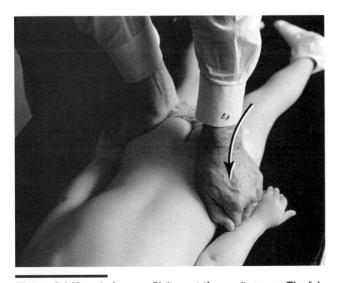

Figure 9.163.   Left prone PI ilium pisiform adjustment. The following adjusting hand points may be used: left thenar eminence on the contact site, with the heel of the stabilization (Rt.) hand (no thrust is made with this hand) contacting the compensating contralateral AS ilium or a left pisiform contact with the caudal (Lt.) hand and the stabilization (Rt.) hand wrapped or resting on the adjusting hand (not shown).

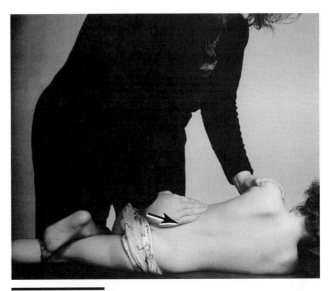

Figure 9.164.   Left ilium pisiform PI push adjustment. The caudal (Rt.) hand will deliver the adjustment. The following adjusting hand points may be used: soft pisiform or finger push. The right pisiform of the caudad hand is applied to the posterior inferior border of the high side PSIS. The cephalad (Lt.) hand will stabilize the upper torso (by holding the toddler's crossed arms) perpendicular.

table, with both arms at the sides of the patient, over the side of the table or with the hands on the hand rests.
Doctor's position: The doctor stands on the opposite side of the PI ilium, remaining close to the patient's thigh and table.
Contact site: The superior posterior aspect of the PSIS on the left ilium. Tissue pull is taken from inferior to superior by the stabilization (Rt.) hand.
Pattern of thrust: The doctor angles the adjusting arm to allow the direction of thrust to be posterior to anterior (+Z) and inferior to superior (+θX) in the direction of the plane of movement of the sacroiliac joint.

PI ILIUM (LEFT) SIDE POSTURE ADJUSTMENT

Name of technique: Gonstead
Name of technique procedure: Side posture PI ilium pisiform push adjustment.
Indications: Left PI (−Z,−θX) subluxation (Fig. 9.164).
Contraindications: All other listings, hypermobility, instability, lytic metastasis in the region, inability to lie in the side posture position, Legg-Calve-Perthes or slipped femoral capital epiphysis of the involved side.
Patient position: The patient is placed in the side posture position on the pelvic bench. The PI listing is involved side up.
Doctor's position: The doctor stands slightly inferior and oblique towards the patient. The patient's left side knee is straddled and moved cephalad until the PSIS is felt to move back into the right pisiform or finger push contact hand. The knee is then brought back slightly until the tension in the joint is felt to release.
Contact site: The superior posterior aspect of the left PSIS.

Tissue pull is taken from inferior to superior by the stabilization (Lt.) hand.

Supportive assistance: The bent and inferior straight leg can be stabilized by the parent. The parent is to assist in preventing lower body rotation.

Pattern of thrust: The doctor angles the adjusting forearm to allow the direction of thrust to be posterior to anterior (+Z) and inferior to superior (+θX) in the direction of the plane of movement of the sacroiliac joint.

Contraindication for the thrust: Inability of the toddler or pre-schooler to maintain a perpendicular position. The doctor is unable to minimize the introduction of y-axis rotation to the upper or lower body region.

PI ILIUM (LEFT) SIDE POSTURE ADJUSTMENT

Name of technique: Gonstead

Name of technique procedure: Side posture PI ilium thumb push adjustment.

Indications: Right PI (-Z,-θX) subluxation (Fig. 9.165).

Patient position: The patient is placed in the side posture position on the pelvic bench. The PI listing is placed involved side up.

Contact site: The superior posterior aspect of the PSIS on the right ilium. Tissue pull is taken from inferior to superior by the stabilization (Rt.) hand.

Pattern of thrust: The doctor angles the adjusting forearm to allow the direction of thrust to be posterior to anterior (+Z) and inferior to superior (+θX) in the direction of the plane of movement of the sacroiliac joint.

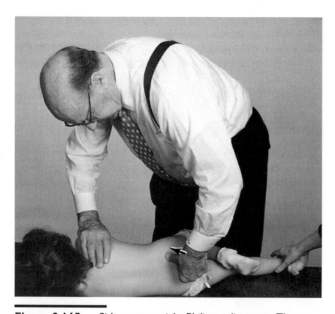

Figure 9.165. Side posture right PI ilium adjustment. The caudal (Rt.) thumb or finger push set-up (not shown) will deliver the adjustment. The thumb or finger push set-up of the caudad (Rt.) hand is applied to the posterior superior border of the high side PSIS. The cephalad (Lt.) hand will stabilize the upper torso (holding the toddler's crossed arms) perpendicular.

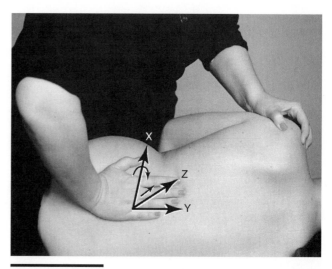

Figure 9.166. The side posture push adjustment is the position of choice for the adolescent. The caudal (Rt.) hand will deliver the adjustment. The following adjusting hand points may be used: soft pisiform or finger push (not shown). The cephalad (Lt.) hand will stabilize the anterior shoulder or holding the smaller pre-adolescent crossed arms. The patient is to be positioned perpendicular.

Pre-Adolescent and Adolescent

PI ILIUM (LEFT) SIDE POSTURE ADJUSTMENT

Name of technique: Gonstead

Name of technique procedure: Side posture PI ilium push adjustment.

Indications: Left PI (-Z, -θX) subluxation (Fig. 9.166).

Patient position: The patient lies in the side posture position on the pelvic bench. The PI ilium is involved side-up.

Contact site: The superior posterior aspect of the PSIS on the left ilium. Tissue pull is taken from inferior to superior by the stabilization (Lt.) hand.

Pattern of thrust: The doctor angles the adjusting forearm to allow the direction of thrust to be posterior to anterior (+Z) and inferior to superior (+θX) in the direction of the plane of movement of the sacroiliac joint.

PI ILIUM (RIGHT) PRONE ADJUSTMENT

Name of technique: Gonstead

Name of technique procedure: Prone PI ilium push adjustment.

Indications: Right PI (-Z, -θY) subluxation (Fig. 9.167).

Contraindications: All other listings, hypermobility, instability, lytic metastasis in the region, inability to lie prone.

Patient position: The patient lies prone on a pelvic or hi-lo table, with both arms at the sides of the patient, over the side of the table or with the hands on the hand rests.

Doctor's position: The doctor stands on the opposite side of the PI ilium, remaining close to the patient's thigh and table.

Contact site: The superior posterior aspect of the PSIS on the right ilium. Tissue pull is taken from inferior to superior by the stabilization (Lt.) hand.

Adjusting and stabilization hand contact: The following adjusting hand points may be used; caudal (Rt.) thenar eminence on the contact site, with the heel of the stabilization (Lt.) hand contacting the compensating contralateral AS ilium or a pisiform contact with the caudal hand and the stabilization hand wrapped or resting on the adjusting hand (not shown). Pattern of thrust: The doctor angles the adjusting arm to allow the direction of thrust to be posterior to anterior (+Z) and inferior to superior (+θX) in the direction of the plane of movement of the sacroiliac joint.

PIEX ILIUM

The ilium has rotated counterclockwise around an oblique axis (–θX) and translated posteriorly (–Z). The second component of this compound listing is lateralward (i.e., EX) movement of the PSIS (±θY).

AP AND LATERAL RADIOGRAPHIC ANALYSIS

An increase in the vertical height of the innominate from the iliac crest to the ischial tuberosity is detected (see Chapter 8). The size of the obturator increases on the AP projection. The PI component increases length of the diagonal measurement, whereas the Ex increases the width at the base of the obturator. The PI and Ex positions both lower the femoral head (see Chapter 8), unless unequal leg lengths are present. Both the PI and Ex positional dyskinesia may increase the lumbar lordosis on the lateral radiograph.

CLINICAL FINDINGS

The sacroiliac joint is opened at its posterior superior aspect with the PI ilium listing. The Ex component rotates away from the posterior joint space opening both the upper and lower

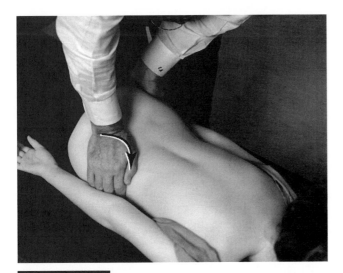

Figure 9.167.   The following adjusting hand points may be used; caudal (Rt.) thenar eminence on the contact site, with the heel of the stabilization (Lt.) hand contacting the compensating contralateral AS ilium or a pisiform contact with the caudal hand and the stabilization hand wrapped or resting on the adjusting hand (not shown).

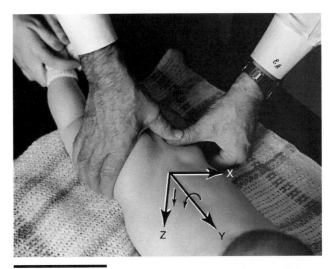

Figure 9.168.   The left PIEx ilium is contacted by a thumb on thumb contact. The doctor places either thumb (or digit for the larger hand) on the contact site. The opposite thumb or pisiform is placed on top of the adjusting thumb or digit.

portions of the SI joint. Fixation dysfunction is detected with motion palpation. There may be ipsilateral internal foot rotation. Skin temperature instrumentation may elicit a reading at the posterior superior aspect of the joint. This listing is uncommon in the very young (e.g., newborn/infant, toddler), unless marked rotational trauma (i.e. from a fall) has occurred.

Newborn and Infant

PIEX ILIUM (LEFT) PRONE ADJUSTMENT

Name of technique: Gonstead
Name of technique procedure: Prone PIEx ilium push adjustment. This position is recommended for the newborn/infant. Indications: Left PIEx (–Z, –θX, –θY) subluxation (Fig. 9.168).
Patient position: The newborn or infant is placed prone across the lap of a parent. A soft cushioned adjusting table may also be used. The involved side is towards the doctor.
Doctor's position: The doctor stands inferior and slightly oblique on the ipsilateral side of the listing facing the patient. Depending on the height of the doctor, kneeling may be required.
Contact site: The lateral border of the left PSIS. Tissue pull by the stabilization hand is inferior to superior and medialward on the involved PSIS.
Supportive assistance: Is given by the parent to stabilize the upper and lower body from activity.
Pattern of thrust: Posterior to anterior (+Z), inferior to superior (+θX), and lateral to medial (+θY) direction.

PIEX ILIUM (LEFT) SIDE POSTURE ADJUSTMENT

Name of technique: Gonstead
Name of technique procedure: Side posture PIEx ilium push

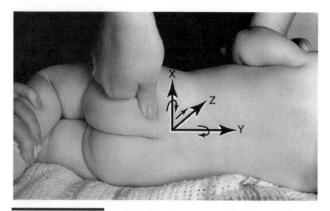

Figure 9.169.   The left PIEx ilium push set-up. The doctor places the caudal (Rt.) thumb or finger push for the larger hand (not shown) on the contact site. Rarely can a pisiform be selected due to the medial to lateral position of the fingers. The doctor's cephalad (Lt.) hand stabilizes the crossed arms of the newborn/infant in front of the patient's chest.

adjustment. Side posture positioning with the involved side up is preferred when the PI component of the listing predominates.

Indications: Left PIEx (-Z, -θX, -θY) subluxation (Fig. 9.169).

Patient position: The newborn/infant is placed left side superior in the side posture position. This occurs on the pelvic bench. The side posture position can be adopted to the parent's lap if necessary.

Doctor's position: The doctor stands on the ipsilateral side of the listing facing the patient. Depending on the height of the doctor, kneeling may be necessary. The doctor (or assistant) will stabilize the superior leg bent and the inferior leg.

Contact site: The lateral border of the left PSIS. Tissue pull by the stabilization hand is inferior to superior and medialward on the involved PSIS.

Pattern of thrust: Posterior to anterior (+Z), inferior to superior (+θX), and lateral to medial (-θY) direction. There is no body drop during the adjustment.

PIEX ILIUM (RIGHT) SIDE POSTURE ADJUSTMENT

Name of technique: Gonstead

Name of technique procedure: Side posture PIEx pull adjustment. This side posture set-up is preferred when the Ex component is greater.

Indications: Right PIEx (-Z, -θX, +θY) subluxation (Fig. 9.170).

Contraindications: All other listings, hypermobility, instability, lytic metastasis in the region, inability to lie in the side posture position, congenital hip dislocation on the contralateral side.

Patient position: The newborn/infant is placed in the side posture position on the pelvic bench with the PIEx ilium involved side down. The parent's lap may be an alternative replacement site.

Doctor's position: The doctor stands facing the patient. Depending on the height of the doctor, kneeling may be necessary.

Contact site: The lateral border of the right PSIS.

Pattern of thrust: Posterior to anterior (+Z), inferior to superior (+θX), and lateral to medial (-θY) direction. There is no torque or body drop during the adjustment.

Toddler and Pre-Schooler

PIEX ILIUM (RIGHT) SIDE POSTURE ADJUSTMENT

Name of technique: Gonstead

Name of technique procedure: Side posture PIEx ilium push adjustment. This procedure is preferred when the PI component is greater.

Indications: Right PIEx (-Z, -θX, +θY) subluxation (Fig. 9.171).

Patient position: The toddler/pre-schooler is placed involved side up in the side posture position. This occurs on the pelvic bench.

Doctor's position: The doctor stands facing the patient inferior and at a slightly oblique angle. The superior bent leg can be straddled by the doctor's legs.

Contact site: Location is detected with bisecting the PI and Ex vector points and contacting the lateral border of the right PSIS. Tissue pull by the stabilization hand is inferior to superior and medial on the involved (Rt.) PSIS.

Pattern of thrust: Posterior to anterior (+Z), inferior to superior (+θX), and lateral to medial (-θY) direction. There is no body drop during the adjustment.

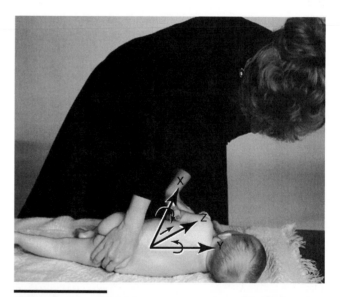

Figure 9.170.   The side posture set-up is preferred when the Ex component is greater. The doctor raises the involved (Rt.) ilium with the cephalad (Lt.) hand until the distal metacarpals of the caudad (Rt.) adjusting hand can be positioned. Tissue pull by the caudad metacarpals are inferior to superior and medial on the involved (Rt.) PSIS. The adjusting forearm is angled slightly to compensate for the listing. If the Ex component is greater the adjusting forearm is lateral, if the PI component is greater the adjusting forearm is angled more cephalad. The doctor's cephalad (Lt.) hand stabilizes the crossed arms of the newborn/infant in front of the patient's chest.

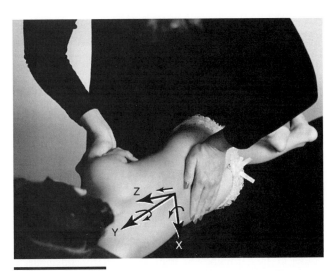

Figure 9.171. The side posture PIEx ilium push adjustment is preferred when the PI component is greater. The doctor places the caudal (Lt.) adjusting pisiform on the contact site. The doctor's cephalad (Rt.) hand stabilizes the crossed arms in front of the patient's chest.

PIEX ILIUM (RIGHT) SIDE POSTURE PULL ADJUSTMENT

Name of technique: Gonstead
Name of technique procedure: Side posture PIEx pull adjustment. This procedure is preferred when the Ex component predominates.
Indications: Right PIEx ($-Z$, $-\theta X$, $+\theta Y$) subluxation (Fig. 9.172).
Patient position: The toddler/pre-schooler is placed in the side posture position on the pelvic bench with the PIEx ilium involved (Rt.) side down.
Doctor's position: The doctor stands inferior at a slight oblique angle facing towards the patient. The superior bent leg can be straddled by the doctor's legs.
Contact site: The lateral border and slightly inferior (from the PI contact site) of the involved PSIS.
Pattern of thrust: Posterior to anterior ($+Z$), inferior to superior ($+\theta X$), and lateral to medial ($-\theta Y$) direction. There is no torque or body drop during the adjustment.

PIEX ILIUM (RIGHT) PRONE ADJUSTMENT

Name of technique: Gonstead
Name of technique procedure: Prone PIEx ilium push adjustment. This positioning is preferred when the PI component is greater.
Indications: Right PIEx ($-Z$, $-\theta X$, $+\theta Y$) subluxation (Fig. 9.173).
Patient position: The patient lies prone on the pelvic or hi-lo table, both arms to the sides, over the side of table or hands resting on the hand rests.
Doctor's position: The doctor stands inferior with a slight oblique angle towards the patient on the involved side.
Contact site: Is slightly inferior (from the PI site) and the lateral border of the (Rt.) PSIS. The stabilization (Lt.) hand tissue pull

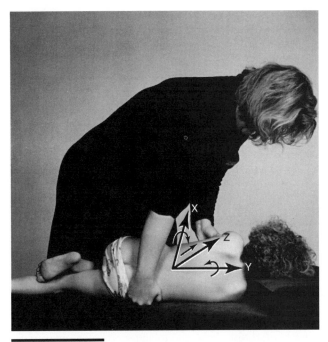

Figure 9.172. The right ilium PIEx ilium pull set-up. The doctor raises the involved (Rt.) ilium with the cephalad (Lt.) hand until the proximal metacarpals of the caudad (Rt.) adjusting hand have been positioned. Tissue pull by the caudad metacarpals are inferior to superior and medial on the involved (Rt.) PSIS. The adjusting forearm is angled slightly cephalad. The doctor's cephalad hand stabilizes the toddler's/pre-schooler's arms that are crossed in front of the chest.

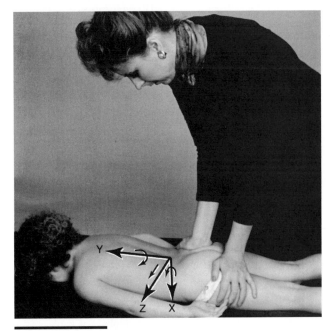

Figure 9.173. The doctor stands on the same side of the PIEx setup. The cephalad (Rt.) adjusting pisiform is placed on the contact site. The doctor's caudad (Lt.) hand stabilizes the opposite ilium at the ischial spine with the heel of the hand.

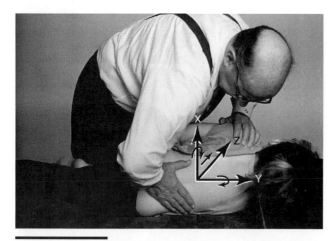

Figure 9.174. Side posture left PIEx ilium push adjustment. The doctor places the caudad (Rt.) adjusting pisiform on the contact site. The doctor's cephalad (Lt.) hand stabilizes the anterior shoulder.

is slightly inferior to superior and lateral to medial direction. Pattern of thrust: Posterior to anterior (+Z), inferior to superior (+θX), and lateral to medial (-θY) direction.

Pre-Adolescent and Adolescent

PIEX ILIUM (LEFT) SIDE POSTURE ADJUSTMENT

Name of technique: Gonstead
Name of technique procedure: Side posture PIEx ilium push adjustment. This procedure is preferred when the PI component is greater.
Indications: Left PIEx (-Z, -θX, -θY) subluxation (Fig. 9.174).
Patient position: The pre-adolescent/adolescent is placed involved side up in the side posture position. This occurs on the pelvic bench.
Doctor's position: The doctor stands slightly inferior and facing the patient at a slight oblique angle. The superior bent leg can be straddled by the doctor's legs.
Contact site: Lateral border of the PSIS. The tissue pull is inferior to superior and lateral to medial.
Pattern of thrust: Posterior to anterior (+Z), inferior to superior (+θX), and lateral to medial (+θY) direction. There is no body drop during the adjustment.

PIEX ILIUM (RIGHT) SIDE POSTURE PULL ADJUSTMENT

Name of technique: Gonstead
Name of technique procedure: Side posture PIEx pull adjustment. This procedure is preferred when the Ex is the larger component.
Indications: Right PIEx (-Z, -θX, +θY) subluxation (Fig. 9.175).
Patient position: The pre-adolescent/adolescent is placed in the side posture position on the pelvic bench with the PIEx ilium placed involved side down.
Doctor's position: The doctor stands facing at a slightly oblique angle towards the patient. The superior bent leg is straddled by the doctor's legs.

Contact site: Lateral border of the involved PSIS.
Pattern of thrust: Posterior to anterior (+Z), inferior to superior (+θX), and lateral to medial (-θY) direction. There is no body drop during the adjustment.

PIEX ILIUM (LEFT) PRONE ADJUSTMENT

Name of technique: Gonstead
Name of technique procedure: Prone PIEx ilium push adjustment.
Indications: Left PIEx (-Z, -θX, -θY) subluxation (Fig. 9.176).
Patient position: The patient lies prone on the pelvic or hi-lo table. Both arms are placed to the sides, over the side of the table or hands resting on the hand plates.
Doctor's position: The doctor stands inferior with a slightly oblique angle towards the contact site on the involved side.
Contact site: Is slightly inferior (from the PI site) and the lateral border of the left PSIS. The stabilization (Rt.) hand applies a tissue pull inferior to superior and lateral to medial.
Pattern of thrust: Posterior to anterior (+Z), inferior to superior (+θX), and lateral to medial (+θY) direction.

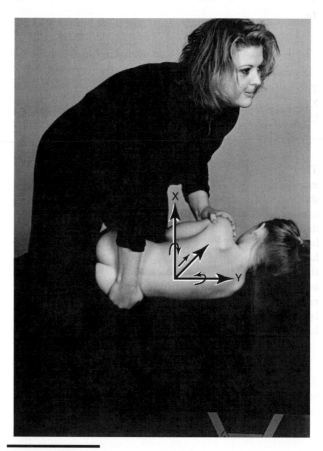

Figure 9.175. Side posture right PIEx ilium pull adjustment. The doctor raises the involved ilium with the cephalad (Lt.) hand until the caudad hand has been positioned. Tissue pull by the caudad (Rt.) adjusting hand is inferior to superior and medial on the involved (Rt.) side of the PSIS. The adjusting forearm is angled slightly cephalad if the PI component is greater. A lateral position for the adjusting forearm is chosen when the Ex component is greater. The doctor's cephalad hand stabilizes the anterior shoulder.

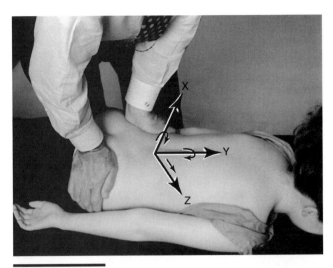

Figure 9.176.   Prone left PIEx ilium adjustment. The left adjusting pisiform contacts slightly inferior (from the PI site) and the lateral border of the left PSIS. The doctor's right hand stabilizes the opposite ilium at the ischial spine with the heel of the hand.

PIIN ILIUM

The PI ilium is a counterclockwise rotation around an oblique X-axis (i.e., -Z, -θX). The PSIS is also subluxated medialward (±θY) opening the SI joint at its anterior aspect.

AP AND LATERAL RADIOGRAPH ANALYSIS

The PI causes an increase in the vertical height of the innominate (iliac crest to the ischial tuberosity). The size and shape of the obturator changes (see Chapter 8). The PI component increases the diagonal measurement and the In decreases the width at the base of the obturator. The femoral head height is influenced. The PI decreases the femoral head height. The In raises the femoral head height. Depending on the combined results (excepting factors such as leg length inequality) the femoral head height will be either lowered or raised depending on which component predominates. On the lateral radiograph the PI fixation may increase the lumbar lordosis and the In may decrease the lumbar lordosis.

CLINICAL FINDINGS

Although the PI opens the joint space at its posterior superior margin, the In opens the anterior and closes the posterior joint space. For this reason, it may be difficult to palpate edema and/or tenderness. The lower limb may be rotated externally on the involved side.

Newborn and Infant

PIIN ILIUM (LEFT) PRONE ADJUSTMENT

Name of technique: Gonstead
Name of technique procedure: Prone PIIn ilium push adjustment.
Indications: Left PIIn (-Z, -θX, +θY) subluxation (Fig. 9.177).

Patient position: The newborn/infant is placed prone on the lap of the parent. A soft cushioned table may also be used. The involved ilium is placed away from the side of the doctor.
Doctor's position: The doctor stands on the contralateral side of the PIIn ilium facing the patient.
Contact site: Medial border of the left PSIS. With the stabilization (Rt.) hand, a tissue pull is made from inferior to superior and medial to lateral.
Pattern of thrust: The thrust is given in a posterior to anterior (+Z), inferior to superior (+θX), and medial to lateral (-θY) direction.

PIIN ILIUM (RIGHT) SIDE POSTURE ADJUSTMENT

Name of technique: Gonstead
Name of technique procedure: Side posture PIIn ilium push adjustment. This patient position is preferred when the PI component predominates.
Indications: Right PIIn (-Z, -θX, -θY) subluxation (Fig. 9.178).
Patient position: The newborn/infant is placed involved side up on the pelvic table. The parent's lap may be used as an alternative.
Doctor's position: The doctor stands in front of the patient.
Contact site: Medial border of the right PSIS. With the stabilization (Lt.) hand, a tissue pull is made inferior to superior and medial to lateral.
Pattern of thrust: The thrust is given in a posterior to anterior (+Z), inferior to superior (+θX), and medial to lateral (+θY) direction.

PIIN ILIUM (LEFT) SIDE POSTURE PULL ADJUSTMENT

Name of technique: Gonstead
Name of technique procedure: Side posture PIIn ilium pull move adjustment. This procedure is preferred when the In component predominates.

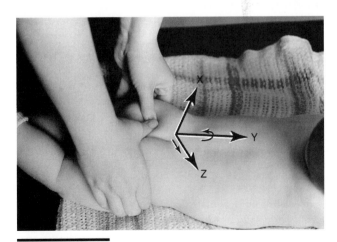

Figure 9.177.   Prone left PIIn ilium adjustment. The distal end of the left adjusting thumb is placed on the contact site. The large-handed doctor may need to substitute this contact with the distal end of the second or fifth digit. The stabilization (Rt.) thumb or hand will rest on the nail bed or wrapped around the adjusting hand.

Indications: Left PIIn (-Z, -θX, +θY) subluxations (Fig. 9.179).

Patient position: The newborn/infant is placed involved side up on the pelvic table. The parent's lap may be used as an alternative.

Doctor's position: The doctor stands in front of the patient.

Contact site: Medial border of the PSIS. The skin is pulled inferior to superior and medial to lateral.

Pattern of thrust: The thrust is given in a posterior to anterior (+Z), inferior to superior (+θX), and medial to lateral (-θY) direction.

Toddler and Pre-Schooler

PIIN ILIUM (RIGHT) SIDE POSTURE ADJUSTMENT

Name of technique: Gonstead

Name of technique procedure: Side posture PIIn ilium push adjustment. This procedure is preferred when the PI component is greater.

Indications: Right PIIn (-Z, -θX, -θY) subluxation (Fig. 9.180).

Patient position: The toddler/pre-schooler is placed involved side up on the pelvic table.

Doctor's position: The doctor stands in front of the patient. The superior bent leg may be straddled on the larger patient.

Contact site: Medial border of the PSIS. The skin is pulled inferior to superior and medial to lateral.

Pattern of thrust: The thrust is given in a posterior to anterior

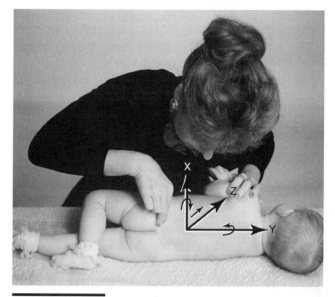

Figure 9.179. Side posture left PIIn ilium finger push adjustment. The fingers of the caudad (Rt.) adjusting hand are placed side by side on the contact site. The stabilization (Lt.) hand will hold the crossed arms of the newborn/infant in front of the chest.

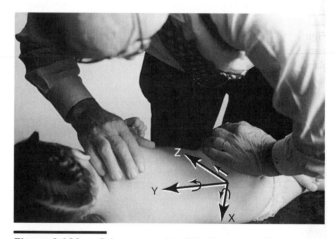

Figure 9.180. Side posture right PIIn ilium push adjustment. The caudad (Lt.) adjusting hand will set up with one of the following contact choices: pisiform (shown), finger push (not shown), or thumb (not shown). The stabilization (Rt.) hand will hold the crossed arms of the toddler/pre-schooler in front of the chest.

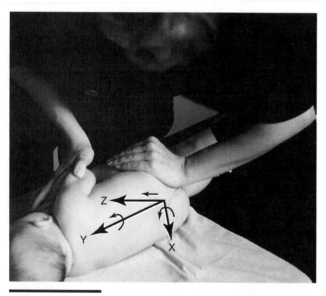

Figure 9.178. Side posture left PIIn ilium pisiform push adjustment. The pisiform of the caudad (Lt.) adjusting hand is placed on the contact site. The left finger or the distal end of the left thumb may be alternative adjusting hand set-ups (not shown). The stabilization (Rt.) hand will hold the crossed arms of the newborn/infant in front of the chest. The parent should stabilize the superior bent leg and the inferior leg in a straight position. Special consideration must be taken not to allow the newborn/infant to rotate around the Y-axis.

(+Z), inferior to superior (+θX), and medial to lateral (+θY) direction. There is no body drop.

PIIN ILIUM (LEFT) SIDE POSTURE PULL ADJUSTMENT

Name of technique: Gonstead

Name of technique procedure: Side posture PIIn ilium pull move adjustment. This patient position is preferred when the In component is greater.

Indications: Left PIIn (-Z, -θX, +θY) subluxations (Fig. 9.181).

Patient position: The toddler/pre-schooler is placed involved side up on the pelvic table.

Doctor's position: The doctor stands in front of the patient. The superior bent leg may be straddled on the larger child.

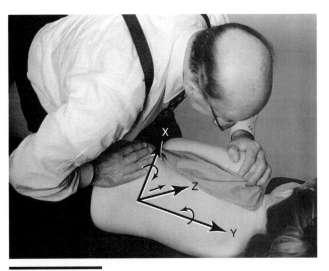

Figure 9.183. Side posture left PIIn push adjustment. The right pisiform or finger push (not shown) is placed on the contact site. The stabilization (Lt.) hand will hold the crossed arms of the smaller patient in front of the chest or the anterior shoulder.

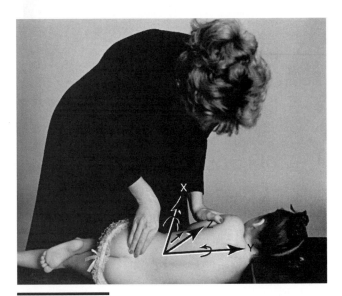

Figure 9.181. Side posture left PIIn ilium finger pull adjustment. The fingers of the caudad (Rt.) adjusting hand are placed side by side on the contact site. The stabilization (Lt.) hand will hold the crossed arms of the toddler/pre-schooler in front of the chest.

Contact site: Medial border of the PSIS. The skin is pulled inferior to superior and medial to lateral.

Pattern of thrust: The thrust is given in a posterior to anterior (+Z), inferior to superior (+θX), and medial to lateral (-θY) direction. There is no body drop.

PIIN ILIUM (LEFT) PRONE ADJUSTMENT

Name of technique: Gonstead

Name of technique procedure: Prone PIIn ilium push adjustment.

Indications: Left PIIn (-Z, -θX, +θY) subluxation (Fig. 9.182).

Patient position: The patient lies prone on the pelvic or hi-lo table, both arms are placed to the side of the patient, over the side of the table or the hands placed on the hand rests.

Doctor's position: The doctor stands inferior (and slightly oblique) to the contralateral side of the ilium.

Contact site: Medial border of the PSIS. The skin is pulled inferior to superior and medial to lateral.

Pattern of thrust: The thrust is given in a posterior to anterior (+Z), inferior to superior (+θX), and medial to lateral (-θY) direction. There is no torque.

Pre-Adolescent and Adolescent

PIIN ILIUM (LEFT) SIDE POSTURE ADJUSTMENT

Name of technique: Gonstead

Name of technique procedure: Side posture PIIn ilium push adjustment. This patient position is preferred if the PI component is greater.

Indications: Left PIIn (-Z, -θX, +θY) subluxation (Fig. 9.183).

Doctor's position: The doctor stands in front of the patient. The superior bent leg is straddled by the doctor's legs.

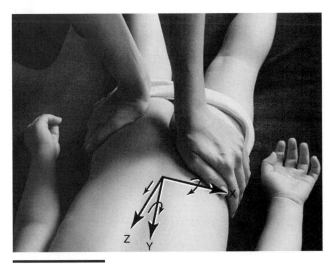

Figure 9.182. Prone left PIIn ilium push adjustment. The left adjusting pisiform or thumb (not shown) of the larger hand is placed on the contact site. The pisiform contact is stabilized when the opposite (Rt.) hand is placed on ischial spine of the contralateral ilium. The stabilization (Rt.) hand is placed on top or wrapped around the adjusting hand on the thumb set-up.

Contact site: Medial border of the PSIS. The skin is pulled inferior to superior and medial to lateral.

Pattern of thrust: The thrust is given in a posterior to anterior (+Z), inferior to superior (+θX), and medial to lateral (-θY) direction. There is no body drop.

PIIN ILIUM (LEFT) SIDE POSTURE PULL ADJUSTMENT

Name of technique: Gonstead

Name of technique procedure: Side posture PIIn ilium pull move adjustment. This procedure is preferred when the In component is greater.

Indications: Left PIIn (-Z, -θX, +θY) subluxations (Fig. 9.184).

Patient position: The pre-adolescent/adolescent is placed involved side up on the pelvic table.

Doctor's position: The doctor stands in front of the patient. The bent superior leg is straddled.

Contact site: Medial border of the PSIS. The skin is pulled inferior to superior and medial to lateral.

Pattern of thrust: The thrust is given in a posterior to anterior (+Z), inferior to superior (+θX), and medial to lateral (+θY) direction. There is no body drop.

PIIN ILIUM (RIGHT) PRONE ADJUSTMENT

Name of technique: Gonstead

Name of technique procedure: Prone PIIn ilium push adjustment.

Indications: Right PIIn (-Z, -θX, -θY) subluxation (Fig. 9.185).

Patient position: The patient lies prone on the pelvic or hi-lo table, both arms are placed to the sides of the patient, over the side of the table or the hands placed on the hand rests.

Doctor's position: The doctor stands inferior and slightly oblique to the contralateral side of the ilium.

Contact site: Medial border of the PSIS. The skin is pulled inferior to superior and medial to lateral.

Pattern of thrust: The thrust is given in a posterior to anterior

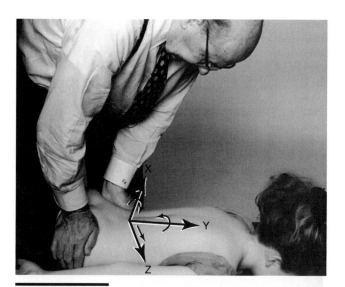

Figure 9.185. Prone right PIIn push adjustment. The adjusting (Rt.) pisiform or thumb (not shown) is placed on the contact site. The pisiform contact is stabilized when the opposite (Lt.) hand is placed on the ischial spine of the contralateral ilium. The stabilization (Lt.) hand is placed on top of or wrapped around the adjusting hand on the thumb set-up (not shown).

(+Z), inferior to superior (+θX), and medial to lateral (+θY) direction.

AS ILIUM

The anterior superior (AS, +θX, +Z) ilium is identified when the innominate has positioned itself in an anterior and superior direction relative to the ipsilateral sacral surface. The adjustment for this type of listing will primarily introduce a -θX motion with a slight -Z vector.

AP AND LATERAL RADIOGRAPH ANALYSIS

The vertical height from the iliac crest to the ischial tuberosity decreases (see Chapter 8). On the AP radiograph the size of the obturator foramen decreases in its diagonal length. The AS ilium causes a functional lengthening of the leg; the femoral head is raised, provided no leg length inequality exits. The lateral radiograph may reveal a decreased lumbar lordosis and/or decreased sacral base angle.

CLINICAL FINDINGS

The position of the AS ilium is caused by trauma to the inferior portion of the SI joint. Tenderness and edema may be palpated at this location. The gluteal fold is higher and flattened on the side of the AS ilium. The functional leg length may be increased, provided there is symmetry of the lower limbs.

Newborn and Infant

AS ILIUM (LEFT) PRONE ADJUSTMENT

Name of technique: Gonstead

Name of technique procedure: Prone AS ilium push adjust-

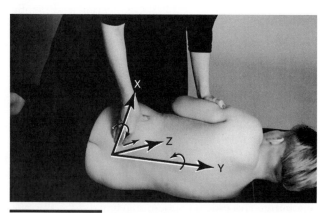

Figure 9.184. Side posture left PIIn finger pull adjustment. The caudad (Rt.) adjusting fingers are placed side by side on the contact site. The stabilization (Lt.) hand will hold the crossed arms of the smaller patient in front of the chest or at the anterior portion of the shoulder.

ment. This position is highly recommended for the newborn/infant.

Indications: Left AS (+θX, +Z) subluxation (Fig. 9.186).

Patient position: The newborn/infant is placed prone across the lap of a parent. A soft cushioned adjusting table may also be used. The involved side is towards the doctor.

Doctor's position: The doctor stands on the ipsilateral side of the listing facing the patient.

Contact site: The left ischial spine (rim of the acetabulum). Tissue pull is performed by the stabilization (Lt.) hand from superior to inferior.

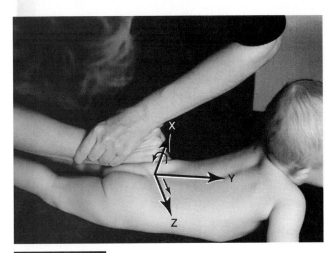

Figure 9.186. Prone left AS prone adjustment. The heel of the doctor's cephalad (Rt.) adjusting hand contacts the left ischial spine. The stabilization (Lt.) hand is wrapped around or placed on top of the adjusting hand.

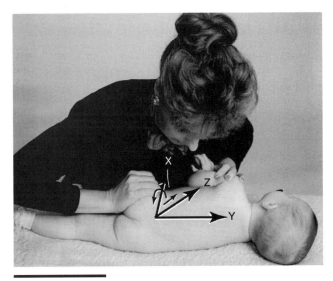

Figure 9.187. Side posture left AS push adjustment. The doctor stands on the ipsilateral side of the listing facing the patient. The doctor places the caudad (Rt.) adjusting pisiform on the contact site. The doctor's cephalad (Lt.) hand stabilizes the newborn/infant arms that are crossed in front of the chest.

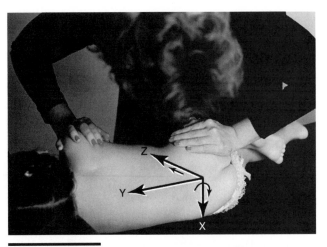

Figure 9.188. Side posture right AS push adjustment. The doctor stands on the ipsilateral side of the listing facing the patient. The doctor places the caudad (Lt.) adjusting pisiform on the contact site. The doctor's cephalad (Rt.) hand stabilizes the arms that are crossed in front of the chest.

Pattern of thrust: Inferiorward (-θX) with a slight posterior to anterior (+Z) movement.

AS ILIUM (LEFT) SIDE POSTURE ADJUSTMENT

Name of technique: Gonstead

Name of technique procedure: Side posture AS ilium push adjustment.

Indications: Left AS (+θX, +Z) subluxation (Fig. 9.187).

Patient position: The newborn/infant is placed involved side up in the side posture position. This occurs on the pelvic bench. The parent's lap may also be chosen as an alternative site.

Doctor's position: The doctor stands on the ipsilateral side of the listing facing the patient. Depending on the height of the doctor, kneeling may be necessary. The doctor or assistant will stabilize the superior leg bent and the inferior leg straight.

Contact site: The contact site is medial to the rim of the acetabulum over the left ischial spine. Tissue pull by the stabilization (Lt.) hand is from superior to inferior, towards the shaft of the femur. It is contraindicated to contact the ischial tuberosity for the push procedure. This long lever contact may result in too much force being applied at the level of the SI joint.

Pattern of thrust: Inferiorward (-θX) and slight posterior to anterior (+Z) movement.

Toddler and Pre-Schooler

AS ILIUM (RIGHT) SIDE POSTURE ADJUSTMENT

Name of technique: Gonstead

Name of technique procedure: Side posture AS ilium push adjustment.

Indications: Right AS (-θX, +Z) subluxation (Fig. 9.188).

Patient position: The toddler/pre-schooler is placed involved side up in the side posture position on the pelvic bench.

Doctor's position: The doctor stands inferior and slightly

oblique to the patient on the ipsilateral side of the listing. The doctor or assistant will stabilize the superior leg bent and the inferior leg straight.

Contact site: The contact site is medial to the rim of the acetabulum over the right ischial spine. The stabilization (Rt.) hand tissue pulls from superior to inferior, towards the shaft of the femur.

Pattern of thrust: Inferiorward ($-\theta X$) with a slight posterior to anterior ($+Z$) vector. There is no body drop.

AS ILIUM (RIGHT) PRONE ADJUSTMENT

Name of technique: Gonstead

Name of technique procedure: Prone AS ilium push adjustment.

Indications: Right AS ($+\theta X$, $+Z$) subluxation (Fig. 9.189).

Patient position: The patient lies prone on the pelvic and hi-lo table, with both arms placed to the side of the patient, over the side of the table or with the hands placed on the hand rests.

Doctor's position: The doctor stands inferior with a slight oblique angle towards the contact site on the involved side.

Contact site: The right ischial spine. The tissue pull is performed by the stabilization hand (Rt.) from superior to inferior.

Pattern of thrust: Inferiorward ($-\theta X$) with a slight posterior to anterior ($+Z$) movement.

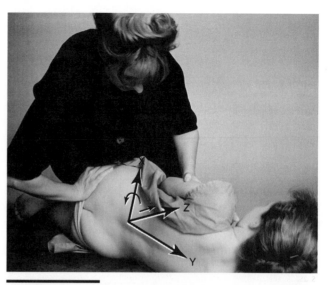

Figure 9.190.　Side posture left AS push adjustment. The doctor stands on the ipsilateral side of the listing facing the patient. The doctor places the caudal (Rt.) adjusting pisiform on the contact site. The patient's superior leg is moved forward until tension is felt under the contact hand. The knee is slightly released. The doctor's cephalad (Lt.) hand stabilizes the arms that are crossed in front of the chest or at the anterior shoulder for the larger patient.

Pre-Adolescent and Adolescent

AS ILIUM (LEFT) SIDE POSTURE ADJUSTMENT

Name of technique: Gonstead

Name of technique procedure: Side posture AS ilium push adjustment.

Indications: Left AS ($-\theta X$, $+Z$) subluxation (Fig. 9.190).

Patient position: The pre-adolescent/adolescent is placed involved side up in the side posture position on the pelvic bench.

Doctor's position: The doctor stands inferior and slightly oblique on the ipsilateral side of the listing facing the patient. The doctor will straddle the patient's legs.

Contact site: The contact site is medial to the rim of the acetabulum over the left ischial spine. The stabilization (Lt.) hand tissue pulls from superior to inferior, towards the shaft of the femur.

Pattern of thrust: Inferiorward ($-\theta X$) with a slight posterior to anterior ($+Z$) movement. The thrust is made down the shaft of the patient's femur and towards the symphysis pubis of the doctor. There is no body drop.

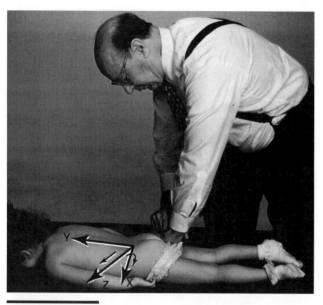

Figure 9.189.　Prone right AS push adjustment. The heel of the doctor's cephalad (Lt.) adjusting hand contacts the right ischial spine. The stabilization (Rt.) hand is wrapped around or placed on top of the adjusting hand. An alternative use of the stabilization (Rt.) hand is placement on the ipsilateral ilium over the ischial spine.

AS ILIUM (RIGHT) PRONE ADJUSTMENT

Name of technique: Gonstead

Name of technique procedure: Prone AS ilium push adjustment.

Indications: Right AS ($+\theta X$, $+Z$) subluxation (Fig. 9.191).

Patient position: The patient lies prone on the pelvic or hi-lo table, with both arms placed to the side of the patient, over the side of the table or hand placed on the hand rests.

Doctor's position: The doctor stands inferior with a slightly oblique angle towards the contact site on the involved side. Contact site: The right ischial spine. The tissue pull is performed by the stabilization hand from superior to inferior. Pattern of thrust: The thrust is made with a straight arm inferiorward (-θX) with a slight posterior to anterior (+Z) movement.

ASIN ILIUM

The anterior superior listing represents a clockwise movement around an oblique X-axis. There may also be varying amounts of anteriorward translation (+Z). This type of positional dyskinesia is associated with trauma at the lower portion of the SI joint. The In component is rotation around the Y-axis and is associated with separation of the SI joint at the anterior.

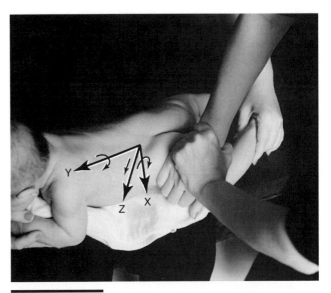

Figure 9.192.   Prone left ASIn pisiform push adjustment. The doctor's caudad (Rt.) adjusting pisiform or thumb (not shown) is placed on the contact site. The cephalad (Lt.) hand will rest on top of or wrapped around the adjusting hand. The doctor achieves the correct line of correction by positioning the contact arm's shoulder vertically over the S2 or S3 sacral segments.

AP and Lateral Radiograph Analysis

The AS causes a decrease in the long axis length of the innominate. The shape of the obturator foramen shows a change on the AP radiograph. The AS decreases the diagonal measurement, and the In decreases the width at the base. The femoral head height is raised, provided no leg length inequality exists. The lumbar lordosis and/or sacral base angle may decrease due to the AS and In components.

Clinical Findings

Although the AS opens the sacroiliac joint at its posterior inferior margin, the In opens the anterior and closes the posterior joint space. Edema and tenderness may be difficult to palpate, especially if the In component of the listing predominates. Groin pain can occur, as can medial knee or hip pain. The patient may also have an external foot flare on the ipsilateral side of involvement.

Newborn and Infant

ASIN ILIUM (LEFT) PRONE ADJUSTMENT

Name of technique: Gonstead
Name of technique procedure: Prone ASIn ilium push adjustment. This procedure is the recommended choice.
Indications: Left ASIn (-θX, +Z, +θY) subluxation (Fig. 9.192).
Patient position: The newborn/infant is placed prone across the lap of a parent with the involved ilium towards the doctor for a pisiform or thumb contact. A soft cushioned adjusting table may also be used.

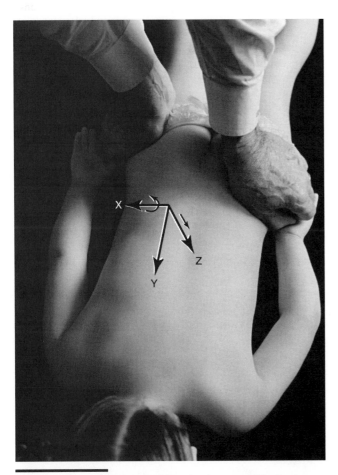

Figure 9.191.   Prone right AS push adjustment. The heel of the doctor's cephalad (Rt.) adjusting hand contacts the right ischial spine. The stabilization (Lt.) hand is to place the heel on the contralateral ilium over the ischial spine. An alternative set-up for stabilization is wrapping the caudad hand around or placed on top of the adjusting hand.

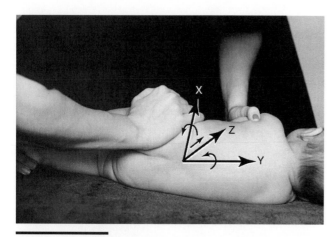

Figure 9.193. Side posture left ASIn push adjustment. The doctor contacts with the cephalad (Rt.) adjusting pisiform the contact site. The stabilization (Lt.) hand will hold the crossed arms of the newborn/infant in front of the chest.

Doctor's position: The doctor stands on the lateral side of the ASIn ilium facing the patient.
Contact site: The location is on the left ischial spine. The stabilization (Lt.) hand will tissue pull superior to inferior and medial to lateral.
Pattern of thrust: The thrust is inferiorward (-θX), slightly posterior to anterior (+Z), and medial to lateral (-θY).

ASIN ILIUM (LEFT) SIDE POSTURE ADJUSTMENT

Name of technique: Gonstead
Name of technique procedure: Side posture ASIn ilium push move adjustment.
Indications: Left ASIn (-θX, +Z, +θY) subluxation (Fig. 9.193).
Patient position: The newborn/infant is placed involved side up on the pelvic table. The parent's lap may also be used as an alternative.
Doctor's position: The doctor stands in front of the patient.
Contact site: The contact point is medial to the rim of the acetabulum, over the left ischial spine.
Pattern of thrust: The direction is inferiorward (-θX), posterior to anterior (+Z) and medial to lateral for the In component. A torque action is included with the thrust. The torque is clockwise for the left ilium (-θY).

Toddler and Pre-Schooler

ASIN ILIUM (LEFT) SIDE POSTURE ADJUSTMENT

Name of technique: Gonstead
Name of technique procedure: Side posture ASIn ilium push move adjustment. This procedure is preferred when the AS component is greater.
Indications: Left ASIn (+θX, +Z, +θY) subluxation (Fig. 9.194).
Patient position: The toddler/pre-schooler is placed involved side up on the pelvic table.
Doctor's position: The doctor stands in front of the patient.

The superior bent leg may be straddled on the larger patient.
Contact site: The medial rim of the acetabulum, over the left ischial spine. The stabilization (Lt.) hand provides a tissue pull from superior to inferior and medial to lateral.
Pattern of thrust: The thrust is inferiorward (-θX), posterior to anterior (+Z), and in a medial to lateral direction. The torque is clockwise for the left ilium (-θY).

ASIN ILIUM (LEFT) PRONE ADJUSTMENT

Name of technique: Gonstead
Name of technique procedure: Prone ASIn ilium push adjustment.
Indications: Left ASIn (+θX, +Z, +θY) subluxation (Fig. 9.195).
Patient position: The toddler/pre-schooler lies prone on the pelvic or hi-lo table, both arms placed to the side of the patient, over the side of the table or with the hands placed on the hand rests.
Doctor's position: The doctor stands slightly inferior and oblique to the patient on either the ipsilateral or the contralateral side of the ASIn ilium.
Contact site: The location is on the left ischial spine. The stabilization (Rt.) hand will tissue pull superior to inferior and medial to lateral.
Pattern of thrust: The thrust is inferiorward (-θX), posterior to anterior (+Z), and medial to lateral (-θY).

Pre-Adolescent and Adolescent

ASIN ILIUM (LEFT) SIDE POSTURE ADJUSTMENT

Name of technique: Gonstead
Name of technique procedure: Side posture ASIn ilium push move adjustment. This procedure is preferred when the AS component is greater.
Indications: Left ASIn (+θX, +Z, +θY) subluxation (Fig. 9.196).
Patient position: The pre-adolescent/adolescent is placed involved side up on the pelvic table.

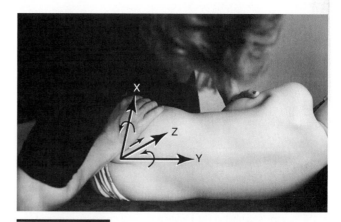

Figure 9.194. Side posture left ASIn push adjustment. The doctor's cephalad (Rt.) adjusting pisiform is placed on the contact site. The stabilization (Lt.) hand will hold the crossed arms of the toddler/pre-schooler.

Doctor's position: The doctor stands inferior and slightly oblique in front of the patient.

Contact site: The medial rim of the acetabulum, over the left ischial spine. The stabilization (Lt.) hand tissue pulls from superior to inferior and medial to lateral.

Pattern of thrust: The thrust is given inferiorward (-θX), posterior to anterior (+Z), and in a medial to lateral direction.

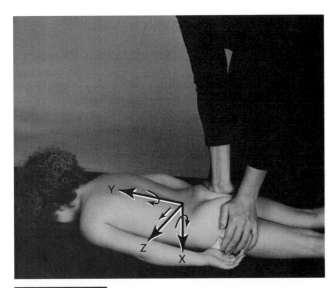

Figure 9.195. Prone left ASIn push adjustment. The doctor's caudad (Lt.) adjusting pisiform or on the larger child the heel of hand is placed on the contact site (as shown). For the pisiform contact the cephalad (Rt.) hand will rest on top or wrapped around the adjusting hand. The stabilization (Rt.) hand for the caudad heel procedure (as shown) is placed on the opposite PSIS.

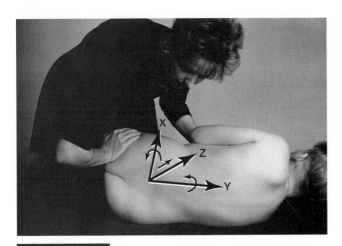

Figure 9.196. Side posture left PIIn push adjustment. The doctor's cephalad (Rt.) adjusting pisiform is placed on the contact site. The stabilization (Lt.) hand will hold the crossed arms of the smaller patient or the anterior shoulder may be contacted. To increase the preload at the joint, the knee is slightly moved forward until tension is felt by the contact hand. Prior to the thrust, a slight release of the knee is made.

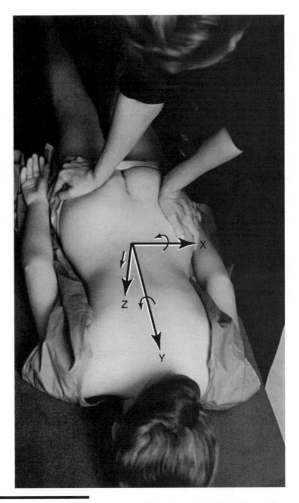

Figure 9.197. Prone right ASIn adjustment. The doctor's cephalad (Rt.) adjusting pisiform is placed on the contact site. The stabilization (Lt.) hand will hold the crossed arms of the smaller patient or the anterior shoulder may be contacted. To increase the preload at the joint, the knee is slightly moved forward until tension is felt by the contact hand. Prior to the thrust, a slight release of the knee is made.

The torque is clockwise for the left ilium (-θY). The thrust is down the shaft of the patient's femur and the towards the pubic symphysis of the doctor.

ASIN ILIUM (RIGHT) PRONE ADJUSTMENT

Name of technique: Gonstead

Name of technique procedure: Prone ASIn ilium push adjustment.

Indications: Right ASIn (+θX, +Z, -θY) subluxation (Fig. 9.197).

Patient position: The patient lies prone on the pelvic or hi-lo table, both arms placed to the side of the patient, over the side of the table or on the hand rests.

Doctor's position: The doctor stands slightly inferior and oblique towards the patient on the contralateral side of the ASIn ilium.

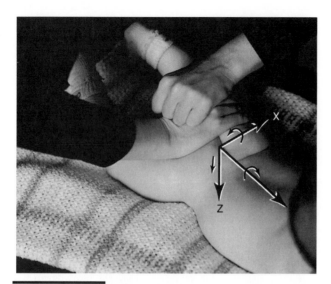

Figure 9.198. Prone right ASEx push adjustment. The doctor places the right thumb or a small pisiform (as shown) on the contact site. The thumb contact should be stabilized with the opposite (Lt.) pisiform resting on top. The pisiform contact can be stabilized two ways: the second hand rests on top of or is wrapped around the wrist of the adjusting hand (as shown) or the stabilization hand is placed on the contralateral PSIS. The doctor's adjusting forearm is vertical and lateral.

Contact site: The location is on the right ischial spine. The stabilization (Lt.) hand will tissue pull superior to inferior and medial to lateral. The heel of the doctor's caudad (Rt.) adjusting hand is placed on the contact site. The smaller patient may be contacted with the caudad (Rt.) pisiform. The stabilization (Lt.) hand is placed on the opposite PSIS. Pattern of thrust: The thrust is inferiorward (-θX), posterior to anterior (+Z), and medial to lateral (+θY).

ASEX ILIUM

The ilium has rotated clockwise around an oblique X-axis. The second component of the listing is external rotation of the PSIS (±θY).

AP AND LATERAL RADIOGRAPH ANALYSIS

A decrease in the long axis length of the innominate is present (see Chapter 8). The AS position decreases the diagonal measurement of the obturator foramen and the "Ex" component increases the width of the base. The AS ilium raises the femoral head height and the Ex lowers it. Depending which listing component predominates, the femoral head height is either raised or lowered. If leg length inequality exists, then the femoral head height will also be influenced by this factor.

CLINICAL FINDINGS

The sacroiliac joint is opened at its posterior inferior aspect with the AS component of the listing. The "Ex" component opens the lower and upper portion of the posterior aspect of the SI joint. Tenderness and edema may be palpated all along

the medial border of the PSIS. The "Ex" may cause internal foot rotation.

Newborn and Infant

ASEX ILIUM (RIGHT) PRONE ADJUSTMENT

Name of technique: Gonstead
Name of technique procedure: Prone ASEx ilium push adjustment.
Indications: Right ASEx (+θX, +Z, -θY) subluxation (Fig. 9.198).
Patient position: The newborn/infant is placed prone across a soft cushioned adjusting table. If the lap of the parent is used, the involved side is towards the doctor.
Doctor's position: The doctor stands on the side contralateral of the listing facing the patient on the adjusting table. If the newborn/infant is on the lap of the parent, the doctor stands facing the ipsilateral side.
Contact site: The lateral right ischial spine. Tissue pull by the stabilization (Lt.) hand is superior to inferior and medialward.
Pattern of thrust: Inferiorward (-θX), slightly posterior to anterior (+Z), and lateral to medial (+θY).

ASEX ILIUM (RIGHT) SIDE POSTURE ADJUSTMENT

Name of technique: Gonstead
Name of technique procedure: Side posture ASEx ilium push adjustment. This patient position is preferred when the AS component predominates.
Indications: Right ASEx (+θX, +Z, -θY) subluxation (Fig. 9.199).
Patient position: The newborn/infant is placed involved side up in the side posture position on the pelvic bench. The parent's lap may be used as an alternative.

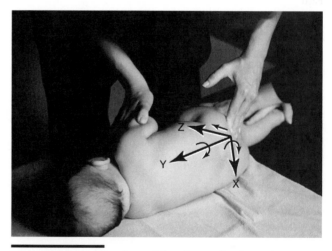

Figure 9.199. The digits of the adjusting hand are placed on the medial aspect of the ischial spine for the ASEx adjustment. The doctor places the small aspect of the caudad (Lt.) adjusting digits (as shown) or pisiform on the contact site. The doctor's adjusting forearm is vertical, slightly inferior and lateral. The stabilization (Rt.) cephalad hand will hold the newborn/infant's crossed arms in front of the patient's chest.

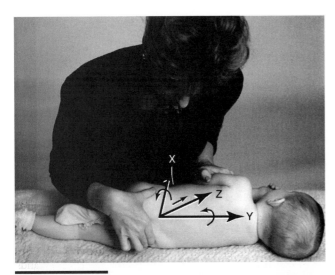

Figure 9.200.   Side posture right ASEx pull adjustment. The doctor raises the involved (Rt.) ilium with the cephalad (Lt.) hand until the distal metacarpals of the caudad (Rt.) adjusting hand can be positioned. Tissue pull by the caudad (Rt.) metacarpals are inferiorward and medial to the rim of the acetabulum. The stabilization cephalad (Lt.) hand will hold the newborn/infant's crossed arms in front of the patient's chest.

Doctor's position: The doctor faces the patient. Depending on the height of the doctor, kneeling may be necessary. The doctor (or assistant) will stabilize the superior leg bent and the inferior leg straight.
Contact site: Slightly medial of the rim of the acetabulum over the right ischial spine. Tissue pull by the stabilization (Lt.) hand is superior to inferior and medialward.
Pattern of thrust: Inferiorward (-θX), slightly posterior to anterior (+Z), and lateral to medial (+θY). The contact hand is torqued clockwise for the right ilium.

ASEX ILIUM (RIGHT) SIDE POSTURE PULL ADJUSTMENT

Name of technique: Gonstead
Name of technique procedure: Side posture ASEx ilium pull move adjustment. This patient position (with the involved side nearest the table-top) is preferred if the Ex component of the listing predominates.
Indications: Right ASEx (+θX, +Z, -θY) subluxation (Fig. 9.200).
Patient position: The newborn/infant is placed with the involved ilium side down in the side posture position on the pelvic bench. The parent's lap may also be used in some incidences.
Doctor's position: The doctor faces the patient. Depending on the height of the doctor, kneeling may be necessary. The doctor (or supportive assistant) will stabilize the superior leg bent and the inferior leg straight.
Contact site: The lateral right ischial spine.
Pattern of thrust: Inferiorward (-θX), slight posterior to anterior (+Z), and lateral to medial (+θY).

Toddler and Pre-Schooler

ASEX ILIUM (RIGHT) SIDE POSTURE ADJUSTMENT

Name of technique: Gonstead
Name of technique procedure: Side posture ASEx ilium push adjustment. This positioning is recommended when the AS component of the listing predominates.
Indications: Right ASEx (-θX, +Z, -θY) subluxation (Fig. 9.201).
Patient position: The toddler/pre-schooler is placed involved side up in the side posture position on the pelvic bench.
Doctor's position: The doctor stands slightly inferior and oblique to the patient. The doctor will straddle the superior bent leg.
Contact site: Slightly medial of the rim over the right ischial spine. Tissue pull by the stabilization hand is superior to inferior and medialward.
Pattern of thrust: Inferiorward (-θX), slight posterior to anterior (+Z), and lateral to medial (+θY) direction with a slight torque. The contact hand is torqued clockwise for the right ilium. There is no body drop.

ASEX ILIUM (RIGHT) SIDE POSTURE PULL ADJUSTMENT

Name of technique: Gonstead
Name of technique procedure: Side posture ASEx ilium pull adjustment. This patient position is recommended when the Ex component of the listing predominates.
Indications: Right ASEx (+θX, +Z, -θY) subluxation (Fig. 9.202).
Patient position: The toddler/pre-schooler is placed in the side posture position on the pelvic bench with the ASEx ilium involved side down.

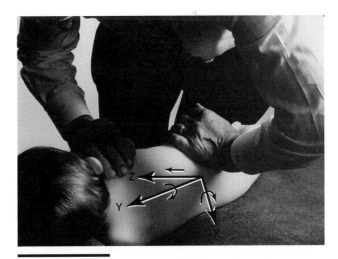

Figure 9.201.   Side posture right ASEx pisiform adjustment. The doctor places the caudad (Lt.) adjusting pisiform on the contact site. The doctor's adjusting forearm is vertical, slightly inferior and lateral. The stabilization (Rt.) cephalad hand will hold the toddler/pre-schooler's crossed arms in front of the patient's chest. The larger child may by stabilized at the anterior shoulder.

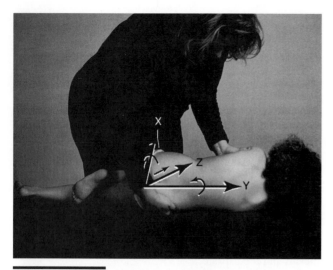

Figure 9.202. Side posture right ASEx pull adjustment. The doctor raises the involved ilium with the cephalad (Lt.) hand until the proximal metacarpals of the caudad (Rt.) adjusting hand can be positioned. Tissue pull by the caudad metacarpals are inferior to medialward to the rim of the acetabulum and lateral to the (Rt.) ischial spine. The stabilization (Lt.) hand will hold the toddler's/pre-schooler's crossed arms in front of the patient's chest. The larger child may be stabilized at the anterior shoulder.

Doctor's position: The doctor stands inferior and at a slightly oblique angle towards the patient. The doctor (or assistant) will stabilize the superior leg bent and the inferior leg straight.

Contact site: Medial to the rim of the acetabulum and lateral to the right ischial spine.

Pattern of thrust: Inferiorward (-θX), slightly posterior to anterior (+Z), and lateral to medial (-θY).

ASEX ILIUM (RIGHT) PRONE ADJUSTMENT

Name of technique: Gonstead

Name of technique procedure: Prone ASEx ilium push adjustment.

Indications: Right ASEx (+θX, +Z, -θY) subluxation (Fig. 9.203).

Patient position: The patient lies prone on a pelvic or hi-lo table, both arms are placed at the sides of the patient, over the side of the table or on the hand rests.

Doctor's position: The doctor stands inferior with a slightly oblique angle towards the contact site on the involved side.

Contact site: The lateral right ischial spine. The ipsilateral ASEx ilium is contacted skin to skin with the heel of the doctor's adjusting (Rt.) hand lateral to the ischial spine.

Pattern of thrust: Inferiorward (-θX), slightly posterior to anterior (+Z), and lateral to medial (-θY).

Pre-adolescent and Adolescent

ASEX ILIUM (LEFT) SIDE POSTURE ADJUSTMENT

Name of technique: Gonstead

Name of technique procedure: Side posture ASEx ilium push

adjustment. This procedure is recommended when the AS is predominate.

Indications: Left ASEx (+θX, +Z, -θY) subluxation (Fig. 9.204).

Patient position: The pre-adolescent/adolescent is placed involved side-up in the side posture position on the pelvic bench.

Doctor's position: The doctor stands slightly inferior and oblique to the patient. The doctor straddles the superior leg and moves it forward until tension is felt under the contact pisiform. Prior to the thrust, a slight release of tension at the leg is made.

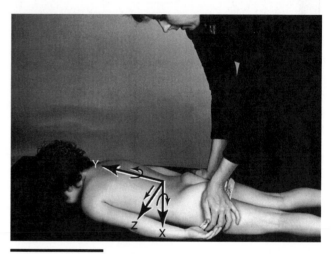

Figure 9.203. Prone ASEx push adjustment. The outside (Rt.) adjusting pisiform is placed on the contact site, the inside (Lt.) hand on the contralateral PSIS.

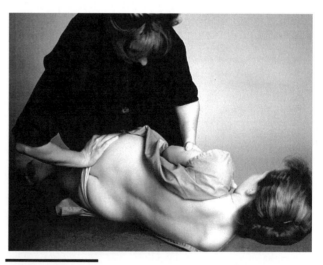

Figure 9.204. Side posture left ASEx ilium adjustment. The doctor places the caudad (Rt.) adjusting pisiform on the contact site. The doctor's adjusting forearm is vertical and lateral. The stabilization cephalad (Lt.) hand will contact the anterior shoulder.

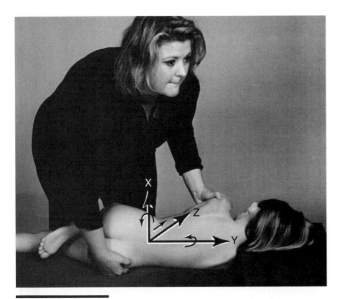

Figure 9.205. Side posture right ASEx pull adjustment. The doctor raises the involved ilium with the cephalad (Lt.) hand so that the caudad (Rt.) adjusting hand can slip under the ilium with the fingers extending around and under the ASIS. The small innominate is contacted by the proximal metacarpals of the caudad hand. Tissue pull by the caudad hand/metacarpals is inferior and medialward to the rim of the acetabulum and lateral to the ischial spine. The stabilization (Lt.) hand will hold the patient's anterior shoulder.

Contact site: Slightly medial of the rim over the left ischial spine. Tissue pull by the stabilization hand is superior to inferior and medialward.

Pattern of thrust: Inferiorward ($-\theta X$), slightly posterior to anterior ($+Z$), and lateral to medial ($+\theta Y$). The contact hand is torqued counterclockwise for the left ilium. There is no body drop.

ASEX ILIUM (RIGHT) SIDE POSTURE PULL ADJUSTMENT

Name of technique: Gonstead

Name of technique procedure: Side posture ASEx ilium pull move adjustment. This patient position is recommended when the Ex component of the listing predominates.

Indications: Right ASEx ($+\theta X$, $+Z$, $+\theta Y$) subluxation (Fig. 9.205).

Patient position: The patient is placed in the side posture position on the pelvic bench with the ASEx ilium involved side down.

Doctor's position: The doctor stands inferior and at a slightly oblique angle towards the patient. The patient's pelvis is stabilized by the doctor resting the caudad knee against the posterior thigh of the patient's bent superior leg.

Contact site: Medial to the rim of the acetabulum and lateral to the right ischial spine.

Pattern of thrust: Posterior to anterior ($+Z$), superior to inferior ($-\theta X$) and lateral to medial ($-\theta Y$). The thrust is performed rapidly by straightening the flexed wrist of the contact hand.

ASEX ILIUM (LEFT) PRONE ADJUSTMENT

Name of technique: Gonstead

Name of technique procedure: Prone ASEx ilium push adjustment.

Indications: Left ASEx ($+\theta X$, $+Z$, $-\theta Y$) subluxation (Fig. 9.206).

Patient position: The patient lies prone on a pelvic or hi-lo table, both arms are placed to the sides of the patient, over the side of the table or on the top of the hand rests.

Doctor's position: The doctor stands inferior with a slightly oblique angle towards the contact site on the involved side.

Contact site: The lateral left ischial spine. The ipsilateral ASEx ilium is contacted skin to skin with the heel of the doctor's outside (Lt.) hand lateral to the ischial spine. The outside (Lt.) adjusting pisiform is placed on the contact site and the inside (Rt.) hand on the contralateral PSIS.

Pattern of thrust: Inferiorward ($-\theta X$), slightly posterior to anterior ($+Z$), and lateral to medial ($+\theta Y$).

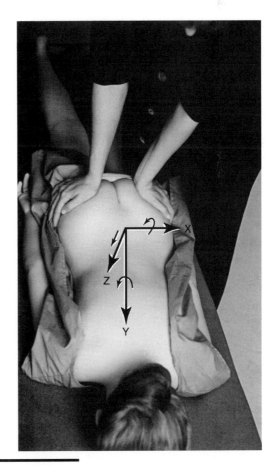

Figure 9.206. Prone left ASEx push adjustment.

IN AND EX SUBLUXATION

The PSIS can rotate laterally or medialward (±θY). The reference point for movement around the Y-axis is the PSIS. An SI joint that is sprained at its anterior aspect is referred to as an "In." If the sprain occurs at the posterior aspect of the SI joint, resulting in an external rotation of the PSIS, then the listing is "Ex." Since both innominates are joined at the symphysis pubis, if one side is In, the other side is Ex. It should be noted that only one of the two ilia is subluxated (i.e., fixated). The other side is considered a compensatory misalignment. Occasionally, a fixation can occur at both SI joints.

AP and Lateral Radiograph Analysis

On the AP projection the vertical height of the innominates from the iliac crest to the ischial tuberosities remains unchanged for both the In and Ex displacements. The AP radiograph may demonstrate that the shapes of the obturator foramenae are altered. The In has a more narrow width at the base of the obturator foramen. The Ex has a wider width at the base. Due to projectional distortion, the femoral head heights may be changed. The femoral head height will be raised with an In and be lowered with an Ex, provided no leg length inequality exists. The In may decrease the lumbar lordosis and the Ex may increase it.

Clinical Findings

The lateral to medial rotation of the In opens the SI joint at the anterior aspect. The tenderness and edema associated with this type of sprain is nonpalpable. The medial to lateral rotation of the Ex opens the joint at its posterior aspect; tenderness and edema are palpated at the posterior upper and lower margins of the joint. The newborn/infant may be held up to observe lower limb rotation associated with different pelvic misalignments. The In will show external lower limb or foot rotation and the lower limb or foot will rotate internally with an Ex ilium. The older patient can be analyzed in the supine position for the presence of foot flare associated with ilium misalignment. The standing position can also be used for the analysis, however foot pronation may also cause external rotation of the foot and must be differentiated. In the prone position, the undiapered infant with an "In" ilium may show a wide and flat gluteus. The Ex creates a narrow width and more protuberant musculature.

Newborn/Infant

IN ILIUM (LEFT) PRONE ADJUSTMENT

Name of technique: Gonstead
Name of technique procedure: Prone In ilium push move adjustment.
Indications: Left In (+θY) ilium (Fig. 9.207).
Patient position: The newborn/infant is placed prone on the pelvic bench. The parent's lap may also be used with the involved side towards the doctor.
Doctor's position: The doctor stands facing the patient. Depending on the height of the doctor, kneeling may be required.

Contact site: The medial border of the left PSIS. Tissue pull is from medial to lateral and is performed by the stabilization (Rt.) hand.
Pattern of thrust: Medial to lateral (-θY) direction.

IN ILIUM (LEFT) SIDE POSTURE PULL ADJUSTMENT

Name of technique: Gonstead
Name of technique procedure: Side posture In ilium finger pull move adjustment.
Indications: Left In (+θY) ilium (Fig. 9.208).
Patient position: The newborn/infant is placed involved side up on the pelvic bench. The parent's lap may be used as a replacement site.
Doctor's position: The doctor stands facing the patient. Depending on the height of the doctor, kneeling may be necessary.
Contact site: The medial border of the left PSIS. Tissue pull is from medial to lateral and is performed by the stabilization (Lt.) hand.
Pattern of thrust: Medial to lateral (-θY) direction.

IN ILIUM (LEFT) SIDE POSTURE ADJUSTMENT

Name of technique: Gonstead
Name of technique procedure: Side posture In ilium push move adjustment.
Indications: Left In (+θY) ilium (Fig. 9.209).
Patient position: The newborn/infant is placed involved side up on the pelvic bench. The parent's lap may be used as an alternative.
Doctor's position: The doctor stands facing the patient. Depending on the height of the doctor, kneeling may be necessary.

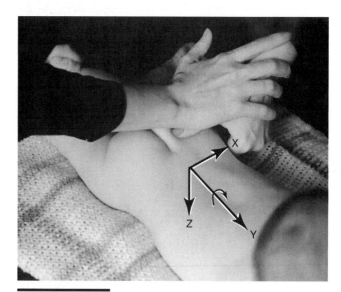

Figure 9.207.   Prone left In thumb push adjustment. The contact thumb (Lt.) is placed on the medial border of the involved (Lt.) PSIS. The stabilization (Rt.) hand will be placed on top of the thumb contact.

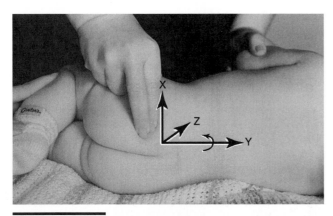

Figure 9.208. Side posture left In finger push adjustment. The second digit (with the third digit placed on top of the nail bed for support) of the caudad (Rt.) adjusting hand is placed on the contact point. The cephalad (Lt.) hand holds the crossed arms of the newborn/infant in front of the chest.

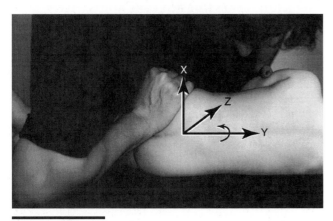

Figure 9.209. Side posture left In push adjustment. The pisiform (smaller handed practitioner) of the caudad (Rt.) adjusting hand is placed on the contact site (as shown). The finger push procedure is recommended for the large-handed practitioner. The cephalad (Lt.) hand holds the crossed arms of the newborn/infant in front of the chest.

Contact site: The medial border of the left PSIS. The tissue pull is from medial to lateral and is performed by the stabilization (Lt.) hand.
Pattern of thrust: Medial to lateral (-θY) direction.

Toddler and Pre-Schooler

IN ILIUM (LEFT) SIDE POSTURE PULL ADJUSTMENT

Name of technique: Gonstead
Name of technique procedure: Side posture In ilium finger pull move adjustment.
Indications: Left In (+θY) ilium (Fig. 9.210).
Patient position: The toddler/pre-schooler is placed involved side up on the pelvic bench.

Doctor's position: The doctor stands slightly inferior towards the patient. The doctor may straddle the superior bent leg or use supportive assistance.
Contact site: The medial border of the left PSIS. The tissue pull is from medial to lateral and is performed with the stabilization (Lt.) hand.
Pattern of thrust: Medial to lateral (-θY) direction.

IN ILIUM (RIGHT) SIDE POSTURE ADJUSTMENT

Name of technique: Gonstead
Name of technique procedure: Side posture In ilium push move adjustment.
Indications: Right In (-θY) ilium (Fig. 9.211).
Patient position: The toddler/pre-schooler is placed involved side up on the pelvic bench.
Doctor's position: The doctor stands slightly inferior towards the patient. The doctor may straddle the superior bent leg or use supportive assistance.
Contact site: The medial border of the right PSIS. The tissue pull is from medial to lateral and is performed by the stabilization (Rt.) hand.
Pattern of thrust: Medial to lateral (+θY) direction.

Pre-Adolescent and Adolescent

IN ILIUM (LEFT) SIDE POSTURE PULL ADJUSTMENT

Name of technique: Gonstead
Name of technique procedure: Side posture In ilium finger pull move adjustment.
Indications: Left In (-θY) ilium (Fig. 9.212).

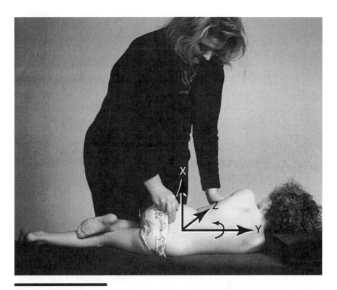

Figure 9.210. Side posture left In finger push adjustment. The second and third digit of the caudad (Rt.) hand is placed side by side on the contact site. The cephalad (Lt.) hand holds the crossed arms of the toddler/pre-schooler in front of the chest. The parent may stabilize the superior leg bent and the inferior leg straight.

Patient position: The patient is placed involved side up on the pelvic bench.

Doctor's position: The doctor stands inferior and slightly oblique, facing the patient and straddles the superior bent leg. On the larger patient or in the case of a smaller doctor, the doctor must straighten their posture upright to position the adjusting forearm for the line of correction.

Contact site: The medial border of the left PSIS. The tissue pull is from medial to lateral and is performed with the stabilization (Lt.) hand.

Pattern of thrust: Medial to lateral (–θY) direction.

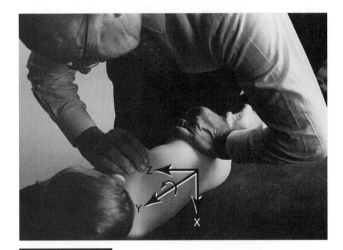

Figure 9.211. Side posture right In push adjustment. The caudad (Lt.) adjusting pisiform of the small-handed doctor is placed on the contact site (as shown). The finger push procedure is recommended for the large-handed practitioner. The cephalad (Rt.) hand holds the crossed arms of the toddler/pre-schooler in front of the chest.

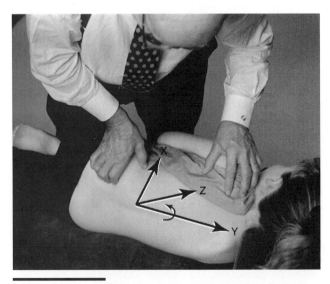

Figure 9.212. Side posture left In pull adjustment. The second digit, and the third digit of the caudad (Rt.) hand, are placed side by side on the contact site. The cephalad (Lt.) hand holds the crossed arms of the smaller patient in front of the chest.

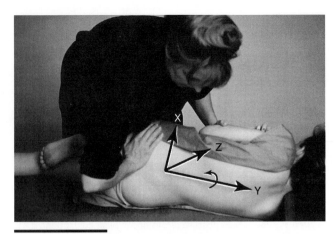

Figure 9.213. Side posture left In push adjustment. The pisiform of the caudad (Rt.) adjusting hand is placed on the contact site. The cephalad (Lt.) hand holds the crossed arms of the smaller patient in front of the chest.

IN ILIUM (LEFT) SIDE POSTURE ADJUSTMENT

Name of technique: Gonstead

Name of technique procedure: Side posture In ilium push move adjustment.

Indications: Left In (+θY) ilium (Fig. 9.213).

Patient position: The patient is placed involved side up on the pelvic bench.

Doctor's position: The doctor stands inferior and slightly oblique towards the patient. The doctor straddles the superior bent leg.

Contact site: The medial border of the left PSIS. The tissue pull is from medial to lateral and is performed with the stabilization (Lt.) hand.

Pattern of thrust: Medial to lateral (–θY) direction.

Newborn and Infant

EX ILIUM (RIGHT) PRONE ADJUSTMENT

Name of technique: Gonstead

Name of technique procedure: Prone Ex ilium push adjustment.

Indications: Right Ex (–θY) subluxation (Fig. 9.214).

Patient position: The newborn/infant is placed prone on the pelvic bench. The lap of the parent may also be chosen.

Doctor's position: The doctor faces the patient on the ipsilateral side of the listing.

Contact site: The lateral border of the right PSIS.

Pattern of thrust: Lateral to medial (+θY).

EX ILIUM (RIGHT) SIDE POSTURE PULL ADJUSTMENT

Name of technique: Gonstead

Name of technique procedure: Side posture Ex ilium pull adjustment.

Indications: Right Ex (–θY) subluxation (Fig. 9.215).

Patient position: The newborn/infant is placed involved side down in the side posture position on the pelvic bench.

Doctor's position: Facing the patient.

Contact site: The lateral border of the right PSIS.
Pattern of thrust: Lateral to medial (−θY).

Toddler and Pre-Schooler

EX ILIUM (RIGHT) SIDE POSTURE PULL ADJUSTMENT

Name of technique: Gonstead
Name of technique procedure: Side posture Ex ilium pull adjustment.
Indications: Right Ex (−θY) subluxation (Fig. 9.216).
Patient position: The toddler/pre-schooler is placed involved side down in the side posture position on the pelvic bench.

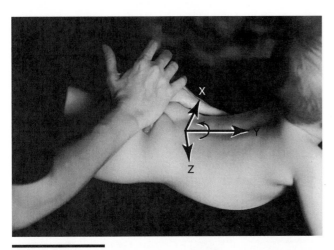

Figure 9.214.   Prone right Ex thumb push adjustment. The contact (Lt.) thumb is placed on the contact site. The pisiform of the stabilization (Rt.) hand is placed on the adjusting hand thumb.

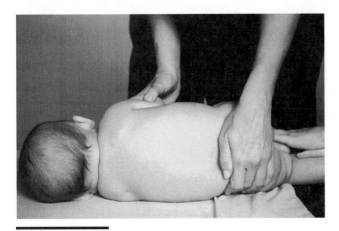

Figure 9.215.   Side posture right Ex pull adjustment. The doctor raises the involved (Rt.) ilium with the cephalad (Lt.) hand until the proximal metacarpals of the caudad (Rt.) adjusting hand have been positioned on the contact site. The ilium is lowered after the contact has been established. Tissue pull by the caudad (Rt.) metacarpals is inferior to superior and medialward to the right PSIS. The cephalad (Lt.) hand will hold the crossed arms of the patient in front of the chest.

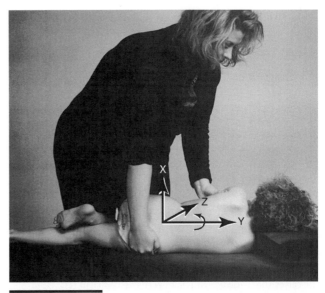

Figure 9.216.   Side posture right Ex pull adjustment. The doctor raises the involved (Rt.) ilium with the cephalad (Lt.) hand until the proximal metacarpals of the caudad (Rt.) hand have been positioned on the contact site. The small-handed doctor may use the distal metacarpals on the contact site. The ilium is lowered after the contact has been established. Tissue pull by the caudad (Rt.) metacarpals is inferior to superior and medialward to the right PSIS. The cephalad hand will hold the crossed arms of the patient in front of the chest.

Doctor's position: The doctor stands slightly inferior and towards the patient.
Contact site: The lateral border of the right PSIS.
Pattern of thrust: Lateral to medial (−θY).

Pre-Adolescent and Adolescent

EX ILIUM (RIGHT) SIDE POSTURE PULL ADJUSTMENT

Name of technique: Gonstead
Name of technique procedure: Side posture Ex ilium pull adjustment.
Indications: Right Ex (−θY) subluxation (Fig. 9.217).
Patient position: The patient is placed involved side down in the side posture position on the pelvic bench.
Doctor's position: The doctor stands slightly inferior and towards the patient. The lower body is stabilized by a gentle, but a definite contact by the doctor's knee against the posterior thigh of the patient. No thrust is given by the doctor's knee during the thrust.
Contact site: The lateral border of the right PSIS.
Pattern of thrust: Lateral to medial (+θY). The thrust is accomplished by extending the flexed wrist of the contact hand.

IN-EX ILIUM

Occasionally both ilia can be subluxated and fixated. Any combination of listings can result, but the most common dual

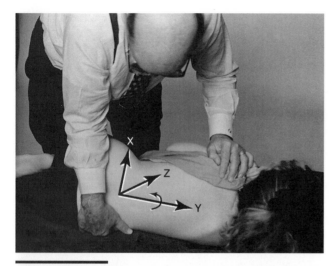

Figure 9.217. Side posture right Ex pull adjustment. The doctor raises the involved (Rt.) ilium with the cephalad (Lt.) hand until the distal metacarpals of the caudad (Rt.) adjusting hand have been positioned at the contact site. The ilium is lowered after the contact has been established. Tissue pull by the caudad (Rt.) metacarpals is inferior to superior and medialward on the right PSIS. The cephalad (Lt.) hand is placed on the anterior shoulder. The smaller patient can be stabilized by holding the crossed arms of the patient in front of her chest.

subluxation is the In-Ex. There is usually no axial rotation of the lumbar spine present. When a bilateral subluxation occurs, both listings are recorded, the left listing first, followed by a hyphen before the right listing.

AP and Lateral Radiograph Analysis

On the AP projection the vertical heights of the innominates from the iliac crests to the ischial tuberosities are unchanged. Further the lumbar spine will reveal no Y-axis rotation. The iliac widths (the alae) will change. The In will have an increased width; the Ex, a decreased width. The obturator foramen will project a more narrow width at the base for the In and a larger width for the Ex.

Newborn and Infant

EX-IN ILIA SIDE POSTURE PULL/PUSH ADJUSTMENT

Name of technique: Gonstead
Name of technique procedure: Side posture In-Ex ilium pull adjustment. This subluxation component is rare with the newborn/infant.
Indications: EX-IN (±θY) subluxation (Fig. 9.218).
Patient position: The newborn/infant lies in the side posture position on the pelvic bench. The In ilium is on the high side, the Ex is on the down side.
Doctor's position: The doctor faces towards the newborn/infant.
Contact site: The lateral border of the left PSIS on the Ex ilium. The medial border of the right PSIS on the In ilium.

Pattern of thrust: Simultaneous bilateral movement; lateral to medial (-θY) on the Ex ilium and medial to lateral (+θY) on the In ilium. The thrust is directed through the oblique orientation of the sacroiliac joints.

Toddler and Pre-Schooler

EX-IN ILIA SIDE POSTURE PULL/PUSH ADJUSTMENT

Name of technique: Gonstead
Name of technique procedure: Side posture Ex-In ilium pull adjustment.
Indications: Ex-In (±θY) subluxation (Fig. 9.219).
Patient position: The toddler/pre-schooler lies in the side posture position on the pelvic bench. The In ilium is on the high side, the Ex is on the down side.
Doctor's position: The doctor stands facing the patient. The doctor's caudad knee is raised and rested against the posterior thigh of the patient's bent superior leg. This will help stabilize the patient's pelvis. No thrust is given by the doctor's knee.
Contact site: The lateral border of the left PSIS on the Ex ilium. The medial border of the right PSIS on the In ilium.
Pattern of thrust: Simultaneous bilateral movement; lateral to medial (+θY) on the Ex ilium and medial to lateral (+θY) on the In ilium. The thrust is directed through the sacroiliac joints by the distal and proximal metacarpals (smaller patient) or the pisiform and forearm (larger patient), to achieve a simultaneous bilateral correction of the Ex and In ilia.

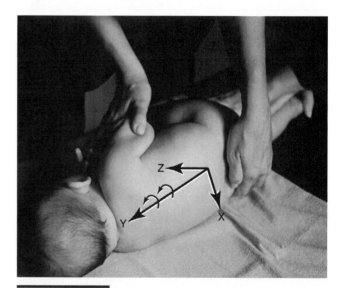

Figure 9.218. Side posture Ex-In ilium adjustment. The doctor's cephalad (Rt.) hand raises the patient's pelvis to enable the distal metacarpals of the caudad (Lt.) adjusting hand to contact the lateral border of the left PSIS of the Ex ilium. The ilium is lowered. The proximal metacarpals contact the medial border of the right PSIS of the In ilium. The stabilization (Rt.) hand will hold the crossed arms of the newborn/infant in front of the chest. The parent should stabilize the superior bent leg and the inferior leg straight.

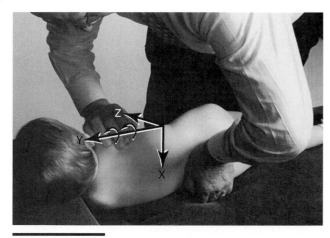

Figure 9.219. Side posture Ex-In ilium adjustment. The doctor's cephalad (Rt.) hand raises the patient's pelvis to enable the distal metacarpals of the caudad (Lt.) adjusting hand to contact the lateral border of the left PSIS of the Ex ilium. The ilium is lowered. The proximal metacarpals contact the medial border of the right PSIS of the In ilium. For the larger patient, a contact is made by the caudad (Lt.) pisiform on the lateral border of the left PSIS on the Ex ilium, the doctor's caudad (Lt.) forearm contacts the medial border of the right PSIS of the In ilium. The stabilization (Rt.) hand contacts the anterior shoulder of the larger patient.

Pre-Adolescent and Adolescent

IN-EX ILIA SIDE POSTURE PULL/PUSH ADJUSTMENT

Name of technique: Gonstead
Name of technique procedure: Side posture In-Ex ilium pull/push adjustment.
Indications: In–Ex (±θY) subluxation (Fig. 9.220).
Patient position: The pre-adolescent/adolescent lies in the side posture position on the pelvic bench. The In ilium is on the high side, the Ex is on the down side.
Doctor's position: The doctor stands facing the patient. The doctor's caudad knee is raised and rested against the posterior thigh of the patient's bent superior leg. This will help stabilize the patient's pelvis. No thrust is given by the doctor's knee.
Contact site: The lateral border of the right PSIS on the Ex ilium. The medial border of the left PSIS on the In ilium.
Pattern of thrust: Simultaneous bilateral movement; lateral to medial (-θY) of the Ex ilium and medial to lateral (-θY) of the In ilium. The thrust is directed through the sacroiliac joints by the distal and proximal metacarpals (smaller patient) or the pisiform and forearm (larger patient), to achieve a simultaneous bilateral correction of the Ex and In ilia.

The sacrum can subluxate at the level of the lumbosacral junction (i.e., base posterior), at the sacroiliac articulations (rotated sacrum, P-L or P-R), or at the segmental level within an unfused sacrum (i.e., posterior S2 or S3). The posterior (-Z) sacral segment (e.g., S2, S3, S4) is a commonly overlooked subluxation. The toddler or pre-schooler who is not closely monitored/examined/treated during their early years, may develop a permanent deformity of the sacrum due to compression trauma and the resultant intersegmental subluxation.

AP and Lateral Radiograph Analysis

For the rotated sacrum (i.e., P-L or P-R), the width of the lateral border of the sacrum is increased on the side of posterior rotation (see Chapter 8). The lower lumbar spine will usually rotate in the same direction as the rotated sacrum. On the lateral radiograph, the intersegmental sacral subluxation will demonstrate varying degrees of retrolisthesis and/or widening

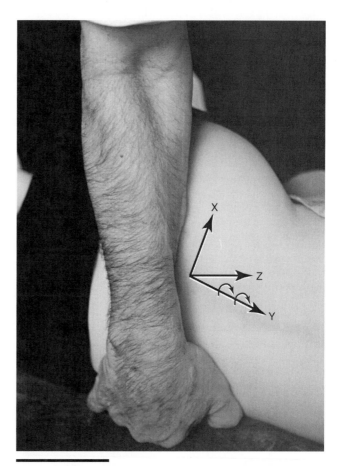

Figure 9.220. Side posture In-Ex pull adjustment. The doctor's cephalad (Lt.) hand raises the patient's pelvis to enable the distal metacarpals of the caudad (Rt.) adjusting hand to contact the lateral border of the PSIS of the right Ex ilium. The ilium is lowered. The proximal metacarpals contact the medial border of the PSIS of the left In ilium. The larger patient is contacted by the caudad (Rt.) pisiform on the lateral border of the right PSIS on the Ex ilium and the doctor's caudad (Rt.) forearm contacts the medial border of the left PSIS of the In ilium. The stabilization (Lt.) hand contacts the anterior shoulder of the larger patient.

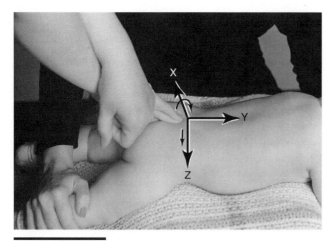

Figure 9.221. Prone posterior sacral push adjustment. Depending on the size of the sacral segment and doctor's contact (Lt.) hand, the smallest distal digit (e.g., fifth, second) is placed on the sacral segment. The thumb contact may be used if the sacral segment is larger or the doctor's thumb is small. Depending on the amount of depth necessary, the doctor will stabilize with the distal end of the opposite digit (e.g., fifth, second, thumb) and place it on the nail bed of the adjusting digit. The doctor's forearms should follow the plane line of correction for the involved joint.

of the posterior aspect of the rudimentary joint space. Occasionally, in the unfused sacrum, there may be a displacement in the sagittal plane (i.e., retrolisthesis) combined with Y-axis rotation at the SI joint.

Clinical Findings

Static palpation will generally demonstrate tenderness and edema along the posterior side of Y-axis rotation. Restriction of motion in the sacroiliac joint on the side of sacral posteriority should also be present. Inspection can sometimes reveal prominence of the lateral border of the sacrum on the side of posterior rotation.

The newborn/infant is palpated for posteriority of a sacral segment in the prone position. The doctor places the distal end of the palpating digit on the sacral tubercle. Tenderness (i.e., flinching of the patient) or edema may be palpated at the level of the sacral tubercle. Skin temperature asymmetry at the level of the sacral segments (e.g., S1-S2, S2-S3, S3-S4) may also be present.

Newborn/Infant

S2 POSTERIOR PRONE ADJUSTMENT

Name of technique: Gonstead
Name of technique procedure: Prone sacral push adjustment.
Indications: Posterior (P, -Z) sacral segment subluxation (Fig. 9.221).
Patient position: The newborn/infant is placed prone across the lap of the parent or on the pelvic table. Depending on the height of the doctor, kneeling may be required.
Doctor's position: The doctor stands inferiorward facing towards the patient for the posterior listing.

Contact site: The involved sacral segment (e.g. S2) for the posterior (P) listing. The tissue pull is performed by the stabilization hand from inferior to superior.
Pattern of thrust: The "P": listing is corrected with a posterior to anterior vector.

ROTATED SACRUM (P-L) PRONE ADJUSTMENT

Name of technique: Gonstead
Name of technique procedure: Prone sacral push adjustment.
Indications: P-L ($+\theta Y$) sacral subluxations (Fig. 9.222).
Patient position: The newborn/infant is placed prone across the lap of the parent or on the pelvic table. Depending on the height of the doctor, kneeling may be required.
Doctor's position: The doctor stands on the side of sacral rotation facing towards the patient.
Contact site: The rotated left sacral ala segment is contacted. Tissue pull is performed by the stabilization (Rt.) hand from inferior to superior and medial to lateral.
Pattern of thrust: Posterior to anterior ($+Z$) (along the oblique orientation of the SI joint) and slightly medial to lateral ($-\theta Y$).

S2 POSTERIOR SIDE POSTURE ADJUSTMENT

Name of technique: Gonstead
Name of technique procedure: Side posture sacral finger push adjustment. Indications: P ($-Z$) second sacral segment subluxation (Fig. 9.223).
Patient position: The newborn/infant is placed either side up in the side posture position on the pelvic bench.
Doctor's position: The doctor adopts the side posture position for the pelvic bench.
Contact site: The second sacral tubercle. The tissue pull is

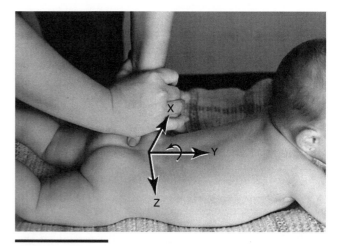

Figure 9.222. Prone P-L sacral push adjustment. Depending on the sizes of the sacral segment and doctor's hand, the smallest distal digit (e.g., fifth, second) is placed on the contact site (sacral ala). The adjusting (Lt.) thumb contact (as shown) may be used if the sacral ala is larger or the doctor's thumb is small. Depending on the amount of depth necessary, the doctor will stabilize with the distal end of the opposite (Rt.) pisiform or digit (e.g., fifth, second, thumb) and place it on the nail bed of the adjusting digit. The doctor's forearms should follow the oblique plane line of correction for the involved joint.

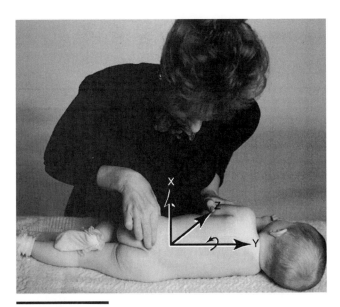

Figure 9.223.   Side posture posterior sacral finger push adjustment. The caudad (Rt.) second digit (supported by the third digit on the nail bed) on the second sacral tubercle. The thumb contact may be used if the sacral tubercle is larger or the doctor's thumb is small. The doctor's forearm should follow the plane line of correction for the involved joint. The cephalad (Lt.) hand holds the cross arms in front of the chest.

performed by the stabilization (Lt.) hand from inferior to superior.

Pattern of thrust: Posterior to anterior (+Z).

Toddler and Pre-Schooler

S2 POSTERIOR PRONE ADJUSTMENT

Name of technique: Gonstead
Name of technique procedure: Prone sacral push adjustment.
Indications: Posterior second sacral segment subluxation (Fig. 9.224).
Patient position: The toddler/pre-schooler is placed prone on the pelvic or hi-lo table, both arms placed to the sides of the patient, over the side of the table, or hands on top of the hand rests.
Doctor's position: The doctor stands inferior facing (cephalad) towards the patient.
Contact site: The second sacral tubercle. The tissue pull is performed by the stabilization hand from inferior to superior.
Pattern of thrust: Posterior to anterior (+Z).

ROTATED SACRUM (P-L) PRONE ADJUSTMENT

Name of technique: Gonstead
Name of technique procedure: Prone sacral push adjustment.
Indications: P-L (-Z, +θY) second sacral segment subluxation (Fig. 9.225).
Patient position: The toddler/pre-schooler is placed prone on the pelvic or hi-lo table, both arms are placed to the sides of the patient, over the side of the table, or on top of the hand rests.
Doctor's position: The doctor stands on the contralateral side facing towards the patient.

Contact site: The left second sacral ala. The tissue pull is performed by the stabilization hand from inferior to superior and medial to lateral.
Pattern of thrust: Posterior to anterior (along the oblique SI joint plane) (+Z) and slightly medial to lateral (-θY).

S2 POSTERIOR SIDE POSTURE ADJUSTMENT

Name of technique: Gonstead
Name of technique procedure: Side posture sacral thumb or finger push adjustment.
Indications: P (-Z), second sacral segment subluxation (Fig. 9.226).
Patient position: The toddler/pre-schooler is placed either side up in the side posture position on the pelvic bench.

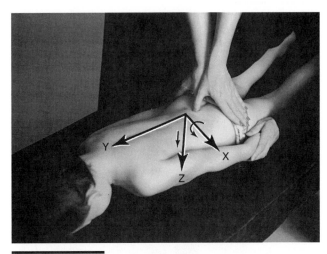

Figure 9.224.   Prone posterior sacral push adjustment. The adjusting thumb contacts the S2 tubercle. The doctor's stabilization thumb (as shown) or pisiform will be placed on the nail bed of the adjusting digit. The doctor's forearms should follow the plane line of correction for the involved joint.

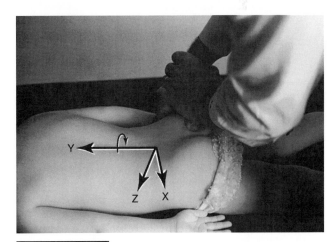

Figure 9.225.   Prone P-R sacral push adjustment. The right adjusting thumb is placed on the contact site. The doctor's stabilization thumb or (Lt.) pisiform (as shown) will be placed on the nail bed of the adjusting digit. The doctor's forearms should follow the oblique plane line of correction for the involved joint.

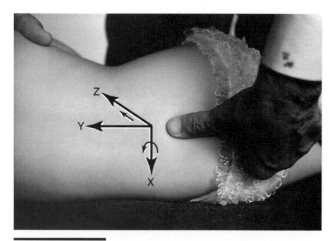

Figure 9.226. Side posture posterior sacral thumb adjustment. The caudad (Lt.) thumb (as shown) or second digit (supported by the third digit on the nail bed) on the second sacral segment. The doctor's forearm should follow the plane line of correction for the involved joint. The cephalad (Rt.) hand holds the crossed arms in front of the chest. The larger patient may be stabilized at the anterior shoulder.

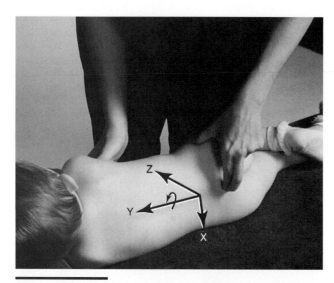

Figure 9.227. Side posture P-L sacral finger push adjustment. The left second digit, supported by the third digit on the nail bed (as shown) or caudad thumb on the right second sacral ala. The doctor's forearm should follow the plane line of correction for the involved joint. The cephalad (Rt.) hand holds the crossed arms in front of the chest. The larger patient may be stabilized at the anterior shoulder.

Doctor's position: The doctor adopts the side posture position for the pelvic bench. The doctor will straddle the superior bent leg.
Contact site: The second sacral tubercle for the posterior (P) listing. The tissue pull is performed by the stabilization hand from inferior to superior.
Pattern of thrust: Posterior to anterior (+Z).

ROTATED SACRUM (P-R) SIDE POSTURE ADJUSTMENT

Name of technique: Gonstead
Name of technique procedure: Side posture sacral finger push adjustment.
Indications: P-R (-θY) sacrum subluxation (Fig. 9.227).
Patient position: The toddler/pre-schooler is placed involved side up in the side posture position on the pelvic bench.
Doctor's position: The doctor adopts the side posture position for the pelvic bench. The doctor will straddle the superior bent leg.
Contact site: The right second sacral ala. The tissue pull is performed by the stabilization hand from inferior to superior and medial to lateral.
Pattern of thrust: Posterior to anterior (+Z) and slightly medial to lateral (+θY).

Pre-Adolescent/Adolescent

S2 POSTERIOR SIDE POSTURE ADJUSTMENT

Name of technique: Gonstead
Name of technique procedure: Side posture sacral pisiform push adjustment.
Indications: P (-Z) intersegmental sacral subluxation (Fig. 9.228).
Patient position: The pre-adolescent/adolescent is placed either side up in the side posture position on the pelvic bench.
Doctor's position: The doctor adopts the side posture position for the pelvic bench. The doctor will straddle the superior bent leg.
Contact site: The second sacral tubercle. The tissue pull is performed by the stabilization hand from inferior to superior.

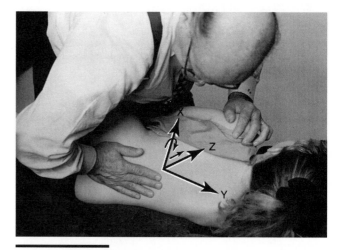

Figure 9.228. Side posture posterior sacral push adjustment. The larger patient is contacted by the right pisiform (as shown) or thenar on the second sacral tubercle. For the smaller patient (or large-handed doctor) the caudad (Rt.) second digit, supported by the third digit on the nail bed is placed on the contact site. The direction of the fingers of the pisiform for the posterior listing is cephalad. The doctor's forearm should follow the plane line of correction for the involved joint. The cephalad (Lt.) hand contacts the anterior shoulder.

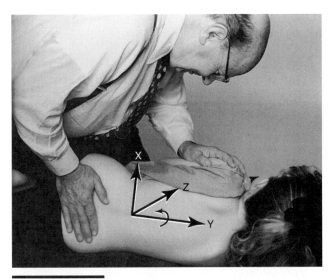

Figure 9.229. Side posture P-L sacral push adjustment. The larger patient is contacted by the (Rt.) pisiform (as shown) or thenar on the left sacral ala. For the smaller patient (or large hand doctor) the caudad (Rt.) second digit, supported by the third digit on the nail bed is placed on the left sacral ala. The direction of the fingers of the pisiform set-up should be towards the table, resting across the sacrum and the contralateral ilium. The doctor's forearm should follow the oblique plane line of correction for the involved joint. The cephalad (Lt.) hand contacts the anterior shoulder.

Pattern of thrust: For the P listing, the thrust is posterior to anterior (+Z). To improve the line of correction, the doctor leans over the patient to lower the elbow to the level of the plane of the sacroiliac joint.

ROTATED SACRUM (P-L) SIDE POSTURE ADJUSTMENT

Name of technique: Gonstead
Name of technique procedure: Side posture sacral pisiform push adjustment.
Indications: P-L ($+\theta Y$) rotated sacrum subluxation (Fig. 9.229).
Patient position: The pre-adolescent/adolescent is placed involved side up in the side posture position on the pelvic bench.
Doctor's position: The doctor adopts the side posture position for the pelvic bench. The doctor will straddle the superior bent leg.
Contact site: The left sacral ala. The tissue pull is performed by the stabilization hand from inferior to superior and medial to lateral.
Pattern of thrust: Posterior to anterior (+Z) and slightly medial to lateral ($-\theta Y$). To improve the line of correction, the doctor leans over the patient to lower the elbow to the level of the plane of the sacroiliac joint.

S2 POSTERIOR PRONE ADJUSTMENT

Name of technique: Gonstead
Name of technique procedure: Prone sacral push adjustment.

Indications: Posterior (-Z) sacral segment subluxation (Fig. 9.230).
Patient position: The patient is placed prone on the pelvic or hi-lo table with both arms placed to the sides of the patient, hanging over the side of the table or on top of the hand rests.
Doctor's position: The doctor stands inferior and slightly oblique towards the patient.
Contact site: The involved sacral tubercle for the posterior (P) listing. The tissue pull is performed by the stabilization hand from inferior to superior.
Pattern of thrust: For the P listing, the thrust is posterior to anterior (+Z).

Coccyx

Due to a fall onto an uneven surface, the coccyx can subluxate with its apex moving anteriorward ($-\theta X$). If the injuring vector is more oblique, the apex may be shifted to the right (AR) ($-\theta X, -\theta Z$) or left (AR) ($-\theta X, +\theta Z$).

AP and Lateral Radiograph

The lateral radiograph should demonstrate that the apex of the coccyx has subluxated anteriorward. Fracture in the region should be differentiated. The AP view may show the apex of the coccyx deviated to the right or left.

Clinical Findings

The most common cause of coccyx subluxation is trauma from a fall onto the buttocks. Often severe pain is manifested in the region. The pain may be aggravated when the patient rises from a seated position, sits or upon defecation. Palpation should reveal marked tenderness and edema at the level of the sacro–coccygeal joint.

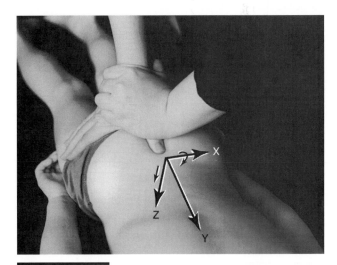

Figure 9.230. Prone posterior sacral push adjustment. The right pisiform or thumb (as shown) is placed on the contact site. The doctor's stabilization (Lt.) hand will rest on top or wrapped around the adjusting hand. The doctor's forearms should follow the plane line of correction for the involved joint.

Newborn/Infant or Toddler/Preschooler

COCCYX ANTERIOR PRONE ADJUSTMENT

Name of technique: Gonstead
Name of technique procedure: Prone coccyx pull/thrust adjustment.
Indications: A (-θX) coccyx (Fig. 9.231).
Patient position: The newborn/infant is placed prone on the lap of the parent. The pelvic table may be selected.
Doctor's position: Inferior to the contact site. For the A listing, the doctor may stand to either side.
Contact site: Slightly inferior to the sacrococcygeal junction. To reduce slippage, a thin cotton fabric (not a diaper) separates

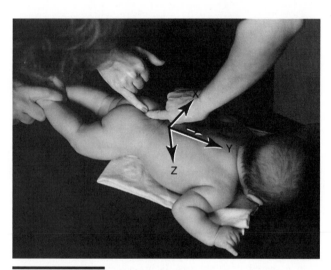

Figure 9.231. Prone anterior coccyx pull/thrust adjustment. The left fifth (as shown) or second digit is placed on the contact site. The doctor must determine which aspect of the stabilization (Rt.) hand (e.g., thumb, pisiform) will be placed on the nail bed of the contact site.

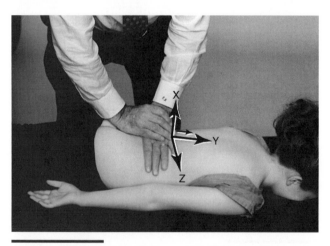

Figure 9.232. Prone anterior coccyx pull/thrust adjustment. The left thumb (as shown) or second digit is placed on the contact site. The doctor's stabilization (Rt.) pisiform is placed on the nail bed or slightly above on the contact thumb.

the digit and patient's skin. The stabilization hand may be used to apply slight pressure from posterior to anterior and inferior to superior.
Pattern of thrust: The movement is a pull thrust from inferior to superior (+θX).

COCCYX ANTERIOR AND LATERALLY FLEXED PRONE ADJUSTMENT

Name of technique: Gonstead
Name of technique procedure: Prone coccyx pull/thrust adjustment.
Indications: AL or AR (-θX, ±θZ) coccyx (not shown).
Patient position: The newborn/infant is placed prone on the lap of the parent. The pelvic table may also be used.
Doctor's position: Inferior to the contact site. The doctor stands on the side of lateral deviation (±θZ).
Contact site: Slightly inferior to the sacrococcygeal junction. To reduce slippage, a thin cotton fabric (not a diaper) separates the digit and patient's skin. The stabilization hand may be used to apply slight pressure from posterior to anterior and inferior to superior. The skin is distracted in such a way as to pull the sacrococcygeal ligament at its left lateral aspect (AR subluxation).
Adjusting and stabilization hand contact: The fifth or second digit is placed on the contact site. The doctor must determine which aspect of the stabilization hand (e.g., thumb, pisiform) is placed on the nail bed of the contact site.
Pattern of thrust: The movement is a pull from inferior to superior (+θX).
Contraindication for the thrust: The newborn/infant is unable to be stabilized in the prone position.

Pre-Adolescent and Adolescent

COCCYX ANTERIOR PRONE ADJUSTMENT

Name of technique: Gonstead
Name of technique procedure: Prone coccyx pull/thrust adjustment.
Indications: A (-θX) coccyx (Fig. 9.232).
Patient position: The patient is placed prone on the pelvic or hi-lo table. A pillow is placed under the pelvis, or the pelvic piece is raised to elevate the coccyx.
Doctor's position: Inferior to the contact site. The doctor stands to either side.
Contact site: Slightly inferior to the sacrococcygeal junction. To reduce slippage, a thin cotton fabric separates the digit and patient's skin. The stabilization hand applies slight pressure from posterior to anterior and inferior to superior.
Pattern of thrust: The movement is a pull from inferior to superior (+θX).

REFERENCES

1. Smith R. Where is the wisdom? The poverty of medical evidence. Br Med J 1991; 303:798-799.
2. Zimmerman AW, Kumar AJ, Gadoth N, Hodges FJ. Traumatic vertebrobasilar occlusive disease in childhood. Neurology 1978; 28:185-8.
3. Graham JM. Smith's recognizable patterns of human deformation. 2nd ed. Philadelphia: WB Saunders, 1988.
4. Dunne KB, Clarren SK. The origin of prenatal and postnatal deformities. Pediatric Clin North Am 1986;33:1277-1297.

5. Anrig C. Chiropractic approaches to pregnancy and pediatric care. In: Plaugher G, ed. Textbook of clinical chiropractic: a specific biomechanical approach. Baltimore: Williams & Wilkins, 1993:383-432.

6. Dunn PM. Congenital postural deformities. Br Med Bull 1976;32:71-76.

7. Paulson J. Accidental injuries. In: Behrman R, Vaughan VC, Nelson WE, eds. Nelson textbook of pediatrics, 13th ed. Philadelphia: WB Saunders, 1987:211-214.

8. Leventhal HR. Birth injuries of the spinal cord. J Pediatrics 1960;56:447-453.

9. Byers RK. Spinal-cord injuries during birth. Develop Med Child Neurol 1975;17:103-110.

10. Towbin A. Latent spinal cord and brain stem injury in newborn infants. Develop Med Child Neurol 1969;11:54-68.

11. Hinwood JA, Hinwood JA. Children and chiropractic: a summary of subluxation and its ramifications. J Aust Chiro Assoc 1981;11:18-21.

12. Patient educational brochure, "Back to sleep". Dept. of Health & Human Services, Bethesda MD, 1995.

13. NEISS Special study. U.S. Consumer Product Safety Commission, Directorate Epidemiology, Division of Hazard Analysis, Wash. D.C., April-December 1988.

14. Menkes JH, Batzdorf J. Postnatal trauma and injuries by physical agents. In: Menkes JH, ed. Textbook of child neurology. 3rd ed. Philadelphia: Lea & Febiger, 1985:493-496.

15. Educational literature. Washington, DC: National Head Injury Foundation, 1991.

16. Fielding JW. Cervical spine injuries in children. In: Sherk HH, Dunn EF, Eismont FJ, eds. The cervical spine. 2nd ed. Philadelphia: JB Lippincott, 1989;199:422-435.

17. Pang D, Wilberger JE. Spinal cord injury without radiographic abnormalities in children. J Neurosurg 1982; 57:114-129.

18. Lewit K. Manipulative therapy in rehabilitation of the locomotor system. London: Butterworth & Co, Ltd., 1985:23-29.

19. Kirkaldy-Willis WH. Managing low back pain. New York: Churchill and Livingstone, 1983:82.

20. Lopes MA, Plaugher G, Walters P, Cremata E. Spinal examination. In: Plaugher G, ed. Textbook of clinical chiropractic: a specific biomechanical approach. Baltimore: Williams & Wilkins, 1993:73-111.

21. Haas M. The physics of spinal manipulation. Part I. The myth of F=ma. J Manipulative Physiol Ther 1990;13:204-206.

22. Plaugher G. Clinical anatomy and biomechanics of the spine. In: Plaugher G, ed. Textbook of clinical chiropractic: a specific biomechanical approach. Baltimore: Williams & Wilkins, 1993:12-51.

23. Haas M. The physics of spinal manipulation. Part II. The myth of F=ma. J Manipulative Physiol Ther 1990; 13:253-256.

24. Haas M. The physics of spinal manipulation. Part III. Some characteristics of adjusting that facilitate joint distraction. J Manipulative Physiol Ther 1990;13:305-308.

25. Plaugher G., Lopes MA. The knee-chest table: indications and contraindications. Chiropractic Tech 1990;2:163-167.

26. Wood J, Adams AA. Comparison of forces used in selected adjustments of the low back by experienced chiropractors and chiropractic students with no clinical experience: a preliminary study. Proceedings: 14th Annual Biomechanics Conference on the Spine. Boulder: University of Colorado, 1983:73-98.

27. Adams AA, Wood J. Changes in force parameters with practice experience for selected low back adjustments. Proceedings: 15th Annual Biomechanics Conference on the Spine. Boulder: University of Colorado, 1984:143-147.

28. Adams AA, Wood J. Forces used in selected chiropractic adjustments of the low back: a preliminary study. Proceedings: 14th Annual Biomechanics Conference on the Spine. Boulder: University of Colorado, 1984:51-71.

29. Hessel BW, Herzog W, Conway PJW, McEwen MC. Experimental measurement of the force exerted during spinal manipulation using the Thompson technique. J Manipulative Physiol Ther 1990;13:448-453.

30. Herzog W. Clinical biomechanics of the sacroiliac joint (Abstract from Low Back'90.) J Manipulative Physiol Ther 1991;14:277.

31. Herzog W, Conway PJ, Zhang EM, Hasler EM, Ladly K. Forces exerted during spinal manipulative treatments of the thoracic spine. Proceedings of the 1991 International Conference on Spinal Manipulation. Arlington, Virginia: Foundation for Chiropractic Education and Research, 1991:275-280.

32. Triano JJ, Schultz AB. Cervical spine manipulation: applied loads, motions and myoelectric responses. Proceedings: American Society of Biomechanics, 1990;14:187-188.

33. Roston JB, Haines RW. Cracking in the metacarpophalangeal joint. J Anat 1947;81:165-173.

34. Lopes MA. Vertebral Subluxation Complex. In: Plaugher G, ed. The textbook of clinical chiropractic: a specific biomechanical approach. Baltimore: Williams & Wilkins, 1993:52-72.

35. Herbst RW. Gonstead chiropractic science and art. Mt. Horeb: Sci-Chi Publications, 1968.

36. Plaugher G, Lopes MA, Melch PE, Cremata E. The inter- and intraexaminer reliability of a paraspinal skin temperature differential instrument. J Manipulative Physiol Ther 1991;14:361-367.

37. Perdew W, Jenness ME, Daniels JS, et al. A determination of the reliability and concurrent validity of certain body surface temperature measuring instruments. Dig Chiro Econ 1976 May/June:60-65.

38. Cremata E, Plaugher G, Cox WA. Technique system application: the Gonstead approach. Chiropractic Technique 1991; 3:19-25.

39. Araghi HJ. Upper cervical spine. In: Plaugher G, ed. The textbook of clinical chiropractic: a specific biomechanical approach. Baltimore: Williams & Wilkins, 1993:303-324.

40. Yochum TR, Rowe LJ. Essentials of skeletal radiology. Baltimore: Williams & Wilkins, 1987.

41. Williams PL, Warwick R, eds. Gray's anatomy. 36th British ed. Philadelphia: WB Saunders, 1980.

42. Lestinini W, Wiesel S. The pathogenesis of cervical spondylosis. Clin Orthop 1989;239:69-93.

43. Peterson CK, Wei T. Vertical hyperplasia of the cervical articular pillars. J Am Chiro Assoc 1987;21(4):78.

44. Stillwagon G, Stillwagon KL. In search of the ideal cervical curve. Am Chiro 1984;Jan/Feb:38-42.

45. Bagnall KM, Harris PF, Jones PR. A radiographic study of the human fetal spine. 1. The development of the secondary cervical curvature. J Anat 1977;123;3:777-782.

46. Plaugher G. Lower cervical spine. In: Plaugher G, ed. Textbook of clinical chiropractic: a specific biomechanical approach. Baltimore: Williams & Wilkins, 1993:279-302.

47. Friedenberg ZB, Miller WT. Degenerative disc disease of the cervical spine: a comparative study of asymptomatic and symptomatic patients. J Bone Joint Surg 1963;45A:1171-1178.

48. Keating JC. Inter-examiner reliability of motion palpation of the lumbar spine: a review of quantitative literature. Am J Chiro Med 1989; 2:107-110.

49. Fracheboud R, Kraus S, Choiniere B. A survey of anterior thoracic adjustments. Chiropractic 1988;1:89-92.

50. Panjabi MM, Yamamoto I, Oxland T, Crisco J. How does posture affect coupling in the lumbar spine? Spine 1989;14:1002.

51. Tanaka S, Plaugher G. Thoracic spine. In: Plaugher G. ed. Textbook of clinical chiropractic: a specific biomechanical approach. Baltimore: Williams & Wilkins, 1993:243-265.

52. Lee M. Mechanics of spinal joint manipulation in the thoracic and lumbar spine: a theoretical study of postero anterior force techniques. Clin Biomech 1989; 4:249-251.

53. Cyriax J. Textbook of orthopaedic medicine. Vol 2. 8th ed. London: Bailliere Tindall, 1974.

54. Ahmed AM, Duncan NA, Burke DL. The effect of facet geometry on the axial torque-rotation response of lumbar motion segments. Spine 1990;14:391-401.

55. White AA, Panjabi MM. Clinical biomechanics of the spine, 2nd. ed. Philadelphia: JB Lippincott, 1990.

56. Giles LGF, Taylor JR. Innervation of lumbar zygapophyseal joint synovial folds. Acta Orthop Scand 1987; 58:43-46.

57. Ho RWH, Chance JA. Lumbar facet study. J Am Osteopath Assoc 1959; 59:257-265.

58. Stokes IAF, Counts DF, Frymoyer JW. Experimental instability in the rabbit lumbar spine. Spine 1989; 14:68-72.

59. Mierau DR, Cassidy JD, Hamin T, Milne RA. Sacroiliac joint dysfunction and low back pain in school aged children. J Manipulative Physiol Ther 1984;7:81-84.

60. Otter R. A review study of the differing opinions expressed in the literature about the anatomy of the sacroiliac joint. Euro J Chiro 1985;33:221-242.

61. Steindler A. Kinesiology of the human body. Springfield: Charles C. Thomas, 1970.

62. Schafer RC. Clinical biomechanics: musculoskeletal actions and reactions. 2nd ed. Baltimore: Williams & Wilkins, 1987.

63. Faye LJ. Spinal biomechanics. Motion Palpation Institute. Seminar notes, 1985.

64. Calliet R. Low back pain syndrome. 3rd ed. Philadelphia: F.A. Davis, 1981.

65. Sandoz R. The choice of appropriate clinical criteria for assessing the progress a chiropractic case. Ann Swiss Chiro Assoc 1985;VII:53-74.

66. Diakow PRP, Cassidy JD, DeKorompay VL. Post surgical sacroiliac syndrome: a case study. J Can Chiro Assoc 1983; 27:9-23.

67. Walters P. Pelvis. In: Plaugher G, ed. The textbook of clinical chiropractic: a specific biomechanical approach. Baltimore: Williams & Wilkins, 1993:150-189.

68. Lecture Notes. Gonstead Seminar of Chiropractic. Mt. Horeb, WI, 1989.

69. Plaugher G, Hendricks AH. The inter- and intraexaminer reliability of the Gonstead pelvic marking system. J Manipulative Physiol Ther 1991; 14:503-508.

70. Schafer RC, Faye LF. Motion palpation and chiropractic technique: principles of dynamic chiropractic. Huntington Beach, USA: Motion Palpation Institute, 1989.

10 Craniosacral Therapy

Carol J. Phillips

Despite how "uncomplicated" a birth may appear, the physical trauma of that event may have its own peculiar dangers to the cranial and spinal structures of the infant (1–3). These injuries, if left unidentified and unattended, may adversely affect the physical, emotional and mental growth and development of the child during one of the most vital periods of his or her life. Identifying and addressing the resultant injuries may be a large challenge especially to the uninitiated. Those who choose to accept the challenge are advised to acquire the knowledge and skills necessary to address both spinal and cranial injuries. This chapter will be limited to the cranial evaluation and will provide the reader with baseline information that may be used as a tool for those who wish to incorporate craniosacral therapy (CST) into their own treatment protocol or as knowledge to be used when a referral to a specialist is more appropriate.

Cranial adjusting procedures have been a part of chiropractic and osteopathic therapeutic repertoires for over 60 years and a small but growing body of literature generated during that time supports the concepts of cranial adjusting (1–19). While many within these two professions have investigated and reported on the effectiveness of cranial therapy, literature describing the efficacy of these practices during the perinatal period is limited and requires further investigation.

This chapter discusses the role of CST during the period from birth through the first year of life. This is a critical period of susceptibility when craniosacral strain patterns may contribute to aberrant neuromusculoskeletal growth and development. Adopting a "wait and see" attitude when an infant presents with possible neuromusculoskeletal (NMS) dysfunction is to allow developmental anomalies of the central nervous system to manifest as a result of an alteration of the basilar bones and membranes of the cranium. For the experienced practitioner who is familiar with the cranial concept and who has the palpatory skills necessary to apply CST during this period, each case will present with challenges and rewards. For others less experienced, treatment may include a referral to a qualified craniosacral practitioner.

While there are many forms of cranial techniques taught within both the chiropractic and osteopathic professions, it is this author's opinion that cranial treatment of the pediatric patient should primarily be limited to a non-force indirect method. The forces of nature alone can cause considerable damage without additional forces being applied by well-meaning health care providers either during the birth process or afterwards.

Craniosacral therapy, as taught by the Upledger Institute, has two very broad goals. First, to improve the patient's level of wellness by restoring optimum cerebrospinal fluid (CSF) physiology. And, secondly, by restoring balance to the reciprocal membranous tension within the cranial system, thus improving neurological function. There are also five very specific goals:

1. To reduce articular restrictions
2. To reduce membranous restriction patterns
3. To improve circulation
4. To reduce the potential for neural entrapment from exit foramen in the cranial base
5. To increase the vitality of the cranial rhythmic impulse (16)

Literature

Research related to the cranial concept began in the 1960s and has focused primarily on the validation of motion within the cranial sutures and the palpable cranial rhythmic impulse. With the technological advances seen in the 1980s and 1990s, objective evidence has demonstrated that the adult sutures are in motion and capable of being influenced by both internal and external forces. While there is little doubt that the pediatric skull continues to mold and change its inherent shape well into adulthood, it is helpful to review the most pertinent research as it relates to the validation of the cranial motion concept.

In 1970, an attempt was made to demonstrate cranial restriction patterns roentgenographically. Greenman found a strong correlation between roentgenographic findings and clinical observations made independently by a physician experienced in the cranial concept (20). It appeared that it was possible to demonstrate side bending, torsion, flexion, and extension patterns of the skull. Occasionally, lateral and vertical strain of the sphenobasilar junction was also demonstrated. Correlation of clinical observations with the finding of low occiput on the side of the low sacrum was excellent, but that with the lumbosacral angle and the angle of the base of the skull was extremely poor.

The hypothesis that the cranial bones move and possess a slow rhythmic motion pattern was investigated by a team of researchers at Michigan State University College of Osteopathic Medicine in 1975 by direct instrumentation of cranial bone displacement in the monkey. Parietal bone displacement patterns were recorded. One corresponded to the respiratory frequency; another of 5–7 cycles per minute corresponded to neither heart rate nor changes in central venous pressure. This was later identified as the cranial rhythmic impulse (CRI) (21).

In 1977, Upledger (22) reported on the interexaminer reliability of cranial examination findings. The examinations were performed on schoolchildren ages 3–5 yr by skilled examiners. An analysis of the data (Table 10.1) derived from the 50 craniosacral examinations on the 25 preschool children indicated high levels of agreement (>.80) on the reproducibility of their findings. The study also helped to establish the CRI as an independent physiologic rhythm.

Upledger (23) reported in 1979 on a study of mechano-electric measurements performed on patients that showed distinct strain gauge, electrocardiography, electromyography, and integrated-electromyography patterns. These patterns corresponded with palpatory sensations perceived by cranially oriented physicians. This correlation far exceeded random probability. This study demonstrated that subjective impressions of various changes in the craniosacral mechanics which are reported by a trained craniosacral practitioner are documentable by objective instruments.

Pederick (4) reported in 1984 on studies conducted to investigate the cranial rhythmic impulse. Computerized tomographic (CT) scans were performed to follow up on telemetry and ultrasound studies which showed brain motion coincident with sinusoidal pressure waves at a frequency of 2–9 cycles per minute. The examiners were able to detect even lower frequency waves suggesting complex peristaltic movement of the brain powered by the flow of blood and CSF through the ventricular cisternal system.

In 1991, Kostopoulos (24) reported on a cadaver study that attempted to validate cranial suture mobility. The study suggested that when a controlled external force was applied to the frontal bone of an embalmed cadaver, the force would be transmitted to the falx cerebri resulting in a relative elongation of that membrane. There was a positive but low correlation between the applied force and the relative elongation of the falx cerebri. This offers validation to the scientific basis of craniosacral therapy and supports the contention that cranial sutures are mobile even after death.

In 1992, an instrument was developed by the research team at the University of Michigan College of Osteopathy to quantify parietal bone motion. The isotonic measuring device was attached to the surgically exposed skulls of anesthetized adult cats in an attempt to measure the bidirectional cranial bone motion relative to the skull's sagittal suture. The resulting data, which was reported by Adams (25) in 1992, indicated that not only did the parietal bones move in reference to one another by forces applied externally to the head, but they were

---

Table 10.1. **Parameters Rated by Skilled Examiners in a Study of the Reproducibility of Craniosacral Examination Findings**

Occiput

    1-Right (restriction of motion)

    2-Left (restriction of motion)

Temporal bones

    3-Right (restriction of motion)

    4-Left (restriction of motion)

Sphenobasilar joint

    5-Restriction towards flexion

    6-Restriction towards extension

    7-Sidebending rotation, restriction towards right

    8-Sidebending rotation, restriction towards left

    9-Torsion, restriction towards right

    10-Torsion, restriction towards left

    11-Compression-decompression restriction

    12-Lateral strain, restriction towards right

    13-Lateral strain, restriction towards left

    14-Vertical strain, restriction towards superior motion

    15-Vertical strain, restriction towards inferior motion

Sacrum

    16-Restriction towards flexion

    17-Restriction towards extension

    18-Restriction towards right torsion

    19-Restriction towards left torsion

The rating system employed is as follows:

1 = easy or "normal" response to induced passive motion

2 = moderate or transient restriction to induced passive motion

3 = severe or complete restriction to induced passive motion

Increments of 0.5 between 1 and 3 on the rating scale were allowed.

---

also displaced by intracranial forces. Cerebrospinal fluid (CSF) pressure increases accompanying induced hypercapnia or injected norepinephrine were closely correlated with lateral, if not rotational, parietal bone movement during both onset of effect and recovery from it. Similar correspondence was demonstrated when intracranial pressure was increased by bolus injections of artificial CSF.

Pick (14) investigated the effects of external maxillary and frontal parietal manipulation on intercranial structures of the human brain and reported his findings in 1994. A 42-yr-old male participated as the subject in the intriguing experiment. Magnetic resonance imaging (MRI) was used to evaluate the

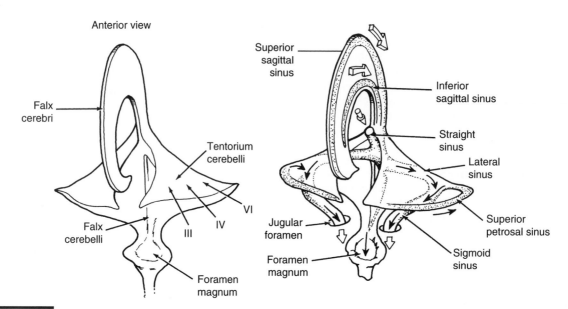

Figure 10.1. The dura mater forms the falx cerebri, tentorium cerebelli, and the falx cerebelli. As the external layer of the meninges, it is fused with the internal aspect of the skull. The dura mater contains the cerebrospinal fluid, houses the venous sinus system, and affords passage for cranial nerves. Modified from Upledger J. CranioSacral Therapy I. Study Guide. The Upledger Institute 1991;129.

internal cranial structures while one investigator applied a light pressure to the subject's parietal/frontal area and a second investigator applied light pressure to the subject's hard palate. A mid–sagittal plane scan was obtained while the investigators touched the contact points and a second scan was made while the investigators applied the appropriate pressure to the contact areas. Gross visible changes in the brain's internal structures were visible following the application of the external manipulation. The study lends support to the theory that external cranial manipulation causes detectable changes in the cranial vault.

In the last two decades, several investigators have conducted large scale clinical trials with newborns and small children in an attempt to validate the correlation between cranial and spinal restriction patterns and neurophysiological findings.

In 1992, Biedermann (2) reported on a study in which he used several thousand case histories and catamneses to investigate the pathogenetic potential of the craniovertebral junction in newborns and young children. He reported that manual therapy cannot be the universal remedy for all children suffering from kinematic imbalances due to suboccipital strain, but it should be considered as one of the most efficient therapies available.

Fryman (3), conducted a retrospective study of several hundred children to investigate the correlation between a distinctive traumatic pattern within the craniosacral mechanism and subsequent learning problems. She discovered that 72.8% of infants in whom learning problems later developed had suffered some considerable trauma before or during birth, compared with 28.3% of those without learning problems.

Upledger (26) conducted a standardized craniosacral examination on a mixed sample of 203 grade school children. The probabilities calculated supported the existence of a positive correlation between elevated craniosacral motion restriction scores and subsequent disabilities.

Clinical Anatomy

The use of CST requires that the practitioner conduct an intense academic study of the osseous cranium, sutures and meninges. For application during the perinatal period, the practitioner is also encouraged to conduct a study of the process of birth so that the presentation of abnormal structure and/or function can be accurately addressed. While it is not within the scope of this chapter to provide such detailed information, an attempt will be made to summarize the most important aspects of newborn anatomy and consequences of birth trauma.

Dural Membranes and Septa

FALX CEREBRI (FC)

A vertical sheet of tough, relatively elastic connective tissue in the newborn, the falx cerebri arises from both the occipital and the frontal bones and attaches to all four clinoid processes of the sphenoid bone. This membrane contributes to the interior ceiling cover and separates the cortical hemispheres as it affords passage for the sagittal and inferior venous sinuses (Fig. 10.1).

It is not difficult to imagine abnormal membrane tensions interfering with normal cranial bone motion and with free blood flow through this venous sinus system which transmits tension from any source through itself in a direction dictated by its geometry and its attachments (16).

TENTORIUM CEREBELLI (TC)

The superior leaves of the TC are continuous with the two layers of the FC as they separate to form the two superior and horizontal walls of the straight venous sinus (Fig. 10.1). The inferior layers of the leaves of the TC are continuous with the inferior walls of the straight sinus and then with the two layers of the falx cerebelli. The inferior layers attach anteriorly to the posterior clinoid processes, and the superior layers attach to the anterior clinoid processes of the sphenoid bone. Lateral to the clinoid attachments, both leaves of the TC attach to the petrous ridges of the temporal bone. Here the tentorium encloses the superior petrosal sinuses.

Moving posteriorly, the attachment of the TC is to the mastoid portions of the temporal bones, then to the parietal bones and finally, to the transverse ridges of the occiput where it affords passage to the transverse venous sinuses. Clinically, rotational dysfunction of the temporal bones may be etiologically related to many visual motor problems. This occurs because rotational dysfunction of the temporal bone places increased tension into the anterior cerebellar tent at the petrous ridges. Cranial nerves III, IV, V and VI all pass between the leaves of the TC. Correction of the anatomico-physiologic dysfunction of the temporal bone often rapidly and dramatically corrects strabismus and nystagmus (16).

FALX CEREBELLI (FC)

The falx cerebelli houses the occipital venous sinus and forms the tough fibrous ring around the foramen magnum (FM). Tension upon this falx can interfere with the free passage of venous blood through that sinus. The FC, TC and spinal dural tube may all transmit tension to the FM and surrounding tissue. This tension along with cervical muscle hypertonus, somatic dysfunction of the occipital condyles and cranial base dysfunction may interfere with normal function of structures within the jugular foramina (Fig. 10.1). This results in intracranial fluid congestion due to venous back pressure, and symptoms resultant to dysfunction of CNIX, CNX, CNXI and CNXII (27).

SPINAL DURA

Relatively elastic in the infant, the spinal dura mater attaches firmly at the FM; to the posterior bodies of C2 and C3; the body of the S2 sacral segment where it becomes the filum terminale externus; passes out the sacral hiatus; and attaches to the coccyx as its periosteum (Fig. 10.2). The endosteal layer of the intracranial dura mater is represented below the FM by the vertebral periosteum which lines this canal. It is considered to be an extension of the inner or meningeal layer of the intra-cranial dura mater (16). With each pair of spinal nerves is a reduplication of the dura which partly fuses with the

periosteum at the intravertebral foramen. Thus, any segmental lesion may adversely affect the function of the craniosacral system.

Newborn Cranium

VAULT BONES

The newborn skull is extremely fragile with no bony sutures. The bones, particularly of the vault, are still floating in membrane which provides flexibility during the molding process. The bones in the base of the skull develop in cartilage. This will provide a stronger and more protective support for the brain as the fetus maneuvers the birth canal. The frontal bone develops in two halves. Its midline suture is obliterated by the eighth year, but it may persist (in some races more often than others), and is then known as the metopic suture. At birth, the mastoid process is still undeveloped, thus exposing both the styloid process and the stylomastoid foramen. Compression or distortion of this foramen may result in facial nerve dysfunction.

The temporal and sphenoid each consist of three membranous segments which will continue to develop and unite during the first year of life. Excessive force applied to these structures during pregnancy, labor or assisted delivery (i.e., forceps, vacuum and/or the Ritgen Maneuver) (Fig. 10.3 A,B) may distort the membranous segments and alter the function of the associated soft tissue. This may go unnoticed until the infant exhibits any number of symptoms, one of which may be chronic otitis media with hyper or hypotonicity of the tensor tympany and tensor vali palatine muscles. This may result in persistent retraction and eustachian tube patency.

The occiput consists of four segments: the squama, two condylar parts and the basilar portion. The occipital squama unites with the condylar segments between 3-5 years of age. The condylar segments unite with the basilar portion between 7-8 years of age. The occiput directs the pattern of the cranium while the sphenoid directs the pattern of the facial bones. If during development there is a malalignment or crowding of these segments, developmental deformity of the cranial base

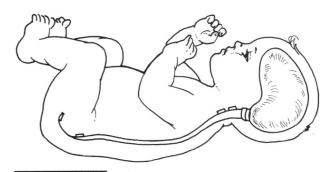

Figure 10.2.   The spinal dura mater attaches firmly at the foramen magnum; to the posterior bodies of C2 and C3; loosely throughout the vertebral canal; the body of S2; and to the coccyx. Thus, any segmental lesion will affect the function of the craniosacral system and associated structures.

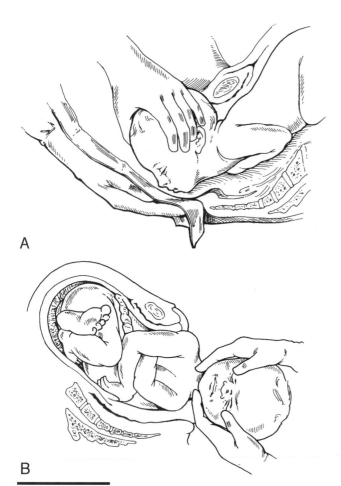

A

B

Figure 10.3.   A, Step 1 of the Ritgen's maneuver: The right hand is used to extend the head, while counterpressure is applied to the occiput by the left hand to allow a controlled delivery of the fetal head. B, Step 2: A downward force is applied to the fetal cranium until the anterior shoulder slides out from under the pubic symphysis. This is followed by a superior traction of the fetal cranium until the posterior shoulder is delivered. With this maneuver the degree of force applied to the fetal cranium varies depending on the position of the attendant's forearm and the amount of counterforce applied. Modified from Willson J. Obstetrics and gynecology. Missouri:CV Mosby Company,1983:501.

will result. This deformity may be obvious with excessive molding and craniofacial deformities or it may go unnoticed until the patient suffers serious sequelae to some minor injury. If severe, a spinal scoliotic compensation may develop (1,13,16).

FONTANELLES

The anterior, posterior, sphenoidal and mastoid fontanelles are membranous gaps of dura mater formed at the corners of the parietal bones (Fig. 10.4 A–C). The anterior fontanelle is the largest of the membranous gaps which are literally small springs, or fountains, which fluctuate with changes in intracranial pressure. At birth, the brain is 25% of its adult size and will grow to 75% by the end of the first year. The fontanelles

located at the bregma, lambda, pterion and asterion allow for this growth. As the cranial bony plates continue to ossify on and across the dura mater, the fontanelles will eventually reduce in size until the cranial plates join to form the moveable cranial sutures.

SPHENOBASILAR (SB) ARTICULATION

The most important of the cranial articulations, the sphenobasilar synchondrosis is formed at the juncture between the occiput and the sphenoid (Fig. 10.5A). During the birth process and with the initiation of breathing, the sphenobasilar plate, consisting largely of cancellous bone surrounded by a very thin layer of dense bone, is capable of flexibility in various directions. Anatomical distortions between the components of the SB synchondrosis are secondary to cranial base suture dysfunctions and/or abnormal membrane tensions within the

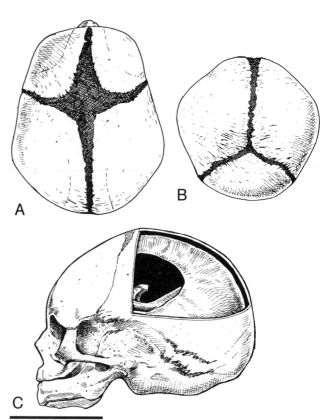

A

B

C

Figure 10.4.   A, The anterior fontanelle is located at the anterior-superior border of the parietal bones (bregma) and is ideally centered between the coronal sutures, metopic suture, and sagittal suture. B, The posterior fontanelle is located at the posterior-medial border of the parietal bones (lambda) and is ideally centered between the sagittal suture and the lambdoid sutures. C, The sphenoidal fontanelle is located at the anterior lateral border of the parietal (pterion). The mastoid fontanelle is located at the posterior lateral border of the parietal (asterion). Modified from Netter F. The CIBA Collection of Medical Illustrations. NJ:Ciba,1983 and McMinn R.M.H. Color Atlas of Human Anatomy. Chicago, IL:Year Book Medical Publishers, Inc.,1977.

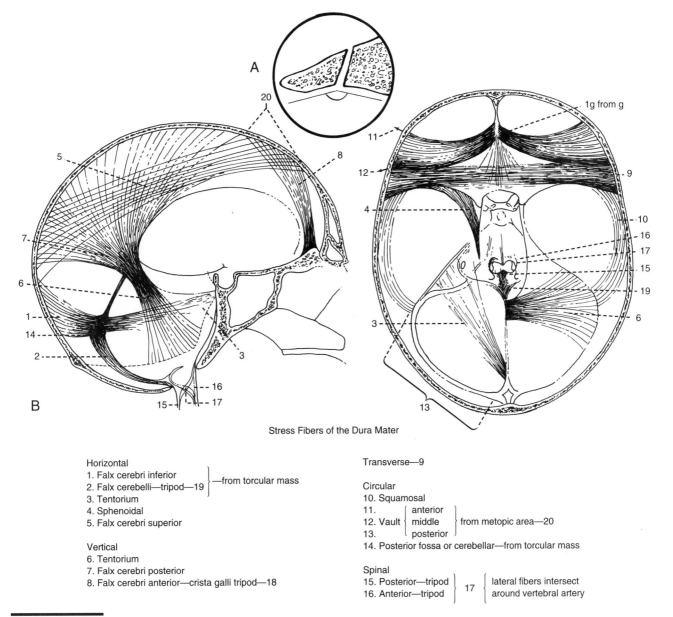

Stress Fibers of the Dura Mater

Horizontal
1. Falx cerebri inferior
2. Falx cerebelli—tripod—19   }—from torcular mass
3. Tentorium
4. Sphenoidal
5. Falx cerebri superior

Vertical
6. Tentorium
7. Falx cerebri posterior
8. Falx cerebri anterior—crista galli tripod—18

Transverse—9

Circular
10. Squamosal
11.   { anterior
12. Vault { middle   } from metopic area—20
13.   { posterior
14. Posterior fossa or cerebellar—from torcular mass

Spinal
15. Posterior—tripod } 17 { lateral fibers intersect
16. Anterior—tripod   }   { around vertebral artery

Figure 10.5. A, Sphenobasilar articulation. B, Stress fibers of the dura mater that guide, control and limit the motion of the whole craniosacral mechanism through their various poles of at-tachment. Modified from Arbuckle B. The Selected Writings of Beryl E. Arbuckle. Indiana: American Academy of Osteopathy, 1994.

dura mater. Therefore, after delivery, the continued flexibility depends upon: 1) the freedom of motion of the petrous portions of the temporal bones and associated sutures and 2) the lack of tension in the dural stress fibers about the base of the skull and throughout the vertebral canal (16) (Fig. 10.5B).

The sphenobasilar and lumbosacral (LS) articulations are in the same plane and may move synchronously to initiate and regulate the rate of the cranial rhythmic impulse (CRI) (6,7,16). During inhalation, both articulations are moved physiologically into flexion, about a transverse axis (Fig. 10.6). At the same time, the paired bones of the periphery are rotated externally. Extension and internal rotation follow in the exhalation phase. Sutural restrictions, soft tissue distortions,

segmental lesions within the skeletal system (see Chapter 7) and imbalance within the reciprocal membranes of the dura mater may all influence the SB and LS articulations as they move in synchrony (14,16,28) (Figs. 10.7, 10.8).

GESTATION

Compressive forces applied to the fetal spine and cranium during the last weeks of pregnancy begin the cranial molding process and prepare the fetus for descent through the birth canal. These forces are influenced by the strength of Braxton Hicks contractions and the degree of maternal pelvic and

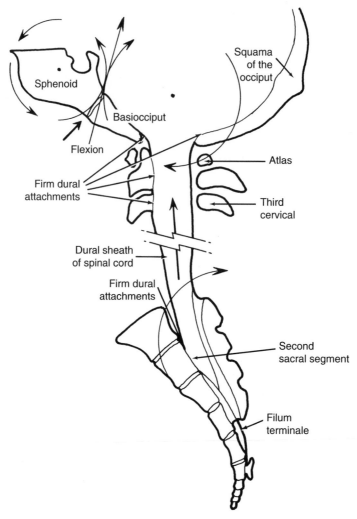

Figure 10.6. Sphenobasilar and lumbosacral articulations move synchronously to initiate and regulate the rate of the CRI. In flexion, the occiput moves posteriorward as the sacral base also moves posteriorward. Modified from Magoun H. Osteopathy in the Cranial Field. Missouri: The Journal Printing Co., 1976.

perineal resistance. In-utero cranial molding is also influenced by the position of the fetus in relation to the placenta, the maternal spine and its degree of lordosis, the inclination and mobility of the maternal sacrum, contour of the bony pelvis, and the innervation of uterine musculature.

In-Utero Constraint

Confining counteractive forces, such as those that occur with constraint or compartment syndromes, alter the plane of the temporal bone, thus altering the tensity of the dura. The force applied to the stress fibers of the dural membranes may then alter 1) the pattern of the cranial base at the craniofacial junction thus, altering the plane of the face, and 2) the craniovertebral junction thus, altering the plane of the sacrum. Should these forces persist throughout labor and delivery, excessive molding may occur. Reinforcing stress fibers within the dural membranes help to prevent severe overriding of the bones which would result in tearing of the venous sinuses (10.5 A,B).

Birth Process

In an uncomplicated natural delivery process, certain basic tenets of childbirth occur during the last month of pregnancy to prepare both the mother and the fetus for delivery. First, there is an increase in maternal compressive force through the fetal spine and upon the cranial base. This leads to an alteration in the various planes of stress fibers throughout the fetal cranium. With each stage and change in position there will be stress placed upon a different plane of the protective intracranial dural membranes (1). By this time, the long axis of the fetal spine is ideally parallel with the long axis of the uterus and the short axis of the cranium is ideally perpendicular to the long axis of the fetal spine. This will allow for forward cervical flexion without rotation.

Second, with each ensuing contraction, fluid is forced out of the skull to reduce its size and to allow cranial molding to begin. This generally consists of the moderate overriding and compression that occur as the cranial segments meet the resistance of the sacral promontory and soft tissue within the pelvic floor. The flexible membranous cranial vault will correct itself after a few days if excessive force was not applied to any particular group of stress fibers.

Following birth, crying balloons out the perimeter of the skull and suckling flexes the sphenobasilar articulation via the vomer. Both of these newborn behaviors will normalize the pull of the intracranial membranes as the associated stress fibers

become balanced within the skull. Thus, in an uncomplicated case, the general morphology, symmetry and mobility of the individual preosseous elements are retained (13).

BIRTH TRAUMA

Birth related trauma may be defined as tissue deformation, distortion, disruption or destruction sustained by the fetus. The origin of obvious birth trauma has been addressed in the literature and may be classified under three headings: 1) gestational, 2) incident to labor and 3) trauma during delivery. These in turn are considered as injuries to the brain, the cord, the peripheral nerves and to the musculoskeletal system. They are reported as:

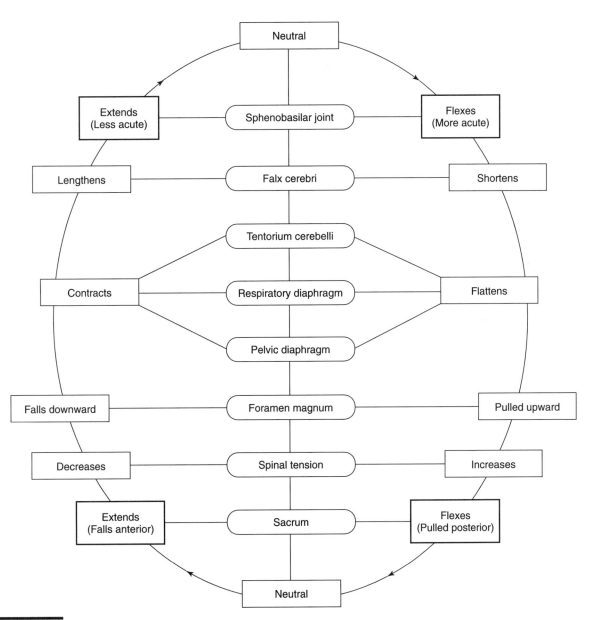

Figure 10.7. Cranial rhythmic impulse. The normal range of frequency for the CRI is 6-12 cycles per minute (cpm). Within each cycle, the craniosacral mechanism influences and is influenced by associated soft tissue and osseous structures.

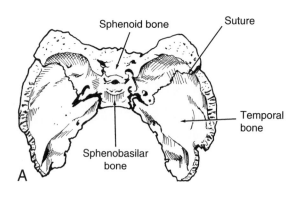

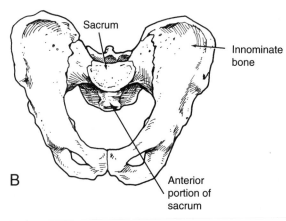

Figure 10.8. A, Sphenoid and temporal articulation. B, Sacrum and pelvic articulation. Note the similar structure. Due to the dural attachments into both the cranial and pelvic structure, an alteration in cranial articulations may adversely affect the synchronous movement of the pelvic articulations. Modified from Mees L.F.C. Secrets of the skeleton. New York: Anthroposophic Press, 1984.

1. Trauma to the bony/cartilaginous skeleton such as skull fractures (29–31), skull depression (32), and nasal trauma (30);

2. Trauma to vascular tissue and fluid dynamics such as cephalhematomas (29), retinal hemorrhages (33–34), intracranial hemorrhages (35–38), intracranial arterial aneurysm (39), extradural hemorrhages (40), and hydrocephalus (41);

3. Trauma to nervous tissue such as spinal cord injury (29–30,42), Erb's Palsy (43), brachial plexus injury (30), and ocular injuries (30);

4. Trauma to soft tissue components such as congenital torticollis (44–57), intra-abdominal trauma (29), and diaphragmatic paralysis (30); and

5. Asphyxia due to anoxia or injudicious use of anesthetics (58).

Asphyxia resulting in fetal mortality is said to be one of the most reported incidents of birth trauma (58). Conversely, it has been reported that newborn brain stem, spinal cord and other musculoskeletal injuries may be the most under-reported cause of infant morbidity (42). A skilled practitioner, therefore, should be prepared to perform an evaluation that includes an assessment of all cranial and spinal structures.

Many forms of birth trauma are evident within the first 24–48 hours after birth. Yet, the more subtle effects of that trauma can go undetected or untreated for months or years. Arbuckle, an osteopathic pediatrician, once wrote, "It has been very interesting to note that some babies treated immediately after birth for very severe cranial conditions, and observed during the first year or two of life, have progressed more rapidly both mentally and physically than those presenting no difficulties and receiving no such treatment" (1).

As chiropractors, we sometimes have infants present with chief complaints that appear to be idiopathic. An investigation of the birth process can oftentimes yield interesting facts that will correlate with the subjective database. Below are described several such cases. The photographs used in this section were either provided by the patient's family or were taken during the actual treatment session for the purpose of documenting treatment and patient progress.

CASE REPORT

Emma

A 31-day-old female presented with a history of severe irritability for approximately four weeks, an inability to maintain head control, an inability to suck on a pacifier, and light sleep cycles of less that 1-2 hr in duration. The patient's parents reported a heightened sense of concern for their baby and felt that her constant screams indicated that she was experiencing a great deal of pain that they were unable to alleviate.

PRENATAL HISTORY

The patient's mother reported that she was involved in a serious motor vehicle accident (MVA) just prior to conception. During the accident, which occurred during a severe snowstorm, she was trapped for approximately one hour in her car with her knees pinned to her chest by the steering wheel. Removal from the vehicle required the use of the Jaws of Life.

BIRTH HISTORY

The first stage of labor was rapid. Due to intense back pain, the mother was given an epidural. Full dilation occurred within that hour. The second stage of labor resulted in dystocia and a second epidural was administered while the mother remained supine and attached to a fetal monitor. Over the next eight hours, multiple attempts were made with a vacuum extractor to help the baby descend through the cervix. When this failed, the mother was scheduled for an emergency c-section. Due to the baby's in-utero malposition, excision into the uterine wall resulted in a facial laceration from the corner of the newborn's mouth up toward the right eye. Plastic surgery was performed immediately.

POSTNATAL HISTORY

This patient was born with a large hematoma and developed jaundice which required five days of continuous phototherapy. Since birth, she reportedly had not slept longer than a few hours at a time. The crying intensified nightly around 9:00 p.m. and continued until morning. She was unable to suck on a pacifier, resisted the right breast and seemed to require constant parental support. When held up against her parent's shoulder, it was reported that her body flopped off to the side with no apparent head control. She cried intensely when placed in the car seat and her head flopped to either side (no preference).

EXAMINATION

The routine physical exam was deferred initially due to the obvious distress of the patient and a cranial evaluation was immediately performed. Due to the nature of the birth injury, the recommended cranial protocol was deferred and treatment began with an evaluation of the cranial base. A contact on the palate initiated a sucking motion as the occiput was gently tractioned posterior and inferior (Fig. 10.9A-C). The patient fell quickly into a deep sleep. This contact was maintained for several minutes as the patient's cervical muscles relaxed and the C0-C1 junction was decompressed. As the

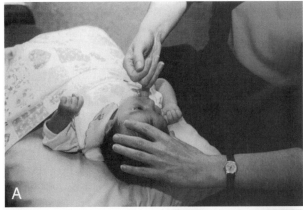
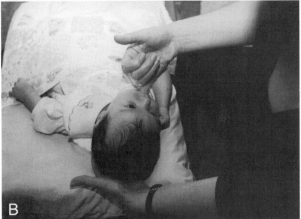
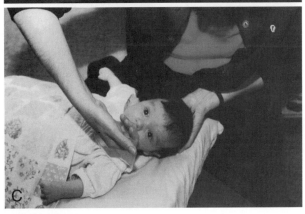

Figure 10.9. A, Parietal Lift: A light contact is made on the parietal tuberosities and they are gently lifted superiorward while the patient is encouraged to suck. B, Occipital Decompression: The base of the skull is cradled lightly in the palm with the third and fourth digits lightly contacting the C0-C1 junction. When the tissue relaxes, a light traction is applied in a posterior-superior direction. C, Dural Tube Release: With the occiput decompressed, the patient will slowly release any abnormal tension or torsion within the dural system. That motion is followed while continuing to decompress the condyles.

soft tissue components elongated, rotational distortions palpated in the mid-cervical region corrected without a direct cervical adjustment.

A spinal evaluation revealed posteriority of T12 and L1. These were addressed while the patient was held vertically and a posterior to anterior and inferior to superior thrust was applied to the transverse processes of those segments. Medial compression of the gluteal musculature revealed a soft tissue distortion with a deviation of the gluteal crease from the area of S2 toward the right iliac crest. This indicated a possible anterior/inferior subluxation of the sacral base on the right ($+\theta Y$, $+\theta Z$). This subluxation was addressed by utilizing a Logan Basic contact on the right sacrotuberous ligament for 1-2 minutes. An inversion analysis was performed by gently suspending the patient by her ankles. This revealed a marked pelvic rotation with no cervical rotation.

A pelvic transverse fascial release was performed by the application of an A/P pressure applied transversely to the abdomen while a supporting hand contacted the posterior aspect of the patient's lumbar region. The patient was nursing during this procedure and continued to nurse while the entire pelvis rotated to the left approximately 100 degrees with a strong flexion of the entire lower body. While maintaining the contact on the pelvic musculature, the patient was allowed to twist and release any fascial restriction patterns within the torso.

TREATMENT OUTCOME

Immediate cessation of crying occurred with the occipital release. The patient was extremely cooperative for the next hour while receiving craniosacral therapy, spinal adjustments and soft tissue work (Fig. 10.9A-C). This patient has continued to be symptom free for over one year during which time she has been evaluated on a once a month basis.

DISCUSSION

Theoretically, the patient's mother may have suffered from trauma to her spine, cranium and associated soft tissue during the MVA. The skeletal and transverse fascial restrictions resulted in an intrauter-

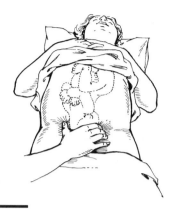

Figure 10.10. In-utero malposition resulting in hyperextension of the occiput and dystocia. Modified from Willson J. Obstetrics and gynecology. Missouri:CV Mosby Company, 1983:501.

ine compartment syndrome (57). The patient was then forced to hyperextend her head with her face pressed tightly against the anterior uterine wall for an unknown period of time prior to delivery (Fig. 10.10). Thus, she was unable to descend down through the open cervix. The hyperextension resulted in anterior compression of the occipital squama into the foramen magnum. Rotation and compression of the occiput would have resulted in distortion of the craniocervical junction. The dural attachment around the entire foramen magnum and at the posterior aspect of the upper cervical spine also resulted in traction of the dentate ligaments (59) and a pull on the sacral dural attachment sites with the resultant sacral anteriority on the right. Multiple potential sites for the production of facilitated spinal cord segments (60) may have resulted in an elevated level of sympathetic nerve activity. Therapeutic intervention with CST and spinal adjustments may have defacilitated the involved segments and reduced the cranial and/or spinal pressure.

CASE REPORT

Lauren

A 9-wk-old female presented with a history of severe irritability. Her parents reported that she had cried excessively since birth with the crying intensifying from 11:00 p.m. until 5:00 a.m. She refused to lie recumbent and had to be held upright against her parent's shoulder at all times. Her parents were forced to sleep upright to maintain that posture. She rarely slept during the day even though she cried throughout the night. Chiropractic spinal adjustments, homeopathic remedies, herbal teas, car rides, and placement on a clothes dryer all failed to alleviate her discomfort. The parents reported that they were "at their wit's end."

PRENATAL HISTORY

This patient's mother reported having been in a MVA at 14 yrs of age. She was not wearing a seatbelt when the car rolled over several times, yet she did not report any injury at the time of the trauma. Her history was negative for any other significant trauma. The pregnancy was unremarkable with no history of nausea or discomfort. She received chiropractic spinal adjustments throughout the pregnancy.

BIRTH HISTORY

During labor this patient's mother suffered from premature rupture of membranes (PROM), severe back pain and dystocia. Labor was managed with prostaglandin gel, oxytocin, Nubain, and morphine. Both an internal and external monitor was utilized throughout the 40 hour labor. Second stage labor required 4 hours of unsuccessful pushing before the patient was delivered with forceps.

EXAMINATION

The patient exhibited extreme bilateral external rotation of the temporals resulting in a marked flaring of both ears (Fig. 10.11 A,B). She had an extremely narrow cranium with the left parietal buckled out at the ossification center. The anterior fontanelle was very small and displaced off to the left. Both coronal and sagittal sutures exhibited overriding lesions. A sacral evaluation demonstrated a marked right anterior sacrum (+θY).

TREATMENT OUTCOME

After the first treatment, which involved utilizing craniosacral therapy to balance the reciprocal membrane tension within her cranium, the patient slept off and on throughout the night both recumbent and on her mother's chest. She was reportedly very "gassy and burpy." Her next evaluation revealed a change in the ear flare with the left now worse than the right. The right coronal suture exhibited less overlapping while the left remained the same.

The second treatment incorporated both CST and spinal adjustments. C6-C7 was adjusted to correct for a posterior subluxation. The patient was then held vertically in a thoracic lift and the area of T3-T9 released. This was followed by a release of L1-L4, also while using a

vertical lift contact. Afterwards, the patient reportedly slept through the night in her cradle. She was fine for three days before she started exhibiting a cranky nature again. Five days after the first adjustment, the patient was reportedly sleeping through the night.

The patient was treated three times the next month and twice the following month. The patient was reportedly doing fine with no aberrant sleep patterns or crying spells. The shape and function of the cranium improved with a decrease in the external temporal rotation (Fig. 10.11C,D). Over the next eight months the patient was seen six times with a chief complaint of constipation.

DISCUSSION

Due to the previous MVA, the patient's mother may have distortion within her pelvic and respiratory diaphragms with dysfunction in her own craniosacral system. Theoretically, distortion of the cross restricting diaphragms would result in chronic distortion of the pelvic and spinal structures that will not correct with spinal adjustments alone. The broad and round ligaments which insert into the pelvic structures would then contort the uterine environment. During the last four weeks of fetal growth, the uterine distortion may force the fetus into an aberrant position. Unable to follow the natu-

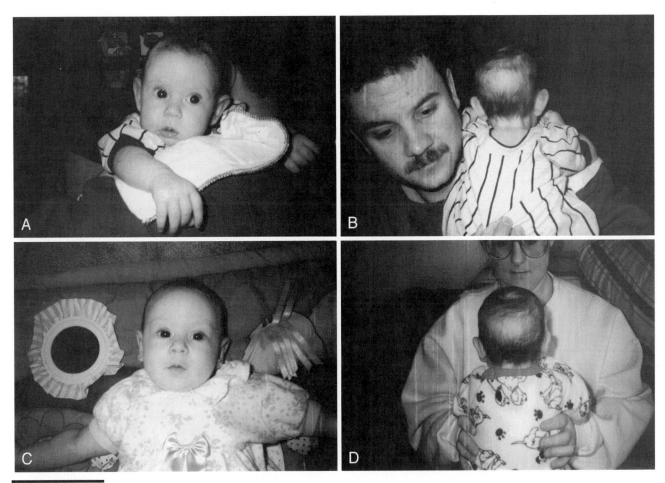

Figure 10.11.   A, Pre-treatment: A/P view of B/L external rotation of the temporals resulting in flaring of the external auricle. B, P/A view. C, Post-treatment: A/P view demonstrating a decrease in auricle flaring as external temporal rotation is reduced and symptoms of irritability resolved. D, P/A view.

ral course of cranial flexion and rotation, either the first or second stage of labor may be inhibited resulting in dystocia. In this case, the use of forceps may have resulted in a successful delivery, but medial compression from the forceps may also have contributed to the existing lesion pattern resulting in a sagittal sutural compression, and a narrow extended skull due to external temporal rotation.

Confining counteractive forces and medial compression may have resulted in hypertonicity of the surrounding musculature thus inhibiting normal cranial molding and craniosacral motion. It is unlikely that

a diagnosis of the exact cause of dysfunction can be described due to: 1) the numerous muscle attachments into the temporal bone, 2) the extensive sutural articulations which are present around their boundaries, and 3) the generous attachment for the tentorium cerebelli. Even though the exact etiology cannot be described, it appears that normal motion was restored to the craniosacral mechanism as the ear flare reduced in conjunction with the reduction in symptomatology. Lying in a recumbent position was apparently no longer uncomfortable and the patient's irritability resolved.

CASE REPORT

Irene

A 9-month-old female presented with a diagnosis of congenital hemihypertrophy. This is a rare condition of unknown etiology, characterized by enlargement of part or all of one side of the body (61-62). Having just started a series of therapeutic treatments with a massage therapist and an acupuncturist, this patient was referred to a chiropractor for spinal adjustments and CST with the hope that a multi-disciplinary approach might have a positive influence on her condition.

PRENATAL HISTORY

The patient is the second sibling in her family. Her mother reports having had an uncomplicated first birth with her son who weighed 9 pounds. She had no medical treatment with the first pregnancy and delivered her baby in Spain. The patient was conceived in the United States and her mother received standard medical prenatal care. At 3 months gestation, the patient's father suffered a heart attack which caused her mother a great deal of emotional stress. At 4 months a routine sonogram revealed a normal fetus. The next two sonograms demonstrated an abnormal growth pattern. Six follow-up biophysical sonograms were performed to monitor the aberrant growth pattern. Initial diagnoses of Down's syndrome and Dwarfism were all eventually ruled out.

BIRTH HISTORY

Labor was induced 4 weeks early when electronic fetal monitoring (EFM) demonstrated possible placental decomposition and fetal distress. The delivery was vaginal and extremely rapid. Weighing only 4 pounds at delivery, the patient spent 5 days in the intensive care unit. Her condition was complicated by low glucose levels and jaundice which required phototherapy.

POSTNATAL HISTORY

Despite the diagnosis of hemihypertrophy with structural anomalies, the patient was considered a very healthy baby (Fig. 10.12A,B). Gross and fine motor skills appeared to be within an expected range. Verbal skills were nonexistent although she had reportedly said "mama" for a few weeks at one time. She never appeared to express

joy or happiness and was described as an "unhappy camper" most of the time by her grandparents who were the day care providers.

Recommended medical therapy for the hemihypertrophy consisted of routine ultrasonography every 3 months. This would be continued until age 7 years to monitor the growth of possible tumors.

EXAMINATION

Analysis of the cranium revealed the following: occiput flattened on the right; frontal flattened on the left; anterior right orbit; externally rotated right maxilla; and an internally rotated right mandible. Facial expression was diminished on the left. Further postural and structural analysis demonstrated a left head tilt; decreased tissue and bone growth on the left side of the body; abnormally shaped radius on the left arm; and syndactyly of the 2nd and 3rd toe on the left. Static palpation of C1 revealed an apparent left lateral subluxation. Medial compression of the gluteal tissue revealed deviation of the tissue to the left indicating an apparent left anterior (-θY) sacral subluxation. Static palpation of the spine revealed tight paraspinal musculature with no other apparent subluxations. Inversion analysis resulted in hyperextension of the cervical spine. There was obvious hypertrophy of all the patient's bones and tissue on the right side of her body and hypopigmentation on the left lower extremity that resembled lightning bolts along the full length of her leg.

It was also noted that the patient habitually sucked on her pacifier which was observed to be resting on a vertical plane approximately 45 degrees from midline.

TREATMENT OUTCOME

The patient was treated seven times over the next 4 weeks. A photo assessment after the seventh treatment (Fig. 10.12C,D) revealed only slight improvement in the facial distortion pattern. The most obvious change came in her ability to smile and show expression.

The patient was very cooperative with cranial/facial contacts and allowed the treatment sessions to last approximately 30 minutes while she sat and played with toys. Verbal skills improved and the patient began going through the normal phases of babbling and imitating. The change in her oral structure was reflected mostly in the position of her pacifier which was now resting on a horizontal plane. Unfortunately, she was not photographed with the pacifier initially for comparison. The change in positioning of the pacifier suggested improvement in the intraoral structure. The action of sucking and smiling appears to temporarily correct the facial asymmetry (10.12D,E). The family reported that she appeared to be happier and more content. This attitude may have been a reflection of in-

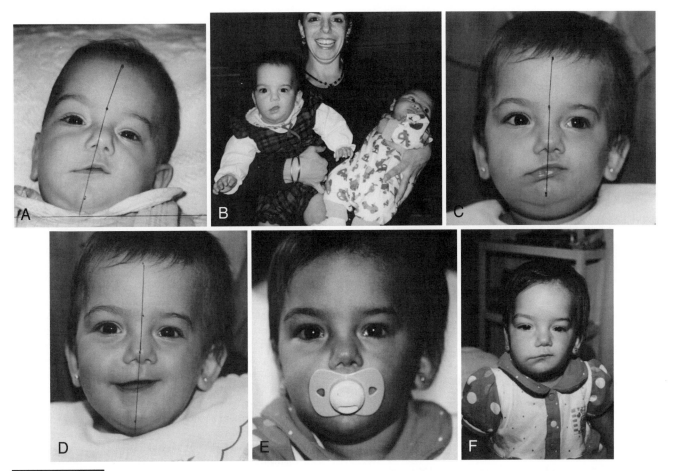

Figure 10.12.   A, Pre-treatment: 4 month old female with right sided hemihypertrophy and facial asymmetry: anterior right sphenoid; externally rotated right maxilla; left lateral deviation of the nasium; internally rotated right mandible; left head tilt. B, At 6 months of age her facial expression is altered with facial neuropathy on the right side. C, Post-Treatment: After 7 treatments: Anterior forward shift of the left sphenoid; right lat-

eral shift of the nasium; decreased external rotation of the right maxilla. D, Improved facial expression on the right and a decrease in right head tilt. E and F, After 25 treatments: The pacifier has moved from a semi-vertical angle that was approximately 45 degrees to the left of midline to a horizontal position (Pretreatment photograph unavailable). The sucking appears to temporarily correct the facial asymmetry.

creased facial expression as the right side of her face began to respond symmetrically when she smiled.

DISCUSSION

While there are multiple variables to be considered in this case, two will be addressed in this discussion. One is the possibility of cellular mutation as a result of the increased exposure to ultrasonic waves. The possibility of this occurring has been studied and reported in the literature. The possibility of in-vitro genetic alterations occurring after ultrasonic exposure was reported by radiologists Liebeskind and Bases (63,64). Animal studies have also revealed delayed neuromuscular development, altered emotional behavior, EEG changes, anomalies, and decreased survival (65). There is no way to determine the amount of ultrasonic energy received by this patient in-utero due to the variable energy output within the different machines and the time constant that changes from patient to patient. Yet, the patient clearly had excessive exposure due to the number of examinations performed. One can also consider the influence

of maternal emotional trauma due to the father's heart attack as this was inflicted simultaneously with the ultrasonic exposure.

The second concern would be the effect of induction on a 4 lb fetus that results in a precipitous delivery. As stated earlier, the newborn skull is extremely fragile, has no bony sutures, and the bones, particularly of the vault, are still floating in membrane. Inducing labor contractions before the fetus has had an opportunity to align its spine with the long axis of the uterus or to align the short axis of the cranium with the long axis of the spine may result in crowding or malalignment of the basilar bones that support the developing brain. Rapid compression and malalignment of the fronto-occipital areas can then distort the facial bones, cranial vault bones, spinal vertebra, and sacrum. Eventually, the individual segments that make up each bone will fuse in their distorted position. This may affect the ultimate shape of the many exit foramina and adversely influence the structures passing through them. Motion distortion of the sphenoid around its transverse axis may result in a flexion, extension or vertical strain lesion. Motion distortion around the vertical axes may result in a sidebending or lateral strain lesion pattern. Ultimately, disrupted motion patterns may distort the tentorium cerebelli attached to the clinoid processes within the sphenoid. This may alter the shape of the sella turcica, the diaphragma sellae, the hypophyseal infundibulum and may eventually disrupt the function of the pituitary gland. This may adversely influence the endocrine system leading to abnormal growth patterns.

Distortion and dysfunction of cranial, spinal and pelvic structures should be addressed as soon as 24 hours after delivery. While craniosacral therapy may influence the function of the craniosacral

mechanism positively, delaying treatment for 8 months, as in this case, may reduce the chance of making significant changes in facial structure.

Abrupt fronto-occipital compression in the course of a precipitous delivery may also cause laceration of the falx cerebri or the free edge of the tentorium cerebelli (66). Though the stretching may not be severe enough to cause an arterial aneurysm or hemorrhage, it may cause a stretching of the tentorium with injury to a small distal branch of the superior cerebellar artery. If this was the case, the full effects of the delivery may be subtle or not present for many decades.

CASE REPORT

Kelsey

A 12-wk-old female presented to the author for a cranial evaluation with a chief complaint of torticollis and irritability. She had received chiropractic spinal adjustments since birth.

PRENATAL HISTORY

The patient's mother reported having been in a motor vehicle collision 10 years prior to conception. This was her first pregnancy, at age 37 years. The pregnancy was positive for pubic bone pain throughout the 2nd and 3rd trimester despite spinal adjustive therapy. She received routine medical pre-natal care with her first sonogram at 14 weeks, a total of 4-5 sonograms and weekly non-stress tests for 6 weeks prior to the patient's delivery.

BIRTH HISTORY

The patient's mother worked very hard at achieving her goal of having a natural childbirth. Labor began spontaneously but failed to progress as planned. During the ensuing 18 hours she suffered severe back pain, hyperemesis and dystocia. Both an internal and external fetal monitor was used as labor was eventually managed with pitocin, morphine, and finally an epidural. The baby suffered from fetal distress on several occasions that required maternal oxygen support.

During the second stage, an episiotomy was performed, a vacuum extractor was applied, and a nurse performed fundal pressure to speed up the process. The patient delivered with the cord wrapped tightly around her neck three times and her body was covered with meconium (Fig. 10.13A,B).

POSTNATAL HISTORY

This patient's history was positive for episodes of severe irritability and congenital torticollis with cranial distortion. At 12 weeks, pressure marks were still prominent on her face in the occipital/cervical region and at the vertex of her head (Fig. 10.13C). She also maintained a right head tilt and an apparent congenital torticollis. Spi-

nal adjustive therapy had only moderate success in reducing her symptomatology.

TREATMENT OUTCOME

During the first treatment session with CST, a transverse fascial release of the pelvic diaphragm and left leg resulted in a somatoemotional response (SER). This is a phenomenon whereby the patient will have a strong release of emotions that appear to be related to the time at which the physical trauma occurred. When the tissue trauma is addressed the tissue memory is released and the patient exhibits the same emotional patterns that were imprinted at the time of injury. This was evident by the high pitched newborn cry that she exhibited while making no attempt to stop the treatment (for more information refer to Upledger's textbook on SER). The second session resulted in a freeing of the craniosacral mechanism as the reciprocal membrane tension was restored. There was an associated decrease in the muscle tension and improvement in the torticollis (Fig. 10.13D,E).

DISCUSSION

While spinal adjustive therapy is the treatment of choice for the reduction of the vertebral subluxation complex, this case demonstrates that birth trauma to the spine and cranium can likely best be addressed with the addition of craniosacral therapy. This case is also an excellent example of how birth trauma can occur even in those families where a great deal of planning and preparation went into ensuring a safe and natural childbirth.

If the mother has a previous history of torsion within the transverse fascial system, such as that which occurs during motor vehicle accidents, both the pelvic and respiratory diaphragms may become hypertonic. This may occur when the pelvis is held stable by the lap belt and one shoulder is held tightly by the harness. On impact, the free shoulder is allowed to twist forward resulting in torsion of all the transverse fascia and associated musculature. This may adversely affect the position of the uterus within the pelvic cavity. At any time in the future, a fetus may then have a very difficult time descending through the hypertonic pelvic floor muscles and the mother may experience dysfunctional labor or dystocia. It is recommended by the author that these mothers also receive craniosacral therapy prior to conception with continued support through delivery to reduce the chance of having a difficult labor and delivery experience.

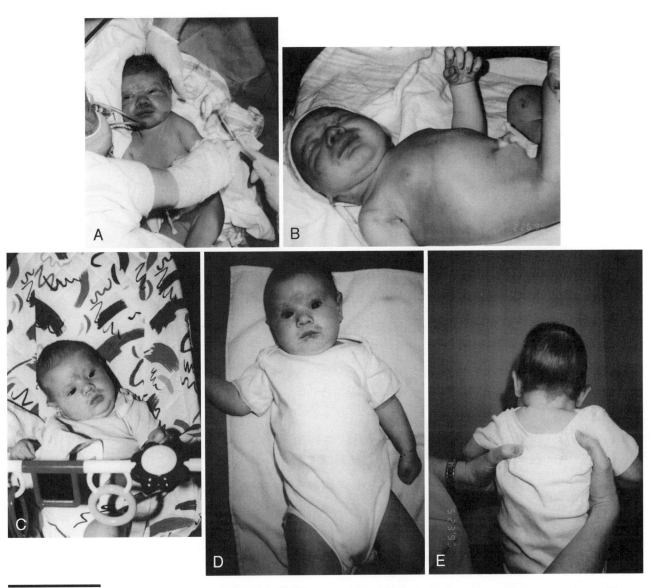

Figure 10.13.   A, Birth trauma evident at 1 minute with facial pressure marks. B, At 10 minutes, facial bruising accompanies marked periorbital edema. C. Pre-CST: Congenital torticollis and persistent facial and cranial pressure marks are evident at 12 weeks. D, Post-Treatment: Pressure marks are beginning to fade as the torticollis resolves at 14 weeks.

EXCESSIVE SKULL MOLDING

The physical exam of a newborn should begin with an evaluation of the cranium for signs of excessive skull molding. Injury to the newborn before, during or after birth may affect the normal process of restitution. The manner in which the skull has been altered will give valuable information as to the source of aberrant neurophysiology. Cranial molding patterns can be classified into three general types:

1. Brachycephalic, which is round
2. Mesocephalic, which is medium
3. Dolichocephalic, which is long and narrow (13)

A look at the family album will help the examiner determine if the presenting skull shape is a genetic predisposition or aberrant skull molding. Excessive skull molding patterns may not become apparent until 3 to 6 months after delivery as the infant skull begins the transformation into the eventual adult form. Since the possibilities for excessive molding are infinite only certain generalizations are included here. For ease in identification, the author has grouped them into Types A, B, C, E, F and O that correspond to the structures of the presenting lesion. Each skull molding pattern will be demonstrated with an associated case report.

Type A is used to identify the average (i.e., normal) skull pattern that will present without excessive molding (Fig.

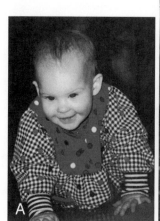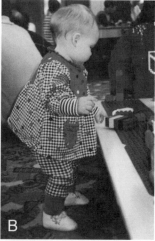

Figure 10.14. A, Type A: A/P view of the average infant cranium. Note the anterior aspect is slightly more narrow than the posterior aspect. B, The lateral view demonstrates that the distance from the mental point to the lambda closely parallels the A/P diameter.

10.14A,B). The anterior skull is slightly narrower than the posterior skull. Laterally the distance from the mental point to the lambda closely parallels the A/P diameter. The infant generally presents with no aberrant symptomatology.

CASE REPORT

Nina

PRENATAL HISTORY

This patient's mother is a chiropractor who was on disability during her pregnancy due to a history of lumbar disc herniation with surgical correction, chronic L5 radicular pain, and Scheuermann's disease with herniation in the area of T9/T10. Hyperemesis predominated during the first trimester and she was hospitalized with weight loss. She received chiropractic care and craniosacral therapy during the last trimester and arranged for labor support during the delivery. No sonograms were performed nor medication used during the delivery.

BIRTH HISTORY

The mother suffered from hyperemesis during the 8 hours of labor but delivered naturally and without manual or surgical assistance.

POSTNATAL HISTORY

The patient received chiropractic and craniosacral therapy immediately after delivery and has had continued care since birth. She has reportedly only suffered from slight cold symptoms associated with teething since birth.

Type B is described as a Buckled Mastoid or Declined Base. On exam, the patient presents with a prominence behind one or both auricles. This prominence is a buckling of the mastoid portion of the temporal bone. One auricle presents higher and flatter than the other due to internal rotation of the temporal on the side of the flattened auricle and external rotation on the side that flares. Correction must be directed to the buckled mastoid portion responsible for obliteration of the mastoid fontanels. This correction must occur within a few days of birth. According to Arbuckle (67,68), if left uncorrected this deformity may later result in chronic sinusitis, migraines, eye defects, malocclusion, crowding of the jugular foramen with irritation of the vagus, and GI symptoms, if not in childhood, then in early adolescence or later in life.

CASE REPORT

Justin

A 3-yr-old male (Fig. 10.15) presented for a consultation with his mother and chiropractor. He had a history of complex partial seizures with episodes of status epilepticus, chronic vomiting, hyperactivity and autistic behavior. MRI studies were reportedly negative for pathology.

PRENATAL HISTORY

This patient's mother reports that her first pregnancy with the patient's sibling was enjoyable and void of complications. Her second pregnancy with Justin was fine until she experienced physical trauma at 6 months gestation. She reportedly pushed a boat into the water, slipped on the mossy rocks and fell extremely hard on her sacrum. Afterwards, she became extremely uncomfortable and experienced chronic indigestion, insomnia, and neuropathy.

BIRTH HISTORY

Justin's mother was so uncomfortable with her pregnancy she requested assistance in initiating labor. The OB stripped her membranes during an exam and labor began the next day. The entire labor lasted only 7 hours. The onset of labor was slow and pain

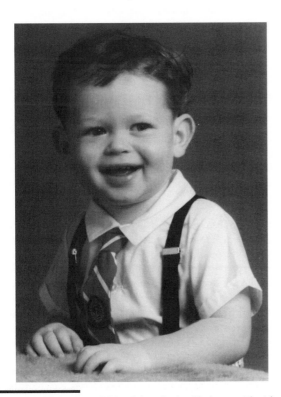

Figure 10.15. This child exhibited a buckled mastoid with symptoms that included seizures, migraines and hyperkinetic behavior.

medication was administered. Six hours after labor began, her water broke spontaneously causing rapid dilation and a precipitous delivery.

POSTNATAL HISTORY

Within hours of delivery Justin's skin broke out in a rash and he began itching and scratching at his body. He appeared to be in pain from the first few days of life. As he grew older, he continually exhibited signs of distress. He refused to be cuddled; responded negatively to even an attempt at touching him when he was in pain; he constantly pulled away if held; and he rejected being nursed. His mother and doctor both suspected that he had recurrent migraine-type headaches due to his extreme behavior of pulling and hitting at his head.

Digestive difficulties included excessive vomiting, which began at birth, and chronic constipation. He rarely slept and always appeared excessively alert. Additional concerns reported by his mother included: 1) that the soft spot would bulge at various times making her fear that there was swelling inside his head, 2) his eyes appeared to change size at various times with one appearing larger than the other; 3) his speech and mental function were grossly deficient; and 4) he appeared to have allergies and/or sensitivities to many foods.

Justin had his first seizure at 4 months of age. He continued to have various types of seizures ranging from mild staring to intense focal seizures. The focal seizures lasted anywhere from 1-2 hours and required that he be hospitalized and heavily medicated. The seizures generally followed a severe bout of vomiting and resulted in one-sided paralysis. After a seizure, Justin appeared to have migraine-type headaches that lasted 1-2 hours causing him to hyperextend his head while screaming. The vomiting that preceded the seizures generally continued for 4-5 days after the seizure activity. At the time of the consult, he was heavily medicated in an attempt to reduce the seizure frequency.

Justin's mother also reported that he took antibiotics for 2 years for chronic otitis media, bronchitis and upper respiratory infections and is now suspected to have severe candidiasis.

EXAMINATION

An exam was almost impossible to conduct due to the hyperkinetic behavior and adversity to touch sensation. Eventually, Justin did allow me to follow him around while rubbing his scalp with my fingertips. There was an immediate awareness of cranial buckling in the area of the mastoid portions of the temporal bones. The left temporal exhibited external buckling where the three segments apparently fused with the right temporal exhibiting internal buckling. The frontal bone exhibited severe overriding onto the parietals with a right lateral shift. The frontal was also anterior on the right.

Craniosacral therapy was eventually completed with Justin sitting in his carseat, as this was the only place he would sit willingly without movement. During the therapy, he sat quietly and eventually fell into a deep sleep. Follow-up therapy by the patient's chiropractor was difficult and again had to be completed in the car seat. Initial response to therapy appeared to be improved sleep behavior and decreased vomiting. After 4 treatments he experienced one episode of status epilepticus that lasted 2 hours and required hospitalization. He has not had another seizure as of the time of this writing.

DISCUSSION

As the infant skull progresses through the normal stages of molding, restitution, the joining of the individual segments into one bone, the ossification of each separate bone, and finally the evolution of the skull into the adult form, it is imperative that distortion and dysfunction of the cartilaginous and membranous structures be addressed early or serious consequences may plague the child throughout his lifetime. Buckling of the mastoid portion of the temporal bone will distort the cranial base and alter the jugular foramen in such a way that symptomatology will most likely increase in severity as the skull evolves into its adult form. If Justin had been treated as an infant prior to the fusing of the individual segments of the temporal bone, the distortion of the jugular foramen may have been avoided. Now, correction of the altered dynamics of the craniosacral mechanism must be the goal of treatment but it must be accepted that the treatment may never fully reduce the effect of the distortion on the contents of the jugular foramen, specifically the cranial nerves. This patient may continue to exhibit symptoms of cranial nerve compression as his skull continues to grow and change into its adult form.

Type C is described in the literature as an extension lesion, cone shaped, elongated or scaphocephalic skull pattern (1,13,14). This is an excessive molding pattern that becomes evident within weeks to months after delivery and may result in craniosynostosis with serious sequelae to the central nervous system. This next case is an example of a Type C skull with aberrant symptomatology so severe that it lead to the child's death at age 3.

CASE REPORT

Brian

*T*his 3-yr-old male presented with his parents for an evaluation with a diagnosis of severe, static central nervous system impairment, most likely acquired, without evidence of a preexisting genetic or chromosomal disorder. Manifestations included profound developmental delays in all areas, spastic quadriparesis, severe microcephaly, a seizure disorder (controlled on medication), impaired swallowing (with functioning GT), irritability, and evidence of at least cortical visual impairment. Neuroimaging demonstrated extensive, bilateral encephalomalacia. Multiple radiographs of the bony calvarium showed no indication of an acute fracture or bone destruction. Changes consistent with craniosynostosis was demonstrated. The patient was maintained with fundoplication, a GT tube and a tracheotomy.

The patient had significant spasticity of all four extremities, with fisting of his hands and decreased movement patterns. Trunk and head control were decreased, and there was significant arching. The patient was unable to roll and had no sitting balance. His parents reported that he appeared to have been in a continuous state of pain from birth until he had the breathing tube inserted about 6 months earlier. Now, unable to utter any sounds, they felt he was generally in less pain. When they arrived after a 2 hour ride in the car, he was unable to utter a sound while his face exhibited signs of anguish and despair as tears rolled down his cheeks.

EXAMINATION

The superior portion of Brian's skull was only a few inches wide with protrusion of both eyes, tongue thrust, excessive drooling and an opisthotonic posture. He was cortically blind and had no gross or fine motor skills and exhibited spastic paralysis. I was told that physical therapy was limited to just a few minutes per day due to his level of pain and rigidity.

PRENATAL HISTORY

The patient's mother reports that she was in three separate motor vehicle accidents prior to his conception but that she never suffered any serious injuries. A seatbelt and harness were worn in 2 of the accidents. Her history is negative for any other serious injury. This pregnancy was negative for any known maternal complications. The mother reports that she received a sonogram at 14 weeks and 29 weeks. Both were negative for pathology. At 34 weeks gestation, she received another sonogram. During the exam, the patient exhibited fetal sinus ventricular tachycardia (SVT). The mother was placed on Digoxin and another sonogram was performed at 35 weeks. The patient had not improved and now exhibited ascites in his arms, hands and scrotum. An emergency C-section was performed that day.

Following delivery, the patient was reported to have apgar scores of 7 and 5, was intubated at labor and delivery and bagged with 100% O_2. The patient was extubated in the nursery and reintubated due to cyanosis. He was placed on a respirator and transferred to a children's hospital for further management.

POSTNATAL HISTORY

The patient continued taking Digoxin for the SVT and had a full complement of immunizations. At three months, Brian began to demonstrate a conical shape to the superior portion of his skull (Fig. 10.16). It was believed that he would grow out of this aberrant molding so a "wait and see" approach was taken by his allopathic health care provider. Instead, his health deteriorated rapidly over the ensuing months and years. While he was evaluated and treated by the medical profession, no chiropractic or alternative therapy had been employed.

TREATMENT OUTCOME

While Brian was examined and treated for 2 hours with craniosacral therapy, he stared silently and intently in my direction. His body relaxed and his crying ceased as the reciprocal membranes within the dural system were balanced. At the end of that session, he sat upright on his father's lap and slowly allowed his head to flex forward while the sphenobasilar articulation was decompressed. This was accomplished with one doctor contacting the greater wing of the sphenoid to gently traction it anteriorward while I performed an occipital lift.

Later, when held upright in his father's arms, Brian's legs relaxed and straightened out as he dropped his head forward on his father's cheek. He appeared comfortable on the two hour ride back home and reportedly smiled the whole way (something he rarely did). The next day he returned after another two hour ride in the car seat

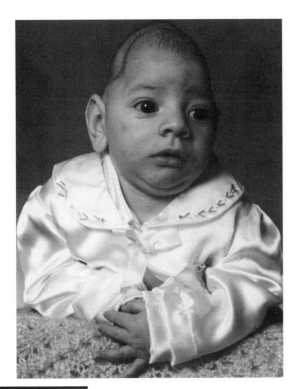

Figure 10.16.   This 3-month-old demonstrates a Type C skull pattern. Note the elongation and coning of the cranium with the narrow superior diameter, overriding sutures, bulging eyes, deviated nasium and ear flare. Eventually, he required a tracheotomy to breath and gastrogavage tube for feeding before he died at age 3 years.

still full of smiles. He presented smiling with decreased tongue thrust and decreased drooling. Brian relaxed into the second treatment session with the same ease as the day before. Unfortunately, the family was unable to bring the patient back for further treatment but

they continued to invert him daily as that seemed to relieve so much of his pain. Two months later the patient died quietly in his sleep.

DISCUSSION

The type C skull pattern is noted for a long A/P diameter and a narrow transverse diameter. Transverse compression results in the condylar portions of the occiput being displaced medially into the foramen magnum with distortion of the craniocervical junction. Internally, the brain is crowded by the altered bone case, its shape elongated and its size lessened by the overriding of the sutures. There is a change in the size, shape and position of the ventricles, the subarachnoid space is crowded and the craniosacral mechanics are definitely disturbed. An upward strain is present in the middle area of the falx cerebri which also elevates the tentorium, compressing the associated venous sinuses. Because of the low occiput and the transverse compression of the skull, the posterior cranial fossa is deeper and narrower. The hind brain is displaced downward causing increased angulation of the junction of the great cerebral vein with the straight sinus as well as tension on the tributaries of the straight sinus with the definite possibility of hemorrhage in the posterior fossa. Further danger of hemorrhage comes from the overriding parietals tending to stretch or shear the tributaries to the sagittal sinus.

Extension of the sphenobasilar is usually present in an exaggerated degree leading to hemiplegia from crowding of the Sylvian fissure or the spastic type of cerebral palsy from pressure on the pyramidal tracts (13).

While craniosacral therapy appeared to improve the quality of this patient's life, it is unlikely that any form of therapy could have prolonged his life. If correction of the excessive molding is not employed during the first year of the child's life, the goal in a case such as this is then to relieve increased pressure within the cranium and decrease the level of the patient's pain, thus improving the quality of life.

Type F skull molding is described as a flexed, flat or oxycephalic skull patterning and is a result of sphenobasilar compression with overriding of the lambdoid and/or coronal sutures.

CASE REPORT

*A*ustin

PRENATAL HISTORY

The patient's mother reported that her pregnancy began with a transvaginal sonogram at 5 weeks followed by abdominal sonograms at 9, 13, and 17 weeks. Each sonogram demonstrated that the baby was maintaining a hyperextended posture deep within the left side of the uterus. The fetus reportedly never moved from that position during the last 2 months of the pregnancy.

The patient's mother had a lengthy history of near constant headaches due to TMJ dysfunction. Surgical correction had been at-

tempted years before but had only increased her level of pain. During the last trimester, she sought help for her pain from a chiropractor who provided chiropractic adjustments and acupuncture. The patient's chiropractor referred her to the author for labor support since her two previous deliveries had been extremely difficult.

BIRTH HISTORY

Labor began with sporadic episodes of contractions that were difficult to endure due to the TMJ discomfort and severe headaches. After several days of intermittent contractions, pitocin was administered and with the assistance of five labor support people she delivered her baby without manual or surgical assistance.

POSTNATAL HISTORY

The patient was extremely irritable from the moment of birth. He demonstrated a marked deviation of his mandible immediately after delivery and received craniosacral therapy within the hour. The deviated jaw quickly resolved but the patient had difficulty nursing and demonstrated apparent pain from the second day of life. His crying episodes would last for an average of 3 hours at a time with sleep periods lasting only minutes to an hour.

EXAMINATION

The patient was treated several days after delivery. At that time, he demonstrated a marked anteriority of the thoracolumbar spine. The patient maintained a hyperextended posture when prone and appeared to have a sympathetic dominant nervous system as he was constantly exhibiting the startle reflex. The patient's mother reported that he was almost impossible to calm and he screamed whenever placed supine. During inversion analysis, his body twisted with the shoulders turning in an A/P orientation to one side while the pelvis twisted in the opposite direction. Relief from his pain appeared to occur only when held in the inverted position. This therapy was then applied daily by his parents with intermittent CST and spinal adjustments.

DISCUSSION

The oxycephalic skull presents externally with an increase in the vertical and transverse diameter of the head. The face is broad and the nose flat, with shallow orbital cavities. The flattened occiput is more nearly vertical causing the condylosquamous junction to more nearly approach a right angle. The superior angle of the occiput may underride the parietals. Jamming of the vault sutures is the rule.

Internally the brain is crowded by the altered brain case. There is a change in the size, shape and position of the ventricles. The subarachnoid space is crowded and the function of the craniosacral system is usually disturbed (possibly resulting in abnormal flow of the cerebral spinal fluid). The falx cerebri is elevated with the vault. The middle and posterior cranial fossae are abnormally deep and the hind brain is pushed deeply into the latter. This leads to altered tension on venus sinuses and blood vessels, altered angulation of the great cerebral vein with the straight sinus and possible hemorrhage. Such tension is further aggravated by extreme internal or external rotation of the temporal bones. With internal rotation the tentorium will be elevated sufficiently to possibly cause a tear at the junction with the great cerebral vein. External rotation leads to a flattened tentorium and decreased venous drainage. In the Type F skull, there may be distortion of the sphenobasilar, the temporals and the condylar parts of the occiput which may then, according to Magoun (13), lead to mental defects.

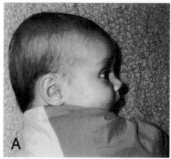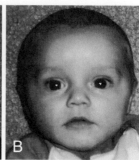

Figure 10.17.   A, 3-month-old with a Type F skull pattern. The patient presents with a flattened occiput, prominent eyes and a short A/P diameter to the cranium. B, The patient presents with a wide transverse diameter.

It is possible that the patient's in-utero malposition contributed to the cranial distortion pattern that resulted in his aberrant skull molding pattern and consequent symptomatology. The patient was seen several times over the first few weeks of life and gradually the patient's symptoms began to resolve. At three months there was a sudden adverse change in his behavior and he was presented for a follow-up evaluation. The excessive skull molding was now apparent with a flattened occiput, wide transverse diameter (Fig. 10.17A,B), and protruding orbits. He was again very uncomfortable in the supine position. An assistant was used to gently stabilize the pelvis and extend the legs while the sphenobasilar articulation was gently decompressed and the reciprocal membrane tension balanced. Symptoms rapidly resolved and at the next visit the flattened occiput had molded into a more normal position. The eyes were less prominent and there was a reduction in the overlapping coronal sutures. At one year of age, the patient has no sign of mental or developmental delays.

The Type O skull is described as the oblique, quadrilateral, plagiocephalic or a scoliosis capitis skull pattern. This type of lesion occurs when the fetal skull is rotated, laterally flexed and compressed in-utero. When force is applied along the fetal spine by the uterine contractions, the cranium is unable to flex forward without rotation. Labor may then be complicated by severe back pain and dystocia as the abnormal fetal positioning results in occipital pressure being applied to the maternal sacrum and associated spinal nerves.

CASE REPORT

Christian

A 5-month-old male presented with congenital torticollis. A pediatrician had followed the progress of this patient's condition since birth. When the torticollis failed to resolve spontaneously, he had warned the parents of the possibility that surgical excision of the cervical musculature would have to be performed unless the torticollis was corrected successfully with cervical traction.

PRENATAL HISTORY

Christian's mother reported that she suffered from chronic TMJ, shoulder and knee pain during her pregnancy. She also had chronic heartburn, a uterine infection, and was put on bedrest due to painful Braxton Hicks contractions. She suffered from rib pain that was so severe she eventually experienced numbness along the border of the rib cage that remained for several weeks post delivery.

BIRTH HISTORY

The first stage of labor was prolonged and marred with severe pain in the mother's back and thighs. Second stage lasted only about one-half hour but the delivery was observed by the grandmother to be traumatic. Two nurses applied fundal pressure while the doctor used rotation and extreme traction of the head to deliver the body. The force necessary to deliver the body was so great that the grandmother reported she feared the baby had been "decapitated."

POSTNATAL HISTORY

Christian not only had torticollis at 14 days old (Fig. 10.18A), but also had difficulty with sucking, sleeping, and breathing. He was unable to remain asleep for any length of time and appeared lethargic for 2-3 months. At birth, his head was perfectly round. At 3-4 months, he began to demonstrate a flattening of the right occiput. He continued

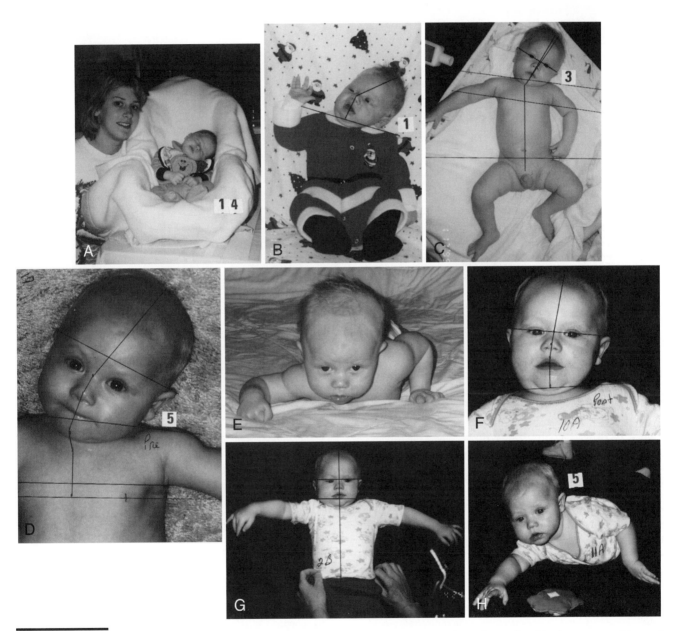

Figure 10.18.   A, Pre-treatment: Congenital torticollis at 14 days. B, At 1 month, the patient also exhibited difficulty in moving the left arm. C, At 3 months, there was no change in the torticollis or arm movement. Sutural distortion was becoming more prominent. D, At 5 months, the patient had no resolution of the torticollis and presented for chiropractic treatment. E, The patient would not tolerate being placed in the prone position and maintained flexion of the left arm. F, Post-treatment after 1 week (4 treatments). G, After 1 month (8 treatments). H, Spasm in left shoulder girdle began to resolve and the patient was more willing to lie prone to play.

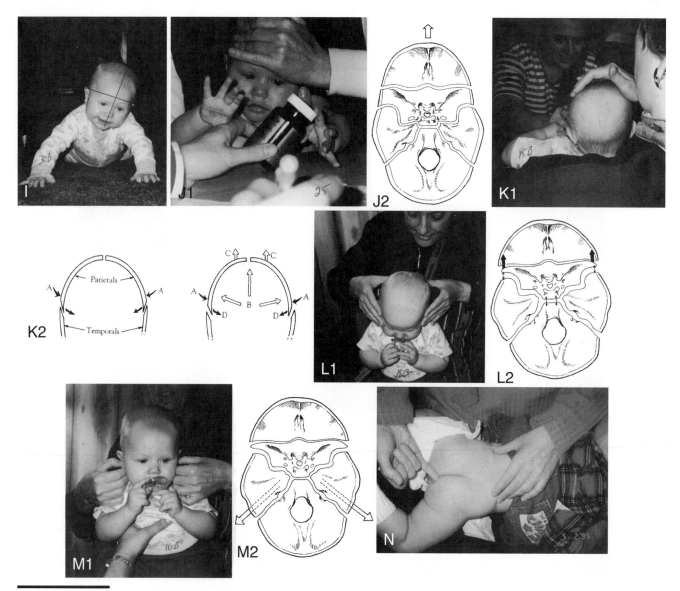

Figure 10.18. *(continued)* I, After 10 treatments the patient would tolerate the prone position long enough to raise himself up. Note how the head tilt would return with the arm forward. Balancing the reciprocal membrane tension. J, The frontal bone is gently tractioned anteriorward while the patient is stabilized in the examiner's lap. K, A contact is made on the parietal tuberosities as they are gently directed medial until they disengage from the temporals, then superiorward. L, The greater wing of the sphenoid bone is gently tractioned anteriorward to decompress it from the temporals and the occiput at the sphenobasilar articulation. M, The temporals are decompressed by directing the auricle inferior and along the plane of the petrous portion of the temporal (anterior in infants). N, Logan Basic Contact lifting the sacrotuberous ligament on the right to correct an anterior/inferior sacral base subluxation.

to demonstrate torticollis for five months and the family was continually encouraged to forcefully stretch out the contracted musculature. Due to his obvious pain, this was not accomplished. He refused to lie prone for more than a few seconds and maintained flexion of his left arm so milestones such as rolling or raising himself up when prone had not been accomplished (Fig. 10.18B–E).

When Christian presented for chiropractic care he was on Albuterol to control wheezing and had been chronically ill with para-influenza. Nursing was unusual insofar as it resulted in loud gulping sounds.

The examination revealed a Type O skull molding pattern and left shoulder girdle dysfunction. The patient had never exhibited bilateral symmetry when lifting the upper extremities and preferred to leave the left arm down at his side. If placed on the floor in the prone position he would pull the left arm back and cry until he was turned over onto his back.

The patient's parents were told that spinal adjustments would not be performed until after an initial trial with craniosacral therapy. If the torticollis did not show improvement after three treatments then all additional treatment would be delayed until a full radiographic evaluation of the spine had been completed.

Treatment Outcome

Improvement was noticed after the second treatment (Fig. 10.18F) with resolution of the head tilt after the seventh treatment (Fig. 10.18G). Dysfunction in the left shoulder girdle gradually resolved by the end of the first month of treatment. As mobility improved, the patient began to demonstrate the appropriate symmetry when moving his arms and he was able to bring the left arm forward when prone. The patient no longer cried in the prone position, raised himself up and finally achieved the expected milestone of lifting his head and chest off the floor (Fig. 10.18H–I).

Treatment was focused on correcting the torsion in the cranial base by balancing the reciprocal membrane tensions (Fig.10.18J–M), balancing the sacral base with Logan Basic (Fig. 10.18N), adjustment of C1 with an activator adjusting instrument (Fig.10.18O), CST release of the transverse fascial tissue (Fig. 10.18P), trigger point

therapy to the muscles of the shoulder girdle (Fig. 10.18Q,R), cervical stretching (Fig. 10.18S), and cranial molding (Fig.10.18T). As the hypertonicity resolved, thoracic spinal adjustments were incorporated into the protocol. The mother was given instructions on how to perform inversion therapy, trigger point therapy, and cranial molding which she completed daily.

Compliance with recommended visits was good with 9 treatments the first month, 7 treatments the second month, and 5 treatments the third month. All signs of wheezing resolved during the third visit and previously prescribed medication was no longer needed. At the 5th visit, Christian's mother reported that his spine had started popping every time he was picked up and the loud gulping was no longer noticeable when he nursed.

Discussion

The cranial obliquity associated with the Type O skull pattern is most frequently due to the position of the fetus in the last weeks or even months of pregnancy. If the head is rotated and then laterally flexed, the forces of uterine contraction carried through the fetal spine will rotate portions of the occiput. The condylar parts will be rotated to one side, one laterally and the other medially, each

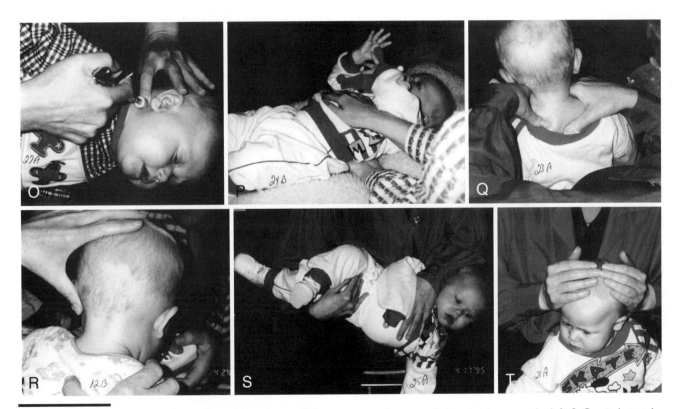

Figure 10.18. *(continued)*   O, C1 is adjusted lateral to medial and A/P with a light force directed through my finger. P, Release of the transverse fascial tissue within the respiratory diaphragm. The second treatment, resulted in a somatoemotional release (SER) as the patient cried with the voice of a newborn. Afterwards, there was an immediate improvement in the torticollis. Q, Trigger point therapy is used to break up spasms in the shoulder girdle while traction is applied to the cervical musculature on the left. R, As the musculature relaxed additional

stretch was applied to the tissues on the left. S, Cervical stretch is accomplished by: 1) lying the cranium down on one thigh with the involved side down, 2) allowing the torso to drop between the treating doctor's legs, 3) stabilizing the anterior chest with one hand and 4) slowly lifting the pelvis superior. (Parents must use toys to distract throughout all procedures) and the lift was only to patient comfort. T, The cranium was molded by gently directing hands over the skull toward the flattened occipital area.

about a vertical axis; the squama will be rotated toward the side of the condylar parts which is in lateral position; the basilar portion will be posterior on that side and anterior on the side on which the condylar is rotated medially. This will be the flat side of the back of the skull. The altered relationship between the anterior part of the basilar portion and the posterior part of the body of the sphenoid bone constitutes the first scoliotic curve in the cranial axis. The second will be at the sphenoethmoid junction.

Because of the altered relationship of the occiput and sphenoid bone, the petrous portions of the temporal bones will be in different planes. The one on the flat side of the skull, the concave side of the sphenobasilar junction, will be nearing the coronal plane, cephalad in relative position, in internal rotation with an added degree of posterior spiraling and probably anteromedial compression. The petrous portion of the temporal bone on the convex side of the sphenobasilar junction (i.e., the side to which the condylar parts was rotated laterally) will be relatively caudad, inclined toward the sagittal plane, externally rotated and further posterior about its apex, with a degree of increased anterior spiraling. Eventually, if not corrected soon enough, the cranial scoliosis will lead to a spinal scoliosis with deviation of the shoulder and pelvic girdles (69).

There are certain warning signs that indicate the possibility that a Type O skull pattern is developing with the resultant scoliotic curves in the sphenobasilar, sphenovomer and eventually cervicothoracic regions. These signs may include:

1. Preference for position;
2. Inability to lie prone;
3. Initially a perfectly round head;

4. Flatness of the occipital bone on one side;
5. Flatness of frontal bone on the opposite side; and
6. Congenital torticollis.

Warning signs in the preschooler include:

1. Neurological symptoms
2. Changes in inclination of the various transverse planes of the body: the petrous ridges, the base of the skull, the shoulder and pelvic girdles
3. Severe symptoms that result from a seemingly minor injury

Cranial obliquity needs to be addressed within 24 hours to avoid subsequent distortion to the membranous vault, basilar bones and cerebellum. If the distortion is not corrected before the condylar portions ossify at one year they will retain the distortion even when the mechanism is freed. These patients should have follow-up evaluations every 4-6 months to avoid severe reactions from occurring after a seemingly minor injury (69) and to avoid a spinal scoliotic compensation from developing.

This patient was exhibiting an in-utero constraint syndrome as evidenced by the mother's unrelenting rib pain and painful Braxton Hicks contractions. Prescribed bedrest may have only exacerbated the problem when the mother restricted her normal movement patterns. This resulted in abnormal force being applied during the delivery process which also may have contributed to the severity of the symptoms.

Craniosacral Examination and Treatment Protocol

An examination and treatment protocol for craniosacral procedures in the pediatric patient is provided in Figure 10.19.

Observe and Palpate

The newborn infant is best observed when placed in the center of a standard chiropractic cervical pillow that has raised lateral borders. The evaluation will be broken down into four basic areas: the vault and face, the mouth, the torso, and the extremities.

VAULT AND FACE

The examiner begins by observing and gently palpating the vault. First, observe the sutures and note any overriding or depressed areas. Next, using an extremely light touch with the palmar aspect of your hand, palpate the membranous vault and note any bony ridges or unusual depressions. The vault should appear and feel smooth and round with obvious membranous intervals at the four angles of the quadrilateral shaped parietal bones in the newborn. Note which of the fontanelles have closed. Note any abnormal bulging or depression of the anterior fontanelle which would indicate possible hydrocephalus or dehydration that must be addressed immediately.

Note any obvious asymmetry of the paired bones of the vault or distortion of the individual unossified segments within each bone. The facial bones may be evaluated for symmetry by carefully observing the symmetry of the more obvious facial features. Keep in mind that the newborn with a Type O (Oblique) skull may present with a perfectly round skull at birth and will only later (>10 weeks) begin to demonstrate the osseous changes in the cranium and spine.

MOUTH

Next, observe and palpate the cranial base by placing the palmar surface of the distal tip of your fifth digit gently against the palate (Fig. 10.20). A high, narrow, arched palate or a ridge palpated along the medial aspect indicates cranial base distortion. Correction may occur while the patient sucks on the examiner's finger, as the opposite hand is used to balance the reciprocal membrane tension within the cranial vault. The palate should have a soft C-shape to it both antero-posterior and side to side. The examiner should never apply force in the mouth of a newborn. The amount of force necessary will be sufficiently applied by the tongue of the infant against the examiner's finger. The examiner's contact is for the purpose of

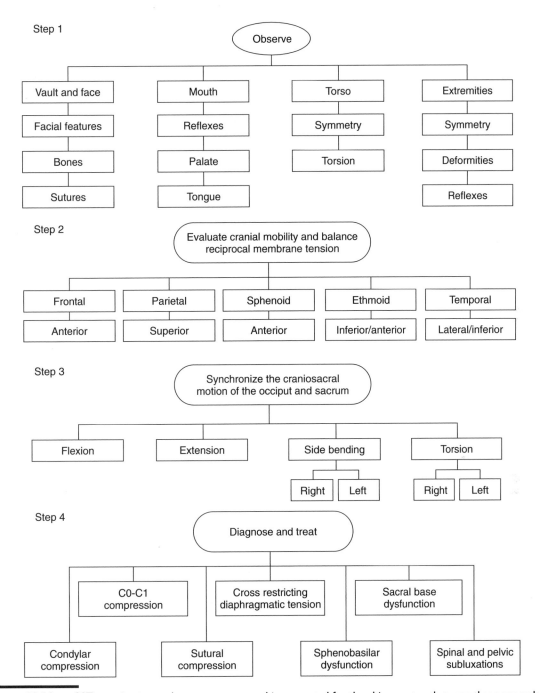

Figure 10.19.   CST examination and treatment protocol is presented for the chiropractor that uses these procedures.

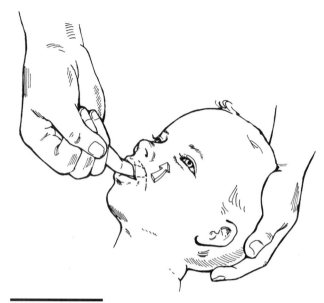

Figure 10.20. Evaluate the contour of the palate as an assessment of the cranial base.

the craniosacral system. That aspect of the examination is thoroughly covered throughout this text and will not be elaborated on in this chapter.

EXTREMITIES

When eliciting the infant reflexes, observe for symmetry of response between the two upper and lower extremities. Observe carefully for subtle anomalies such as a palmar crease, syndactyly of the fingers or toes, or abnormally large or small digits. These are all indicators alerting the examiner to possible skeletal or organ anomalies that should be investigated.

Evaluate Cranial Base Mobility and Balance

RECIPROCAL MEMBRANE TENSION

History alone is not a valid determination of either the presence or absence of adverse cranial compression. It is imperative that each newborn be carefully evaluated for restricted cranial base mobility and that abnormal membrane tension within the dural system be corrected by using the vault bones as handles to evaluate and correct distortion

evaluating for asymmetry, compression, or distraction of the paired palatine bones; evaluating the strength, weakness, and motor control of the tongue; and to elicit the sucking reflex. If this contact is placed correctly and elicits the gag reflex, the infant may be having neurological difficulties and this portion of the exam should be quick and brief until further treatment has been completed.

TORSO

Observe the torso for abnormal shape or symmetry of the ribs, clavicles, and scapula; the nipples; and the umbilicus. Next, palpate the cross restricting diaphragms (i.e., thoracic, respiratory, and pelvic) by placing the palmar aspect of your left hand flat and under the posterior aspect of the diaphragm and the second and third digits of the right hand over the anterior aspect. Very gently apply a light A/P vector of force into the diaphragm and monitor the subtle tissue response (16).

The pelvic floor muscles and the respiratory diaphragm are said to exhibit a powerful influence on the longitudinal fascial mobility and the delivery of fluid through these transverse structures (14). It is, therefore, imperative that muscular hypertonus and fascial tension imbalances be successfully treated before abnormal alterations in the craniosacral physiological motion can be corrected.

Due to the nature of craniosacral therapy, the very act of palpating these diaphragms correctly will also allow you to release or restore abnormal torsion or tone within the muscles and their fascial coverings. If this occurs, go back and re-evaluate any skeletal asymmetry noted earlier before moving on to the examination of the extremities.

The chiropractic examiner should complete the examination of the torso with a thorough examination of the spinal and pelvic structures as subluxations may cause tension or abnormal change in the character of the dural sleeve. If this occurs, it will produce a "dural drag" upon the free motion of

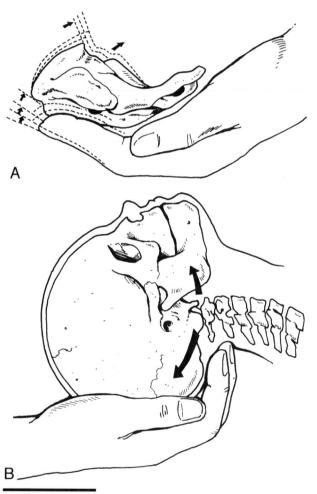

A

B

Figure 10.21. A, The sacral base is moving anteriorward during sacral extension. B, The occiput is gently tractioned posteriorward during cranial flexion.

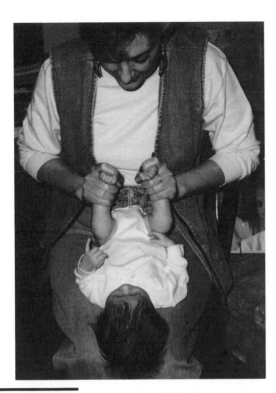

Figure 10.22.   Inversion Analysis: With the infant resting face up on the parent's lap, the ankles are grasped with the index finger placed over the sole of the foot.

within the stress fibers of the dural membrane. If this is not achieved prior to the ossification of the individual segments of the cranial bones, not only will the various components fuse in an aberrant position, but the elasticity of the associated membranes will be impaired and the stress fibers within will thicken. According to Arbuckle (1), the associated thickening will make correction at a later date difficult if not impossible. See Fig. 10.18 J-M for a demonstration of this procedure.

SYNCHRONIZING THE MOTION BETWEEN THE OCCIPUT AND SACRUM

When evaluating the mobility of the spinal dural tube in a small child it is imperative that it be done only when the infant/child is comfortable and relaxed. If the baby is crying or fighting the treatment it will lead to incorrect diagnostic impressions and, ultimately, to ineffective treatment.

To balance the occiput and the sacrum, one hand cups the occiput while the other hand is placed under the sacrum (Fig.10.21A-B). Evaluate the synchronous movements of the occiput and sacrum by simultaneously putting them into flexion (the occiput and sacral base drop posterior as the forehead and sacral apex move anterior), extension (the occiput and sacral base both move anterior as the forehead and sacral apex move posterior) sidebending (both the cranium and the sacrum are laterally flexed to the same side as the torso becomes concave on the side of lateral flexion) and torsion (the cranium rotates to one side as the pelvis rotates to the opposite side). Any restrictions noted are mobilized

by holding gentle pressure against the restriction barrier until a relaxation is felt. This should be followed by symmetrical movement of all the associated tissues. If this does not achieve correction, then the patient should be evaluated further for spinal or sacroiliac subluxations. Following adjustive therapy, the patient should be reevaluated to insure that correction of the restricted motion between the occiput and sacrum has been achieved.

Patient Education

A chiropractor's role in patient care does not end with the treatment. As a doctor, we should help all parents understand how they can prevent spinal injuries, recognize spinal distortion patterns and perform daily exercises that reduce minor subluxations and fixations before they become chronic problems. One way to achieve these goals with the newborn is by performing an inversion analysis daily.

To perform this exercise, the infant is placed face up on the parent's lap with the infant's head resting on the parent's knees. The ankles are grasped gently, but firmly, with the index finger over the bottom of the foot (Fig.10.22). In a larger child, the leg can be grasped firmly around the calf muscle. The other parent or a sibling will now stand directly in front of the infant so that they do not become alarmed as the parent slowly stands up. With the infant in the vertical position (Fig.10.23), the weight of the head will place a gentle traction on the muscles of the body and will allow the CSF to flow in the direction of the cranium. A gentle back and forth swaying of the body will then allow the parents to visualize the symmetry of the pelvis

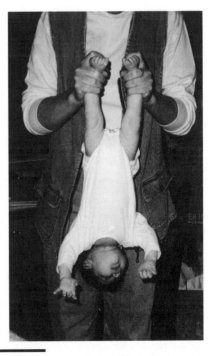

Figure 10.23.   In the vertical position, aberrant posturing is indicated if the infant maintains any structural deviation away from the center of gravity.

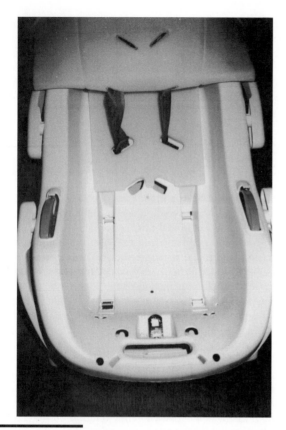

Figure 10.24. Parents are encouraged to inspect all infant carriers and car seats. Most carriers have no form of support below a piece of foam on the upper aspect of the carrier. This has the potential to induce spinal or pelvic subluxations.

the infant appears centered and relaxed. Then, an extremely slight downward impulse is directed through the feet to help the muscles set the alignment of the spine. If the infant does not move into a vertically relaxed position, no downward thrust should be performed and further evaluation and treatment is indicated. While this author is not aware of any contraindications to conducting this procedure, the analysis should be applied carefully and slowly. Should an infant have any indication of possible hip dislocation, he or she may be held upright by gently but firmly grasping the pelvis and the analysis can be restricted to the upper torso, spine and cranium. Parents can be taught to perform this analysis daily as they can decrease minor subluxations as they occur. The parents will also become adapt at noticing asymptomatic distortions within their child's structure and may then take a more proactive position in determining the frequency of treatment.

Parents of a newborn or small child should also be taught how to prevent spinal subluxations from occurring by having them investigate their child's infant carrier. Most carriers are made with a piece of foam placed on the upper aspect of the hard plastic seat (Fig. 10.24). Parents are encouraged to replace that with a piece of foam that covers the entire seat and gives the infant spine full support. Figure 10.25 demonstrates what the seat looks like with the additional piece of foam that fits the entire seat.

and spine. This procedure is performed for approximately 20 seconds. This analysis is less accurate when the child is old enough and strong enough to forcefully twist their body to look at someone. Aberrant posturing is indicated if the infant:

1. Rotates or laterally flexes their head to one side and maintains that posture
2. Rotates or laterally flexes the shoulders or pelvis
3. Maintains flexion of one or both legs
4. Does not demonstrate symmetry of arm motion
5. Maintains a hyperextended spinal posture

If properly prepared for inversion prior to being lifted into this position, a child will generally laugh and relax when the procedure is performed. If they begin to cry during the procedure, stop immediately and observe the cranium. It should appear flushed with no white areas over the sutures. If this occurs, it is an indication that there may be a restriction within one or more sutures and CST is indicated. Re-evaluate after the patient has received CST and spinal adjustments to insure that the restrictions have been reduced.

During the 20–30 seconds of inversion, the infant should be allowed to move his or her body and/or rotate the head until

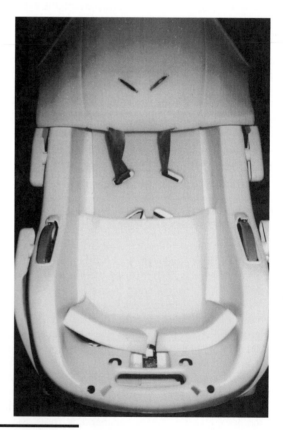

Figure 10.25. This infant seat has a piece of foam inserted that matches the existing foam. Note the depth needed to level out the back support.

General Considerations in Case Management

Chiropractic spinal adjustive therapy and craniosacral therapy, when applied during the perinatal period, should be non-intrusive and indirect (except in the case of balancing the motion between the occiput and sacrum which uses a gentle direct pressure). Upledger defines the indirect technique as one that releases a restriction or abnormal barrier to motion within the cranium by encouraging motion in the direction of ease (which is usually opposite to the direction of the restriction). The therapeutic effect will be one of tissue softening or releasing which will result in an ease of cranial motion and restoration of symmetry.

The inherent mobility and energy of the craniosacral mechanism has a much smaller range and amplitude in the newborn. Moreover, the levers (cranial vault bones) with which we perceive much of the motion are significantly smaller, and the movement of the membranous regions more subtle (14). Therefore, in order to apply this manual technique with the required precision, depth, and dexterity, the practitioner should become proficient in assessing craniosacral dysfunction first in the adult, next in the teenager, the adolescent and finally the child prior to treating the newborn.

Also, for desired results, the carefully applied examining forces should always be carried away from, never toward, foramina or fontanelles. These force vectors must be understood, for the misapplication of forces or management of stresses may add further insult to the original injury. Last of all, before treating a newborn, it is necessary to understand the immature structure to be handled, the details of the mechanism, and the needed alterations. When a practitioner is asked to treat a newborn or small child prior to the achievement of these necessary skills, they should consider referring the patient to a Craniosacral therapist in their area. Craniosacral therapy is a rapidly growing profession with therapists in almost all of the healing arts such as: chiropractic, osteopathy, occupational therapy, physical therapy, massage therapy, dentistry and medicine. A directory of craniosacral therapists is available through the International Association of Healthcare Practitioners (IAHP) and can be acquired through the Upledger Institute in Palm Beach, Florida. Currently, training in CST is offered, on a regular basis, in more than 50 cities throughout the United States. At this time, there are more than 20,000 people around the world who have completed the training.

While it is inadvisable to begin learning CST on a small pediatric patient, the therapy has been applied by many chiropractors who have received the information, as it has been presented in this chapter, with positive results reported to this author.

REFERENCES

1. Arbuckle B. The Selected Writings of Beryl E. Arbuckle. Indiana: American Academy of Osteopathy, 1994.
2. Biedermann H. Kinematic imbalances due to suboccipital strain in newborns. J Manual Medicine 1992;6:151-156.
3. Frymann V. Learning difficulties of children viewed in the light of the osteopathic concept In: The Cranium and Its Sutures. Germany: Springer-Verlag, 1987.
4. Pederick F. For debate: cranial adjusting-an overview. Chiropr J Aust 1993; 23:106-12.
5. Retzlaff EW, Michael DK, Roppel RM, Mitchell FL. The structures of cranial bone sutures. J Am Osteopath Assoc 1976;75:607-608.
6. Boyd R. An introduction to bio cranial therapy. United Kingdom: International Bio Cranial Academy, 1991.
7. Cohen D. The craniosacral rhythmic impulse. Am Chiropractor 1989;Mar:
8. Bilgrai Cohen K. Clinical Management of Infants & Children. Calif: Extension Press, 1988.
9. Cottom N. Cranial and facial adjustment step by step. Self-published, 1987.
10. DeJarnette B. Cranial technique. Nebraska:Self-published, 1979.
11. Goodheart GJ. Applied kinesiology 1981 Workshop Procedure Manual-Vol. 1, 1981.
12. Freedman B. The biodynamical aspect of cerebrospinal fluid in disease and health. J Manipulative Physiol Ther 1979; 2:79-83.
13. Magoun H. Osteopathy in the cranial field. Missouri: The Journal Printing Co., 1976.
14. Pick M. A preliminary single case magnetic resonance imaging investigation into maxillary frontal-parietal manipulation and its short-term effect upon the inter-cranial structures of an adult human brain. J Manipulative Physiol Ther 1994; 17:168-173.
15. Sutherland A. The cranial bowl. Minnesota:Self-published,1939.
16. Upledger J. Craniosacral therapy. Seattle: Eastland Press, 1983.
17. Walther D. Applied kinesiology. Colorado: Systems DC, 1988:343-393.
18. Smith GH. Cranial Dental Sacral Complex. Pennsylvania: Self-published, 1983.
19. Denton D. Craniopathy and dentistry. California: Self-published, 1979.
20. Greenman P. Roentgen findings in the craniosacral mechanism. J Am Osteopath Assoc 1970;70:60-70.
21. Retzlaff E. A preliminary study of cranial bone movement in squirrel monkeys. J Am Osteopath Assoc 1975;74:866-869.
22. Upledger J. The reproducibility of craniosacral examination findings: a statistical analysis. J Am Osteopath Assoc 1977;76:890-899.
23. Upledger J. Mechano-electric patterns during craniosacral osteopathic diagnosis and treatment. J Am Osteopath Assoc 1979; 78:782-91.
24. Kostopoulos D. Changes in magnitude of relative elongation of falx cerebri during the application of external forces on the frontal bone of an embalmed cadaver. Physical Therapy Forum 1991;April 5:9-11.
25. Adams T, et al. Parietal bone mobility in the anesthetized cat. J Am Osteopath Assoc 1992; 92:599-622.
26. Upledger J. The relationship of craniosacral examination findings in grade school children with developmental problems. J Am Osteopath Assoc 1978; 77:738-54.
27. Upledger J. Beyond the dura. Seattle, Washington: Eastland Press, 1987.
28. Karni Z, Upledger JE, Mizrahi J, et al. Examination of the cranial rhythm in long-standing coma and chronic neurologic cases. In: Upledger JE, Vredevoogd JD, eds. Craniosacral therapy. Seattle, Washington: Eastland Press, 1983: 275-281.
29. Gresham E. Birth trauma. Ped Clin North America 1975; 22:317-328.
30. Donn S, Faix R. Long-term prognosis for the infant with severe birth trauma. Clinics in Perinatology 1983; 10:507-520.
31. Beyers N, Moosa A. Depressed skull fracture in the newborn. SA Medical J 1978; Nov:830-832.
32. Eisenberg D. Neonatal skull depression unassociated with birth trauma. AJR 1984; 143:1063-1064.
33. Bergen R, Margolis S. Retinal hemorrhages in the newborn. Ann Ophthalmol 1976; Jan:53-56.
34. Kaur B, Taylor D. Fundus hemorrhages in infancy. Surv Ophthalmol 1992; 37:1:1-17.
35. Wigglesworth JS, Husemeyer RP. Intracranial birth trauma in vaginal breech delivery: The continued importance of injury to the occipital bone. Br J Obst Gyn 1977; 84:684-691.
36. Govaert P. Traumatic neonatal intracranial bleeding and stroke. Arch Dis Child 1992; 67:840-845.
37. Takage T. Posterior fossa subdural hemorrhage in the newborn as a result of birth trauma. Child's Brain 1982; 9:102-113.
38. Sugai M. Four autopsy cases of neonatal giant cell hepatitis died suddenly and unexpectedly from intracranial hemorrhage. Acta Path Jap 1978; 28:185-191.
39. Piatt J. Intracranial arterial aneurysm due to birth trauma. J Neurosurg 1992; 77:799-803.
40. Takagi T. Extradural hemorrhage in the newborn as a result of birth trauma. Child's Brain 1978; 4:306-318.
41. Coupland S. Visual evoked potentials, intracranial pressure and ventricular size in hydrocephalus. Documents Ophthalmologica 1987; 66:321-330.
42. Gottlieb M. Neglected spinal cord, brain stem and musculoskeletal injuries stemming from birth trauma: review of the literature. J Manipulative Physiol Ther 1993; 16:537-543.
43. Weiselfish S. An overview of Erb's Palsy with case history documenting treatment with manual and craniosacral therapy. Physical Therapy Forum 1990; IX:12.
44. Bilkey WJ. Cranial suture manipulation in the treatment of torticollis. J Manual Medicine 1992; 6:212-214.
45. Poole, Briggs M. The cranio-facio-cervical scoliosis complex. Br J Plastic Surg 1990; 43:670-675.
46. Bredenkamp JK. Congenital muscular torticollis. A spectrum of disease. Arch Otolaryngol Head Neck Surg 1990; 116:212-216.

47. Lawrence WT. Congenital muscular torticollis: a spectrum of pathology (Review). Ann Plastic Surg 1989; 23:523-530.
48. Wolfort FG. Torticollis (Review). Plastic Reconstructive Surg 1989; 84:682-692.
49. Binder H. Congenital muscular torticollis: results of conservative management with long-term follow-up in 85 cases. Arch Phys Med Rehab 1987; 68:222-225.
50. Jacobson RI. Abnormalities of the skull in children (Review). Neurol Clin 1985; 3:117-145.
51. Suzuki S. The aetiological relationship between congenital torticollis and obstetrical paralysis. International Orthopaedics 1984; 8:175-181.
52. Cheng JC. Infantile torticollis: a review of 624 cases. J Pediatric Orthop 1994; 14:802-808.
53. Emery C. The determinants of treatment duration for congenital muscular torticollis. Phys Ther 1994; 74:921-929.
54. Toto BJ. Chiropractic correction of congenital muscular torticollis. J Manipulative Physiol Ther 1993; 16:556-559.
55. Slate RK. Cervical spine subluxation associated with congenital muscular torticollis and craniofacial asymmetry. Plastic Reconstructive Surg 1993; 91:1187-1195.
56. Ferguson JW. Cephalometric interpretation and assessment of facial asymmetry secondary to congenital torticollis. The significance of cranial base reference lines. International J Oral Maxillofacial Surg 1993; 22:7-10.
57. Davids JR. Congenital muscular torticollis: sequela of intrauterine or perinatal compartment syndrome. J Pediatr Orthop 1993; 13:141-147.
58. Mukasa G.K. Birth trauma among liveborn infants in Mulago hospital, Uganda. East African Med J 1993; 70:438-440.
59. McAlpine J. A discussion of the dentate ligament and neural traction mechanism. Int Rev Chiro 1980; Oct-Dec:35-37.
60. Upledger J. The facilitated segment. Massage Ther J 1989; Summer:22-25.
61. Bueno I. Congenital hemihypertrophy. Genetic Counseling 1993; 4:231-234.
62. Stoll C. Twelve cases with hemihypertrophy: etiology and follow up. Genetic Counseling 1993; 4:119-126.
63. Haire D. Fetal effects of ultrasound: a growing controversy. J Nurse-Midwifery 1984; 29:241-244.
64. Taylor K. A prudent approach to ultrasound imaging of the fetus and newborn. Birth 1990; 17:218-222.
65. Ziskin M. Update on the safety of ultrasound in obstetrics. Seminars in Roentgenology 1990; 25:294-298.
66. Piatt J. Intracranial arterial aneurysm due to birth trauma. J Neurosurg 1992; 77:799-803.
67. Arbuckle B. The value of occupational and osteopathic manipulative therapy in the rehabilitation of the cerebral palsy victim. In: Selected Writings of Beryl E. Arbuckle. Indiana: The American Academy of Osteopathy, 1994.
68. Arbuckle B. Effects of uterine forces upon the fetus. In: The Selected Writings of Beryl E. Arbuckle. Indiana: The American Academy of Osteopathy, 1994.
69. Arbuckle B. Scoliosis Capitis. In: The Selected Writings of Beryl E. Arbuckle. Indiana: The American Academy of Osteopathy, 1994.

11 Pediatric Nutrition

Susan M. St. Claire and Ronald J. Picardi

Most chiropractors recognize the importance of good nutritional practices in health promotion. Although historically nutritional factors have been well-described for a variety of disease states (e.g. scurvy, starvation), only relatively recently has the importance of optimal nutrition in disease prevention been recognized. This change in perspective comes at a time when in the U.S., eight of the ten leading causes of death have diet-related components (1).

This chapter focuses on several key areas of pediatric nutrition. The importance of breast feeding during the first 6 months of life is discussed in some detail, as are the topics of food allergy, hyperactivity syndrome, vegetarian diets, childhood obesity, sports nutrition, and supplementation. It is beyond the scope of this chapter to present all issues of pediatric or adult nutrition. The reader is referred to other sources (2,3) to supplement the information discussed here.

General Considerations

The common divisions of nutritional changes occur in the following age groups:

1. Infants: age 0-6 months
2. Infants: 6 months-1 year
3. Toddlers: age 1-3 years
4. Children: 4-10 years
5. Adolescents: 11-18 years
6. Adults: 18 or 19+

The oldest form of assessment is the calorie count which was based on the erroneous assumption that malnutrition was due to a reduced consumption of nutrients. Actual malnutrition or deficiency is based on five factors as described by Herbert in 1973 (4):

1. Inadequate intake
2. Impaired absorption
3. Impaired utilization
4. Increased excretion
5. Increased requirements

Monitoring dietary intake is important, but does not measure nutritional status. The most important functional index of nutriture in children is growth. The velocity of growth requires serial measurement (see Chapter 14; growth charts).

Growth of infants during the first two years of life is of particular interest because recent studies indicate that most growth faltering in disadvantaged populations occurs during that period (5-7).

Pediatric nutritional deficiency is not uncommon in the US. In one study, 18% of admitted pediatric patients were found to have two or more indices indicating nutritional deficiency (6). Nutritional deficiency commonly impairs immune responses prior to clinical signs, making judgments of nutritional status without adequate knowledge of the child's nutritional history incomplete (6). There are many signs and symptoms associated with nutritional deficiencies. Early identification can prevent more severe problems later.

Breast Feeding vs. Formula and Cow's Milk

The preferred first food for infants during the first 6 months of life is human breast milk. The benefits of breast feeding are biochemical (nutritional), immunological, psychological, and socioeconomic. In the late 1960s and early 1970s formula feeding exceeded breast feeding by about four-fold. This was followed by a steady increase in the incidence of breast feeding which peaked at about 55% at birth in the mid-1980s. Presently, about 48% of newborns and 80% of infants at 6 months receive infant formula rather than human milk (8).

Although the psychological benefits will not be discussed in this chapter, it is notable that infants have fewer feeding problems (whether bottle or breast) when the mother is happier and more comfortable with her child. The infant grimaces and gags less during feeding when the mother smiles and vocalizes more frequently during feedings (9).

Immunity

Increased immunity occurs in infants who are breast fed. Sepsis, which is the presence of pathogenic organisms or their toxins in blood or tissues, is a major cause of morbidity and mortality in infants. Among neonates, breast feeding protects against neonatal sepsis (10). Intestinal sepsis often leads to diarrhea, which can dehydrate the child. Severe dehydration can cause death.

DIARRHEA

Severe diarrhea is a major cause of morbidity and mortality in infants and young children in developing countries or in children in developed nations who are immunocompromised (e.g., AIDS), attend day-care centers, or travel to other countries. There is no safe or effective vaccine for many important intestinal pathogens. Antibodies in human milk provide protection against diarrheal disease in breast-fed infants (11,12). *Bifidobacterium bifidum* and *S thermophilus* are the main intestinal flora of breast-fed children. These organisms appear to reduce the incidence of acute diarrhea and rotovirus shedding.

A double-blind placebo controlled study of children receiving a standard formula and one supplemented with the normal flora found that the supplemented group had less diarrheal disease populations (13). These organisms can be cultivated cheaply and the recommendation was to routinely add them to foods for children and adults as a practical means to reduce diarrheal disease, especially in hospitalized or immuno-suppressed populations.

Non-breast-fed infants can receive passive immunity through bovine colostrum when the cow has been immunized with a retrovirus. The immunoglobulin concentrates in the cow's milk can be fed to infants. However, not enough of the antibodies survived the gastric PH or trypsin (pancreatic enzyme). Petschow and Talbott (14) have suggested administering the bovine antibodies via microencapsulation or in combination with a trypsin inhibitor as an economical and safe method of providing immunity.

LUNG DISEASE

Bronchitis, bronchiolitis, and pneumonia cause four times more deaths in infants who are not breast fed. Bottle feeding increased the risk of Hemophilus influenza, bacteremia, and meningitis by four to sixteen-fold in North American infants (15).

DIABETES

Breast feeding seems to play a marginal role in the prevention of insulin-dependent diabetes mellitus (16).

OTITIS MEDIA

Otitis media and allergies are less common in breast-fed children. Exclusive breast feeding for at least 4 months protects against otitis media (17). The incidence was decreased by half when compared to non-breast fed infants and 40% less than infants supplemented with other foods prior to 4 months. The recurrence rate was 10% in breast-fed infants and 20.5% in non-breast fed infants (17,18).

Growth

Breast fed children put on weight more slowly than formula fed, are leaner (less body fat), and take in fewer kcals. It appears that the breast-fed are able to regulate food intake better (19,20).

Length and head diameters are almost identical for breast-fed and formula-fed infants during the first 2 years, but the formula-fed children are on the average heavier than breast-fed children between 7 and 18 months (5). The breast-fed child continues to put on weight at a constant or even increasing rate (change in weight in grams/month) between ages 8 and 21 months, whereas the formula-fed infant slows in rate of change in weight. Between 21 and 24 months, both groups show an abrupt decline in weight gain and merge on the same path.

NEUROLOGICAL DEVELOPMENT

Breast-fed infants appeared to have an improved neurological development than formula-fed children (21). Lanting et al. (21) report on a study of 135 breast-fed and 391 formula-fed infants who at birth received neurological tests and were subsequently classified as normal, slightly abnormal, or frankly abnormal. At the age of 9, the children were re-examined. The breast-fed infants had higher neurological outcomes. The longer chain poly-unsaturated fatty acids (PUFA) present in breast milk, but not in most formulas, may have a role since they are vital for brain development. Previous studies (21) have reported less learning disorders and behavioral problems in the breast fed.

INTELLECTUAL DEVELOPMENT

Breast feeding appears to influence the intellectual development of the child based on psychomotor skills. In one study (22), 229 healthy infants were either breast-fed or bottle-fed. Skills were measured between the ages of 18 and 29 months. Those performing the poorest were bottle-fed, lower middle and lower social class, low maternal education, had more temper tantrums, and were more likely to have siblings (22).

Contraindications

There are some potential risks with mother's milk since it may be a carrier of contaminants—both dietary (alcohol) and environmental (smoke residue/drugs). Most women in the US use at least 2 drugs during lactation (23).

Contraindications to breast feeding include galactosemia, active maternal TB, AIDS, and possibly familial hypercholesterolemia. Additional supplementation may be required for infants with malabsorption and low body weight. With the preceding caution, mother's milk is the food of choice (23).

COMPOSITION

Human breast milk is designed to meet the nutritional needs and physiologic limitations of human infants (24). Several factors must be considered:

1. Is the composition of the milk adequate?
2. Should you supplement with a formula?

3. Should you introduce complementary foods?

4. What are the nutritional needs of the child?

The composition of each species' milk reflects its needs to ensure optimal growth, development, and survival. Human milk needs vary among infants and human milk composition varies among mothers. Breast milk contains 8-10% protein, 45% fat, and 45% carbohydrates (25). What the mother eats influences both the sensory qualities (odor and flavor) and the composition of her milk. Infants will drink more or less milk depending on these factors. For example, when mothers ingested garlic capsules, infants responded by sucking more and for a longer period than following a placebo (26). The composition of milk can be affected by:

1. Stage of lactation
2. Premature delivery
3. Age of the mother
4. Timing of milk release during a feeding
5. Baby's demand for milk
6. Mother's nutritional status
7. Geographical region (soil content)

Formulas are designed to mimic mothers milk plus additional supplementation like vitamin D and iron thought to be low in breast milk. The typical base is cow or soy (protein isolates or hydrolysates) and most of the fat is from vegetable oils (human milk is high in long chain PUFAs to supply the EFA). Lactose or sucrose and corn syrup are the usual carbohydrates. The cow protein ratio of whey to casein is usually modified to match human breast milk.

Human milk compared to cow's has higher lactose. Alpha-lactalbumin, a key protein involved in the synthesis of lactose, represents 25-30% of total human milk protein. Bifidobacterium flourish well in this environment (27). Human milk has lower protein and mineral content, but it is more bioavailable than cow's milk. This reflects the slower rate of growth and longer duration of infancy in humans compared to cows. Formulas are based on general analysis of human milk composition. Left out are the known, but unidentified, binding proteins and transfer factors which are necessary for optimum uptake, distribution, and utilization of nutritional components as well as identified factors such as prostaglandins, epidermal growth factor, prolactin and other milk-borne hormones (8).

IRON SUPPLEMENTATION

Iron supplementation is typically recommended since human milk is low in iron, but may be unnecessary or even hazardous. Human milk is rich in lactoferrin, an iron-chelating protein that makes iron available to the gut while sequestering it from iron-dependent gut flora. The high rate of red blood cell salvage of heme iron combined with a small but steady supply from maternal milk, may create optimal ecology. Transferrin is also found in human breast milk.

Excess iron in the gut has been associated with gastrointestinal tract disturbances and a risk factor for later colorectal cancer and heart disease (28). Excess iron intake has been known to increase bacterial replication during infections in tissue and in the gut (29,30). Iron may compete with the uptake of other essential nutrients such as zinc (31).

Iron may also retard growth of anemic infants. During a 4 month study on 12-18 month old children, the supplemented group gained less weight than the placebo group although length and arm circumference remained the same. The group was not analyzed for lean vs. fatty muscle mass (32).

The American Academy of Pediatrics recommends withholding cow's milk until at least one year of age. Infants receiving whole cow's milk during the first year of life developed iron deficiency because cow's milk is a poor source of iron, is not bioavailable, lacks adequate vitamin C and causes occult gastrointestinal bleeding (33).

VITAMIN D

Vitamin D fortified milk and infant formulas are the norm, but may cause toxicity. Vitamin D has been added to cow's milk since the 1930s to decrease the incidence of Rickets. Hypervitaminosis D may occur from drinking as little as ½ cup daily of milk that has been incorrectly or excessively fortified. This causes excessive loss of calcium compromising bone integrity and muscular function. In one reported case of hypervitaminosis D, a 15-month-old girl had a history of failure to thrive, anorexia, constipation, irritability, and vomiting after weaning to whole milk. Renal ultrasound revealed nephrocalcinosis (34). An evaluation of milk and infant formulas revealed that none had the amount of Vitamin D shown on the label. Some samples had none and seven out of ten had 200% of the listed amount while one had 419% of the amount on the label. Both too little and too much vitamin D is hazardous to health (35).

ZINC

Zinc is usually supplemented in formulas at an amount higher than in human milk. Human milk has small doses of zinc and over the first few months of lactation decreases significantly. Zinc deficiencies are common in premature infants, malabsorption syndromes, and in parenteral fed infants, but uncommon in breast-fed infants. Recently zinc deficiencies have been reported in breast-fed infants. Zinc is essential for protein synthesis. Signs and symptoms appear in rapidly growing tissue as skin lesions (appearing similar to diaper rash or candida), diarrhea, growth failure, alopecia, irritability, and anorexia. The zinc deficiencies are most likely due to inadequate amounts in the breast milk due to poor intake by the mother or through a defective uptake by the mammary gland from the plasma (36).

A study done on 200 exclusively breast-fed infants who lost rather than gained weight during the first 6 months of life were found to be zinc deficient. The mothers were supplemented with 0, 20, or 40 mg zinc sulfate daily. Supplements helped maintain the zinc concentrations in milk and improved the mothers' serum values. Supplementation had no effect on the growth rates of the infants. In fact, those with the lowest zinc levels grew the fastest. There was no correlation with birth weight or length and infant or mothers' zinc concentration (37).

VITAMIN A SUPPLEMENTATION

Children deficient in vitamin A are more likely to die from measles, a common childhood disease (38,39). Vitamin A is available in low cost liquid formulations and is supplemented in infant formulas (2000 u/L). The current recommendation for children diagnosed with measles is to receive 100,000 IU oral vitamin A if younger than 12 months and 200,000 IU for older children if there is any reason to suspect vitamin A deficiency. If there are also signs and symptoms of vitamin A deficiency, the World Health Organization (WHO) recommends a repeat dose 24 hours and 4 weeks later. At this time, no reported cases of acute vitamin A toxicity have occurred with this protocol since it was initiated in 1987 by the WHO (38,39).

Vitamin A has also been shown to reduce severe diarrhea in a double-blind placebo controlled trial of 1240 children in Brazil aged 6-48 months. Those under age 12 months received 100,000 IU while older children received 200,000 IU as oral gelatin capsules given at the start and every 4 months for 4 total doses. Of school aged children, about 16% had a biochemical deficiency of vitamin A. There was no reduction in respiratory tract infections in the vitamin A group (40).

VITAMIN K

Hemorrhagic disease of the newborn (HDN) and late HDN occur as unexpected bleeding in previously healthy appearing neonates and infants as a result of vitamin K deficiency. This occurs primarily in breast-fed infants who did not receive prophylatic vitamin K at birth or in infants with malabsorption syndromes. Oral vitamin K is currently not available in the U.S. so intramuscular doses are administered. In 1990, a researcher suggested a correlation between IM vitamin K at birth and an increased incidence of childhood leukemia. Recent data does not support that conclusion (41).

Caloric Requirements

As the child grows, it needs more nutrients. In most situations, the mother's milk production increases to meet the demand. In most of the world, the mother continues to nurse for as much as two years. According to Konner (42), the Kune Bush people breast feed 4-5 times per hour for 2-3 years. The child develops its own immunity by age 3-5 years. If breast feeding stops too soon (before age one), the child will not get the mother's passive immunity resulting in high infant death rates. If the child is not growing as expected, or the mother cannot produce adequate milk, then additional foods may be needed. The energy requirements at different ages are as follows:

1. Infants (80-140 kcal/kg/day)
2. Children (40-90 kcal/kg/day)
3. Adolescents (30-50 kcal/kg/day)

The protein requirements for infants are 2-4 g/kg/day. For children, 1.5-2.5 g/kg/day is needed and for adolescents 1-2 g/kg/day is required.

If switching to cow's milk, use a formula and keep it to no more than one third the day's total kilocalories. Never use non-formula cow's milk for infants. Non-formula cow's milk should not be used until at least one year of age. It causes allergies, contains almost no iron, essential fatty acids, or vitamins, and may cause gastrointestinal tract bleeding. The quantity of minerals and the high protein content and osmolality may be harmful to some infants. Skim milk provides too few calories in an inappropriate distribution of protein, carbohydrates and fats (25,43).

Complementary Foods

It is recommended to wait to introduce the first complementary food until about 6 months. The child's development of the gastrointestinal tract and immune system is usually able to handle some foods. The introduction of foods and liquids increases the risk of diarrheal disease due to ineffective and immunological/allergic complications. Because of this, foods are typically introduced one at a time. There appears to be no advantage to starting complementary foods prior to 6 months in terms of growth (weight and length). The infant takes in the same amount of kcals whether on breast milk, complementary foods, or a combination, and the growth rates (weight and height) remain within normal (44,45).

The child appears more likely to try a new, solid food if it has been pre-exposed through mother's milk. Animal studies indicate that the weanling will be more likely to try foods mom ate or passed into her feces or got caught in her fur (46). In a study of 36 infants age 4 to 6 months, those that were breast fed showed greater acceptance of solid foods (vegetables) and greater levels of intake than formula fed infants (46). Although the breast fed infants took in more vegetables, they did not gain any more weight than the formula fed infants eating vegetables.

The introduction of vegetables should begin one at a time. Begin with yellow vegetables (e.g. carrot, squash), followed by the greens. The introduction of vegetables may take several weeks to months. The vegetable item may be prepared with a food processor. The parent should present the vegetable for several days, prior to introducing the next item. Whole grains (e.g. rice, millet, etc.) and legumes can be prepared by softening the grain/legume with added water and simmering. This produces the whole grain/legume in a texture that may be swallowed.

Many parents are choosing to avoid or limit dairy products in their children's diet. Replacing dairy (e.g. milk, cheese) with rice or soy products is an alternative. Tofu and Tempe products can also be added to diets that have reduced or eliminated dairy and/or meat products but need to maintain protein intake.

FRUIT JUICES

Excessive fruit juice intake (and it could conceivably be any sugar-rich liquid like soda or Kool Aid) has been associated with failure to thrive. Children under age 5 consume more fruit than any other age group at approximately 9 gal/child/year. Apple juice is the main one. Fruit juices are popular with children because they are sweet and popular with parents because they are "natural." They are naturally rich in simple sugars (sometimes added), have no protein, fat, or fiber and are naturally very low in vitamins and minerals. Juices cause failure to thrive (defined as lack of growth) for a variety of reasons.

1. Dietary imbalances (replaces foods containing protein and EFAs)
2. Nutrient deficiencies (iron being most common)
3. Diarrhea/abdominal pain/bloating due to malabsorption of fructose and sorbitol
4. Lack of adequate kcals (fill up on sugar and so is not hungry) (47)

It should be recommended that parents avoid introducing fruit juices into the infant-toddler diet. Rather, parents should use water for fluid intake requirements. If a parent insists on the use of fruit juice, the doctor can recommend adding 2-3 tablespoons of the juice to water, rather than diluting the juice with water. The parent should be made aware that concentrates require large quantities of fruit. The quantity far exceeds the infant/toddler's ability to ingest this fruit if it was given in whole portions. It should also be discouraged to give the infant/toddler fruit drinks prior to going to bed. This may contribute to dental caries.

Food Allergies and Intolerances

Intolerance reactions to food components are common among infants and children, whose gut mucosal barrier system is confronted with a wide variety of potentially harmful food substances. Protein intolerances and allergies are the most common (48).

Cow's milk protein allergies are usually the first and most common seen among infants. The beta-lactoglobulin, the major whey protein, has the highest immunogenic potential. Casein is the second most common protein allergy. More than 25 cow's milk proteins are known to cause allergies in humans. In most cases the allergy is produced by more than one cow's milk protein.

There is the possibility that heat treatment of milk during pasteurization generates new antigens by unfolding polypeptide chains and by rupturing disulfide linkages.

There is an almost endless list of foods reported to cause allergies in infants and children, including soy (from infant formulas), eggs, pork, fish, citrus fruits, nuts, wheat, food additives, food contaminants, gluten (wheat, rye, barley), and yeast.

Allergies can be related to multiple food antigens. A pre-existing food allergy to a single food can cause increased absorption of other proteins with the potential for secondary allergies to multiple antigens. This has been suggested as the cause of gluten-sensitive enteropathy (celiac disease) as a subsequent event to a cow's milk allergy with a genetic predisposition.

Clinical manifestations of milk induced enteropathy in infancy include diarrhea, vomiting, and failure to thrive. These manifestations may lead to colic and bleeding from the bowel. The symptoms may be immediate or delayed. Malabsorption of other nutrients then occur leading to additional symptoms. The child may also have respiratory (runny nose and sneezing with the later development of bronchial asthma and wheezing) and skin (swelling of the lips, trachea, urticaria, angiodema) symptoms.

Foods should be added one at a time as a whole product (not mixed with anything else) to an infant's diet starting about age 6 months. After a few days of use, check for signs and symptoms of allergies. This is the basis of the elimination challenge diets used to identify allergies after multiple foods have been introduced (48).

Elimination and challenge diets must be used cautiously in children and adolescents. The main problem is the development of nutrient deficiencies due to the stringent diets. But this is considered the test of choice. The treatment would then be to avoid the offending food (48,49).

The skin prick test for foods is not very reliable and should not be done in a child under age 3. Some of the allergies are transient in infants and will disappear by age 2 or 3. However, some require lifetime restriction. Breast feeding will greatly reduce the development of many allergies (48).

Attention Deficit Hyperactivity Disorder

Attention deficit hyperactivity disorder (ADHD) is a disturbance of behavior of at least 6 months duration that:

1. Begins before 7 years of age
2. Does not meet the criteria for a pervasive development disorder
3. Is associated with at least 8 of the following behaviors

The behaviors, in descending order of discriminating power are:

1. Often fidgets with hands or feet or squirms in seat (in adolescents, may be limited to subjective feelings of restlessness)
2. Has difficulty remaining seated when required to do so
3. Is easily distracted by extraneous stimuli
4. Has difficulty awaiting turn in games or group situations
5. Often blurts out answers to questions before they have been completed
6. Has difficulty following through on others' instructions (e.g., fails to finish chores). This difficulty is not due to failure of comprehension or oppositional behavior
7. Has difficulty sustaining attention in tasks or play activities
8. Often shifts from one uncompleted activity to another
9. Has difficulty playing quietly
10. Often talks excessively

11. Often interrupts or intrudes on others (e.g., "butts" in on other children's games)

12. Often does not seem to listen to what is being said to him or her

13. Loses things necessary for tasks or activities at school or at home (e.g., toys, pencils, books, assignments)

14. Engages in physically dangerous activities without considering the possible consequences (e.g., runs into the street without looking). The child does not engage in these activities for the purpose of thrill-seeking.

No single therapy program is ideal (see Chapter 17). The child needs family counseling, realistic goal setting, small classes with specific educational goals, and nutritional changes. Many children are given drugs such as Ritalin. Nutritional and non-drug approaches have been proposed by many authors (50). The child does not appear to outgrow the problem, and it has been associated with later disruptive and illegal behaviors (51).

In 1973, allergist Dr. Benjamin Feingold proposed a diet for hyperactivity (52). The main idea was to remove allergy provoking foods and food additives gradually from the diet. A variety of researchers studied his diet including the National Institutes of Health. It does have a positive effect on some children and should be considered as an initial treatment in the management of hyperactivity.

Others have been examining children to see if nutritional deficiencies may lead to hyperactivity. Although many children show deficiencies, no clear cut pattern has emerged. Studies on disruptive behavior in adolescents before and after supplementation have been done. The studies appear promising, but cannot be correlated with hyperactivity syndrome (51).

Vegetarian Diets in Children

Most of the world's population exists almost exclusively on vegetarian diets with few ill effects (49). In North America, some groups such as the Seventh Day Adventists routinely follow well-established vegetarian regimens. There are three types of vegetarian diets (53):

1. Vegan: no animal products
2. Lacto-vegan: dairy included
3. Lacto-ovo: dairy and eggs included

Vegetarian diets offer several nutritional benefits:

1. High in fiber, vitamins, and essential fatty acids
2. Low in cholesterol, fat, and calories

Even pure vegan diets can provide all the nutrients necessary for children, including infants, if planned well. A child needs adequate kcals for growth. If the child does not get adequate energy intake, the muscle mass will be used for energy. A child also needs adequate protein. Most vegetarian diets provide adequate protein, but a small child may have difficulty getting enough legumes or grains to supply the protein. They simply cannot eat that much since legumes and grains are so filling and these sources are not easily bioavailable. Thirty-seven percent of the protein must contain the essential amino acids in an infant, 32% in a child, and 16% in an adult (49,53).

The lacto and lacto-ovo vegetarians have no problem meeting protein needs. Plant proteins (except perhaps soy) are low in one or more essential amino acids. Cereal grains are low in lysine. Legumes are low in methionine. When eaten together, they supply all the amino acids. The parent and child must learn proper food-combining techniques. The plant proteins are not as bioavailable so more may be needed (49,53).

Vitamin B12

The child is born with adequate stores of vitamin B_{12} to last for the first year of life (49). During pregnancy and lactation, B_{12} must come from the diet of the mother. In humans, B_{12} is made by gut flora or ingested. Mother's stores are not readily mobilized (unlike calcium or iron) to be given to the fetus/infant. B_{12} is not found in plant foods. Some can be obtained from fermented soy products, tempura, and seaweed (bacteria). A B_{12} deficiency can occur in infants who are breast-fed by vegan mothers who do not supplement. Vitamin B_{12} supplements are highly recommended for vegan mothers and their children (49).

Minerals

Minerals may be deficient in the vegetarian child for two reasons (49):

1. Phytates, primarily in cereal grains, bind calcium, zinc, iron, and other minerals limiting their absorption and decreasing their bioavailability; and

2. These three minerals are also low in vegan diets and iron is low in dairy.

Iron deficiency anemia is common among vegan children since most is found in animal flesh. Non-heme iron can be obtained from other sources, but it is not as bioavailable.

Vitamin D

Vitamin D stores may be low in infants of vegetarian mothers whose breast milk has low content (49). Sun exposure will provide adequate amounts. Supplementation is recommended in breastfed infants of vegetarian mothers if sunlight exposure is limited. Older vegan children may be deficient since they are not ingesting fortified milk. Fortified soy milk can be given.

Childhood Obesity

Obesity is a prevalent condition in childhood and is associated with an increased risk of becoming an obese adult (54). From 1963 to 1980 childhood obesity increased significantly. Twenty-seven percent of 6 to 11 year olds are now obese compared to 18% in 1963. The 12 to 17 year old group went from 16% being obese up to the current 22%. The older the child is when obese, the more likely the obesity will continue as an adult. Forty percent of children obese at age 7 will become obese adults. About 70% of obese 10-13 year olds become obese adults, whereas, only 10% of non-obese 10-13 year olds become obese as adults. Risk factors for childhood obesity include:

1. Being born to obese parents;
2. Being born obese (high fat mass);
3. Having obese siblings;
4. Being an only child; and
5. Being bottle fed.

Adult obesity does not respond well to treatment so it is important to treat and prevent obesity in the child. Obesity is defined as 20% or more above the IBW or the median weight for age. One method of testing is skin fold thickness. For adolescence, a skin fold greater than the 85th percentile for the American population is considered obese. The thickness correlates well with body fatness.

Childhood obesity is related to many of the same cardio-vascular risk factors as is adult obesity. The kids have elevated blood pressure, elevated total cholesterol, higher LDL, and decreased HDL cholesterol relative to thinner children. Arteriosclerosis begins in childhood. Fatty streaks in the aorta have been found beginning at age 3 and increase as the child ages. By the second decade of life, more than half of children have coronary lesions and about 10% have atherosclerotic-like plaques. Prevention of atherosclerosis and heart disease should begin in children.

Diet has a strong influence on serum cholesterol levels during the first year of life. Those children who have high cholesterol and LDL levels during their first year also have high levels at age five. Breastfed infants receive much cholesterol and saturated fat and have markedly higher cholesterol levels than formula fed children. This difference disappears by 12 months. After the weaning process is completed, children's relative serum cholesterol levels become established and remain stable into adulthood (55).

The mechanisms for the development of obesity may be fat exposure during pregnancy, modeling behavior, food and exercise availability (53). There is some evidence that obese children have more fat cells than non-obese. Researchers are now looking for a "fat gene" similar to the one found in mice. Overweight children tend to be less active than normal weight kids. Calorie intake may be significantly increased; although, some studies show the same or fewer Kcals are eaten compared to lean children.

Treatments have been developed for adolescents. Little has been done for younger children. One group surveyed mothers as to their preschoolers' favorite foods. They then did a computer analysis of fat content and tried to substitute low and moderate fat foods that would be acceptable and reach the 30% total fat guideline. They noted difficulty in planning diets for 2-5 year olds. The best suggestion was to use lean cuts of meat and switch to skim milk. Getting enough kcals was noted as a major concern. Once they modified the diet to provide adequate kcals and still be 30% fat, the vitamin and mineral intake was appreciably increased (due to more use of plant products). If a child chose too many low fat foods, it might not get the amount of fat needed. This was not actually tried with the children (53,56).

Programs assist about 20% of adolescents to keep the weight off. Infants and toddlers can be managed when the parents are educated in proper food choices and the children are encouraged to exercise. If the parents are not the only caregivers (daycare or relatives), then eating patterns are usually disrupted.

Treatment should produce a significant reduction in body weight to below 20% over IBW while getting the appropriate nutrition for growth and development. The program must take into consideration the child's age, developmental level, and parental influence. The program includes the following components:

A. Diet
    1. Will produce weight loss
    2. Is easy to follow and adhere to
    3. Will promote growth
    4. Can be done by entire family to some degree
B. Exercise
    1. Fun
    2. Easy to do (no special equipment or other people)
    3. Aerobic
    4. Appropriate to the age/developmental level
C. Behavior Modification
    1. Includes entire family
    2. Indirectly includes other caregivers (teachers)
    3. Involves rewards, not punishments
    4. May include more traditional therapy

Forty-four obese 10-11 year olds were divided into two groups: one group received dietary counseling for 14-18 months and the other group received dietary and family counseling. A control group was comprised of 50 obese children who received no intervention. One year later, the family counseling group showed the greatest progress toward leanness determined by a decreased body mass index than the other two groups. They also had decreased skin fold thickness (decreased fat mass) and better physical fitness. One important aspect of family therapy was that the therapist emphasized personal responsibility by the child and the family (57). Implementation of the plan is as follows:

1. The adolescent records daily food intake.
2. A dietary plan is designed around common, available, and liked foods with modifications.
3. Parents are put on a dietary plan.
4. Child and parents are weighed in at each session.
5. Group sessions are held for ongoing support/education.
6. Family members praise one another for meeting goals and healthy choices.

7. Quizzes and lessons are given at each session.

8. Contracts and incentives are decided each week.

9. Family is educated in nutrition and given menus and lists of foods.

The traffic light diet is as follows:

1. green: eat as much as you like;

2. yellow: caution, eat in moderation; and

3. red: stop, do not eat.

Currently American children consume 35% fat with 14% being saturated. Adults' programs usually achieve weight reduction by decreasing caloric intake. For a child to grow and develop, an adequate amount of calories must be provided. See charts of exchanges made to achieve a moderate fat diet. The current recommendations for fat in the diet are as follows:

1. Infants: 45% of kcals;

2. Children: 30% (only 10% saturated); and

3. Adolescents and adults 20% or less with little saturated.

Niacin

Niacin has been tried as a treatment in hypercholesterolemic children (age 4-14) with good results, but significant adverse effects. Twenty-one children received 500 to 2250 mg daily in a graduated dose until either LDL levels decreased or adverse effects increased. Those receiving greater than 1000 mg daily had significant decreases in total cholesterol and LDL without affecting HDL and triglycerides. Eight discontinued therapy due to flushing, abdominal pain, vomiting, headache, or elevated serum aminotransferase levels. Niacin is as equally effective as the two most commonly used drugs cholestyramine and cholestipol. The drugs are routinely used for children although the compliance rate is often poor due to side effects and unpalatability (58). Niacin is palatable and is a fraction of the cost of drugs.

Fast Foods

Obesity is a problem in those who routinely eat at fast food establishments: a hamburger, fries, and shake provide more than half the day's calories for children plus most of the day's sodium allowance. The calories are primarily as fat or simple sugars. The foods are also low in many vitamins, essential fatty acids, and fiber. However, a McDonald's hamburger has about the same caloric, fat, sodium content as a tuna fish sandwich with mayonnaise or a peanut butter and jelly sandwich. Junk foods are those that have no nutritional value other than calories. All are typical in kids' diets. The families are educated in limiting ingestion of these foods. They should not be thought of as a reward (59).

School Lunches

Children consume one-fourth to one-third the daily kilocalories during the school lunch. The school lunch program has an impact on the overall nutrition of US children and tends to provide high fat foods as the only choices. In one study elementary school children were provided an entree of either 30% fat or the typical high fat entree (>40% fat). A consistent 29% of the students voluntarily chose the lesser fat entree over an 8 month period. There was more food wastage of this entree and there was no division in groups (high vs. less fat). The kids randomly selected what they wanted that day. The researchers noted flaws in the design (amount of kcal wastage not determined, other food items consumed not included, etc.), but it clearly showed almost one-third of children would choose a lower fat entree when given the opportunity (59).

Sports Nutrition

Most young athletes regularly make poor nutritional choices (60). They tend to follow poor dietary practices/fads, have inadequate nutrition knowledge, and take inappropriate supplements/drugs. High school male athletes tend to eat too much while female athletes eat too little. Even with adequate calories, many may be deficient in micronutrients like iron, magnesium, and zinc which are essential for optimal performance. Weight manipulation has been associated with non-recommended dietary practices. Adolescents report that peer pressure, convenience, affordability, and taste are more important than exercise and recovery needs of the body. Good nutrition can have the following positive effects:

1. Increase the level of performance;

2. Decrease the healing time after injury;

3. Optimize physical development;

4. Increase the athlete's self-concept; and

5. Establish long-term eating patterns.

Amphetamines and anabolic steroids are the two most commonly used drugs among adolescent athletes (61). These are to be discouraged. Amphetamines are associated with increased risk of injury, cardiac failure, aggressive brutality, or paranoia. Female virilization, oligospermia, testicular atrophy, infertility, and gynecomastia, premature closure of the epiphyses, acne, increased blood cholesterol and hepatocellular carcinoma are seen with the use of anabolic steroids.

Bulimia, anorexia, use of laxative, etc. are reported in as much as 25% of all adolescent athletes. These are very dangerous practices.

Vitamin deficiencies are related to poor athletic performance and many children may be deficient, but there is no evidence that megadosing with any vitamin will improve athletic performance.

Energy Requirements

The child should be encouraged to avoid any major weight restrictions during the adolescent growth spurt. The adolescent should begin to follow the adult requirements:

1. 12-15% protein;

2. 20% dietary fat mainly of essential fatty acids; and

3. 55-75% carbohydrates.

Adolescent males need about 1 gram protein/kg body weight and females need 0.8 grams/kg. Protein should be increased if muscle wasting is evident. 20% is maximum in a healthy athlete following a strenuous exercise plan. If the child shows weight loss leading to poor appearance, poor performance, 10% or more below IBW, or a significant decrease in body mass index, then increase caloric intake. Extremely athletic children age 7-10 may need 3,000-4,000 kcals per day. Adolescent athletes with rigorous workout schedules may need as many as 5,000 kcals a day. Adding more complex carbohydrates is the best way to increase caloric amounts. Fat should not be increased.

Mineral Supplementation

Mineral supplementation should include calcium and iron for female athletes (62). Iron should only be given to males when iron deficient or with blood loss. Zinc is recommended for all teenagers at about 15 mg a day. When prolonged activity results in significant perspiration, sodium and potassium should be replaced with water. Sports drinks are usually too high in sugars.

Hydration

Water is the best drink unless exercising at a high intensity continuously for more than one hour (63). Children are more susceptible to adverse affects of dehydration. They should be reminded to replenish water frequently to avoid weakness, fatigue, and exhaustion.

Endurance Competitions

Children are rarely involved in long term endurance competition, however, adolescents may be (63). The guidelines for pre-event, event, and post-event meals are the same as for adult athletes. Food should be familiar and well-tolerated focusing primarily on easily digested complex carbohydrates before the event. Fluids with combinations of glucose polymers and fructose during a long event, especially in the form of blended fruit drinks are well-tolerated. The post-event meal should contain high quality protein up to 20% and carbohydrates up to 75% of the total caloric intake.

High Fat and Sugar Diets

Li et al. (64) studied the effect of a high fat-sucrose diet on bone-ligament-bone junction in growing rats compared to low fat-complex carbohydrate diet. After 10 weeks, the fat-sugar diet resulted in decreased ability to carry loads and load failure with less weight. It weakens the bone compartment due to a loss of calcium/magnesium and high blood glucose mimicking diabetic associated osteopenia. Cell density was less in medial collateral ligaments of fat-sucrose rats.

Supplementing Children

Infant supplements are normally in formulas. A few liquid supplements are available for sale. When the child can chew, a chewable supplement is recommended. Many pharmaceuticals, including supplements, contain allergy provoking inert ingredients. The most common additives are: saccharin and sucrose followed by sorbitol, glucose, fructose, aspartame, and lactose. The type of artificial flavoring is not identified in most. Cherry, vanilla, and lemon are the most common in those identified. Many different dyes and coloring agents are used with red dye #40 being most common followed by yellow #6. Of the preservatives used, sodium benzoate and methylparabens were most common (65).

As long as the child is not allergic to the above additives, a well-tolerated chewable is best. Many reputable companies try to avoid many of the additives. By the time the child is a teenager, most can swallow adult supplements. Adult formulations can be easily found without all the additives above.

Infants usually receive vitamin D and an injection of vitamin K at birth. Infant formulas are usually supplemented. When weaned from the breast, infants need additional iron, usually from fortified cereals. Infants on formulas of evaporated milk need additional vitamin C. All B vitamins and zinc, are essential for normal growth.

Children eating an entirely plant based diet (i.e. vegans) need additional supplements of iron, vitamin D (if not exposed to the sun), and vitamin B_{12}.

Children with diets high in polyunsaturated fats should be encouraged to supplement with vitamin E.

Adolescent females should supplement with additional calcium and iron.

Athletes' requirements vary with the intensity of the activity. They may need to increase electrolytes consumption, water and calories.

Children with lactose intolerance should be supplemented with additional calcium.

If a child is exposed to antibiotics, then intestinal flora should be reinoculated with lactobacillus and acidophillus.

Food and Water for Thought

With the many controversies surrounding diet and its contributions to health, there are some truths that many practitioners consider reasonable. Among them is the role our genetic predisposition plays in our ability to resist disease. An example would be the happy, healthy 87-year-old great-grandfather who smokes ten cigars a day and survives on waffles and ice cream. Although this is by and large the exception rather than the rule, it must be acknowledged. While we cannot change our genetic inheritance, we can influence our health with some basic dietary guidelines.

Dietary guidelines considered to contribute to health promotion would include the following. Parents and children should choose foods which are nutrient-dense. Eating foods that are as close to their natural state allows for increased bioavailability as well as better absorption and assimilation.

Eating plenty of live foods allows our body to utilize enzymes and other co-factors which are sensitive to heat and some cooking methods (66).

Eating fruits, vegetables, and whole grains which are certified to be organically grown will reduce the risk of exposure to herbicides and pesticides. Growing children with rapid cell differentiation are at a higher risk. Free range animals and their byproducts are preferred over commercially-raised brands because of the more limited use of drugs, additives and hormones. With popular demand rising, these alternatives are becoming increasingly available and affordable.

Beans, legumes, nuts and seeds should be a significant part of a growing child's diet. Legumes combined with grains provide all the essential amino acids that are the building blocks of protein. Beans such as soy provide the body with a high quality protein source. Studies have demonstrated that new-born animals gain three times as much weight on a diet of the same percentage of protein when legumes are combined with grains as compared to given separately (67). Combining legumes such as lentils with whole grains such as brown rice or millet, provides the framework for growth and repair as well as dietary fiber to keep the digestive system at optimum health.

Nuts and seeds are nutritious whole foods that contain high quality fat and protein. They should be stored in a cool place or frozen to protect the essential fatty acids. The food becomes rancid when exposed to heat and air. Essential fatty acids (EFA) are crucial to the development of the endocrine, immune and neurological systems. Supplementation to the diet with EFA's from flax seed or borage oil is a beneficial way to ensure that the body receives the healthy fat it needs (68).

One commonly overlooked aspect of optimizing health and preventing disease is the quality and quantity of water consumed. Good quality water should not be substituted by sugar-filled soft drinks or fruit juices. Water flavored with fresh fruit juice in diluted concentrations is recommended for younger children but pure water is best. The industrial age has brought new challenges in maintaining the purity of our water supply. Federal standards allow minute levels of certain contaminants such as chlorine and other industrial chemical byproducts. The cumulative effects of these substances on the health of children is unknown and remains very controversial. Many people feel that you either buy a filter or act as one. With the body composed of over 70% water, purchasing a filter for bathing, cooking, and drinking is reasonable and could prove to be beneficial to health. Again, rapidly differentiating cells in an infant or small child would be most at risk to any exposure.

When creating a healthy diet, avoiding "antinutrients" is just as important as including beneficial nutrients. An antinutrient is considered to be anything consumed that places a negative stress on biological systems. An example would be refined white sugar or white flour which places a burden on the body to then donate vitamins and trace minerals such as B_6 and magnesium from its reserves. Whole foods, complete the way nature intended, add to nutrient reserves (69). Trace minerals are essential for many enzyme systems to function properly.

The tsentieth century has placed very unique stresses on metabolic systems of both the young and old. A high quality vitamin and mineral supplement can be helpful in ensuring that the body has all adequate co-factors for metabolism. Superior supplements would be ones that combine their nutrients with other co-factors, increasing bio-availability. The monetary cost is generally higher for these types of supplements but the biological benefit is also increased.

Finally, it is wise for children as well as adults to eat in a peaceful and relaxed environment to ensure proper digestion as well as to experience the social benefits of eating with loved ones.

REFERENCES

1. U.S. Department of Health and Human Services. The Surgeon General's report on Nutrition and Health. BH (PHS) Publication No. 88-50210, 1988.
2. Mahan LK, Escott-Stump S. Krause's food, nutrition and diet therapy. 9th ed. Philadelphia: WB Saunders Co., 1996.
3. Pressman AH, Adams AH. Clinical assessment of nutritional status: a working manual. 2nd ed. Baltimore: Williams & Wilkins, 1990.
4. Herbert V. The five possible causes of all nutrient deficiency: illustrated by deficiency of vitamin B_{12} and folic acid. Am J Clin Nutr 1973; 26:77-86.
5. Peerson JM, Heinig MJ, Nommsen LA, Lonnerdal B, Dewey KG. Use of growth models to describe patterns of length, weight, and head circumference among breast-fed and formula-fed infants: the DARLING study. Human Biology 1993;65: 611-626.
6. Puri S, Chandra RK. Nutritional Regulation of Host Resistance and Predictive Value of Immunologic Tests in Assessment of Outcome. Pediatric Clin North Am 1985; 32:499-516.
7. Solomons N. Assessment of nutritional status: functional indicators of pediatric nutriture. Pediatric Clin North Am 1985; 32:319-334.
8. Ellis LA, Picciano MI. Milk-borne hormones: regulators of development in neonates. Nutrition Today 1992; Sept/Oct:6-14.
9. Meyer EC, Coll CT, Lester BM, Boukydis FZ, McDonough SM, Oh W. Family-based intervention improves maternal psychological well-being and feeding interaction of preterm infants. Pediatrics 1994;93(2):241-246.
10. Ashraf RN, Jalil F, Zaman S. Breast feeding and protection against neonatal sepsis in a high risk population. Arch Dis Child 1991; 66:488-490.
11. Cunningham AS. Morbidity in breast-fed and artificially fed infants. J Pediatrics 1977; 90:726-729.
12. Glass RI, Svennerholm A, Stoll B, et. al. Protection against cholera in breast-fed children by antibodies in breast milk. N Engl J Med 1983; 308:1389-92.
13. Saavedra JM, Bauman NA, Oung I, Perman I, Yolken RH. Feeding of bifidobacterium bifidum and streptococcus thermophilus to infants in hospital for prevention of diarrhea and shedding of rotovirus. Lancet 1994; 344 (Oct 15):1046-1049.
14. Petschow and Talbott. Reduction in virus-neutralizing activity of a bovine colostrum immunoglobulin concentrate by gastric acid and digestive enzymes. J Pediatric Gastroenterology and Nutrition 1994;19:228-235.
15. Cunningham AS, Jelliffe DB, Jelliffe EF. Breast-feeding and health in the 1980's: a global epidemiological review. J Pediatrics May 1991; 118: 659.
16. Samuelsson V, Johansson C, Lodvigssun J. Breast feeding seems to play a marginal role in the prevention of insulin-dependent diabetes mellitus. Diabetes Research and Clinical Practice 1993; 19:203-210.
17. Duncan B, Ey J, Holberg CJ, Wright AL, et al. Exclusive breast-feeding for at least 4 months protects against otitis media. Pediatrics 1993; 91:867-872.
18. Sheard NF. Breast feeding protects against otitis media. Nutr Reviews 1993; 51:275-277.
19. Dewey KG, Heinig MJ, Nommsen LA, Peerson JM, Lonnerdal B. Growth of breast-fed and formula-fed infants from 0 to 18 months: the DARLING study. Pediatrics 1992; 89:1035-1041.
20. Roche AF, Guo S, Siervogel RM, Khamis HJ, Chandra RK. Growth comparison of breast-fed and formula-fed infants. Revue Canadienne de Sante Publique 1993; 84:132.
21. Lanting CJ, Fidler V, Huisman M, Touwen BC, Boersma ER. Neurological differences between nine year old children fed breast milk or formula milk as babies. Lancet 1994; 344(Nov 12):1319-22.
22. Temboury MC, Otero A, Polanco I, Arribas E. Influence of breast-feeding on the infant's intellectual development. J Pediatric Gastroenterology Nutrition 1994; 18:32-36.
23. Frank JW, Newman J. Breast-feeding in a polluted world: Uncertain risks, clear benefits. Canadian Med Assoc J 1993; 149:33-37.
24. Anderson GH. Human milk feeding. Pediatric Clinics North Am 1985; 32:335-353.
25. Barnes L. Infant feeding: formulas, solids. Pediatric Clin North Am 1985; 32: 355-362.
26. Mennella JA, Beauchamp GK. Maternal diet alters the sensory qualities of human milk and the nursling's behavior. Pediatrics 1991;88:737-744.
27. Milliman WB. Childhood immunity. J Naturopathic Med 1993;5(1):44-50.

28. Gutteridge JMC. Iron and oxygen: a biologically damaging mixture. Acta Paediatr Scan 1990; 365(suppl):78-85.
29. Dallman PR. Upper limits of iron in infant formulas. J Nutr 1989; 119:1852-55.
30. Oppenheimer SJ. Iron and infection: the clinical evidence. Acta Paediatr Scand 1990; 365(suppl):53-62.
31. Fairweather-Tait SJ, Southon S. Studies of iron: zinc interactions in adult rats and the effect of iron fortification in two commercial infant weanling products on iron and zinc status of weanling rats. J Nutr 1989; 119:599-606.
32. Idjradinata P, Watkins WE, Pollitt E. Adverse effect of iron supplementation on weight gain of iron replete young children. Lancet 1994; 343:1252-54.
33. Fuchs. Iron status and intake of older infants fed formula vs. cow's milk with cereal. Am J Clin Nutr 1993; 58:343-348.
34. Jacobus CH, Holick MF, Shao Q, et. al. Hypervitaminosis D associated with drinking milk. N Engl J Med April 30; 1992; 326:1173-7.
35. Holick MF, Shao Q, Liu W, Chen TC. The vitamin D content of fortified milk and infant formula. N Engl J Med April 30, 1992;326:1178-1181.
36. Khoshoo V, Kjarsgaard J, Krafchick B, et. al. Zinc deficiency in a full-term breast-fed infant: unusual presentation. Pediatrics 1992; 89:1094-1095.
37. Nanto V, Siimes MA. Low zinc intake during exclusive breast-feeding does not impair growth. J Pediatric Gastroenterology Nutrition 1994; 18:361-370.
38. Hall CB, Granoff DM, Gromsich DS, et. al. Vitamin A treatment of measles. Pediatrics 1993; 91:1014-1015.
39. Butler JC, Havens PL, Sowell AL, et. al. Measles severity and serum retinol (vitamin A) concentration among children in the United States. Pediatrics 1993; 91:1176-1181.
40. Barreto ML, Santos LM, Assis AM, et. al. Effect of vitamin A supplementation on diarrhea and acute lower-respiratory tract infections in young children in Brazil. Lancet 1994; 344(Jul 23):228-31.
41. Israels LG. Controversies concerning vitamin K and the newborn. Pediatrics 1994; 93:156-7.
42. Melvin Konner, International Symposium of Functional Medicine, March 1994.
43. The use of cow's milk in infancy. Pediatrics 1992; 89:1105-1109.
44. Cohen RJ, Brown KH, Canahuati J, Rivera LL, Dewey KG. Effects of age of introduction of complementary foods on infant breast milk intake, total energy intake and growth: a randomised intervention study in Honduras. Lancet 1994; 344 (Jul 30):288-93.
45. Hendricks KM, Badrudden SH. Weaning recommendations: the scientific basis. Nutr Rev 1992;50:125-133.
46. Sullivan SA, Birch LL. Infant dietary experience and acceptance of solid foods. Pediatrics 1994; 93:271-277.
47. Smith MM, Lifshitz F. Excess fruit juice consumption as a contributing factor in nonorganic failure to thrive. Pediatrics 1994; 93:438-443.
48. Stern M, Walker WA. Food allergy and intolerance. Pediatric Clin North Am 1985; 32;471-492.
49. Hanning RM, Zlotkin SH. Unconventional eating practices and their health implications. Pediatric Clin North Am 1985; 32:429-445.
50. Crook WG. Help for the hyperactive child. Jackson, TN: Professional Books, 1991.
51. Baker S, Baker R. Parents' Guide to Nutrition. Ch.7: Alternative diets: the good, the bad and the ugly. Reading, MA: Addison-Wesley Publ Co, 1987:205-206.
52. Feingold B. Why your child is hyperactive. New York: Random House, 1975.
53. Neinstein LS. Adolescent health care: a practical guide. Baltimore: Urban & Schwarzenberg, 1984.
54. Epstein LH, Wing RR, Valoski A. Childhood obesity. Pediatric Clin North Am 1985; 32:363-379.
55. Kallio MJT, Salmenpera L, Siimes MA, Perheentupa J, Miettinen TA. Tracking of serum cholesterol and lipoprotein levels from the first year of life. Pediatrics 1993; 91:949-954.
56. Sigman-Grant M, Zimmerman S, Kris-Etherton PM. Dietary approaches for reducing fat intake of preschool-age children. Pediatrics 1993; 91:955-960.
57. Flodmark CE, Ohlsson T, Ryden O, Svger T. Prevention of progression to severe obesity in a group of obese schoolchildren treated with family therapy. Pediatrics May 1993; 91:880-884.
58. Colletti RB, Neufeld EJ, Roff NK, et al. Niacin treatment of hypercholesterolemia in children. Pediatrics 1993; 92:78-82.
59. Whitaker RC, Wright JA, Finch AJ, Psaty BM. An environmental intervention to reduce dietary fat in school lunches. Pediatrics 1993; 91:1107-1111.
60. Hackman RM, Katra JE, Geertsen SM. The athletic trainer's role in modifying nutritional behaviors of adolescent athletes: putting theory into practice. Journal of Athletic Training 1992; 27:262-267.
61. Dyment P. Drug misuse by adolescent athletes. Pediatric Clin North Am 1982; 29:1363-1368.
62. Eichner ER. Sports anemia, iron supplements, and blood doping. Medicine Science Sports Exercise 1992; 24(9)(suppl.): S315-S323.
63. Houtkooper L. Food selection for endurance sports. Medicine Science Sports Exercise 1992; 24(9)(suppl.):S349-S359.
64. Li K-C, Zernicke RF, Barnard RJ, Li A F-Y. Response of immature bone-ligament junction to a high-fat-sucrose diet. Clin Biomech 1993; 8:163-165.
65. Kumar A, Rawlings RD, Beaman DC. The mystery ingredients: sweeteners, flavorings, dyes, and preservatives in analgesic, antipyretic, antihistamine/decongestant, cough and cold, antidiarrheal, and liquid theophylline preparations. Pediatrics 1993; 91:927-933.
66. Ballentine R. Diet and nutrition-a holistic approach. Himalayan Publishers, 1978: 42-48.
67. Geiger E. The role of the time factor in feeding supplementary proteins. J Nutrition 1988; 36:813-819.
68. Erasmus V. Fats and oils. Alive Publishing, 1986.
69. Crayhon R. Nutrition made simple. New York: M. Evans and Co., 54-58.

Case Management

12 Spinal Subluxation

Joel Alcantara, Gregory Plaugher, Mark A. Lopes,
and David L. Cichy

*T*he reduction of the subluxation is the cornerstone of the art, science and philosophy of the chiropractic profession. An examination of all facets of this topic is beyond the scope of this chapter but its clinical application is discussed in some detail. The meaning of *subluxation* has been gradually expanded upon over the years by chiropractic authors and has resulted in a more modern terminology for the clinical modeling of this disorder, the *vertebral subluxation complex* (VSC). It is the intention of the authors to discuss selected topics of the VSC and provide the reader not only an overview into this complex disorder but also an insight as it applies to the clinical practice of chiropractic pediatrics.

Historical Perspective

Subluxation is defined as a partial dislocation, a sprain (1). According to the Oxford English Dictionary (1), subluxation was first used in writings from the year 1688, "Sublaxation [sic], a dislocation, or putting out of joint." As the term is currently defined, joint surface malalignment is not the only area of concern but also the sprain of the ligaments supporting the joint. Thus subluxation as a clinical finding associated with a trauma that caused a sprain of the joint has been supported since the beginning of the term's usage. According to D.D. Palmer (2), partial or incomplete separation of spinal joints called sub-luxations (as opposed to displaced or luxated joints

where the joint surfaces are entirely separated) caused associated nerves to be too tense or too slack. In so doing, they caused a variation of "tone resulting in disease," the term "tone" being the expression of nervous system activity to maintain homeostasis. Palmer's original hypothesis of "bone out of place," or sub-luxation, thus laid the foundation for the chiropractic profession by establishing the chiropractic lesion.

Terrett (3), in an investigation of the medical literature, put forth that the fundamental hypotheses of chiropractic as originated by D.D. Palmer had been in existence in the medical literature well before the existence of chiropractic. Citing the works of Harrison (4–6) and Brown (7), the term subluxation was used in the context of neurology (i.e., spinal irritation), spinal biomechanics and manual correction of subluxations. The development of the chiropractic subluxation as a clinical entity reducible with a specific adjustment, however, is uniquely chiropractic. It is beyond the scope of this chapter to outline the term's entire historical development and the reader is referred to other sources (1).

Clinical Concepts of Vertebral Subluxation Complex

Spinal trauma has been categorized into meaningful clinical entities by a variety of health care professionals. For example, the same injury may be classified as having a primary neurological component (e.g., sciatica) by neurologists or bony abnormality (e.g., canal stenosis) by medical orthopedists, as sprain/strain by a general practitioner, as somatic dysfunction by the osteopathic doctor, and finally, the VSC by chiropractors. Each of these models has application to the various respective specialties. Insofar as this discussion is concerned, the authors' concept of the VSC is as a conglomeration of physical signs and symptoms as a result of injury.

Pediatric spinal trauma is underestimated and underreported due to a variety of factors (8). Children with fatal injuries are usually not included in clinically based studies of spinal trauma, nor are those who sustained mild forms of trauma. For example, half of all children with a spinal cord injury die immediately or within the first hour of injury. Twenty percent of those who survive the first few hours of injury die of complications within 3 months. Spinal trauma can result from birth injury (8), physical abuse (see Chapter 2), motor vehicle accidents (9) (see Chapter 4), sports and recreational injuries (10), and daily scrapes, falls and tumbles of everyday childhood experiences. Since many of these types of trauma do not result in hospitalization, conclusions as to the incidence of these injuries are based on sharply circumscribed clinical experiences (8).

Spinal trauma termed subluxation has gradually evolved into the concept of the vertebral subluxation complex. According to the International Chiropractors Association (11), the VSC is defined as, "...any alteration of biomechanical and physiological dynamics of the contiguous spinal structures which can cause neuronal disturbances." The American Chiropractic Association defines the VSC as "any aberrant relationship between two adjacent structures that may have functional or pathological sequelae, causing alteration in the biomechanical and/or physiological reflections of those articular structures, their proximal structures and/or body systems that may be directly or indirectly affected by them" (12).

Outside the chiropractic profession, the osteopaths conceptualize the manipulable lesion as somatic dysfunction; that is, altered or impaired function of the components of the somatic system (e.g., musculoskeletal, arthrodial and myofascial structures) and related vascular, lymphatic and neural elements (13–15). Allopathic and manual medicine's conceptualization of the manipulable spinal lesion exists as articular dysfunction that contributes to complex neurologic reflexes that affect the musculoskeletal system (13,14,16,17).

Models of the Vertebral Subluxation Complex

According to Dishman (18,19), the VSC model as developed by Faye consists of five components. They are: 1) kinesiopathology; 2) neuropathology; 3) myopathology; 4) histopathology; and 5) biochemical abnormalities. The model was refined by Lantz (20) to include a hierarchy of importance with respect to the etiology of the chiropractic lesion and the addition of connective tissue pathology, vascular abnormalities and inflammatory response as components of the model. Further modification of this model was proposed by Lantz (21) by eliminating the "patho" term in the nomenclature and including the components "anatomy" and "physiology."

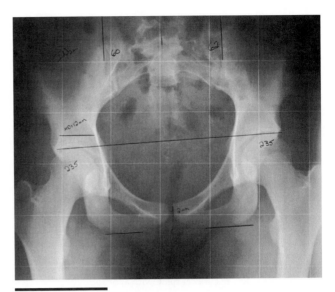

Figure 12.1. AP pelvis demonstrating leg length insufficiency on the left of 12 mm with associated pelvic obliquity.

KINESIOPATHOLOGY

In the realms of anatomy and physiology, one of the fundamental criteria that defines life is motion (22). Kinesiopathology includes global posture (i.e., scoliosis; see Chapter 15), torticollis, spondylolisthesis with sway back, postural tilt due to leg length inequality (Fig. 12.1), intersegmental posture or alignment (e.g., KISS Syndrome, positional dyskinesia) (Fig. 12.2), fixation dysfunction, compensatory hypermobility, and changes in the pattern of movement of the functional spinal unit (FSU) as it moves through its range of motion. Lantz's model of the VSC corroborates this by placing the kinesiology/kinesiopathology component at the zenith of the hierarchy (20,21). For brevity of discussion, we will focus mainly on the pediatric spine. In particular, we will examine kinesiology/kinesiopathology of the FSU. The FSU, as proposed by White and Panjabi (23), is the fundamental spinal motion segment in the biomechanics of the spine. It consists of two adjacent vertebrae and all the ligaments and other soft tissue structures that connect them and are contained within them. Motion dysfunction of the typical FSU results from aberrant motion of the three joint complex consisting of the two facet joints and the intervertebral disc (24). The center of axial rotation is located close to the intervertebral disc. Aberrant motion of the FSU alters this center of rotation leading to unequal loading of the three joint complex. This results in segmental dysfunction and eventually, global dysfunction of the spine and related structures. Deviation from normal motion may lead towards the two poles of hypomobility and hypermobility in the motion spectrum resulting in motion dysfunction.

The clinical entity of vertebral subluxation may exist anywhere within the spectrum of abnormal motion. An interrelatedness of these components exists such that hypomobility or hypermobility may result in vertebral malpositioning or vice-versa. Cineroentgenological studies of the spine by

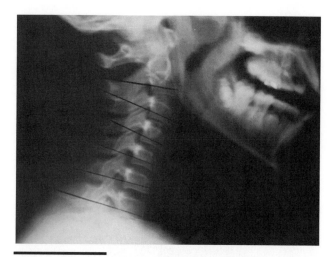

Figure 12.2. Lateral cervical radiograph demonstrates a mild kyphosis of the lower cervical spine with a lordotic configuration in the upper cervical spine.

Howe (25), however, found no correlation exists between vertebral malposition as demonstrated on x-ray and motion studies indicating hypomobility or hypermobility. Also, apparently well-aligned vertebra may at times exhibit abnormal motion. At the stage of current knowledge, it is probably wise to not conclude too much about the dynamics of the spine from a static x-ray.

VERTEBRAL MALPOSITION

D.D. Palmer's original chiropractic lesion described spinal segments in vertebral malposition leading to altered tone resulting in disease. In the practice of chiropractic pediatrics, possible mechanisms leading to vertebral malposition are interarticular soft tissue disruption from traumatic (macrotraumatic and microtraumatic) and nontraumatic events. This is discussed in more detail later.

Severe cervical spine injuries are considered rare in children. In a study by Evans et al. (26), only 24 consecutive cases were found from a review of patients treated for traumatic cervical spine injuries in a period of 20 years — a rate of 1.2 cases per year. This does not differ significantly from findings of 1.3 cases per year by Rang et al. (27) or 1.9% in a series of 631 cervical lesions in a 20-year period as stated by Henrys et al. (28). When cervical spine injuries do occur, they are located most commonly above the fourth cervical vertebra (29). In the chiropractic realm of evaluation and treatment of the pediatric patient, there are several reasons why the numbers of injuries appear at first glance to be underreported. It is likely that pediatric occupants of an automobile involved in a collision to be considered unscathed, when the adult occupants are diagnosed with serious conditions and treated at length. In the case of very young children, those unable to speak, symptom complexes involving increased crying and disturbed sleep patterns should alert the family and doctor that further evaluation is needed. If radiographs are not a part of this assessment, then a low reported incidence of injuries will be the result. One cannot find pediatric problems if thorough evaluations are not made.

Traumatic dislocation of the occiput-atlas-axis articulation may be due to several events. Motor vehicle accidents account for a majority of the injuries but they may also result from falls, violent manual shaking as in physical abuse and obstetrical injuries. Farley et al. (30) report atlanto-occipital dislocation resulting in a near total transection of the spinal cord with brainstem edema and prevertebral soft-tissue swelling. De Beer et al. (31) reported 4 cases of an atlanto-axial subluxation with an intact odontoid. The authors reported good results with conservative treatment consisting initially of halter traction followed by a Minerva brace for 8–12 weeks. Orenstein et al. (32) reported 9 cases of delayed diagnosis of pediatric spine injuries. Six of the 9 cases were in the first and second cervical vertebrae and were the result of a motor vehicle accident or fall. Pennecot et al. (33) reported 16 cases of traumatic ligamentous instability of the cervical spine in children. In those cases where pronounced neurological deficits were ruled out, the symptomatology consisted of only a stiff neck and pain when the C2 spinous process was palpated. A predilection towards misdiagnosis was present in such cases and a careful analysis of the radiographs is recommended by the authors.

Vertebral malpositioning in the thoracic and thoracolumbar spine in pediatrics is exemplified from the study by Hellstrom et al. (34). Radiographic studies were performed on athletes (Figs. 12.3, 12.4) ages 14–25 years and non-athletes ages 19–25 years. Scoliosis and spondylosis were two to three times more common among athletes as a group compared with non-athletes. Abnormalities such as scoliosis (Fig. 12.5), spondylosis, spondylolisthesis (Fig. 12.6), decreased disc height, Schmorl's nodes (Fig. 12.7), and apophyseal abnormalities; were, not surprisingly, more common in athletes than non-athletes. Trauma was suggested to be an important mechanism

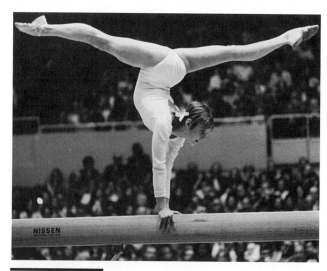

Figure 12.3. Olga Korbut on the beam at the 1976 Montreal Olympics. Courtesy: AP/Wide World Photos.

microtrauma of hyperflexion, hyperextension or twisting in gymnastics and the dynamic turning, jumping and/or lifting of the dancer (36,37). Repetitive high loading of the spine in gymnasts and dancers resulted in higher rate of fatigue fractures of the pars interarticularis when compared with the normal population (38,39). Repetitive microtrauma is also involved in the progression of the phases of the degenerative process.

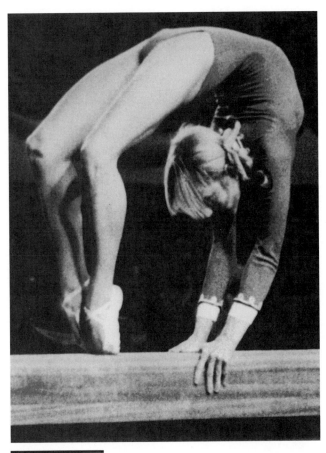

Figure 12.4.   Olga Korbut on the beam in 1975. Courtesy: AP/Wide World Photos.

of injury and should be more closely monitored and hopefully prevented to minimize the effects of its occurrence.

Macrotrauma and Microtrauma. As initially put forth above, traumatic events are subdivided into macrotraumatic and microtraumatic events (35). Trauma occurs as a result of failure of the muscular and ligamentous systems in resisting a load. Macrotraumatic events are those situations in which the spine is subjected to sudden damaging forces. These damaging forces, whether compressive, distractive, shearing, torsional or a combination of forces, are defined as the major injuring vectors or MIV (23). Macrotraumatic events such as cervical spine injuries to children are relatively underreported. Epidemiology studies found that of those patients presenting to hospitals with cervical spine injuries, less than 14% were children (9). Microtraumatic events are those situations in which the spine is subjected to subthreshold forces over a long period (i.e., the effects of gravity on the mass of the individual in combination with unbalanced contraction of postural muscles) that eventually results in an injury (35). Examples of macrotraumatic events resulting in potential injury are those cited above for the cervical spine. Examples of events resulting in injury to the young are exemplified in the repeated

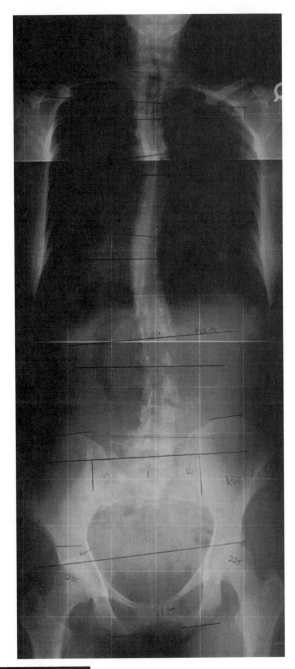

Figure 12.5.   AP full spine radiograph. Scoliosis is demonstrated with convexities in multiple spinal regions. A leg length insufficiency of 19 mm is present on the left.

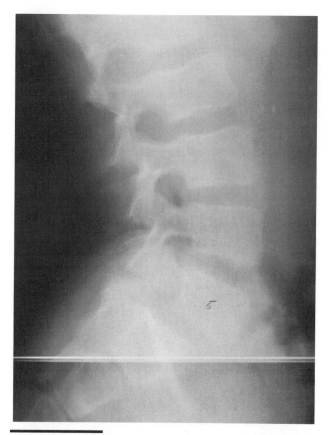

Figure 12.6. Lateral lumbar radiograph with spondylolisthesis of L5.

Nontraumatic events associated with or capable of causing vertebral malposition in pediatric patients may be from the following causes: 1) an inflammatory process such as acute tonsillitis, acute mastoiditis and retropharyngeal abscess; 2) tuberculosis, syphilis, osteomyelitis, rheumatic fever, rheumatoid arthritis and destructive growths destroying supporting structures; 3) paralysis of the muscles of the neck in anterior poliomyelitis or diphtheria. Due to any of the above, vertebral malposition such as forward dislocation of the atlas, atlanto-axial rotation, and occipito-atlantoid dislocation may occur in the cervical spine. The only symptomatology in the patient may be torticollis (40). Marar and Balachandran (41) reported 12 cases of spontaneous atlanto-axial dislocation. Infection around the neck is implicated as the etiological factor. The pathogenesis is controversial but transverse ligament laxity and laxity in the ligaments around the facet joints are implicated. Hunter (42) reports similar cases of atlanto-axial dislocation. The patient with otitis media may present with no obvious history of trauma, yet display signs of vertebral malposition or fixation dysfunction at the upper cervical motion segments (43).

The most common method by which vertebral malposition is identified is spinography defined as a roentgenological diagnostic procedure that uses weight bearing, postural radiographs for the principal purpose of evaluating the spinal column and pelvis for evidence of clinically significant biomechanical irregularities. It is beyond the scope of this writing to describe the various spinographic methodologies or discuss their validity, reliability and clinical relevance (see Chapter 8) (44). Various chiropractic contributions to these methodologies include those by Thompson (45), Winterstein (46), Hildebrandt (47), Gonstead (48) and Logan (49). Examples of intersegmental malalignment are depicted in Figures 12.8 to 12.10.

Analysis of cervical spine posture can be performed by qualitative and quantitative evaluation of the cervical lordosis (Fig. 12.11). The spinal cord must adapt to changes in length of the spinal canal during physiological motion and quasistatic positional changes (i.e., kyphosis). The reader is referred to the work of Breig (50) on the effects of postural and motion disturbances in creating mechanical tension in the central nervous system. Due to the marked range of the cervical spine and the powerful influences of the righting reflex, many

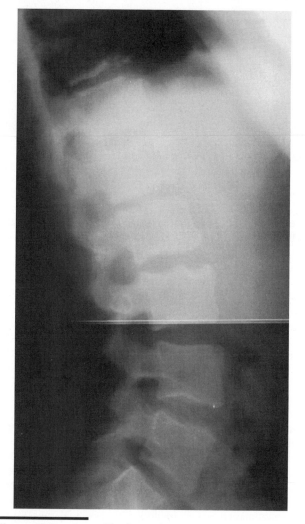

Figure 12.7. Lateral lumbar radiograph of a 16-year-old male with Schmorl's nodes present at L3, L1 and T11.

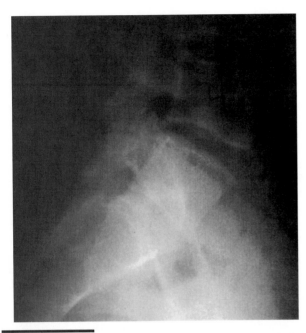

Figure 12.8.   Lateral lumbar radiograph. Sacralization of L5 present with retrolisthesis of L4.

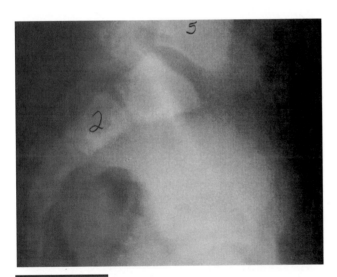

Figure 12.9.   Lateral lumbosacral radiograph. There is a widening of the rudimentary disc between S1 and S2.

cervical spines of children, the following pseudosubluxations and normal variations were observed. 1) Variations due to displacement of vertebrae resembling a subluxation. For example, marked anterior displacement of C2 on the C3 vertebra and less frequently, C3 on the C4 vertebra. Also, there exists an overriding of the atlas on the odontoid process on lateral views during extension resulting in an increase in the atlanto–dental interspace. 2) Variations of curvature of the cervical spine resembling spasm and ligamentous injury to that region. For example, loss of the normal lordotic curve in the cervical spine in neutral and flexion lateral views. Again changes in the posture of the cervical spine and its mobility may be compensatory for other regional and intersegmental dysfunctions. 3) Variations resembling fractures due to the presence of the ossification centers. For example, vestigial basilar epiphyseal plates resemble fractures of the odontoid process. Chapter 7 includes clinical radiologic case studies to

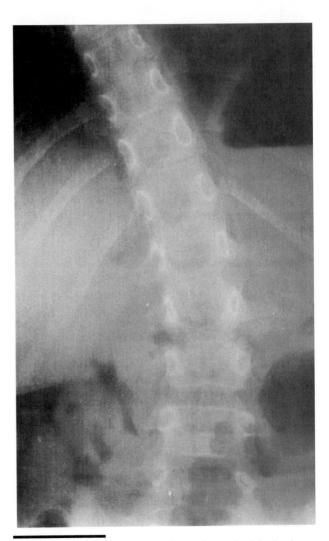

Figure 12.10.   Left lateral bending radiograph of the lumbar and lower thoracic spine. Fixation dysfunction is evident at L4-L5 with restriction of lateral flexion motion towards the left side.

changes in head and neck posture can be due to postural compensatory changes in other spinal regions (54).

Physicians utilizing radiographs for children suspected of serious neck injuries should be aware of normal roentgenographic variations in these patients. According to Cattell et al. (52), incomplete ossification, epiphyseal variations, unique osseous architecture and relative hypermobility of the cervical spine in children may lead to errors in radiographic interpretations. In a roentgenographic study of 160 clinically normal

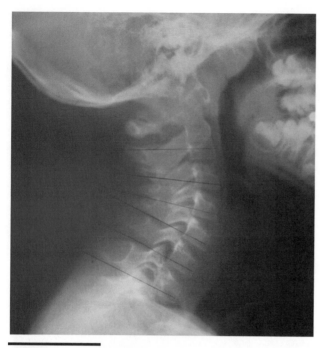

Figure 12.11.   Lateral cervical radiograph. Hypolordosis is present in the lower cervical spine with retrolisthesis at C4 and C3. Notice the break in Georges line at the involved levels.

further describe the misalignment components (i.e., postural dysfunction) of subluxation.

HYPOMOBILITY

Hypomobility, as applied to the spine and in particular to the FSU, means restriction or decrease in range of motion in any or all of its six degrees of freedom. Fixation dysfunction, one clinically relevant form of hypomobility may result from a variety of mechanisms. One involves fixations as a result of contractures and adhesions. Adhesions and contractures are due to scar tissue formation in wound healing and prolonged immobilization (53–55). Another cause of fixation may be due to meniscoid entrapment and disc derangement. In the meniscoid entrapment model, intra-articular synovial tabs or meniscoids are trapped between articular surfaces resulting in derangement and restriction and irritation of certain receptors causing pain and muscle spasms (56–58). In the disc derangement model, the nucleus pulposus extrudes beyond its normal constraints and into the annulus fibrosis. This expropriation of the nucleus pulposus causes restriction in motion and subsequent fixation (59–62). Some of the mechanisms put forth are not without criticisms; the presence of meniscoids as well as their role in causing fixation have been questioned (54) and in disc derangement, fixation can occur in joints without discs (63). Rahlman (64) has summarized the multifactorial nature of intervertebral joint fixation.

Clinical Considerations. Intra-articular edema due to capsular injury could be a plausible mechanism for fixation dysfunction in the upper cervical joint complexes and other synovial joints.

At the sacroiliac joint, connective tissue adhesions have been identified as well as other signs of degenerative joint disease in post-mortem evaluations (65). In addition to fibrous changes in the sacroiliac ligaments, other mechanisms by which fixation dysfunction at this articulation could possibly arise would be misalignment of the joint surfaces due to the presence of various undulating ridges in the joint architecture.

In the practice of chiropractic pediatrics, fixation dysfunction may occur as described above. A fixation dysfunction phenomenon that occurs in children is atlantoaxial rotatory fixation (AARF). The diagnosis of AARF is made when a persistent torticollis exists and there is demonstrated fixation of the atlas on the axis from physical examination and radiographic findings (66). The radiographs should show rotation of the atlas in the APOM view while in the lateral view, the wedge shape mass of the atlas rotates forward to occupy the position normally held by the anterior arch of the atlas (67).

The etiology put forth for AARF are many; synovial joint inflammation (68), impingement of the atlantoaxial articular capsule (69), excessive muscle spasm (66), inflammation (70), and rupture of the transverse or alar ligament (71). According to Kawabe et al. (67), meniscoid-like synovial folds were found at the atlanto-axial and atlanto-occipital joint capsules and it is thought that rupture, infolding and inflammation of these structures may be the cause of AARF. Ono et al. (72) investigated the mechanism of AARF by computed tomography (CT). In the acute stage, rotation between the atlas and axis takes place with facet dislocation in the anteriorly subluxated lateral mass of the atlas. The occiput rotates with the atlas. In later stages, the atlas becomes interlocked with a unilateral dislocation in the atlanto-occipital and atlanto-axial joint. The key mechanism suggested was thought to be a combination of muscle spasms causing extreme neck rotation, laxity of the lateral mass articulation and hypermobility of the atlanto-occipital joint in children. Although atlanto-axial subluxations should be suspected in a patient with torticollis, subluxations in the lower cervical and upper thoracic spine can also cause torticollis presentations and should not be overlooked in the examination (73).

In addition to torticollis presentations, the patient with cervical spine joint and postural abnormalities may present with postural head tilt (74), headache, stiff neck or pain.

HYPERMOBILITY

Hypermobility is the increase in range of motion of any joint. As applied to the FSU, there is an increase in any or all of its six degrees of freedom of motion. To the clinician, this may present in a variety of disorders from congenital dislocations of the hip to connective tissue disorders. Hypermobility is common in children (75). Hypermobility is often associated with instability. The problem lies not in their association but in the confusion that they are synonymous. Instability is defined by White and Panjabi (23) as, loss of the ability of the spine under physiologic loads to maintain relationships between vertebrae in such a way that there is neither damage nor subsequent irritation to the spinal cord or nerve roots, and in addition, there is no development of incapacitating deformities or pain due to structural changes. The confusion may exist due to the fact that one of the manifestations of instability is hypermobility (76). Diagnostic criteria based on clinical examination and radiographs have been put forth (10,77).

In the care of children, one must be cognizant of the idea that due to hypermobility, normal variants and pseudosubluxations may exist. On radiographs, the C2 vertebra may seem anteriorly displaced with respect to the C3 vertebra secondary to normal mobility of the upper cervical spine in children. This is at times difficult to differentiate from pathological displacement. In pathological dislocations of C2 on C3, the posterior cervical line misses the posterior arch of C2 by 2 mm or more. In normal variants, the posterior cervical line may pass through the posterior arch of the C2, touch the anterior aspect of the cortex of the posterior arch of C2 or come to within 1 mm of the anterior cortex of the posterior arch of C2 (78).

Finally on this topic, the issue of infantile atlanto-occipital instability is also another form of hypermobility. Based on the neonate and cadaver studies of Gilles et al. (79), adventitious side-to-side, anteroposterior and/or rostrocaudal motion of the atlantooccipital articulation have been found. The occipital condyle was hypoplastic and flat allowing considerable anteroposterior movement. The apical ligament is absent or poorly developed, the alar ligaments are directed horizontally instead of rostrally, combined with a cartilaginous odontoid tip, this allows for rostrocaudal motion in the atlantooccipital articulation. The foramen magnum is ellipsoid in shape while the atlas is smaller and more circular in structure in the neonate and infant. This allows for atlantal arch inversion on extension and compromise of the vertebral artery. This is consequential when adjusting children with hyperextension. Gilles et al. (79) further point out that these anatomic abnormalities may contribute to unanticipated death in the following three groups.

1. Sleep apnea
2. Sudden infant death syndrome (SIDS)
3. Stillbirths

Schneier and Burns (80) performed a triple blind radiographic study of SIDS and non-SIDS infants. They found that relative measurements suggest that a correlation exists between instability in the atlanto-occipital joint and SIDS (see Chapter 8: Atlas Inversion).

We now describe the syndrome of kinematic imbalances due to suboccipital strain (KISS Syndrome) in newborns. The work of Biedermann (74) is presented. Children with histories of birth trauma such as prolonged labor, the use of extraction aids and multiple fetuses have a propensity to develop KISS Syndrome. The syndrome is characterized by signs and symptoms of C-scoliosis, torticollis, lateral microsomy, impaired motor development and unilateral maturation of the hip joints, sleeping disorders, extreme sensitivity of the neck, and fever of unknown origin. Pathogenesis models include myogenic as in ischemic contraction of the sternocleidomastoid muscles, intracerebral damage and proprioceptive signal blockage in the suboccipital region due to suboccipital strain. According to the description by Biedermann, the main treat-

ment consists of manipulation; it consists of a short thrust with the proximal phalanx of the medial edge of the second finger. The direction to adjust is determined primarily from radiographs.

NEUROPATHOLOGY

Nerve compression is historically known as D.D. Palmer's foot-on-the-hose theory (2). Today, the neuropathology component of the VSC has evolved and is much more complex and sophisticated. Neurological models now include nerve, nerve root and dorsal root ganglion compression or traction, spinal cord compression, somatosomatic reflexes, somatovisceral and viscerosomatic reflexes, motor system degeneration and psychoneuroimmunology, to name but a few (13,14).

SPINAL CORD COMPRESSION AND TRACTION

Spinal cord compression or traction was first proposed by B.J. Palmer (81). It provided the foundation for his hole-in-one technique. Compression of the spinal cord is termed compressive myelopathy and has been implicated in SIDS as a result of trauma and cervical subluxation (82). Leach (83) defines compressive myelopathy as subluxations resulting in irritation, compression and disturbance of the spinal cord. More subtle examples of spinal cord traction could result from changes in the cervical lordosis (50) or meningeal stretch from the dentate ligaments (84).

Clinical Biomechanics. Spinal cord injury in children may be the result of trauma, infection, congenital anomalies and neoplasms. The relatively greater elasticity of the pediatric spinal column results in greater tractional and torsional force requirement to cause a deformation of the column. Unfortunately, the spinal cord is not as resilient to deformation forces and will easily be damaged. This is observed in accidents causing marked and sudden hyperextension and hyperflexion injuries as in motor vehicle accidents (see Chapter 4), vertical compressions from diving accidents or falls, athletic injuries, and even from violent shaking of the child as in child abuse (76, 85–92) (see Chapter 2).

SPINAL CORD INJURY WITHOUT RADIOGRAPHIC ABNORMALITY

The vertebral columns of neonates and infants have greater elasticity than their spinal cords. Leventhall (93) showed that the vertebral column can be stretched 2 inches but the spinal cord can be stretched only one-quarter of an inch before rupturing. Spinal cord injury without radiographic abnormality (SCIWORA) describes a ruptured or injured spinal cord with no corresponding fracture or dislocation in the vertebral column. SCIWORA accounts for 16–19 % of all spinal cord injuries and occurs almost exclusively in children 8 years of age or younger (94). SCIWORA includes mechanisms of injury such as hyperflexion and hyperextension, distraction, rotation and crush injuries. Neurological symptomatology include complete and partial cord syndrome, Brown-Sequard syndrome, and central cord syndrome. Children younger than 8 years presented with more serious injuries and had a higher incidence of upper cervical and thoracic cord injuries (90,95).

Yngve et al. (96) examined 16 patients with spinal cord injury without osseous spine fractures and 55 patients with spine fractures. They proposed that the spinal cord may be injured via vascular compromise and mechanical tension or compression. As for the lack of the spinal column injury, the immature spinal column may deform in a relatively stable fashion through multiple small displacements of the vertebral end plates. The cumulative displacements may cause the spinal cord injury. Since the endplates are cartilaginous in the immature spine, the injuries may not be apparent on radiographs resulting in SCIWORA.

CERVICAL CANAL STENOSIS

Torg et al. (97) report a distinct clinical entity in children resulting in cervical spinal cord neuropraxia with transient quadriplegia. The sensory signs include burning pain, numbness, tingling and loss of sensation. Motor signs ranged from weakness to complete paralysis. The neuropraxia may be the result of decreased antero-posterior diameter of the spinal cord as a result of intervertebral disc herniation, degenerative changes, post-traumatic instability and congenital anomalies. Ladd et al. (98) provide two case reports of children with congenital cervical stenosis presenting as transient quadriplegia.

Saleh et al. (99) present a case study of hyperflexion injury in a 9-year-old male resulting in central cord syndrome; characteristic findings included a disproportionately greater motor impairment in the upper extremities, urinary retention and varying degrees of sensory loss below the level of the lesion.

NERVE AND NERVE ROOT TRACTION AND COMPRESSION

Nerve root injuries are classified into three types (100,101):

1. Neuropraxia
2. Axonotmesis
3. Neurotmesis

Neuropraxia involves an impaired functioning in conduction but no observable structural damage to the axon. This may be due to acute nerve ischemia or demyelination. Intact Schwann cells reestablish myelination for full recovery in weeks to months. Axonotmesis involves biochemical apparatus damage to the axons but the anatomical structure is left intact. Axons distal to the site will undergo Wallerian degeneration but the intact Schwann cells will regenerate eventually. These can occur due to crushing injuries. Neurotmesis involves damage to the nerve such that the axon and connective tissues are anatomically discontinued. Surgical reanastomosis is usually indicated to avoid neuroma disruption to repair. Functional recovery is poor due to poor guiding mechanisms to reestablish original sensory and motor tracts. To address this subject in the realms of chiropractic pediatrics, we limit our discussion to findings in children with brachial plexus, lum-

bosacral plexus and nerve compression injuries. More subtle types of neuropathologies exist but will not be discussed in this chapter. The reader is encouraged to review the works of Gunn (102) on denervation supersensitivity, Korr (103) for facilitative dysfunction, and Slosberg (104) for a discussion of spinal learning or neuroplasticity.

BRACHIAL PLEXUS INJURY

Brachial plexus injury can occur as a result of obstetrical delivery and hence the pseudonym—obstetric palsy. Upper segments of the brachial plexus are injured (Erb's Palsy) when the head presents during delivery and is used to distract the rest of the fetus from the mother's womb. Lower brachial plexus (Klumpke's Palsy) occurs in breeched deliveries - the arm presents first and is used to traction the rest of the body for delivery (see Chapter 5). Erb's Palsy results in abduction of the shoulder, extension and pronation of the elbow and flexion of the wrist and fingers producing the waiter's tip deformity (105,106). Klumpke's palsy is a posture of flexion and supination of the elbow, extension of the wrist, hyperextension of the metacarpophalangeal joints and flexion of the interphalangeal joints producing the claw-hand deformity (106,107).

Clinical Considerations. Larkin-Thier and Hendricks (108) report a case study involving the presentation, chiropractic treatment and outcome of a female infant with unilateral brachial plexus palsy resulting from birth trauma. The patient presented with a flaccid left upper extremity, limited shoulder abduction and absent shoulder extension and flexion during active range of motion (ROM) on the left side. Passive ROM was performable without restriction on the affected side. The grasp reflex was delayed and a positive reversed fencer's reflex was elicited on the affected side. Palpable findings included hypertonicity in the left upper cervical musculature and hypertonic upper thoracic paraspinal musculature, bilaterally. Subluxation findings included an atlas listing of anterosuperior with left laterality and posterior rotation (ASLP). The second thoracic vertebra had a listing of spinous process right (PR). Treatment involved a specific contact, short lever arm, high velocity, low amplitude adjustments to the atlas and second thoracic vertebra over two visits. The mother was instructed to perform passive ROM to the upper extremity and return for follow up within 3 days after the second visit. Objective findings on the second visit included increased resistance in the left upper extremity, positive left reverse fencer's reflex and palpable hypertonicity in the left upper cervical musculature. On the third visit, ROM studies were within normal limits and without resistance to both arms, equal grasp reflex and negative reverses fencer's reflex.

Harris and Wood (109) report a case of a 5-week-old male patient who suffered obstetrical trauma during delivery and was born with a brachial plexus injury (i.e., Erb's palsy). After a course of specific contact short lever-arm adjustments directed at the level of subluxation (i.e., C5) combined with electrical stimulation of the involved extremity musculature, there was a near complete resolution of symptomatology. Twenty-two treatments were provided over 3 months.

LUMBOSACRAL PLEXUS NEUROPATHY

Awerbuch et al. (110) report a distinct clinical entity called lumbosacral plexus neuropathy (LSPN). The clinical criteria for LSPN includes onset within hours to days, pain in the extremity (often severe without back pain exacerbated by Valsalva's maneuver), weakness and muscle atrophy in the distribution of the nerves as well as paresthesia. Lumbosacral plexus neuropathy must be differentiated from neuropathy due to neoplasms, trauma, infection or toxins. Clinical and laboratory investigation must also rule out diabetes, vascular lesions, amyloidosis, sarcoidosis and heavy metal poisoning. Radiographic studies were unremarkable by medical interpretation but electromyography (EMG) shows denervation in muscles innervated by the lumbosacral plexus at several levels. Awerbuch et al. suggest that LSPN should be considered in children with acute pain and weakness of one lower limb when EMG demonstrates evidence of denervation in the lumbosacral plexus with sparing of the paraspinal musculature in that region. Lumbosacral plexus neuropathy is a benign syndrome with a favorable prognosis.

NERVE COMPRESSION

Gutmann (111) reports a syndrome present in infants and small children due to blocked nerve impulses at the atlas. This syndrome is called blocked atlantal nerve syndrome. The clinical picture for this syndrome includes disturbance in motor responses, a brain-stem net central disturbance of negative regulatory systems and inclination to infections in the throat, nose and ear region. Examination findings include torticollis, disturbance in postural development, disturbed and asymmetrical motor responses, scoliosis, hip joint impairment and dysplasia and growing pains. The patient reacts with massive pain and flight reactions to palpation. According to Gutmann, there is muscular fixation and blockage in the atlanto-occipital articulation and treatment consists of a directed manual impulse to the atlas (i.e., an adjustment).

MYOPATHOLOGY

Joint dysfunction mediated through the arthrokinetic reflex following an injury results in reflex muscular spasms (112). Injury occurs when muscular and ligamentous systems fail to support an applied external load. Clinicians have attempted to reduce the muscle spasms due to the notion that since they are a source of symptoms, they must have caused the joint injury. Spinal models suggest that muscles cannot exert enough force to suddenly damage ligaments (113). If this were so, this would result in self-destruction to the body. Prolonged asymmetrical muscle contractions, however, can result in ligamentous deformation of the motion segment. Fixation dysfunction could result in immobilization degeneration.

Myopathology such as spasm or hypertonicity, in the context of pediatric chiropractic, will be examined from the perspective of immobilization of a joint. Joint immobilization will not only affect the muscle structures associated with that joint but also the ligaments and tendons, vasculature and neural elements (21). Immobilization causes the muscles to undergo degeneration known as disuse atrophy (114) and connective tissue structures undergo contractures (115). Intervertebral discs receive nutrients and removal of waste products via imbibition. Immobilization interferes with the imbibition process and impedes the flow of fluids into and out of the intervertebral joint resulting in disc degeneration (10). Interarticular motion is also important for the prevention of haphazard orientation of collagen fibers, dehydration and glycosaminoglycan loss (19). Immobilization effects on the zygapophyseal joints can be seen from discectomy surgeries. Within 6 months, the zygapophyseal joints were fused after discectomy (116).

Toto (117) reports a case of congenital muscular torticollis in a 7-month-old male. The patient received specific adjustments at the level of subluxation in the mid and upper cervical spine. Passive stretching and postural recommendations were also a component of the management plan. The patient was treated at a frequency of three visits per week during the first 3 months of care. As the patient gradually improved, the visit frequency was reduced accordingly. Near complete resolution of the torticollis occurred after about three and a half months of care. These results were maintained at follow-up examination when the infant was 12 months old.

HISTOPATHOLOGY AND BIOCHEMICAL ABNORMALITIES

Histopathology is defined as the science concerned with the study of the abnormal or diseased structure of cells, tissues and organs in relation to their function (118). In reality then, any of the components of the VSC described above are histopathologic components of the VSC. The designation neuropathology and myopathology are terms denoting specific tissue involvement and the inclusion of a histopathology model is nothing more than semantics.

The biochemical component of the VSC model will be addressed by examining the inflammatory response. Inflammation is a biochemical response at the molecular and cellular level as a response to trauma. The classic cardinal signs of inflammation are rubor (redness), tumor (swelling), calor (heat), dolor (pain) and altered or loss of function (119). Inflammation is insidious in the presence of the various tissue pathologies. If macrotrauma is involved, then the acute inflammatory response occurs with the presentation of the classic cardinal signs. Acute inflammatory responses are well characterized (53).

If microtrauma is involved such as that observed in prolonged immobilization, the chronic inflammatory response occurs. Chronic inflammatory response includes alteration of tissue structures and function due to prolonged exposure to macrophages. In muscle structures, muscles atrophy (114), their structure and function are altered (120,121), and muscle contractures occur (122). In connective tissue structures, there is a loss of proteoglycan and increase collagen cross-linking resulting in contractures (123,124). Neural tissue can undergo inflammation resulting in hyperexcitability (125). The effects are dependent on whether the neural structure is motor (i.e., spasms) or sensory (i.e., pain) in function (126). Ossification is also a byproduct of inflammation which can be seen as osteophyte formation (127).

Certain chemicals can play a role in tissue injury and inflammation and have been characterized. For example, connective tissues release substances called autocoids (128) and mast cells release histamine (129) in response to tissue injury and inflammation. Substance P, a mediator of neurogenic inflammation as well as in the perception of pain, is produced in the dorsal root ganglia and transported to the periphery via axoplasmic transport (130). The above are but a few examples of specific chemicals involved in histopathology. Many more substances exist and many more will be discovered. Biochemical abnormalities and histopathology are interrelated.

CLINICAL CONSIDERATIONS

The chiropractor should recognize the signs of inflammation when performing the spinal examination. The findings of tenderness, edema, redness (readily identifiable in the infant) and altered mobility are important changes in superficial tissues that are manifestations of trauma. Their identification will lead to a more specific application of the adjustment at the site of the subluxation and can serve as outcome measures of treatment.

VASCULAR ABNORMALITIES

The local microvasculature, especially the venular vessels, supplying the nerve roots are most susceptible to compressive lesions in the area of the intervertebral foramen lateral recess. Microcirculatory changes, especially venular congestion, occur at very low pressures (131). Nerve root nutrition via direct intraneural vessels and also via diffusion from the vasculature through the cerebrospinal fluid may be impeded due to compressive lesions. Compressive lesions are relatively less common than mechanical dysfunction or irritant lesions of the spine and therefore other mechanisms must be considered in relation to the vascular component of the VSC.

Immobilization may lead to venous stasis, retrograde venous flow and decreased venous return (132). Eventual degenerative articular changes and radiculitis may speculatively be considered as secondary to this type of venous alteration.

Local inflammation secondary to trauma is mediated through the vasculature. Inflammatory fragments of collagen and proteoglycans may spill over into the surrounding tissues and lead to chemical radiculitis. Spillover of hyaluronic acid may stimulate new growth of capillaries (132).

Segmental and suprasegmental autonomic nervous system dysfunction leading to vasomotor disturbances may occur secondary to the VSC. Mechanically traumatized spinal articulations create kinesiologic disorders that generate distorted sensory information which is relayed through the intraarticular sensory apparatus. Sustained "sympathicotonia" has been associated with these disorders (103). Local and distal vascular and skin temperature changes have been postulated as being the physiologic results of this sustained sympathicotonia. Vasoconstriction induced lower skin temperature caused by autonomic nervous system dysfunction has also been associated with denervation supersensitivity (133). These findings have been reported in low back sprain patients without otherwise obvious clinical findings (102).

Noxious stimuli from lumbar interspinous ligament and other somatic locations elicit somatovisceral changes that have been experimentally shown to alter sciatic nerve blood flow (134). This reflex activity may facilitate or cause changes that lead to symptoms or asymptomatic dysfunction of the neural elements.

Suprasegmental vascular changes secondary to autonomic dysfunction and/or noxious afferent reflexes may be responsible for microcirculatory induced ischemia which may be involved in theoretical models for hibernation (135), optic nerve ischemia (136), and other similar intracerebral microcirculatory changes.

CLINICAL CONSIDERATIONS

The clinical assessment of the pediatric patient should include vascular parameters. Paraspinal hyperemia or the "red reflex" is often evident of other VSC segmental concomitant findings (137). Palpation or other physical contact over the involved area often stimulates this redness of the paraspinal skin.

VSC induced vasomotor disturbances of the superficial blood vessels may be revealed with thermographic assessment of the skin. Paraspinal and full body skin temperature assessment may be useful in such investigations (see Chapter 9). The potential results from a chiropractic adjustment directed at reducing malalignment and fixation dysfunction could be decreased edema and venous congestion, and decreased reflex nervous system dysfunction which may, in turn, lead to normalization of local and systemic vascular changes.

Summary

Models of the VSC are constructs of the various tissue alterations. Research suggests that the components of kinesiopathology, neuropathology, myopathology, vascular abnormalities, histopathology, and biochemical abnormalities are part of an integrated system giving rise to the clinical entity of the VSC. This integration is reflected in the phases of spinal degeneration. Major links exist between the components so that a hierarchy placed upon them serves only cosmetic purposes.

In the physical and biological sciences, scientists attempt to rebuild a system with model constructs available to them. In this attempt, limitations certainly exist due to a lack of total knowledge about the true system. Nonetheless, in constructing the model, the attempt is made to maintain fidelity with respect to the true system as much as possible. In so doing, one hopes to account for a large variety of observations and predict new ones from the model system. In chiropractic, our models of the VSC serve the same function with respect to the chiropractic lesion and chiropractic treatment. As our knowledge of the human body increases, our model of the VSC will be refined and developed accordingly and as a result enhance patient care. The model of the VSC then manifests our current state of knowledge in who we are and what we do. This is critical in today's ever-changing environment of health care as chiropractic doctors assume a preeminent role. It was our goal to provide the reader with an insight into the VSC and an impetus to further explore the relationship of the various models of the VSC with their academic and clinical implications.

It is also the authors' hope that further research will be conducted to gain a greater understanding of the complex issues facing the chiropractor in the assessment of the pediatric patient. Although the issues of macro and microtrauma have been explored in detail in this chapter, it should be understood that trauma in all of its apparent and occult forms plays a regular role in every child's life. With the processes of learning to crawl, walk, run, or ride a bike the doctor should have an appreciation for the reality of spinal trauma in our young. There is no such thing as a simple pediatric case. The combined effects of repeated macro and microtrauma to the same child present a complex scenario, one for which little substantive research exists from which to base our clinical applications. Further clinical chiropractic research in the area of pediatrics is sorely needed. Our hope is that this chapter will serve as an impetus for further research to enhance the quality of care to our most precious commodity, our children.

REFERENCES

1. Simpson JA, Weiner ESC. The Oxford English Dictionary, 2nd ed. Oxford: Clarendon Press, 1989; XVII:42.
2. Palmer DD. The science, art and philosophy of chiropractic. Portland Printing House, Portland, Oregon. 1910.
3. Terrett A. The search for the subluxation: an investigation of medical literature to 1985. Chiro History 1987; 7:29-33.
4. Harrison E. Remarks upon the different appearances of the back, breast and ribs, in persons affected with spinal diseases: And on the effects of spinal distortion on the sanguineous circulation. London Med Phys J 1820; 44:365-378.
5. Harrison E. Observations respecting the nature and origin of the common species of disorders of the spine: With critical remarks on the opinions of former writers of this disease. London Med Phys J 1821; 45: 103-122.
6. Harrison E. Observations on the pathology of spinal diseases. London Med Phys J 1824; 51: 350-364.
7. Brown T. Irritation on spinal nerves. Glasg Med J 1826; 131-160.
8. Dickman CA, Rekate HL. Spinal Trauma. In: Eichelberger MR, ed. Pediatric trauma. St. Louis: Mosby Year Book, 1993;362-377.
9. Lebwohl NH, Eismont FJ. Cervical spine injuries in children. In: Weinstein SL, ed. The pediatric spine: principles and practice. New York: Raven Press Ltd. 1994; 725-741.
10. Junghanns H. Clinical implications of normal biomechanical stresses on spinal function. Rockville, Maryland: Aspen Publishers, Inc., 1990.
11. ICA International Review of Chiropractic definition. Nov 1987.
12. Luedtke KL. Chiropractic definition goes to world organization. ACA J Chiropractic 1988; 25(6):5.
13. Mootz RD. Chiropractic models: Current understanding of vertebral subluxation and manipulable spinal lesions. In: Sweere JJ, ed. Chiropractic family practice: a clinical manual. Gaithersberg, Maryland: Aspen Publishers, Inc., 1992;2.1-2.12.
14. Mootz RD. Theoretic models of chiropractic subluxation. In: Gatterman M. Foundations of chiropractic subluxation. St. Louis: Mosby, 1995;175-189.
15. Greenman PE. Principles of manual medicine, 2nd ed. Baltimore: Williams & Wilkins, 1989.
16. Mennel JM. History of the development of medical manipulation concepts-medical terminology. In: Goldstein M, ed. The research status of spinal manipulative therapy. Bethesda, MD. National Institute of Neurologic and Communicative Disorders and Stroke, 1975.
17. Cyriax J. Treatment of pain by manipulation. In: Goldstein M, ed. The research status of spinal manipulative therapy. Bethesda, MD. National Institute of Neurologic and Communicative Disorders and Stroke, 1975.
18. Dishman RW. Review of the literature supporting a scientific basis for the chiropractic subluxation complex. J Manipulative Physiol Ther 1985; 8: 163-174.
19. Dishman RW. Static and dynamic components of the chiropractic subluxation complex: A literature review. J Manipulative Physiol Ther 1988;11:98-107.
20. Lantz CA. The vertebral subluxation complex. ICA Review of Chiropractic. 1989; Sept./Oct :37-61.
21. Lantz CA. The vertebral subluxation complex. In: Gatterman M, ed. Foundations of chiropractic subluxation. St. Louis: Mosby, 1995.
22. Tortora GJ, Grabowski SR. Principles of anatomy and physiology. 7th ed. New York: HarperCollins College Publishers, 1993.
23. White AA, Panjabi MM. Clinical biomechanics of the spine. 2nd ed. Philadelphia: JB Lippincott, 1990.
24. Farfan HF. Biomechanics of the lumbar spine. In: Kirkaldy-Willis WH, ed. Managing low back pain. New York: Churchill Livingston, 1983.
25. Howe JW. Observations from cineroentgenological studies of the spinal column. J Am Chiro Assoc 1970; 7:65-70.
26. Evans DL, Bethem D. Cervical spine injuries in children. J Ped Orthop 1989; 9:563-568.
27. Rang M. Children's fractures. 2nd ed. Philadelphia: JB Lippincott, 1983: 333-345.
28. Henrys P, Lyne D, Lifton C, Ssalciccioli G. Clinical review of cervical spine injuries in children. Clin Orthop 1977; 129:172-176.
29. Jones ET, Hensinger RN. C2-C3 dislocation in a child. J Ped Orthop 1981; 1:419-422.
30. Farley FA, Graziano GP, Hensinger RN. Traumatic atlanto-occipital dislocation in a child. Spine 1992; 17:1539-1541.
31. DeBeer J de V, Hoffman EB, Kieck CF. Traumatic atlantoaxial subluxation in children. J Ped Orthop 1990; 10:397-400.
32. Orenstein JB, Klein BL, Ochsenschlager DW. Delayed diagnosis of pediatric cervical spine injury. Pediatrics 1992; 89:1185-1188.
33. Pennecot GF, Leonard P, Peyrot Des Gachons S, Hardy JR, Pouliquen JC. Traumatic ligamentous instability of the cervical spine in children. J Ped Orthop 1984; 4:339-345.
34. Hellstrom M, Jacobson B, Sward L, Peterson L. Radiologic abnormalities of the thoraco-lumbar spine in athletes. Acta Radiologica 1990; 31:127-132.
35. Lopes MA, Plaugher G. Vertebral subluxation complex. In: Plaugher G, ed. Textbook of clinical chiropractic: a specific biomechanical approach. Baltimore: William & Wilkins, 1993:52-72.
36. Micheli LJ. Back injuries in gymnastics. Clinics Sports Med 1985; 4:85-94.
37. Micheli LJ. Back injuries in dancers. Clinics Sports Med 1983; 2:473-484.
38. Jackson DW, Wiltse LL, Cirincione RL. Spondylolysis in the female gymnast. Clin Orthop 1976; 117:68-73.
39. Micheli LJ. Overuse injuries in children's sports. Orthop Clin North Am 1983; 14:337-360.
40. Englander O. Non-traumatic occipito-atlanto-axial dislocation. Br J Radiol 1942; 15: 341-345.
41. Marar BC, Balachandran N. Non-traumatic atlanto-axial dislocation in children. Clin Orthop 1973; 92:220-226.
42. Hunter GA. Non-traumatic displacement of the atlanto-axial joint. J Bone Joint Surg 1968; 50:44-51.
43. Fysh P. Otitis media: a report of five cases. J Clin Chiro Pediatr 1996; 1(2).
44. Plaugher G. The role of plain film radiography in chiropractic clinical practice. Chiro J Australia 1992; 22:153-161.
45. Thompson EA. Chiropractic spinography. 2nd ed. Davenport, Iowa: Palmer College of Chiropractic 1919:15-27.
46. Winterstein JF. Chiropractic spinographology. Lombard: National College of Chiropractic, 1970.
47. Hildebrandt RW. Chiropractic spinography. 2nd ed. Baltimore: Williams & Wilkins 1985:1-259.
48. Herbst RW. Gonstead chiropractic science and art. Mt. Horeb, WI. Sci-Chi Publications, 1968.
49. Logan HB. In: Logan VF, ed. Textbook of Logan basic methods. St. Louis: Logan Chiropractic College, 1950.
50. Breig A. Adverse mechanical tension in the central nervous system. Stockholm: Almqvist & Wiksell Int, 1978.
51. Voutsinas SA, MacEwen GE. Sagittal profiles of the spine. Clin Orthop 1986; 210:235-242.
52. Cattel HS, Filtzer DL. Pseudosubluxation and other normal variations in the cervical spine in children. J Bone Joint Surg 1965; 47A:1295-1309.
53. Robbins SL, Cotran RS, Kumar V. Inflammation and repair. In: Pathologic Basis of Disease. Philadelphia:WB Saunders, 1984:30-86.
54. Akeson WH, Amiel D, Woo S. Immobility effects of synovial joints: The pathomechanics of joint contracture. Biorheology 1980; 17:95-110.
55. Grieve GP. Common vertebral joint problems. New York: Churchill Livingstone, 1981.
56. Bogduk N, Engle R. The menisci of the lumbar zygapophyseal joints: A review of their anatomy and their clinical significance. Spine 1984; 9:454-460.
57. Giles LGF. Lumbar apophyseal joint arthropathy. J Manipulative Physiol Ther 1984; 7:21-24.
58. Kirkaldy-Willis WH, Burton CV, eds. Managing low back pain. 3rd ed. New York: Churchill Livingstone, 1992.
59. Zamani M, MacEwen GD. Herniation of the lumbar disc in children and adolescents. J Orthop Ped 1982: 2: 528-533.
60. Herring JA, Asher MA. Intervertebral disc herniation in a teenager. J Orthop Ped 1989; 9:615-617.
61. Cox JM. Low back pain: mechanism, diagnosis and treatment. 5th ed. Baltimore: Williams & Wilkins, 1990.
62. Plaugher G, ed. Textbook of clinical chiropractic: a specific biomechanical approach. Baltimore: William & Wilkins, 1993.

63. Good AB. Spinal joint locking. J Manipulative Physiol Ther 1985; 8:1-8.
64. Rahlman J. The mechanism of intervertebral joint fixation. J Manipulative Physiol Ther 1987; 10:177-187.
65. Bowen V, Cassidy JD. Macroscopic and microscopic anatomy of the sacroiliac joint from embryonic life until the eighth decade. Spine 1981; 6:620-628.
66. Fielding JW. Atlanto-axial rotatory fixation. J Bone Joint Surg 1977; 59: 37-44.
67. Kawabe N, Hirotami H, Tanaka O. Pathomechanism of atlantoaxial rotatory fixation in children. J Ped Orthop 1989; 9:569-574.
68. Coutts MB. Atlanto-epiphyseal subluxation. Arch Surg 1934; 29:297-311.
69. Wortzman G, Dewar FP. Rotatory fixation of the atlantoaxial joint: Rotational atlanto axial subluxation. Radiology 1968; 90:479-487.
70. Watson-Jones R. Spontaneous hyperaemic dislocation of the atlas. Proc R Soc Med 1931; 25:586-590.
71. Firrani-Gallotta G, Luzzatti G. Sublussazione laterale e sublussazione rotatorie dellallente. Arch Orthop 1957; 70:467-484.
72. Ono K, Yonenobu K, Fuji T, Okada K. Atlantoaxial rotatory fixation: Radiographic study of its mechanism. Spine 1985; 10:602-608.
73. Plaugher G, Doble RW, Lopes MA. Lower cervical spine. In: Plaugher G, ed. Textbook of clinical chiropractic: a specific biomechanical approach. Baltimore: Williams & Wilkins, 1993:293-294.
74. Biedermann H. Kinematic imbalances due to suboccipital strain in newborns. J Manual Medicine 1992; 6:151.
75. Cheng JCY, Chan PS. Joint laxity in children. J Ped Orthop 1991; 11:752-756.
76. Weinstein SL, ed. The pediatric spine: principles and practice. New York: Raven Press Ltd., 1994.
77. Peterson CK. The nonmanipulable subluxation. In: Gatterman M, Foundations of chiropractic subluxation. St. Louis: Mosby, 1995.
78. Swischuck LE. Anterior displacement of C2 in children: physiologic or pathologic? Pediatric Radiology 1977; 122:759-763.
79. Gilles FH, Bina M, Sotrel A. Infantile atlantooccipital instability. Am J Dis Child 1979; 133:30-37.
80. Schneier M, Burns R. Atlanto-occipital hypermobility in sudden infant death syndrome. Chiropractic: The Journal of Chiropractic Research and Clinical Investigation 1991; 7(2):33-38.
81. Palmer BJ. The subluxation specific: The adjustment specific. Davenport, Iowa: Palmer College of Chiropractic, 1934.
82. Valdes-Dapena MA. Sudden infant death syndrome: a review of the medical literature 1974-1979. Pediatrics 1980; 66: 597-614.
83. Leach RA. The chiropractic theories. A synopsis of scientific research. 3rd ed. Baltimore: Williams and Wilkins, 1995.
84. Grostic JD. Dentate ligament-cord distortion hypothesis. Chiro Research J 1988; 1:47-55.
85. Sneed RC, Stover SL, Fine PR. Spinal cord injury associated with all-terrain vehicle accidents. Pediatrics 1986; 77:271-274.
86. Linssen WHJP, Praamstra P, Gabreels FJM, Rotteveel JJ. Vascular insufficiency of the cervical cord due to hyperextension of the spine. Pediatr Neurol 1990; 6:123-125.
87. Ahmann PA, Smith SA, Schwartz JF, Clark DB. Spinal cord infarction due to minor trauma in children. Neurology 1975; 25:301-307.
88. Scher AT. Trauma of the spinal cord in children. SA Med J 1976; 27:2023-2025.
89. Tator CH, Edmonds VE, Lapczak L, Tator IB. Spinal injuries in ice hockey players, 1966-1987. Can J Surg 1991; 34: 63-69.
90. Kewalramani LS, Tori JA. Spinal cord trauma in children: Neurologic patterns, radiologic features and pathomechanics of injury. Spine 1980; 5:11-18.
91. Gotlieb MS. Neglected spinal cord, brain stem and musculoskeletal injuries stemming from birth trauma. J Manipulative Physiol Ther 1993; 16: 537-543.
92. Swischuck LE. Spine and spinal cord trauma in the battered child syndrome. Radiology 1969; 92: 733-738.
93. Leventhall, HR. Birth injuries of the spinal cord. J Pediatr 1960; 56:447-453.
94. Pang D, Wilberger JE. Spinal cord injury without radiographic abnormalities in children. J Neurosurg 1982; 57:114-129.
95. Chambers HG, Akbarnia BA. Thoracic, lumbar, and sacral spine fractures and dislocations. In: Weinstein, SL, ed. Pediatric spine: principles and practice. New York: Raven Press, Ltd., 1994.
96. Yngve DA, Harris WP, Herndon WA, Sullivan JA, Gross RH. Spinal cord without osseous spine fractures. J Ped Orthop 1988; 8:153-159.
97. Torg JS, Pavlov H, Genuario SE, Sennett B, et al. Neuropraxia of the cervical spinal cord with transient quadriplegia. J Bone Joint Surg 1986: 68A:1354-1370.
98. Ladd AL, Scanton PE. Congenital cervical stenosis presenting as transient quadriplegia in athletes. J Bone Joint Surg 1986; 68A:1371-1374.
99. Saleh J, Raycroft JF. Hyperflexion injury of cervical spine and central cord syndrome in a child. Spine 1992; 17:234-237.
100. Eichelberger MR. Pediatric trauma. St. Louis: Mosby Year Book, 1993.
101. Kimura J. Electrodiagnosis in diseases of nerve and muscle: principles and practice. 2nd ed. Philadelphia: FA Davis, 1989.
102. Gunn C, Milbrandt W. Early and subtle signs in low back pain. Spine 1978; 3:267-281.
103. Korr I, ed. The neurobiologic mechanisms in manipulative therapy. New York: Plenum Press, 1978:229-268.
104. Slosberg M. Spinal learning: central modulation of pain processing and long-term alteration of interneuronal excitability as a result of nociceptive input. J Manipulative Physiol Ther 1990; 13:326-336.
105. McFarland L, Raskin M, Daling J, Bendetti T. Erb/Duchennes Palsy: a consequence of fetal macrosomia and method of delivery. Obstet Gynecol 1986; 68: 784-788.
106. Alfonso I, Papazian O, Reyes M, Sanchez GL, et al. Obstetrical brachial plexus injury. Intl Pediatr 1995; 10: 208-213.
107. Hardy A. Birth injuries of the brachial plexus. J Bone Joint Surg 1981; 63B:98-101.
108. Larkin-Thier SM, Hendricks CL. Chiropractic care of brachial plexus palsy: A case study. Palmer J Res 1994; 1(2):45-47.
109. Harris SL, Wood KW. Resolution of infantile Erb's palsy utilizing chiropractic treatment. J Manipulative Physiol Ther 1993; 16:415-418.
110. Awerbuch GI, Nigro MA, Dabrowski E, Levin JR. Childhood lumbosacral plexus neuropathy. Pediatr Neurol 1989: 5:314-316.
111. Gutmann G. Blocked atlantal nerve syndrome in infants and small children. ICA Intl Rev Chiropractic, July/August 1990.
112. Farfan HF. Biomechanics of the lumbar spine. In: Kirkaldy-Willis WH, ed. Managing low back pain. New York: Churchill Livingstone, 1983: 9-21.
113. Gracovetsky S, Farfan HF, Lamy C. The mechanism of the lumbar spine. Spine 1981; 6:249-262.
114. Tomanek RJ, Lund DD. Degeneration of different types of skeletal muscle fibers. II. Immobilization. J Anat 1974; 118:531-541.
115. Akeson WH, Amiel D, La Violette D. The connective tissue response to immobility: A study of the chondroiten -4 and 6- sulfate and dermatan sulfate changes in periarticular connective tissue of control and immobilized knees of dogs. Clin Orthop 1967; 51:183-198.
116. Tarlov IM. Cyst (perineural) of the spinal roots. Another cause (removal) of sciatic pain. JAMA 1948; 138:740-744.
117. Toto BJ. Chiropractic correction of congenital muscular torticollis. J Manipulative Physiol Ther 1993; 16:556-559.
118. Hensyl WR, ed. Stedmans pocket medical dictionary. Baltimore: Williams & Wilkins, 1987.
119. Warren CG. The use of heat and cold in the treatment of common musculoskeletal disorders. In: Kessler RM, Hertling D, eds. Management of common musculoskeletal disorders: physical therapy principles and methods. Cambridge: Harper & Row, 1983:115-127.
120. Esaki K. Morphological study of muscle spindle in atrophic muscle induced by immobilization. Nagoya Med J 1966; 12:185-201.
121. Maier A, Eldred E, Edgerton V. The effects on spindles of muscle atrophy and hypertrophy. Exper Neurol 1972; 37:100-123.
122. Stauffer ES. Rehabilitation of the spinal cord-injured patient. In: Rothman RH, Simeone FA, eds. The Spine. Philadelphia: WB Saunders, 1982:1118.
123. Troyer H. The effect of short-term immobilization on the rabbit knee in joint cartilage. Clin Orthop 1975; 107:249-257.
124. Akeson WH, Amiel D, Mechanic GL, et al. Collagen cross-linking alterations in joint contractures: Changes in the reducible cross-links in periarticular connective tissue collagen after nine weeks of immobilization. Connect Tissue Res 1977; 5:15-19.
125. Howe JF, Loeser JD, Calvin WH. Mechanosensitivity of dorsal root ganglia and chronically injured axons: a physiological basis for the radicular pain of nerve root compression. Pain 1977; 3:25-41.
126. Waxman SG, deGroot J. Correlative neuroanatomy. 22nd ed. Norwalk: Appleton and Lange, 1995.
127. Lussier A, DeMedicis R. Correlation between ossification and inflammation using a rat experimental model. J Rheum 1983; 11:114-117.
128. Castor C. Regulation of connective tissue metabolism by autocoid mediators. J Rheum 1983; 11:55-60.
129. Chakravarty N. Histamine release from mast cell granules. Agents Actions 1982; 12:94-110.
130. White D, Helme R. Release from substance P from peripheral nerve terminals following electrical stimulation of the sciatic nerve. Brain Res 1985; 336:27-31.
131. Rydevik B. Physiology of spinal nerve compression. Conference proceedings of the Chiropractic Centennial Foundation, 1995:89-109.
132. Lantz CA. The vertebral subluxation complex. In: Gatterman MI, ed. Foundations of chiropractic: subluxation. St. Louis: Mosby-yearbook, 1995:149-174.
133. Axellson J, Theslett S. A study of supersensitivity in denervation mammalian skeletal muscles. J Physiol 1959; 147:178-193.
134. Sato A. Somatovisceral reflexes. Conference proceedings of the Chiropractic Centennial Foundation, 1995:111-134.
135. Terrett AGJ. The cerebral dysfunction theory. In: Gatterman MI, ed. Foundations of chiropractic: subluxation. St. Louis: Mosby, 1995:340-352.
136. Gorman R. The treatment of presumptive optic nerve ischemia by spinal manipulation. J Manipulative Physiol Ther 1995; 18:172-177.
137. Wright HM, Korr IM, Thomas PE. Local and regional variations in cutaneous vasomotor tone of the human trunk. Neural Transmission 1960; 22:34-52.

13 Clinical Neurology

Steven T. Tanaka, Charles J. Martin, and Peter Thibodeau

A Completed Birth…
It was December 28, 1979. There were no movements and no intent, just a limp baby. Seconds before, the mother lay depleted from hours of pushing with barely any gain in the position of her child through the birth canal. The child's skull had been pushed and locked into the mother's bony pelvis, and the canal would open no further. Craniosynostosis is a condition in which one or more plates of the skull are fixed. They cannot mold and flex upon themselves; the head blocks its own exit into the world. Paralyzed by exhaustion through the last several urges, the child's mother stirred and rose to her elbows, forcefully folding at the abdomen. The perineal skin tore and the pelvic bones yielded. The newborn's body slipped out. The new baby was quiet, limp, and blue.

The central nervous system was in shock. The child's eyes did not open to acknowledge this world. She did not have the urge to feed on the antibodies of her mother's colostrum. To thrive at birth is the absolute birthright of every new child entering the world. She was failing this test. The pediatrician waited in reserve for the disorder to manifest pathologically. Behaviors become automatic in these times, instinctive. The child's father, a chiropractor, simply let his hands do what his hands had been trained to do, as he had done previously for his son who was yellow upon birth four years earlier.

When palpating the small bones of her spine, there was no resistance. Each bone felt like a starred nugget. Each felt similar … except for one, the third cervical vertebra. It was more prominent on the pad of the chiropractor's forefinger. The contact seemed to cause a stirring in the child. By it, the child knew about the outside world, much more so than by the tremendous forces of birth itself. The child seemed to

know that the outside world could reach her. The outside world knew about her and could help her.

Like any good spinal adjustment, it was completed before it began. Like all good adjustments, it made a difference. In this case, the child's eyes flashed as if a light had been turned on. The child's arms reached out waving to touch and to hold. The child's mouth went instinctively to the breast. The child's skin received the wash of her mother's joyous tears and toiled sweat. The birth was now complete. In that moment, the child had claimed her birthright—the right of every new child who enters this life in complete health.

That child still claims her birthright. The natural relationship she has always had with herself and the many people she lets into her life continues. Her life is healthy, vital and whole—nothing added, nothing taken away. That first chiropractic spinal adjustment was the most important event that a 10 minute old spine could have had.

The development of a complex organism, such as Homo sapiens from the union of two cells, is truly a celebration of the "miracle of life." Nature recognizes the need to control and organize the rapidly developing and differentiating protoplasm, Therefore, the first system to begin forming is the nervous system. To protect the core aspect of the nervous system, nature protects it with the skull and vertebral column.

Introduction

Chiropractors have always been awed by the entire process which creates and sustains life. Chiropractors have labeled this

479

scientifically unmeasurable power, innate intelligence, and the all-encompassing organizing power, universal intelligence. They have long recognized the power of this intelligence to self-correct. The key to this process is the nervous system. The other systems of the body help to sustain it. The spine is a major part of the nervous system.

Chiropractors have taken care of people from birth to old age, i.e., "womb to tomb." The importance of the pediatric period can never be overstated as this is the period of time when the vital nervous and musculoskeletal systems are maturing. Alterations at this stage will have an effect later in life. Nuturing a healthy nervous system as it is maturing is a key to developing a fully functional mature nervous system which will have an optimal effect on all systems and functions. This level of integrity is called health.

The purpose of this chapter is to present a review of the nervous system including central processing, somatic control, and, of major importance to chiropractors, the functional neurology and pathophysiology of the autonomic or visceral nervous system. The key to the somatovisceral and viscerosomatic anatomy and function of the primary interconnecting structure is the autonomic nervous system. Lastly, we will review selected neurological and visceral disorders with an emphasis on their characteristics and any case reports utilizing chiropractic management.

Functional Neuroanatomy

From the neonate to the geriatric patient, a working knowledge of neuroanatomy and neurophysiology is necessary when you, as a chiropractor, are studying the integrity of a patient's nervous system. You can then custom design a neurological evaluation for each patient based upon the presenting history. This is particularly valuable in wellness care as it helps you to monitor the integrity of your patient throughout the course of his life. If abnormalities such as subtle neurological changes are found, then you can narrow down the structures that may be affected in a systematic manner.

The "safety pin cycle" was a simple model used by early chiropractors as a model to explain the effectiveness of the chiropractic adjustment and the effects of the vertebral subluxation complex. Ongoing developments in modern neurosciences have shown that this model is oversimplistic, but it does not deny its basic concept of a feedback loop—it is not as oversimplistic as the orthodox, linear cause-effect model that is still being used in mainstream healthcare. There are numerous additions that must be added to the cycle, such as neurotransmitters, multi-level synaptic connections, receptors, and other chemicals and structures. An interference in this cycle, such as that caused by the chiropractic vertebral subluxation complex, would undoubtably cause a disturbance in this system. It gives one pause to consider the effects of an interruption in the normal flow of information among the growing cells and systems in a child, particularly noxious signals to the nervous system, and the ramifications that those noxious signals have on the future health of the individual in light of the concept of cellular memory.

Postnatal Development of the Nervous System

Postnatal growth of the nervous system is greatest during the infant's first two years. Most prominent is the growth of the brain. The brain grows two and one-half to three times its birth size in the first year of life—the brain is about 350 grams at birth and grows to about 1000 grams by the first birthday. There is marked proliferation of supportive structures, such as glial cells. Growth slows after this time. At puberty, the brain weighs about 1250 grams in females and 1375 grams in males (1). At birth, the brain exceeds 10% of the entire body weight compared to about 2% in the adult (1). At birth, water constitutes about 85% of the brain's weight but by age four, this figure drops to about 75% (2).

An active area of neurological research is how the growing nerves reach their specific end organs in the periphery. The current speculation centers on chemicals that repel the growing neuron and chemicals that attract specific neurons. As the neuron grows it may be repelled by the surrounding tissues until it finds the tissues with the attracting chemicals. This helps explain the individual differences in the course and area of innervation of the various nerves. Studies of peripheral motor nerves show that there is a "growing cone" on the end of the axon that seems to be involved in leading it to its target muscle. The process by which specific axons branch off from the nerve bundle to go to their target muscle is unknown. The axons have been found to continue with the nerve bundle past their target muscle when a couple of recently identified proteins have been removed. A protein has been found that tells the nerve to stop at the target muscle. Other proteins set up the neuromuscular connection (3). It is a marvel to consider how specific nerves find their end organs.

Myelination of the spine begins in the cervical spine and progresses caudally (2). Myelination of the ventral root occurs before that of the dorsal root (2). Myelination of most of the axons of the major spinal tracts and the cerebrum are largely completed by the end of the second year of postnatal life (4). The cerebrum completes its myelination from the anterior to the posterior (4). Full myelination is completed after the tenth year of life (4). An illustrative demonstration of myelination is that gray matter represents 35% of the matter in the cervical spinal cord's matter of a newborn; in the adult, this is reduced to 19% when full myelination is completed (5).

At birth, the cerebellum continues to grow with further cellular differentiation and migration and continued myelination. By adulthood, the surface area of the cerebellum has grown four-fold (5).

Structures such as the reticular formation, commissural neurons, and intercortical association areas mature after the tenth year of life (4).

The dendrites of the cortical neurons are quite rudimentary at birth. During the first year of life, each cortical neuron develops 1,000 to 100,000 connections with other neurons (2).

At birth, the caudal end of the spinal cord is at the L3 vertebral level (2,5,6)—the cord is about 15 to 17 cm in length (2). By adulthood, the growth of the spinal column has moved the conus medullaris to the level of the inferior margin of L1 and the filum terminale has its cephalic end at the L2 level (5,6). This changes the angulation of the nerve roots exiting the intervertebral foramina.

In the neonate, the nervous system has yet to fully develop and integrate. This is apparent because of the presence of primitive reflexes. These signs may show up in later life when there is a high level lesion or disorganization or degenerative changes. As each sign disappears in the infant and as the infant is able to perform more tasks and control more of its physical and mental functions, the evaluator knows that there is increasing organization of the nervous system—the "wiring" is connecting up. The integration usually occurs at a similar time in most infants so charts have been developed that have chronologically recorded these "milestones."

Overview of the Primary Structures of the Nervous System

Following is a brief review of the functional neuroanatomy of the central and peripheral somatic nervous system. Knowledge of the neurological structures and their function is important in evaluating the nervous system. When a lesion is suspected in the nervous system, the first step is to pinpoint the location(s) and/or structure(s) that is damaged or dysfunctional. This section focuses on the "somatic" portion of the nervous system. As most readers will be fairly well acquainted with this portion of the nervous system, the description will be brief. Following that will be an in-depth description of the autonomic or visceral portion.

Brain

Cerebrum

The cerebrum includes the cerebral cortex, subcortical white matter, corpus callosum, basal ganglia, internal capsule, hippocampal formation, olfactory tracts and bulbs, and the diencephalon, i.e., the thalamus, epithalamus, hypothalamus, and metathalamus. It forms most of the structures that most people consider the brain. The major regions of the cerebrum are reviewed (Fig. 13.1).

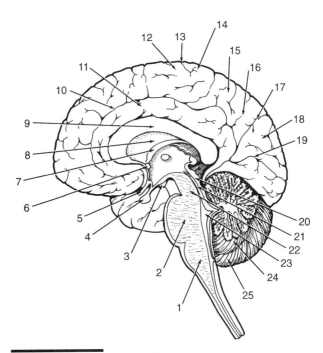

Figure 13.1. Medial surface feature of the brain.
1. Medulla oblongata
2. Pons
3. Mammillary body
4. Pituitary body
5. Optic nerve and chiasma
6. Anterior commissure
7. Fornix
8. Septum Pellucidum
9. Corpus callosum
10. Cingulate sulcus
11. Cingulate gyrus
12. Precentral gyrus
13. Central sulcus
14. Postcentral gyrus
15. Superior parietal lobule
16. Precuneus
17. Parieto-occipital sulcus
18. Cuneus
19. Calcarine fissure
20. Superior and inferior colliculi
21. Cerebral adjunct
22. Midbrain
23. IV ventricle
24. Vermis of the cerebellum
25. Cerebellar hemisphere
Modified from Martin JG. Neuroanatomy Text and Atlas. Norwalk, CT: Appleton & Lange, 1989, p. 405.

Cerebral Cortex

The cerebral cortex is characterized by the myriads of folds over its surface which greatly expands the surface area in a limited size container, the skull. An estimated fourteen billion

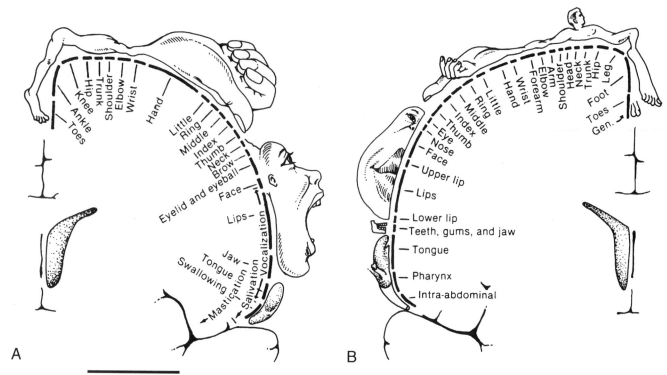

Figure 13.2.   A, Motor homunculus. B, Sensory homunculus. Reprinted with permission from Nolte J. The Human Brain, 3rd ed. St. Louis, MO: Mosby Year Book, 1993.

neurons reside in the adult cerebral cortex (7). Combine the number of neurons with the seemingly infinite number of potential and actual interconnections between dendrites and axons, the power of the brain is beyond comprehension.

The cortex has gyri with the infolding sulci. The cortex is divided into lobes. The anterior portion is the frontal lobe which is separated from the middle region, parietal lobe by the fissure of Rolando. The temporal lobe is separated superiorly by the fissure of Sylvius and an artificial line posteriorly from the occipital lobe. An artificial line separates the parietal lobe from the occipital lobe.

A knowledge of the particular function of each cortical area is invaluable in localizing suspected cortical lesions. The precentral gyrus is concerned with motor control. Posterior to that is the postcentral gyrus or sensory cortex. Together they form the primary sensorimotor cortex. The sensorimotor cortex is somatotopically organized. The medial aspect of these regions which is located cephalically and within the central fissure controls the lower extremities and the lateral aspect, progressively higher regions of the body—this is the well known "homunculus." Although the "homunculus" is a valuable aid in localization, modern neurobiologists have found that the areas representing each region of the body in the motor cortex is not distinct as is classically illustrated as each neuron has an influence over various muscles because movements usually involve multiple muscles and joints rather than a one-to-one relationship between neurons and muscles (Fig. 13.2). The homunculus is fuzzy. The posterior aspect, the

occipital lobe, is associated with vision. There are also association areas that integrate sensory inputs and motor responses. The temporal lobe is located in the inferolateral region of the cerebral cortex and is separated from the upper regions by the lateral cerebral fissure or fissure of Sylvia and functionally from the posterior regions. The hippocampal and parahippocampal regions are prominent parts. The insula is located deep within the fissure of Sylvius. The major activities of the temporal lobe are speech, auditory association, and memory.

There is asymmetrical cortical control for some functions, such as speech. This is an aid in localizing some cortical lesions. An example is Broca's or expressive aphasia which is associated with a lesion to Broca's area 44 or motor speech area in the left inferior frontal lobe.

The association and commissural fibers connect different areas of the cortex. They are the primary components of the white matter of the cerebral hemispheres (8). The afferent and efferent connecting fibers between the cortex and other central structures—i.e., brain stem and spinal cord—are the corona radiata. These fibers converge to form the internal capsule as they pass between the thalamus and caudate nucleus and the lentiform nuclei (7).

Basal Ganglia

The basal ganglia are composed of three subcortical gray nuclei—the caudate nucleus and the lenticular nucleus (putamen and globus pallidus) (9). The basal ganglion integrates complex motor activities into previously learned behavior performance (10). In children, a lesion of the basal ganglion may cause Sydenham's chorea, a disorder often associated with rheumatic fever (9). Children with a familial history of Huntington's chorea may be victims in their thirties or forties from this disease that affects the cerebral cortex and basal ganglion (9).

Thalamic Structures

The thalamic structures are located in the diencephalon and contain many nuclei. Thalamic structures are involved in the integration of neural impulses and secretion of many of the neurohormones.

Thalamus

The thalamus is a relay station which is composed of nuclear groups that integrate the sensory impulses other than those of olfaction. It is also the major source of afferent impulses traveling to the cerebral cortex (11,12). Afferent projections to the thalamus come from a variety of other sources which include peripheral input from the spinothalamic and trigeminothalamic tracts, brainstem, cerebellum, and other thalamic structures (12). Efferent impulses from the thalamus project to the cerebral cortex, cerebellum, striatum, and other thalamic structures (12). It processes sensory information, such as hearing, vision, proprioception, and exteroception (13). Emotions and pain perception are associated with the thalamus (11).

The anterior thalamic nuclei are elements in the "emotional circuit of Papez." Impulses from the hippocampus pass through the fornix and the mammillary body to the thalamus before continuing on to the cingulate gyrus. Impulses continue onward to the parahippocampal gyrus before returning in a feedback loop back to the hippocampus. This circuit appears to be involved in short term memory (11).

Subthalamus

The subthalamus is a structure which lies anterior and caudal to the thalamus and is adjacent to the internal capsule and hypothalamus. It is composed of the subthalamic nuclei, zona incerta, and nuclei of the tegmental fields of Forel (7). Its function is vague, but it appears to have excitatory influence on its targets. It is part of the extrapyramidal system (7).

Epithalamus

The epithalamus is an area of mystery. It is composed of the habenular nuclei, the pineal gland and the habenular and posterior commissure (12). The pineal gland or epiphysis secretes melatonin among other hormones. The quantity of secretion of melatonin has been associated with the amount of light that the organism receives and amount of stress that the organism perceives. Science is constantly speculating about or finding new effects of melatonin in the body. The habenula is associated with autonomic responses to olfaction. The habenula is attached by three connections—stria medullaris thalami, habenular commissure, and habenulointerpeduncular fasciculus (11,13).

Hypothalamus

The hypothalamus is part of the diencephalon and surrounds the third ventricle. There is an anterior, middle, and posterior region. The subependymal gray connects the hypothalamus to the rest of the CNS (13). It is associated with responses to emotions and the maintenance of homeostasis. Hunger, fullness, and thirst are expressions of the hypothalamus (11). Many of the neurohormones produced in the hypothalamus are produced in a portion called the hypophysis cerebri or pituitary gland (11).

Other components of the cerebrum include the commissures which interconnect different parts of the cerebrum, the ventricles (described later), and the internal capsule which is the passageway for many of the fibers traveling to and from the cerebral hemispheres.

Cerebellum

The cerebellum resides in the posterior fossa (14). It is best known as the center for regulating fine movements, muscle tone, and posture (10). Dysfunction degrades movement (10). Ataxia and dysmetria (overshooting or undershooting movements) are signs of cerebellar lesions (8). Lesions of the cerebellum are also associated with asthenia (mild weakness), atonia (diminished resistance to limb manipulation) or hypotonia (flaccidity of the muscle with diminished resistance to passive limb manipulation), and astasia (jerky movements) (15). Some cases of dysarthric speech and ocular movement problems may be associated with cerebellar lesions (8).

Afferent impulses enter the cerebellum from the spinal cord through the middle and inferior cerebellar peduncles. Much of the input arrives from the pontine nuclei (13). Efferent impulses leave the cerebellum through the superior cerebellar peduncle (13).

Brain Stem

The brain stem is the part of the brain minus the cerebrum and the cerebellum. It includes the medulla, pons, midbrain, fourth ventricle, and diencephalon (7). It is an area of critical clinical importance. The "vital centers" are located in the brain stem. Some of the spinal tracts synapse, divert to terminal structures, or make horizontal crossovers (decussate) in this area. Most of the cranial nerves arise in the brain stem. The vertebral arteries, basilar artery, circle of Willis, and their tributaries feature prominently in this area. Compromise of any of these arteries may have a devastating effect on adjacent brain stem structures.

In the neonate, the brain stem has an oblique orientation and must bend in order to pass through the foramen magnum. It becomes more vertically oriented as the nervous system matures (2). The caudal end of the brain stem forms the beginning of the spinal cord.

Limbic System

Although not a specific region of the central nervous system but rather a functional designation, the limbic system or "visceral brain" (16) must be included. The limbic lobe or cortex, which includes the subcallosal, cingulate, and parahippocampal gyri, insula, hippocampal formation, and dentate gyrus and other structures, such as the amygdaloid complex, hypothalamus, epithalamus, parts of the thalamus, and septal nuclei, part of the midbrain, form the limbic system (7,16). The limbic system is associated with emotions and behavior. It is concerned with the basic drives for individual and species preservation (7,16). Lesions of the limbic system are thought to include schizophrenia, depression, amnesia, anxiety states, and phobias (16).

SPINAL CORD

The spinal cord has a white matter periphery surrounding an inner gray matter core. The spinal cord is covered in pia, arachnoid, and dura mater. The white matter periphery of the spinal cord is composed primarily of myelinated nerve fibers. These form the ascending and descending spinal tracts. The inner "H"-shaped portion is the region of gray matter consisting of neuron cell bodies, dendrites, and glia (13). In the center of the cord is the central canal. Cerebrospinal fluid passes through this vertically-oriented canal. A blockage may cause enlargement of this canal in a condition known as syringomyelia whose classical clinical presentation is neurological deficits of those structures lining the canal, in particular, the spinothalamic tract (pain and temperature).

The gray portion of the spinal cord is largest in the thoracic and lumbar portions of the spine because of the innervation to the extremities. The gray is divided into several sections. The anterior horn is the location of motor neurons. These are arrayed somatotopically. The upper body and upper extremities are located laterally, the lower extremities have a more medial location. Extensor muscles are located towards the anterior region while flexor muscles are located towards the posterior portion of the anterior horn (7). The dorsal horn is the entry point of the sensory fibers from the dorsal root. Processing of much of the sensory input occurs in the dorsal horn. A central section is a crossover region between the two sides and surrounds the central canal. In the thoracic and lumbar spine, there is a lateral horn which is the location of the cell bodies of autonomic nerves. Rexed divided the gray matter into nine laminae with a tenth lamina surrounding the central canal (7).

The cervical cord has a large cross-section because of the considerable amount of white matter formed by all of the ascending and descending tracts that pass through it to travel to all regions of the spinal cord. The two enlargements of the spinal cord are associated with innervation to the extremities. The cervical enlargement (cord levels C5 to T1) is associated with the upper extremities (brachial plexus) while the lumbar enlargement (cord levels L1 to S2) is associated with the lower extremities (lumbar and sacral plexi) (7).

At the caudal end of the spinal cord is the conus medullaris. The last of the nerve roots continue on in the cauda equina, each exiting the spine at their respective levels. An extension of the pia mater along with a sheathing of dura mater constitute the filum terminale and provides the caudal anchor for the spinal cord at the coccyx.

SPINAL TRACTS

In the evaluation of peripheral pathological manifestations of the nervous system, the clinician must have a working

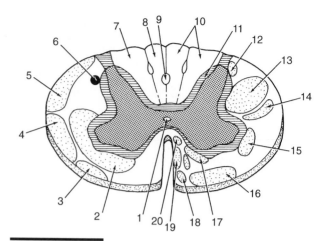

Figure 13.3.   Spinal cord tracts.
1. Central canal
2. Anterolateral spinothalamic and spinoreticular tracts
3. Spino olivary and spinotectal tracts
4. Anterior spinocerebellar tract
5. Posterior spinocerebellar tract
6. Spinocervical tract
7. Fasciculus cuneatus
8. Fasciculus gracilis
9. Fasciculus septomarginalis
10. Posterior/dorsal columns
11. Fasciculus proprius
12. Raphespinal tract
13. Lateral corticospinal tract
14. Rubrospinal tract
15. Lateral (medullary) reticulospinal tract
Modified from Sierra-Romeo C: Neuroanatomy: A Conceptual Approach. New York: Churchill Livingstone, 1986, p. 226.

knowledge of the spinal tracts which connect the peripheral nervous system to the higher centers. Below is a brief review of the major tracts and their primary functions (Fig. 13.3).

Efferent/Motor Tracts

CORTICOSPINAL TRACT

The corticospinal tracts are the main descending pathways and form what is called the pyramidal system. They terminate in synaptic connections onto motor neurons and sensory interneurons. The corticospinal tracts are responsible for voluntary movement and modulation of spinal motor neuron activity (13).

Lesions in the tract or at higher levels are considered upper motor neuron lesions. The typical clinical signs of upper motor neuron lesions include hyperreflexia, muscle hypertonicity, and the presence of the Babinski sign (13). Lesions from the anterior horn cells to the peripheral terminus are considered lower motor neuron lesions—muscle flaccidity and loss of deep tendon reflexes. The neurons from the anterior horn cells to the periphery are referred to as the "final common pathway."

OTHER IMPORTANT DESCENDING TRACTS

Vestibulospinal, reticulospinal, rubrospinal and tectospinal tracts are among the tracts forming the extrapyramidal system. The reticular formation forms a large part of the extrapyramidal system (5). Muscle hypertonicity and involuntary movement disorders are associated with extrapyramidal lesions (5).

Ascending Afferent/Sensory Tracts

DORSAL COLUMNS: FASCICULI GRACILIS AND CUNEATUS

The dorsal columns occupy the posteromedial region of the spinal cord. They transmit proprioception, fine touch, vibration, and two-point discrimination (16,17). The more laterally positioned f. cuneatus innervates the upper body and occupies the lateral aspect of the dorsal columns from T6 cephalically while the more medial f. gracilis innervates the lower body (13,17). The fibers ascend without interruption to the medulla oblongata and synapse in their respective nuclei (7). At this point the second-order fibers cross and form the medial lemniscus. The medial lemniscus ascends to the thalamus. From the thalamus, the impulses are projected to the somatosensory cortex (16).

ANTERIOR SPINOTHALAMIC TRACT

The anterior spinothalamic tracts carry "light touch" sensations to the ventral posterolateral nucleus of the thalamus (7). The fibers synapse and cross over in the anterior white commissure immediately upon entering the cord (7).

LATERAL SPINOTHALAMIC TRACT

The lateral spinothalamic tracts transmit pain and temperature sensations to the ventral posterolateral nucleus of the thalamus. Like the anterior spinothalamic tract, these fibers cross over immediately at their respective cord level (7,16).

SPINOTECTAL TRACT

Fibers of this tract cross over immediately in the cord and ascend with the anterior spinothalamic tract. It carries nociceptive impulses to the superior colliculus and the periaqueductal gray area (7).

POSTERIOR SPINOCEREBELLAR TRACT

The posterior spinocerebellar tracts carry ipsilateral unconscious proprioception to the cerebellum (7). This tract arises in the dorsal nucleus of Clarke and ascends uncrossed to the inferior cerebellar peduncle (7,13). It is important in fine coordination of the extremity muscles of posture and movement (7). Lesion to the spinocerebellar tracts is difficult to isolate (7).

ANTERIOR SPINOCEREBELLAR TRACT

The fibers of the anterior spinocerebellar tract cross over before ascending the cord. It carries unconscious proprioception from the lower extremity (7). Impulses arrive at the cerebellum through the superior cerebellar peduncle (7). The proprioceptive and exteroceptive sensory information is important in coordinating movement and posture of the lower extremities (7,13).

MIXED AND ASSOCIATION TRACTS

There are mixed and association tracts. The medial longitudinal fasciculus (MLF) originates in the brainstem. The fibers arise from several nuclei. In Lissauer's fasciculus, dorsal nerve root fibers ascend or descend up to six levels of the cord (7,18). The multi-level dispersion diffuses the sensory impulses (18). Lissauer's Zone is considered part of the structure involved in the "gate control" theory of Melzack and Wall (48). Fibers in the Lissauer's Zone also merge with the spinal root of the trigeminal nerve (48). There are association tracts that are formed by the ascending or descending branches of the dorsal roots (7,14,18).

SPINAL NERVES

Thirty-one pairs of spinal nerves branch off of the cord. There are typically eight cervical, twelve thoracic, five lumbar, five sacral, and one coccygeal paired nerves (7).

The ventral root of the spinal nerve roots carry motor or efferent impulses. The sensory impulses enter the cord via the dorsal roots. Both somatic and visceral information travels through the dorsal root. The dorsal root ganglion contains the cell bodies of the sensory neurons.

The two roots join together forming a mixed spinal nerve that splits into ventral and dorsal rami. The dorsal ramus further divides into lateral and medial branches. The ventral ramus has a lateral branch. The spinal nerves also carry autonomic fibers to and from the sympathetic chains (see the next section on the functional neuroanatomy of the autonomic nervous system) (9). The somatic spinal nerves continue onward to the musculature and skin of the body with motor and sensory fibers.

SOMATIC PERIPHERAL NERVES

The somatic peripheral system and autonomic peripheral system have intermingling fibers which confound many attempting to follow their pathways. The spinal roots carry both somatic and autonomic fibers. Some of the description of the functional anatomy of the somatic peripheral nerves is in the autonomic nervous system section because of the intermingling of fibers.

There are four major plexi formed by the ventral primary rami of the spinal nerves. They are the cervical, brachial, lumbar, and sacral plexi.

The cervical plexus is formed by the ventral rami of the C1 to C4 spinal nerves (19). The muscular branches innervate many of the muscles of the anterior neck. The strap muscles of the neck via the ansa cervicalis arcs around the internal jugular vein. The phrenic nerve is a branch of the cervical plexus and provides both motor and sensory supply to the diaphragm. Cutaneous branches supply sensory fibers to the skin and underlying tissues from the area of the clavicle over the head to the posterior scalp (19). Injury to the cervical plexus may cause disorders, such as respiratory problems, neck aches, neck stiffness, cervical syndrome, or atrophy of the neck muscles (17).

The brachial plexus is formed by the C5 to T1 spinal nerves and often some fibers from C4 and T2 (19). From the spinal roots, the plexus is divided into trunks, divisions, cords, and then nerves, such as long thoracic, dorsal scapular, axillary, radial, ulnar, musculocutaneous, and median nerves which innervate the upper torso and upper extremities (19). The long thoracic and dorsal scapular nerves innervate the interscapular muscles which are important in scapular position. Lesions may cause Erb-Duchenne paralysis, Klumpke's paralysis, Horner's syndrome (17).

The lumbar plexus is formed by the ventral rami of the L1 to L4 spinal nerves and some fibers from T12 (19). The major branches of the lumbar plexus include the iliohypogastric, ilioinguinal, genitofemoral, lateral cutaneous, obturator, and femoral nerves. They give cutaneous and muscular branches to the abdominal wall down to the lower extremities (19). Lesion to the femoral nerve is called meralgia paresthetica.

The sacral plexus is formed by the spinal nerves from L4 to S3. It transmits somatic, motor and sensory, and also sympathetic fibers to the pelvis, lower abdomen, and lower extremity (19). The most notable branch of the sacral plexus is the sciatic nerve. Other major branches include the common peroneal, pudendal, posterior femoral cutaneous, tibial, and muscular nerves (17,19). The best known lesion of the sacral plexus is sciatica or sciatic neuritis.

There is also a coccygeal plexus. It give cutaneous branches to the skin in the area around the coccyx (7,19).

The thoracic spinal nerves do not form plexi but the spinal nerve sends cutaneous and muscular branches along one intercostal space with some branches to adjacent intercostal spaces. This gives each intercostal space a nerve supply from two to four spinal nerves. The thoracic spinal nerves supply the skin and muscles of the chest and thoracic wall (19). A common manifestation of thoracic nerve lesion is shingles (herpes zoster).

Afferent sensory fibers transmit impulses from receptors and nerve endings. The cell bodies of peripheral somatosensory nerves are in the dorsal root ganglion. Somatic receptors include the proprioceptors and exteroceptors. Pacinian corpuscles, muscle spindles, and Golgi tendon organs are the major proprioceptors. Free nerve endings, Meissner's corpuscles (light touch), Pacinian corpuscles (deep pressure), Krausse end bulbs, Golgi-Mazzoni receptors, and Ruffini endings are the major exteroceptor receptors and endings (19). The area that the sensory neuron responds to is the receptive field. Areas where receptive fields are small and occur in large numbers are fields with high sensory acuity. The fingertips are an example of an highly sensitive region with a large number of small receptive fields (19).

The primary somatic efferent neurons are the motor neurons. There are two major types of motor neurons: the alpha motor neurons which send out A-alpha (Aa) and A-beta (Ab) fibers to the striatal skeletal muscles, and the gamma motor neurons which send out fibers to the intrafusal fibers of the muscle spindles (19). The primary tracts influencing the motor neurons from higher centers are the corticospinal, vestibulospinal, rubrospinal, and reticulospinal tracts (19). A motor unit is composed of a single anterior horn cell and the muscle fibers that it innervates. In muscles where only crude or gross movement is required, one axon innervates hundreds or thousands of muscle cells. In areas where muscles engage in fine movements, one axon innervates ten or less muscle cells. Thigh or chest wall muscles are an example of the former while extraocular muscles are an example of the latter (16,19).

When there is damage to the motor neurons, there are more motor units created upon regeneration but this number diminishes to the original number with further tissue repair (19).

An important function of the peripheral nerve are the reflex arcs. The simplest is the monosynaptic reflex arc. Stretch of the muscle spindle causes afferent impulses to travel up the involved peripheral afferent nerve to the dorsal root of the spinal nerve and into the spinal cord. The neuron synapses with motor neurons in the anterior horn of the spinal cord sends impulses back to the muscle causing contraction of the affected muscle. There are much more complex reflex arcs involving agonist muscles and muscles of the opposite limb.

Upper Motor Neuron Lesions vs Lower Motor Neuron Lesions

When evaluating alterations to the integrity of the somatosensory nervous system that manifests in peripheral structures, the initial determination made is whether the lesion is in the peripheral nervous system or in the central nervous system. Clinical manifestations differ according to the location of the lesion in classical ways. The peripheral nerve in the somatomotor system begins in the anterior horn of the spinal cord. As noted, this is called the "final common pathway." The peripheral somatosensory neurons have their cell bodies in the dorsal root ganglion.

The classical clinical signs of lesions of the spinal nerves tend to cause dermatomal sensory loss, hyporeflexia, motor weakness, and muscle atrophy. The hyporeflexia is due to interruption of the reflex arc. The motor weakness and muscle atrophy is due to interruption of the direct nerve supply to the muscles.

The classic clinical signs of upper motor neuron lesions are hyperreflexia, clonus, and muscle atrophy.

Blood Supply of the Nervous System

The nervous system requires a substantial portion of the blood supply during the fetal and postnatal stages because of its rapid growth. It continues to require a major proportion of the vascular supply in adulthood as well.

Brain

The high metabolic rate of the brain demands a disproportional percentage of the total oxygen and nutrient-rich blood flow required by the entire body. Seventeen per cent of the oxygen-rich blood from the heart and one-fifth of the total oxygen is required by the brain in order to function. This is in spite of the fact that the brain only constitutes 2% of the body's weight. Normal cerebral blood flow is about 50 ml/100 g brain tissue/minute and consumes about 3.3 ml of oxygen/100g brain tissue/minute (7). The arterial supply to the brain is via the vertebral and internal carotid arteries (17).

The primary blood supply to the brain is through the two internal carotid and two vertebral arteries (7,9). These arteries join in a complex of arteries called the Circle of Willis. Branches from this complex go to the brain and adjacent structures. The cerebral arteries course over the surface of the cerebrum with branches dropping perpendicularly into its interior. This contrasts with most other organs which have a hilus where the arteries supplying the organ enters (6).

Veins emerge from the brain and form pial plexi. These join to form the valveless deep and superficial cerebral veins which pass through the subarachnoid space to the sinuses of the dura mater. The sinuses converge and eventually drain into the internal jugular veins (7). Of special importance is the superior sagittal sinus which is vulnerable to head trauma. The veins of the brain stem and cerebellum tend to follow the arterial supply. The cerebellar veins drain into the veins and sinuses that also drain the cerebral hemispheres. Those of the brain stem drain into the great cerebral vein or internal cerebral veins (7).

Spine

The arterial supply to the spinal cord is from the radicular arteries and the posterior spinal and anterior spinal branches of the vertebral arteries. The largest of the anterior radicular arteries supplies the lower thoracic and lumbar cord and is called the artery of Adamkiewicz (7,9). The thoracic spine has a relatively poor blood supply and relies upon a single radicular artery (9).

The venous distribution tends to follow that of the arterial supply. The venous branches drain into the epidural venous plexus (7). The valveless venous plexus of the spine is quite fascinating. If intra-abdominal pressure is increased, venous flow from the pelvic plexus passes to the spinal plexus. Drainage from the brain may also enter the spinal plexus. Tremendous work was done by Batson on correlating the metastasis of neoplasms of the prostate, brain, and breast to the spine. From the studies by Batson and others, it has been found that because of the valveless nature of the spinal venous system, venous blood flow can reverse. This is the mechanism which allows circulating cancerous cells to enter the spine from remote primary sites (20,21).

Ventricle System—Cerebrospinal Fluid Flow

The ventricle system is composed of the two lateral ventricles, the interventricular foramen of Munro which connects the lateral ventricles to the third ventricle, the third ventricle, the cerebral aqueduct connecting the third and fourth ventricles, the fourth ventricle, the Foramen of Magendie, and the central canal which traverses down the spinal cord. CSF (cerebrospinal fluid) flows throughout the ventricle system and the subarachnoid space.

The lateral ventricles are located in the cerebral hemispheres. The lateral ventricles have five parts. These are the anterior or frontal horn, the ventricular body, the collateral trigone, the inferior horn, and the posterior horn (7). CSF passes from the two lateral ventricles via the interventricular foramen of each respective ventricle to the third ventricle. The third ventricle lies between the thalami and hypothalami. Structures such as the optic chiasma, the posterior perforating substance, and mamillary bodies lie at the floor of the third ventricle and the stalk of the pineal gland to the posterior (14). From the third ventricle, CSF passes through the singular cerebral aqueduct of Sylvius to the fourth ventricle. The fourth ventricle lies between the brainstem and medulla oblongata and the cerebellum. Many cranial nerve nuclei and tracts passing to and from the spinal cord are adjacent to the anterior aspect of the fourth ventricle. CSF in the fourth ventricle passes through openings such as the foramina of Luschka and Magendie into the subarachnoid space surrounding the brain and spinal cord and into the central canal of the spinal cord (7,14).

Cerebrospinal fluid is a clear, colorless fluid that protects, cushions and supports the central nervous system (9,22). It fills the extracellular interstitial spaces and CSF cavities (22). There is about 50 ml of CSF in infants and 150 ml in adults (22). CSF is thought to be composed of an ultrafiltrate of plasma with secondary processing which makes it effective at isolating nervous tissue (22). The choroid plexus, a blood vessel rich network in the pia mater that projects into the ventricular cavities of the CNS, appears to be a primary origin of CSF (9). A large percentage, possibly up to 50%, is formed by the cerebral endothelium (22). The choroid plexus receives its nerve supply from vagal, glossopharyngeal, and sympathetic branches (23). CSF returns to the venous system through arachnoid villi in the superior sagittal sinuses (9,22).

Innervation of the Spine

A very controversial issue concerns nerve supply to the intervertebral disc. In contrast, innervation to the other structures of the spine, e.g., facets, ligaments, muscles, is fairly well established. Jinkins has done some research into the innervation of the intervertebral disc as has Mendel et al and Bogduk et al. Studies have found nerve fibers in the anulus, particularly in the middle one-third of the disc. Mendel et al have found small Pacinian corpuscles-like receptors and also Golgi tendon organ-like receptors in the posterolateral, upper one-third of cervical discs (23). Bogduk et al found branches of the sinuvertebral and vertebral nerves and ventral rami of the cervical spine innervating the discs. The latter have found nerve fibers and nerve endings in the anterolateral portion of the discs (26). Much of the nerve supply to the disc appears to be autonomic in origin, but some somatic innervation is suspected (26). Whether or not nociceptive information is obtained from these nerves has not been established (26).

The recurrent meningeal or sinuvertebral nerve innervates the structures in the area of the posterior vertebral body (18,28). It arises from the ventral root and the gray rami communicans (18,27,29) and returns to the spinal canal via the intervertebral foramen (28,5). Branches may ascend or descend one or two levels (18).

Functional Neuroanatomy of the Autonomic Nervous System

The plethora of names that have been given to the visceral nervous system suggests its anatomical complexity, its physiological uniqueness, and its wide variety of effects. These include the vegetative, involuntary, autonomic, plexiform, or major sympathetic nervous system. Its striking configuration of chains, cords, ganglia, nuclei, plexi, nerves, and filaments do not lend themselves to effortless understanding. The map of the cerebrospinal system appears to be relatively simple in comparison.

The autonomic nervous system (ANS) has often been said to make nothing but be responsible for everything. Korr noted that stimulation of the autonomic nervous system alone does not introduce new qualities, but modifies (by increasing, decreasing, accelerating, retarding, stimulating, or inhibiting) the inherent physiological properties of the target tissue. The modified effect on each of these tissues has its own particular effect on total body physiology (30). The ANS influences all unconscious operations, leaving little that it does not control except the direct voluntary movement of striatal muscles. Yet, even the latter receives its metabolic support and tone from ANS activities.

The chiropractic clinical and philosophical position on health has often been popularly stated as, "health comes from above down, inside out," "health comes from within," and "chiropractors do not cure diseases but remove the 'nerve interferences' which allows innate intelligence to be more fully expressed." The ANS may provide the primary neurological pathway for health and "innate intelligence," and is likely not distinguishable from it. This section of the chapter is devoted to both the anatomical and functional considerations of the ANS.

Anatomy of the Autonomic Nervous System

Like the cerebrospinal nervous system (CSNS), the ANS has central processes and peripheral processes with efferent and afferent fibers and effector and receptor terminals. The central processes of both systems are located in the gray regions of the spinal cord and brain. The peripheral processes are those structures which are peripheral to the spinal cord and brain. The ANS is distinguished from the CSNS by virtue of an additional layer of complexity, namely, the peripheral ganglia. In the ANS, the equivalent of the "final common pathways" of the CSNS arise from these peripheral ganglia as post-ganglionic nerves (Fig. 13.4).

Although afferent and efferent nerve fibers are the peripheral components of both the cerebrospinal and autonomic nervous systems, communication between the autonomic central nuclei and the terminal receptors or effectors is via either sympathetic or parasympathetic pathways. The sympathetic and parasympathetic each have a unique design with distinct central origins, peripheral distributions, and responses to stimuli (31). In most viscera, however, they do have overlapping influences.

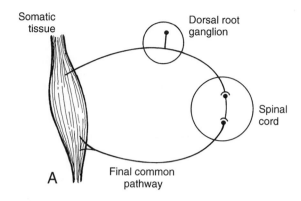

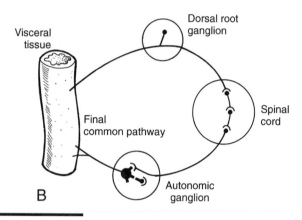

Figure 13.4. Modulation prior to final common pathway. Simple reflex arcs of somatic neurons (cerebrospinal nervous system) (A), visceral neurons (autonomic nervous system) (B). Note: there is an extra level of processing prior to the final common pathway. Modified from Sierra-Romeo C. Neuroanatomy: A Conceptual Approach. New York: Churchill Livingstone, 1986, p. 170.

CENTRAL PROCESSES OF THE AUTONOMIC NERVOUS SYSTEM

PARASYMPATHETIC NUCLEI

There are three regions which contain the central nuclei and gray matter of the parasympathetic division. The most cephalic region is within the anterior and paraventricular region of the diencephalon (in the rostral hypothalamus). These centers are linked to the frontal cortex and limbic system. Caudal to this are regions in the mid brain, pons, and brainstem which contain the nuclei for cranial nerves 3, 7, 9, and 10. The caudal most region is located in the middle horn or intermediolateral gray matter of the S2 to S4 levels of the spinal cord. The location of these central origins of the parasympathetic nervous system lead anatomists to call the parasympathetic system the "craniosacral" nerve system.

SYMPATHETIC NUCLEI

There are two regions which contain the central nuclei and gray tissues associated with the sympathetic nervous system. The cephalicmost region is in the diencephalon (in the caudal hypothalamus) which is linked to the frontal cortex and limbic systems. The lower region is in the intermediolateral and intermediomedial columns of the lateral gray horns of the spinal cord from the T1 to L3 cord levels. A type of somatotopic organization is present in the spinal cord—the nuclei of the medial column represent the viscera of the trunk, and the nuclei of the lateral column represent the trunk wall and extremities. The central location of these origins of the sympathetic system in the spinal cord has given this system the designation of "thoraco-lumbar" nerve system.

The parasympathetic (cranio-sacral) and sympathetic (thoraco-lumbar) designations of the autonomic nerve systems make clear that these systems are two anatomically distinct systems arising from anatomically isolated central origins.

PERIPHERAL OUTFLOW OF THE AUTONOMIC NERVOUS SYSTEM

PARASYMPATHETIC OUTFLOW— PARASYMPATHETIC GANGLIA, PLEXI, AND NERVES

Parasympathetic nerves run a relatively direct route to and from their central origins and their visceral terminations (Fig. 13.5). Both the vagus nerve (cranial nerve 10) and the sacral parasympathetic nerves (pelvic splanchnic nerves) synapse within ganglia that are in or immediately adjacent to the organ being innervated—they terminate as local visceral plexi.

SYMPATHETIC OUTFLOW—SYMPATHETIC GANGLIA, PLEXI, AND NERVES

Sympathetic nerves provide the communicating link between the viscera and the spinal cord via much more complex, integrated, multiple-level routes (Fig. 13.6). The sympathetic afferent nerves typically synapse in the spinal cord. The sympathetic efferent nerves synapse in peripheral ganglia which are distant from their viscera, unlike the parasympathetic ganglia. Sympathetic fibers form independent autonomic nerve and vascular nerve plexi and also join spinal and cranial nerves (32).

Sympathetic neurons leaving the spinal cord are called pre-ganglionic sympathetic neurons. They may first synapse in one of the paired chains of ganglia which are positioned along the entire length of the spinal column (para vertebral ganglionic chain), or more peripherally, in an abdominal ganglia (pre-vertebral ganglia). After synapsing in either location, fibers become postganglionic sympathetic neurons. The thoracic portion of the paravertebral sympathetic ganglion chain is positioned against the costotransverse joints, while the lumbar portion is positioned against the anterolateral portion of the vertebral body.

Some pre-ganglionic nerves will synapse at the same level that they enter the paravertebral chain. Some pre-ganglionic neurons enter the chain but travel cephalically or caudally several segmental levels (up to three to five levels) before synapsing within a paravertebral chain ganglion. Finally, some pre-ganglionic neurons pass through the paravertebral ganglia, without synapsing, directly into the abdomen and synapse in individual, remote, pre-vertebral ganglia.

The ganglia of one side are functionally isolated from those of the contralateral side except by interconnections within the spinal cord and brain. In the sacral region, the ganglionic chains often connect at the coccyx and terminate as a single, small, midline ganglion—the ganglion impars (32).

CONNECTION OF THE SYMPATHETIC GANGLIA AND THE SPINAL CORD VIA THE SYMPATHETIC NERVE ROOTS

Sympathetic nerves exit from the anterior horn with other neurons of the primary anterior spinal nerve root (Fig. 13.7). In the intervertebral foramen, a distinct sympathetic bundle emerges from the anterior root. Because it is myelinated, it is termed the *white ramus communican* or *ramus albus*. This small bundle exits the intervertebral foramen and travels anteroinferiorly along the perimeter of the vertebral body before joining the paravertebral sympathetic chain ganglia at that level.

The white rami of the sympathetic nervous system contain both afferent and efferent sympathetic fibers. The afferent fibers join white rami after travelling from their visceral terminus to the sympathetic ganglia. They enter the white communicating rami from the ganglia without synapsing, enter the anterior division of the spinal nerve, and converge to become indistinguishable with the somatosensory fibers of the dorsal root. They course through the dorsal root ganglion to the posterior horn of the spinal cord. The entire length of the sympathetic chain, which extends from the occiput to the coccyx, is supplied by white communicating rami even though these rami only exit from the intervertebral foramina of the T1 to L3 vertebral levels.

A bundle comprised of efferent sympathetic fibers leaves the paravertebral ganglia to join spinal nerves. These sympathetic fibers are unmyelinated post-ganglionic fibers and are called *gray ramus communican* or *rami griseus*. Unlike the white rami, the gray communicating rami emerge from all levels of the chain to supply each of the spinal nerves from the occiput to the coccyx. They accompany both the ventral and dorsal primary divisions of the spinal nerves. Gray rami innervate the skin, blood vessels, sweat glands, piloerector muscles, and somatic tissues. It has been reported that 15% of the spinal nerve is of sympathetic origin. The discrepancy between the entry points of the autonomic sensory nerves into the spinal cord at levels T1 to L3 and S2 to S4, and the entry point of the somatic sensory nerves into the spinal cord at each level from the occiput to the fourth coccygeal nerve accounts for the referral of a visceral stimulus to a somatic structure far removed from the actual site of autonomic irritation.

Spinal cord centers have been found to have specific topical outflows. The preganglionic sympathetic efferent neurons of the upper thoracic spine have a fixed relationship with the postganglionic sympathetic fibers of the cervical sympathetic trunk of the vertebral and inferior cardiac nerves and the sympathetic fibers of the vagus (33).

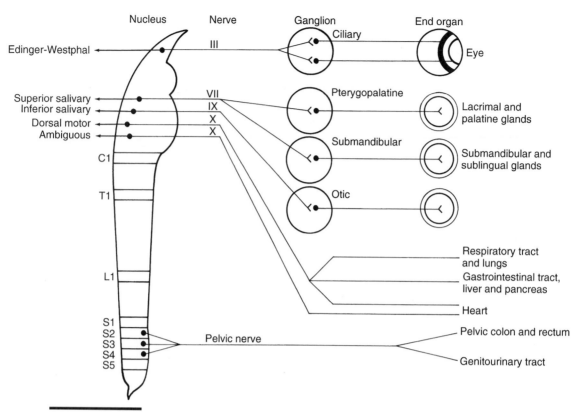

Figure 13.5.   The outflow of the parasympathetic nervous system. Modified from Low PA. Clinical Autonomic Disorders. Boston: Little, Brown & Co., 1993.

Extensive paravertebral synapsing occurs. Each sympathetic preganglionic neuron generally innervates 15 to 30 post-ganglionic fibers (1:30). Each of these in turn innervate many effector cells. This divergence is in great contrast to that of the parasympathetic system (34).

Parasympathetic Ganglia, Plexi, and Nerves

Parasympathetic pre-ganglionic nerves synapse after a long run from their CNS nuclei to ganglia at or in the target viscera. Post-ganglionic fibers are short and few in number—typically, a pre-ganglionic axon innervates only two post-ganglionic nerves (1:2 ratio) which in turn innervate a only few effector cells (13).

Many of the organs that are under parasympathetic control are largely self-regulating and controlled by local, intrinsic reflexes. The gastrointestinal tract is regulated by its own nerve system—the enteric or intramural nerve system. Local reflexes generated by the presence of food cause both smooth muscle contraction and secretion of digestive fluids. Auerbach's (mes-enteric) plexus regulates peristalsis (chopping, mixing, and passing of the food bolus), and Meissner's (submucous) plexus regulates digestive fluid secretion (32). These function under normal circumstances with little central autonomic control (35), although profound effects on those functions can occur when extraordinary circumstances exist (34).

Four Functional Regions of the Sympathetic Nervous System

The configuration of components within the autonomic nervous system varies greatly. However, the components of the SNS are contained within two natural divisions. These two divisions can roughly be further subdivided. The divisions correspond to the visceral cavities or fields of the body, namely a lower abdominal/pelvic field and an upper thoracic/cervi-cocranial field. The diaphragm separates the two fields.

The viscera of the abdominal and pelvic compartment are innervated by 11 pairs of splanchnic nerves. These nerves exit the spinal column from segmental levels T6 to L3. Splanchnic nerves are pre-ganglionic and pass through the paravertebral chain without synapsing until they terminate in the large, remote abdominal ganglia. These ganglia supply two func-tional plexi. One serves the abdominal compartment and the other serves the pelvic compartment.

The viscera of the thoracic cavity and cervicocranial field—those above the diaphragm—are innervated by sympa-thetic nerves which exit from T5 to T1. There are no splanchnic nerves or prevertebral ganglia as in the lower division. All of the sympathetic nerves synapse in the paraver-tebral chain. Like the lower visceral compartment, the upper compartment collectively forms two functional plexi, one serving cardiopulmonary functions associated with the tho-racic cavity and the other, the head.

The somatic tissue fields of the upper and lower extremities receive sympathetic somatic innervation from the upper and lower portions of the sympathetic chains, respectively (32,36).

The lower functional region of the sympathetic nervous system includes the abdominal and pelvic fields. The two collective plexi within the lower trunk are associated with several large ganglia. The largest and most cephalic ganglia are the celiac ganglia. The two ganglia overlie the aorta beneath the diaphragm. They generally innervate the GI tract from the lower esophagus to the proximal large intestines and are involved with accessory functions of the liver, gall bladder, pancreas, adrenal gland, as well as the vascular supply to these organs. The celiac ganglia are supplied by the splanchnic nerves which exit from the T5 to T11 spinal levels. The splanchnic nerves from T5 to T11 converge to form the greater splanchnic nerve. Nerves from T9 and T10 often form the lesser splanchnic nerve. The least splanchnic nerve, when present, is usually formed by the roots of T12.

Caudal to the celiac ganglion is the superior mesenteric ganglion. It is associated with innervation of the small and large bowels. The greater and lesser splanchnic nerves also innervate the superior mesenteric ganglion. The lesser splanchnic nerve generally contributes to a pair of small ganglia—the aortico-renal ganglia (32).

The most caudal ganglion is the inferior mesenteric ganglion. It receives fibers from the least splanchnic nerve. The inferior mesenteric ganglion is involved in the sex organs and in elimination functions—the rectum, kidneys, bladder and ureter. The T12 cord level also supplies the renal ganglion and plexus.

The upper splanchnic nerves exit the spinal column and overlie the spine as they descend along the posterior midline wall of the thorax (37). They pierce the diaphragm in order to reach the abdominal ganglia. The lumbar splanchnic nerves from the T10 to L3 cord levels synapse in four to six smaller unnamed ganglia. The post-synaptic fibers from these ganglia form the superior and inferior hypogastric plexi which influence the lower abdominal and pelvic functions.

The splanchnic nerve arising out of the T10 spinal cord level innervates the adrenal medulla. Unlike other sympathetic pathways, its pre-ganglionic fibers synapse directly on the organ itself—the chromaffin cells in the adrenal medulla.

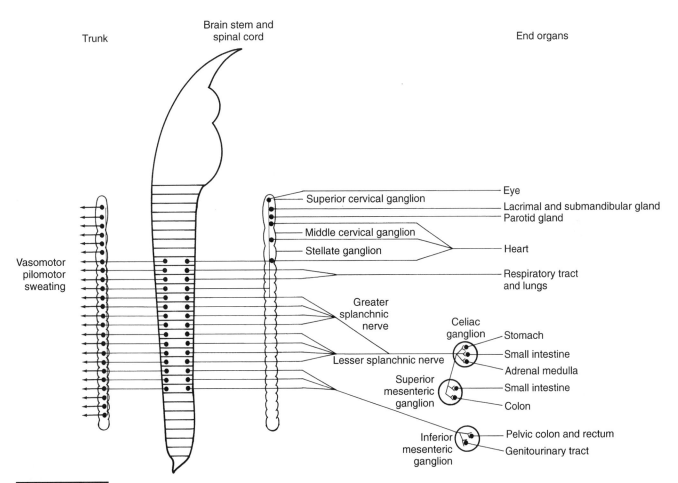

Figure 13.6.   The outflow of the parasympathetic nervous system in the thoracolumbar spine. Modified from Low PA. Clinical Autonomic Disorders. Boston: Little, Brown & Co., 1993. Korr IM: The Spinal Cord as Organizer of Disease Process II: The Peripheral Autonomic System. In: Peterson B (ed). The Collected Works of Irvin M. Korr. Colorado Springs, CO: American Academy of Osteopathy, 1979.

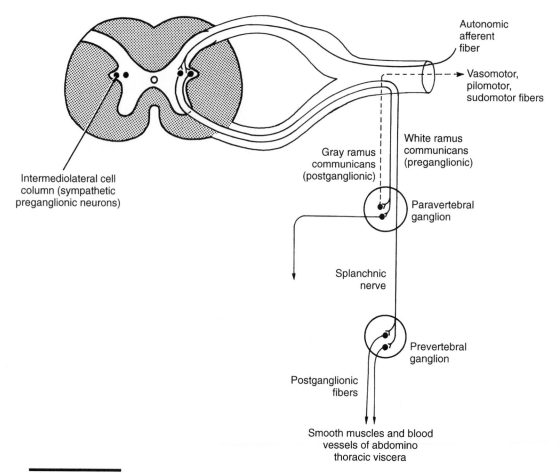

Figure 13.7. The sympathetic outflow of the spinal cord. Modified from Low PA. Clinical Autonomic Disorders. Boston: Little, Brown & Co., 1993.

Stimulation causes a systemic release of epinephrine and norepinephrine from the adrenal medulla sufficient to dramatically influence the sympathetic nervous system throughout the entire body (16)

Autonomic tone of the lower extremities is regulated by the post-ganglionic fibers of T12 to S4 (36). These fibers usually follow the course of the major arteries. They are not part of splanchnic nerve system.

The upper functional region of the sympathetic nervous system includes the cardiopulmonary and cranial fields. The postganglionic nerves from T1 to T5 control viscera of the thorax and head and somatic tissues of the upper extremities. In the thoracic and lumbar spine, a pair of sympathetic ganglia are associated with each vertebral level. Only three or four pairs of sympathetic ganglia are located in the cervical portion of the sympathetic chain. Each of these ganglia is a fusion of two or three ganglia and is significantly larger than the thoracic or lumbar ganglia. In this way, these ganglia may have a greater integrative capacity. The superior cervical ganglia are the largest and are located anterolateral to C2/C3. The middle cervical ganglia are usually located anterolateral to C5/C6.

The inferior cervical ganglia are located at the cervicothoracic junction. A variant of the inferior cervical ganglia is the stellate ganglia which is the fusion of the inferior cervical ganglion with the first thoracic ganglion (14).

The cervical ganglia receive preganglionic fibers from T1 to T5 only. No preganglionic sympathetic nerves emerge from the cervical or cranial regions. Therefore, there are no cervical or cranial preganglionic sympathetic nerves. The cervical and upper thoracic ganglia provide postganglionic plexi innervation to the cardiopulmonary field. The superior cervical sympathetic ganglion provides postganglionic plexi that accompany arteries and arterioles to innervate the head. Autonomic tone of the upper extremities is largely supplied from the thoracic ganglia of T1 to T3 and the inferior and middle cervical ganglia (32,36) (Table 13.1).

Upper thoracic sympathetic nerves and cervical nerves communicate with cranial structures and the sympathetic nervous system influence over the parenchyma of the brain and head. While the course of sympathetic nerves to the cardiopulmonary axis is conceptually rather straightforward, sympathetic innervation of the facial and intracranial tissues is worthy of special review.

The upper five thoracic sympathetic nerves, the upper five cervical spinal nerves, and the lower cranial nerves converge on one another to influence the cranial structures.

Communications of upper thoracic, cervical, and cranial nerves. Sympathetic nerves have their origin in the upper thoracic spinal cord and form the cervical sympathetic trunk. Innervation continues into the head as three arterial plexi—the vertebral, internal carotid, and external carotid artery plexi (32) (Table 13.2).

The vertebral sympathetic plexus arises from the T1 to T5 cord levels (32), ascends in the paravertebral chain, and contributes in the formation of the inferior cervical sympathetic ganglia. The fibers leave the ganglia, attach to the vertebral arteries as a plexus, ascend through the transverse foramen of the cervical transverse processes, and enter the skull through the foramen magnum. Fibers then invest the cerebellar, basilar, and posterior cerebral arteries and their branches. They innervate the lower cranial nerves, brain stem, cerebellum, occipital lobe of the cerebral cortex, and diencephalon.

The internal carotid plexus arises from the T1 to T5 spinal cord levels. These fibers pass through the paravertebral chain to enter the superior sympathetic ganglia. From this point, the fibers invest the internal carotid artery as a plexus which then enters the skull through the carotid canal. After the internal carotid arteries reach the Circle of Willis, sympathetic fibers form the cavernous plexus. Fibers follow the anterior and middle cerebral arteries and their branches before terminating in the ocular orbit (opthalmic artery), choroidal tissues, and pia mater.

Fibers of the external carotid sympathetic plexus arise from the T1 to T5 spinal cord segments, ascend the chain, and exit via the superior cervical ganglion. The fibers of this plexus wrap around the external carotid artery before innervating the oral cavity, facial structures, and tissues of the external cranium.

Cervical sympathetic nerves arise from T1 to T5 cord levels and exit from the middle and superior sympathetic ganglia to form plexi for the pharynx and throat (32). Some sympathetic fibers join the spinal nerves of C1 to C4 via the gray communicating rami.

Cervical spinal nerves containing both sympathetic and somatic nerves communicate with cranial nerves 7, 9, 10, 11, and 12 (32). Proprioceptive input from the upper cervical spine is integrated with input from the vestibular (cranial nerve 8) and ocular (cranial nerves 2, 3, 4, and 6) stimulatory fields within the cranium (38).

INFLUENCES TO CRANIAL PARENCHYMA AND GENERAL VASOTONIC INFLUENCES: A SUMMARY

Cranial nerves and the sympathetic nervous system influence sensory and motor functions which produce the movements and accommodation of the eye and the secretions and vasoregulation of the eye, nasal and oral cavity, middle ear, pharynx, larynx, and skin (32). The sympathetic plexi from the cavernous plexus innervate the intracranial tissues of the hypothalamus, hypophysis (pituitary gland), and pineal gland. Sympathetic fibers extend to the terminal branches of the anterior, middle, and posterior cerebral arteries to innervate the cortical pia mater. The choroid plexi are richly innervated with sympathetic fibers which influence the production of cerebrospinal fluid (32).

In the cervical spine, the superior cervical ganglion communicates directly with the vagus and glossopharyngeal ganglia and the hypoglossal nerve (32). Cervical sympathetic plexi innervate and communicate with the pharyngeal plexi. The somatic and sympathetic (gray rami) fibers of the upper four cervical spinal nerves communicate directly with cranial nerves 7 through 12 (32). Indirect relationships between cranial nerves and cervical nerves exist because somatic and parasympathetic fibers of the lower cranial nerves generate impulses from their terminations on the parenchyma of the throat and neck. Those same tissues receive innervation from somatic and sympathetic nerves of the cervical spine.

Autonomic regulation of the head is similar to that of the rest of the body; that is, control is exerted largely by a dual innervation of the parasympathetic and sympathetic systems. The eye and the parotid, submaxillary, sublingual, lacrimal, and mucosal glands receive dual innervation. While the parasympathetic nuclei and pathways are fully contained within the skull the sympathetic nuclei and pathways are not. The sympathetic system has its origin in the thoracic spine from

---

Table 13.1.   Sympathetic Nervous System (Segmental Origins and Peripheral Distribution)

Cord Levels	Ganglionic Relays	Peripheral Distribution
T1–T2	Superior cervical	Eye, brain, head, neck
T1–T5	Superior, middle & inferior cervical, upper 5 thoracic	Heart
T2–T7	Middle cervical, stellate	Upper extremity
T2–T3	Upper thoracic chain	Lungs, trunk wall
T5–T12	Preaortic	GI tract, adrenal medulla
T12–L3	Lumbosacral chain	Trunk wall, lower extremity, perineum
T12–L3	Pelvic	Bladder sphincter, ductus deferens, rectum

Adapted from FitzGerald MJT. Neuroanatomy Basic and Applied. Philadelphia PA: Baillière Tindall, 1985.

Table 13.2. **Association of the Cranial Nerves 3 through 12 and the Nerves of the Thoracic and Cervical Origin Based On Direct Neurologic Associations and Tissue Over Which They Have Common Influence**

The functions of cranial nerves 3 to 12 are listed below. Their origins and actions on target tissue/organs (sensory and motor fields) are compared to the origins and course of sympathetic nerves associated with the cranial nerves 3 to 12 and the targets that they have in common.

OCULOMOTOR FUNCTION
Oculomotor nerve (Cranial Nerve 3)
Origin: Nuclei in the midbrain.
Action:
Somatic: motor control of eye movements/ position.
Autonomic: parasympathetic, motor—changes in the diameter of the pupil and lens via ciliary ganglia.
Sympathetic Nerve Plexus
Origin: Sympathetic centers of the upper thoracic spinal cord.
Course: Fibers travel to the ganglionated chain, superior cervical ganglion, internal carotid artery, cavernos plexus, the ciliary ganglia (cranial nerve 3), and the vascular supply of the extraocular muscles.

TROCHLEAR FUNCTION
Trochlear Nerve (Cranial Nerve 4)
Origin: Nuclei in the mid brain.
Action: Somatic: motor control of the eyes/position.
Sympathetic Nerve Plexus
Origin: Sympathetic centers of the upper thoracic spinal cord
Course: Fibers travel to the ganglionated chain, superior cervical ganglion, internal carotid artery, cavernos plexus, and then to cranial nerve 4.

TRIGEMINAL NERVE FUNCTION
Trigeminal Nerve (Cranial Nerve 5).
Origin: Arises from nuclei in the mid brain, pons, medulla, and cervical spine.
Action:
Somatic (sensory)—to the face (eyes, skin, membranes of oral sinus and nasal cavities, teeth, and meninges of middle fossa).
Somatic (motor)—mastication (muscles of jaw and upper pharynx).
Sympathetic Nerve Plexus
Origin: Sympathetic centers in the upper thoracic spinal cord
Course:
1). Fibers travel to ganglionated chain, superior cervical ganglion, internal carotid artery, internal carotid plexus, the trigeminal (sensory), ganglia.
2). Fibers travel to the ganglionated chain, superior cervical ganglion, internal carotid artery, cavernous plexus, the ophthalmic division of the trigeminal general distribution and nasociliary nerve to the iris and bulb of the eye. Branches of cranial nerve 5 communicate with and share function with the ganglia, nerves and glands innervated by cranial nerves 3, 4, 6, 7, and 9.

ABDUCENS FUNCTION
Abducens Nerve (Cranial Nerve 6).
Origin: Nuclei in the pons.
Action: Somatic—motor control of the eyes and eye position.
Sympathetic Nerve Plexus
Origin: Sympathetic centers in the upper thoracic spinal cord.
Course: Fibers travel to ganglionated chain, superior cervical ganglion, internal carotid artery, internal carotid plexus, and to cranial nerve 6.

FACIAL NERVE FUNCTION
Facial Nerve (Cranial Nerve 7)
Origin: Nuclei in the pons/medulla.
Action:
Somatic (sensory)—to external ear and meatus.
Somatic (special sensory)—taste to anterior 2/3 tongue.
Somatic (motor)—face, scalp and neck floor of mouth.
Autonomic (parasympathetic, secretomotor)—to the submandibular, sublingual, lacrimal, nasal glands and all mucous glands of the oral, nasal, auditory and sinus cavities.
Sympathetic Nerve Plexus
Origin: Sympathetic centers in the upper thoracic spinal cord.
Course:
1). Fibers travel to ganglionated chain to superior cervical ganglion to external carotid artery. It then has the following branches:
a). Middle meningeal artery and then the geniculate ganglia (sensory ganglia for taste, sense of the mouth, throat, nose and external ear/mastoid).
b). To facial and lingual arteries to innervate the sublingual and submandibular glands.
2). Internal carotid artery, internal carotid plexus and has the following branches:
a). To the maxillary artery and onto to sinus cavities.
b). To the deep petrosal nerve, pterygopalatine ganglia, and innervates lacrimal and nasal/oral mucous glands and vascular tissue.
c). To the tympanic plexus to innervate the middle ear.
Branches of cranial nerve 7 communicate with and share function with the ganglia, nerves and glands innervated by cranial nerves 5, 9, and 10 and cervical cutaneous nerve of the cervical plexus.

Table 13.2. *(continued)* **Association of the Cranial Nerves 3 through 12 and the Nerves of the Thoracic and Cervical Origin Based On Direct Neurologic Associations and Tissue Over Which They Have Common Influence**

GLOSSOPHARYNGEAL NERVE FUNCTION
Glossopharyngeal nerve (Cranial Nerve 9)
Origin: Nuclei in the medulla.
Action:
Somatic (general sensory)—sensation of middle ear, tongue and pharynx.
Somatic (special sensory)—taste posterior 1/3 tongue and throat
Autonomic (parasympathetic, secretomotor)—to pharynx and parotid gland, and middle ear.
Autonomic (general sensory)—to carotid body and sinus for cardiotensive/chemovascular sense.
Brachiomeric, motor—swallowing/phonation
Sympathetic Nerve Plexus
Origin: Sympathetic centers in the upper thoracic spinal cord.
Course:
1). Ganglionated chain, superior cervical ganglion, and inferior ganglia of cranial nerve 9.
2). Internal carotid plexus, and continues on with the following branches:
   a). To tympanic plexus for sensory to mucous membrane of mastoid, auditory tube, tympanic membrane, fenestra ovalis and rotunda.
   b). To pharyngeal plexus
   c). To carotid body and sinus and cranial nerve 9 (10)
3). External carotid, middle meningeal plexus and onto the parotid gland.
Branches of cranial nerve 9 communicate with and share functions with ganglia, nerves and/or glands innervated by cranial nerves 7 and 10 and shared plexi with cervical spinal nerves (26)

VAGAS NERVE FUNCTION
Vagus nerve (cranial nerve 10)
Origin: nuclei in the medulla.
Action:
Somatic (special sensory)—taste in the throat.
Somatic (general sensory)—meninges, posterior fossa, external ear, and auditory meatus.
Parasympathetic (general sensory)—to the glands and organs of the throat to the proximal large intestine. Cardiotensive and chemovascular sense.
Autonomic (parasympathetic, motor)—to glands and muscular walls of the organs of the throat, thorax, and most of the abdomen (the pharynx, larynx, bronchi, lungs, heart, esophagus, stomach, intestines, and kidney).
Brachimeric (motor)—muscles of the larynx, pharynx, and palate for swallowing/phonation.

Sympathetic Nerve Plexus
Origin: Sympathetic centers in the upper thoracic spinal cord
Course:
1). Fibers travel to ganglionated chain, superior cervical ganglion, superior, and on to the inferior ganglia of cranial nerve 10.
2). Ganglionated chain or sympathetic nerves, autonomic plexi associated with each organ innervated by the vagas nerve from the pharynx down to the proximal large intestine.
Branches of cranial nerve 10 communicate and share function with ganglia, nerves and/or glands innervated by cranial nerves 7, 9, 11, and 12, superior cervical sympathetic ganglia, sympathetic plexi of the pharynx, larynx, trachea heart, bronchi, lungs, abdominal viscera and first and second cervical spinal nerves.

ACCESSORY NERVE FUNCTION
Accessory nerve (cranial nerve 11)
Origin: Nuclei in the medulla.
Action: Somatic, motor-laryngeal and pharyngeal muscles and neck muscles.
Sympathetic Nerve Plexus
Origin: Sympathetic centers in thoracic spine
Course: Fibers travel to ganglionated chain and on to cervical spinal nerves.
Branches of cranial nerve 11 communicate or share function with ganglia of cranial nerve 10 and the first through fifth cervical spinal nerves.

HYPOGLOSSAL NERVE FUNCTION
Hypoglossal nerve (Cranial nerve 12)
Origin: Nuclei in the medulla.
Action:
Somatic (motor)—to the muscles of the tongue.
Somatic (sensory)—dura of posterior fossa of the cranium.
Sympathetic Nerve Plexus
Origin: Sympathetic centers in the upper thoracic spinal cord.
Course: Fibers travel to the gangliated chain, superior cervical ganglia and onto cranial nerve 12.
Branches of cranial nerve 12 communicate with or influence the sympathetic system (superior sympathetic cervical ganglion), parasympathetic system (inferior ganglion of vagas nerve), the pharyngeal and lingual plexus, and the first through third cervical spinal nerves.

Adapted from Goss AB (ed). Gray's Anatomy (29th ed). Philadelphia: W.B. Saunders Co., 1973.

which its fibers exit and traverse complex tissue systems within the neck before innervating the glands in the head. They are therefore exposed to somatic insult.

Further, general vasomotor regulation of the brain and head is influenced by sympathetic system tone. Though the sympathetic influence on cranial blood flow is not thought to have the extensive influence that it has on other tissues of the body (particularly striated and cardiac muscles), it does exist. Vascular ischemia, vascular headaches, and seizure disorders are attributed to vasoregulatory abnormalities.

PARASYMPATHETIC NERVOUS SYSTEM OUTFLOWS—GANGLIA, PLEXI, AND NERVES

The parasympathetic outflow has less anatomical complexity and extends to fewer tissues than does the sympathetic outflow.

In the head, parasympathetic innervation balances sympathetic innervation to control pupil size and lens accommodation via the third cranial nerve (oculomotor nerve). Lacrimation, salivation, and mucus secretions in the oral, nasal, and auditory cavities are controlled by the seventh cranial nerve (facial nerve). Salivation and swallowing are controlled by the ninth cranial nerve (glossopharyngeal nerve). (Note: swallowing is a complex, multi-step event and involves a coordinated sequence of opening and closing of the oral, nasal, auditory, and esophageal passages). Swallowing is controlled by cranial nerve 10 (vagus nerve) and esophageal plexus.

Parasympathetic visceral outflow to the body is largely via the paired tenth cranial (vagus) nerves. The vagus nerve is enclosed in the carotid sheath along with the internal jugular vein and internal carotid artery until it enters the thoracic cage. The name vagus, which is Latin for "the wanderer," aptly describes the long journey that it takes as it innervates the organs of the throat, thorax, and abdomen (32).

Two pairs of ganglia are associated with the vagus nerve—the superior or jugular and the inferior or nodose ganglia. The superior ganglion is located within the jugular foramen on the cranial floor. It receives afferent impulses from the dura of the posterior fossa and the external ear. The inferior or nodose ganglion is located immediately external to the jugular foramen lateral to the occipital condyles. It is adjacent to and communicates with the superior sympathetic cervical ganglion, branches of the facial nerve branches, ganglion of the glossopharyngeal nerve, accessory nerve, hypoglossal nerve, and C1 and C2 spinal nerves. Unlike the sympathetic ganglia which contain synapses, the vagal ganglia contain the cell bodies of afferent nerve fibers.

The cervical spine, particularly the upper cervical spine, contains several large parasympathetic and sympathetic ganglia, as well as extensive plexi of parasympathetic, sympathetic, and somatic origin. The influences of the ganglia and plexi extend into the head and organs of the abdomen.

The lower outflow of the parasympathetic nervous system originates in spinal cord nuclei from the S2 to S4 cord levels. It largely innervates organs of the pelvic cavity, the descending large intestine and rectum, bladder, ureter, and sex organs via the pelvic plexus.

PARASYMPATHETIC AND SYMPATHETIC AUTONOMIC PLEXI

Distinct sympathetic and parasympathetic central and peripheral pathways exist. As they travel to their target tissues, both the sympathetic (pre- and post-ganglionic) and parasympathetic (pre-ganglionic) nerves meet on the walls of vascular structures with an extensive intermingling of fibers. The great autonomic plexi created are more complex and extensive than are the brachial or lumbosacral plexi. In fact, these great autonomic plexi are considered an independent, third division of the autonomic system. The sympathetic and parasympathetic systems are the other two (32). Within these great autonomic plexi, extensive axo-axonal interactions occur and usually result in overall inhibition.

Functional Considerations of the Sympathetic Nervous System

The primary function of the nervous system is to control and coordinate all of the organs and structures within the body and relate the individual's body to the external environment (32). The autonomic nervous system is usually described as having a distinct functional identity within the nervous system which distinguishes it from the somatic portion of the nervous system in the following ways. The function of the somatic portion of the nervous system is to regulate the musculoskeletal system, particularly the striatal muscles that are under voluntary control. The somatic system specializes in the movement of the body or resistance to movement in the external environment which presumably allows the organism to gain an advantage by moving towards or remaining in (resisting movement) a more beneficial position in the environment, or by moving away from a hazardous one. The autonomic portion of the nervous system regulates all of the other functions of the body including the underlying tone and metabolism of the somatic system and the autonomic nerve system itself. Cannon describes the autonomic system as the system that senses the internal environment and initiates all internal adjustments in order to maintain homeostasis. He calls it the "interofective system" to distinguish it from what he calls the "exterofective system" or the somatic system which senses and responds to the external conditions (36). The autonomic nervous system has the following basic functions:

1. The support of somatic responses to environmental conditions, such as temperature changes, deprivation of water, gravitational pull, physical threat, and microbial/toxic challenges. The ANS responds by maintaining constant temperature, creating and releasing energy reserves, regulating cardiac and pulmonary functions, augmenting striatal muscle contractions, and regulating blood resources (34); and

2. The influence of internal organ function and coordination. Organ functions are controlled by the extent of the contraction or relaxation of the smooth muscles in organs, the secretion of the contents of both exocrine and endocrine glands, and the control of the

circulatory system (34). Organs and systems which receive autonomic influence include the digestive tract (glands, sphincters and tubes and the biliary tract—liver and gall bladder), kidney, spleen, cardiovasculopulmonary system, reproductive tracts, and the nervous system (Table 13.3).

Distinct functional characteristics of the autonomic nervous system are suggested by the divided anatomical pathways of the parasympathetic division with cranio-sacral origin and the sympathetic division with thoraco-lumbar origin. Functionally, activities of the ANS are classified as parasympathetically-dominant, sympathetically-dominant, or parasympathetically-sympathetically balanced.

The functional characteristics of sympathetic and parasympathetic activity arises from the organism's need to direct its finite resources in two opposing physiological processes. Energy and materials can be considered to be the "currency" of the body. They are generated, stored, and then expended appropriately in the healthy organism. If too much energy or materials are expended on external demands at the expense of internal needs, or vice versa, the organism's health is jeopardized.

The primary function of the parasympathetic nervous system is to optimize digestion/assimilation of materials and rest. Thus, it creates and preserves materials and energy. The primary function of the sympathetic system is to optimize somatic movements (or resistance to it) and expend materials and energy to augment skeletal muscle contractions.

Actions of the Parasympathetic and Sympathetic Divisions of the Autonomic Nervous System

Stimulation of the parasympathetic system:

1. Increases peristalsis.
2. Stimulates secretion of the glands associated with digestion and respiration.
3. Diminishes tone in the sphincters.

Secondary effects of parasympathetic stimulation include the following:

1. Diminishes cardiac output.
2. Lowers blood pressure.
3. Diminishes striatal muscle activity.

The secondary functions create generalized quiescence (including closure of the pupils) by antagonizing sympathetic stimulation, thus conserving resources for the primary activity of digestion and assimilation. Stimulation of the sympathetic system includes the following:

1. Dilates cardiac and skeletal muscle arterioles.
2. Increases efficiency of cardiac and skeletal muscle systems.

3. Dilates the bronchi.
4. Increases "alertness."

Secondary effects of sympathetic stimulation are as follows:

1. Diminishes blood flow to smooth muscles.
2. Closes sphincters.
3. Diminishes peristalsis.
4. Diminishes secretions of glands except the sweat glands and the thick mucous secretions of the nose and mouth.

When a major external hazard is present, the sympathetic activities may significantly inhibit, even halt, parasympathetic activity. The sympathetic system has extensive interconnections via the ganglion chains by nearly every part of the body. The gangliated chains control both the cardiopulmonary and musculoskeletal systems and antagonize parasympathetic stimulation (34). Sympathetic effects are amplified and supported by the systemic release of the powerful sympathetic neurotransmitter adrenaline (epinephrine) from the adrenal medulla which literally floods the body's sympathetic synapses with adrenaline. This release of adrenaline produces the classic "flight or fight" state (34) (Table 13.4).

Review of Parasympathetic and Sympathetic System Effects

Stimulation of parasympathetic activities increases resource creation and storage. Specifically, it stimulates gastrointestinal peristalsis and secretion and slows the heart rate, reduces blood pressure, and institutes rest or relaxation of the body (36).

Stimulation of sympathetic activities mobilizes stored energy and materials for immediate use. Specific effects include elevation of the cardiac output (the rate and force of contraction), constriction of arterioles in the skin and intestines, reserve arterioles, dilation of blood vessels to the striatal muscles (via increased blood volume and pressure to somatic tissue), and release of red blood corpuscles from the spleen (36).

Because the two systems have opposing effects on their target organs, most tissues have both sympathetic and parasympathetic innervation. The exceptions to this are the somatic tissues; namely, skin, bone, voluntary muscle, and most blood vessels. The sympathetic system has very direct influence over these tissues while the parasympathetic system has little, if any. The adrenal medulla receives only sympathetic innervation. It functions like an oversized post-synaptic sympathetic terminal (34).

Under normal conditions, energy use and creation are finely coordinated by the two systems. Coordination of these two systems in the periphery is extensive and occurs at two sites: 1) within mixed autonomic plexi and 2) at the neuro-effector junctional gap (16). The proximity of the sympathetic nervous system and parasympathetic nervous system in the great autonomic plexi allows side by side "contact modulation" as fibers pass en route to target terminations. Axoaxonal, dendrodendritic, axodendritic, and axosomatic exchanges

Table 13.3.   Sympathetic and Parasympathetic Innervation of Organs and Effects

Organ	Sympathetic			Parasympathetic		
	Preganglionic Neuron	Postganglionic Neuron	Action	Preganglionic Neuron	Postganglionic Neuron	Action
Eye	T1–T2	Superior cervical ganglion	Mydriasis; dilated pupil	Edinger–Westphal nucleus (oculomotor nucleus)	Ciliary ganglion	Miosis (contraction of ciliary muscle) (accommodation) Constriction of the pupil
Lacrimal, Sublingual, Submandibular glands	T1–T2	Superior cervical ganglion	Vasoconstriction; viscous secretion	Superior salivary nucleus	Pterygopalatine & Submandibular ganglion	Secretion of tears; secretion of watery saliva; vasodilatation
Mucous membranes of the head	T1–T2	Superior cervical ganglion	Vasoconstriction	Cranial nerve 7	Pterygopalatine ganglion	Vasodilatation
Parotid glands	T1–T2	Superior cervical ganglion	Vasoconstriction, secretion	Inferior salivary nucleus	Otic ganglion	Secretion of saliva
Thyroid gland	T1	Middle cervical ganglion	Increases secretion	Vagus nerve (cranial nerve 10)	Thyroid plexus	Decreases secretion
Heart	T1–T4 (T5)	Superior, middle, inferior cervical, & superior thoracic ganglia	Dilatation of bronchi; inhibition of secretion	Dorsal nucleus of vagus nerve	Cardiac plexus	Bradycardia; constriction of coronary arteries; decrease force of contraction
Bronchi/Lungs	T2–T7	Inferior cervical ganglion/superior thoracic ganglion	Dilatation of bronchi/inhibition of secretion	Dorsal nucleus of vagus nerve	Bronchial & pulmonal plexus	Serous & mucous secretion/constriction of bronchi
Stomach	T6–T10; superior splanchnic nerve	Celiac ganglion	Inhibition of peristalsis & secretion; contraction of sphincter	Dorsal nucleus of vagus nerve	Gastric plexus	Peristalsis; relaxation of sphincter; evacuation
Gall bladder	T4–T8		Relaxes muscle; constricts sphincter	Vagus nerve (cranial nerve 10)	Gall bladder plexus	Constricts muscle; relaxes sphincter

Organ	Spinal level	Sympathetic ganglia	Sympathetic effect	Parasympathetic source	Plexus	Parasympathetic effect
Small intestine & ascending colon	T6–T10	Celiac & superior mesenteric ganglia	Inhibition of peristalsis & secretion	Dorsal nucleus of vagus nerve	Myenteric plexus/Auerbach's plexus & submucosal plexus/Meissner's plexus	Secretion; peristalsis; evacuation
Spleen	T6–T8	Celiac ganglion	Contracts smooth muscle	Vagus nerve (cranial nerve 10)	Plexus of the spleen	Relaxes smooth muscle
Pancreas	T6–T10	Celiac ganglion	Decreased secretion	Dorsal nucleus of vagus nerve	Periarterial plexus	Secretion
Liver	T8–T10		Increases glycogen to glucose; increases protein metabolism; vasoconstriction	Vagus nerve (cranial nerve 10)	Hepatic plexus	Relaxes smooth muscle
Descending colon; rectum	L1–L2	Inferior mesenteric & hypogastric ganglia	Inhibition of peristalsis & secretion	S2–S4	Myenteric plexus/Auerbach's plexus; submucosal plexus/Meissner's plexus	Secretion; peristalsis; evacuation
Anal sphincter	L3	Celiac ganglion	Contracts	S3–S5	Anal plexus	Relaxes
Kidney	T10–L1		Vasoconstriction; inhibition	Vagus nerve (cranial nerve 10)	Renal plexus	
Urinary bladder	L1–L2	Celiac ganglion; renal & hypogastric plexus	Stimulation of internal sphincter muscle; relaxation of wall	S2–S4	Hypogastric plexus (vesical plexus)	Relaxation of internal sphincter muscle; contraction of detrusor muscle; vasodilatation
Prostate gland	T10–L1		Contracts muscle & spermatic vein	S2–S4	Prostate plexus	Increases secretion
Adrenal glands	T11–L1	Adrenal cells	Secretion (norepinephrine, epinephrine)	—	—	—
Male sex organs	L1–L2; pelvic splanchnic nerves	Superior & inferior hypogastric plexi (pelvic plexus)	Ejaculation; vasoconstriction	S2–S4	Hypogastric plexus (pelvic plexus)	Erection; vasodilatation; secretion
Fallopian tubes	T10–L1	Inferior mesenteric ganglion	Contracts muscle	—	—	—
Uterus	L1	Inferior mesenteric ganglion	Contracts body	S2–S4	Uterine plexus	Relaxes body; contracts cervix

Table 13.3. *(continued)* **Sympathetic and Parasympathetic Innervation of Organs and Effects**

Organ	Sympathetic			Parasympathetic		
	Preganglionic Neuron	Postganglionic Neuron	Action	Preganglionic Neuron	Postganglionic Neuron	Action
Skin of head & neck	T2–T4	Superior & middle cervical ganglia	Vasoconstriction; sweat secretion; piloerection	—	—	—
Arms	T3–T6	Inferior cervical & upper thoracic ganglia		—	—	—
Legs	T10–L2	Lower lumbar & upper sacral ganglia		—	—	—

Adapted from Duus P. Topical Diagnosis in Neurology (2nd ed). New York: Thieme Medical Publishers. pp. 214–215.

Table 13.4.   Sympathetic Responses to External "Fight or Flight" Threat

Pale skin	Vasoconstriction of skin
Wet skin	Secretion of sweat glands
Raised hair	Constriction of piloerector muscles
Dilated pupils, mydriasis	Dilatation of pupillae muscles
Raised upper eyelid	Constriction of tarsal muscle
Redistribution of blood from the skin and viscera to the brain, heart muscle, and skeletal muscles	Vasodilatation of skeletal muscle vessels
Increased heart rate	Activation of heart muscle
Increased blood pressure	Increase in peripheral resistance of arterioles
Dilated bronchi	Dilatation of bronchial smooth muscles
Diminished intestinal activity and closed sphincters	Constriction of intestinal smooth muscles and glands
Raised blood sugar level	Adrenal medulla release of adrenalin, acting on the liver
	Glucogen conversion into glucose
Dry mouth	Constriction of salivary glands

Adapted from: Duus P. Topical Diagnosis in Neurology (2nd ed). New York: Thieme Medical Publishers 1989.

occur. The overriding effect is mutual inhibition which allows refinement of nerve impulse traffic (16).

The terminal neuroeffector junctional gaps at organ sites accumulate the nervotransmitters that both the sympathetic and parasympathetic fibers release. The organ activity that results is based upon the respective concentrations of the ANS branches in these terminal clefts.

Synapses of the Autonomic Nervous System

The autonomic neuroeffector terminal cleft differs from those of the somatic myoneural terminal cleft. The autonomic terminal gap is considered to be the simplest class of synapse (35). They are up to ten times wider than a somatic cleft. They are non-directional and are distributed over long, branching chains which cover a wide area of effector tissue. Neurotransmitter substances are therefore released over a large area of the terminal or organ tissue (35). For example, stimulation of a sympathetic nerve would affect a lengthy terminal to influence numerous branchings of a blood vessel which is comprised of many smooth muscle cells (35). The somatic counterpart typically stimulates a short and narrow cleft which influences a number of individual muscle cells.

Neurotransmitters of the Autonomic Nervous System

A limited number of neurotransmitters are associated with the ANS. Epinephrine (or adrenaline), norepinephrine (or noradrenaline), and acetylcholine are, by far, the predominant ones. Cholinergic transmitters (acetylcholine) are found throughout the nervous system—in the parasympathetic, sympathetic, and somatic nerve system. But in the ANS, cholinergic substances are called parasympathetic mediators. The adrenergic transmitters, epinephrine and norepinephrine, influence only the sympathetic postganglionic terminal gaps. Adrenergic substances cause sympathetic effects on the tissues and are called sympathetic mediators.

Some postganglionic sympathetic nerves secrete cholinergic transmitters at their neuroeffector junction and can be said to have a cholinergic or parasympathetic effect. The vasodilatation of the blood vessels that supply somatic muscles, the skin, external genitalia, and sweat glands is considered a cholinergic effect. In this response, cholinergic effects support sympathetic functions by increasing the vascular supply to the muscles and helping to cool the body (39).

The two types of adrenergic transmitters have two types of effects: 1) Norepinephrine or noradrenaline increases blood pressure by increasing vascular peripheral resistance; and 2). Epinephrine or adrenaline increases blood pressure by increasing cardiac output and also increases metabolism. The adrenal gland secretes both types (34), but about 80% of its secretions are epinephrine and 20% norepinephrine. Sympathetic nerve terminals release only norepinephrine (not epinephrine). In the CNS, norepinephrine is produced primarily in the locus ceruleus which is located in the pons region of the brain (40) (Table 13.5).

The adrenergic effects of epinephrine and norepinephrine are dependent on the type of adrenergic receptors present in the tissues. Alpha (a) and beta (b) tissue receptors are stimulated by neurotransmitters in different ways and cause different tissue activities. In general, stimulation of alpha (a) receptors supports a mild facilitation which is associated with mental alertness, and heightened sensory acuity. Beta (b) receptors generally support intense muscular actions.

The number of neurotransmitters is small compared to the number of neuromodulator substances. Researchers are continually finding more substances which are observed to modulate the effect that neurotransmitters have in the neuro-effector gap, greatly enhancing or even ultimately cancelling in its entirety, all of the post-cleft visceral effects.

Factors in Abnormal Reflex/ Referral Cord Processing

Under normal conditions, afferent stimulation from tissue receptors is transmitted to appropriate visceral and somatic efferent nerves integrating the responses of both the visceral and somatic tissues. An absence of interrelating reflexes to soma and viscera represents a significant breakdown in organization. When the spinal cord functions abnormally, abnormal relationships occur between soma and viscera. For example, when a primary lower back dysfunction produces back pain and leg pain, additional inappropriate somatovisceral reflexes, such as local trophic skin changes, and even constipation, may be present. These abnormal reflexes with their additional pathophysiological manifestations do not improve the primary spinal disorder, and in fact, only make the original neuromusculoskeletal problem more complex.

Spinal cord processing errors cause abnormal referral/reflex relationships. Some authors have noted that the central nervous system will misread, misrepresent, mis-register, mis-map, imagine, or imperfectly localize a stimuli (41). It has been called garbled and generalized (42,43) or obscure (44). The resulting reflexes often suggest those of a more primitive or embryological nervous system, i.e., that of a less complex organism (41,44).

Tissues of similar embryological origin often maintain functionally distinct relationships in the mature human being

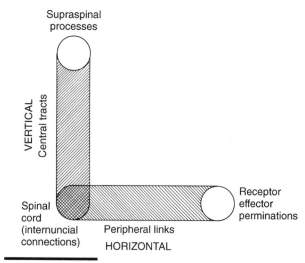

Figure 13.8. Safety pin cycle—horizontal and vertical neuronal loops.

(Fig. 13.8). The spinal cord, by extensive central inhibition, is the site of reflex refinement. Loss of specific and developed patterns of inhibition result in vestigial somatotomal and viscerotomal reflexes. It is important to understand spinal cord processing in the autonomic nervous system.

Dysfunction of the spinal cord will establish a particular segmental reflex based upon the following generalized schema:

1. Horizontal or peripheral pathway connections: this includes all input from the peripheral sensory receptors (both autonomic and somatic) and adjacent horizontal spinal cord internuncial connections.

2. Vertical or central tract connections: this includes input from descending tracts originating in the brain and internuncial connections from adjacent vertical levels of the spinal cord.

A given segmental level of the spinal cord is an intermediary link between the vertical and horizontal connections. The amount of pre-processed or unmodulated afferent peripheral input to the spinal cord is enormous. The spinal cord limits conversion of sensory (peripheral horizontal) and descending (vertical) impulses to a select number of efferent nerve impulses. Specifically, the spinal cord is a site of generalized inhibition, except in a relatively few well-established internuncial circuits.

Extensive inhibition must take place because internuncial neurons in the spinal cord are characteristically short, multisynaptic (46), highly excitable, and fire spontaneously up to 1500 times per second (34). They are 30 times more numerous than efferent neurons.

Table 13.5. **Adrenergic Receptors and Their Functions**

Alpha (a) Receptor	Beta (b) Receptor
Vasoconstriction	Vasodilatation (b2)
Iris dilatation	Cardioacceleration (b1)
Intestinal relaxation	Increased myocardial strength (b1)
Intestinal sphincter contraction	Myometrial relaxation (b2)
Pilomotor contraction	Intestinal relaxation (b2)
Bladder sphincter contraction	Uterus relaxation (b2)
	Bronchodilatation (b2)
	Calorigenesis (b2)
	Muscle glycogenolysis (b2)
	Lipolysis (b1)
	Bladder wall relaxation (b2)

Adapted from Guyton AC. Textbook of Medical Physiology, 8th ed. Philadelphia PA: W.B. Saunders Co. 1991. p. 671.

Impulse inhibition begins before the first synapse through presynaptic inhibition. There is further impulse inhibition in the posterior and middle portions of the spinal cord, and to a lesser extent, in the anterior horn. Impulses follow the "routes of least resistance" (45) or through circuits in which the least inhibition exists for either a peripheral motor response (horizontal) and/or a second-order central sensory transmission (vertical). Inhibition may completely halt impulse transmissions.

The concept of neurological "gates" has been developed by Melzack and Wall (16,47). When the gates are closed, vertical (ascending) passage of afferent impulses is inhibited. When the gates are "open," there is little resistance to impulse passage. While Melzack's "gates" in the substantia gelatinosa of the spinal cord's gray matter are thought to inhibit c-fiber transmission, there are probably similar gating effects which balance transmission of neural impulses in other CNS locations.

Patterns of Impulse Transmission Within the Spinal Cord—Reflexes and Referrals

The spinal cord, acting as an intermediary link, establishes internuncial routes of transmission (reflexes and referrals). These routes are based upon: 1) the properties inherent to spinal cord neurons and their specialized cell functions; and 2) the quantity and types of converging afferent nerve stimulation from the present and the past (16,34).

Inherent Properties of Spinal Cord Neurons

a. Habituation/fatigue: the nerve transmissions following a prior nerve transmission are reduced (47).
b. Sensitization: the nerve transmissions following a prior nerve transmissions are increased (47).
c. Facilitation by summation: the multiple sub-threshold impulses from neurologically related sources converge and reach threshold (34).
d. Divergent amplification: (34) the increased stimulation caused by an increased axon to dendrite ratio.
e. Synaptic after-discharge: reverberating circuits (34).
f. Cross-modal sensory translation: stimulation of a sensory path crosses to another sensory path, as in allodynia (light pressure or mild temperature changes on the skin are experienced as excruciatingly painful) (47).

The inherent properties of nerve fibers listed above are necessary for spinal cord processing. They do not operate equally in all types of nerve tissues. Habituation tends to be associated with large fiber afferent excitation (mechanoreception), whereas sensitization is a characteristic of small fiber afferent excitation (nociception and visceroreception). Consequently, large fiber excitation (mechanoreception) tends to depress subsequent transmissions while small fiber excitation (pain) tends to perpetuate subsequent transmissions. Both habituation and sensitization may last for minutes, days, or even weeks (47). These inherent properties play a role in spinal learning and spinal memory (detailed explanation appears in section on spinal learning).

Convergent Afferent Nerve Stimulation from the Present and Past

Converging stimulation will affect how transmission patterns develop in the spinal cord based on the fiber types present, the frequency of the impulse, the location of the fiber's terminal branchings in the spinal cord, and the prior levels of excitation.

Afferent stimulation of a body's receptive sensory field converges on a corresponding excitatory internuncial or terminal field in the spinal cord (34). Branches of functionally and/or topically related nerve endings converge and terminate in designated spinal cord fields. Changes in the excitatory terminal fields will alter spinal cord processes and change subsequent reflexes/referral transmissions.

The changes in excitatory fields are a result of two factors:

1. The quantity of internuncial stimulation (facilitation or inhibition) in a given stimulatory field—i.e., the amount of presynaptic neurotransmitter/neuromodulator within multi-neuronal synapse pools. These increase or decrease the threshold needed for subsequent transmission. When facilitated, the CNS can be stimulated in a way that is entirely out of proportion to the stimulus causing it (46). This leads to repetitive hyperactivity of efferent neurons, including the autonomic outflow (46,48).

2. The three-dimensional spatial area of the stimulatory field (36,34) changes in size both horizontally and vertically (46). Spatial expansion of a stimulatory field follows a nerve action potential because additional or stronger stimuli will not cause further excitation of that neuron, but it will excite other neurons and thus expand the field of excitation (45). A subsequent signal passing through a facilitated neuronal pool could diverge so widely that the source within the receptive field may be completely obscured at its terminus in the excitatory field (34). This causes the reflex action and referrals to be expressed more widely (45).

Types and Effects of Convergent Horizontal and Vertical Input on Spinal Cord Processes

Horizontal Input—Afferent Stimulation from the Periphery

The type and quantity of nerve stimulation reaching the spinal cord establishes not only *what* the spinal cord processes but *how* it will process that input. Korr wrote that there is a "proper" ratio of large to small fiber afferent excitation that is needed for appropriate spinal cord processing to create a "balance" of neural activity. He states that excessive pain stimuli (stimuli carried on small fibers) causes a "jamming" of spinal cord processes. Further, abnormal spinal cord reflexes will "freeze" in place and produce an altered communication in the CNS (49).

Table 13.6. **Classifications of Peripheral Nerve Fibers using ABC and Type Systems**

ABC	Type	Diameter (mm)	Source/Function
Aa	I a & b	12–22	Motor to skeletal muscles, muscle spindles (annulospiral) & Golgi tendon organs
Ab	II	5–13	Meissner's, Paccinian & Ruffini corpuscles
Ac	II	3–8	Muscle spindles fusimotor, large hair receptors
Ad	III	1–5	Pain, temperature
B		1–3	Preganglionic autonomic sympathetic receptors
C (unmyelinated)	IV	0.3–1.5	Postganglionic sympathetic pain, temperature

Adapted from Barr M, Kiernan J. The Human Nervous System (5th ed). Philadelphia: J.P. Lippincott Co. 1988.

The large fiber group contains the A alpha (Aa), beta (Ab), and gamma (Ag) (also called types Ia, Ib, and II) (Table 13.6). They are 22.0 to 5.0 (mm) micrometers in size, myelinated, have a high threshold, are fast conducting and fast adapting. They are found in the somatic nerve system. The sensory fibers are exteroceptive and proprioceptive. The motor fibers are the efferent nerves to striate muscles.

The small fiber classification includes A delta (Ad), B and C, or types III and IV. They are 0.3 to 5.0 micrometers in size and are thinly myelinated or unmyelinated, have a low threshold, are slow conducting, and are slow adapting. They are found in the somatic (protopathic) and visceral systems. They tend to be interoceptive and affect vegetative functions. The small fibers are typically less specialized, poly-synaptic, poly-modal fibers with a wide dynamic range. They may respond to mechanical, chemical, or thermal stimulation (46). The difference between the small somatic and autonomic nerve fibers are their different terminations and not their cytoanatomy (41). Most small fiber excitations, particularly those in the ANS, are sub-cortically processed and not consciously perceived (46). When consciously perceived, stimulation of a ANS nerve fiber is perceived as crude, diffuse sensations of temperature, pressure, and chemical irritation. As stimulation increases, the modalities produce protopathic pain, often with a sensation of alarm and/or overall un-pleasantness.

Because small fibers are characteristically poly-modal, less specialized, and have a wide dynamic range, they are particularly suited to transposed or cross sensory stimulation. When small neurons are hyperpathic or neuropathic, they can register light touch or mild temperature changes as severe pain. They have a lowered "cross modality threshold (70)." Damaged nerves have been seen to readily communicate with adjacent nerves (particularly unmyelinated neurons) both for axonal support and as an outlet for transmission (ephapsis and cross-talk). See earlier discussion on inherent properties.

Expansion and Facilitation of Spinal Cord Internuncial Fields by the Imbalance of Large-to-Small Fiber Stimulation Ratios

Excited receptor fields expand and/or facilitate spinal cord internuncial excitability and referral/reflex relationships.

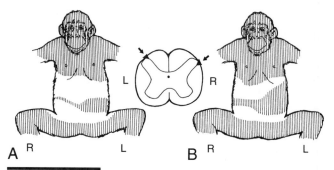

Figure 13.9. LI Dermatomes of the monkey. A, A medical section of the left Lissauer's tract results in near total contraction of the left LI dermatome. B, Lateral section (right Lissauer's tract) results in an almost two-fold expansion of the LI right dermatome. Modified from Fitzgerald MJT. Neuroanatomy: Basic and Applied. Philadelphia: Balliere Tindal, 1985, p. 108.

Maximum excitability is seen when small fiber input (pain, temperature, automonic) increases while simultaneously the large fiber input (proprioception) decreases (50).

One understanding of the influence that small and large fiber stimulation has on the spinal cord has been developed in pain transmission studies. Large fiber stimulation (proprioceptive) shuts the pain "gates" pre-synaptically and synaptically in the substantia gelatinosa and inhibits subsequent pain transmission (46,47).

When large fiber input (touch). is suppressed by restricting the peripheral stimulation of touch, a remarkable build-up of C-fiber neuron activity results in that field. If C-fibers are subsequently stimulated, a prolonged after-discharge and facilitation results (47). Further, when type A (large) fibers of a single nerve root were inactivated, the dermatomal pain receptive field for that nerve root nearly doubles in size (16). When expression of large fiber stimulation increases, small fiber facilitation and the size of the excitatory field in the spinal cord decreases (Fig. 13.9).

Studies of spinal cord excitatory fields show that they can be expanded by deep tissue C-fiber excitation (51). In one study, increasing C-fiber excitation to a limited region of the semitendinosus muscle lowered the threshold of response to a subsequent innocuous pressure within that field. It also expanded the receptor field such that a lowered threshold was found not only in the stimulated region but also anywhere in the entire muscle and its functional partner, the gastrocnemius-soleus muscle (51).

Functionally, nociception causes a general excitement in both the dorsal and intermediolateral horn of the spinal cord. There is a simultaneous and associated increase in somatic effects (isotonic muscle hypertonicity and vasodilation) and visceral effects (vasoconstriction). Proprioception, however, inhibits non–specific dorsal and intermediolateral horn inter-nuncial excitation, reduces pain, releases vasoconstriction of muscles, and promotes lateral inhibition of muscle activity which restores discrete movements (46).

Currently, gating better explains the phenomenon of inhibition than it does the mechanism of inhibition. It accounts for why stimulating the skin (rubbing) often reduces the sense of a deeper connective tissue irritation; why rocking in a chair temporarily reduces pain by reducing the suppressed propriocep-tive stimulation resulting from muscle contractures; and possibly, the beneficial effects of various electrical stimulators.

Well-applied, non-traumatic chiropractic adjustments may restore suppressed mechanoreceptor activity (due to hypomo-bility) and increase proprioception—large fiber stimulation without increasing pain (small fiber) stimulation (50,52). Conservative management of RSD, even non-chiropractic treatments, such as graduated exercise, movement, and restoration of function, increase proprioceptive stimulation. Sedentary behaviors, e.g., bed rest, suppress proprioception which promotes further small fiber excitation, nociception, and sympathetic hyperactivity. The diminished overall pain is realized from a more complete proprioceptive stimulation even though there may be an initial transient increase of pain.

Regardless of its source, large fiber stimulation has a normalizing effect on spinal cord pain and efferent sympathetic transmission by restoring a balance of large to small afferent fiber stimulation within spinal cord stimulatory fields.

Spinal Learning—Local Spinal Cord Reflexes That Are Changed by C-Fiber Excitation

"Unconditioned stimuli" cause "inborn" responses such as the autonomic withdrawal reflex from a painful (nociceptive) stimulus (flexor response). A "conditioned stimulus" is learned when a neutral or slightly innocuous stimulus is paired with an unconditioned response. A study was made in which a spinal-ized cat received a low intensity electrical stimulus which produced a marked response if a previous low intensity stimulus was paired with a high intensity stimulus (51). Unconditioned stimulus must be of sufficient intensity or duration, or both, to establish the new reflex or "learned response" within the inter-nuncial pathways. Learning is maximal when C-fibers are excited to create the new conditioned stimulus (51). Learning does not occur if C-fibers are blocked (51).

Spinal cord reflexes that are conditioned by the C-fiber excitation of an injured tissue establish not only a vigorous response to any subsequent minor afferent input (51), but the reflex pattern persists without spontaneously decaying even

after the C-fiber excitation (healing) ceases. The residual new interneuronal pathways were probably localized to one or two spinal cord levels (51).

Presumed Effects of Stimulating Large and Small Fibers under Different Conditions

For simplicity, small fiber stimulation will be called "pain" and large fiber stimulation "proprioception." Balanced afferation will be called "2/2" (Table 13.7).

Sources of Large and Small Fiber Afferent Impulses

While dermatomes are perhaps the best understood of the different types of receptor fields, all tissues of the body reside within a neurological receptor field. Receptive fields are topical regions of the body that are innervated by a common afferent nerve or nerve bundle and have a corresponding excitatory field of representation in the spinal cord. Tissue fields, a source of small and large afferent fiber stimulation, can be divided into those that are local and those peripheral to the spinal axis (41). The local tissues have a direct role in the physiology of the vertebral column. Those that are the peripheral tissues do not.

1. The tissues in the receptor fields of small afferent fibers
   a. Somatic tissues. Joints, muscles, bones, fascia, and skin. When conscious, there are sensations of pain, cold, heat, pressure, and itch.
   b. Autonomic tissues.
      (1) Viscera and organs, namely, the splanchnic, vascular, cardiopulmonary, and nerve tissues.
      (2) Innervation of somatic tissues are by an autonomic afferent nerve supply which may be either distinct from or in parallel system with or integrated with the somatic supply.

LOCAL TISSUE RECEPTOR FIELDS (VERTEBRAL COLUMN)

1. Local somatic tissue receptor fields include the spinal muscles, bones, joints, ligaments, intervertebral discs, fascia, and skin.
2. Local autonomic tissue receptor fields include spinal vascular and neural tissues—chain ganglia, cords, splanchnic nerves, vagus and hypoglossal nerves, and nerve filaments (autonomic plexi). The autonomic receptor fields of local somatic tissues are also included and represent the spinal muscles, bones, joints, ligaments, intervertebral discs, fascia, and skin.

PERIPHERAL TISSUE RECEPTOR FIELDS

1. Peripheral somatic tissue receptor fields include muscles, bones, joints, ligaments, fascia, and skin peripheral to the spine.
2. Peripheral autonomic tissue receptor fields include viscera, sheaths, skin, blood vessels, and the nerves and their ganglia and plexi which are not directly associated with the spine.

Table 13.7.   Presumed Effects of Stimulating Large and Small Fibers Under Different Conditions

Normal ratio of pain: proprioceptive is 2:2 or	If pain increases to:	And proprioception . . .	Then . . .	Because small to large fiber ratio is . . .
1	3	increases to 3	OK	maintained at 3:3 1
1	3	remains 2	increased pain is felt	increases to 1.5
1	3	decreases to 1	greatly increased pain is felt	increased to 2
Normal ratio of pain:proprioception is 2:2 or	If proprioception decreases . . .	And pain . . .	Then . . .	Because, small to larger fiber ratio is . . .
1	1	decreased to 1	OK	increased to 1:1, or 1
1	1	remains the same 2	increased pain is felt	increased to 2:1, or 2
1	1	increased to 3	greatly increased pain is felt	maintained at 3:1 3

For simplicity, small fiber stimulation is called "pain," and large fiber stimulation is called proprioception. The normal balance between afferent impulses will be considered to be 2/2.
Adapted from Wyke BD. Articular Neurology and Manipulative Therapy. In: Glasgow EF, et al. Aspects of Manipulative Therapy (2nd ed). New York: Churchill Livingstone 1985. pp. 72–80.

TISSUE RECEPTOR FIELDS OF LARGE AFFERENT FIBERS

Large afferent nerves supply only somatic tissue fields. Peripheral and local tissue receptor fields include the muscles, joints, ligaments, fascia, and skin. Local tissue receptor fields include the anulus of the intervertebral disc, spinal muscles, joints, ligaments, fascia and skin.

DISTURBED SMALL TO LARGE FIBER AFFERENT SUPPLY RATIO FROM THE LOCAL TISSUE RECEPTOR FIELDS

Both the peripheral and local afferent fiber stimulation influences spinal cord processing. Of special interest to chiropractors is the effect of altered afferent input from local or spinal receptor fields on spinal cord processing. This will be described below.

SMALL FIBER IRRITATION FROM THE SPINAL COLUMN

Most somatic and autonomic spinal tissues are richly innervated by small fiber nerves. Somatic irritations (pain) have been extensively studied (50) while autonomic irritations have received little attention.

All nerve fiber transmissions are initiated in one or both of two ways—by their receptors or by nonreceptor depolarizations. Receptor-initiated impulses result from excitation at the tissue receptor junction and produce a "true representation" of the receptor field at the spinal cord. Non-receptor-initiated impulses are a result of an ectopic depolarization somewhere along the course of the nerve fiber and consequently register a "false representation" of the receptor field at the spinal cord. In other words, depolarization of the afferent fiber can be initiated at the tissue giving a true representation of that tissue or be caused by neuropathophysiological changes resulting from a disturbance of the fiber's membrane giving a false representation of the innervated tissue. Either way, the spinal cord may register an identical stimuli.

The spinal column, in particular, is a site of both non-receptor and receptor-based impulse production. Depolarizations at the non-receptor (membrane) sites are not uncommonly caused by three types of aberrant sources—pathobiomechanical, pathobiochemical, or pathobioelectrical irritations.

Pathobiomechanical irritations are due to compression, traction or torsion of nerve tissues, including autonomic nerves, at the anterior or lateral disc margins, or posterior joint and spinal canal. There may be irritation at the anterior and lateral intervertebral disc due to protrusions of the disc and/or osteophytes (29,37,43). Nathan found direct compression on paraspinal sympathetic cords, splanchnic nerves and ganglia in 65% of the 1000 adult cadavers studied which were caused by disc protrusions and osteophytes. Giles found similar direct distortion of sympathetic tissues as well (Fig. 13.10).

There may be irritation of the posterior joint from capsule swelling and laxity/hypertrophy of posterior spinal canal ligaments. These affect the dorsal root or the tract of Lissauer (entry point of most small nerve fibers to the spinal cord). The dorsal root ganglia are very sensitive to mechanical pressure (53). Somatic and autonomic nerve fiber cell bodies within the ganglia (35) are located in the lateral canal. Not only is this a common site for mechanical irritations but the ganglia is the most common site of ephapsis or cross-communications between fibers. Robuck reports that vertebral lesions have a more serious effect on the sympathetic chain ganglia than they have on the dorsal root ganglia (54).

Mechanical traction on a nerve produces intraneural venous stasis when it is stretched more than 8% of its original length. Complete intraneural circulatory stasis occurs when the nerve is tractioned an additional 15% of its original length (55). Stasis produces hyperexcitability and spontaneous discharge.

Biochemical irritations are due to a pooling of neurokinins (56), congestive ischemia (edema), vascular disturbances, and lymph stasis (43). Fibrosis with or without inflammation is a common sequel of longstanding biochemical irritations.

In addition to mechanical pressures, Giles found that autonomic reflex dysfunction results from abnormal microvascular circulation in neural structures. A secondary disturbance results from a disruption of axoplasmic transport and the manufacture of important neurotransmitters, precursors, and enzymes (29).

Korr found that damage from vertebral trauma or herniated discs was less disruptive to local ANS tissues than long term subtle pressures produced by circulatory changes (edema, congestion, compression, angulation, ischemia) associated with spinal pathomechanics (42). Characteristically, the osteophytes and disc damage causing biomechanical irritation are the terminal stages of long established spinal pathomechanics. Early spinal pathomechanics are accompanied by subclinical pathochemical and ischemic conditions which may exist for many years before the characteristic signs of spinal degeneration become evident.

Pooled vasoactive substances and neurokinins increase permeability of the capillary walls. Increased permeability results in vascular congestion and intraneural ischemia, disruption of the intraneural microvessels with local demyelination, enhanced axonotmesis, (57) and replacement of neural tissue by infiltration of connective tissue with fibrotic tissue (58). Fibrosis has been found in sympathetic ganglia (37). These conditions lead selectively to hyperexcitability and spontaneous discharge in small fiber, nociceptive, afferent neurons (55,59).

Korr found biochemical changes were also produced by sustained local muscle activity which was more significant than those produced by biomechanical pressures. He found that spontaneous nerve activity was produced in sympathetic nerve trunks (42). Vasospasm, secondary to sympathetic irritations

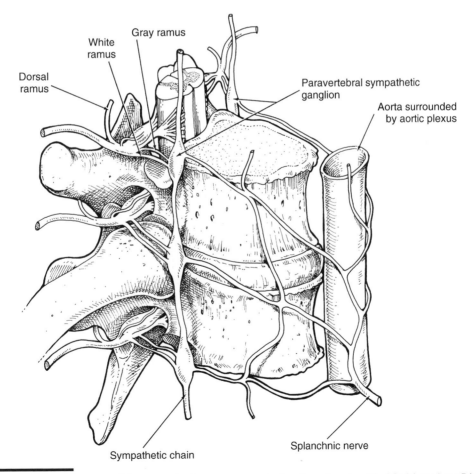

Figure 13.10.   Elements of the sympathetic nerve system in the thoracic spine. Modified from Low PA. *Clinical Autonomic Disorders.* Boston: Little, Brown & Co., 1993.

led to further ischemia and chemical imbalances in the vascular nerve plexi (58). Blumberg found that in these conditions, afferent sympathetic fibers develop "abnormal chemosensitivities" to noradrenalin (59) disrupting the autoregulatory correction of sympathetic excitation.

Sympathetic nerve fibers are usually repaired by denervation supersensitivity which can occur anywhere in the ANS system—in smooth muscles, glands, autonomic ganglia, spinal and cortical neurons (60). Supersensitivity in any autonomic pathway increases blood vessel tone in virtually any tissue in the body and may lead to further structural disintegration of that tissue and even more stimuli (44).

ISCHEMIA

Ischemia has a selective effect on the different nerve fiber types. Ischemia diminishes excitatory properties of the larger neurons before that of the smaller neurons. In other words, ischemia has a selective excitatory effect on small nerve fibers and has a lesser or delayed effect on the larger A delta (Ad) mechanoreceptor nerve fibers (44). The combined effect is particularly disruptive to the balance of the small/ large fiber ratio in the spinal cord, expanding and facilitating the somatic/sympathetic excitatory terminal fields. This leads to abnormal reflex and referral patterns.

Though not a reflex, irritation of the vertebral column will directly stimulate the efferent arm of autonomic nerve pathways—including splanchnic and paravertebral ganglia (37). Either through direct efferent excitation or afferent reflexive excitation, automonic nerve function is affected by local pathobiomechanical and pathobiochemical spinal damage. Jinkins writes that distant autonomic referred effects from pathophysiological conditions of the spinal envelope (its local adjacent tissue) encompass such viscerosomatic reactions as blood pressure changes, changes in heart rate, respiratory rate and elevations in alertness and nausea. These effects do not reflect in direct proportion to the severity and extent of spinal irritations (41).

Local effects (clinical signs) of hypersympathecotonia include the classic autonomic changes of tissue swelling, trophoedema (diaphoresis), sudomotor (dry or sweating) activated pilomotor activity (goose flesh) vasomotor instability (red reflex/blanching, temperature changes), and muscle facilitation. These are physical findings that chiropractors often use for determining the location of the vertebral subluxation complex. They pre-exist spondylosis detectibility or x-ray findings. Any chronic, nutritional, and neurotrophic inadequacies of the spinal column and its enveloping tissues produce progressive, cyclic, pathophysiological failures, both locally (spinal deterioration) and peripherally (organ disregulation) as a reflex of the disturbed autonomic disregulation.

Large Fiber Irritations from the Spinal Column

Large fibers are intrinsic within the musculoskeletal system and dermis overlying the vertebral column. The effects of large fiber stimulation have been developed with the concept of gating mechanisms. Lowered basal levels of large afferent fiber transmission is often due to segmental spinal fixation (suppressed mobility). This promotes the size and excitability of the associated small fiber terminal field in the spinal cord. Decreased large fiber stimulation creates a hyperresponsiveness to afferent sympathetic stimulation and somatic and sympathetic sensitization of muscle spindle apparatus. Increased striatal muscle tone further increases contracture which decreases mobility further. This results in degradation of the biochemical vascular environment, as previously noted. The neuropathophysiology of ischemia results in expansion and fixing of the facilitory fields which alters spinal cord reflex and referral transmissions (42,43)

Unconscious Small Fiber Autonomic Afferent Input—Silent Pain?

Research tends to be driven by the possibility that new findings will be applied to the clinical understanding and control of symptoms. However, 90% of all somatic and autonomic sensory input is unconscious (26) or silent. Autonomic afferent impulses rarely register a sensation but yield extensive autonomic physiological changes.

Peripheral "Silent" Pain

Interoceptive sensory stimuli are rich subcortically (below the conscious level). Rosen et al used dynamic positron-emission tomography (PET) to monitor cerebral blood flow in patients following the induction of an angina attack with intravenous dobutamine. Afferent ANS impulses from the induced attacks presumably transmit along sympathetic pathways and through vagal fibers to the posterior hypothalamus. All of the induced angina attacks resulted in chest pain with variable left arm pain (referred) and decreased blood flow in the brain in a pattern typically seen during cardiac ischemia.

High levels of thalamic activity continued for hours after cardiac ischemia, pain, and cortical (conscious) patterns ceased. Myocardial tissue distress produced afferent autonomic transmission for a much longer period of time than the time period in which the patient reported symptoms, both before and after the symptomatic period. This study verifies the observation that pain is an inconsistent and variable feature of severe cardiac crises. Rosen suggests that high levels of subcortical, visceral afferent impulses are present in other nonsymptomatic "silent" visceral diseases. Viscera produce ANS afferent impulses which can be described as a form of silent visceral pain (61).

Local "Silent Pain"

Local ANS irritations cause unconscious afferent stimulation of ANS pathways and the spinal cord. The stimulation may remain unconscious or present as variable and inconsistent symptoms often out of proportion to the severity and extent of the spinal irritations (41,44,46). A major role of the paravertebral sympathetic plexus is to mediate unconsciously local autonomic function within the segmental autonomic reflex arcs of the spinal cord. Local segmental autonomic reflexes within the paravertebral envelope may "spatially misregister" the conscious perception of pain, as is seen by nondermatomal referrals into the Zones of Head. Unconscious, excessive, local autonomic function can be misregistered but have functional visceral consequences (62). Locally, prespondylosis (44) and peripherally, latent trigger points (46) are common, silent, physiological manifestations of ANS disorders.

Vertical Link—The Nature of Supraspinal Influences on Local Spinal Reflexes

The horizontal spinal cord reflexes are, in turn, heavily influenced by higher CNS levels (41). The integrity of signal transmission (61) is maintained by supraspinal centrifugal nerve fiber stimulation, primarily as an "inhibitory blanket" to intermediary spinal cord internuncial pools. Inhibition is consistently provided by higher centers at every cord level (45).

An autonomic dysreflexia of the spine is defined as an excitatory disorder of local autonomic homeostasis caused by the failure of supraspinal inhibition to traverse a spinal cord lesion, and therefore, fail to restore an autonomic equilibrium (63). A disruption of descending ANS spinal tracts can allow sympathetic hyperreflexias within local sympathetic arcs. This may be what contributes to the "roar" of small fiber afferents which "garble" the communication within the neuronal spinal cord processes as Korr had researched (42,43).

Vertical autonomic longitudinal neuronal spinal tracts of Rexed lamina 7, the intermediolateral and intermediomedial tracts, not only influence synaptic transmission in autonomic reflex arcs, but literally, complete, with their short axons and dendrite processes, the local horizontal links of the sympathetic circuitry (59).

The supraspinal influences on the musculoskeletal system are much better understood than are the supraspinal influences on visceral systems. The chief modulating influence on the musculoskeletal system of man is one of inhibition or modification of inappropriate unconditioned or inborn spinal reflexes. Supraspinal inhibition allows local afferent/efferent reflexes to be remarkably plastic. Conditioned or learned reflexes become possible at local spinal cord segmental levels. Spinal learning or local spinal "memory" has shown, at least in the corticospinal system, how supraspinal centers influence some local spinal cord reflexes. The following studies elucidate the plasticity of the interneuronal circuitry in the spinal cord, the role of small fiber irritations in conditioning local reflexes, in "spinal cord learning," and how supra spinal processes direct or compensate for nonadaptive local spinal cord reflexes.

Supra-Spinal Compensation

Internuncial circuits of local somatic reflexes are under a flood of supraspinal inhibitory stimulation. When inhibition is removed or inadequate, general states of excitability create an exaggerated myotatic (stretch) reflex. According to Cook, the myotatic reflexes, as monosynaptic arcs, are not affected by small fiber (C-fiber) conditioning (134).

Unconditioned stimuli in spinal cord reflexes (see previous text on conditioned and unconditioned stimuli) are inhibited or subordinate to supraspinal impulses. In a study by Chamberlain, dogs were given cerebellar lesions. After a minimum of 45 minutes, a new "fixed" spinal cord reflex was produced which was secondary to the effects of the cerebellar lesion (51). When the spinal cord was transected, removing the influence

of the lesioned cerebellum, the spinal fixation remained. Supraspinal control can alter spinal reflexes in a way that is self-perpetuating at the spinal reflex level.

Frankstein produced pathological nerve excitation in cats. He injected turpentine into the foot pads which resulted in noxious C-fiber stimulation. This caused the animals to limp until they recovered. They regained a normal gait following recovery. When the animals were decerebrated, the original noxiously-induced spinal arc returned producing the characteristic limp. Supraspinal control had compensated for the traumatic C-fiber-induced excitation of local spinal cord "gait" reflex internuncials. The effect of traumatic, noxious excitations at the terminal field in the foot pad remained as a reflex entity for an extended period. When supraspinal compensations were removed, the pathophysiological reflex was re-expressed (51). Patterson suggested that some traumatic reflexes may be permanent and never completely reverse (51). This has also been demonstrated in rats.

The precise mechanism of hypothalamic modulation of local sympathetic arcs is very difficult to study. There have been reports of patients who experience visceral symptoms such as ulcers and cardiac distress when they become fatigued or stressed. Presumably, the effectiveness of supraspinal inhibition is dependent in some way on the general physical reserves of the body (Fig. 13.11).

SUPRASPINAL AUTONOMIC INFLUENCE

DESCENDING TRACTS

1. Reticulospinal tract: the reticulospinal tract is composed of the raphespinal tract and the hypothalamospinal tract.
   a. The raphespinal tract descends in the dorsolateral funiculus of the spinal cord and terminates in laminae 1 and 3. It modulates C-fiber transmission in order to modulate pain.
   b. The hypothalamospinal tract terminates in laminae 7 and modulates pre-ganglionic autonomic transmission.

Descending tracts originating in the limbic system or hypothalamus relay to the reticular formation or pass without synapsing to the spinal cord. The intermediolateral cell column is an uninterrupted extension of the reticular formation and carries descending impulses (26).

2. Parasympathetic pathways from the nucleus dorsalis provide supraspinal control over a course (vagus nerve) which is parallel to and independent of the spinal cord.

ASCENDING TRACTS

Ascending tracts include the spinothalamic and spinoreticular tracts. The spinothalamic and spinoreticular tracts ascend in the ventral and ventrolateral fasciculi to terminate in the reticular formation, thalamus and hypothalamus (26).

The spinothalamic tract ascends in the spinal cord with neurons from laminae 5, as well as laminae 1, 7, and 8 (Fig. 13.12). Ascending transmission is based upon the interplay of large and small fiber dendrites within laminae 2, 3 and 4. The

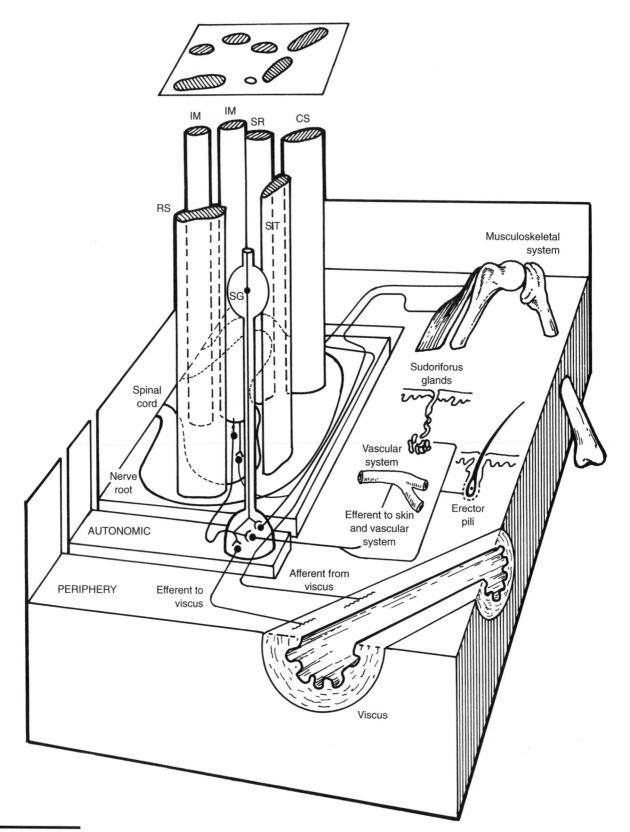

Figure 13.11. Neuroanatomicophysiological regions. Autonomic regions include not only chain ganglia but also autonomic nerves and prevertebral ganglia and plexi. Autonomic tracts: IM, intermediomedial tracts; SR, spinoreticular and spinomesencephalic tracts; ST, lateral spinothalamic tract; RS, medullary pontine and reticulospinal tracts; SG, sympathetic ganglion and paravertebral chain. Somatic tracts: CS, corticospinal tracts.

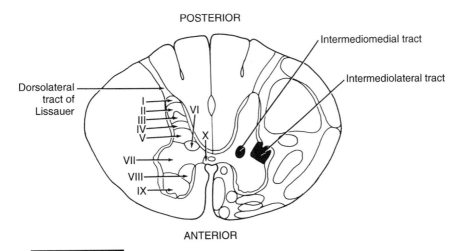

Figure 13.12.   Laminae and tracts of the midthoracic spine. Modified from Low PA. Clinical Autonomic Disorders. Boston: Little, Brown & Co., 1993.

tract gives off numerous collateral branches in the reticular formation of the medulla, pons, and mid brain (periaqueductal grey region). This tract carries the sensations of pain and related stimuli.

The spinoreticular tract arises from laminae 5, 6, 7, and 8 and branches extensively in the medullary and pontine reticular formation. It transmits impulses from internal organs.

SPINAL CORD (REXED). LAMINAE— EXCITATORY FIELDS WITHIN THE SPINAL CORD AND ASCENDING AND DESCENDING PATHWAY TERMINATIONS ON THOSE FIELDS

Specific laminae of the cord have been described by Rexed. Below are those laminae that have a significant role in ANS function:

Lamina 1 (tract of Lissauer) contains arborizations of both autonomic (visceral) (41) and somatic afferents. Some fibers enter lamina 2 and 5 (16). At its rostral end, this column along with lamina 2, 3, and 4, is continuous with the spinal tract of cranial nerve 5 (trigeminal tract) which extends into the brain stem (26).

Lamina 2 (substantia gelatinosa) is important in editing sensory input and transmission of pain impulses to the thalamus. It contains many internuncial synapses of neurons from laminae 1 2, 3, 4 and 5. This is influenced by the descending recticulospinal tract (from raphe nucleus) (26).

Lamina 3 contains many axons of primary afferent fibers from the dorsal root including small fibers from laminae 1 and 2. It receives numerous dendrites of large fiber neurons which arise from laminae 4, 5, and 6. Therefore, large and small fiber communicate in lamina 3 (26).

Lamina 4 contains even more primary afferent fiber axons from the dorsal root than does lamina 3 and synapses with dendritic synapses of larger nerve fibers. Lamina 4 contains many corticospinal tract fibers. There is substantial contact between large and small fiber in lamina 4 (26).

Lamina 5 contains larger afferent neurons than lamina 4 and a significant number of descending fibers, primarily of the

corticospinal tract. Most of the spinothalamic tract fibers originate in this area (26).

Lamina 6 is associated with the limb enlargements of the cord. It receives neurons of the corticospinal tract (26).

Lamina 7 is the largest region of the grey matter of the cord. It contains many of the internuncial neurons of the spinal cord. The chief autonomic tracts—the intermediolateral (cell bodies of preganglionic sympathetic neurons) and intermediomedial (primary visceral afferent fibers) columns are within lamina 7. Local ANS circuitry of the horizontal or segmental arc is completed by branchings with axons of vertically-directed interneurons (26). Some spinothalamic fibers arise in this lamina.

Lamina 8 contains the terminations of some descending fibers including the recticulospinal tract . It projects to laminae 7 and 9. Some spinothalamic fibers arise in lamina 8 (26)

Lamina 9 is embedded in laminae 7 and 8. It contains cell bodies of alpha motor neurons (26).

Lamina 10 is the midline region which surrounds the central canal and is the region where neurons crossover or decussate (26).

Impulses associated with conscious temperature, pain and touch sensations have cell bodies in lamina 5. (41). Sympathetic afferent neurons terminate in laminae 2, 3, 4, 5, 6 and 7. The visceral sympathetic terminations are most concentrated in laminae 1, 5, 6 and 7. Somatic sympathetic terminations are most concentrated in laminae 2, 3 and 4 (41,64). A distinct sympathetic viscerosomatic region of overlap lies in laminae 5 and 6. These two laminae contain both somatic and visceral branchings (Figs. 13.13, 13.14).

Local Afferent Supply—The Spine as an Afferent Impulse Driver

The somatic and autonomic tissues of the vertebral column have extensive sympathetic receptor fields, which include the paravertebral autonomic neural plexus itself. Anteriorly, this plexus innervates the anterior longitudinal ligament, periph-

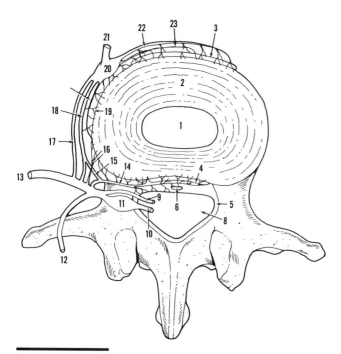

Figure 13.13. Innervation of anterior spinal canal and structures of the anterior and lateral aspect of the spinal column.

1. Nucleus pulposus
2. Anulus fibrosus
3. Anterior longitudinal ligament
4. Posterior longitudinal ligament
5. Leptomeninges
6. Epidural vasculature
7. Filum terminale
8. Intrathecal lumbosacral nerve root
9. Ventral root
10. Dorsal root
11. Dorsal root ganglion
12. Dorsal ramus of spinal nerve
13. Ventral ramus of spinal nerve
14. Recurrent meningeal nerve
15. Sympathetic branch to the recurrent meningeal nerve
16. Direct somatic branch from ventral ramus of spinal nerve to lateral disc
17. White ramus communicans (from L2 cephalad)
18. Gray ramus communicans
19. Lateral sympathetic efferent branches projecting from gray ramus communicans
20. Paraspinal sympathetic ganglion (SG)
21. Paraspinal sympathetic chain
22. Anterior paraspinal afferent sympathetic ramus projecting to SG
23. Anterior sympathetic efferent branches projecting from SG
Modified from Jinkins JR, Whittemore AR, Bradley WG. The anatomic basis of vertebrogenic pain and the autonomic syndrome associated with lumbar disk extrusion. Am J Neuroradiol 1989;10:219-231.

ery of anulus fibrosus, vertebral body, periosteum, meninges, nerva nervosa, and vasa nervosa. Posteriorly, through the recurrent meningeal nerve, the lateral and posterior periphery of the disc and connective tissues are innervated. With the

combined plexi, the entire vertebral column is innervated (41). Afferent fibers from the paravertebral sympathetic plexus pass through the paraspinal sympathetic ganglia to reach the spinal cord by way of the white communicating rami and the posterior sensory nerve root and enter the lateral horn. There are conscious and unconscious autonomic manifestations and reflexes (41).

A "tissue sensitivity index" for the spinal tissues was developed by Kuslisch. The most sensitive tissues, in descending order, are the supraspinous ligament and the lateral and central region of the intervertebral disc (i.e., endplate ruptures or Schmorl's nodes). Joints and muscles were moderately pain-generating. Where nerves were stretched or compressed, extreme irritation was produced. Interestingly, normal nerves are almost completely insensitive to pain (65).

Jinkins studied lumbar disc extrusions in 145 subjects. He found that those subjects with anterior or central disc extrusions (vertebrogenic and discogenic but not neurogenic irritations) had referred pain into the somatosomal "Zones of Head." The referral patterns correlated to where the sympathetic sensory nerve fibers entered the spinal cord, and not with the level where the disc was actually irritated

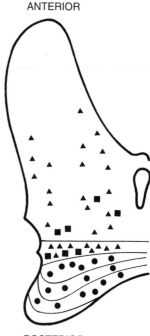

Figure 13.14. Overlapping afferent terminations. Points of visceral, somatic, and indeterminate terminations in the right gray matter of the spinal cord. Circles: terminations of sympathetic somatic tissue afferent fibers on somatic spinal cord neurons. Triangles: terminations of sympathetic visceral tissue afferent fibers or viscerosomatic spinal cord neurons. Squares: terminations of sympathetic somatic tissues afferent fibers or viscerosomatic spinal cord neurons. Modified from Jinkins JR, Whittemore AR, Bradley WG. The anatomic basis of vertebrogenic pain and the autonomic syndrome associated with lumbar disk extrusion. Am J Neuroradiol 1989;10:219-231.

unlike what is seen when a somatic sensory nerve is irritated (41). Younger patients had a higher incidence of central disc extrusions, i.e., endplate fractures or Schmorl's Nodes, than adults because the anulus is less damaged by accumulated traumas (41). This accounts for the rarity of radiculopathy in youth and the common occurrence of diffuse somatosomal extremity pain ("growing pains").

Somatic, somatosympathetic, and visceral sympathetic nerve fibers terminate on specific laminae within the spinal cord—many having the same or some of the same central connections on "viscerosomatic terminal fields" in the spinal cord (41). Further, some "indeterminate" somatic afferent fibers terminate in visceral excitatory fields. Somatic and autonomic afferent fibers run in parallel to their spinal cord terminations or may converge to a single afferent fiber which synapses on spinal cord internuncial neurons and register viscerosomatic stimulation. Internuncial thresholds and field areas are modulated by a convergence of spinal nerve afferent stimulation and supraspinal compensations. Viscerosomatatopic representations of the CNS and consequent modifications of reflexes are dependent upon "adequate" neuronal tone. "Adequate" tone is derived from the broad spectrum of afferent stimulation generated by adequate function of healthy tissue.

It is rare that the human spinal column shows no sign of degenerative changes, particularly in the adult population. Back and neck pain is a chief human complaint and is a leading cause of impairment and disability.

The spinal column is the chief organ of posture. It is the sole agent against gravity and it supports an almost unlimited range of physical activities. Despite its segmented design of over 100 joints, it protects the spinal cord. Vertebrogenic afferent stimulation from the somatic and autonomic paravertebral plexi provides the critical input to the brain and cerebellum upon which the support and protection function of the spinal column is orchestrated. The paravertebral plexus innervates all of the components of the spinal column except the nucleus pulposus, though even the nucleus is purported to have nerve filaments (41). The spinal column is itself a rich source of afferent spinal cord stimulation.

Healthy spinal function excites balanced somatic and autonomic nerve system activity and stabilizes efficient spinal cord reflexes. Healthy spinal function has a tonic effect on nerve and somatic tissues of the spine. Biochemical and biomechanical damages associated with poor spinal function at specific spinal levels stimulate spinal cord excitability by concurrently producing heightened C-fiber activity and suppressed levels of large fiber (proprioceptive) stimulation. This alters local spinal cord reflexes which, to varying degrees, may or may not be compensated for by supraspinal inhibition. Altered local reflexes may be acute and conscious, or "silent" and unconscious, as is typically the case in chronic spinal biomechanical degeneration. Specific chiropractic adjustments appear to affect regional afferent input, introducing a sudden wide range of fiber stimulation which, for a variable period of time, destabilizes established abnormal pathophysiological reflexes and referrals within the spinal cord and the respective receptive and motor fields in its local tissues (51).

Dysfunction of the Autonomic Nervous System

The dysfunctioning nervous system fails not only itself but fails its targets as well. Thus, the entire body is involved. The diversity of effects resulting from ANS dysfunction is not the simple result of stimulation to the sympathetic pathways but is the response of abnormal stimulation by the innervated tissues and organs (86). Once dysfunctioning, the disrupted targets create afferent impulses which, in turn, disturb subsequent central processes and the resulting efferent nerve responses. Each activity of the ANS provides progressive cyclical corrections or failures.

Despite the early recognition that the autonomic nervous system (ANS) is responsible for the integration, regulation, coordination, and adaptation of the organism, ANS function research has always lagged behind that of the somatic nervous system. According to Calaresu, the reason for the paucity of studies on the ANS is that there are major conceptual and technical difficulties in forming the models which are both sufficiently comprehensive and/or specific enough to account for the diverse and complex interactions (66).

The study of the relationship between improvements of visceral health and function and chiropractic spinal adjustments has largely been derived from clinical reports. Although very few studies are at the level of the so-called scientific gold standard, this should not deter our interest in this area. Many chiropractors and others using spinal adjustments or manipulation have speculated upon and written about this relationship for decades. In recent years, as chiropractors have begun to use the tools of recognized scientific protocol, this neurovisceral connection has begun appearing in respected, peer-reviewed chiropractic journals, as well as allopathic and manual medicine journals. Since the turn of the century, osteopathic journals have included a wealth of information on the effects that spinal adjustments have on various visceral disorders. Unfortunately, much of this information is not easily accessed.

Significant Components and Mechanisms of Disturbed ANS Activity

Reflex sympathetic dystrophy (RSD) can be viewed as a simple model of autonomic reflex dysfunction in even more complex ANS/tissue disturbances. The literature suggests that the classic neurological disturbances of RSD—hypersympatheticotonia, neurovascular dysregulation, and atrophy occur to visceral targets with differing degrees of similarities (67). (RSD will be described later in this section).

There are four characteristic neurological disturbances seen in RSD and similar ANS disturbances, the precise neuropathophysiology manifestation of which is always a composite of 4 varying degrees. The first three neurological disturbances will be briefly mentioned below but are outside the scope of this chapter's outline. The fourth is at the center of our work in ANS neuropathophysiology.

1. Abnormal nerve impulse transmissions (impulse-based) in otherwise normal nerve tissues are seen as either a decrease or increase in impulse traffic. This results

in dystonic distension or hypertonic hypertrophy in smooth and cardiac muscles. Both result in:

a. Decreased vascular perfusion and congestion of tissues.
b. Abnormal supplies of synaptic neurotransmitters, co-transmitters and neuromodulators at the neuro-effector sites.

Tissue atrophy is a result of persistent abnormal volume of nerve impulse transmission and a degraded biochemical and metabolic environment.

2. Abnormal neurotrophic transmissions (nonimpulse-based) in otherwise normal nerve tissue.

Neurotrophic substances give physiological support to the parenchyma of target organs and the neuron itself. A decrease in production of nerve cell substances or a disturbance of their intracellular distribution causes tonic, nutritive, modulative, and/or genetic/growth disturbances. The substances distributed in both orthograde (in the direction the normal impulse travels) and retrograde (in the direction opposite to the normal impulse travel) axoplasmic flow are themselves or will be a part of the at least 60 known substances described as neurokinins, cotransmitters, neuromodulators, neuroenzymes, and precursors which regulate the way that the nerve system and soma biochemically interrelate (47).

The structure of the nerve cell (cytoskeleton), nerve cell metabolism, neuron secretion, and absorption of neurochemical substances of which only a fraction are true neurotransmitters, are affected by the manufacture and distribution of intracellular substances in the neuron (47).

Because most neurochemical substances or their precursors are produced in the cell body, the ability of the neuron to transport these substances is critical, particularly when the eccentricities of the cell's shape is considered. The ratio of the size of the nerve cell body to the size of the axon (the width to length) is not seen in any other type of cell. The size of the typical neuron body is about 100 microns in diameter, but its axon process can be up to 1000 mm in length. In other words, if a neuron had a cell body diameter of four inches, its axon would be eight miles in length (55). Disruption to the microcirculation anywhere along the length of the axon may result in degraded nerve structure and function, atrophy (neuropathy), and effector tissue dysfunction and atrophy.

3. Regeneration/repair in damaged tissue. The following adaptations take place in damaged neurons:

a. Denervation supersensitivity (proliferation of post synaptic receptor sites) (44).
b. Synaptic hypereffectiveness (pre-synaptic hypertrophy of healthy intact transmitter boutons).
c. Neo-synapsis including ephaptic transmission (side to side axon-axonal and or axono-dendritic transmission increases).
d. Persistence of hyperinnervation.
e. Recruitment of silent synapses.
f. Regenerative and collateral axonal sprouting-reactive synaptogenesis in CNS.
g. Vicarious function.

These regenerative responses may be adaptive or non-adaptive (16). Alterations in function or structure following repair take place anywhere in the nerve system—peripheral, central, or autonomic systems (16). As an example of a regenerative response, about 90% of the myocardial norepinephrine normally required by the heart is produced by sympathetic terminals in the heart. When the local production of norepinephrine is lost, as in congestive heart failure, the heart becomes supersensitized to exogenous norepinephrine which results in a loss of discrete local control (68).

To isolate a primary tissue source or phenomenon as a single initiating cause of neuropathology is an interesting exercise but is usually therapeutically unproductive (as in the case of RSD). Once an abnormal neurophysiological reflex is established, its point of origin often becomes insignificant. The continuity of the neuropathic reflex is itself the root of pathology. Favorable clinical outcomes are based upon disrupting the isolated cycles of failures so that the aberrant neurophysiological processes can be re-influenced by the inherent, normalizing organizational activities, i.e., the innate restorative resources of the brain and nervous system.

The remainder of this section will examine, in light of the fourth mechanism of disturbed ANS function, the reflex/referral abnormalities, and specific normal and abnormal neurophysiological processes. It will conclude by considering some common neurologically influenced visceral conditions.

4. Neurological Reflex/Referral Abnormality—the fourth mechanism of disturbed ANS function. The spinal cord, and to an extent, the paraspinal ganglia, are points where both the ascending and descending vertical tracts (longitudinal axis) of the nerve system intersect and interact with the peripheral neural pathways (horizontal axis). Impulse transmission is profoundly modified at these neural intersections.

REFLEX/ REFERRAL RELATIONSHIPS

The improvements seen in ANS disorders treated with spinal adjustments result from the improving neurophysiological relationship between soma (spine principally) and viscera. The "soma" in chiropractic care consists of spinal tissues (bones, muscles, ligaments, spinal cord, and nerve roots) and the "viscera" (the smooth muscles and glands and their nerves). Neurophysiological relationships of soma and viscera are described by listing the tissue generating the impulse followed by the tissue to which the impulse travels (Table 13.8). The four neurophysiological relationships are:

1. Somatosomatic—from soma to soma
2. Somatovisceral—from soma to viscera
3. Viscerosomatic—from viscera to soma
4. Viscerovisceral—from viscera to viscera

These relationships are further designated as a referral or a reflex relationship. A referral occurs when sensory excitation originating in one system or functional pathway stimulates sensory nerves of another system or pathway. This occurs

Table 13.8.   Head Zones: Viscerosomatic Referrals to the Head and Body

Inflamed Viscera	Associated Hyperalgesia in Trunk and Extremity Distributions	Location of Hyperalgesia in the Spine	Location of Hyperalgesia in the Head
Heart	C3–C4, T2–T8	L, B	Ventricles & aorta—N, FN, MO, FT Auricles–FT, T, V, P
Lungs	C3–C4, T4–T9	C, S	N, FN, MO, FT, T, V, P
Stomach	T7–T9	B	FN, MO, T, V, P
Intestine	T9–T12	B, L	V, P, O
Rectum	S2–S4		
Liver	C3–C4, T7–T10	R, C	FN, MO, T, V, P, O
Gall bladder	T8–T9		T, V
Kidney and urethra	T11–L2	C, S	
Urinary bladder	S3–S4	C	
Detrusor muscle	T11–L2		
Prostate	T10–T12, S1–S3	C	
Testicle	T10	C	O
Ovary	T10	C	O
Uterus	T10–L1		
Neck of uterus	S2–S3	C	
Breast	T4–T5	C	
Spleen	T6	L	

Laterality

B	Bilateral		S	Ipsilateral
R	Right		C	Centrally over spine
L	Left			

Areas of the head

N	Nasal or rostral area		FN	Frontal-nasal area
MO	Medio-orbital area		FT	Fronto-temporal area
T	Temporal area		V	Vertical area
P	Parietal area		O	Occipital area

The zones of head are based on:

1) Cases of cutaneous hyperasthesia in the coincident visceral affection.

2) Topography of eruptions in 52 cases of herpes zoster.

3) Mapping of analgesic areas in organic diseases on the spine and nerve roots.

Modified from Pottenger S. Symptoms of Visceral Disease (6th ed). St. Louis: C.V. Mosby. 1994.

where both systems or pathways have sensory nerve terminals juxtaposed in the spinal cord. Thus, sensory excitement from one system causes an expansion of a sensory event into another system or path. A reflex occurs when sensory excitement at a termination point in the spinal cord stimulates a juxtaposed motor nerve or its pathway. Thus, sensory excitement of a system causes motor excitement.

Referred sensation, by definition, is a perception of the CNS and not a true representation of the tissue (41). In studies of referred sensation, the source of a referred leg pain—the spinal tissue—was anesthetized. Both the spinal pain and extremity pain associated with the nerve abated. Anesthetizing only the area of extremity pain produced no change in pain (Projections of sensations even occur in an extremity which has been amputated—"phantom limb pain"). The CNS is subject to being "tricked" under certain conditions. Afferent stimulation from one system of the body can affect sensory information, a referral, and/or motor activity, a reflex, in a system entirely different from the source.

SOMATIC AND VISCERAL RELATIONSHIPS DEFINED

Somato-somatic relationship: when nerve impulses which have originated from the sensory receptors of one somatic tissue stimulate the adjacent spinal cord terminations of another somatic tissue. This stimulates a referral termed somatosomatosensory excitement or a reflexed termed somatosomatomotor excitement in the nerves of the other somatic tissue. Example: 1) somatosomatosensory referral: vertebrogenic back pain impulses stimulating the sensory terminals of the leg in the spinal cord which causes referred leg pain; and 2) somatosomatomotor reflex: vertebrogenic back pain causing hypertonicity (spasms) of regional back muscles.

Somato-visceral relationship: when nerve impulses which originated in the sensory receptors of a somatic tissue (e.g., spine, trunk, or extremities) stimulates the terminations of adjacent visceral tissue neurons in the spinal cord. This somatic stimulation may produce in the visceral nerve system a somatovacerosensory referral, somatovisceromotor reflex, or both. Examples: 1) somatovacerosensory referral: lower back pain stimulating testicular pain; and 2) somatovisceromotor reflex: spinal disturbances causing cardiac arrhythmia/hypotension (69).

Viscero-somatic relationship: when nerve impulses originate in the sensory receptors of a visceral tissue stimulate terminations of adjacent somatic tissue neurons in the spinal cord. This visceral sensory stimulation produces a viscerosomatosensory referral or viscerosomatomotor reflex, or both. Examples: 1) viscerosomatosensory referral: cardiac distress which refers pain to the left arm and chest wall; and 2) viscerosomatomotor reflex: appendicitis stimulating abdominal rigidity.

Viscero-visceral relationships: when nerve impulses originate in the sensory receptors of visceral tissue stimulate the terminations of adjacent visceral tissue neurons in the spinal. This produces a response in those other visceral nerve systems that will be viscerovacerosensory referral, viscerovisceromotor reflex, or both. Examples: 1) viscerovacerosensory referral: gall bladder dysfunction producing gastric pain (70); and 2) viscerovisceromotor reflex: appendicitis causing pylorospasms (36).

SOMATIC VS. VISCERAL PAIN AND MOTOR FUNCTION

Somatic sensory registrations, particularly pain and paresthesias, characteristically manifest within a finite distribution.

Typically, they are easy for the patient to pinpoint. There is certainty when a patient says, "It is here," and with a finger or two fingers spread like calipers, points to a specific area or "map." The classic somatic pain is sciatica causing a sharply linear, 1-1/4 inch wide painful strip in the posterolateral thigh and calf.

Sensory disturbances, on the other hand, do not produce discrete localization of pain. Quantitatively, patient descriptions are vague. For example, the visceral pain of angina is often demonstrated with the fist or palm held broadly over the chest and is accompanied by a general feeling of uneasiness, a sense of "sickness," or a display of affect.

The motor disturbances of the somatic and visceral nerve systems are distinctive in similar ways. Somatomotor function can be fast and discrete with a highly developed start/stop mechanism. This ability allows for adaptative responses to sudden changes in the external environment. The viscera do not function in this way. Classically, the visceromotor nervous system creates broad physiological responses to a relatively well-controlled internal environment, particularly when the nerve system is functioning in a healthy manner.

ILLUSTRATION OF SOMATIC AND VISCERAL FUNCTIONAL INTEGRATION

Stepping barefooted upon a piece of glass normally causes an immediate withdrawal of the foot—a flexor response (34). This is a purely somatomotor reflex. Also initiated is an autonomic sensory and motor reflex which causes vasoconstriction, immune cell responses, and the initiation of the healing process. Pain continues in the foot even though the glass is no longer present; one puts less weight on that foot. This lingering pain (protopathic) allows the internal conditions at the injured site to be conducive to healing—a function of the ANS.

A single stimulus (glass puncture) produces two integrated responses in two nerve systems. The sharp pain in the injured tissue causes a change in the foot's relationship to the piece of glass in the external environment—a function of the somatic system. This "quick response system" has dedicated, specialized, rapidly-transmitting nerve tissues (types I and II or A-alpha, -beta, and -gamma). The dull pain from tissue damage and the pain that remains during the healing process come from changes in the condition of the internal environment—a function of the ANS. The optimum response entails rapid withdrawal from the external source of injury (somatic) so as to avoid further damage and the establishment of optimum healing of the damaged tissue (visceral).

Together the somatovisceral and viscerosomatic reflexes integrate somatic and visceral responses and provide and promote optimal preservation organism as a whole.

ADDITIONAL SPECIFIC NERVE/TISSUE INTERRELATIONSHIPS

Some reflexes and referrals between soma and viscera have been investigated in specific tissues. Examples of organ-specific somatovisceral reflexes include the following:

Cutaneovisceral reflexes:

1. Cutaneocardiac reflex: stimulation of the skin causes a cardiac response (70); and
2. Cutaneo-intestinal: pinching the skin of the abdomen inhibits peristalsis (70,71).

Because the spinal cord is the site of intermediary processing between a horizontal cortical link (afferent and efferent peripheral fibers) and vertical links (centrifugal/centripetal influences towards and away from the brain) to the brain, a special significance is placed on the brain's role in regulating the reflex/referral interrelationships. Psychovisceral, psychosomatic, visceropsychic, and somatopsychic reflexes describe the relationships between local referral/reflex circuits and supraspinal control. The following referrals and reflexes have been described:

Psychovisceromotor: gastrointestinal ulcers, diarrhea, constipation, hives (70), etc.

Psychoviscerosensory: "aching heart;" "butterflies in the stomach."

Psychoviscerosomatosensory: "I feel my heart beating in my throat."

Pyschosomatosensory: "I feel ants crawling on me."

Pyschosomatomotor: "feigned paralysis"

Somatopsychosensory: a sick or uneasy feeling with bodily stimulation

Reflex Sympathetic Dystrophy

Perhaps the best understood ANS dysfunction is reflex sympathetic dystrophy (RSD). RSD is an ideal conceptual model for understanding ANS dysfunction, and, in its own right is an important clinically topic.

As is typical of ANS disorders, RSD does not fit into a simple, unified, or even consistent model. Its multitude of presentations are due to the diversity of tissues affected which accounts for the wide variety of symptoms and courses (72). The large number of synonyms demonstrates RSD's complex and variable presentations. Among these include: Sudeck's atrophy, post-traumatic pain syndrome, shoulder-hand syndrome, algodystrophy, causalgia, peripheral acute trophoneurosis, atypical post-traumatic pain syndrome, postinfarctional sclerodactyly, traumatic angiospasm, acute atrophy of bone, algoneurodystrophy, and post-traumatic osteoporosis (73,74).

Note: Causalgia is typically used if the condition is caused by direct injury to a peripheral nerve and it usually requires the following criteria: burning pain which occurs spontaneously or is evoked by stimulation, including, touch, heat, dryness, excitement, emotion, or the thought of being touched (75).

Although the pathophysiology of RSD is little understood, the sympathetic nervous system is almost universally implicated. Scores of medical clinical studies have demonstrated a full tissue and physiological restoration of atrophied tissue following chemical or surgical ablation or blocking of one or more sympathetic nerve ganglia (59). It appears that an overreaction of the sympathetic nervous system may be the mechanism behind this disorder.

Key characteristics of RSD found in one or more of the extremities include the following:

- Unilateral extremity hyperesthesia (hyperpathia and allodynia), burning, edema, hyperhidrosis, and trophic changes.
- Alternating warm, then cold extremity (vasomotor dysequilibrium).
- Alternating dry, then damp skin (sudomotor dysequilibrium).
- Sequela to injury, visceral irritation, or an increasingly painful reaction to a mild sustained or repetitive irritation (facilitation)
- A psychological component may accompany the disorder, although it is unknown whether the component precedes or merely follows RSD.
- The most successful allopathic medical treatment for RSD is a spinal cord block. The efficacy and outcomes of this procedure have come under question (47).

Stages of Reflex Sympathetic Dystrophy (25,73)

Stage 1—Sympathetic denervation in the affected structure. This stage is characterized by diminished sympathetic activity, increased temperature, redness, edema, dry skin, rapid growth of hair and nails, decreased range of motion.

Stage 2—Dystrophic sympathetic hyperactivity. This stage is characterized by increased sympathetic activity, decreased skin temperature, cyanotic or colorless hue, moist skin, exacerbations by cold and relief with warmth, bone and joint degeneration, and muscle atrophy.

Stage 3—Atrophy. This stage is characterized by a loss of sympathetic control, a decrease in pain, hyperesthesia, temperature changes, and permanent tissue changes. The skin is smooth, glossy, and drawn; tendinous contractures and fibrosis occurs; muscles are wasted; and osteoporosis and joint ankylosis occurs.

Ganglionectomy or ganglion block procedures have proclaimed up to a 87% success rate in reducing the symptoms of RSD (47). The best surgical results appear to require complete severance of all of the sympathetic rami from multiple, contiguous levels of the spine—in effect, severing all sympathetic connections to the central nervous system. The therapeutic goal is, with a "broad brush," interruption of all neural transmissions in the afferent/efferent reflex loop (59). This interrupts hyperstimulation; indeed, all stimulation within the sympathetic nerve reflex pathway without regard to any specific neuropathic point(s) of origin in that reflex, including nebulous supraspinal influences of psychological and emotional origin. RSD is conceived and treated as an overall event in the sympathetic nervous system which should be stopped rather than a reaction of the sympathetic nervous system to a subset of specific but variable neurophysiological abnormalities within it.

The treatment model utilizing ganglionectomy is drastic and dangerous (72). Despite their popularity, these procedures have never been subjected to proper clinical trials. Ochoa reports that the entire diagnosis is dangerous and the permanence of the procedures has come into serious question (72). Once the diagnosis is made, it is difficult to disprove and commonly progresses to an unchecked escalation of highly invasive, and marginally effective interventions. Serious warnings exist regarding the significant residual effects (72).

Mechanism of RSD

Sympathetic dysfunction does not cause RSD. More correctly, a "trigger point" initiates a central disturbance. A central process in turn stimulates the sympathetic nerves which initiate further peripheral responses in the sympathetic nervous system. The subsequent secondary peripheral effects initiate more afferent impulses adding to and reinforcing the original "trigger point" disturbance. The secondary peripheral effects and central activity support the sustained pathophysiological reflex (59,72).

The classical myofascial "motor points" are included in the group of RSD trigger points. Triggers may also be any noxious stimulation, conscious or unconscious, at any point in one or more of the major ANS loops—within the cortex-hypothalamus-spinal cord; within the spinal cord; and from the spinal cord-ganglion-tissue. Triggers may be present in visceral organs. Ashwal describes myocardial infarct as an RSD trigger (76).

The locations and tone of RSD triggers are difficult to determine. However, if found, they are a more accurate predictor of RSD than is the severity of any antecedent trauma, if one had occurred. Often severe traumatic chemical or psychic insults result in routine recovery. Conversely, a relatively minor insult commonly initiates a progressively worsening response significantly out of proportion to the initial insult or injury. The progressive, secondary responses may perpetuate or even replace the initial insult with advanced, intractable neuropathology. The manifestations of RSD seem to be based more upon the condition of the nervous system than a pure effect of peripheral or central nervous system injury (76).

Reflex Sympathetic Dystrophy in Children

In children, RSD tends to be more benign, resolves more quickly, and has fewer complications than it does in adults. Trauma plays a lesser role in juvenile RSD. Its incidence is more common than was previously thought because many cases are undiagnosed or misdiagnosed (77). Commonly overlooked is a childhood fall (e.g., falling off of a swing) or involvement in a relatively minor auto accident. There may be a momentary loss of consciousness or disorientation with headaches, neck pain, and nausea which clear up after a few days. Later in life, complaints of vascular-type headaches may arise due to irritation of the sympathetic fibers within the now further degenerated cervical spine (46).

Because vague or mild insults are typical causative factors in childhood RSD, obtaining the history of trauma is difficult. Only persistent questioning of siblings, parents, or the child will elicit the cause. A minor sprain or twist may precede the condition (77). Wilder reports that half of his pediatric patients with RSD had traumatic episodes during supervised sports activities (77). Lower extremities were involved in up to 80% of the cases. Although only 44% of the plain x-ray films showed abnormalities (76,77), Laxer found abnormal radionuclide bone scans in 70% of the RSD cases.

Conservative management is almost always successful (76-78). Conservative medical treatment typically consists of physical therapy. Spinal and extremity exercises are usually given. The therapeutic goal is to improve function. Often, there is an initial transient increase in the severity of the pain (77). In spite of the rare failures of conservative care, the prognosis does not appear to be worsened by the initial course of conservative, non-invasive therapies (77).

Langweiler presented a 24-year-old female with RSD who sought chiropractic care. The initial symptoms were stiffness and tenderness in the thoracic spine that progressively worsened in the affected areas. This patient initially complained of pain upon cervical rotation in the cervical and thoracic spine and scapular region. Cervical distraction produced a C5/6 radicular pain pattern. Adjustments of T3/T4 and C5/C6 were given. Adjunctive treatments of electroacupuncture and muscle rehabilitation were also given. There was complete recovery (73).

Ellis treated a 13-year-old patient with a severe case of RSD in the lower extremity complicated by muscle paralysis. The patient required the use of crutches. Clinical findings included scoliosis and lumbar hyperlordosis. Specific chiropractic adjustments (Gonstead technique) were used. After one year of chiropractic care, the extremity was 95% of normal as assessed by a chiropractic pediatric specialist (79).

As noted above, childhood RSD has a quicker and more complete resolution than does adult RSD. Hinwood and Hinwood postulated that the young spine has made fewer compensatory adaptations because postural and traumatic insults are less chronic (80). In experiments which induced minor postural stresses using heel lifts and a tilt-chair, Thomas induced local hyperactivity of segmental sympathetic nervous system. When tipping the horizontal base of the spine, the increased tone of axial muscles of one side caused a sympathetic facilitation. This was determined by measuring sudomotor activity (81).

Dystrophy and Development

Rush (77) noted that three of his pediatric cases had significant uneven leg lengths that may have resulted from RSD. Discrepancy in leg lengths was thought to be due to the dystrophic effect of RSD on growing tissues, specifically at the epiphysis and in muscles. Gunn reported that following sympathetic nerve denervation, the total collagen in soft tissue and skeletal tissues is reduced. Further, the replacement collagen is weaker, and this may lead to many degenerative conditions associated with weight-bearing. Idiopathic scoliosis may be a structural sequel to uneven leg lengths, altered weight-bearing, and gait asymmetries associated with pain avoidance. Altered weight-bearing positions could conceivably cause a sympathetic facilitation near or in the vertebral column suggesting that improper structural development of the axial skeleton may be a component of sympathetic dystrophy (44).

Gunn further reported that supersensitivity in autonomic pathways can lead to an increase in blood vessel tone. This may affect a wide variety of tissues and cause secondary structural disintegration (44). Cannon and Rosenblueth (law of denervation supersensitivity) found effects of denervation supersensitivity not only in striate and smooth connective tissues, but also in the salivary glands, sudorific glands, autonomic ganglia, and spinal and cortical neurons. They noted that a physical interruption of the autonomic pathways was not required for supersensitivity to occur (60).

If development of bone and muscle are disturbed by interrupted or oversensitivity of autonomic pathways and cause an increase of peripheral vascular resistance in most tissues, then dystrophic or developmental deficiencies can be expected in organs and other systems. In other words, childhood sympathetic dystrophic disorders may cause incomplete development of the internal organs and systems.

Postural problems are seen in association with disturbances in visceral function. Ruggeri cites a case of childhood RSD with lower extremity pain including heel pain accompanied by abdominal pain (82). Insult to regional sympathetic structures may be the common feature (80)

The classic dystrophies of RSD are changes to bone, muscle, hair, nails, and skin, such as osteopenia, joint damage including Charcot's joints, muscle atrophy, alopecia, hypertrichosis, ridging of nails, hyperkeratosis, and mottling of the skin (59). These have been accepted as characteristic signs of RSD primarily because they are readily observable changes that may be viewed either visually or by x-ray. The internal signs of oversensitive autonomic pathways are not directly observable and are therefore difficult to assess except through a consideration of very subtle topical changes.

Fortunately, the potential for harm by initiating conservative management of RSD is nearly non-existent compared to the risks associated with radical interventions such as ganglionectomy or ganglion blocks (72). Short of rare and fatal infectious diseases, there is no other disease in which prevention is a more important consideration than in the treatment of sympathetic reflex dystrophy. Although early treatment and prevention are preferable, in the event that RSD becomes clinically established, the more severe stages of the disease must be avoided. The more aggressively the illness is treated in its early stages (the stage of reflex sympathetic temporary dysfunction or RSTD), the better are the chances of preventing the progression to the second, more serious dystrophic stage of RSD. Preventing the development of the third or atrophic stage of RSD is necessary. In this stage, the chance of a successful resolution drops off dramatically. The third stage exposes the patient to risks associated with surgical procedures including amputation, sympathectomy, and, in susceptible individuals, a profound emotional despair and suicide.

The manifestations of this autonomic nervous system disorder are complex, numerous, and variable as the disorder involves both peripheral and central processing, including a supraspinal link. The mechanism involved in reflex sympa-

thetic dystrophy will require further scientific exploration into the organization of the spinal cord and paraspinal tissues of the autonomic nervous system and the tissues that it innervates. Clearly, chiropractors are provided with the background to favorably influence the outcome of this autonomic disorder.

SYMPTOMATIC CONDITIONS

An early study of the influence of the sympathetic nervous system on visceral organ health and function was done by Henry Windsor, MD. In his 1921 "Medical Times" article, he found 221 diseased organs in 50 cadavers. Of these diseased organs, 212 were innervated by sympathetic fibers with origins in regions of the spine which were rigid and demonstrated minor curvatures. He implicated "vaso-motor spasm" as the likely cause of disease in these organ tissues (83).

Because of their associations with hospitals and their access to funding, osteopathy has provided many of the detailed studies of the relationship between the nervous system and the viscera. Today, however, chiropractic has begun taking a greater role in the study of this relationship.

The experienced clinician quickly concedes that there is no prescriptive or "cookbook" approach to treating visceral disturbances. There are too many variables and interactions in the body for any single conceptual approach to work for the wide spectrum of visceral disorders. The following will help provide a framework within which one can rule in or out the clinical involvement of a given spinal segment in aberrant ANS reflexes.

RULING IN OR OUT VERTEBRAL SUBLUXATION COMPLEX INVOLVED WITH VISCERAL PATHOPHYSIOLOGY

Most authorities agree that some if not all pathological changes in the viscera have an impact on impulse traffic within the nervous system, whether conscious or not. This produces variable but detectable changes in the tissues of the spinal column. Therefore, the entire spine must be considered when studying its role either as initiator or sustainer of visceral neuropathophysiological states. ANS stimulation is considered to produce two general categories of visceral responses:

1. Sympathetic stimulation (usually increased stimulation or sympathicotonia) stops the flow and/or absorption of the contents of most hollow organs. It causes relaxation of the hollow organs, vessels, ducts, and bladders, and closes the sphincters. Sympathetic stimulation withholds blood from the digestive tissues and their metabolic processes but increases blood flow to the skin, striated muscles, and heart (84); and

2. Parasympathetic stimulation (usually increased stimulation or parasympatheticotonia) promotes passage and/or absorption of contents to most hollow organs. It contracts tubes, ducts, bladders, and vessels and opens their sphincters (84).

Adaptation is perhaps the single most important function of the nervous system. Consequently, the physiological manifestations of spinovisceral dynamics are often obscure. For example, vagal dysfunction may initiate a pathophysiological condition in the viscera that it innervates. The viscera, via sympathetic or somatic afferent pathways to the thoracic spine, may cause a compensatory alteration in local sympathetic activity by perhaps increasing sympathetic tone and adapting to the primary hyperparasympathetic disorder. Correcting the altered sympathetic function in this situation would not restore normal visceral function. Vertebral subluxation complexes appear to have a variety of effects on nerve function. Some

subluxations appear to be facilitory and produce a hyperirritation of efferent nerves while other subluxations appear to have dystonic effects which suppress nerve function. The chiropractic premise is that effective correction of a subluxation will reduce the subluxation and restore a more optimal neural and paraneural environment that will, in turn, improve nerve health and function, as well as that of the target organs served. A viscera with an established primary disease process, though manifesting viscerosomatic spinal signs and even symptoms via viscerosomatic referral, if aggressive, warrants consultation by a specialist.

The chiropractor must assess all regions of the spine for indications of vertebral subluxation complex and establish a clinical prognosis and a time frame necessary for recovery based upon the complexity and chronicity of the visceral and spinal disturbances. Fortunately, in a pediatric patient, many conditions have not reached the level of complexity and chronicity typically seen in the adult.

ON BRAIN FUNCTION/ LEARNING DEVELOPMENT—"BRAIN HIBERNATION"

Slow learning in children has been attributed to autonomic dysregulation. "Brain hibernation" is a sub-optimal level of brain function characterized by diminished cortical ability. Terrett has investigated the effects of regionally diminished cerebral blood flow and notes that a host of dysfunctions appear to be attributable to altered CSF production or circulation (85) (Table 13.9). "Brain hibernation" occurs when there is diminished vascular irrigation of regions of the brain. The result is suspension of function without cellular death. The tissues most susceptible to this are the higher order brain tissues (cortical), rather than those concerned with the brain's regulation of basal functions (85) (Table 13.10).

Outer brain tissues are supplied by extra-parenchymal blood vessels—the core regions have intraparenchymal and pial blood supplies. The outer and pia supplies have been seen to be influenced by vasoconstriction as a result of sympathetic

---

Table 13.9. Signs and Symptoms That Are Theorized Could Be Caused by Decreased Cerebral Performance

Giddiness/dizziness	Lethargy/excessive tiredness
Difficulty sleeping/ insomnia	Depression
Nervousness	Restlessness/anxious
Miserable/irritable	Disoriented
Personality change	Hyperkinesia in children
Whining child syndrome	Tantrums
Headache	Problems with memory
Learning disabilities	Poor concentration
Difficulty thinking	Clumsiness
Changes in visual acuity	Visual disorders
Auditory disorders	Mixing up words
Losing track of conversation while talking	Loss of interest in sex in adults

Adapted from Terrett AGJ. Cerebral Dysfunction: A Theory to Explain Some of the Effects of Chiropractic Manipulation. Journal of Chiropractic Technique 1993 November; 5(4):168–173.

Table 13.10. Disorders That Are Proposed May Be Produced by Progressive Decrease in Cerebral Blood Flow (CBF)

Normal CBF (Oxygen Normal) All Cerebral Units Operational	Decreased CBF (Less Oxygen than Normal) Not All Cerebral Units Operational	Further Decrease in CBF (Poor Oxygen Supply) Few Cerebral Units Operational
No giddiness	Giddy with use of the arms, or postural changes	Giddy all or most of the time
Normal visual field	Some loss of peripheral vision	Tunnel vision
Able to read fine print	Some visual difficulty	Only able to read large print
Happy	Irritable under stress	Irritable all of the time
Able to cope with calculations	Difficulty with calculations	Unable to cope with calculations
Well rested	Easily tired	Feels continually tired
Well coordinated	Problems with manual tasks under stress	Clumsy
Never or rarely suffers headaches	Headaches under stress	Commonly suffers headaches

Adapted from Terrett AGJ. Cerebral Dysfunction: A Theory to Explain Some of the Effects of Chiropractic Manipulation. Journal of Chiropractic Technique 1993 November; 5(4):168–173.

discharges and by vasodilatation as a result of parasympathetic discharges. The core regions with their intraparenchymal supply are the least affected by a reduced blood flow. Though cerebral vessels largely "autoregulate" in response to carbon dioxide levels, cervical sympathetic nerves change the way they autoregulate by altering their sensitivity to carbon dioxide level (86).

Interestingly, the cervical sympathetic ganglia modulate the production of CSF through vasomotor effects on the choroid plexus (87). Increased vasomotor tone of the choroidal regions decreases CSF production (87).

Alterations in the blood supply of the brain cause many of the pathological processes that affect the brain. Branches of the sympathetic autonomic system innervate and control the internal carotid arteries, carotid plexus, cavernous plexus and circle of Willis, and generally influence brain hemodynamics and neuroregulatory functions (88).

Burns found extensive circulatory disturbances in the brain which are associated with upper cervical lesions, particularly the C1 vertebra (54). Burns noted the relation between the vascular perfusion of the pituitary, the subsequent influence on the hypothalamus, and the resulting influence on the rest of the body (54).

The true incidence of headaches in children is not known. The role of headaches in children's learning difficulties has not been considered, although, in adults, headaches make attentive learning difficult. Migraine headaches and associated transient symptoms, such as nausea, vomiting, irritability, photophobia, visual field disturbances, speech disorders, and paraesthesias, are associated with vascular overreaction (28).

Further, vascular disease in the brain may establish a susceptibility to erroneous autonomic discharge swings causing mild petite mal seizures (86).

Burns experimentally induced C1 lesions in rats. They had fewer successful runs through a maze and were more "frustrated" than non-lesioned rats. When autopsied, they had an accumulation of cerebrospinal fluid sufficient to flatten the surface of the brain (54,89).

Becker found that children with attention-deficit disorder (ADD) can benefit significantly from osteopathic manipulative therapy (54).

In conclusion, upper cervical spinal nerves innervate the superior sympathetic ganglion. This ganglion has a tonic/trophic influence on the irrigation of cerebral tissues. The cervical spine also innervates the last three cranial nerves (sensory portion) and a cranial nerve sensory tract (cranial nerve 5) within the spinal cord (see previous text). The thoracic spinal nerves influence the sympathetic ganglionated chain which, in turn, influences vasoregulators and cranial nerve targets. Thoracic spinal nerves also influence the ascending spinoraphe or reticular tracts in the spinal cord. This influences the excitation levels of the reticular formation in the mid brain.

Systemic Immune System

Axons of the sympathetic nervous system innervate the parenchyma of the spleen, lymphoid tissue, bone marrow, and thymus. Nerve endings contact T-lymphocytes, monocytes and to a lesser degree, B-lymphocytes. This is verified by the presence of numerous types of neurotransmitter receptors on T-cells, B-cells, suppressor cells and macrophages. Most of these receptors are specific for norepinephrine and epinephrine—the chief transmitters of the sympathetic nerve system (2). In addition to these, receptors sites have been found for histaminic substances, somatastatin, VIP, and other active peptides (90).

The effects of catecholamines (sympathetic neurotransmitters) on T-lymphocytes at low concentrations is stimulatory, but at high concentrations, catecholamines are inhibitory. Control by the sympathetic nervous system exists in the conventional sense as its neurotransmitters affect receptor sites (90). Further, a trophic influence is expected by the sympathetic system to help manufacture the cytokines which influence lymphocyte responses. Nerves supply not only their own cellular processes with essential biochemicals, but also those of their end organs. Both "cytokines" (chemical regulators of immune cell responses) as well as "neurokines" (chemical regulators of the nerve cell activity) are found within the nerve system (91). Evidence even suggests that cytokines and neurokines are transmutable (91).

High-weight molecular proteins within sympathetic ganglia inhibit lymphocyte cell production. Because the SNS plays a major role in inhibiting the immune response, autoimmune disorders have been associated with sympathetic hypoactivity, either regionally or systemically. Recently, myasthenia gravis and MS have been added to the list of autoimmune disorders. Arnason and Byto associated these two conditions with diminished sympathetic control (92).

Fidelibus claims that the neuropeptides and neurohormones—adrenocorticotrophic hormone (ADH), endorphins, encephalins, vasoactive intestinal peptides and substance P—are stored or synthesized in white blood cells. There have now been more than 50 neuropeptides recognized in the body (93). When released from the white cells, some are believed to generate afferent stimulation according to how the immune response is progressing. Fidelibus states that these "immunotransmitters" produce a type of unconscious nerve stimuli as a result of sensing the fine events or microchanges of the internal environment.

Regionally, sympathetic ablation studies suggest that the SNS orchestrates the progression of cellular and humoral responses. The effects of severing sympathetic innervation on immunological function was studied by Stein-Werblowsky. Stein-Werblowsky found that sympathetic nerves are concerned primarily with the initiation of the immune or inflammatory reaction, setting off a chain of reactions which leads to cell-mediated, homograft immunity. It was found that tissues which were previously tumor-resistant became receptive hosts to grafts of transplanted tumor conjugates following sympathetic denervation. Two-thirds of the animals (24 of 38) with the destroyed sympathetic nerves supported the tumor preparations whereas only one of the 30 intact normal animals supported the tumor implant (94).

Systemically, macrophages release a neuromodulator that binds to sites in the hypothalamus and initiates fever and depresses appetite. The symptoms of hypotension, lassitude, fatigue, myalgia, and headache which characterize systemic viral illness may partially depend upon the actions of circulating cytokines on sympathetic nerves systemically (92).

Clinically, Allen lists a half dozen studies indicating increases in lymphocyte levels with adjustments (91). Brennan et al found that chiropractic spinal adjustments increased both polymorphonucleocytes (PMN) and monocytes if the adjustment was of sufficient force and impulse (95). It is apparent that the nervous system "talks" with the immune system via the SNS, and possibly via the PNS as well, though there are fewer studies on the latter (95). Obviously, any significant organ disregulation, in particular, those of the adrenals, liver, and pancreas, generally causes a lowered tissue resistance (88).

GI Tract

Most intestinal functions are intrinsically controlled by the "third" nervous system, the enteric nervous system. The enteric nervous system is composed of local simple reflex arc. As contents fill a cavity, juices are secreted which causes the tube to squeeze rhythmically in transverse and longitudinal waves, "chopping and passing" materials (peristalsis). The parasympathetic system is most active during maximum peristalsis. The sympathetic nerve system modulates parasympathetic nerves ephaptically and synaptically at the ganglia, plexi, and terminal gaps.

While the enteric nerve system has a dominating influence on peristalsis through most of the approximately 25 feet of intestinal tubing, the central autonomic control significantly influences each end, namely, the entrance beginning with the lips, mouth, esophagus, stomach and duodenum, and the exit, beginning near the proximal large intestine (ileocecum) through the descending colon and anus.

In the work-up of a patient complaining of intestinal disturbances, look for any changes in stool color and consistency. This is to determine the general motility and water content. Increased motility and fluid indicates imbalanced, unchecked parasympathetic tone.

The GI tract receives sympathetic innervation from T8 to L2 and parasympathetic innervation from the brain stem (vagus nerve) and S2 to S4 sacral roots. Lawrence states that a C1 subluxation may affect, either directly or indirectly, the vagus nerve (88). This may be due to the inferior vagal ganglion being exposed to the occipitoatlantal dynamics (88). In generalized gastrointestinal disease, a study by Nicholas found palpatory findings of subluxations in the region of T7 to T12, the vertebral sympathetic supply (84). See the appendix on selected visceral disorders for the neurology of specific conditions and chiropractic management as described in the literature.

Pediatric Neurologic Evaluation

The clinician must be relaxed and patient and have keen observational skills when examining the neonate, infant, child or adolescent. The examiner must also bear in mind that the level of maturity and integrity of the nervous system and the level of communications skills that the child possesses will alter elements of the neurological examination.

A period of neurological shock has been observed in the newborn immediately after birth and may last up to 24 to 60 hours (96). The most prominent neurological finding during this period of birth shock is poor muscle tone, although not as extreme as is found in pathological cases of shock, atonia, or mongolism (96–97). When the examiner palpates the skin of a newborn whose muscle tone is still poor, the sensation is not unlike that of a feather quilt or the skin of an overripe fruit. There may also be findings of minimal resistance to movement and postural attitudes which may be characterized as pretonic in nature (96).

The birth shock period is considered physiological by some. Others feel that it is due to anoxia and traumatizing mechanical factors that inhibit the normal functions of the nervous system. Escardo and De Coriat found that appropriate psychoprophylactic care given to the mother during pregnancy may decrease this period of birth shock by allowing the mother to concentrate and consciously direct her muscular efforts without fear. This would shorten the uterine contractions that impinge against the newborn's body, particularly the head. These researchers speak of the "painless childbirth" as a benefit of appropriate psychoprophylactic care (96).

Avoiding sedatives and anesthesia, decreasing muscle tension, and perhaps improving the emotional attitudes of the mother and others attending the birth may stimulate the receptors of the newborn which may influence the activity of the central nervous system beginning in early intrauterine life. Because intensification of the birth shock to pathologic levels may threaten the neurologic future of the newborn, reducing the duration of this shock period may assure a better prognosis (96).

After the period of birth shock, the examiner begins the evaluation by observing the infant at rest for spontaneous movements, palpebral fissure equality, and eye abnormalities such as the "setting sun sign" and Marcus-Gunn sign (elevation of the lid with jaw movements) or other signs of neurological deficits, such as writhing baby syndrome, myoclonus, flaccidity, jitteriness, and irregular development among others (Figs. 13.15, 13.16).

In the normal newborn, the purposeless movements of the extremities are associated with well-defined muscle tone in spite of the lack of motor skills. In addition, the normal newborn has a well-developed ability to suck and swallow.

Neurological Development in Infancy and Early Childhood

The neonatal child's nervous system is not a simple system spontaneously changing from its original level of immaturity to its final mature state. It matures in a specific pattern which is constantly subject to self-regulating mechanisms. Each stage must be passed through in sequence. If there is a failure in the self-regulating mechanism, the organism, when confronted by a new situation, can only respond by modifying the current stage of maturation through a mechanism of adaptation. The

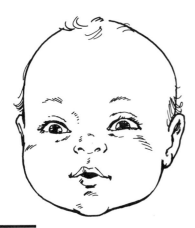

Figure 13.15. Setting sun sign. Modified from Haynes U. A developmental approach to case finding. Washington, DC: U.S. Department of Health, Education, and Welfare, 1967.

system attempts to make optimal adaptation. This is often referred to as the brain's "plasticity" or "dynamism."

The developmental and neurologic examination of the infant and young child differs in several respects from that of an adult. Initially, a neurologic abnormality in an infant is usually diffuse rather than localized, and there may be a continuum of damage that ranges from minimal to severe. The sequelae may be a variety of neurological and possibly psychological abnormalities.

Neurological integrity and maturation or development are intertwined. A mere cataloguing of abnormal signs without reference to the developmental level of the infant is inadequate for making a decision as to the individual's level of health. The process of maturational development itself may cause compensatory changes so that seemingly significant deviations from normal in infancy may leave no discernible residuals in later examinations. An analogous event is the orthopedic case of scoliosis. The chiropractic doctor has the clinical experience of understanding the adaptability of the scoliotic spinal condition based upon the principle of dynamic homeostasis. Highly invasive intervention without regard to this principle may produce disastrous results. In most of these cases, proper management with little or no invasive intervention to aid the natural process of adaptation allows the child to grow into a normal healthy individual. The static and dynamic development from neonate into adulthood depends upon the maturation process and integrity of the central and peripheral nervous systems. This process of development is determined by genetically established patterns of behavior and stimulation from the environment and the individual's ability to adapt to the environment. The chiropractor is clearly interested in the CNS and PNS as it relates the growing child to its environment.

Assessment and Neurologic Screening

A chiropractic clinician must conduct neurological screening tests when evaluating an infant. These may include, but are not limited to, positioning, spontaneous and induced movements,

crying, knee and ankle jerk, and elicitation of the rooting, grasp, tonic neck, and Moro automatisms. Neonates with neurological abnormalities and those at risk for central nervous system interference require comprehensive neurological evaluations at frequent intervals.

Findings during the neurologic examination differ significantly as the child develops and the nervous system matures. At birth, the undeveloped central nervous system functions at subcortical levels. Cortical functions develop slowly and cannot be fully tested until early childhood. Therefore, in the neurologic evaluation during the newborn and early infancy period, establishing whether there is normal brainstem and spinal function does not necessarily imply an intact cortical system as cortical abnormalities may exist without concomitant brainstem or spinal cord abnormalities (98).

A number of infantile automatisms are found in the normal neonate and should disappear in early infancy. Absence of infantile automatisms in the neonate or persistence of these beyond the expected time of their disappearance may indicate nerve system interference (98–100).

Intracranial central nervous system lesions may lead to postural abnormalities, particularly, persistent asymmetries—e.g., predominant extension of the extremities and constant

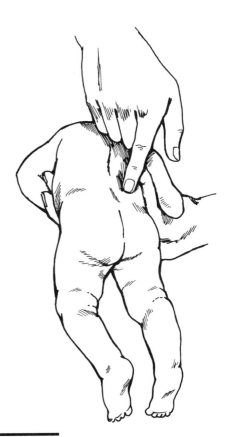

Figure 13.16. Trunk incurvation response to a finger running down the paravertebral area. Modified from Paine RS. Neurologic examination of infants and children. Ped Clin North Am 1960;7(3):490.

turning of the head to one side (98–100). Marked extension of the head, stiffness of the neck, and extension of the extremities (opisthotonus) is indicative of significant meningeal or brainstem irritation as is seen in intracranial infection or hemorrhage (97,101,102).

SENSORY EXAMINATION

The usefulness of the sensory examination in the child is limited. Thresholds for touch, pain, and temperature are high in older children, and reactions to these stimuli are relatively slow. Gross sensory testing can be useful. Absence of the withdrawal response when a painful stimulus applied to an extremity is indicative of paralysis. If a painful stimulus produces a facial change or crying without a withdrawal response, the examiner would suspect paralysis rather than anesthesia. Interference in the spinal cord may cause a withdrawal response to a painful stimulus without a change in facial expression or crying, i.e., anesthesia rather than paralysis (98–100,103,104).

CRANIAL NERVE TESTING

Cranial nerve testing is performed as in an adult, although there may be some difficulty in assessing the optic and auditory nerves. The hypoglossal nerve (cranial nerve 12) is easily tested in the infant by pinching the nostrils. There should be a reflexive opening of the mouth and a raising of the tip of the tongue. If a 12th cranial nerve paresis is present, the tip of the tongue will deviate towards the affected side (99).

REFLEXES

Corticospinal pathways are immature in the child leading to variable spinal reflexes—i.e., deep tendon reflexes and plantar response. Their exaggerated presence or their absence has little diagnostic significance unless the response is different from those observed in previous testing (99).

Mastering the Pediatric Neurological Examination

Responses to stimuli form a large part of the neurological examination of an infant. These responses include the Moro response, Dazzle reflex, dorsal reflex, Landau sign, Babinski sign, plantar and palmar grasp response, rooting reflex, extension reflex of the fingers, stepping response, placing response, tonic neck response, neck righting reflex, blink reflex, jerking reflex to sound, knee jerk, clonus, and the parachute response, among others. To master the examination, the chiropractic doctor must constantly practice these procedures. A clinician well versed in these procedures will be able to recognize the importance of these tests and will be able to recognize altered responses.

It is important to give that part of the exam least disturbing to the child first. Observation is the least invasive part of the evaluation. Observe the infant's position movements for normal automatic reactions. The infant is placed prone with the upper extremities alongside to the torso. One or both arms will normally and spontaneously be brought forward so that the hands lay level with a shoulder or the face. Initially, this position usually occurs, and often solely occurs, on the side that

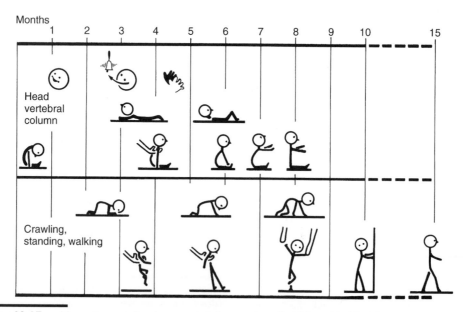

Figure 13.17.   Normal motor development in infants and small children. Modified from Mumenthaler M. Neurology (3rd ed.) New York: Thieme Medical Publishers, Inc., 1990, p. 2.

the face is turned towards. This reaction may be facilitated by applying pressure to the opposite buttocks. The examiner may also notice the infant turning his/her head to one side or alternately rotating the head side to side. The infant may attempt to raise the head and/or perform a creep or crawl motion with the lower extremities. The creep motion may be stimulated by gentle pressure on the soles of the feet. The response may be vigorous enough to propel the baby forward. These movements are expected in a normal infant (101–105).

NORMAL TONE

In order to understanding the evolving neurological patterns during the perinatal period (from the twentieth to twenty-eighth week of gestation to 7 to 28 days after birth) and later, the examiner must become familiar with the changes occurring in the tonus and the consistency of primary or automatic reactions of the growing infant. Flexor tonus of the extremities increases with maturation from the more caudal muscles to those more cephalic. The posture of the most premature infant of about 28 weeks gestation is commonly one of extension (or deflexion) of all limbs. With further maturation, tonus increases in the lower extremities. By the thirty-fifth week, the infant lies primarily with the legs flexed and the arms extended in the "frog position" (104). The normal developing pattern progresses to increased upper extremity flexor tonus. As tonus increases, the range of spontaneous movement diminishes. Brett states that the free windmill-like movements of the early premature infant will gradually diminish to the relative immobility of the term infant who may be described as "a prisoner of his/her own tone" (101,102,104,105) (Fig. 13.17).

Primary and Automatic Reactions

Most of the repertoire of primary or automatic reactions observed in the normal infant are mediated at the subcortical level; some are even obtainable in the anencephalics (104). An exception is the placing response—described as flexion followed by extension of the leg which occurs when the normal infant six weeks of age and younger is held erect, and the examiner allows the dorsum of the foot to be drawn along the under edge of a tabletop. The placing reaction is typically absent in all four limbs of children with mental ages of less than four months (IQs less than 28) (105). Animal studies show that the placing reflex is dependent upon the presence of a considerable amount of cortex, particularly the parietal lobe area 4 of the post-central gyrus (note that this area is sensory) (105). Establishing the neuroanatomical location in the cerebral cortex helps to explain this peculiar association between a postural reflex and cognitive development. Therefore, it has been concluded that the absence of the placing reaction is an index of severe mental retardation (101,102,104) (Fig. 13.18).

NEUROLOGICAL RESPONSIBILITIES
OF THE EXAMINER

The primary concern of the examining chiropractor is the evaluation of the health status of his/her patient. The importance and uniqueness of the chiropractic neurological assess-

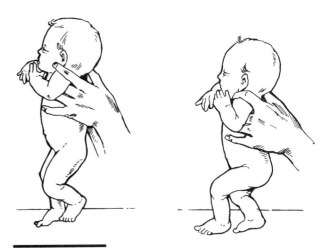

Figure 13.18. Placing response. Modified from Bates B. A guide to physical examination and history taking (5th ed). Philadelphia: J. B. Lippincott Co., 1991, p. 630.

ment is demonstrated by the fact that most chiropractors obtain clinical information related to the overall level of health expression, not merely the presence or absence of a disease state. To recognize that human beings can always achieve a higher expression of health is somewhat unique to the chiropractic profession. Therefore, it is imperative for the chiropractic examiner to understand and obtain the neurologic responses.

The chiropractic examination begins with the examiner asking: "Is there interference with the function of the nervous system?" If so, where is it? What is it? And, what can be done about it? In addition, the examiner must ask, "Has the nervous system matured appropriately for the child's age?" Anatomic orientation is, of course, an intellectual exercise. Yet, knowing the suspected or actual location of the interference or lesion aids the doctor in planning a course of care that may lead towards the expression of optimum health.

An ideal starting point is hypotonia, a condition that is easily recognized. It is a nonspecific sign and may be a result of dysfunction at any point along the entire neuraxis. The cerebral cortex, basal ganglia, cerebellum, spinal cord (including the anterior horn cell), nerves, and even muscles and ligaments are suspect. During the observation phase of the examination, a finding of unusual joint laxity may accompany the hypotonia/"floppiness" of differing etiologies and is occasionally quite dramatic to the point of becoming the chief complaint. This laxity may even be confused with Ehlers-Danlos syndrome, a collection of inheritable collagen diseases with hyperextendable joints and skin but usually near normal strength (107,108). Differentiation must also be made from infantile spinal muscular atrophy or Werdnig-Hoffman disease, a condition affecting the anterior horn cells of the spinal cord without involvement of the cerebral cortex. Werdnig-Hoffman disease is marked by delayed motor "milestones" (99,105–107,109,110). Oppenheim, in 1900, described a condition, "amyotonia congenita," which is a congenitally diffuse muscular weakness with atrophy of the muscles and decreased or absent deep tendon reflexes that tended to improve. This condition can be differentiated from Werdnig-Hoffman disease by electromyography (EMG) studies and the fact that Werdnig-Hoffman disease is progressive and is usually fatal by age five years (62). These few examples show that there are many forms of hypotonia.

Hypotonia is a generalized decrease in muscular activity and can be measured by the overall amount of muscular activity. Hypotonia can be concluded if an infant presents with little or no spontaneous movement, does not adjust to postural demands, and has little resistance to passive extremity movements (62,107,110). In contrast, the hypertonic state may result in spasticity and rigidity in response to postural changes and passive movements, as well as increased spontaneous activity (62,99,111,112). Muscle tone and floppiness should be graded as weakness or true hypotonia. For accuracy, tone must be assessed in the alert but not overaroused infant. Resistance offered to passive movements is a subjective finding and must be correlated to the state of arousal. Bilateral comparisons of extremities, trunk, and neck should be evaluated.

Diminished tone occurring with normal strength is indicative of central nervous system involvement (Fig. 13.19). Many infants with central hypotonia will later develop excessive tone. The hypertonia may be localized to specific areas with other areas remaining hypotonic. When this is seen, the examiner should pay particular attention to the thumb adductors, wrist pronators, and hip adductors which are often the first to stiffen—cortical thumb and leg scissoring is often observed in early cerebral palsy (107,108,110,112).

STRENGTH

In the assessment of strength, the crying baby will usually provide the most accurate information. Bilateral comparison is important. In the adult and older child, the 5-point motor strength grading scale can be used, but this scale cannot be applied to the infant and younger child. In this case, strength can be documented by noting the heaviest toy or other object

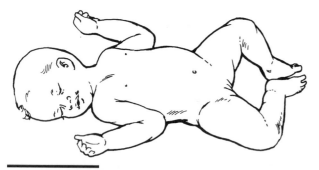

Figure 13.19. A hypotonic infant at rest. The thighs are in a fully abducted "frog leg" position and arms are in a flaccid position alongside the head. Modified from Fenichel GM. Clinical pediatric neurology. Philadelphia: W.B. Saunders Co., 1988, p. 147.

that the infant can pick up (62,107,110). The distance that a particular extremity can be extended or the amount of truncal tilt before the head loses support should be noted. A uniquely chiropractic procedure is for the examiner to hold the infant up under the armpits, face-to-face, and slowly tilt the trunk to the left, right, forward, and backwards. Note any asymmetries in head support.

WEAKNESS

The presence of weakness must be graded as it generally implies motor unit involvement. Central involvement may be present since weak infants are also hypotonic. In the previously mentioned Werdnig-Hoffman disease, the muscles of the face, diaphragm, and pelvic sphincters are classically spared (107,110,113). In general, infantile myasthenic syndromes preferentially affect the bulbar and oculomotor muscles. Most myopathies tend to affect proximal limb muscle function more than fine distal movements of the digits (107,110,113).

DEEP TENDON REFLEXES

Generally, deep tendon reflexes are easily obtained at the biceps, knees, and ankles. Other reflexes may be more difficult to obtain. The floppy child with hyperactive reflexes almost certainly has central nerve system dysfunction as in the case of the hypotonic infant with normal strength (107,110,113). Muscle disease is characterized by both hyporeflexia and weakness (107,110,113). If the reflexes are completely absent and not proportional to the amount of weakness, neuropathy or central nerve system disease is suspected. Hyperreflexia implies interference between the cortex and anterior horn cells in the spinal cord (so-called upper motor neuron), and hyporeflexia implies interference between the anterior horn of the spinal cord and the muscle (lower motor neuron).

HYPERACTIVE REFLEXES (HYPERREFLEXIA)

Frequently, the examiner will find children with exaggerated reflexes that might be considered hyperactive, but hyperactive reflexes in the presence of downgoing toes upon plantar stroking are usually normal (107,110,111,114). If hyperactive reflexes truly reflect pyramidal tract interference, the toes should also respond abnormally, i.e., upgoing. Using plantar reflex (Babinski sign) to determine the reaction of the toes does not always yield good results, despite the popularity of this test. Chaddock maneuver (stroking the dorsolateral aspect of the foot) (111,114) may be used to elicit a Babinski-like response with much more accuracy (111,114). Contraction of the tensor fascia lata following stroking of the sole of the foot suggests pyramidal tract dysfunction (111,114). It should not be confused with contraction due to withdrawal of the foot. Abdominal reflexes (stroking the skin adjacent to the umbilicus) may be absent on the side of pyramidal tract dysfunction (111,114). In children with hyperactive reflexes, it is important to check for the presence of a jaw jerk. Its presence suggests bilateral interference above the midpons which would affect the motor division of the fifth cranial nerve (111,114).

Unilateral upgoing toe (using Babinski or Chaddock maneuvers) or hyperreflexia suggests interference to one side of the nervous system. The examiner must determine whether this is indicative of an old lesion or a recent one. The history becomes important. Was the birth difficult? Had there been neonatal complications? An otherwise normal appearing child may have unilateral hyperreflexia due to birth injury or mild cerebral palsy. Looking for asymmetry in extremity development or handedness may reveal a clue (107,111,114). Left handedness may indicate left hemisphere involvement. Unilateral hyperreflexia may be a result of an old neurologic lesion, meningitis, head trauma, or even uncomplicated subdural hematoma (107,111,114). Other than cerebral palsy, hydrocephalus, or parasagittal intracranial mass, hyperreflexia in the extremities suggests interference or lesion at the cervical cord or higher (107,111,114). Hyperreflexia in the lower extremities suggests interference at cord levels below the cervical cord; bilateral hyperreflexia suggests bilateral interference in the pyramidal tract (107,111,114). Tumors, bony abnormalities, and perhaps non-CNS tumors, among other space-occupying masses may be etiological factors (107,111,114).

HYPOACTIVE REFLEXES (HYPOREFLEXIA)

Hyporeflexia is usually indicative of peripheral nerve interference; although it is seen when any component of the reflex pathway is abnormal. It may be necessary to perform the Jendrassik maneuver (have the child clasp his/her hands together and try to pull them apart, make a fist, or bite down) to elicit a response or reinforce the reflex (98,77,111,115). Occasionally, the examiner may be presented with an otherwise normal child who displays hyporeflexia without an obvious cause. Areflexia may be seen in the initial stages of cord damage which may be traumatic, vascular, or neoplastic in origin. Hyperreflexia may be seen in later stages (112). Hyporeflexia may be seen in later stages of myopathies (98,100,112). Weakness from muscle disorders is generally proximal (hip and shoulder) while weakness from peripheral nerve involvement is usually distal (hand and foot) (98,100,112).

GENERAL MOVEMENTS

When observing an infant, the examiner may notice changes in general movements (GM). One study videotaped the spontaneous motility in the supine position of a group of 22 full term healthy infants aged 2 to 18 weeks at four week intervals. Each follow-up session included a neurological examination. In the newborn infant, the GM had a "writhing" quality to it; the movements were characterized as tight in quality, slow speed, and of limited amplitude. The "writhing" character gradually evolves into a so-called "fidgety" character. This "fidgety" character was almost constant by the age of 8 to 12 weeks. In the third month, very rapid hand movements ("swipes" and "swats") were seen. The developmental changes in the form of the GM and those of the neurological repertoire showed no significant correlation. However, studies on the development of head and eye movements in early infancy illustrated that the communication between the visual, vestibular, head and eye movement systems showed a marked shift between the second and third month of life. It has been suggested that the changes in visuomotor behavior, including

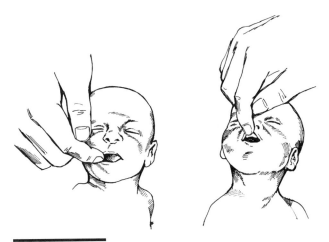

Figure 13.20. Rooting reflex. Modified from Paine RS. Neurologic examination of infants and children. Ped Clin North Am 1960;7(3):483.

the appearance of steady fixation and brisk orienting reactions, reflected the establishment of functional connections between different cortical areas and between the cerebral cortex and the tectum (116,117).

The following testing procedures can easily be understood so long as the examiner masters the understanding of the mechanisms involved. The names given to these tests are not always reported as the same; i.e., authors have given identical or similar tests other names.

REFLEX TESTING (BEHAVIOR PATTERNS)

Feeding behavior is best demonstrated and exhibited by the infant after spontaneous awakening (known as the Gentry-Aldrich Rooting Reflex) (118). Gentry and Aldrich have demonstrated that the newborn infant who is in deep sleep did not exhibit the rooting reflex The rooting reflex is opening of the mouth and rotating the head toward the side of constant light pressure or light stroking on the cheek. It should not be confused with the side to side head movement or the head turning from the preferred side upon stroking (118). Sleeping, dozing, and crying will interfere with the rooting reflex (Fig. 13.20).

The sucking response is elicited by touching the infant's lips. Drowsiness depresses the sucking response. Gentry and Aldrich found that the best time for feeding is after spontaneous awakening, and is essentially governed by real need. The infant always awakens when he/she needs to eat, but will not always need to eat when awakening.

CORRELATION OF REFLEX TESTS WITH CENTRAL NERVOUS SYSTEM DEVELOPMENT

Note: The following testing procedures can be easily understood if the examiner understands the mechanisms involved. Some of these tests have more than one name.

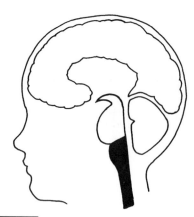

Figure 13.21. Spinal cord level.

SPINAL LEVEL

Reflexes at the spinal level are mediated in the CNS by Deiters' nucleus which is located in the lower one-third of the pons (114). Spinal reflexes are considered "phasic" because there is movement which coordinates muscles of the extremities in either total flexion or extension (114). During the first two months of life, positive or negative reactions to spinal reflex testing may be present in the normal child (98,100,114). After two months of age, persistence of positive reactions may be indicative of delayed maturation of the CNS. At this point, negative reactions are normal (98,100,114). Apedal (prone or supine-lying) positions are a result of complete domination by these primitive spinal reflexes (98,100,114) (Fig. 13.21).

TESTS

WITHDRAWAL RESPONSE TO STIMULUS

The infant is placed in the supine position. An irritating stimulus is applied to the foot. A negative response is volitional withdrawal or a controlled maintenance response. A positive reaction consists of uncontrolled flexion of tested leg which is not to be confused with a reaction to tickling. A positive reaction is normal up to two months of age. Delayed reflexive maturation is suspected if a positive reaction continues after two months of age (98-100,106,114) (Fig. 13.22).

EXTENSOR RESPONSE TO STIMULUS

The child is tested in the supine position. The head is kept in the neutral position and one leg is extended and the other flexed. A stimulus is applied to the sole of the foot on the side of the flexed leg. A negative reaction is the leg maintained in controlled flexion. A positive reaction is an uncontrolled extension of the stimulated leg. Do not confuse this with a tickling reaction. A positive reaction is normal only up to age two months; after that, it is indicative of delayed reflexive maturation (98–100,114) (Fig. 13.23).

CONTRALATERAL EXTENSION TO STIMULUS

The infant is positioned as per the extensor thrust response. In this test, the stimulus is applied by flexing the extended leg. A negative response is the continuation of the flexed position of the contralateral leg. A positive reaction is extension of the contralateral flexed leg. A positive reaction is normal up to the age of 2 months and is abnormal after that (98–100,114).

There is an alternate method of testing this response. The infant is in the same position. The stimulus is applied by tapping the medial surface of one leg. There should be no

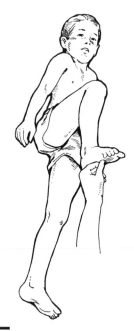

Figure 13.22. Flexor withdrawal test—positive reaction. Modified from Fiorentino MR. Reflex testing methods for evaluating CNS development (2nd ed). Springfield, IL: Charles C Thomas Publishers, 1973, p. 9.

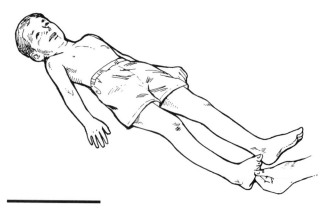

Figure 13.23. Extensor thrust—positive reaction. Modified from Fiorentino MR. Reflex testing methods for evaluating CNS development (2nd ed). Springfield, IL: Charles C Thomas Publishers, 1973, p. 10.

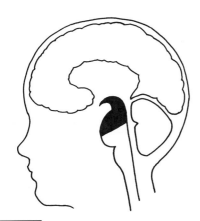

Figure 13.24.   Brain stem level.

response. A positive reaction is adduction and internal rotation of the contralateral leg along with plantar flexion of the foot. This is typical of the scissor position. A positive reaction is normal up to age two months; a positive reaction beyond this point is indicative of delayed reflexive maturation (98–100,114).

Brain Stem Level

From the caudal level of the basal ganglia down to Deiters' nucleus is an area of the brain stem where the following reflexes are mediated (Fig. 13.24). These brain stem reflexes are "static." They are postural responses—a response to changes in the position of the head and body in space (responding to stimulation of the labyrinths) or in the head position relative to the body (proprioception in the cervical spine) (98–100,114). During the first 4 to 6 months, positive or negative reactions to the brainstem responses are normal. Positive reactions persisting beyond 6 months of age suggests delayed motor maturation of the central nervous system. Negative responses are normal. Complete domination by these response results in apedal posture (98,100,114).

TESTS

EXTREMITY RESPONSE TO HEAD ROTATION

This test is performed with the child in the supine position, head is in the neutral position, and all extremities are extended. The testing stimulus is provided by rotating the infant's head one side. A negative reaction is no reaction. A positive response occurs when there is extension of the ipsilateral arm and leg on the side the face is turned towards or an increase in extensor tone and flexion of the contralateral arm and leg or an increase in flexor tone. A positive reaction is normal up to four to six months of age, beyond that point, a positive reaction may be indicative of delayed reflexive maturation (98,100,102,106,114) (Fig. 13.25).

EXTREMITY RESPONSE TO HEAD FLEXION

This test is performed with the child lying prone in the quadruped position over the examiner's knees. The test stimulus is provided by forward flexion of the head. A negative reaction is no change in tone of the extremities. A positive reaction is flexion or an increase in tone of the upper extremities and an increase in tone or extension of the lower extremities (98,100,102,106,114).

EXTREMITY RESPONSE TO HEAD EXTENSION

The positioning of the patient is identical to Extremity Response to Head Flexion. In this test, the head is dorsiflexed. A negative reaction is no change in tone of the extremities. A positive response is extension or increased tone in the upper extremities and flexion or increased tone in the lower extremities (98,100,102,106,114).

SUPINE PROPRIOCEPTIVE RESPONSE (TONIC)

The child is supine with the head in the neutral position and all extremities are extended. A negative response is no increase in extensor tone of the extremities even when they are passively flexed (Fig. 13.26). A positive reaction is indicated when extensor tone dominates when the extremities are passively flexed. A positive reaction is normal up to four months of age. A positive reaction after four months of age may indicate delayed reflexive maturation (98,100,102,106,114).

PRONE PROPRIOCEPTIVE RESPONSE (TONIC)

In this test, the infant is lying prone, and the examiner observes the head position. A negative reaction is extension of the head without an increase in flexor tone (Fig. 13.27). A positive reaction is an inability to dorsiflex the head, retract the shoulders, or extend the trunk or extremities. Positive reactions are normal up to four months of age and may be indicative of delayed reflexive maturation after that (93,100,114).

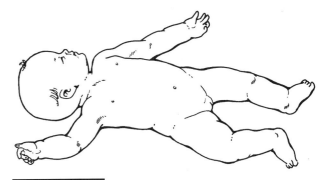

Figure 13.25.   Extremity response to head rotation or asymmetric tonic neck reflex. Modified from Brett EM (ed). Pediatric neurology. New York: Churchill Livingstone, 1991, p. 8.

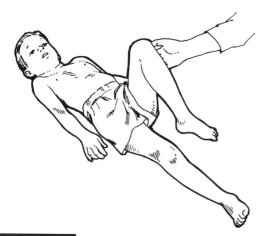

Figure 13.26. Tonic labrynthine supine—negative reaction. Modified from Fiorentino MR. Reflex testing methods for evaluating CNS development (2nd ed). Springfield, IL: Charles C Thomas Publishers, 1973, p. 17.

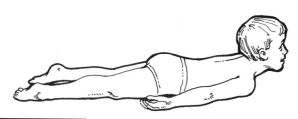

Figure 13.27. Tonic labrynthine prone—negative reaction. Modified from Fiorentino MR. Reflex testing methods for evaluating CNS development (2nd ed). Springfield, IL: Charles C Thomas Publishers, 1973, p.18.

RECIPROCAL REACTIONS

This test is performed with the infant lying in the supine position and, if old enough, asked to squeeze an object. If the infant is hemiplegic, have the infant squeeze with the uninvolved side. A negative reaction consists of minimal or no reaction or increased tone in parts of the body other than the tested limb. A positive reaction consists of reciprocal squeezing in the contralateral hand and/or increased tone in other parts of the body. A positive sign along with other abnormal signs is indicative of delayed reflexive maturation (114).

EXTENSOR SUPPORTING REACTION (POSITIVE)

The examiner stands behind and holds the infant under the axillae in an upright position. The stimulus is bouncing the infant several times on the soles of his/her feet. A negative response is no increase in tone and volitional flexion of the lower extremities. A positive test is increased extensor tone in the lower extremities; plantar flexion of the feet and genu recurvatum may be observed. Positive reactions are considered normal in infants of three to eight months of age (98,100,102,114).

EXTENSOR SUPPORTING REACTION (NEGATIVE)

The examiner raises the infant up to a standing position. Weight-bearing is the stimulus for the test. The negative reaction is the release of extensor tone from positive support which allows plantigrade feet and flexion of the legs. The positive reaction is no release of the extensor tone and the persistence of positive support. The normal reaction consists of sufficient release of the extensor tone to allow flexion for reciprocation. The abnormal reaction is the continuation of positive support beyond eight months of age. A reaction of excessive flexion upon weight-bearing is abnormal beyond four months of age (98,100,114).

Midbrain Level

TESTS

These reflexes are integrated in the midbrain level (Fig. 13.28) above the red nucleus but do not include the cerebral cortex. These responses are the first to develop after birth and reach their maximum concerted effort about age 10 to 12 months. These righting reflexes interact with each other and work towards the establishment of normal head and body relationships in space as well as in relation to each other. As maturation progresses and cortical control increases, these reflexes are gradually modified, inhibited, and eventually disappear towards the end of the fifth year. Their combined actions enable the developing child to roll over, sit up, get up onto his hands and knees, and make him an upright quadrupedal being (98,100,102,114).

REFLEXIVE MATURATION (BODY ROTATION RESPONSE)

The infant is in the supine position with the head in the neutral position and all extremities extended. The infant's head is actively or passively rotated to one side. The body does not rotate in a negative response. A positive reaction is rotation of the entire body to the same side as the head. Positive reactions

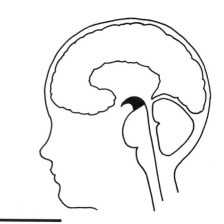

Figure 13.28. Midbrain level.

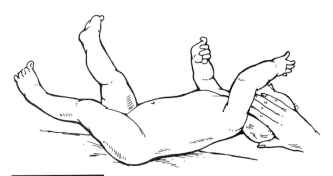

Figure 13.29. Neck righting reflex. Modified from Haynes U. A developmental approach to case finding. Washington, DC: U.S. Department of Health, Education, and Welfare, 1967.

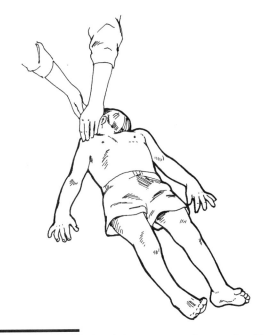

Figure 13.30. Neck righting test—negative reaction. Modified from Fiorentino MR. Reflex testing methods for evaluating CNS development (2nd ed). Springfield, IL: Charles C Thomas Publishers, 1973, p.23.

are normal to age six months. A positive reaction beyond six month of age or a negative reaction beyond one month of age is suggestive of delayed reflexive maturation (98,100,102,114) (Figs. 13.29, 13.30).

REFLEXIVE MATURATION (SEGMENTAL TORSO RESPONSE)

This test is performed with the infant supine, head in the neutral position, and all four extremities extended. The stimulus is rotating the infant's head to one side as in the previous test. The change in body position is observed. In a normal infant, the body rotates as a whole. A positive response is segmental rotation of the torso between the shoulders and the pelvis; i.e., following head rotation, the shoulders rotate

followed by rotation of the pelvis. Positive responses should appear between the ages of 6 month and 18 months. Negative reactions after age 6 months are considered to be abnormal (98,100,102,114) (Fig. 13.31).

PROPRIOCEPTIVE HEAD RAISING RESPONSE (PRONE)

The infant is blindfolded and held up in the air in the prone position. A negative reaction to this position consists of no automatic head raising to the level position. A positive reaction consists of head raising to the extended position with the face vertical and the mouth horizontal. A positive reaction is normal from about age six months and should continue throughout life. Negative reactions after age six months are considered abnormal (98,100,102,114) (Fig. 13.32).

PROPRIOCEPTIVE HEAD RAISING RESPONSE (SUPINE)

This test is performed blindfolded in the supine position. A negative reaction to this position is an inability to raise the head automatically to the flexed position. A positive reaction is the head being raised automatically to the flexed position with the face vertical and the mouth horizontal. A positive reaction should be seen from 6 months of age and continue throughout a lifetime. Negative reactions after the age of 6 months are considered abnormal (98,100,114).

PROPRIOCEPTIVE HEAD RAISING RESPONSE

This test is performed with the child blindfolded. The examiner holds the child at the pelvis and laterally tilts the child to the right and left (Fig. 13.33). In a negative reaction, the head does not automatically right itself. In a positive reaction, the head rights automatically. The positive reaction should be seen from age six to eight months and continue throughout a lifetime. A negative reaction continuing past eight months of age is considered abnormal (98,100,114).

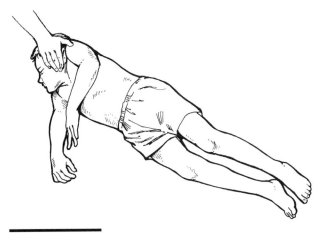

Figure 13.31. Body righting acting on the body test—negative reaction. Modified from Fiorentino MR. Reflex testing methods for evaluating CNS development (2nd ed). Springfield, IL: Charles C Thomas Publishers, 1973, p. 24.

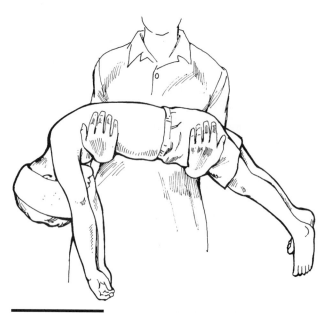

Figure 13.32. Labrynthine righting acting on the head #1—negative reaction. Modified from Fiorentino MR. Reflex testing methods for evaluating CNS development (2nd ed). Springfield, IL: Charles C Thomas Publishers, 1973, p. 29.

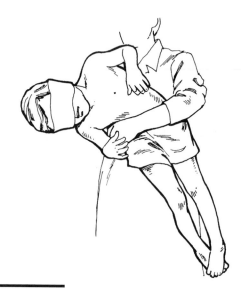

Figure 13.33. Labrynthine righting acting on the head—negative reaction. Modified from Fiorentino MR. Reflex testing methods for evaluating CNS development (2nd ed). Springfield, IL: Charles C Thomas Publishers, 1973, p. 27.

A variation is used by chiropractors using the Gonstead system which does not require a blindfold. A young infant's cervical spine can be examined for upper cervical fixation (usually C2) by grasping the infant under the axillae and tilting him laterally to each side. If the infant cannot allow the head to initially lateral flex to the ipsilateral side of tilting, it is thought that the upper cervical spine, particularly C2, may be fixated.

VISUAL RIGHTING REFLEXES (PRONE)

The child is held in the prone position (Fig. 13.34). The negative reaction is noted when the child remains in the downward position and does not automatically raise itself to the extended position. In a positive reaction, the head is raised automatically so that the face is vertical and the mouth horizontal. The positive reaction is seen soon after the labyrinthine righting acting on the head response is observed (1 to 2 months of age) and continues on throughout a lifetime. (The optical righting tests in all positions are only valid if the labyrinthine righting is not present). Negative reactions after this time are abnormal (98,100,114).

VISUAL RIGHTING REFLEXES (SUPINE)

In this variation, the child is held in the supine position (Fig. 13.35). A negative reaction is the head extending down towards the floor; the head is not automatically raised. A positive reaction is flexing the head so that the face is vertical and the mouth horizontal. A positive reaction is normal from about the age of six months. A negative reaction after this time is considered abnormal (98,100,114).

VISUAL RIGHTING REFLEXES (UPRIGHT)

The child is held at the pelvis in an upright position (Fig. 13.36). The child is tilted laterally to each side. A negative response is the inability to automatically right the head and torso. A positive sign is an automatic righting of the head and

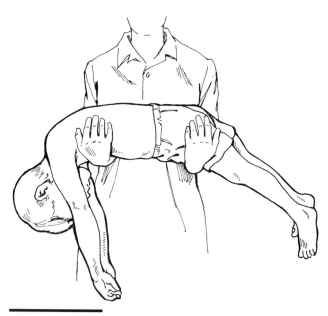

Figure 13.34. Optical righting #1. Modified from Fiorentino MR. Reflex testing methods for evaluating CNS development (2nd ed). Springfield, IL: Charles C Thomas Publishers, 1973, p. 29.

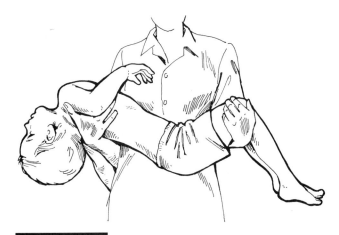

Figure 13.35.   Optical righting #2. Modified from Fiorentino MR. Reflex testing methods for evaluating CNS development (2nd ed). Springfield, IL: Charles C Thomas Publishers, 1973, p. 30.

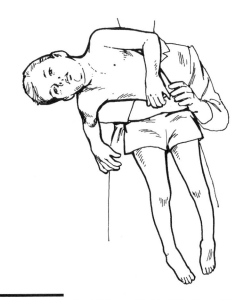

Figure 13.36.   Optical righting #3. Modified from Fiorentino MR. Reflex testing methods for evaluating CNS development (2nd ed). Springfield, IL: Charles C Thomas Publishers, 1973, p. 31.

trunk. A positive reaction is normal from the age of 6 months. A negative response is considered abnormal after 8 months of age (98,100,114).

Extremity Reaction to Pelvic Tilt Stimulus

The child is prone with the head in a neutral position, the legs are extended, and the arms are extended over the head. The pelvis is lifted on one side. A negative response is an inability to flex the ipsilateral arm, hip and knee. A positive response is automatic flexion of the ipsilateral arm, hip, and knee. A

positive response is normally seen from the age of six months; a negative response should not be seen after that age (98,100,114).

Subcortical Automatic Movement Reactions

TESTS

These reflexes are responses observed in infants and young children. They are not righting reflexes, per se, but are reactions produced by changes in the position of the head. In theory, they involve the semi-circular canals, the labyrinths, and/or the proprioceptors in the cervical spine. As in the righting reflexes, they appear at certain stages of maturation and their persistence, or absence, can be observed in patients under conditions which interfere with normal nervous system function (96,102,114,119). These reflexes are described later.

The proper response to these tests requires efficient interaction of the cerebral cortex, basal ganglia, and cerebellum (98,100,102,114) (Fig. 13.37).

The upright bipedal stage of motor development is brought about by maturation of motor development at the cortical level. These responses occur when muscle tone is normalized and provide the adaptation necessary to respond to changes in the center of gravity of the body. Emerging at the age of 6 months, a positive response at any one level indicates the ability to progress to the next higher level of motor activity.

Supine Test

The child lies supine on a tiltboard. The board is tilted, and the child's response is observed. A negative reaction is non-righting of the head and torso, i.e., no equilibrium or protective reactions. A positive response is for the child to right the head and torso while simultaneously abducting and extending the limbs on the raised side. This is the equilibrium reaction. The protective reaction occurs on the lowered side of the board. This response also includes abduction and extension of the arm and leg (98,114).

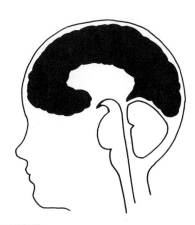

Figure 13.37.   Cortical level.

PRONE TEST

The patient lies prone on a tiltboard. As the board is tilted, the child's response is noted. A positive response is righting of the head and torso and abduction and extension of the arms and legs on the raised side—equilibrium reaction. The protective reaction occurs on the lowered side of the board. Positive reactions reach normal at about 6 months of age and continue on throughout life. Negative reactions after 6 months of age are considered abnormal (98,114).

FOUR-FOOT KNEELING TEST

On the tiltboard, the child is in a crawling or quadruped position and is tilted to one side. A negative response is non-righting of the head and torso—no equilibrium or protective reactions. A positive reaction shows righting of the head and torso and abduction and extension of the arm and leg on the raised side—equilibrium reaction. Protective reactions occur on the lowered side. Positive reactions normalize at about 8 months of age and continue on throughout life. Negative reactions should not persist after 8 months of age. Positive reactions may be selective to some body parts rather than the entire body (98,114).

SITTING TEST

The patient is seated in a chair and is pulled or tilted to one side. A negative response is non-righting of the head and torso—no protective reactions. A positive reaction is righting of the head and torso, abduction and extension of the arm and leg on the raised side (equilibrium reaction), and a protective reaction on the lowered side. Positive reactions may not be global but may occur in some body parts. Positive reactions should be established at 10 to 12 months of age and continue throughout life. Negative reactions should not persist after the age of 12 months (114).

KNEEL-STANDING TEST

The patient is upright in the kneeling position and is pulled or tilted to one side. A negative reaction occurs when the patient's head and torso do not right themselves—no equilibrium or protective reaction occurs. A positive reaction appears as righting of the head and torso with abduction and extension of the arm and leg on the raised side (equilibrium reaction) and a protective reaction on the lowered side. Positive reactions may be selective to some body regions rather than global. Positive reactions should peak at 15 months of age and continue on throughout a lifetime. Negative reactions should not persist after the age of 15 months (98,114).

HOPPING TEST

This test should be done in several positions. With the child standing and attempting not to move his feet, the examiner shifts the child to one side and watches for a response before shifting the child to the other side, then forward and backwards. A negative reaction is the inability to right the head and torso; i.e., no hopping steps are made to maintain balance.

Positive reactions normalize by the age of 15 to 18 months. Negative reactions beyond this age are probably abnormal (98,114).

DORSIFLEXION TEST

The child stands and the examiner stands behind and holds the patient under the axillae. The child is tilted backwards. A negative response is no righting of the head and torso and no dorsiflexion of the feet. A positive response is righting of the head and torso. There should be a positive response by the age of 15 to 18 months, which should continue throughout a lifetime. Continuation of a negative response after this age is considered abnormal (98,114).

SEE-SAW MANEUVER

This test can be performed once the child is able to maintain a standing position. While the child is standing, the examiner holds the hand and the foot of the same side. The arm is pulled gently forward and laterally. A negative response is the inability to right the head and torso or maintain balance. A positive response is self-righting of the head and torso and slight abduction and extension of the flexed knee to maintain equilibrium. Positive reactions should be seen by the age of 15 months (98,114).

SIMIAN POSITION

The child squats down and is tilted to one side. Non-righting of the head and torso is a negative response—the child cannot maintain the squatting or "simian" position, maintain equilibrium, or provide a protective reaction. The positive reaction is righting of the head and torso and extension and abduction of the arm and leg on the raised side (equilibrium reaction), and protective reaction simultaneously on the lowered side. Positive reactions should be attained by the age of 15 to 18 months (98,114).

Primitive Reflexes: Reflexes That Normally Disappear with Maturation

REFLEXES

The Landau, Moro, and Tonic Neck reflexes are primitive movement patterns that can be demonstrated in healthy infants. These reflexes are demonstrative of primitive movement patterns. The disappearance of these movement patterns demonstrates that higher cerebral pathways have established dominance over the primitive reflexes as the nervous system matures (120). These reflexes may return in the elderly as cerebral function diminishes (98,120,121).

LANDAU REFLEX

The infant is held in one hand at the abdominal level in the horizontal prone position. The examiner's other hand flexes the infant's head forward. The normal response is flexion of the legs onto the trunk. This response normally occurs several weeks after birth and persists for up to the age of one or two (120,121).

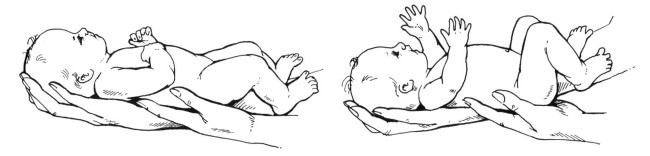

Figure 13.38.   Moro reflex. Modified from Bates B. A guide to physical examination and history taking (5th ed). Philadelphia: J.B. Lippincott Co., 1991, p. 632.

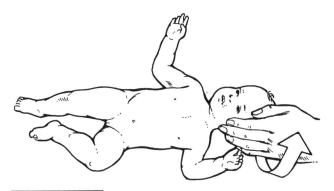

Figure 13.39.   Tonic neck reflex test. Modified from Blasco PA: Primitive reflexes: Their contribution to the early detection of cerebral palsy. Clin Ped 1994; 37(7):391.

MORO REFLEX

The infant is propped up into a sitting position and is leaning slightly backwards. The support against the back is suddenly removed (120,121). An alternative is to lie the infant supine on a table and give a sharp, loud slap to the tabletop (120,121). The former is preferable as it requires the use of cervical spine proprioceptors while the latter method is considered to be inappropriate by some authorities (121,122). The normal response is extension of the arms followed by their flexion with spreading of the fingers. There should be also be flexion of the femurs on the pelvis. A variety of afferent pathways may be involved especially if variations on the test are performed. Testing by making a sharp, loud noise (the original Moro test) must be distinguished from the startle response. Testing is sometimes done by grasping the infant's hand, extending the arms, and releasing them, and by lifting the head of the bassinet and suddenly dropping it. This response is missing or incomplete in the young premature infant, but it should be present in the normal, full-term infant. The Moro reflex (Fig. 13.38) should begin fading by the fourth to eighth week, at which point it may become incomplete or asymmetrical. Prolonged retention of the Moro reflex is occasionally seen in cerebral palsy (120,122).

CERVICAL PROPRIOCEPTIVE, TONIC NECK, OR FENCER REFLEX

This reflex has its origin in the proprioceptor endings in the neck muscles and joints and the brainstem representation at the level of the red nucleus in animals (120) (Fig. 13.39). If an infant is supine and rotates its head actively to one side or if the head is rotated passively by the examiner, there should be extension of the arm and leg on the side of facial rotation and flexion of the contralateral arm and leg. A constant pattern does not usually occur in the newborn. The reflex normally achieves its physiological peak between two and four months of age (123). This pattern can, in part, be prompted by the examiner actively rotating the infant's head against which the infant should be able to overcome by vigorous struggling. Complete obligatory tonic neck patterns (in the obligate response, the infant maintains the tonic neck posture as long as his head is turned to the side) are abnormal at any age. The tonic neck reflexes should disappear by six months of age. Retention of the reflex may indicate general psychological retardation, but retention in a strong form is a major sign of motor postural disability (123). McMullen has described this reflex along with the Reverse Fencer's Response and digital palpation when assessing the upper cervical spine (124,125).

A reflex with a similar response is the Reverse Fencer Reflex. In this case the infant is supine. The examiner grasps both feet and ankles of the infant, one in each hand, and gently elevates legs and buttocks until the infant is vertical with the head free. If there are no obvious signs of distress, transfer the weight of the body onto one leg by relaxing the weight off of the other. Up to the age of 6 months, the infant should turn the head away from the weightbearing side. Persistence of this sign beyond the age of 6 months may indicate a cerebral lesion (123,124) (Table 13.11).

MATURATIONAL REFLEXES AND SIGNS; THOSE THAT NORMALLY APPEAR WITH MATURATION

PASSIVE CERVICAL PROPRIOCEPTIVE OR NECK RIGHT REFLEX

The infant is in the supine position. The examiner rotates the infant's head to one side which should result in the shoulders and torso rotating towards the same side. This reflex appears

Table 13.11.   **Summary of Reflexes and Signs During the First Year**

Reflex/Response	Appears	Disappears
Moro	Birth	4–5 months
Stepping and Placing	Birth	Persists as voluntary standing
Positive Supporting	Newborn–3 months	Persists voluntarily
Tonic Neck★	2–3 weeks	4–6 months (never obligatory or sustained)
Crossed Adductor†	2–3 months	7–8 months
Neck Righting	4–6 months	Persists voluntarily
Parachute	6–7 months	Persists
Grasp		
Palmar Grasp	Birth	3–4 months
Voluntary Reach	4–5 months	
Palmar Grasp (voluntary)	4–5 months (entire hand)	
	6–7 months (pincer)	
Ankle Clonus	(8–10 beats in newborn)	Gradually disappears by the age 2 months

★*The tonic neck reflex, when consistently asymmetrical, may be an early sign of hemiparesis on the side of increase response. Sitting is often impossible until this reflex disappears. The obligate response precludes rolling over. [PAINE]*
†*The crossed adductor reflex applies when there is contraction of both hip adductors when the knee jerk is elicited. Persistence of the reflex is a sign of pyramidal tract interference.*
Adapted from Weiner HL et al. Pediatric neurology for the house officer (3rd ed). Baltimore: Williams & Wilkins. 1988. p. 5.

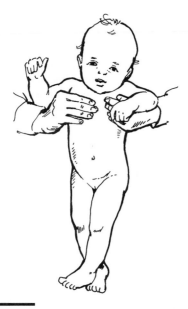

Figure 13.40.   Vertical suspension placing. Scissoring of the legs (fixes adduction and extension of the legs) indicates spastic paraplegia or diplegia. Reprinted with permission from Bates B. A guide to physical examination and history taking (5th ed). Philadelphia: J.B. Lippincott Co., 1991, pp. 629-260.

when the tonic neck reflex disappears—usually about four months when the baby is beginning to turn over. It should be present by age 8 to 10 months and become a part of voluntary activity (98,110).

POSTURE IN HORIZONTAL OR PRONE SUSPENSION

This is a test of head control and motor function. A 5-month-old infant held horizontally should begin to arch their back and hold their head above the horizontal plane (see Landau Reaction) (98,110).

POSTURE IN UPRIGHT OR VERTICAL SUSPENSION

During the first half year of life when the infant is suspended vertically or in the upright position, flexion is apparent and is followed by extension (Fig. 13.40). Persistent extension and adduction or "scissoring" of the lower extremities is always abnormal and is a sign of spasticity. An infant attempting to stand on its own provides a normal positive supporting reaction, but too much positive supporting is often the first sign of spasticity. In atonic diplegia, there may be withdrawal of the extremities and lack of a positive supporting reaction. Parents may describe this reaction as an "unwillingness" to bear weight, when in fact, the infant is actually flexing the hip and extending the knee (98,110).

HANDGRASP AND FOOT OR PLANTAR GRASP

The normal handgrasp of the infant should be present at the age of 4 or 5 months (Figs. 13.41, 13.42). The infant is able to reach and grasp at this time. Thumb and finger or pincer grasp begins at 6 to 7 months of age and should be present in normal infants by their first birthday. By 7 to 8 months, the infant should be able to shift objects from one hand to

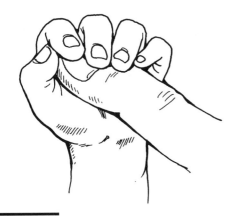

Figure 13.41. Palmar grasp. Reprinted with permission from Haynes U. A developmental approach to case finding. Washington, DC: U.S. Department of Health, Education, and Welfare, 1967, p. 23.

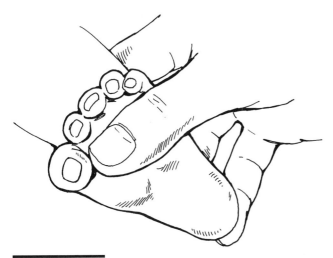

Figure 13.42. Plantar grasp. Reprinted with permission from Haynes U. A developmental approach to case finding. Washington, DC: U.S. Department of Health, Education, and Welfare, 1967, p. 23.

the other. Handedness usually does not appear before the age of 1 year, but should be apparent at that time. Ambidexterity in writing after 3 years of age should be further evaluated (98,110,120,126).

In the neonate, the plantar grasp should be strong. It is elicited by placing a finger or thumb firmly into the area of the base of the toes. This response should disappear at age 8 to 9 months. Asymmetry of the response should be noted. The persistence of edema in the feet should also be noted. Persistent edema in the feet of a female infant may be indicative of a chromosomal abnormality (126).

PARACHUTE REFLEX

The parachute sign is sometimes described as two tests. The typically described sign is sometimes known as the upper

parachute reflex or reaction. A lower extremity reflex is sometimes described and is known as the lower parachute reflex or reaction (127).

The normal infant should begin demonstrating the parachute reflex at 6 to 7 months of age, and it should be well developed by 1 year of age. It is produced by suspending the infant prone and horizontally, then suddenly plunging the baby downwards. The eyes must be open. The reflex consists of arm extension to "break the fall" (98). This is sometimes called the upper parachute response (127).

For the lower parachute response, the evaluator holds the infant under the axillae. With the infant's eyes open, the infant is suddenly brought down vertically. The positive response is downward extension of both legs (127).

The parachute response is an excellent test of upper extremity pyramidal tract function, and if asymmetrical, may be a sign of hemiparesis (98) (Fig. 13.43). One study found that in the infants who developed the ability to sit late and the appearance of the parachute reflex, particularly the upper extremity response, was late (after the age of 10 months), the ability to independently walk was delayed. Those who were late in sitting but had the parachute reflex by the age of 10 months were largely able to walk by 15 months of age (127).

TRACTION RESPONSE

The examiner raises the supine infant by the hands into the seated position. The head will lag and then come forward. In the newborn, there should be sufficient strength for the infant to bring the head to an unright position. Asymmetrical response may indicate brachial palsy or hemiparesis. Absence of the response will be seen in hypotonia, e.g., Down syndrome (126).

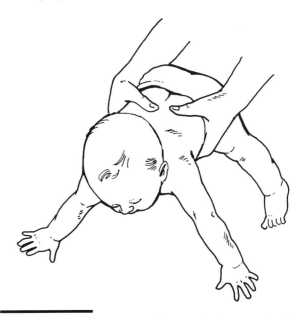

Figure 13.43. Parachute sign. Reprinted with permission from Haynes U. A developmental approach to case finding. Washington, DC: U.S. Department of Health, Education, and Welfare, 1967, p. 22.

Developmental Milestones Screening Tests

The Denver Development Screening Test may be used to assess, in percentage form, fine motor, language, and personal-social milestones during the course of the first 6 years. Fine motor and "conceptual" developmental progress can be tested when the child is able to use a pencil and do Gesell, Binet, and Bender-Gestalt drawings. If a more definitive assessment is required, formal neuropsychological testing is done (98,110).

WALKING

Most children are able to walk well by age 14 to 15 months. If a child does not walk by 18 months, there is probably an abnormality (obesity is not a cause of late walking). When presented with a child who is a late walker, the examiner should consider certain clues, such as abnormal reflexes (e.g, Babinski and/or Chaddock), head circumference below 3% of normal, history of perinatal distress, delayed speech, creatinine phosphokinase (CPK may be increased in muscular dystrophies), and thyroid function. A familial history of late walking is a normal variant (98,110).

Pelvic and spinal misalignments may contribute to the difficulty or inability to walk. Much of the evidence in this connection is anecdotal. Grice has written an excellent article on this connection (128).

LANGUAGE

Most children say single words by the age of 14 months and are combining words by 20 to 24 months of age. By age 2 years, a child should be able to combine two different words and point to named body parts. If language is delayed, the examiner should consider an evaluation for the previously mentioned signs and the possibility of mental retardation, hearing or visual deficit, autism, aphasia, oral-motor problems (problems with sucking, blowing, and excessive or prolonged drooling are signs of articulatory dyspraxia, especially where understanding outshines expressive abilities). Always check hearing in a child with delayed language development (110).

Prematurity may retard developmental "milestones." However, a child born four weeks premature generally "catches up" by age one year. Normal developmental milestones may not apply to the child with systemic illnesses. Illnesses such as cardiac disease, cystic fibrosis, and celiac disease may affect developmental progress (110,113,129).

Neurological Examination of the Older Child

The neurologic examination of a child older than two years of age should be as unceremonious as possible while at the same time maintaining a basic flow pattern designed to complete a full and relevant evaluation. By this time, a child should have acquired a large repertory of skills. Many neurologic functions of 2- to 4-year-old children are evaluated in much the same manner as those under 2 years of age. It has been the experience of many chiropractors that the most comfortable placement for a child is in the parent's lap. Observation and play techniques are essential means of monitoring intellectual and motor skills. One of the authors has found that a very large picture book (2 to 3 feet in height and width) placed in the vicinity of a child requires the child to demonstrate motor and intellectual skills if it wishes to explore such as large object. Motors skills are readily observed as the child moves to the book and opens it. The child's ability to relate to printed material provides some insight into intellectual skills (130).

Observation of the child is important while conducting the history-taking session. Older children will often sit in a chair or performs tasks such as reading or drawing. If the child actively participates in the history-taking, the child's understanding and contributions to the session are an aid to the clinician when making valid judgments about the child's intellectual and language skills. Problems with dysarthria, dysphonia, or ataxic speech patterns can be assessed. Aberrant head and facial movements including lip tremors, eye blinking, and staring may be evidence of epilepsy. Movement disorders involving the face such as chorea or tic, as well as other movement disorders involving the neck, trunk, or limbs may be noticed—e.g., athetosis, chorea, dystonia, myoclonus, tics, and spasms (126).

Most children 4 years and older will easily participate in gross motor function screening examinations (130). The child should first stand before the examining clinician and be told to carefully observe the examiner demonstrate the desired motor acts. The child is asked to walk forward and backward on his/her heels and toes. He/she is asked to arise from a squatting position, hop in place on each foot, and tandem walk forward and backward. The child is then asked to stand with his/her feet close together with arms outstretched on front. After watching the posture for a few seconds, the child is then asked to maintain the position and to close the eyes, i.e., Romberg sign. The child can then relax for a moment. Once again, the eyes are closed and the same position is maintained, the child is instructed to abduct and stretch the arms out at shoulder height. The child is then told to touch one index to the other and to alternately touch the nose with each index finger. These movements assess proprioception and adventitious movements (130).

Following the screening procedure, the examiner can begin a more detailed evaluation. Any abnormalities observed during the screening examination requires further evaluation during the rest of the evaluation.

DEEP TENDON REFLEXES

Deep tendon reflexes, more accurately known as muscle stretch reflexes, should be done after assuring the child that there is no discomfort associated with the test. Most children are amused by these tests. The deep tendon stretch reflex screen usually involves the biceps, triceps, brachioradialis, patellar, and Achilles. Each reflex is mediated at a specific spinal segmental level(s).

Hyperactive reflexes or a clonic response to stroking or tapping the tendon is usually a result of corticospinal dysfunction (upper motor neuron). Hyperreflexia may also be a result of an aberrant "spread" of responses. These include contraction of muscle groups which usually do not contract when a reflex is being established (crossed thigh adductor and finger flexor responses). Unilateral hyperreflexia is almost always a sign of a lesion; bilateral brisk reflexes may be normal, particularly if only one reflex is involved (103,110,113).

Hyporeflexia or diminished or absent reflexes are usually associated with lower motor neuron involvement, e.g., anterior horn cell disease, peripheral neuropathy, or myopathy. On occasion, hyporeflexia may be found in central nervous system depression, poor central control of the gamma-loop (central hypotonia), or involvement of the posterior or dorsal root (either intramedullary or extramedullary). Anterior horn cell involvement, such as seen in infantile spinal muscular atrophy, may present with diminished or absent patellar reflexes in the early stage as the cells innervating the more proximal muscles are usually affected first. Sensory involvement, particularly peripheral, is often detectable in the presence of neuropathies. Correspondingly, the distal deep tendon stretch reflexes tend to be involved earlier and to a greater degree than those proximal (103,110,114,131). With certain myopathies, the reflexes may be normal in the early stages but become absent in later progression of the disease course. Cerebellar disease may cause decreased reflexes by affecting gamma-loop responsiveness.

Cerebellar disease usually decreases muscle tone and may decrease tendon reflexes because of the gamma-loop responsiveness. The Jendrassik maneuver may enhance the tendon reflexes when these reflexes seem to be absent.

Other reflexes that should be considered are the plantar toe sign (this is normal while the Babinski sign is always abnormal), Hoffman's reflex, cremasteric reflex, and abdominal reflex. The up-going toe sign is called the Babinski and is produced by a firm, slow stroke along the lateral margin of the sole of the foot from anterior to posterior with a blunt, smooth object. The stimulus should not be painful. Flicking the child's fingernail (second or third finger) downward with the examiner's nail (Hoffman's reflex) results in flexion of the distal phalanx of the thumb. No response or a muted response may occur in a normal child. Stroking the inner thigh in a caudal-rostral direction (cremasteric reflex) and observing the contraction of the scrotum is normally present and symmetrical. Asymmetry or absence indicates corticospinal tract involvement. In the current climate, you should explain to the parent(s) any tests in "sensitive" areas prior to conducting those tests. Having the parent(s) present is important. If anything, explaining the tests that you are going to do on a child helps to dispel anxiety of the parent and/or child and shows them the thoroughness of your evaluation, and they can help you with some of the tests requiring a child to be still or requiring more than two hands.

Overview of Muscle Spindle Function

An understanding of the deep tendon reflexes/muscle stretch mechanism begins with the structure of the muscle spindles. Muscle spindles contain up to 12 intrafusal muscle fibers; in this context, ordinary muscle fibers are extrafusal. The larger, intrafusal fibers extend beyond the ends or poles of the spindle and attach to the connective tissue (perimysium) or to a tendon. The smaller ones are anchored to the collagenous capsule of the spindle. At the center of the spindles (equators),

the sarcomeres are replaced almost entirely by nuclei, in the form of "bags" (in large fibers) or "chains" (in small fibers) (16,98,103).

Muscle spindles have a motor and sensory nerve supply. The motor fibers, fusimotor, are in the A gamma size range, in contrast to the A alpha axons supplying extrafusal muscle fibers (this is important to remember when using the Jendrassik Maneuver as the gamma motor system is facilitated). Each fusimotor axon in humans forms a discrete "plate and trail" on each end of an intrafusal fiber (16,98,103).

The sensory supply is often double (like the "plate and trail"). A single, primary sensory axon supplies all of the equators in a single spindle. The axon is type Ia. Its equatorial endings in the human are called annulospiral but are often claw-like. Secondary sensory endings (if present) are juxta-equatorial on one or both sides of the primary endings. They are type II fibers (16,100).

Because muscle spindles are stretch receptors, the sensory endings are activated by stretching the equator. The receptor action potential travels to the final heminode where the nerve impulses are generated. Equatorial stretching may be active or passive.

In passive stretch, the entire muscle belly is passively lengthened. Such momentary lengthening is produced when the tendon reflexes are elicited by striking tendons with a neurological hammer.

When the patellar or other tendon is struck, the muscle spindles are stretched and discharged synchronously to the spinal cord. Here, the type Ia and II afferents synapse directly upon an alpha motoneurons (they give rise to A alpha axons). The alpha motoneurons respond by causing the extrafusal muscle fibers to contract. This is a monosynaptic reflex (16,100).

In active stretch (elicited by the Jendrassik maneuver), the striated segments of the intrafusal muscle fibers are made to contract by gamma motoneurons. Active contraction greatly increases the sensitivity of the muscle spindle to passive stretching (16,98,100).

Cerebellar Function

Cerebellar dysfunction may be evidenced by head tilt (131). The tilt is usually ipsilateral to the involved cerebellar hemisphere, but exceptions are common (131). Herniation of the cerebellar tonsils through the foramen magnum secondary to increased intracranial pressure may cause head tilt. Neoplasms other than those of the cerebellum that induce increased intracranial pressure may cause downward pressure on the cerebellum, which may result in head tilt. Station and gait testing may be used to evaluate cerebellar function also.

Tremor occurring with action (intention tremor) may be seen in cerebellar dysfunction. Handpatting (alternating pronation and supination of one hand on the thigh while the other hand remains stationary on the other thigh) is a valid method for assessing dysdiadochokinesis. Finger and toe tapping finger-to-nose or finger-to-examiner's finger are other valid methods of assessing the cerebellum. Any breaks in rhythm and nonfluidity of movement are noted.

Cranial Nerve Examination

The older child presents an easier subject for cranial nerve examination compared to an infant or younger child; the assessment can proceed in an orderly fashion from cranial nerve I through XII. The younger child usually requires some modification and ingenuity depending upon the degree of the willingness and interaction granted on the part of the child.

CRANIAL NERVE I – OLFACTORY NERVE

In children, the olfactory nerve function is rarely impaired (131). The olfactory nerve can be assessed by having the child smell pleasant aromas—e.g., vanilla, chocolate, coffee, or peppermint—through each individual nostril. Cranial nerve I sensation is intact if the child can appreciate a change in odor without necessarily identifying the particular odor. Anosmia may occur in children with upper respiratory involvement or head trauma, particularly to the occipital region. Neoplasms in the cribriform plate or inferior frontal lobe may cause anosmia. Unilateral anosmia may be more worrisome than bilateral anosmia (131).

CRANIAL NERVE II – OPTIC NERVE

One of the most critical portions of the neurological examination is the evaluation of the optic nerve. Visual acuity testing with a Snellen chart or "near card" is appropriate in older children. Visual field and acuity tests should be performed in a well-lit room with glare minimized. Occasionally, it is necessary to detect subtle changes which is aided by holding the visual field test object against a background of less contrast increasing the difficulty of identification.

The very young child poses difficulty in visual evaluation. Gross vision can be assessed in children less than 3 or 4 years of age by their ability to recognize familiar objects of varying sizes, shapes, and colors. Beyond four years of age, the "E" test is useful. The child is taught to recognize the "E" and instructed to indicate the direction in which the three "arms" are pointing by a finger accordingly. "E's" of varying sizes and directions of orientation are shown.

The visual field of each eye is examined. The child is confronted with an object that is moved from temporal to nasal along the radii of the field. A small (3mm) red test object or a toy may be used (119,132). Double simultaneous testing may be employed by moving two test objects or pen lights simultaneously from the temporal to the nasal fields, then from the superior to the inferior regions of the temporal and nasal fields. In this test the child is instructed to look directly at the examiner's nose. If visual acuity is grossly distorted, finger counting may be used—the examiner holds up one or more fingers and asks the child the number of fingers displayed. In extreme impairment, perception of a rapidly moving finger can be used (131,132).

Ophthalmoscopic evaluation of the optic disc of the older child normally shows a sharply defined and usually salmon-colored optic disc. In the infant, the optic disc is usually a pale gray color (131,132). If the cup of the optic disc is deep, the color may appear pale. The pallor is localized to the center of the disc. In optic atrophy, the pallor encompasses the entire disc, and there is a decreased number of arterioles in the disc margins.

Papilloedema or "choked disc" is of particular importance in the ophthalmoscopic examination of the optic disc as it is associated with raised intracranial pressure. Papilloedema is most commonly associated with elevation of the optic disc as well as distended veins and a lack of venous pulsations (131,132). Hemorrhages may also surround the disc (131,132). In papilledema, visual acuity is rarely affected until there is scarring of the nerve head (optic disc). This is in sharp contrast to the early loss of visual acuity that accompanies inflammation of the optic nerve (131,132).

The room light level when observing the pupils should allow the pupils to remain slightly mydriatic or dilated. The diameter, regularity of the contour, and responsiveness of the pupils are examined. A fixed, dilated pupil is usually associated with other signs of oculomotor or cranial nerve III dysfunction. A Horner syndrome is a result of sympathetic dysfunction manifesting itself with a miotic pupil, mild ptosis, and loss of sweating on the ipsilateral side of the face. Dragging a finger over the child's forehead may aid in the recognition of anhidrosis (131). The fixed, dilated pupil is usually associated with other signs of oculomotor nerve dysfunction and may be a sign of cerebellar tonsillar herniation (131). The absence or presence of the pupillary light reflex differentiates between cortical and peripheral blindness. Lesions of the anterior visual pathway (i.e., retina to the lateral geniculate body) result in the interruption of the afferent limb of the pupillary light reflex which results in absent or decreased reflex. Anterior visual tract interruption can cause amblyopia (dimness of vision) in one eye. In this case, the pupil fails to constrict when stimulated with direct light; thus, the consensual pupillary response (contralateral light response) is intact. The full response to direct stimulation is delayed because of varying degrees of visual loss, but the consensual reflex is brisk (119). The deficient pupillary response can be revealed by alternately aiming the light source at each eye—swinging light response. On the side with diminished vision, consensual pupillary constriction is greater than the reflex to the direct light stimulation (Marcus-Gunn pupil) allowing the pupil of the affected eye to dilate slightly during direct stimulation.

CRANIAL NERVES III, IV & VI—OCULOMOTOR, TROCHLEAR, AND ABDUCENS NERVES

Cranial nerves III, IV, and VI control extraocular motor movements so as to produce synchrony and single vision with two eyes.

The oculomotor nerve (CN III) innervates the superior, inferior, and medial recti, the inferior oblique, and levator palpebral superioris muscles. The trochlear nerve (CN IV) and the abducens nerve (CN VI) innervate the superior oblique and lateral rectus muscles, respectively. The cardinal directions of gaze test the function of these extraocular muscles. The lateral and medial recti muscles are abductors and adductors, respectively. The superior rectus and inferior oblique muscles are elevators; the inferior rectus and superior oblique muscles are depressors. The oblique muscles act in the vertical plane when the ocular globe is adducted while the recti muscles serve a similar function when the ocular globe is abducted. When the globe is directed forward, the oblique muscles provide torsion or rotation around the z-axis (longitudinal or anteroposterior axis) (131,133).

The heterophorias or phorias are a misalignment of the eye from the visual axes. In heterophoria, when the patient is instructed to look directly forward and fixate on near or far objects, one or both ocular globes deviate upon occlusion of one eye. Forcing fixation of the uncovered eye and alternately covering each eye allows the identification of heterophorias. The febrile or fatigued child tends to predispose towards the phorias. Esophoria is a predisposition to convergence while exophoria is a predisposition to divergence (131).

The heterotropias or tropias are found during binocular vision. Abduction tropias are exotropias and adduction tropias are esotropias. The tropias are most often associated with compromised extraocular muscle innervation (131). Observation of eye movements are useful for detecting extraocular palsies. A red glass is placed in front of one eye. A focused, relatively intense white light is shown in both eyes from various regions of the visual fields while the child fixates on the light. A merged, solitary red-white image is perceived if extraocular movements are normal. If muscle paresis is present, the child reports a separation of the red and white images when looking in the direction of action of the affected muscle. Delayed eye movements may demonstrate or indicate minimal extraocular muscle palsies. Volitional rotation of the head accompanies paresis of the lateral rectus muscle to forestall diplopia. The head appears to deviate towards the paretic muscles, and the eyes are directed straight ahead. In superior oblique or superior rectus muscle palsies, tilting of the head towards the shoulder opposite the side of the paretic eye muscle occurs (131).

Extraocular muscle dysfunction is usually indicative of brainstem, nerve, neuromuscular function, or muscle involvement from conditions such as ophthalmoplegic migraine, cavernous sinus thrombosis, brainstem glioma, myasthenia gravis, and congenital myopathy (131). Cranial nerve VI or abducens function may be impaired by increased intracranial pressure regardless of the cause. Squint (usually esotropia) often accompanies decreased visual acuity in infants and young children (131).

Paralysis or paresis of the extraocular muscles or ptosis is usually the result of dysfunction of cranial nerve III (131,133). The appearance of a slight ptosis may be a result of interference of the sympathetic supply to Mueller's muscle. This muscle, when hyperexcited, causes the ocular globe to protrude (Grave's disease due to hyperthyroidism causes Mueller's muscle to contract and push the eye ball forward; interruption of the sympathetic supply causes Mueller's muscle to relax and allows the eye ball to sink back into the orbit giving the appearance of a slight ptosis). Ptosis as a result of oculomotor compromise tends to be more pronounced than is malposition of the eyelid in Horner's syndrome. This is a helpful feature in the differentiation of these conditions. Complete oculomotor nerve paralysis is rare. If it does occur, the eye will assume a downward and outward gaze (131).

Version (change of direction) eye positioning may accompany either irritative or destructive brainstem lesion and cerebral hemispheric lesions. The conjugate eye movement (version) deviation in destructive brainstem conditions is towards the opposite side (131). Destructive cerebral hemispheric lesions will cause the eyes to deviate ipsilaterally towards the side of lesion (103,133). Irritative cerebral hemispheric lesions will cause the eyes to deviate contralaterally from the lesion (103,133).

Eye movement deviations of the binocular disconjugate (nonparallel) type secondary to brainstem dysfunction may also occur in children (131). Lesions in the tectal area of the midbrain may result in vertical gaze paresis (131). A pineal tumor or hydrocephalus may cause an inability to elevate the eyes for upward gaze (131). Brainstem lesions, especially those in the midbrain or pons, may disrupt the medial longitudinal fasciculus (MLF) resulting in impaired conjugate eye movements known as internuclear ophthalmoplegia (133). These lesions result in weakness of the medial rectus muscles. Usually, there is paresis of the lateral rectus muscle in the abducting eye (131,133). MLF involvement may be unilateral or bilateral and may be associated with hemoglobinopathies, demyelinating disease, or brainstem vascular disease (131).

A fully dilated pupil that is unreactive to light or accommodation but normal functioning of extraocular muscles when tested individually may indicate internal ophthalmoplegia (131). The oculomotor nerve, oculomotor nucleus, or ciliary ganglion are possible sites of involvement (131).

External ophthalmoplegia results in ptosis and paralysis of all extraocular muscles (131). Pupillary reactivity is normal. These features may accompany myesthesia gravis, hyperthyroidism, ocular myopathy, Moebius syndrome, tumors or vascular lesions of the brainstem, Wernicke's disease, botulism, and lead intoxication (131).

Opticokinetic nystagmus (OKN) may be a useful test in evaluating the eye movements in children. When watching a moving object (e.g., the passing landscape from a car window or a rotating drum with vertical stripes), a rhythmic jerk nystagmus or OKN normally appears (1). The generally accepted explanation for this phenomenon is that the slow component of the nystagmus represents an involuntary pursuit movement to the limit of comfortable conjugate gaze. The eyes then make a quick saccadic movement (jerky eye movement) in the opposite direction and fixate on a new target coming into the visual field. A drum or tape with stripes may be drawn or slowly rotated before a child's eyes. With fixation, the child should visually track the object in the direction of movement. A rapid, rhythmic movement (refixation) of the eyes in the reverse direction allows the eyes to fixate on the next figure or stripe. Absence of the response may be due to failure of fixation, amaurosis (blindness without apparent lesion of the eye), or disturbed saccadic eye movements (103,131).

A child who appears to be clinically blind because of a conversion reaction (emotions become transformed into physical 'motor or sensory' manifestations) will exhibit a normal OKN response. Children who present with congenital nystagmus and have a OKN response will likely have adequate functional sight (103,131). Congenital nystagmus without the presence of the OKN response is indicative of reduced visual acuity (103,131). If the OKN response is asymmetrical, lateral lesions in the posterior half of the cerebral hemisphere are suspected—i.e., posterotemporal, parietal, or occipital areas (103,131). The lesion is ipsilateral to the side of reduced or absent OKN reactivity (103,131). Hemianopic field defects may be present (103,131).

A patient may exhibit spontaneous nystagmus (involuntary oscillatory movements of the eye) which may be horizontal, vertical, or rotatory. The movements may consist of a slow and fast phase called jerk nystagmus (103,131). The phases may be of equal duration and amplitude giving it a pendular appearance (103,131).

Nystagmus, especially vertical nystagmus, is most commonly induced by medications such as barbiturates, phenytoin, alcohol, and other sedative/hypnotic drugs. Vertical nystagmus often has a jerk component and is usually most prominent in the direction of gaze (103,131). Vertical nystagmus that is not associated with drugs is indicative of brainstem involvement (103,131). Horizontal nystagmus is indicative of dysfunction of the cerebellum or brainstem vestibular system components. Nystagmus may be coarser (i.e., the amplitude of movement greater) when the direction of gaze is towards the side of lesion (103,131).

CRANIAL NERVE V – TRIGEMINAL NERVE

Cranial nerve V or the trigeminal nerve has both sensory and motor function. The sensory portion of the cranial nerve V is responsible for sensations of the face and the anterior half of the scalp. Brainstem compromise can create sharply delineated patterns of sensory deficits, but the mapping of such deficits may be quite a challenge in children. The corneal response, whose sensory component is the trigeminal nerve, may be diminished or absent as a result of trauma, brainstem tumors, childhood mesenchymal diseases, or cerebellopontine angle tumors (131).

The trigeminal nerve is responsible for motor functions including the muscles of mastication, i.e., masseter, pterygoid, and temporalis muscles. Temporalis muscle atrophy is visually apparent as scalloping of the temporal fossa (131). The masseter muscle may be palpated for bulk while the jaw is firmly closed. The pterygoid muscle strength may be evaluated by having the patient slide the open jaw side to side while the examiner resists the motion and looks for weakness. The jaw reflex or jaw jerk is tested by the examiner placing a finger on the patient's chin. The patient's mouth is slightly opened, and the examiner taps the finger. A rapid muscle contraction with closure of the mouth is the normal response. This stretch reflex receives both afferent and efferent nerve control from the trigeminal nerve (103,131). The segmental level of this reflex is the midpons (103,131). Absence of this reflex response is indicative of motor nucleus and peripheral trigeminal lesion (103,131). An overactive response is indicative of supranuclear lesions. Jaw clonus is rarely present (131). Unilateral impairment of the trigeminal nerve may cause deviation of the jaw towards the side of lesion due to weakness of the ipsilateral pterygoid muscle (131).

CRANIAL NERVE VII – FACIAL NERVE

The facial nerve has sensory fibers responsible for taste sensation over the anterior two-thirds of the tongue and motor fibers responsible for parasympathetic secretory to the lacrimal and salivary glands and control of facial muscles (103,133). Complete motor dysfunction on one side of the face is a result of disruption of the facial nerve pathway in the nucleus, pons, or peripheral nerve. Clinically, the child is unable to elevate the forehead, close the eyes forcefully, or elevate the corner of the mouth on the side of the lesion. Central or supranuclear facial nerve lesions produce only paresis of the muscles of the lower face which results in drooping of the angle of the mouth, absent or diminished nasolabial fold, and increased palpebral fissure. Since the muscles of the forehead receive bilateral innervation, they are unaffected. The cardiofacial syndrome is a congenital weakness that results in an inability to depress the angle of the mouth and is unrelated to facial nerve palsy (131).

The lingual nerve relays afferent impulses from the anterior two-thirds of the tongue to the chorda tympani nerve which carries the taste sensations to the rostral portion of the nucleus solitarius or gustatory nucleus. Testing of taste sensation of younger children is difficult to nearly impossible. When examining the tongue, the examiner requires the tongue to be extended, holds the tongue with a gauze, and places salt, sugar, vinegar, or quinine on the anterior portion of the tongue. The tip of the tongue is more sensitive to sweet and salt; the lateral tongue is more sensitive to sour and bitter (103). The tongue must remain extended until this procedure is completed (131).

CRANIAL NERVE VIII – AUDITORY NERVE

The auditory nerve relays both auditory and vestibular input. Gross auditory impairment may be suspected during the history-taking process. The child may not respond directly to questions or to directions from the parents. Further testing with whispered words, the ticking of a watch, a party noise maker, or a tuning fork may be used to gain more information (131).

Audiometric testing may not be possible for the younger infants, but brainstem auditory-evoked potentials may confirm the hearing impairment and the level of dysfunction in the nervous system (131). Older children can be evaluated with audiometric testing.

Children who do not develop speech or who have slow speech development, as well as those who have difficulties with fluency and articulation, should be suspected of having hearing impairment and tested (131).

Clinical history and caloric testing can be used for gross assessment of vestibular function. More complex evaluation may be necessary when positive findings are noted on gross screening tests. Complaints of nausea, ataxia, vertigo, or unexplained vomiting, singly or in combination, may indicate both labyrinthine and vestibular lesions (131). Caloric testing can be preformed relatively easily, although it is a very unpleasant test. The child is placed supine, and the head is flexed 30°. Ice water is injected into the external auditory canal for a period of 30 seconds. The conscious child develops a coarse nystagmus towards the ipsilateral ear; no eye deviation occurs (131). If the patient has some degree of obtundation (ability to dull sensations), there is modification of the response (131). The eyes become tonically deviated ipsilaterally which is accompanied by contralateral nystagmus. When done on a comatose child, tonic deviation occurs ipsilaterally without nystagmus present (131). If the coma is moribund, no eye changes occur (131). Multiple examinations will help to provide a more accurate assessment and objective monitoring of changes in the level of consciousness.

CRANIAL NERVES IX AND X – GLOSSOPHARYNGEAL AND VAGUS NERVES

In evaluating the function of cranial nerves IX and X, testing the larynx, pharynx, and palate will provide most of the information (131). Unilateral paresis of the soft palate will cause an ipsilateral droop even when the patient is expelling air through the open mouth or gagging in response to a tongue blade (131). Bilateral involvement causes a bilateral flaccid, soft palate (131). With bilateral paresis, the voice becomes nasal and regurgitation of fluids occurs when drinking (131). In the assessment of swallowing, the child should be asked to swallow up to ten times to determine not only the ease or difficulty of swallowing but also stamina (131). The clinician can evaluate the difficulty of swallowing as well as the relative movements of the hyoid bone during the examination.

The gag response is mediated through the glossopharyngeal nerves and is stimulated by touching the posterior pharyngeal mucosa with the tongue blade (131). Because the response of the normal child may range from absence to a seemingly disproportionately violent response, the evaluation of changes in the gag reflex is difficult in the absence of other positive findings. The larynx can be studied under direct or indirect laryngoscopy, but the presence of stridor, hoarseness, or dystonia suggests the need for a more detailed evaluation (131).

CRANIAL NERVE XI – SPINAL ACCESSORY NERVE

The trapezius and sternomastoid muscles are innervated by the spinal accessory nerve. Cranial nerve XI is tested by having the child shrug the shoulders against resistance. Atrophy of the muscle as well as a drooping of the shoulders, are additional tests for the trapezius (131). The sternocleidomastoid muscle is tested by resisted head rotation (131). Paresis of the sternocleidomastoid muscle results in an inability to rotate the head towards the contralateral side (131). The bulk of the sternocleidomastoid muscle is easily palpated and moderate to severe atrophy is readily visible (131). Congenital or acquired lesions in the area of the foramen magnum are the most common cause of spinal accessory nerve dysfunction (131).

CRANIAL NERVE XII – HYPOGLOSSAL NERVE

The hypoglossal nerve innervates the tongue muscles. Lesions to the hypoglossal nucleus or hypoglossal nerve cause ipsilateral atrophy and fasciculation of the tongue. The protruded tongue will deviate towards the side of lesion. The child cannot push the tongue against the cheek of the unaffected side (131). Speech may be muffled or dysarthric (131). Bilateral involvement of cranial nerve XII or the hypoglossal nuclei may be severely incapacitating (131). There will be marked atrophy of the tongue, and fasciculations may be quite apparent. The child may be unable to protrude the tongue beyond the lips. There is marked dysarthria with unintelligible speech produced

(131). Unilateral tongue weakness may affect chewing and swallowing; bilateral involvement may cause considerable difficulty (131). Hypoglossal nerve dysfunction may be a result of supranuclear bulbar palsy secondary to unilateral or bilateral corticospinal tract dysfunction. Although the signs and symptoms may resemble those of hypoglossal nuclei or nerve lesions, lower motor unit signs such as fasciculations and atrophy are absent (131).

Skeletal Motor System

The examination of the child's muscular system includes the evaluation of muscle tone, bulk, and strength. Motor strength against resistance is an integral part of the neurological evaluation. The strength of the child's limb and trunk muscles is determined by the child's ability to counteract resistance imposed by the examiner. Testing of older children is conducted using the same protocol as in adults.

Strength can be measured by a variety of techniques. One such technique is to have the older child place both hands against the wall, lean forward, and perform a push-up-like maneuver. Arm and shoulder strength can be assessed in this manner. Scapular "winging" will be evident with this maneuver. The "wheel barrow" maneuver can also be used to evaluate the older child—the child walks on his hands while the examiner holds both legs up (103,110,131).

Problems with cooperation or coordination of the younger child may require the examiner to play games such as the "wheel-barrow" maneuver (131).

Anterior horn cell lesions may result in weakness of both neck flexor and extensor muscles. Weakness of the neck flexor muscles is evident early in progressive muscular dystrophies, polymyositis, and dermatomyositis (103).

During the examination of gait, the examiner must be aware of the presence of normal movements as well as associated movements such as circumduction of the legs, foot drop, unusual positioning of the feet, and waddling. Note the presence of a limp.

Muscle bulk is evaluated by gentle palpation and observation. Abnormalities, such as atrophy and fasciculations, may accompany anterior horn cell disease and muscle hypertrophy, particularly of the gastrocnemius and deltoid muscles (associated with Duchenne muscular dystrophy and other dystrophies and myotonia congenita). Palpation also serves to evaluate muscle tenderness, nerve tenderness, and nerve hypertrophy. Myotonia can be elicited by tapping over the thenar eminence and deltoid muscles (131). Tapping the individual muscles with the reflex hammer elicits the myotatic reflex (stretch reflexes producing prolonged asynchronous discharge of motor neurons which cause sustained muscle contraction—tonic reflex) which may produce intense muscular contraction These contractions may last for several minutes (103). The range of motion of limbs may be evaluated by shaking the limb and observing the limits of motion.

Tone may be decreased in the presence of cerebellar disease and anterior horn cell disease (103,131). Tone may be increased because of the rigidity associated with basal ganglia lesions and spasticity associated with corticospinal tract lesions (103).

Sensory System

The cooperation of the child during the examination of the sensory system is of paramount importance. Vibration, joint, and position sense are easily tested in all four limbs. The ability to localize touch (topagnosis) is monitored by touching the patient. The eyes should be closed during this part of the examination. The child should be asked to verbally identify the area being touched. The inability to localize the stimulus is associated with cortical parietal lobe dysfunction.

A more complex test, simultaneous touch (double simultaneous stimulation test) can be performed. Extinction is the term applied to denote loss of the ability to perceive both stimuli. The contralateral parietal lobe to the side on which the stimulus was not perceived is the site of dysfunction (131). Double stimulation touching on two areas of the skin can be used to identify extinction of perception over an involved area. Pain should always be tested with gentle stimulus, especially when using the pinprick or pinwheel (single use pinwheels, toothpicks, or safety pins should be used in this era of concern for blood transmitted pathogens). It may be necessary to repeat testing for segmental sensory deficits as attention and cooperation may affect the findings (131). Cortical sensory testing is more easily performed on the older child as testing requires maturity and intactness of the relevant regions of the parietal lobe.

"Soft" Neurological Signs

The term "soft" neurological sign refers to the integrative neurological functions of the child (134). These signs have been used to assess a variety of conditions, such as low birth weight children, mental retardation, children emotionally designated as brain-injured, those malnourished during the first two years of life, and those considered to have minimal brain dysfunction (103,134). The ages 8 to 12 are the ideal ages for conducting this type of evaluation (134). If there are two or more nonfocal signs present, these signs can be found on examination 5 years later.

The "soft signs" are nonfocal and are differentiated from localizing signs. Localizing signs include such typical findings of central nervous system lesions as cranial nerve dysfunction, presence of pathological reflexes, and lateralized dysfunction (hemiparesis). Assessing the presence or absence of nonfocal signs is more involved than the assessment of localizing signs. In the assessment of nonfocal signs, performance of the tasks given to a child are rated as within normal limits, mildly impaired, or markedly impaired. Tasks are grouped in such a way so that the examiner can better develop judgments about the integrity of the broader functional areas. In other words, these tasks provide an understanding of the collective functioning of the nervous system to produce coordinated quality of speech, quality of balance, and other functions as listed below.

TESTING FOR "SOFT SIGNS"

1. The quality of speech: the clarity, intelligibility, and word sound production is rated according to the difficulty that the examiner has in comprehending the child.

2. The quality of balance: balance is considered a nonfocal sign if at least two of the following three are markedly defective.
   a. Balance while standing: the child is asked to stand still with eyes closed, feet together, arms extended forward, and the fingers spread apart. Have the child maintain the position for at least 30 seconds. Swaying back and forth more than one inch at least three times is considered to be marked impairment (135).
   b. Hopping on one foot: The child should be able to hop ten consecutive times on each foot. Inability to hop at least five times on each foot is considered to be marked impairment (135).
   c. Tandem walking in a straight line: the child is asked to walk taking ten steps, placing the heel of one foot directly in front of the toes of the opposite foot. If the child cannot perform at least five steps in this manner, marked impairment is considered (135).

3. Coordinated movements: these are considered a nonfocal sign if at least two of the following four signs are markedly impaired.
   a. Finger-to-nose: the child is asked to extend both arms laterally at shoulder height and alternately touch the nose with each index finger. This is repeated five times. The sequence is then repeated with the eyes closed. If the child cannot perform this task at least three times with the eyes closed, marked impairment is considered (135).
   b. Rapid pronation and supination of the hand (adiadokokinesis): The child is instructed to stand, flex the elbow to 90° and then rapidly alternate the hand in pronation and supination at least five times. Repeat with the opposite hand. Marked impairment is considered if the elbow deviates more than four inches while performing the task (135).
   c. Foot tapping: the child sits in a chair and is instructed to tap the toe of each foot in succession ten times with the heel remaining on the floor. The child is then instructed to tap both feet simultaneously an additional ten times. Marked impairment is considered if the child cannot perform at least five repetitions of this task (135).
   d. Heel-to-shin: the child is seated and the legs are extended. The child is asked to flex the knee of one leg and rub the heel along the opposite leg from the knee to the toes without losing contact. This task should be done twice on each leg. Marked impairment is considered if there is a loss of contact at least two times out of the four attempts (135).

4. Double simultaneous stimulation: the child is seated with the hands on the thighs and the eyes closed. The child is told: "I am going to touch you, and I want you to show me where." The examiner lightly touches the right cheek and left hand. If the child only responded to one of the touches, the examiner asks, "Anywhere

else?" The left cheek and left hand followed by both cheeks and both hands are touched. Repeat the sequence. In order to avoid confusion, the child may be asked to point to the side being touched in order to avoid confusion about left or right side. Any mistake on the second attempt is considered a nonfocal sign (135).

5. Gait assessment: the child is instructed to walk back and forth a distance of 20 feet. The nonfocal sign is denoted if two of the following are present: feet more than 10 inches apart, a lack of smoothness in alternating flexion and extension of the knees, absence of a heel-toe gait, or immobility of the arms (lack of arm swing) (135).

6. Finger-thumb opposition performed sequentially: the child is instructed verbally and by example to oppose the thumb to each finger of the same hand. Each hand is evaluated. At least two errors that are not spontaneously corrected on either hand constitutes a nonfocal sign (103,135).

7. Muscle tone: the assessment of muscle tone has been previously described in the chapter. In addition to motion palpation of the wrists, elbows, hips, knees, and ankles, the examiner should hold the child's forearms and gently but rapidly flap the wrists and then hold the lower leg and flap the knees to assess tone and range of motion. Tone is considered separately in each extremity. Marked hypertonia or hypotonia in all four extremities is necessary for abnormal tone to be noted as a nonfocal sign (135).

8. Graphesthesia: the child is seated with hands on the thighs, palms up, and eyes closed. The child is then asked to identify the letters or numbers that he feels is being written on the palms. A bluntly pointed pencil-like object is used for "writing." The figures "118," "2," "3," "C," and "R" can be used. Each hand is tested. If mistakes are made, he is asked to identify the symbols visually. A nonfocal sign is indicated if there are at least two failures on each hand in the presence of accurate visual identification (135).

9. Astereognosis: the child is asked to identify objects by feeling them in each hand with the eyes closed. Objects may include a pocket comb, key, quarter, and a penny. The child is not allowed to transfer objects from one hand to the other, although manipulation of the object is permitted. After the tasks are completed, the child is asked to visually identify each object. The inability to identify by feel of at least two objects is a nonfocal sign (135).

10. Choreiform movements are assessed by asking the child to mimic the position previously described for the evaluation of standing balance. The examiner watches for small jerky twitches in the fingers, wrists, arms, or shoulders. Choreiform movements are nonfocal signs if ten or more twitches are observed within a 30 second period (135).

Clinical Evaluation of the Child's Skull

Head circumference is an important neurological tool for the pediatric neurologic examiner. A normal increase in skull size reflects a growing brain. Serial measurements will identify a head that is growing rapidly. Not all rapidly growing heads indicate pathology, however. If the child is asymptomatic and the presence of abnormalities is not present, the patient can be followed until several percentile lines are crossed.

When the skull becomes too large, there is usually an underlying intracranial pathology (110). Most children with abnormally large heads have either hydrocephaly or subdural collections of fluid. Rarely, megalocephaly (excessive brain mass) may cause an enlarged head (110).

Transillumination is done in total darkness by tightly placing a flashlight with a rubber adapter throughout the skull. Obviously, a knowledge of skull and suture morphology is necessary. A normal skull transilluminates more in the frontal region (110). Skulls of premature infants transilluminate more than those of full term infants. False transillumination from extravasated intravenous fluids may obscure the findings. Diffuse transillumination is seen in hydranencephaly (complete or near complete absence of the cerebral hemispheres whose space is filled with cerebrospinal fluid), in severe hydrocephalus which is accompanied by marked thinning of the cerebral mantle, bilateral subdural effusions, and occasionally in diffuse cerebral atrophy with enlargement of the subarachnoid spaces (110). See Chapter 10 for further information on abnormalities of the cranium.

REFERENCES

1. Noback CR, Demarest RJ. The Human Nervous System. San Juan: McGraw-Hill Book Co. 1981. pp.137-149.
2. Crelin ES. Functional Anatomy of the Newborn. New Haven: Yale University Press. 1973. pp.7-8, 11-12, 22-25.
3. Roush W. New neurons use "lookouts" to navigate nervous system. Science 1996; 271:1807-1808.
4. McKnight T. "Pediatric and Geriatric Neurology" lecture notes. LACC Chiropractic Neurology course. Palo Alto, California, January 11-12, 1992.
5. Lemire RJ, et al. Normal and Abnormal Development of the Human Nervous System. Hagerstown MD: Harper & Row, Publishers, Inc. 1975.
6. Martinez PFA. Neuroanatomy: Development and Structure of the Central Nervous System. Philadelphia: W.B. Saunders Co. 1982.
7. Carpenter •. Core Text of Neuroanatomy (4th Ed). Baltimore: Williams & Wilkins, 1991.
8. Nieuwenhuys R, Voogd J, van Huijzen C. The Human Central Nervous System: A Synopsis and Atlas, (3rd ed.) New York: Springer-Verlag. 1988.
9. Pansky B, Allen DJ, Budd GC. Review of Neuroscience (2nd ed). New York: Macmillan Publishing Co. 1988.
10. Brooks VB. Cerebellar functions in motor control. Hum Neurobiol 1984; 2(4):251-260.
11. Cramer GD. Clinical Neuroanatomy Session II seminar notes. LACC sponsored Chiropractic Neurology course. Berkeley CA. July 14-15, 1990.
12. Kee LS. An Introduction to the Human Nervous System. Singapore: Singapore University Press, 1986.
13. Romero-Sierra C. Neuroanatomy: A Conceptual Approach. New York: Churchill Livingstone, 1986.
14. Netter FH. The CIBA Medical Collection: Volume 1 Nervous System. Part I: Anatomy and Physiology. West Caldwell NJ: CIBA Pharmaceutical Co., 1986.
15. DeJong RN. The Neurologic Examination (4th Ed). Philadelphia: Harper & Row, Publishers. 1979, pp.304-328.
16. FitzGerald MJT. Neuroanatomy: Basic and Applied. Philadelphia: Bailliere Tindall, 1985.
17. deGroots J, Chusid JG. Correlative Neuroanatomy (20th Ed). East Norwalk CT: Appleton & Lange, 1988.
18. McKechnie B. Low Back Pain in the 90s: A Neurological Perspective notes. ACA Symposium. Los Angeles, California, November 23-24, 1991.
19. Mathers LH. Peripheral Nervous System. Boston: Butterworth Publishers. 1985.

20. Batson VL. The vertebral vein system. Am J Roentgenol Radium Ther Nucl Med 1957; 78(2):195-212.
21. Crock HV, Yoshizawa H, Kame SK. Observations of the venous drainage of the human vertebral body. J Bone Joint Surg 1973; 55-B(3):528-533.
22. Mihorat TH, Hammock MK. Cerebrospinal Fluid as Reflection of Internal Milieu of Brain. In: Wood JH (ed). Neurobiology of Cerebrospinal Fluid, Volume 2. New York: Plenum Press. 1983.
23. Wood JH. Physiology, Pharmacology, and Dynamics of Cerebrospinal Fluid. In: Wood JH. Neurology of Cerebrospinal Fluid. Part I. New York: Plenum Press, 1980; pp.1-14.
24. Mendel T, Wink CS, Zimny ML. Neural elements in human cervical intervertebral discs. Spine 1992; 17(2):132-135.
25. Giles LGF. Spinal fixation and viscera. J Clin Chiropractic 1973; Archive Ed #3:144-165.
26. Bogduk N, Windsor M, Inglis A. The innervation of the cervical intervertebral discs. Spine 1988; 13(1):2-8.
27. Bogduk N, Tynan W, Wilson AS. The nerve supply to the human lumbar intervertebral discs. J Anatomy 1981; 132(1):39-56.
28. Haldeman S. The Neurophysiology of Spinal Pain. In Haldeman S (ed). Principles and Practice of Chiropractic. Norwalk CT: Appleton & Lange. 1992; pp.165-184.
29. Giles LGF. Paraspinal autonomic ganglion distortion due to vertebral body osteophytosis: a case of vertebrogenic autonomic syndromes? J Manipul Physiol Therapeut 1992; 15(9):551-555.
30. Korr IM. Sustained Sympatheticotonia as a Factor in Disease. In: The Collected Papers of Irvin M. Korr. Colorado Springs CO: American Academy of Osteopathy, 1979; pp.77-91.
31. Korr IM. The spinal cord as organizer of disease processes: III. Hyperactivity of the sympathetic innervation as a common factor in disease. J Am Osteopath Assoc 1979; 79(4):232-237.
32. Goss AB (ed). Gray's Anatomy (29th ed). Philadelphia: W. B. Saunders Co., 1973.
33. Kamonsinska B, et al. Spinal segmental sympathetic outflow to cervical sympathetic trunk, vertebral nerve, inferior cardiac nerve and sympathetic fibers in the thoracic vagus. J Autonomic Nerv Syst 1991; 32(3):199-204.
34. Guyton AC. Textbook of Medical Physiology (5th ed). Philadelphia: W.B. Saunders Co. 1976.
35. Barr M, Kiernan J. The Human Nerve System (5th ed). Philadelphia: J.P. Lippincott Co. 1988.
36. Best C, Taylor N (eds). Physiological Basis of Medical Practice (4th ed). Baltimore: Williams & Wilkins, 1945.
37. Nathan H. Osteophytes of the spine compressing the sympathetic trunk and splanchnic nerves in the thorax. Spine 1987;12(6):527-532.
38. Wyke BD. Articular Neurology and Manipulative Therapy. In: Glasgow EF, et al. (eds). Aspects of Manipulative Therapy (2nd ed). New York: Churchill Livingstone, 1985; pp.72-80.
39. Guyton AC. Textbook of medical physiology (5th ed.) Philadelphia: WB Saunders, 1976.
40. Diamond MC, Scheibel AB, Elson LM. The Human Brain Coloring Book. New York: Harper & Row Publishers, 1985.
41. Jinkins JR, Whittemore AR, Bradley WG. The anatomic basis of vertebrogenic pain and the autonomic syndrome associated with lumbar disk extrusion. Am J Neuroradiol 1989; 10:219-231.
42. Korr IM. The Segmental Nervous System as a Mediator and Organizer of Disease. In: Peterson B (ed). The Collected Papers of Irvin M. Korr. Colorado Springs CO: American Academy of Osteopathy, 1979; pp.178-181.
43. Korr IM. The spinal cord as organizer of disease processes: I. Some preliminary perspectives. J Am Osteopath Assoc 1976; 76:35- And in: Peterson B (ed). The Collected Papers of Irvin M. Korr. Colorado Springs, CO: American Academy of Osteopathy, 1979.
44. Gunn CC. Prespondylosis and some pain syndromes following denervation supersensitivity. Spine 1980; 5(2):185-192.
45. Pottenger S. Symptoms of Visceral Disease (6th ed). St. Louis: C. V. Mosby, 1994.
46. Hooshmand H. Chronic Pain, Reflex Sympathetic Dystrophy: Prevention and Management. Boca Raton: CRC Press, 1993.
47. Kandel ER, Schwartz JH. Principles of Neural Science (2nd ed). New York: Elsevier, 1985.
48. Leach RA. The Chiropractic Theories (2nd ed). Baltimore: Williams & Wilkins, 1986.
49. Korr IM. The Trophic Functions of Nerves and Their Mechanisms. J Am Osteopath Assoc 1972; 72: 163-171 and in: Peterson B (ed). The Collected Papers of Irvin M. Korr. Colorado Springs, CO: American Academy of Osteopathy, 1979; pp.182-187.
50. Slosberg M. Effects of altered afferent articular input on sensation, proprioception, muscle tone and sympathetic reflex response. J Manipulative Physiol Ther 1988; 11(5):400-408.
51. Slosberg M. Spinal learning: Central modulation of pain processing and long-term alteration of interneuronal excitability as a result of nociceptive peripheral input. J Manipulat Physiol Therapeut 1990; 13(4):326-336.
52. Korr IM. Proprioceptors and the behavior of lesioned segments. Osteopath Ann 1974; 2:12-32.
53. Cox JM. Low Back Pain: Mechanism, Diagnosis and Treatment (4th ed). Baltimore: Williams & Wilkins, 1985.
54. Hoag JM. Theoretical analysis of osteopathic lesions. In: Yearbook of the Academy of Osteopathy, Colorado Springs: American Academy of Osteopathy 1970.
55. Cohn RE. Ischemic contraction of microvessels and nerve root dysfunction. Chiropractic 1989; 2(3):77-81.
56. Saal J, et al. High levels of inflammatory phospholipase A2 activity in lumbar disc herniations. Spine 1990; 15(7):674-678.
57. Saal J, et al. The role of inflammation in lumbar pain. Phys Med Rehabil: State Arts Rev 1990; 4:191-199.
58. Hoyland JA, Freemont AJ, Jayson MI. Intervertebral foramen venous obstruction. A cause of periradicular fibrosis? Spine 1989; 14:558-68.
59. Blumberg H, Janig W. Changes of reflexes in vasoconstrictor neurons supplying the cat hindlimb following chronic nerve lesions: A model for studying mechanisms of reflex sympathetic dystrophy. J Autonom Nerv Syst 1983; 7(3-4):399-411.
60. Cannon WB, Rosenblueth A. The supersensitivity of denervated structures. NY: MacMillian Co. 1949.
61. Rosen S, et al. Central nervous system pathways mediating angina pectoralis. Lancet 1994; 344:147-150.
62. Jebsen RH, et al. Differential diagnosis of hypotonia. Am J Dis Child 1961; 101(1):8-17.
63. Finestone H, et al. Autonomic dysreflexia after brainstem tumor resection: A case report. Am J Phys Med Rehabil 1993; 72(6):395-397.
64. Van Buskirk R. Nociceptive reflexes and the somatic dysfunction: A model. J Am Osteopath Assoc 1990; 90(9):792-809.
65. Williams RW, McCullough JA, Young PH, eds. Microsurgery of the lumbar spine. Gaithersburg, MD: Aspen Publishers. 1990.
66. Calaresu FR. Introduction: Autonomic preganglionic neurons—The final common pathway of physiological regulations. J Autonom Nerv Syst 1982; 5(1):3-7.
67. Korr IM. Andrew Taylor Still Memorial Lecture: Research and Practice—A Century Later. In: Peterson B (ed). The Collected Papers of Irvan M. Korr. Colorado Springs, CO: American Academy of Osteopathy, 1979; pp.190-199.
68. Braunwald E. The sympathetic nervous system in heart failure. Hospital Practice 1970; 5(12):31-39.
69. Regan JJ, et al. The induction of cardiac arrhythmia and hypotension from spinal cord monitoring. Spine 1986; 11(10):1031-1032.
70. Shafer RC. Basic Principles of Chiropractic. Arlington VA: American Chiropractic Association, 1990.
71. Koizumi K. Autonomic System Reactions Caused by Excitation of Somatic Afferents: Study of Cutaneo-Intestinal Reflex. In: Korr IM (ed). The Neurobiological Mechanisms in Manipulative Therapy. New York: Plenum Press, 1977; pp.219-227.
72. Ochoa J. Reflex Sympathetic Dystrophy: Definitions and History of the Ideas with Critical Review of Human Studies. In: Low PA (ed). Clinical Autonomic Disorders. Boston: Little, Brown & Co, 1993; pp.473-492.
73. Langweiler M, et al. Reflex sympathetic dystrophy syndrome: A case report. J Neuromusculoskeletal Syst 1993; 1(2):69-73.
74. Van Houdenhove. Etiopathogenesis of reflex sympathetic dystrophy: A review and biopsychological hypothesis. Clin J Pain 1992; 8(4).
75. Richards RL. Causalgia. Arch Neurol 1967; 16(4):339-350.e
76. Ashwal S, et al. Reflex sympathetic dystrophy syndrome in children. Pediatr Neurol 1988; 4(1):38-42.
77. Wilder RT, et al. Reflex sympathetic dystrophy in children. J Bone Joint Surg 1992; 74A(6):910-919.
78. Berstein BH, et al. Reflex neurovascular dystrophy in childhood. J Pediatr 1978; 93(2):211-215.
79. Ellis WB, Ebrall P. The resolution of chronic inversion and plantar flexion of the foot: A pediatric case study. Chiropractic Technique 1991; 3(2):55-59.
80. Hindwood JA, Hindwood JA. Children and chiropractic: A summary of subluxation and its ramifications. J Aust Chiropract Assoc 1981; 11(9):18-21.
81. Thomas PE. An approach to the analysis of spinal stress through its physiological manifestations. J Am Osteopath Assoc 1951; 50:403-406.
82. Ruggeri SB, et al. Reflex sympathetic dystrophy in children. Clin Orthop Rel Res 1982; 163:225-230.
83. Windsor H. Sympathetic segmental disturbances. Med Times 1921:266-271.
84. Wiles M. Visceral Disorders Related to the Spine. In: Gatterman MI. Chiropractic Management of Spine Related Disorders. Baltimore: Williams & Wilkins, 1990; pp.379-396.
85. Terrett AGJ. Cerebral dysfunction: A theory to explain some of the effects of chiropractic manipulation. Chiropractic Technique 1993; 5(4):168-173.
86. Haldeman S. The influence of the autonomic nervous system on cerebral blood flow. Intl Rev Chiropractic 1975; 29(5):12-13.
87. Edvinsson L, et al. Autonomic Nervous System Control of Cerebrospinal Fluid Production and Intracranial Pressure. In: Wood JH (ed). Neurobiology of Cerebrospinal Fluid. New York: Plenum Press, 1980; pp.661-666.
88. Lawrence D. Fundamentals of Chiropractic Diagnosis and Management. Baltimore: Williams and Wilkins, 1991.
89. Korr IM. The Sympathetic Nervous System as Mediator Between the Somatic and Supportive Process. In: Peterson B (ed). The Collected Papers of Irvan M. Korr. Colorado Springs, CO: American Academy of Osteopathy, 1979; pp.170-174.

90. Fidelibus J. An overview of neuroimmunomodulation and a possible correlation with musculoskeletal system function. J Manipulat Physiol Therapeut 1989; 12(4):289-292.

91. Allen J. The effects of chiropractic on the immune system: A review of the literature. Chiropract J Aust 1993; 34(4).

92. Arnason BGW. The Sympathetic Nervous System and the Immune Response. In: Low PA (ed). Clinical Autonomic Disorders. Boston: Little, Brown & Co., 1993; pp.143-154.

93. Pert C. The wisdom of the receptors: Neuropeptides, the emotions, and body mind. Advances 1986; 3(3):8.16.

94. Stein-Werblowsky R. The sympathetic nervous system and cancer. Exp Neurol 1974; 42:97-100.

95. Brennan P, et al. Enhanced phagocytic cell respiratory burst induced by spinal manipulation: potential role of substance P. J Manipulat Physiol Therapeut 1991: 14(7):399-408.

96. Escard E, de Coriat LF. Development of postural and tonic patterns in the newborn infant. Pediatr Clin North Am 1960; 7(3):511-525.

97. Amiel-Tison C. Neurological evaluation of the maturity of newborn infants. Arch Dis Childhood 1968; 43(227):89-93.

98. Flehmig I. Normal infant development and borderline deviations. New York: Thieme Medical Publishers, Inc. 1992; pp.8-265.

99. Bates B. A Guide to Physical Examination and History-Taking (5th ed). Philadelphia: J.P. Lippincott Co. 1991; pp.626-635.

100. Mumenthaler M. Neurology (3rd ed). New York: Thieme Medical Publishers, Inc., 1990.

101. Beintema DJ. A neurological study of newborn infants. Clin Develop Med 1968; 28:99-110.

102. Blasco PA. Primitive reflexes: Their contribution to the early detection of cerebral palsy. Clin Pediatr 1994; 33(7):385-397.

103. Adams RD, Victor M. Principles of Neurology (4th ed). New York: McGraw-Hill. 1989; pp.273-290.

104. Dargassies SS. Neurological development in the full-term and premature neonate. New York: Excerpta Medica 1977; pp.68-109, 154-173.

105. Brett EM. Chapter 2: Normal Development and Neurological Examination Beyond the Newborn Period. In: Brett EM (ed). Pediatr Neurol 1991; pp.27-51.

106. Capute AJ. Primitive Reflex Profiles. Baltimore: University Park Press. 1978; pp.1-91.

107. Crawford TO. Clinical evaluation of the floppy infant. Pediatr Ann 1992; 21(6):348-354.

108. Prechtl HFR. Qualitative changes of spontaneous movements in fetus and preterm infant are a marker of neurological dysfunction. Early Hum Develop 1990; 23(3):151-158.

109. Deuel RK, Robinson DJ. Chapter 5: Developmental Motor Signs. In: Tupper DE (ed). Soft Neurological Signs. Orlando FL: Grune & Stratton, Inc. 1987; pp.95-121.

110. Weiner HL, Urion DK, Levitt LP. Pediatric Neurology for the House Officer (3rd ed). Baltimore: Williams & Wilkins, 1988.

111. Dietrich HF. A longitudinal study of the Babinski and Plantar grasp reflexes in infancy. Am J Dis Childhood 1957; 94:265-271.

112. Fenichel GM. Clinical Pediatric Neurology. Philadelphia: W.B. Saunders Co., 1988; pp.147-149.

113. Cowell DH. Chapter 3: Infant Motor Development. In: Brackbill Y (ed). Infancy and Early Childhood. New York: The Free Press, 1967.

114. Fiorentino MR. Reflex Testing Methods for Evaluating C.N.S. Development.

Springfield IL: Charles C. Thomas Publishers 1973; pp.8-49.

115. Brett EM. Chapter 1: Neurology of the Newborn. In: Brett EM (ed). Pediatric Neurology. 1991; pp.4-26.

116. Hadders-Algra M, Prechtl HFR. Developmental course of general movements in early infancy. I. Descriptive analysis of change in form. Early Hum Develop 1992; 28(3):201-213.

117. McGrew MB. The Neuromuscular Maturation of the Human Infant. New York: Hafner Publishing Co., 1969; pp.24-85

118. Gentry EF, Aldrich CA. Rooting reflex in the newborn infant: Incidences and effect on it of sleep. Am J Dis Child 1948; 75(4):528-539

119. Swaiman KF. Chapter 3: Neurologic Examination After the Newborn Period Until 2 Years of Age. In: Swaiman KF (ed). Pediatric Neurology. St. Louis: C.V. Mosby Co. 1989; pp.35-44.

120. Paine RS. Neurologic examination of infants and children. Pediatr Clin North Am 1960; 7(3):471-510.

121. Parmelee AH. A critical evaluation of the Moro reflex. Pediatrics 1964; 33(5, Part 1):773-788.

122. Fredrickson WT, Brown JV. Gripping and Moro responses: Differences between small-for-gestational age and normal weight term newborns. Early Hum Develop 1980; 4(1):69-77.

123. Paine RS. The neurologic examination of the child with minor nervous dysfunction. Clin Develop Med 1966; 20/21:30-212.

124. McMullen M. Assessing upper cervical subluxations in infants under six months: Utilizing the reverse fencer response. ICA Intl Rev Chiropract 1990; 46(2):39-41.

125. Rome PL. Case report: The effect of a chiropractic spinal adjustment on toddler sleep pattern and behavior. Chiropract J Aust 1996; 26(1):11-14.

126. Haynes U. A Developmental Approach to Case finding with Special Reference to Cerebral Palsy, Mental Retardation, and Related Disorders. Washington, D.C.: U.S. Department of Health, Education, and Welfare, 1967.

127. Jaffe M, et al. The parachute reactions in normal and late walkers. Pediatr Neurol 1996; 14(1):46-48.

128. Grice AS. The mechanics of walking development and clinical significance. J Can Chiropract Assoc 1972; 16(3): 15-23.

129. Amiel-Tison C. Neurological Assessment During the First Year of Life. Oxford University Press, 1986; pp.18-43.

130. Forslund M, Bjerre I. Follow-up of preterm children: I. Neurological assessment at 4 years of age. Early Hum Develop 1989 20(1):45-66.

131. Swaiman KF. Chapter 2: Neurological Examination of the Older Child. In: Swaiman KF (ed). Pediatric Neurology. St. Louis: C.V. Mosby Co., 1989; pp.15-32.

132. Meyer S, Gibb T, Jurkovich GJ. Evaluation and significance of the pupillary reflex in trauma patients. Ann Emerg Med 1993; 22(6):1052-1057.

133. Goldberg S. Clinical Neuroanatomy Made Ridiculously Simple. Miami FL: Medmasters, Inc., 1989.

134. Peters JE. A Special or Soft Neurological Examination for School Age Children. In: Tupper DE (ed). Soft Neurological Signs. Orlando FL: Grune & Stratton, Inc., 1987; pp.369-379.

135. Hertzig ME. Appendix B: Neurologic Evaluation Schedule. In: Tupper DE (ed). Soft Neurological Signs. Orlando FL: Grune & Stratton, Inc., 1987; pp 355-379.

APPENDIX 13.1

Summary of the Pediatric Neurologic Evaluation

The primary purpose of the neurological examination is to screen for neurological abnormalities or lesions. When a pathology or disorder is suspected, the neurologist's initial exploration is not so much to name a disease or disorder but to localize the lesion. In other words, the neurologist begins with a broad scan and attempts to narrow down the location and nature of the lesion.

The typical neurological evaluation following a history begins with a neurological screen. As chiropractors, we are usually looking for peripheral nerve alterations. The evaluation includes sensory, motor, and deep tendon reflex of the peripheral nervous system. The cranial nerve evaluation is conducted if the history warrants it. In the very young child or infant, some aspects cannot be conducted as in an adult. More subtle variations must be sought.

The worse case scenarios, neurologically speaking, are a child presenting with comatose state, severe headaches and/or neck pain, particularly if there is a history of recent fever, or abnormal neurological signs with indications of trauma. These cases need to be evaluated carefully. Cases such as these usually go to an emergency room, but on occasion, may show up in your office—or the parents may request your assistance when faced with these symptoms. More subtle cases with an seemingly unremarkable history but with a serious underlying neurological disorder may end up in your office. A suspicious history and examination warrants a thorough evaluation, and in some cases, you may need to share the case with a specialist versed in the area of suspicion, such as a chiropractic neurologist.

The pediatric neurological examination must take into account the age of the child. This will help you design an examination for the child and to evaluate the proper maturation of the nervous system. The periods of maturation may be divided in the following way:

1. *Neonate*
   Note the gross nervous system function, primitive reflexes, and "milestones."
2. *Infant*
   Note delays in development such as persisting primitive reflexes. This is a good time to observe play and social interactions as well as movements such as the development of walking, crawling, gait, and the ability of the infant to sit upright.
3. *Pre-school*
   Note the speech patterns, motor development, and hyperactivity or hypoactivity.
4. *Early School*
   Note social activity, ability to learn and grasp concepts, and also observe developing motor skills. Intellectual impairment may be present. In some cases the latter has

been associated with maternal smoking during pregnancy (1).

5. *Adolescent*
   Because there is sufficient maturing of the nervous system, an adult-like evaluation is possible. Some nervous system immaturity may alter some signs.
6. *Preteen*
   Preteens are evaluated much like adults. The primary concern would be orthopedic problems, such as scoliosis.
7. *Teen*
   Teens are evaluated like adults. The nervous system is nearly fully matured. The primary concern would be orthopedic problems, such as scoliosis.

SEQUENCE OF EXAMINATION STEPS FOR THE MOTOR EXAMINATION OF INFANTS

Case History: history as related by parents, all documents of previous examinations, family photographs. Videotapes of the patient can be of extreme importance.

Neurologic examination, gestational age, and other examination results.

Motor examination: coordinated movements eventually leading to these movements can be stimulated by toys, eye contact, gestures, speech, etc.

AGE-RELATED NEUROLOGIC EXAMINATION SEQUENCE

NEWBORN
The exam begins with the infant at rest:

1. Observations:
   a. Spontaneous movements
   b. Palpebral fissures (symmetry)
   c. The "setting sun" sign
   d. Marcus Gunn sign (elevation of the eyelid with jaw movements)
   e. Moro Reflex
   f. Abnormal movements: e.g., writhing baby, myoclonus, flaccidity, irregular movements, jittery movements, asymmetrical movements
   g. Position of the arms should be noted as the asymmetry of brachial palsy is obvious (hemiparesis is uncommon in the newborn period unless there is trauma or anoxic insult at birth. In cases of congenital cerebral lesions, the earliest sign may be a poverty of movement of one arm with the infant maintaining a clenched fist to a degree greater than the opposite hand).

2. Response to stimuli
   a. Blink reflex (reaction to light)
   b. Dazzle reflex, reaction to sound (jerk or jump reflex)
   c. Moro sign
   d. Palmar grasping
   e. Plantar grasp
   f. Knee jerk (head should be in the midline when conducting this)
   g. Clonus of ankle

PEDIATRIC NEUROLOGIC EXAM

FORMAT

Date: _____   Name: _____   Gender: _____

Temperature: _____   Height: _____   Weight: _____

Birth date: _____   Age: _____   Blood Pressure: _____

Previous Chiropractic   Pulse: _____   Respiratory Rate: _____

  Care? Yes   No   Premature? Yes   No   If yes, weeks: _____

Previous analysis and/or diagnosis (brief comment): _____

GENERAL BEHAVIOR

Cooperative _____   Uncooperative _____

Comments _____

SPEECH

Absent _____   Stutters _____   Stammers _____

Lisps _____   Echolalia _____   Incomprehensible _____

Expressive Aphasia _____   Receptive Aphasia _____

Comments _____

LEFT-RIGHT SIDE AWARENESS

Right hand _____   Left hand _____   Right eye _____

HAND DOMINANCE

Throw an object _____

Turn a door knob/handle _____

Use scissors _____

Write _____

EYE DOMINANCE

(Have the patient look at an object through a circle formed by both hands with both eyes, then each eye. Note the eye that still sees the object on one eye viewing)

FOOT DOMINANCE

Kicking _____

CRANIAL NERVES

Eye movements (cranial nerves 3,4,6) _____

Snellen chart: L   R   Both

Pupils

    R ___mm L ___mm

    Light reflex _____

    Accommodation _____

    Nystagmus _____

    Comments _____

E.O.M.

    Intact _____

    Abnormalities _____

Visual field by confrontation

Single stimulation _____

Intact _____

Abnormalities _____

Double stimulation

Intact _____

Abnormalities _____

Fundi

Disc _____ Normal _____ Abnormalities _____

Retina _____ Normal _____ Abnormalities _____

Corneal sensation

Right: _____ Intact _____ Absent _____

Left: _____ Intact _____ Absent _____

Facial nerve (CN 7)

Facial asymmetry _____

Acoustic nerve (CN 8)

Gross hearing _____ Intact _____ Abnormal _____

Double simultaneous stimulation _____ Intact _____ Abnormal _____

Vagus nerve (CN 10)

Gag reflex _____ Present _____ Absent _____

Hypoglossal nerve (CN 12)

Tongue _____ Midline _____ Right deviation _____ Left deviation _____

Standing balance (30 seconds):   Normal _____ Mildly impaired _____ Markedly impaired _____

Comments _____

Hopping (10 times per foot):   Normal _____ Mildly impaired _____ Markedly impaired _____

Comments _____

Choreiform movements

	None	Slight	Marked
Shoulder	_____	_____	_____
Arm	_____	_____	_____
Finger	_____	_____	_____
Comments	_____	_____	_____
Arm drifts	_____	_____	_____

(patient holds both hands and arms extended with eyes closed for 30 seconds)

Muscle tone (note normal, hypertonic, or hypotonic)

Upper extremities

	Right	Left
Hand flapping	_____	_____
Wrist flexion/extension	_____	_____
Elbow flexion/extension	_____	_____
Hyperextension of fingers	_____	_____

Lower extremities

Knee flapping _____

Ankle _____

Comments _____

Muscle strength

Upper extremities _____

Lower extremities _____

Reflexes

Biceps _____

Triceps _____

Radial _____

Abdominal _____

Knee _____

Achilles _____

Clonus (Absent, Sustained, or Rhythmic)

Note: there may be as many as twelve beats in the first few weeks of life which is considered to be normal (2).

Right _____

Left _____

Plantar response (Flexion, Extension, or equivocal)

Right _____

Left _____

Finger-to-Nose (Normal, Mildly impaired, or Markedly impaired)

	Right	Left
Eyes open	_____	_____
Eyes closed	_____	_____
Comments	_____	

Finger-to-Finger (Normal, Mildly impaired, or Markedly impaired)

	Right	Left
Eyes open	_____	_____
Eyes closed	_____	_____
Comments	_____	

FINGER-THUMB OPPOSITION

1 2 3 4   4 3 2 1   Consecutive movement _____ Overflow movement _____

Right _____

Left _____

Comments _____

PRONATION-SUPINATION OF THE HANDS (NORMAL, MILDLY IMPAIRED, MARKEDLY IMPAIRED)

Right _____

Left _____

FOOT TAPPING (NORMAL, MILDLY IMPAIRED, MARKEDLY IMPAIRED)

	One foot	Both feet
Right	_____	_____
Left	_____	_____
Overflow movement	_____	_____

Comments _____

HEEL-TO-SHIN (NORMAL, MILDLY IMPAIRED, MARKEDLY IMPAIRED)

Right _____

Left _____

Comments _____

SENSORY

Note: Preliminary sensory testing of the limb leads to withdrawal of the stimulated limb if the stimulus is of sufficient force whereas a feeble pricking may produce an extension (1)

Comments _____

Sensation

Pinpricks _____

Light touch _____

Position _____

Graphesthesia

Right hand _____ 3 _____ a _____ 2 _____

Left hand _____ 8 _____ c _____ R _____

Astereognosis

	Right	Left
Key	_____	_____
Quarter	_____	_____
Penny	_____	_____
Comb	_____	_____
Pencil	_____	_____

Gait: Normal _____ Mildly impaired _____ Markedly impaired _____

    Base _____

    Knee flexion/extension _____

    Heel-toe-gait _____

    Arm movements _____

    Comments

Tandem walking: Normal _____ Mildly impaired _____ Markedly impaired _____

Comments _____

Neurological DX:

    Localizing findings _____

    Non-localizing findings: Number of signs

	Positive	Negative
Speech	_____	_____
Balance	_____	_____
Coordination	_____	_____
DSS	_____	_____
Finger-Thumb/Mult finger opposition	_____	_____
Muscle tone	_____	_____
Graphesthesia	_____	_____
Astereognosis	_____	_____
Choreiform movements	_____	_____

    Normal

---

    h. Rooting response
    i. Fasciculations of the tongue.
3. Special senses
    a. Visual fields
    b. Eye movements and conjugate gaze
    c. Reaction to light, strabismus (pinpoints of light)
    d. Hearing (turning eyes or head towards sound)
    e. Sensation of touch (movement away from, turning eyes towards, or turning head toward the touched point)
4. Tests
    Clonus
    Locomotion (asymmetries should be noted)
    Posture when suspended (vertical and horizontal)
    Landau
    Vestibular nystagmus (labyrinthine stimulation, e.g., irritation to the external auditory canal with warm or cold water produces nystagmus). This establishes the OKN (optokinetic nystagmus) which appears within minutes or hours after birth.

    Placing reflex
    Supporting reaction (when feet touch, legs should extend)
    Parachute reflex
    Superficial reflexes
    Tonic righting reflexes
    Tonic neck reflexes
5. ENT: eyes, eye grounds, throat, gag reflex, and ears.
6. Tone of anal sphincter.
7. Transillumination of the head (halo effect done laterally and A-P)

    INFANT WHO ASSUMES THE WEIGHT-BEARING POSITION—ABOUT 1 YEAR OF AGE

The examiner must pay particular attention to the following:
    Balance (sitting and standing by themselves)
    State of consciousness
    Orientation
    Symmetrical face and eye movements

Hand movements and preference (athetosis appearing in the first years of life is usually the result of congenital or postnatal conditions such as hypoxia or kernicterus) (3).

Problem-solving

Test for mental ability and motor skills: e.g., ring and string, stacking cubes, placing cubes in a cup, unwrapping a wrapped cube, observing the child's reaction to a large picture book.

Motor Functions and Adaptation, Grasping, Speech, Social Contact

Normal: Abnormal:

Age: Comments:

Speech

Social Contact

Hearing and localizing noises, phonation while the examiner watches breathing, sucking, and swallowing: state normalities, abnormalities, age, and comments.

Vision and eye movements: routines of daily life, emotional behavior, development (with consideration of sensory integration).

Comment

The maturation process is continuous. However, the integrity of the developing nervous system is paramount. It is a dynamic developmental process. Any disruption, interference, or lack of

Table 13.12. **Gross Motor Ability**

Position	Normal	Abnormal	Age	Comment
Supine				
Prone				
Raising up from the supine position				
Pulling upwards to a sitting position				
Sitting down unaided				
Sitting				
Pulling upwards to a standing position				
Standing up unaided				
Standing				
Rolling, creeping				
Crawling				
Walking				
Posture and muscle tone				
Test of postural patterns in all positions				
(horizontal and head down position, lateral displacement, etc.)				
Reaction to balance				
Symmetry				
Tonic postural patterns and reflexes as well as reactions to early infancy (primary reactions)				

Table 13.13.   **Motor Functions and Adaptation**

	Normal	Abnormal	Age	Comment
Visual				
Acoustic				
Tactile, Kinesthetic, Vestibular				

Table 13.14.   **Examination within the First Year**

Reflex	Present	Absent	Appears	Disappears
Moro			Birth	4–5 months
Stepping and placing			Birth	Persists as voluntary standing
Positive supporting			Newborn to 3 months	Persists voluntarily
Tonic neck			2–3 weeks	4–6 months (never obligatory or sustained)
Crossed adductor			2–3 months	7–8 months
Neck righting			begins 4–6 months	Persists voluntarily
Parachute			begins 6–7 months	Persists
Palmar grasp reflex (at birth)			Birth	3–4 months
Voluntary reach			4–5 months	Persists
Palmar grasp			4–5 months (entire hand)	Persists
Ankle clonus			8–10 beats in newborn	Generally disappears by age 2 months

continuous development should, in itself, already be considered a suspicious sign (4).

Despite numerous studies carried out by various research groups, it has not been possible to come up with generally accepted definition for the characteristics of cerebral palsy (4). The noxious agent of infantile brain injury, e.g., lack of oxygen, diffusely affects the still completely immature brain in an unpredictable manner and with various degrees of intensity (4). The following sequence of thinking may help in the diagnosis of cerebral palsy and will help to differentiate cerebral palsy form other conditions.

Brief Definitions

Spasticity: muscle hypertonicity leads to poor coordination of movement and sustained posture.

Athetosis: oversteering within the locomotor system leading to movements that are undirected, useless, and quite bizarre-looking movements.

Ataxia: feedback mechanism of the central regulating system has been damaged by disturbances of the movement control apparatus of the cerebellum and its nerve tracts leading to permanent co-contraction which is an expression of oversteering in the central nervous system. Walking is with a "stilted" stride. The upper extremities demonstrates patterns of extension. Loss of fine motor movements.

Central hypotonia: coordinated regulation seems completely impossible. The control mechanism is at a complete standstill. Movements are rough, abrupt, and produce extreme effects. Attaining as well as maintaining posture becomes impossible.

Mixed forms: difficult, but are found in children with motor disturbances. They exhibit faulty coordination of movements. The motor disturbance is only part of the overall injury. There are multiple handicaps.

Gait and Movements

Observation of gait and movement is a valuable part of both the musculoskeletal and neurological examination. Careful observation of superficial structures such as the skin and musculature may reveal underlying neurological disorders. Autonomic and spinal nerve disorders may alter the appearance of the skin. These can include color changes or dermatological lesions (e.g., neurofibromatosis). Muscle atrophy may also be of autonomic or spinal nerve origin. Malformations may be observable from visual examination. Klippel-Feil Syndrome, spina bifida, and neurofibromatosis are a few of the developmental disorders that may be revealed upon visual evaluation.

As the child becomes mobile and develops the ability to walk and run, observation of gait must be part of the chiropractor's pediatric examination. Gait disturbances may be an indication of an underlying neurological disorder or vertebral subluxation complex or joint dysfunction (5). A child who smoothly articulates movement on one side but throws the ipsilateral hip forward on the other may have a joint dysfunction or vertebral subluxation complex which does not allow the sacroiliac, hip, or a lower back joint to function properly or may be causing a myotendinous problem, an ataxic gait, a spastic gait.

Overall movements are observed for smooth, symmetrical (except those associated with handedness) movements.

Deep Tendon Reflex Status

Reflex patterns constitute some of the most important findings in a neurological examination. Most commonly, improper procedures, interpretation, and significance is given to these extremely helpful responses.

Deep tendon/muscle stretch reflexes can be graded by a couple of methods:

Descriptive Method:

Equal			Hypoactive
Absent	Hyperactive		
			Wexler Scale
0			Absent with reinforcement
1	+1 1+	+	Hypoactive
2	+2 2+	++	Normal (sluggish or brisk)
3	+3 3+	+++	Hyperactive
4	+4 4+	++++	Hyperactive with transient clonus
5	+5 5+	+++++	Hyperactive with sustained clonus

PALPATION

The palpatory examination is one of the most important parts of the examination for all ages of children. The upper cervical spine may reveal tenderness which may stimulate the infant to cry or withdraw. This is a clear finding which may require x-ray examination.

OPTIC EXAMINATION

The measurement of the optic field affords the examiner an enormous amount of information. Normal functioning of very large regions of the brain is required for a fully intact visual field. Below are several conditions which lead to a better understanding of the visual examination.

1. Pupillary response abnormalities: due to lesions of the fibers proximal to the lateral geniculate body, in the midbrain, or the third cranial nerve.
2. Homonymous hemianopsia: implies a lesion posterior to the optic chiasma. It may involve the optic tract or both the optic radiations emanating from the lateral geniculate body. Because the tract converges near the lateral geniculate body, a smaller lesion is necessary to create homonymous hemianopsia in its vicinity than in more distal regions of the tract.

Table 13.15. **Factors in Cerebral Palsy Diagnosis**

		Present	Not Present	Comment
Spasticity				
	Quadriplegia			
	Diparesis			
	Hemiparesis			
	Bilateral hemiparesis			
Hyperkinesis				
	Athetoid (dystonic, choreo-athetotic, rigid form)			
	Dystonia			
	Tremor			
Rigidity				
	Ataxia			
	Central hyptonia			
	Mixed forms			

Table 13.16.   **Cranial Nerve Tests for the Infant**

Cranial Nerve		Test
I	Olfactory	Non-noxious fragrant substances are used. In young children or infants, this nerve is very difficult or impossible to test.
II	Optic	Visual acuity is tested in the older child as in an adult. An infant is difficult to test.
III	Occulomotor	Pupillary light reflex. In older children, the cardinal eye movements can be checked. In younger children, watch spontaneous eye movements.
IV	Trochlear	In older children, conduct the cardinal eye movements. In younger children, watch for movements associated with the superior oblique muscle.
V	Trigeminal	
VI	Abducens	In older children, conduct the cardinal eye movements. In younger children, watch for movements associated with the lateral rectus muscle.
VII	Facial	Rooting and sucking
VIII	Acoustic	Doll's eye maneuver or Moro reflex
IX	Glossopharyngeal	
X	Vagus	Observe swallowing
XI	Spinal Accessory	
XII	Hypoglossal	Cranial nerve XII can be tested by pinching the infant's nostrils. This produces a reflexive opening of the mouth and raising of the tip of the tongue. Paresis of cranial nerve XII causes deviation of the tip of the tongue to the affected side. [BATES p627]

3. Bitemporal hemianopsia: classically found in craniopharyngiomas or pituitary tumors secondary to pressure on the optic chiasma. Nonhomonymous field defects usually imply a chiasmal lesion. Concentric "tunnel-like" vision may be seen in hysterical blindness.

4. Blindness in one eye: represents retinal or optic nerve dysfunction. The optic nerve is involved in optic neuritis which produces a unilateral blindness. It may also be involved with a tumor (optic glioma) or undergo atrophy secondary to prolonged raised intracranial pressure.

In examining the visual fields, it must be remembered that the optic radiations fan out from the lateral geniculate body and travel in the temporal and parietal lobes before reaching their destination in the occipital lobe. Lesions in the temporal lobe may give a homonymous superior field defect if the optic radiations are affected. Similarly, a lesion in the parietal lobe may show an inferior homonymous field defect.

Cranial Nerves
In an infant, arousal provides an opportunity to evaluate many of the cranial nerves. Crying and grimacing tests some of the nerves—corners of the mouth are displaced and the nasolabial folds are deepened (6). Vision, hearing, and smell are difficult to properly assess in an infant. The vestibular portion of cranial nerve VIII can be tested by the doll's eye maneuver and the Moro reflex (6). Rooting and sucking are partial tests for cranial nerves V, VII, and XII (6). Cranial nerves IX and X can be tested by observing swallowing (6). Older children can be tested like an adult.

ELECTRODIAGNOSIS
There are a multitude of neuroelectrodiagnostic tests that can be ordered. It is important to know which test to order. If in doubt, a specialist in neurology, chiropractic or medical, may be able to advise the doctor.

Many of these tests are used in situations that the doctor of chiropractic may not be presented with, but the chiropractor may be confronted with a young patient whose past work-up had one or more of these tests done. The doctor should have an understanding of the purposes of each of these tests when formulating a clinical opinion.

Electromyography
Electromyography (EMG) records the electrical activity of the muscles. This test is used to evaluate the peripheral motor system.

Nerve Conduction Velocity Test (NCV)
Nerve conduction velocity studies are used to evaluate peripheral nerves for lesions. It is used to confirm other findings of peripheral nerve injury and the extent of the lesion. The NCV studies can be done on motor or sensory neurons. Typically, sensory tests are run to see if the lesion is below the dorsal root ganglion. The studies are useful when evaluating children

where a physical evaluation of peripheral neurological function may be difficult (4).

SOMATOSENSORY-EVOKED POTENTIAL

Somatosensory-evoked potential (SEP/SSEP) uses percutaneous electrical stimulation to measure waveforms from peripheral nerves. By age three, infants should be attaining adult ranges of peripheral conduction velocities. Adult values of spinal cord velocities are not attained until age five (7).

SEP is used to test the integrity of the dorsal columns/medial lemniscus system (7). It is used in evaluating the spinal cord for disorders with etiologies such as trauma, degeneration, or inflammation (7). It can also evaluate for diffuse cerebral disorders with changes in consciousness or mental status (7). SEP has a prognostic value. In those suspected of hemiplegia or a preterm with periventricular hemorrhage, an abnormal SEP carries a poor prognosis (7).

BRAINSTEM AUDITORY-EVOKED RESPONSE

Auditory-evoked potentials of brainstem activity (BAER) measures brainstem activity in response to auditory stimulation (7). It is useful in evaluating the brainstem of a comatose neonate (70). It is also useful in determining hearing loss (7). It is useful in evaluating children who are too young or have a disorder precluding responses in other visual processing tests (7).

VISUAL-EVOKED RESPONSE

Visual-evoked response (VER) is a means of evaluating visual processing (7). Responses of the visual cortex are measured by pick-ups placed over the occiput (7).

ELECTROENCEPHALOGRAPHY

Electroencephalography (EEG) records the electrical activity of the brain (8). It has been used when evaluating for organic brain disease. With the development of CT scanning and MRI, EEG use is diminishing. EEG records the electrical activity of the cerebral cortex, primarily the superficial layers (8).

BRAIN ELECTRICAL ACTIVITY MAPPING

Brain electrical activity mapping (BEAM) or "brain mapping" is done in the resting state and during behavioral or cognitive activity (9). Its usefulness is still controversial because of its low sensitivity and specificity (9).

DIAGNOSTIC IMAGING

The plethora of diagnostic imaging systems have been a boon to the neurologist. The uses and diagnostic accuracy with the new procedures are progressing almost daily. Those who require the procedures in order to evaluate patients can be overwhelmed as they try to keep up with the latest developments.

Neuroimaging studies are anatomical or physiological. X-ray and CT scanning are anatomical studies. PET and most of the other studies are physiological. There is much concerning which study to use. Image selectivity, patient cooperation (very important in children), and cost are important factors.

PLAIN X-RAY

Plain x-ray films are useful for observing osseous structures and soft tissues that have calcified. High density soft tissue can also be imaged with the appropriate technique. Plain x-rays have limitations in the ability to image structures and no ability to assess function directly. They are a useful tool for many osseous anomalies and malformations such as Klippel-Feil syndrome, basilar impression, block vertebrae, and platybasia. Tumors displacing bone or eroding bone and other conditions such as infection that may erode bone may be visualized on the plain film. In this way, it can be a useful tool for determining the necessity for or type of further studies that may be required.

For the chiropractor, it can confirm misalignments or intersegmental motion aberrations in addition to the above noted anomalies, malformations, and pathology.

COMPUTER-AIDED TOMOGRAPHY (CT SCAN)

The practice of neurology has been revolutionized with the development of CT scanning and magnetic resonance imaging (MRI). CT scanning is usually chosen when imaging intracranial disorders (9). Other developing imaging systems have further enhanced the study of structural and physiological processes of the nervous system and related structures.

MAGNETIC RESONANCE IMAGING

Magnetic resonance imaging (MRI) is a structural imaging study. In young children, sedation is often used because of the need for prolonged immobility (9).

The image varies greatly as the nervous system matures. During the first 12 months after birth, five observable stages have been described based upon myelination maturation (9). It has been found useful in imaging white matter disorders, developmental cerebral dysplasias, cerebral infarcts, and brain manifestations of neurocutaneous disorders (9). Contrast agents are being used to visualize tumors and demyelinating diseases (9).

Functional MRI is a physiological imaging system that can map changes in cerebral venous oxygen concentrations as a study of neuronal activity. Images can be obtained in 40 milliseconds (10).

MAGNETIC RESONANCE ANGIOGRAPHY (MRA)

MRA produces three dimensional digital images of medium and large diameter arteries and veins. Because they are digitized, they can be combined with MRI images to form a single combined image of the vascular and the brain structures (16). This is a far less invasive procedure than traditional angiography which can have fatal consequences.

POSITRON EMISSION TOMOGRAPHY (PET)

Positron Emission Tomography (PET scan) is a physiological study. Using positron-emitting isotopes, regional metabolic rates and cerebral blood flow can be measured (9). Cerebral metabolism, blood flow, blood volume, oxygen use, neurotransmitter synthesis, and receptor binding are studied (10). At present, it is being used to study epilepsy (9). It has also been used to image neurodegenerative diseases such as Parkinson's, Alzheimer's, Huntington's, as well as some psychiatric disorders (10).

SINGLE PHOTON EMISSION COMPUTED TOMOGRAPHY

SPECT scans give an indirect assessment of cerebral perfusion via the use of radioisotope tracers in the cerebral blood flow. A variety of tracers are utilized such as Ceretec (Tc hexamethylpropylene) and Spectamine (I-radiolabeled iodoamphetamine) (11).

A study by Kumar, et al. attempted to correlate abnormal SPECT findings in neonates with abnormal neurological and developmental outcomes. They were unable to make a correlation for either. They did conclude that normal SPECT scans tended to predict a normal neurodevelopmental outcome (11). It has been used to image normal brain function, epilepsy, cerebrovascular disease, degenerative diseases, and psychiatric disorders (10).

CRANIAL ULTRASONOGRAPHY

Cranial ultrasonography is done through the anterior fontanelle (9,12). It is noninvasive, does not utilize ionizing radiation, and is easier to use on noncooperative patients than would be the case with CT scan or MR imaging (9). It is used to visualize intracranial structures. It is useful in studying hemorrhage, ventricular appearance, anomalies, and for evaluating neurological sequelae of hypoxic–ischemic encephalopathy (9). It does not have the clarity for smaller lesions that MR imaging or CT scanning would image (9). There are no known risks with the procedure (12). The procedure ceases to be useful after the anterior fontanelle (about age 12 months), and also requires both an experienced operator and a clinician experienced in interpreting the image (12).

TRANSCRANIAL DOPPLER IMAGING

Doppler sonography is done through the anterior fontanelle or transtemporally (9). It is used to study intracranial vascular structures (9).

MYELOGRAPHY

Myelography uses radiopaque dyes and plain x-rays. It is used for gross blockages in the flow of CSF that caused by space-occupying masses such as protrusion of the intervertebral disc, osteophytes, and intracanial neoplasms. It has been largely supplanted by MR imaging and CT scanning.

OTHER PROCEDURES

LUMBAR PUNCTURE

This is an important procedure when there is a high degree of suspicion of central nervous system infection or there is increased intracranial pressure.

PSYCHOLOGICAL/PSYCHIATRIC EVALUATION

Suspicion of or further evaluation for mental disorders may require evaluation by a specialist who is well versed and equipped in this field. Children who have gone through physical or mental trauma may show changes in behavior and/or personality that require evaluation and appropriate care.

LEARNING AND BEHAVIOR TESTING

Numerous forms of tests have been developed to evaluate the learning ability or behavior of children at different ages. These include tests such as Dallas Development Screening Test (13), Bayley Scales of Infant Development, Cattell Infant Intelligence Scale, Wechsler Intelligence Scale for Children - III, Peabody Picture Vocabulary Test - Revised and Stanford-Binet Intelligence Scale IV. The Stanford-Binet Intelligence Scale, Fourth Edition tests the cognitive abilities). It studies crystallized ability (verbal reasoning ability and quantitative reasoning ability), fluid-analytic ability (abstract/visual reasoning), and short-term memory (14).

APGAR SCORE

The Apgar Score depends upon the integrity of the autonomic nervous system. The APGAR Score is a test of neurophysi-

Table 13.17. **Apgar Score**

Criteria	Score		
	0	1	2
Color	Blue	Body pink	All pink
	Pale	Extremities blue	
Heart rate	Absent	<100	>100
Respiration	Absent	Irregular/Slow	Good/Crying
Reflex response to nose catheter	None	Grimace	Sneeze/Cough
Muscle tone	Limp	Some flexion of extremities	Active

Adapted from Berkow R (ed). "The Merck Manual of Diagnosis and Therapy" (14th Ed). Rahway NJ: Merck & Co. 1982. pp. 1756–57.

Table 13.18.   **Glasgow Coma Scale, Pediatric Modified**

Regular Scale		Pediatric Scale	
Eyes open			
Spontaneously	4		
To Speech	3		
To Pain	2		
None	1		
Best Verbal Response			
Orientated	5	Orientated	5
Confused	4	Words	4
Inappropriate words	3	Vocal sounds	3
Incomprehensible sounds	2	Cries	2
None	1	None	1
Best Motor Response			
Obeys commands	5		
Localize pain	4		
Flexion to pain	3		
Extension to pain	2		
None	1		

Adapted from Simpson D, Reilly P. Paediatric Coma Scale. Lancet 1992; II(8295):450.

ological function of the brainstem and spine—an estimation of the severity of asphyxia at birth. First presented in 1953, it took the objective factors that could easily be determined and did not interfere with the care. Prior to that time, numerous haphazard procedures were utilized, many of dubious value (2). A numerical value is given after evaluating breathing, heart, color, skin tone, and response to stimuli. A mnemonic for remembering the components are Appearance, Pulse, Grimace, Activity, and Respiration (15). The APGAR is conducted one minute and five minutes after birth.

The maximum score is ten. A score of ten is not common. Descending numbers indicate the severity of asphyxia. Zero is the worst score and two is normal (2). Scores of 4 are indicative of severe asphyxia. If low Apgar scores continue at the five minutes evaluation, there is a likelihood of neurological damage or neonatal death, although, there are many who survive and live normally (16). Continued low scores after 10 minutes increases the likelihood of a poor outcome (17). If the Apgar scores are very low and a major neurological problem is suspected, there will probably be other clinical signs within days or weeks (18).

GLASCOW COMA SCALE, PEDIATRIC MODIFIED

The Glascow Coma Scale assesses consciousness impairment following head injury. Table 13.18 is a brief summary to help you in its interpretation.

The verbal scale must be modified for children below age 10 because the language skills are still developing. In the infant, the verbal section must be further modified to account for a rudimentary verbal response.

REFERENCES

1. Olds DL, Henderson CR, Tatelbaum R. Intellectual impairment in children of women who smoke cigarettes during pregnancy. Pediatrics 1994; 93(2):221-7.
2. Apgar V. A Proposal for a New Method of Evaluation of the Newborn Infant. Current Researches in Anesthesia and Analgesia July-August 1953; 32(4): 260-267.
3. Adams RD, Victor M. Principles of Neurology. 4th ed. New York: McGraw-Hill. 1989.
4. Greenberg DA, Aminoff MJ, Simon RP. Clinical Neurology, 2nd ed. Norwalk CT: Appleton & Lange. 1993.
5. Grice AS. The Mechanics of Walking Development and Clinical Significance. Journal of the Canadian Chiropractors Association. October 1972; 16(3): 15-23.
6. Fenichel GM. Neonatal Neurology, 3rd ed. New York: Churchill Livingstone. 1988. pp.1-16.
7. Scher MS. Pediatric Electroencephalography and Evoked Potential. In: Swaiman KF, ed. Pediatric Neurology: Principles and Practice. St. Louis MO: C. V. Mosby Co. 1989. pp.97-100.
8. deGroots J, Chusid JG. Correlative Neuroanatomy. 20th ed. East Norwalk CT: Appleton & Lange. 1988.
9. Ferry PC. Pediatric Neurodiagnostic Tests: A Modern Perspective. Pediatrics in Review July 1992; 13(7):248-255.
10. Mazziotta JC. Mapping Human Brain Activity in Vivo. Western Journal of Medicine September 1994; 161(3):273-278.
11. Kumar P, et al. Post Extracorporeal Membrane Oxygenation Single Photon Emission Computed Tomography (SPECT) as a Predictor of Neurodevelopmental Outcome. Pediatrics June 1994; 93(6):951-955.

12. Filipek PA, Blickman JG. Neuroimaging Techniques. In: David RB. Pediatric Neurology for the Clinician. Norwalk, CT: Appleton & Lange. 1992.

13. Bates B. A Guide to Physical Examination and History Taking, 5th ed. Philadelphia: J.B. Lippincott Co. 1991.

14. Hollinger CL, Baldwin C. The Stanford-Binet, Fourth Edition: A Small Study of Concurrent Validity. Psychological Reports June 1990; 66(3, Part 2):1331-1336.

15. Fysh P. Self-published seminar notes.

16. Berkow R (ed). The Merck Manual of Diagnosis and Therapy, 14th ed. Rahway NJ: Merck & Co. 1982. pp. 1756-57.

17. Menkes JH. Textbook of Child Neurology, 3rd ed. Philadelphia: Lea & Febiger. 1985. p.285.

18. Nelson KB. Cerebral Palsy. In: Swaiman KF, ed. Pediatric Neurology: Principles and Practice. St. Louis MO: C. V. Mosby Co. 1989. p.366.

APPENDIX 13.2

Selected Neurological Disorders

Pediatrics is an expanding part of the modern chiropractic practice as parents are finding the benefits of the chiropractic adjustment not only for themselves, but also their children. With this increasing utilization comes the necessity for proper evaluation as is expected of a pediatric primary care physician. It is very important to rule out neurological disorders, although this may have been done prior to the child being presented to your office. This section gives a brief summary of selected neurological disorders so that you can have some understanding of a disorder that a patient may have been previously diagnosed with or that you may suspect.

Each disorder includes a description, its typical features, the typical medical management, and any documented chiropractic management. The medical management is the latest that can be ascertained from medical literature. It is included to help you understand what has been done, what is being done, or what may be done to your pediatric patient. Unfortunately, there are few chiropractic studies on many neurological conditions. Many chiropractors are learning the accepted research protocols and style of writing and are beginning to document cases so that more of the beneficial effects of chiropractic on even so-called incurable and serious neurological disorders are appearing in the literature.

Those who specialize in the chiropractic care of the pediatric patient or whose practice has a large population of pediatric patients must keep up with the latest research on pediatric health. Of great importance is the growing and improving chiropractic research on the care of children who have a variety of pediatric disorders. The dramatic demonstration of the effects of vertebral subluxations and their reduction by the chiropractic adjustment is dramatically emphasized by pediatric disorders. References are given with each disorder in order to facilitate further study.

ATTENTION-DEFICIT HYPERACTIVITY DISORDER (ADHD)

Many learning difficulties often fall under the category of attention-deficit disorder with or without hyperactivity. Current focus tends to be on those associated with hyperactivity or hyperkinesis. Without a distinct clinical picture, learning disorders in this category depend upon a list of somewhat vague behaviors that have been agreed upon by specialists in this area.

Attention-deficit hyperactivity disorder (ADHD) or attention-deficit disorder with hyperactivity (ADDH) affects 1% to 10% of school-aged children (1). Baren states that the clinical prevalence may be about 6% to 8% (2). Males are most likely to be affected, 3:1 to 9:1 (1). The characteristic signs are inappropriate hyperactivity, impulsiveness, and inattentiveness (3). Girls tend to have more cognitive problems and fewer disruptive behaviors than do boys (2).

The cause of ADHD is unknown (1). Researchers have looked at genetics, neurotransmitter abnormalities, insult to or slow maturation of the central nervous system, heavy metal poisoning, thyroid abnormalities (4), artificial chemicals in foods, and minimal brain damage-inducing encephalitis following pertussis vaccination (5). There appears to be a familial occurrence (6). Some subtypes may be associated with depleted supplies of neurotransmitters, such as the catecholamines dopamine and norepinephrine (2). Alterations in the prefrontal and striatal-limbic system and the locus ceruleus may be involved in hyperactive-impulsive ADHD. The cortices of the temporal and parietal lobes may be involved in the inattentive form of ADHD (2). Positron emission tomographic or PET scans have found decreased metabolic activity in the frontal lobes and basal ganglion (caudate nucleus) and increased metabolic activity in the primary sensory and sensorimotor regions (7).

Complicating the understanding of any neuroanatomical, neurophysiological, and/or neurochemical mechanism to ADD/ADHD is that the diagnostic criteria for it is not clear cut.

Some have listed hyperactivity under the term, "minimal brain dysfunction," because of the presence of "soft" neurologic signs. The problem of attaching "brain dysfunction" to this diagnosis is that many of these signs are also seen in otherwise normal children (8).

Allergies to food and other elements in the environment have been studied by some as a possible factor in some cases of hyperactivity. Positive clinical responses have been noted when offending substances were removed (9). Feingold has advocated reducing or removing artificial/synthetic additives (e.g., flavoring and coloring) from food (10). Others have not been able to establish the connection (11,12). Some implicate red and yellow food coloring (13). Eliminating salicylate-containing foods and drugs have also been recommended (9,14).

Weiss, et al have attempted to determine if thyroid abnormalities were prevalent in ADHD children but were not able to find a correlation (1,4). Some feel that indoor light quality without a full natural outdoor spectrum may be related to attention deficit or learning difficulties.

Other neurological disorders may be complicated by ADD or ADHD. For example, many of those diagnosed with Gilles de la Tourette Syndrome have ADHD as well (4,15).

CLINICAL FEATURES

Many behavioral observations have been connected to ADHD. The three primary features of attentional disorders are inattention, impulsivity, and hyperactivity (16).

As noted above, there are no hard factors in the diagnostic work-up for ADHD. The clinician should find the area of learning that the child has difficulties in. Considerations in the history include any prenatal or postnatal factors that may have an influence on the central nervous system, familial history of learning disorders or unusual jobs, and factors that have been associated with learning difficulties such as autoimmune disorders, premature graying, and nondextrality, late appearances of motor or language milestones, oromotor difficulties during infancy, hearing problems, seizures, motor hyperactivity, and psychological or social problems in the family (17).

Scales that are commonly used in the work-up for ADHD include the Conners Teacher and Parent Scales, Revised; the Achenbach Child Behavior Checklists; the ADD-H Comprehensive Teacher Rating Scale, Revised; the ADHD Scales; SNAP-IV; and the Conners, Loney, and Milich scale (2). The "freedom from distractibility" factor which is based upon the Wechsler Intelligence Scales for Children subtests, Digit Span and Arithmetic and from WISC-Revised, the subtest Digit Span, Arithmetic, and Coding, has been used in the work-up for ADHD but does not specifically identify it. Evaluation of the frontal, parietal and temporal lobes have been noted to be helpful in determining the treatment (2).

Diagnosis of ADHD is often based upon the criteria that were developed for the DSM-IV (Diagnostic and Statistical Manual of Mental Disorders, Fourth Edition). There are three basic types of ADHD: predominately inattentive type; ADHD: predominately hyperactive-impulsive type; and ADHD: combined type (2).

A complete physical examination including neurologic and neurodevelopmental evaluation are very important, although apparently often neglected. This will help rule out other conditions that may cause ADHD-like behavior. No laboratory testing, imaging, or electroneurodiagnostic studies can diagnose ADHD but they might be indicated if other neurological disorders are suspected. The diagnostic criteria can include almost any child.

In Europe, the prevalence for hyperkinetic behavior is much lower (1:200 vs 1:20 in the U.S.) as they use the more stringent ICD-10 diagnostic criteria rather than the DSM-IV criteria used in the U.S. In Europe, the diagnosis is based more on interviews by trained interviewers rather than based upon complaints by teachers and parents (18).

MEDICAL MANAGEMENT

Drug treatment is the typical approach. The use of stimulants seems contradictory, but it is thought to work by increasing the threshold to environmental stimuli (19). A controversial but very commonly-used drug in the treatment for ADHD is the drug methylphenidate hydrochloride (brand name Ritalin). Drugs such as dextroamphetamine sulfate (brand name Dexedrine) and Cylert (pemoline) are used in some cases (1). Methylphenidate tends to have dopaminergic effects while dextroamphetamine tends to have noradrenergic effects (20).

The drugs can cause appetite loss, headaches, irritability, emotional lability, insomnia, transient growth impairment, and other symptoms. There is a possibility of tics that may progress to Tourette syndrome (19). There may also be rebound phenomenon (6).

Too many times, there may be inadequate evaluation (sometimes only teacher or parent complaints) with positive effects of the drug as confirmation of the diagnosis. There may be inadequate monitoring of the drug treatment program (19).

Other interventions include schooling in small-group, structured and orderly classrooms with few distractions and stimulations (1) and behavior modification (1). Fifty to seventy percent continue to have symptoms of ADHD regardless of the treatment being used. Hyperactivity tends to diminish with time, but other behavior problems may arise (1).

CHIROPRACTIC MANAGEMENT

Hospers, et al describe a case of a 15-year-old male who had a history of hyperactivity since infancy and was placed in special classes because of learning difficulties. In the interim, he had a series of four falls causing head injury. Prior to this study, he was placed on Dexadrine and Mellaril which caused side effects but no improvement. EEG showed abnormal findings. Upper cervical adjustments were done and EEG readings improved following the adjustments (21).

Webster had patients keep diet diaries. He suspected that foods may trigger vertebral subluxations. Using an instrument not described, they found "readings" reduced when hyperactive children changed their diet. Unfortunately, no mention was made of any changes in behavior, activities, or improvements in learning (13).

An 11-year-old male who presented at Kentuckiana Children's Center had a history of disruptive behavior and hyperactivity. These continued despite the use of Ritalin which was withdrawn by the mother as no positive behavioral changes were noted. He had been in foster care during part of his infancy before being adopted. He had a history of repeated ear infections, allergies, TMJ dysfunction, recurring headaches, enuresis, and epistaxis. He received nutritional supplementation which reduced high levels of aluminum, lead, and cadmium that were noted in his evaluation. He received chiropractic care by "manual and activator methods" primarily to the upper cervical spine. Counseling was also done for a period of one year. During three years of care, he has improved academically, learned that he can control his behavior, and his mother noted an improvement in his attentional span and temper. The TMJ dysfunction is not common nor are the headaches. Enuresis had abated (22).

A 10-year-old male was seen at Northwestern Chiropractic College with a history of ADHD. He also had a history of chronic otitis media for which he had bilateral tympanostomies at ages 4 and 6, as well as a history of chronic and severe headaches and allergies. Previous history included a difficult birth and colic (23).

Anderson and Partridge present a case of a 6-year-old male who presented to the Kentuckiana Children's Center with seizures and attention deficit hyperactivity disorder. He has a family history of ADHD—father and paternal grandmother. On the day he received a DT shot at age three, his temperature rose and he began having seizures. The seizures that followed were absence and post temporal. A pediatric neurologist diagnosed his condition as atypical absence seizures and prescribed Cylert and Depakene. Two months later, EEG studies found abnormalities. Also, an adenoidectomy was performed and ventilation tubes placed. Allergy shots were prescribed. A year later, a psychiatrist diagnosed ADHD. Catapres was prescribed as was family counseling and antidepressants for the father. A few months later he was placed in special education after a visit to a neuropsychological department in a hospital. The medications caused a variety of side effects. He also became very violent. A couple of months later, his parents took him to Kentuckiana with presenting com-

Table 13.19.   Attention Deficit Hyperactive Disorder (ADHD) DSM-IV Diagnostic Criteria

A. Either 1 or 2:

1. Six or more of the following symptoms of *inattention* have persisted for at least six months to a degree that is maladaptive and inconsistent with developmental level:
    a. Often fails to give close attention to details or makes careless mistakes in schoolwork, work, or other activities
    b. Often has difficulty sustaining attention in tasks or play activities
    c. Often does not seem to listen when spoken to directly
    d. Often does not follow through on instructions and fails to finish schoolwork, chores, or duties in the workplace (not due to oppositional behavior or failure to understand instructions)
    e. Often has difficulty organizing tasks and activities
    f. Often avoids, dislikes, or is reluctant to engage in tasks that require sustained mental effort (such as schoolwork or homework)
    g. Often loses things necessary for tasks or activities (toys, school assignments, pencils, books, or tools)
    h. is often easily distracted by extraneous stimuli
    i. is often forgetful in daily activities

2. Six or more of the following symptoms of *hyperactivity-impulsivity* have persisted for at least six months to a degree that is maladaptive and inconsistent with developmental level:
    Hyperactivity
    a. Often fidgets with hands or feet or squirms in seat
    b. Often leaves seat in classroom or in other situations in which remaining seated is expected
    c. Often runs about or climbs excessively in situations in which it is inappropriate (in adolescents or adults, may be limited to subjective feelings of restlessness)
    d. Often has difficulty playing or engaging in leisure activities quietly
    e. is often "on the go" or often acts as if "driven by a motor"
    f. Often talks excessively
    Impulsivity
    g. Often blurts out answers before questions have been completed
    h. Often has difficulty awaiting turn
    i. Often interrupts or intrudes on others (such as butting into conversations or games)

B. Some hyperactivity, impulsive, or inattentive symptoms that caused impairment were present before age 7 years

C. Some impairment from the symptoms is present in two or more settings (such as in school or work or at home)

D. There must be clear evidence of clinically significant impairment in social, academic, or occupational functioning

E. The symptoms do not occur exclusively during the course of a prevasive developmental disorder, schizophrenia, or another psychotic disorder and are not better accounted for by another mental disorder (such as mood, anxiety, dissociative, or personality disorder)

Adapted from Baren M. What ADHD is—and isn't. Patient Care 1995;29(20):59.

plaints of violent and threatening behavior, hyperactivity, and absence seizures. Adjustments and nutritional supplements were begun. Frequency was thrice weekly for 18 months, then decreased to once per two weeks. After one year of care, seizures abated, but later returned after a severe fall which resulted in an elbow fracture. A later fall caused another upper extremity fracture. At the time of the report, some seizures persisted. The mother stated that his behavior improved with adjustments. He was able to control violent behavior (24).

A study was conducted on seven hyperactive children. A Werry-Weiss-Peters parental rating scale was completed by the parents. Skin resistance level was measured. Chiropractic evaluation and radiographic studies were done. Motion recorders were worn by the patients. When an activity was being done by one hand, motion measurements were made of the resting arm. The acetometer also was used while the child was engaged in school-type activity while an observer was hidden. In the initial phase, a mock adjustment was given using an Activator instrument set to zero. During the active adjustment phase, Gonstead and diversified type adjustments were given. After the active care, four of seven showed improvements in radiographic findings (the criteria was not given for improvement). Chiropractic physical findings were improved to some degree in all cases. Acetometer measurements improved in five of seven cases. Four of seven showed improvements in autonomic measurements using the skin conduction instrument. Four of seven also had improvements in the parental scale (25).

In the early 1970s, Walton studied two groups of children with a variety of learning and behavioral problems. Many were diagnosed with hyperkinetic behavior. The students received chiropractic adjustment, often to the upper cervical and thoracic spine. Cross-crawl exercises (as per Goodheart) and vitamin B complex were given as needed. In the first group of 13, most responded very well to the chiropractic care given. The second group consisted of 12 receiving chiropractic care and 12 receiving medication. Nine of those on drugs initially benefited and the medication controlled hyperkinesis and attention span but later, increasing doses were required. One half had adverse effects from the drugs such as loss of appetite, insomnia, and personality changes. There was equal initial reduction in hyperkinesis and improved attention span in the group receiving chiropractic care. The benefit was sustained in the chiropractic care group, and the latter group also had much improvement in lowered nervous tension, better effort and motivation, and improved coordination (26–29).

Lemeshow stated that chiropractors should find the hyperkinetic child a natural and logical challenge. He noted that structural changes may induce changes in the internal environment by reducing muscular tension and improving neural function. Adjunctive care such as nutritional supplementation and psychotherapy were thought to be important in a comprehensive approach (30).

Hammerich indicated that in addition to chiropractic adjustments, dietary modification and nutritional supplementation/vitamins can also be very important. She found insulin dysfunction to be an important part in the picture, particularly as related to hypoglycemia (31).

REFERENCES

1. Leung AKC, et al. Attention-deficit hyperactivity disorder. Postgrad Med 1994; 95(2):153-160.
2. Baren M. What ADHD is—and isn't. Patient Care 1995; 29(20):56-62+.
3. Waldrop RD. Selection of patients for management of attention deficit hyperactivity disorder in a private practice setting. Clin Pediatr 1994; 33(2):83-87.
4. Weiss RE, et al. Attention deficit hyperactivity disorder and thyroid function. J Pediatr 1993; 123:539-545 (also described in the "Literature Review" section of Clinical Pediatrics February 1994; 33(2):124.)
5. Coulter HL, Fisher BL. A Shot in the Dark. Garden City Park, NY: Avery Publishing Group, Inc. 1991.
6. Taylor MA. Evaluation and management of attention-deficit hyperactivity disorder. Am Family Physician 1997; 55(3):887-901.
7. Riccio CA, et al. Neurological basis of attention deficit hyperactivity disorder. Exceptional Children 1993; 60(2):118-124.
8. Adams RD, Victor M. Priniciples of Neurology, 4th ed. San Francisco: McGraw-Hill, Inc. 1989, p. 483.
9. Null G. Hyperactivity and learning disabilities. ACA J Chiropractic 1988; 25(12):34-38.
10. Feingold BF. Hyperkinesis and learning disabilities linked to the ingestion of artificial food colors and flavors. J Learning Disabilities 1976; 9(9):551(19)-559(27).
11. Conners CK. Food Additives and Hyperactive Children. New York: Plenum Press. 1980.
12. Spring C, Sandoval J. Food additives and hyperkinesis: A critical evaluation of the evidence. J Learning Disabilities 1976; 9(9):560-569.
13. Webster L. The hyperactive child and chiropractic. Today's Chiropractic 1988; 17(1):73-74.
14. Backman ZM. The relationship between learning disabilities and behavioral manifestations with toxicity and cerebral allergy. Dig Chiropractic Economics 1985; 27(6):18-19.
15. Como PS, Cui L, Kurlan R. The early course of the Tourette's clinical spectrum. Neurology 1993; 43:1712-1715 (also reviewed in Literature Reviews: Neurology. Clinical Pediatrics February 1994; 33(2):123.
16. Culbert TP, Banez GA, Reiff MI. Children who have attentional disorders: Interventions. Pediatr Rev 1994; 15(1):-14.
17. Weiner HL, Urion DK, Levitt LP. Pediatric Neurology for the House Officer. 3rd ed. Baltimore: Williams & Wilkins. 1988. pp.109-111.
18. Bonn D. Methylphenidate: US and European views converging? (News). Lancet 1996; 348(9022):255.
19. Morgan AM. Use of stimulant medications in children. Am Family Physician 1988; 38(4):197-202.
20. Baren M. Multimodal treatment for ADHD. Patient Care 1995; 29(20):77+
21. Hospers LA, Zezula L, Sweat M. Life upper cervical adjustment in a hyperactive teenager. Today's Chiropractic 1987; 15(16):73-76.
22. Barnes TA. A multi-faceted chiropractic approach to attention deficit hyperactivity disorder: A case report. ICA Intl Rev Chiropractic 1995; 51(1):41-43.
23. Phillips CJ. Case study: The effects of utilizing spinal manipulation and craniosacral therapy as the treatment approach for attention deficit-hyperactivity disorder. Proceed Natl Conf Chiropractic Pediatr, November 1981.San Diego, CA. pp. 57-74.
24. Anderson CD, Partridge JE. Seizures plus attention deficit hyperactivity disorder: A case report. ICA Intl Rev Chiropractic 1993; 49(4):35-37.
25. Giesen JM, Center DB, Leach RA. An evaluation of chiropractic manipulation as a treatment of hyperactivity in children. Journal of Manipulative and Physiological Therapeutics October 1989; 12(5):353-363.
26. Brzozowske WT, Walton EV. The effect of chiropractic treatment on students with learning and behavioral impairments resulting from neurological dysfunction. ACA Journal of Chiropractic December 1977; 14(12):S127-S140.
27. Brzozowske WT. Treatment of the hyperkinetic child. Archives of the California Chiropractic Association 1977; 4(2):17-21
28. Koren T. Learning disorders and chiropractic. Digest of Chiropractic Economics November/December 1991; 34(3):40-41.
29. Walton EV. Chiropractic effectiveness with emotional, learning and behavioral impairments. International Review of Chiropractic September 1975; 31(5):2-5, 21-22.
30. Lemeshow S. The hyperactive child. ACA Journal of Chiropractic July 1974; 11(7):S107-S110.
31. Hammerich KF. Megavitamin therapy: personality, hyperkinesis and allergy in the deficient child. ACA Journal of Chiropractic March 1974; 11(3):S45-S48.

AUTISM

Autism is a behavioral developmental disorder with abnormal social interaction, communications, and activities (1). There are three main criteria that must be met: 1) disturbances of reciprocal interaction; 2) disturbance of communications which includes language comprehension and spoken language; and 3) disturbances of normal variations in behavior and imaginative activities which results in extreme restriction in the behavioral repertoire (2).

The prevalence ranges from 5 to 15 per 10,000 children (1,3). It is four times more likely to occur in males (3). Mental retardation is common in autism. It affects 70% of autistic people (4).

MR imaging and autopsies of autistic children have shown that many have evidence of cerebellar, parietal lobe, and/or corpus callosum abnormalities. A common finding in autopsy and MR imaging was hypoplasia of the posterior vermis and hemispheres of the cerebellum. Autopsy finding on the cerebellum of 12 autistic cases showed Purkinje neuron losses, particularly in the posterior vermis (5). The abnormalities are thought to occur prenatally. The cerebellar abnormalities are thought to affect the abilities to orient spatially and to efficiently shift attention between multiple sensory foci (6). In MR imaging studies, a large group of autistic patients had parietal lobe abnormalities or abnormalities in a posterior area of the corpus callosum cells of the parietal lobes send their projections (5,6). Parietal lobe abnormalities may be causing narrowed visual attention (5).

Autism may be associated with other conditions such as Rett syndrome, schizophrenia, and Fragile X syndrome, among many others (2). Asperger syndrome has some signs similar to autism. Those with Asperger syndrome cannot conceptualize the mental state of others; i.e., they cannot empathize with others (2).

CLINICAL FEATURES

The classical picture of autism is a child with a blank expression sitting on the floor, rocking back and forth or twirling, and constantly rotating the hands. They often display abnormal postures, such as toe walking, unusual postures, arching of the back, and extreme extension of the neck (7).

The characteristic behaviors associated with autism change with age (1). As with any behavior-related disorders, assessment is difficult and requires someone with extensive experience in its diagnosis.

Courchesne found that abnormal cerebellar test findings were significantly more frequent in autistic patients than in normal controls. The most significant were alternating movements, gait, and sequential movements (5).

Stone et al stated that when children under age four are evaluated, screening for autism can also be done at that time. They found the following signs to be relatively consistent in the diagnosis of autism: abnormal social play, lack of awareness of others, poor imitation of others, deficient nonverbal communications, and impaired imaginative play (1).

MEDICAL MANAGEMENT

Medical management is primarily via psychoactive drugs and behavior modification. Fenfluramine is used in some cases as one-third of autistic children have serum serotonin levels three to four times normal levels and fenfluramine has been shown to reduce the levels. Temporary improvements have been noted (8). Early diagnosis and intervention have been found to reduce the signs and symptoms (1).

CHIROPRACTIC MANAGEMENT

Rubinstein described a 7-year-old female who was living in a foster home. She had a history of sexual and physical abuse. The physical examination was unremarkable. She did not respond to verbal commands and was observed to turn around in slow circles, sing an "incomprehensible" song, and have a glazed stare and blank expression on her face. She was seen twice weekly and adjustments were made to C1 based on the chiropractic examination. After two weeks of care, she ceased turning in circles and singing gibberish. After ten months of care, she could converse, follow commands, as well as dress and groom herself. She was also able to go to public school and to read and learn. The doctor lost track of this patient following Hurricane Andrew. When he refound her, the turning in circles and singing had resumed. After adjusting her, she immediately ceased these activities (8).

Sandefur and Adams described a study of autistic children in a local school who received chiropractic care. Interns at a chiropractic college adjusted the four children twice weekly, four for six months and two for three months after x-ray and physical examination. The teachers charted the behavior of each child. Positive changes in behavior were noted. One child had an eight times improvement in using the correct verb tense. A second had fewer reported incidences of noncompliant behavior while a third had fewer charted episodes of self abuse, made more requests to play, and cried less (3).

A 6-year-old was seen at Kentuckiana Children's Center. His birth was difficult and a caesarean section was done after a 10 hour labor. He developed quickly but at 14 months of age, his verbal skills deteriorated, and he began to react violently to loud noises. Antibiotics were given, and at age 15 months, bilateral tympanostomy was done after fluid was found in his ears. At age 2-1/2 years, a referral was made to a speech therapist. A referral was made for physical and psychological evaluation. He was diagnosed with high functioning autism. He does not have the typical mannerisms of autism, i.e., rocking or self-abusive behavior. He has difficulty communicating. He had a history of falls where he struck his head. Chiropractic examination found subluxations. After several

---

Table 13.20. DSM-III-R Diagnostic Criteria for Autistic Disorder

A. Qualitative impairment of awareness of the existence or feelings of others
  1. Marked lack of awareness of the existence of feelings of others
  2. No or abnormal seeking of comfort at times of distress
  3. No or impaired imitation
  4. No or abnormal social play
  5. Gross impairment in ability to make peer friendship

B. Qualitative impairment in communication and imagination
  1. No mode of communication
  2. Markedly abnormal nonverbal communication
  3. Absence of imaginative activity
  4. Marked abnormalities in the production of speech
  5. Marked abnormalities in the form or content of speech
  6. Marked impairment in the ability to initiate or sustain a conversation, despite adequate speech

C. Markedly restricted repertoire of activities and interests
  1. Stereotyped body movements
  2. Persistent preoccupation with parts of objects or attachment to unusual objects
  3. Marked distress overchanges in trivial aspects of environment
  4. Unreasonable insistence on following routines in precise detail
  5. Markedly restricted range of interests

From Stone WL, et al. "Early Recognition of Autism." *Archives of Pediatric and Adolescents Medicine* February 1994; 148(2):174–179.

chiropractic adjustments, he quit standing on his head for prolonged periods of time and made more eye contact. Dietary and nutritional changes were made (9).

ALTERNATIVE MANAGEMENT

Some promising work has been done by the Kaufman family. This was chronicled in books such as, "Son Rise" and "A Miracle to Believe In." "Son Rise," also turned into a made-for-television movie, is about how they helped to heal their autistic son. They created a loving and supportive environment and used mirror-image patterning—they imitated the child's activities such as rocking and spinning objects (10). They have successfully used the same techniques on other autistic children as well. Others have also claimed to have success with a variety of methods. One woman reported constructing a devise to limit the sensory stimuli in her environment to overcome autism.

Another aid that has been used is a special typing pad in a technique called facilitated communication. A "facilitator" moves the hand or arm of the patient who spells out words. This technique has come under much controversy as the facilitator may be unconsciously spelling out words with little or no input from the patient.

REFERENCES

1. Stone WL, et al. Early recognition of autism. Archives of Pediatric and Adolescents Medicine February 1994; 148(2):174-179.
2. Aicardi J. Diseases of the Nervous System in Childhood. Clinics in Developmental Medicine 1992; 115/118:1295-1318.
3. Sandefur R, Adams E. The effect of chiropractic adjustments on the behavior of autistic children: a case review. ACA Journal of Chiropractic December 1987; 24(12):21-25.
4. Edwards DR, Bristol MM. Autism: early identification and management in family practice. American Family Physician November 1991; 44(5):1755-1764.
5. Courchesne E. Infantile autism. part 1: MR imaging abnormalities and their neurobehavioral correlates. International Pediatrics 1995; 10(2):141-154.
6. Kohen-Raz R, Volkmar FR, Cohen DJ. Postural control in children with autism. Journal of Autism and Developmental Disorders September 1992; 22(3):419-432.
7. Courchesne E. Infantile Autism. Part 2: A new neurodevelopmental model. International Pediatrics 1995; 10(2):155-165.
8. Rubinstein HM. Case study–autism. Chiropractic Pediatrics April 1994; 1(1):23.
9. Barnes T. The story of John ... a little boy with autism. ICA International Review of Chiropractic November/December 1996; 52(6):43-46.
10. Kaufman BN. Son Rise. San Francisco: Harper & Row, Publishers. 1976.

BACK PAIN

The incidence of back pain in children is little known and reports of its incidence range widely (1). A 1994 study found the incidence in France of children ages 6 to 20 to be 51.2%. The most common areas of complaint were the low-back and a leg and the thoracic spine. The risk of back pain increased substantially with age. Among smokers, 83.1% had back pain (2). In one study of children and adolescents, spondylolisthesis or spondylolysis were found in one-third of those with back pain. Of the remainder, one-third had Scheuermann's disease/kyphosis, 18% had spinal tumors (see tumors) or infections, and a cause was not found in the remaining 15%. The study by Davids et al. found that 5% had intra-abdominal visceral conditions (3).

Plexopathy of the lower and upper extremities (see brachial plexus injury) have been associated with vaccinations. Extremity neuropathy may be caused by poliomyelitis as a result of oral live polio vaccine. Plexopathy or neuropathy has been associated with DTP and tetanus toxoid vaccinations as well (4).

Beyond a chiropractic vertebral subluxation complex which is discussed elsewhere, other factors should be considered, especially if an adequate evaluation and a reasonable course of chiropractic care do not produce a satisfactory result. Many other disorders cause back pain. As noted, spondylolisthesis and/or spondylolysis were found to be common radiographic findings. The reportedly high incidence of back pain associated with infection or tumor is of obvious concern. The history must uncover any recent or concurrent infection or fever, and a good neurological examination is vital when there is suspicion of an underlying condition. An atypical and/or painful scoliosis may be indicative of a tumor in the posterior element of the vertebra (3). Acute neck pain and rigidity of the neck, especially if preceded by or accompanied by fever, requires careful evaluation as these are classical signs of meningitis.

MANAGEMENT

Gutmann found atlantal "blockage" in a 10-month-old child with congenital torticollis who was developing facial and skull asymmetries as well. Following manual correction of the blockage, the infant gained improvements in posture, motor responses, mental and linguistic development, and facial and skull asymmetries (5).

Chiropractic care by spinal adjustments to reduce or correct vertebral subluxations to children with back pain is quite common. There are few, if any case reports except in those with other disorders where back pain is typically a secondary finding.

DISKITIS

Diskitis is an inflammatory process of the intervertebral disc. It destroys the disc giving the appearance of narrowing at the affected disc space. Diskitis usually occurs in children and adolescents (6). Some feel it is due to trauma, others to infection (6). Some have cultured organisms, primarily *Staphylococcus aureus* (6). Twenty-five percent have positive cultures of bacteria (7). Symptoms vary which may include fever, irritability, abdominal pain, back pain, hip or leg pain, limp, and a refusal to sit, stand, or walk (6). Meningeal signs may be present (6). Of the various signs seen, limited range of motion and paravertebral muscle spasms seem to be most characteristic (6). Bone scan with Technetium-99 is the diagnostic modality of choice if diskitis is suspected (6). Lab findings associated with infection may be present (6).

INTERVERTEBRAL DISC SYNDROME

Disc herniation appears to be rare in children under age 12 with only a handful of cases reported (8). The incidence increases in adolescence (7). The fear in a presentation of back pain and radicular symptoms is neoplasm, infection, or spondylolisthesis (8). Childhood disc herniation is thought to be due to trauma or an anular defect caused by a congenital defect or early degeneration. The case presented by Callahan et al. found upon postsurgical pathological study of the protrusion, a mix of fibrocartilage and bone fragments from the superior S1. Their opinion is that some cases of pediatric disc herniation are due to apophyseal fracture or, in their words, a slipped vertebral apophysis (8).

NERVE ROOT DYSFUNCTION

Nerve root dysfunction is classically characterized by hyporeflexia, motor weakness, and sensory loss or lower motor neuron signs. These do not appear to be very common in children (see brachial plexus injury).

SCHEUERMANN'S KYPHOSIS

This is a relatively common cause of pediatric back pain and is of unknown etiology. It is usually associated with increased thoracic kyphosis (9). Some cases are thought to be hereditary. Some feel that deficiencies in vitamin A and D might be part of the factors involved (10).

There is usually mild backache in the thoracic or thoracolumbar spine. The patient cannot voluntarily posturally reduce the kyphosis unlike those with postural roundback who can. Standing lateral x-rays of the thoracic spine show a thoracic kyphosis of at least 45°, narrowing of the disc space, irregularities of the vertebral body endplates, wedging of the vertebral bodies, and, in some cases, Schmorl's nodes (9).

MEDICAL MANAGEMENT OF SCHEUERMANN'S

The medical care for the kyphosis appears to be bracing and symptomatic drug therapy. Surgical rods have been used but complications are not uncommon (11).

CHIROPRACTIC MANAGEMENT OF SCHEUERMANN'S

Beyeler stated that chiropractic care should begin at an early stage. He felt that much of the progression of the condition is preventable with early intervention. He stated that chiropractic care should be directed to improving the circulation to the spine (10).

Lemire et al. present two adolescents with Scheuermann's kyphosis. The first case was a 13-year-old boy. He had back pain that was aggravated by prolonged sitting and standing, as well as stooping and trunk flexion. In a 10-month period he had worsening of the vertebral plates in the upper lumbar spine. He received eight chiropractic adjustments over a 2 week period as well as stretching exercises and postural advice. Subjective complaints and flexibility of the spine improved, e.g., initial forward flexion reached its maximum with the fingertips at the knee level while the postcare flexion had the fingers approximating the floor. The second case was a 14-year old boy who was sent to a scoliosis clinic for a longstanding painless thoracic kyphosis. He had a 72° thoracic kyphosis. A brace was given but was rarely used over a 10-month period. The kyphosis increased to 92°. Twelve months after the initial presentation, anterior fusion was done from T3 to T9 with Harrington rods inserted. Seventeen months later he had back pain which was attributed to problems with the rods. These were removed. Six years later, he did not have back pain. The kyphosis was 65° (12).

REFERENCES

1. Olson TL, et al. The epidemiology of low back pain in an adolescent population. American Journal of Public Health April 1992; 82(4):606-608.
2. Troussier B et al. Back pain in school children: a study among 1178 pupils. Scand J Rehab Med 1994; 26:143-146.
3. Davids JR, Wenger DR. Back pain in children and adolescents: an algorithmic approach. Journal of Musculoskeletal Medicine March 1994; 11(3):19-21, 25-26, 29-32.
4. Marin R, Bryant PR, Eng GD. Lumbosacral plexopathy temporally related to vaccination. Clinical Pediatrics 1994 March. 33(3):175-177.
5. Guttmann G. Blocked atlantal nerve syndrome in infants and small children. ICA International Review of Chiropractic July/August 1990; 46(4):37-39, 41-43.
6. Moskel MJ, Villar LA. Childhood diskitis: report of 2 cases and review of the literature. Journal of the American Osteopathic Association 1986; 86(3):169-174.
7. Kent C. Radiology in pediatric spine pain. Chiropractic Pediatrics April 1994; 1(1):7-12.
8. Callahan DJ, et al. Intervertebral disc impingement syndrome in a child: report of a case and suggested pathology. Spine 1986; 4:402-404.
9. Winters RB, Lipscomb PR. Back pain in children. Minnesota Medicine March 1978; 63(3):141-147.
10. Beyeler W. Scheuermann's disease and its chiropractic management. Annals of the Swiss Chiropractors' Association 1960; 1:170-178.
11. Murray PM, Weinstein SL, Spratt KF. The natural history and long-term follow-up of Scheuermann kyphosis. Journal of Bone and Joint Surgery February 1993; 75A(2):236-248.
12. Lemire JJ, et al. Scheuermann's juvenile scoliosis. Journal of Manipulative and Physiological Therapeutics March/April 1996; 19(3):195-201.

BRACHIAL PLEXUS INJURIES

Brachial plexus injuries are a complication during birth. They appear to be due to lateral traction of the head and neck or downward traction of a shoulder which adducts causes adduction and internal rotation of the shoulder and forearm (1). High birth weight increases the risk of brachial plexus birth injuries. A 4001 to 4500 gram birth weight infant has a 2.5 times the risk to a normal (2500 to 4000 gram) infant, and a 4500 gram or larger infant has a ten times greater risk (1). Maternal age and maternal diabetes or obesity are risk factors (1). The incidence is 2-3 per 1000 births (2). Injection of foreign substance or vaccines may cause a form of brachial plexus paralysis (1). Erb's or Erb-Duchenne palsy is the most common brachial plexus injury and involves C5 to C6 root levels (2,3). The next most common is C5 to T1 injury (4). An isolated C8 to T1 injury is rare and is often associated with root avulsion. Its clinical feature is Klumpke or Dejerine-Klumpke paralysis (2,3) (See also Chapter 12).

CLINICAL FEATURES

C5-C6 brachial plexus paralysis presents with the affected arm hanging limply at the side in internal rotation with extension of the elbow. Hand motion is normal (3). The muscles of the shoulder girdle are primarily affected. In lower brachial plexus paralysis, weakness and wasting is seen in the small muscles of the hand with a claw-hand deformity. Hypoesthesia occurs on the ulnar hand and forearm (3). In the event that T1 root is involved, there can be sympathetic disturbances, such as Horner's syndrome (3).

Erb-Duchenne palsy is upper brachial plexus paralysis occurring at birth. The fifth and sixth cervical cords are affected (5). Recovery is usually not forthcoming. If upper brachial plexus paralysis occurs later, there may be spontaneous, but not always complete, recovery (3). There is retention of the ability to grasp with the fingers but the arm is flaccid, hangs alongside the trunk, and is maintained in adduction and internal rotation with forearm pronation. There may be extension of the elbow and wrist flexion or the "waiter's tip" position. The shoulder cannot function. If the phrenic nerve is also affected, there may be unilateral paralysis of the diaphragm and scapular winging (5).

Djerine-Klumpke paralysis is due to birth injury of the lower brachial plexus. It is usually the result of a breech birth (3). It is associated with C8 and T1 involvement. The elbow is maintained in a flexed position. Due to paralysis of the muscles of the hand, there is an inability to grasp. There is clawing of the hand. There may also be a Horner syndrome if T1 is affected. The prognosis is poorer than for upper brachial plexus paralysis (5)

CHIROPRACTIC MANAGEMENT

Larkin-Thier and Hendricks describe a 14-day-old female who presented with a limp left arm which was previously noted at birth. The pediatrician told the mother that the child was within normal limits. Other than oxytocin inducement, the delivery was normal. The infant had a limp left arm and could actively abduct the shoulder to 45° but could not flex or extend it. She did not approximate the left hand to the face. There was a delayed grasp reflex and a positive reversed fencers reflex on the left. Passive range of motion (PROM) was normal bilaterally. There had been some improvement in the use of the left hand. Palpation findings included left upper cervical muscle hypertonicity, decreased cervical rotation, and upper thoracic muscle hypertonicity. Subluxation complexes were determined to be at C1 and T2.

Following the chiropractic evaluation, C1 was adjusted in a modified cervical break and T2 was adjusted as a prone transverse process contact on the first visit. The mother stated on the second visit three days later, the arm appeared to be improving and the infant began to grasp objects. C1 was again adjusted, and the mother was advised to perform PROM exercises to the arm. On the third visit two weeks later, the mother stated that the arm was normal. There was increased resistance in arm motion, the reverse fencer's reflex was positive, hypertonicity was present upon palpation of the left upper cervical muscles. The grasp reflex was equal and reverse fencer's reflex was negative. No adjustments were made (1).

A one-year-old Down infant presented with brachial plexus injury caused at birth. Care prior to beginning chiropractic care was 11 months of physical therapy without significant improvement. He required support when sitting up, had moderate hypotonia, lacked upper extremity movement, and had upper body weakness. Chiropractic examination and x-rays were taken. He received global spinal adjustments as per the procedures of Chiropractic Biophysics Techniques and light thrusts on the atlas transverse process. After three adjustments, he was able to move his arms and his coordination had improved to the point where he could place food in his mouth. His sleeping habits had also improved. After 4 months, his posture improved and he was able to sit up (4).

REFERENCES

1. Larkin-Thier SM, Hendricks CL. Chiropractic care of brachial plexus palsy: a case study. Palmer Journal of Research December 1994; 11(2):45-47.
2. Shelov SP. Brachial plexus injuries. Pediatrics in Review February 1992; 13(2):77-78.
3. Adams RD, Victor M. Principles of Neurology, 4th ed. San Francisco: McGraw-Hill, Inc. 1989.pp.1064-65.
4. Peet J. Brachial plexus injury in an infant with down's syndrome: a case study. Chiropractic Pediatrics August 1994; 1(2):11-14.
5. Green M. Pediatric Diagnosis. 5th ed. Philadelphia: W. B. Saunders Co. 1992. pp.109-110.

BRAIN ABSCESS

Infectious processes occasionally occur in the brain causing abscess formation. Abscesses may be single, multiple, or multiloculated lesions. The etiological factors include meningitis (36%), penetrating head trauma (16%), congenital heart disease (9%), other disorders (5%), and no known causes (5%) (1). Males tend to predominate (1). The most common areas of involvement are supratentorial sites in the frontal, parietal, and temporal lobes (1,2). Blood cultures have found streptococci, staphylococci, and Proteus mirabilis but one study found the majority to be sterile (1,2). Mortality is 20% (1). The more neurologic deficits present at initial evaluation, the worse the prognosis (1). The mortality rate was higher in those under 2 years of age—up to 50% (1,2). The use of the CT scan has helped to reduce the mortality rate (1,2).

CLINICAL FEATURES

Symptoms include headaches, vomiting, seizures, fever, and a diminished level of consciousness. Other signs may be present, such as hemiparesis, papilloedema, coma, cerebellar signs, cranial nerve dysfunction depending upon the area of involvement.

MANAGEMENT

Surgical intervention via drainage through burr holes or excision is used. Repeat operations are common, especially for those treated by aspiration (2). Treatment is also via antibiotics, occasionally without surgical procedures (2).

REFERENCES

1. Ersahin Y, Mutluer S, Güzelbag E. Child's nervous system 1994 April; 10(3): 185-189.
2. Tekkök IH, Erbengi A. Management of brain abscess in children: review of 130 cases over a period of 21 years. Child's Nervous System 1992 October; 8(7):411-416.

CEREBRAL PALSY

A working definition of cerebral palsy (CP) is a persistent but not unchanging disorder of movement and posture which is due to a non-progressive disorder of the immature brain (1). The lesion is non-progressive but the maturation of the nervous system affects the presentation over time (2). CP covers a variety of disorders of motor function. The incidence of CP seems to be about 2 - 4 per 1,000 live births (1,3).

The etiology of CP is often thought to be due to acute intrapartum asphyxia, but studies have not been able to substantiate this (4). Two large scale studies have found less than 5% of the CP cases may be associated with intrapartum asphyxia in birth (5). A multifactor etiology is more likely in most cases (4). Prematurely born infants make up a large proportion of the CP population (6). It has been noted that the frequency of CP decreases as the gestational age and birthweight increases. A marked rise in CP was noted for newborns with a birthweight of under 1500 grams—more preterm babies are surviving (7). An interesting side-finding was noted in this last study: a statistically reduced risk of CP was associated with pre-eclampsia (7).

Apgar scores at 20 minutes of 3 or less have been associated with a 250-fold increase in the risk of CP (6). Other risk factors in the neonate include birth weight of less than 2,000 grams, head circumference of greater than 3 standard deviations above normal, diminished activity or diminished crying which lasts for more than one day, thermal instability, need for gavage feeding, either hypotonia or hypertonia, single or multiple apneic episodes, or a hematocrit of less than 40% (8).

There is considerable difficulty in classifying the variety of clinical presentations of CP because the diagnosis is clinical rather than based upon a neuroanatomical lesion. Classification is often by the particular movement disorder and the limbs affected. The classifications for the movements are spastic, dyskinesia or athetoid, and ataxia. Others classify the movements as spastic, hypotonic, dystonic, athetoid, or a combination/mixed (9). The divisions of limbs affected are hemiparesis, hemiplegia, and quadriplegia or tetraplegia (10,11). Currently, the following is a commonly accepted form of diagnostic classification: diplegia, tetraplegia (or quadriplegia), hemiplegia, dyskinetic, and ataxic (6).

Because of the central nervous system location of the lesion(s), other neurological disorders often accompany cerebral palsy. Epilepsy is present in one-third of the children with CP (9). One-half have hemiplegia (9).

Studies of the life expectancy of those with CP find that 10% tend to die by 10 years of age, usually those with severe mental retardation (12).

DESCRIPTION OF THE TYPES OF CEREBRAL PALSY

Spastic Diplegia

The spastic form of CP makes up most of the cases and is associated with abnormalities in the pyramidal or corticospinal tracts. MRI studies have found the underlying mechanism of the diplegic form is associated with hemorrhagic venous infarction in the periventricular area. Birth asphyxia does not appear to be the cause of this form of CP (6).

The primary feature is hypertonicity and spasticity in the lower extremities. Some have a more severe form and have quadriplegia, mental retardation, speech and swallowing problems, often drool, and many are unable to walk (13). Intelligence is usually preserved (14). In the neonatal period, some may present with hypotonia, along with lethargy and difficulties in feeding (14).

Common presentations include "scissoring" gait (due to adduction, extension, and internal rotation of the legs), tightened Achilles tendons, hypertonicity and hyperreflexia in the lower extremities, and ankle clonus and upgoing toes. If the upper extremities are involved, these may show clumsy movements and abnormal postures (13).

Spastic Hemiplegia

This is the second most common form of CP in the preterm infant and the most common in term infants. In term infants, it is usually the result of hypoperfusion during the early third trimester. In the preterm, there appears to be some association with problems during birth (6). A postnatal etiology which includes stroke, trauma and infection often involves the upper extremities rather than the lower (2).

The primary feature is unilateral spasticity in both the upper and lower extremity. It is the most common postnatal form of acquired cerebral palsy. Pathological and imaging findings have found signs of injury in the cerebral regions supplied by the middle cerebral artery (9).

In the early stages, hypotonia and hyporeflexia are seen on the affected side. As it progresses, hypertonicity and spasticity are seen. Most eventually walk. Compare the toe and thumb nail sizes as underdevelopment is common to the affected side. If there is an associated seizure disorder, mental retardation is common. One-third of the those affected have normal intelligence (13).

Spastic Quadriplegia

Typically these are low birth-weight, full-term infants. The infant usually has multiple disabilities. A significant degree of spastic paresis is present in all four limbs and dystonia may be present as well. There may be severe mental retardation, absent or minimal speech, feeding or respiratory problems due to pseudobulbar palsy, microcephaly, hip dislocation, contractures, and scoliosis (2).

Dyskinetic or Extrapyramidal

This form composes 10-15% of the CP cases (14) and appears to occur primarily in term infants during the perinatal period. There is often acute circulatory failure and birth asphyxia. Basal ganglia damage is usually seen, although there may also be cortical and subcortical damage if there is prolonged and severe asphyxia at birth (6).

There is a hyperkinetic form with athetosis and chorea, and a dystonic form (2). Emotions, postural changes, and intentional movements often bring on the abnormal movements (2). Primitive reflexes persist (e.g., righting and tonic neck reflexes) and facial grimacing and oropharyngeal difficulties are present. There may be dysarthria and motor and intellectual problems which are usually worse in the dystonic form. Pyramidal signs are often present in the dystonic form. Fifty percent of those with the dystonic form have difficulty speaking (2). The hyperkinetic form shows significant involuntary movements (14).

Ataxic CP

Ataxic CP may have genetic or acquired hemorrhagic cerebellar damage (6). They tend to be full term infants (2). The diagnosis comes from the predominance of clinical signs of cerebellar lesion (14). Ataxic CP is often difficult to distinguish clinically from other causes of ataxia (6). There tends to be hypotonia, hyporeflexia, and ataxia (13).

Formulating a Diagnosis

When developing a clinical diagnosis of CP, the clinician approaches from several directions. Several means of assessing motor function have been developed. These include motor assessment inventory, limb by limb approach, gross motor function measure, and motor performance measure. The latter two are new research assessment techniques rather than commonly used clinical assessment tools (6).

MEDICAL MANAGEMENT

The primary management appears to be physical therapy, the goal of which is to help the person reduce his physical disabilities, such as, walking and speech problems. Hip stability and scoliosis detection and management are important (6). Magnesium sulfate administered to mothers of very low birth weight infants during labor was associated with a protective effect against cerebral palsy (15).

CHIROPRACTIC MANAGEMENT

Sweat and Ammon presented a case of spasmodic cerebral palsy. This was a 40-year-old woman presenting with thoracic and cervical pain. After nearly a month of chiropractic care, the patient stated that symptoms were 80% improved which was confirmed by the clinical findings. Another month later, the symptoms had abated for the first time in her life (16).

McMullen found that atlanto-occipital region was the most common area for vertebral subluxation complexes in CP cases that she treated. She describes a 14-year-old CP patient who, following a series of spinal adjustments, had less clonic activity, was able to get out of a wheelchair and walk with crutches, had less problem with drooling and urinary incontinence, and was able to enter college (10). Cranial and TMJ joint problems have also been found, and adjustments to those regions have been found to be beneficial (10).

Collins, et al. tested brainstem evoked potential (BSEP), balance, surface electromyography (SEMG), and grip strength in eight patients before and after chiropractic adjustments to the upper cervical spine (17). They stated that they found an overall decrease in muscle activity and a "tendency towards symmetry." BSEP was improved after one adjustment on two of the three with grossly abnormal waveforms. Of the three adults in this study, all had improved eyes closed balance (less postural sway) after chiropractic adjustments. One child who had four unsuccessful surgeries for strabismus had no apparent strabismus after two adjustments. Speech and hearing problems improved. Children were able to hold their heads up longer and were able to crawl or stand with support more than they were able to do prior to the initiation of chiropractic care (17).

Golden and Van Egmond describe a 22-month old male who presented with cerebral palsy, seizures, mental retardation, congenital deformities to the lower extremities, recurrent otitis media, and a history of spinal meningitis at birth. He had optical and verbal disorders as well. He was receiving medication for seizures and ear infections. Evaluation of the child prior to presenting at Kentuckiana chiropractic center included CT scans of the patient which showed ventricular enlargement and multiple focal areas of parenchymal hemorrhage, and neurological examinations which were relatively unremarkable. EEG was mildly abnormal. After chiropractic examination, x-ray, and lab work-up, a course of chiropractic adjustments, nutritional supplements, and crawl patterning was initiated. Podiatric and optometric appliances were also employed. Care continued over an eight year period. Subsequent EEG studies were considered within normal limits. Follow-up CT scans showed mild ventricular dilatation and no other abnormalities. X-ray studies showed a reduction in misalignments. Psychological and intelligence testing at age 3 years 2 months showed a mental, intellectual, and social age well below the chronological age. At age 6 years 4 months, cognitive skills were those of a 4-5 year old, fine motor evaluation was that of a 4 year old, language skills was that of a 6 to 7 year-old, Early Language Development Test

was above his chronological age. Visual problems caused him to work slowly but obvious signs of mental retardation were not present. Otitis media and enuresis ceased with the initiation of chiropractic care. At the time the paper was presented, he was mainstreamed into regular school at the fifth grade level (18).

A 6-year-old male with mental retardation and cerebral palsy presented for chiropractic care. Prior to age 30 months, development appeared to be normal. After that time, development deteriorated. Falls became frequent. Birth was via caesarean section after a breech presentation. At the time of presentation, he was difficult to handle and made a constant, high pitched sound. Adjustments given were to the atlas. After three adjustments, he got on the adjusting table by himself and stayed on the table. After one month of care, the teacher noted much improvement. After five months, he followed verbal commands and had fewer toilet accidents. The high pitched sound diminished and he was able to vocalize more words (19).

A 4-year-old female deaf mute with cerebral palsy was presented for chiropractic care. From her premature, low-weight birth, she had been under near-constant medical care. She was unable to walk. Surgical intervention was recommended in the lower extremities. When the mother was unable to lift her, a relative recommended a chiropractor. She was adjusted 11 times in a one and one-half month period. She was able to take her first steps and then able to run and play. At the time the report was written, it was recommended that she receive care and speech therapy at the Kentuckiana Chiropractic Children's Clinic. The type of cerebral palsy (possibly spastic diplegia) is not listed nor are the vertebral levels or chiropractic findings presented (20).

In a 1955 article in the Journal of the American Osteopathic Association, Arbuckle describes the evaluation and manipulation of the cranial bones in CP afflicted infants. After cranial manipulation, he recommends upper thoracic manipulation in order to improve cranial circulation by stimulating the autonomic nervous system. He also describes the comprehensive care of older children and adults with a variety of therapies including osteopathic manipulative treatments. He states that the osteopathic manipulation aids in correcting the cause of CP symptoms and effects; occupational therapy benefits muscular patterns and behavior, particularly during the early developmental years (21).

Other activities that may help the child is to develop biocular vision and biaural hearing. Alternately feeding from one side and the opposite side is beneficial (10). Developing the cross-crawl pattern is also beneficial. It may have to be done passively. Two-handed object handling is also encouraged (10).

REFERENCES

1. Brett EM. Cerebral Palsy, Perinatal Injury to the Spinal Cord and Brachial Plexus Birth Injury. In: Brett EM. Pediatric Neurology. New York: Churchill Livingstone 1983.
2. Miller G, Couch S. Cerebral Palsy. In: Hoekelman RA (ed). Primary Pediatric Care. 2nd ed. St. Louis, MO: Mosby Year Book. 1992. pp.1179-1183.
3. Hall DMB. Birth asphyxia and cerebral palsy. British Journal of Medicine 299(6694): 279-283.
4. Shields JR, Schifrin BS. Perinatal antecedents of cerebral palsy. Obstetrics & Gynecology June 1988; 71(6, Part 1):899-905.
5. Nelson KB. What proportion of cerebral palsy is related to birth asphyxia? Journal of Pediatrics April 1988; 112(4):572-574.

6. Rosenbloom L. Diagnosis and management of cerebral palsy. Archives in Disease in Childhood April 1995; 72(4):350-354.
7. Murphy DJ, et al. Case-control study of antenatal and intrapartum risk factor for cerebral palsy in very preterm singleton babies. The Lancet December 2, 1995; 346(8988):1449-1454.
8. Nelson KB, Ellenberg JH. Neonatal signs as predictors of cerebral palsy. Pediatrics August 1979; 64(2):225-232.
9. Kuban KCK, Leviton A. Cerebral palsy. New England Journal of Medicine January 30, 1994; 330(3):188-195.
10. McMullen M. Chiropractic and the handicapped child. Part II: Cerebral palsy. ICA International Review of Chiropractic September/October 1990; 46(5):39, 41-43, 45.
11. Netter FH. The CIBA Collection of Medical Illustrations. Volume I: Nervous System. Part II: Neurologic and Neuromuscular Disorders. West Caldwell NJ: CIBA Pharmaceutical Co. 1986.pp. 15-16.
12. Crichton JU, MacKinnon M, White CP. The life-expectancy of persons with cerebral palsy. Developmental Medicine and Child Neurology July 1995; 37: 567-576.
13. Weiner HL, Urion DK, Levitt LP. Pediatric Neurology for the House Officer, 3rd ed. Baltimore: Williams & Wilkins. 1988.
14. Aicardi J, Bax M. In: Aicardi J. Diseases of the nervous system in childhood. Clinics in Developmental Medicine 1992; 115/118:330-356.
15. Nelson KB, Grether JK. Can magnesium sulfate reduce the risk of cerebral palsy in very low birthweight infants? Pediatrics February 1995; 95(2):263-269.
16. Sweat RW, Ammons DL. Case study: treatment of a cerebral palsy patient. Today's Chiropractic November/December 1988; 17(6):51-52.
17. Collins KF, et al. The efficacy of upper cervical chiropractic care on children and adults with cerebral palsy: a preliminary report. Chiropractic Pediatrics April 1994; 1(1):13-15.
18. Golden LM, Van Egmond CA. Longitudinal Clinical Case Study: Multi-Disciplinary Care of Child with Multiple Functional and Developmental Disorders. Proceedings of the National Conference of Chiropractic and Pediatrics. November 1992:24-39.
19. Webster LL. Case study—mental retardation/cerebral palsy. Chiropractic Pediatrics August 1994; 1(2):15-16.
20. The Cindy Beaty story. ICA International Review of Chiropractic July 1963; 18(1):8-10.
21. Arbuckle BE. The value of occupational and osteopathic manipulative therapy in the rehabilitation of the cerebral palsy victim. J Am Osteopath Assoc 1955; 55(4):227-237.

CONGENITAL/ DEVELOPMENTAL DISORDERS

There are many neurological maldevelopments or anomalies that may occur. Most of the most severe forms will probably not be seen in the chiropractic office as the child may not survive infancy or may be institutionalized. A few of the many forms of congenital and developmental disorders of the nervous system are described below.

Arnold-Chiari Malformation (ACM)

Chiari or Arnold-Chiari malformations are considered to be the most common anomalies of the cerebellum (1). ACM is a major cause of hydrocephalus due to blockage of the fourth ventricle (2). Some studies indicate that the cause of the herniation of the cerebellum may be due to a small posterior cranial fossa which may be due to insufficient pressure of fluid in the cranial vault (2,3). Syringomyelia is a common finding associated with ACM (3). The anomalies are categorized into types I to IV. Occasionally the types are described in reverse order.

Type I: Elongation of the cerebellar tonsils with a portion of the cerebellum displaced into the cervical spinal cord (3).

Type II: It is associated with meningomyelocele with the pons and medulla distorted and elongated and the cerebellar vermis displaced inferiorly into the spinal canal (6); there is progressive hydrocephalus; there are abnormalities associated with abnormalities of the lower cranial nerves (4).

Type III: The major characteristics are cerebellar dysplasia, brainstem displacement, and elongation of the 4th ventricle (1).

Type IV: Cerebellar hypoplasia (4).

In severe cases, surgical intervention is done. Surgical procedures include shunting if hydrocephalus or decompression is present (3). In one study, 65% benefited from surgical procedures with 20% becoming asymptomatic. If a syrinx or central cord syndrome was present, two-thirds were unchanged or worse. If only a dural decompression was done, 75% deteriorated post-surgically (3).

Klippel-Feil Syndrome

A wide variety of neurological disorders may result from or be associated with Klippel-Feil syndrome. The characteristic triad of Klippel-Feil is short neck, low posterior hairline, and severe restriction of cervical spine motion due to fusion of cervical vertebrae (5). The prevalence is estimated to be 1:40,000 with females predominant (5).

Pediatric neurological disorders which may be associated with Klippel-Feil syndrome are spinal stenosis, nerve root compression or irritation, syringomyelia, hemiplegia or quadriplegia, motor, sensory, or pain in the extremities, deafness, and extraocular muscle palsies, among others (5).

Hydrocephalus

Hydrocephalus is caused by enlargement of the ventricles. This is due to a disorder which causes an excess of CSF to accumulate in the ventricles (6). There are two forms of hydrocephalus, communicating and noncommunicating. The most common form, the communicating type, presents with normal CSF circulation but a blockage in its absorption. It may be due to meningitis or subarachnoid hemorrhage or may be due to congenital causes. The noncommunicating form presents with a blockage in the ventricular system. It may be due to congenital malformations, such as myelomeningocele, aqueductal obstruction or stenosis, aneurysmal dilatation of the Great Vein of Galen, or a subarachnoid cyst in the posterior fossa, or it may be due to tumors, particularly in the posterior fossa, or, occasionally, due to inflammation (6).

The presentation depends upon the cause and age. Older children may show signs of increased intracranial pressure. Infants may be irritable and miss milestones (6). In advanced forms in infants, there may be an increase in the circumference of the skull, distention of the veins of the scalp, and "sunset eyes," a downward deviation of the eyes (4,7).

When suspected, hydrocephalus is confirmed by imaging studies such as plain skull x-rays, MRI, CT scan, and ultrasonic imaging. Lumbar puncture is contraindicated when there is increased intracranial pressure (6).

Spina Bifida

Spina bifida refers to a failure in the closure or fusion of the posterior portion of the vertebrae. Its simplest form, spina bifida occulta, usually occurs in the lumbosacral region. Its superficial presence is usually noted by a tuft of hair over the area. No neurological or abnormalities to the spinal cord or nerves are noted (8). In its more severe form, multiple spinal levels are affected. The incidence is 1 per 1,000 (9).

A meningocele may be present which is a bulging of the cord meninges through the opening seen as a superficial skin-covered sac. A meningomyelocele occurs when the cord and spinal nerves are included in the sac. In this case, there are usually neurologic findings. Failure of the neural tube to close may expose neural tissue to the surface in a myelocele or rachischisis. Myelomeningoceles are usually associated with severe Arnold-Chiari malformation in which there is caudal displacement of the medulla oblongata and a portion of the cerebellum into the spinal canal (8).

In order to reduce the risk of fetal neural-tube defects, the U.S. Public Health Service recommends that women who may become pregnant consume folic acid, either through food rich in it or fortified with it or through supplementation (10). The recommendation is an intake of at least 0.4 mg/day which is twice the average dietary intake. In Great Britain, it is estimated the ingestion of extra folic acid could prevent more than 1000 of the 1500 children born with neural tube defects each year (11).

REFERENCES

1. Carmel PW. The Chiari Malformations and Syringomyelia. In: Hoffman HJ, Epstein F, eds. Disorders of the Developing Nervous System: Diagnosis and Treatment. Palo Alto CA: Blackwell Scientific Publications. 1986.
2. Hensinger RN. Osseous anomalies of the craniovertebral junction. Spine May 1986; 11(4):323-333.
3. Raynor RB. The Arnold-Chiari malformation. Spine May 1986; 11(4):343-344.
4. Adams RD, Victor M. Principles of Neurology. 4th ed. New York: McGraw-Hill, Inc. 1989. pp.968-980.
5. McBride WZ. Klippel-Feil syndrome. American Family Physician February 1992; 45(2):633-635.
6. Weiner HL, Urion DK, Levitt LP. Pediatric Neurology for the House Officer. 3rd ed. Baltimore: Williams & Wilkins. 1988. p.25-28.
7. Netter FH. The CIBA Collection of Medical Illustrations. Volume 1: Nervous System. Part II: Neurologic and Neuromuscular Disorders. West Caldwell NJ: CIBA Pharmaceutical Co. 1986. pp.8-9.
8. Pansky B, Allen DJ, Budd GC. Review of Neuroscience, 2nd ed. New York: Macmillan Publishing Co. 1988.
9. Liptak GS. Spinal Bifida. In Hoekelman RA, et al (eds). Primary Pediatric Care (2nd ed). St. Louis: Mosby Year Book. 1992. pp.1512-1517.
10. Cordero JF. Finding the cause of birth defects. New England Journal of Medicine July 7, 1994; 331(1):48-49.
11. Ward NJ, Bower C. Folic acid and the prevention of neural tube defects. British Medical Journal April 22, 1995; 310(6986):1019-1020.

DOWN SYNDROME

Down syndrome is due to autosomal trisomy resulting in 47 somatic chromosomes rather than the usual 46 (1) (See also Chapter 17). The chromosomal defect is associated with chromosome 21 (2). Although it is not a neurological disorder per se, neurological deficits are common.

The U.S. incidence is 1 per 800-1000 live births or roughly 0.8 to 1.4% (1,3). Forty to sixty percent of the Down children are born to women over age 35 (1,4). Twenty to thirty percent have the extra chromosome from the father (1).

Congenital heart defects afflict about 40% of Down children (1,2). Congenital gastrointestinal defects afflict 12% (1,5). Ten to twenty-five percent die in the first year of life but the survivors have a shortened life expectancy (3). Today, over 80% survive past the age of 30 years (2).

Refractive errors or other visual problems, such as glaucoma or cataracts, are noted in 75% of Down children (5). Auditory problems are also common and often due to fluid accumulation in the middle ear (2). Language difficulties tend not to be associated with cognitive skills (2).

People with Down syndrome account for one-third of all cases of moderate to severe mental retardation.

Atlanto-axial instability has been associated with Down syndrome and is of much concern. The reported incidence in Down syndrome ranges from 9.5% to 50% (6,7), although 15% to 20% seems to be closer (1,6). The instability can be due to osseous abnormalities or ligamentous laxity (7).

Injury during physical activity has been of concern in cases of atlanto-axial instability. Over a 15 year period, the Special Olympics had not had a single incidence of a significant injury related to atlanto-axial instability (6). They only allow participation in some "risk" sports with a doctor's certificate indicating no atlantoaxial instability (8). A comparison of Down's children with ADIs of 4 mm or more who were divided into two groups, one continuing their normal activities and the other was told to refrain from "risky" activities was made after a one year period of time. There were no differences between the two groups in their functional motor scale scores, the rate of neurological signs, or changes in the ADI. There were no differences with a control group of Down's children with normal ADI. The conclusion was that there is no need to restrict Down's children from sports nor was it necessary to take radiographs prior to initiating sports activities (8).

CLINICAL FEATURES

The characteristic physical feature of Down syndrome include changes to the following structures (1,2):

1. Skull: Bradycephaly; flattening of the occiput.

2. Eyes: Epicanthal folds; slanting palpebral fissures; Brushfield spots.

3. Ears: Small and dysplastic.

4. Nose: Flattened nasal bridge.

5. Mouth: Down-turned corners; furrowed, protruding tongue; markedly arched palate.

6. Teeth: Small, pointed, irregular shapes or absent dentition.

7. Visceral, anatomical, and developmental changes often seen in Down are heart defects (approx. 50% risk), ophthalmolic disorders, duodenal atresia, increased susceptibility to respiratory tract infections, congenital hypothyroidism (1% risk), and leukemia (greater than in general population but less than 1%) (9).

Cervical x-rays are recommended as the atlantodental space has been found to be increased in 15% to 20% of children with Down syndrome (1,6). Neutral lateral views only do not seem to be enough if instability is suspected. Studies have found patients where a neutral lateral was taken which appeared to be normal and a later view showed an increased space. The converse has been found as well (10). Neutral lateral/flexion/extension views can determine if there is atlanto-axial instability which is found in 14% of Down patients; 1-2% develop some evidence of spinal cord compression (2).

Table 13.21.   Down Syndrome: Prevalence of Complicating Factors

Concern	Clinical Expression	Prevalence
Congenital heart disease	Endocardial cushion defect, septal defects tetralogy of Fallot	40%
Hypotonia	Hypotonia, hypermobility, motor function problems	100%
Delayed growth	Typically at or near the third percentile of general population	100%
Developmental delays	Some global delays—degree varies, specific processing problems, specific expressive language delay	100%
Hearing problems	Serous otitis media, small ear canals, conductive impairments	50–70%
Ocular problems	Refractive errors	50%
	Strabismus	35%
	Cataracts	15%
Cervical spine problems	Atlanto-axial instability	
	Skeletal cervical anomalies	10%±
	Possible spinal cord compression	1–2%
Thyroid disease	Hypothyroidism (rare: hyperthyroidism) Decreased growth, activity	15%+?
Obesity	Excessive weight gain	Common
Seizure disorder	Primarily grand mal (generalized); also myoclonic, hypsarrhythmia	5–10%
Emotional problems	Inappropriate behavior, depression	Common
Premature senescence	Behavioral changes, functional losses	Increases with age

Modified from Cooley WC, Graham JM. Down syndrome—an update and review for the primary pediatrician. Clin Pediat 1991;30(4):239.

If the atlantodental interval (ADI) is less than 3 mm, it is considered low risk. If the interval is 3 to 5 mm, risk is intermediate; an ADI greater than 5 mm is considered to be great risk (7). An extensive neurological evaluation is necessary with special emphasis on deep tendon reflexes and clonus, motor and sensory function, gait, muscle tone and size, and Babinski sign or similar signs as pyramidal or long tract signs may be present.

MEDICAL MANAGEMENT

Findings of altanto-axial instability and significant neurological signs of spinal cord compression warrant neurosurgical consultation. Surgical procedures have been performed to stabilize this region but this surgical intervention is controversial. Unfortunately, success with surgical stabilization has been mixed and ranges from reportedly successful stabilization to catastrophic complications which may result in quadriplegia or death (7,11). The study sizes tend to be small. The natural history of the progression of asymptomatic atlanto-axial instability has not been established (11).

Medical management also is towards any congenital defects or other problems that may arise. Help may be rendered for mental retardation.

Nutritional supplements and sicca cell therapy have been tried, but no benefits have been noted in studies conducted to date (2). Plastic surgery for the facial features of Down is being used in Europe (2).

Attempts have been made to do prenatal screening for Down syndrome (See Chapter 17). Increased maternal age and having previous children with Down tends to increase the risk for Down children (3). Maternal serum levels of a-fetoprotein, human chorionic gonadotropin, and unconjugated estriol have been tested but the sensitivity for these tests is poor. Used together rather than singly as a "triple-marker" screening during the second trimester, the sensitivity improves significantly among older women (3,5). During the second trimester, physical characteristics of Down may be seen on ultrasound images. The sensitivity of ultrasound imaging is good for at risk fetuses but is probably lower for low risk fetuses (3). The accuracy of amniocentesis is very good but carries a risk of fetal loss (3). Chorionic villus sampling can be done earlier than amniocentesis or the "triple-marker" screening. It is very accurate as long as there is no contamination by maternal cells, but it has a higher risk of fetal loss, fetal limb deficiencies, and maternal complications than amniocentesis (3).

CHIROPRACTIC MANAGEMENT

Vertebral subluxation complexes in the upper cervical spine are common, followed by the cranial base subluxations (1). McMullen describes two cases. One was a 10-month-old female who was "fussy" and had difficulty sleeping. After the first adjustment, she was able to sleep a full night. Muscle tone improved and head growth stabilized (1). The other case was a 3-year-old female with cardiac and GI tract involvement, as well as behavioral problems. Eating and GI tract complaints improved after adjusting. This patient was lost to follow-up after dying following complications in exploratory cardiac surgery (1). Other changes noted in Down syndrome infants were improvement in muscle tone in hypotonic infants, the disappearance of strabismus in most cross-eyed infants, and reduction in upper respiratory infections and otitis media (1).

Dyck describes a 22-year-old female with Down syndrome who presented for chiropractic care with 2-year history of neck pain. Neurological examination was unremarkable except sensory changes in the left C7 dermatome. X-rays of the cervical spine found a neutral lateral atlanto-dental space (ADI) of 5 mm which increased to 6 mm on flexion and decreased to 1 mm on extension. The upper thoracic spine was adjusted and some trigger point work done on the neck. Cervical spine complaints abated (12).

Craniosacral manipulation has been proposed as being beneficial but no studies appear to have been done to date (2).

There are many resources available to health professionals or parents of Down children. These include periodicals, newsletters, books, and support groups dedicated to these children (2).

REFERENCES

1. McMullen M. Handicapped infants and chiropractic care. Part I: Down syndrome. ICA International Review of Chiropractic July/August 1990; 46(4):32-25.
2. Cooley WC, Graham JM. Down syndrome—an update and review for the primary pediatrician. Clinical Pediatrics April 1993; 30(4):233-253.
3. Dick PT. Periodic health examination, 1996 update: I. Prenatal screening for and diagnosis of Down syndrome. Canadian Medical Association Journal February 15, 1996; 154(4):465-479.
4. Fry T, Mackay RI. Down syndrome: prevalence at birth, mortality and survival. A 17-year study. Early Human Development March 1979; 3(1):29-41.
5. Hayes A, Batshaw ML. Down syndrome. Pediatric Clinics of North America June 1993; 40(3):523-535.
6. Clum GW. Atlanto-axial subluxation in Down's syndrome. Today's Chiropractic May/June 1985; 14(2):33-36.
7. La Francis ME. A chiropractic perspective on atlantoaxial instability in Down's syndrome. Journal of Manipulative and Physiological Therapeutics March/April 1990; 13(3):157-160.
8. Cremers MJ, et al. Risk of sports activities in children with Down's syndrome and atlantoaxial instability. Lancet August 28, 1993; 342(8870):511-514.
9. American Association of Pediatrics. AAP Issue Guidelines on Health Supervision for Children with Down Syndrome. American Family Physician September 1, 1994; 50(3):695-697.
10. American Association of Pediatrics. Atlantoaxial instability in Down syndrome: subject review. Pediatrics July 1, 1995; 96(1):151-154.
11. Doyle JS, et al. Complications and long-term outcome of upper cervical spine arthrodesis in patients with Down syndrome. Spine May 15, 1996; 21(10):1223-1231.
12. Dyck VG. Upper cervical instability in Down's syndrome: a case report. Journal of the Canadian Chiropractors Association June 1981; 25(2):67-68.

HEAD INJURY

Falls may lead to head trauma. In one study, 22% of falls resulted in head injury. A wide spectrum of injuries can occur from abrasions and contusions to skull fractures, concussion, and intracranial hemorrhages (1). In the U.S., 100,000 children under age 15 are admitted to hospitals, 90% due to mild head injury (2).

Closed head injuries are more common in children than open head injuries (penetration of the dura mater) (3). The sequelae of closed head injuries tend to be worse due to increased intracranial pressure (3).

In some cases, relatively minor head trauma may lead to a delayed deterioration in the level of consciousness. One study found that 4% of children with head injury had late deterioration of consciousness and in this study of 42 children, three died. A small epidural hematoma may cause a deterioration of consciousness after 24 to 48 hours after the injury even though the child had been showing clinical improvements. In this case, the primary problem is diffuse brain swelling. In infants under age one year, minor head injury may lead to pediatric concussion syndrome. This is characterized by the child becoming pale, sweating, irritability, sleepiness, and sometimes vomiting. This condition is self-limiting fortunately. Over the age of one year, a similar concussion syndrome may have a progression to coma accompanied by pupillary changes, apnea, and sometimes death (4).

A more forceful blow to the head may produce bleeding in the subgaleal or subperiosteal space which results in the formation of a cephalohematoma. This is relatively common in neonates (5). A severe cephalohematoma may cause a significant decrease in the infant's hematocrit. A lab work-up with blood volume and watching for hyperbilirubinemia may be necessary (5).

In addition to the neurological risks of head injuries, one study found that there was immune system suppression following head injury. This study evaluated 11 children who had a Glasgow Coma Scale of 7 or less. T-cell response and quantity were found to be diminished following head trauma (6).

Skull fractures come in several forms. A linear fracture produces a radiographically distinct straight line with parallel margins. Comminuted fractures produces fracture fragments. If the fragments are driven into the osseous tissue, it is termed depressed. A fracture line that runs into a cranial suture may split a suture which is called a diastasis. A basilar fracture is a fracture of the base of the skull which may be difficult to see on routine skull radiographs. Blood or CSF in the auditory canal, postauricular ecchymosis or Battle sign, CSF rhinorrhea, "raccoon eyes" or periorbital ecchymosis and/or cranial nerve palsies are signs to investigate for a basilar fracture (7). If a skull fracture communicates with the scalp laceration, the parasinuses, or the middle ear cavity, it is termed a compound fracture (5).

Fractures of the skull are less commonly seen in children compared to adults due to greater elasticity of the skull. The most common fracture seen in children are linear fractures (7). Because of the elasticity of the skull, a significant force is required which increases the likelihood of brain injury, as well as cervical spine injury.

Hematoma and intracranial hemorrhage must be ruled out in cases of head injury. Subdural and epidural hematomas can be life-threatening as they may cause compression of the brain stem (8).

SOME ETIOLOGICAL FACTORS

In neonates, one cause of head trauma is due to forceps birth which can distort the malleable cranium.

A new and growing concern is brain injury caused by playing football/soccer. Common images of soccer players around the world are the sights of the player striking the ball with his head or players striking their heads into opponents. Imaging of the brains of a group of soccer players found the presence of lesions in their brains. Soccer is becoming very popular among North American youths. A great concern is what is occurring to the developing brains of these youths who play soccer and try to emulate their professional idols.

A large majority of bicycling deaths are due to head injuries. About one-half of these occur to children (9). In many cases, head injuries due to bicycle accidents might be avoided or the damaged minimized by the use of a properly fitted and designed helmet. A study in Washington state found that there is a significant reduction in head injury, brain injury, and severe brain injury in bicycle crashes involving helmeted riders compared to unhelmeted riders. Helmeted riders involved in crashes had a 69% reduction in head injuries, a 65% reduction in brain injuries, and a 74% reduction in severe brain injuries (10). There is no excuse for not wearing a helmet as they are now comfortable, lightweight, and well-ventilated, and many are quite inexpensive and have trendy colors and graphics. In some states, it is mandatory for children to wear helmets while bicycling. The tragedy is that many states still do not mandate the use of helmets. Make certain that the helmet has been tested and approved by a certification organization like Snell or ANSI.

Inappropriate use of misuse of child car seats may cause severe injuries in an automobile accident. Head injuries caused by impact with a part of the car due to car seat failure are of particular concern. It has been established that rearward facing car seats seem to cause less injury to the child.

"SHAKEN BABY" SYNDROME

"Shaken baby syndrome" is the leading cause of head injury in infants (See also Chapter 2). Usually there are signs or a history of previous suspicious injuries. Some signs include bruising, retina injury, and fracture of long bones. There may be a history of colic or other feeding problems or incessant irritability or crying (11). An important consideration if head trauma is suspected is subdural hemorrhages which is almost always due to trauma (11,12).

CLINICAL FEATURES

Signs of significant head injury, particularly those of hematomas, include altered level of consciousness, altered behavior, severe headache, vomiting and/or nausea, visual changes (particularly those related to compression of the third cranial nerve), sleepiness, hemiparesis or hypertonia, and focal neurological signs (13). There may be signs of concussion and possibly amnesia. Children with head injuries often are drowsy, have headaches, and may vomit (14). The Glascow Coma Scale for children or infants is used in the emergency evaluation of head injury. If the child is stabilized, an extensive neurologic examination is needed.

If the child's head injury is considered to be minor or not requiring extensive testing or observation, the first 24 hours is critical for observing any changes that may occur (see parent's instructions).

MEDICAL MANAGEMENT

The medical management depends upon the type, location, and severity of the injury. It can range from bandages and non-steroidal inflammatory drugs to major surgical procedures.

CHIROPRACTIC MANAGEMENT

Araghi presented a case of a 2-year-old male with a history of vomiting and energy loss following a head injury due to a head first fall from a shopping cart. Immediately after falling, the child's eyes rolled back and vomiting commenced. Subsequently, he had periodic episodes of loss of consciousness; the parents had to arouse him by shaking him or tapping his head. The parents took the child to the emergency room where an examination and CT scan were done. A diagnosis of mild concussion was given and pain medication prescribed. The following two weeks after beginning medical treatment, the vomiting episodes continued and his behavior became "strange" according to the parents. He was a very active child before the fall but became sedentary and quiet and had low energy. Chiropractic evaluation revealed abnormal palpation findings at the atlanto-occipital region. The atlanto-axial articulation was hypermobile and tender. Visualization in the closed eyes, standing position showed elevation of the head, shoulder, and hip on the left side. Full spine and cervical flexion x-rays were taken utilizing shielding, collimation, and extremely fast film/screens. A decrease in the normal spinal

---

Table 13.22. Signs and Symptoms Leading to Suspicion of Severe Child Abuse

Subdural hematoma in the posterior intrahemispheric region without a history of significant accidental trauma.

Retinal hemorrhages.

Unexplained bruises or bumps.

Cigarette burns.

Lacerations or bruises in various stages of healing.

Specific patterns of bruising seen with whipping injuries from belts or cords.

Posterior lesions.

"Finger" bruises, such as grab marks, encirclement bruises, choke marks, and bilateral bruises.

Injuries to bone, e.g., posterior rib fractures, spiral fractures, metaphyseal "chip" fractures, and multiple fractures of different ages.

Modified from Goldstein B, Powers KS. Head trauma in children. Pediatr Rev 1994;15(6):213–219.

Table 13.23.   Pediatric Head Injury Instruction Sheet University of Rochester Medical Center

---

What should I watch for in my child?

Watch your child for 24 hours.

If your child is awake, a constant watch should be maintained.

If your child is sleeping, awaken her/him every 3 hours.

Your child should awaken easily.

Is her/his talking and moving of arms and legs normal?

When further attention is required, call the doctor:

1. Will not wake up or is more sleepy than usual.

2. Vomits more than two times.

3. Has headaches, which get worse or last more than a day.

Modified from Goldstein B, Powers KS. Head trauma in children. Pediatr Rev 1994;15(6):213–219 and originally from University of Rochester Medical Center.

---

curves were noted as was approximation of the posterior upper cervical elements. There was fixation on the flexion view. The atlanto-occipital articulation was adjusted as per the Gonstead System AS-LS-LP listing. Three days later, the child was seen again. The parents stated that the child's energy level had returned, behavior normalized, and no vomiting had occurred (there was no vomiting for the two days prior to the initiation of chiropractic care). A neutral lateral cervical x-ray revealed a normal cervical curve and separation of the posterior atlas from the occiput. Within a four week period, the occiput was adjusted three more times (15).

REFERENCES

1. Rivara FP, et al. Population-based study of fall injuries in children and adolescents resulting in hospitalization or death. Pediatrics July 1993; 92(1):61-63.
2. Snoek JW. Mild Head Injury in Children. In: Levin HS, Eisenberg HM, Benton AL. Mild Head Injury. New York: Oxford University Press. 1989. pp. 103-132.
3. Johnston MV, Gerring JP. Head trauma and its sequelae. Pediatric Annals June 1992; 21(6):362-368.
4. Bruce DA. Delayed deterioration of consciousness after trivial head injury in childhood. British Medical Journal September 22, 1984; 289(6447):714-715.
5. Netter FH. The CIBA Collection of Medical Illustrations. Vol.1 Nervous System. Part II. Neurologic and Neuromuscular Disorders. West Caldwell NJ: CIBA Pharmaceutical Co. 1986. pp.90-105.
6. Meert KL, et al. Alterations in immune function following head injury in children. Critical Care Medicine January 1994; 22(1):A180.
7. Goldstein B, Powers KS. Head trauma in children. Pediatrics in Review June 1994; 15(6):213-219.
8. Weiner HL, Urion DK, Levitt LP. Pediatric Neurology of the House Officer. 3rd ed. Baltimore: Williams & Wilkins. 1988. pp.195-197.
9. Weiss BD. Bicycle-related head injuries. Clinics in Sports Medicine January 1994; 13(1):99-112.
10. Thompson DC, Rivara FP, Thompson RS. Effectiveness of bicycle safety helmets in preventing head injuries: a case-control study. JAMA December 25, 1996; 276(24):1968-1973.
11. Committee on Child Abuse and Neglect. Shaken baby syndrome: inflicted cerebral trauma. Pediatrics December 1993; 92(6):872-875.
12. Caffey J. On the theory and practice of shaking infants. American Journal of Diseases of Children August 1972; 124(2):161-169.
13. Bruce DA. Head injuries in the pediatric population. Current Problems in Pediatrics February 1990; 20(20):67-107.
14. Adams RD, Victor M. Principles of Neurology, 4th ed. New York: McGraw-Hill, Inc. 1989. pp.693-717.
15. Araghi HJ. Post-traumatic Evaluation and Treatment of the Pediatric Patient with Head Injury: A Case Report. Proceedings of the National Conference on Chiropractic and Pediatric. November 1992. pp.1-8.

HEADACHE

Headaches are quite common in children. A Swedish study of 9,000 children found that over 70% have had headaches by 15 years of age (1). A survey in 1988 found that the prevalence of severe or frequent headache in those under age 18 years to be 25.3 per 1000 population—the rate was 9.9 per 1000 for children under age 10 years old and 45.8 per 1000 for those from ages 10 to 17 years (2).

Headaches may be primary (tension headaches, migraines, etc.) or secondary to, or a manifestation of, another disorder. The fear in childhood headaches is intracranial masses, such as tumors or other serious and underlying disorders. Suspicion of an underlying organic disease or a recent history of trauma warrants an in-depth evaluation.

The differentiation of the various types of primary headaches can be difficult, although there are classical features to most. Typically, the differentiation is between migraine, tension, and cluster headaches. The International Headache Society revised its classification system in 1988.

MIGRAINE HEADACHES

Migraines are classified with or without aura—classical or common migraines respectively in previous classification systems. Migraines are the most common headaches in children (3,4). Studies have shown that at least 5% of children are afflicted (4). The highest incidence of childhood migraines are in males aged 10 to 14 (4). One study of 13-year-old schoolchildren which was conducted in Finland found a higher prevalence in females but a companion study of 7-year-olds found a higher incidence among males (5,6).

The classic features of migraine headaches with aura are auras preceding the headache and focal localization of the headache. These occur 15 to 30 minutes prior to the headache and can manifest as homonymous visual auras, unilateral paresthesia and/or numbness, unilateral weakness, and aphasia or other difficult speech problems (7).

A higher percentage of children with atopy, i.e., asthma, rhinitis, or eczema, had a history of headaches when compared to children without a history of atopy (8).

TENSION HEADACHES

Children with tension or muscle contraction headaches tended to have more nausea and photophobia than adults (9). Duration may be minutes or days. Pain tends to be bilateral and may feel like a pressure or band (7).

CLUSTER HEADACHES

The childhood incidence of cluster headache is rare (10). They are unilateral, have a rapid onset, and the duration is brief, but they may occur up to several times a day (7). Most tend to begin after the age of 20. Males tend to predominate. In one study of 35 patients, 31 had pain in the area of the eye. Many also had pain radiating to the temple or ipsilateral maxilla or forehead. Ocular symptoms were common and included lacrimation, conjunctival injectio, photophobia, ptosis, and meiosis. Nasal congestion, rhinorrhea, nausea, sweating of the face and/or other parts of the body, phonophobia, and facial flushing were common as well. The frequency and duration of headaches may increase with time (11).

CERVICOGENIC OR VERTEBROGENIC HEADACHES

This form of headache is not commonly reported. The childhood incidence is unknown. If there is a well-delineated form, it does not appear to be described. Referral from dysfunction in the cervical spine appears to be a common cause (12,13). In one reported case, analgesics injected in a cervical joint relieved the headaches (14). Muscle contraction or tension headaches probably describe most of its manifestations. There are numerous reports of migraine headaches benefitting from spinal manipulation or adjustments. Would these be considered to be cervicogenic migraine headaches?

MEDICAL MANAGEMENT

Medical management is primarily drug oriented. If there is no underlying organic disease or history of trauma, symptomatic relief drugs are usually given. Analgesics and non-steroidal anti-inflammatory drugs are commonly given. Antiemetics may be given if there are gastrointestinal symptoms. Ergotamines and other 5–HT agonists and dopamine antagonists have been used to relieve headache symptoms. It is well known that daily or frequent headaches can be caused by the overuse or frequent use of drugs that are being used to relieve the headache. A self-perpetuating cycle is formed.

Table 13.24. International Headache Society—Headache Classification

Migraine

1.1	Migraine without aura
1.2	Migraine with aura
1.3	Ophthalmoplegic migraine
1.4	Retinal migraine
1.5	Childhood periodic syndromes that may be precursors to or associated with migraines
1.6	Complications of migraine
1.7	Migrainous disorder not fulfilling the above criteria

Tension-type headache

2.1	Episodic tension-type headache
2.2	Chronic tension-type headache
2.3	Headache of the tension type not fulfilling the above criteria

Cluster headache and chronic paroxysmal hemicrania

3.1	Cluster headache
3.2	Chronic paroxysmal hemicrania
3.3	Cluster headache-like disorder not fulfilling the above criteria

Miscellaneous headaches unassociated with structural lesion

Headache associated with head trauma

Headache associated with vascular disorders

Headache associated with a nonvascular intracranial disorder

Headache associated with substances or their withdrawal

Headache associated with noncephalic infection

Headache associated with a metabolic disorder

Headache or facial pain associated with a disorder of the cranium, head, eyes, ears, nose, sinuses, teeth, mouth, or other facial or cranial structures

Cranial neuralgias, nerve trunk pain, and defferentation pain

Headache; not classifiable

Silberstein SD. Differential diagnosis of headache. Hospital Med 1994;30(1):49–54, 59–60.

Table 13.25.   Diagnostic Criteria for Migraine International Headache Society (1988)

Migraine without aura

　At least 5 headache attacks.

　Untreated duration of at least 4 to 72 hours.

　Characteristics (at least 2 of 4):

　　1. Unilateral location.

　　2. Pulsating quality.

　　3. Moderate or severe in intensity interfering with or interrupting daily activities.

　　4. Aggravated by physical activities.

　Concomitant features (at least 1 of 2):

　　1. Nausea and/or vomiting.

　　2. Photophobia and phonophobia.

Migraine with aura

　At least 2 headache attacks.

　Characteristics (at least 3 of 4):

　　1. Aura indicating focal cerebral or brainstem dysfunction.

　　2. Aura developing gradually over 4 minutes or several symptoms that occur in succession.

　　3. Aura lasting less than 60 minutes.

　　4. Headache appears before, with, or within 60 minutes of the aura.

Modified from Singer HS. Migraine headaches in children. Pediatr Rev 1994; 15(3):94–101.

Trigger identification and avoidance, behavioral modification, such as biofeedback and relaxation training, and avoidance of triggering foods are among other therapies that may be used (4).

CHIROPRACTIC MANAGEMENT

Hewitt presented a case of a 13-year-old female suffering from intermittent headaches and neck pain which she experienced for at least one year. There were no complaints of prodromal symptoms prior to the onset of headache attacks nor were there visual problems associated with it. The history noted two neck injuries which occurred during gymnastics several years prior to the evaluation, as well as another gymnastic injury which caused a pedicle fracture of L3. No monthly patterns were noted—she recently began her menses. She had been taking acetaminophen, resting, and using a heat pad on her neck and cold pack on her forehead. These gave temporary relief. Her pediatrician recommended a chiropractic evaluation. The chiropractic analysis noted restriction in right cervical lateral flexion and hypertonia in the cervical and upper thoracic muscles. The neurological evaluation was unremarkable. Thoracic fixations were adjusted using anterior thoracic adjustments and single transverse process contact. A modified rotary break adjustment was given in the cervical spine. Soft tissue work and trigger point therapy were also used. On the day of the first chiropractic treatment, she saw the pediatrician who prescribed Tylenol 3 with codeine which helped her to sleep and a CAT scan which was negative. When she returned for the

third visit, the headaches had improved, and she discontinued taking the Tylenol 3. Two weeks after the initial evaluation, she stated that she did not have headaches or neck pain. On a four-week telephone follow-up, headaches or neck pain had not returned (1).

Lewit found manipulation to be effective in the treatment of headaches (15). In a group of children with both headaches and eye pain, palpation of the atlas transverse process was found to reproduce the ipsilateral retro-orbital pain. Treatment was relaxation exercises to the neck and head muscles. Seventy-four children were treated. Within six months, 57 improved and after one year, only 10 showed no improvement. In another group of 30 children with non-migrainous headaches, Lewit stated that manipulation gave "excellent" results in 28 (13). In a group of 27 with migraine headaches, there were three failures and "excellent results in 24 (15)."

Anderson-Peacock presented five cases. All of these cases had secondary problems in addition to the headache, e.g., back and/or extremity pain and sinus and GI tract problems. All were adjusted using the Diversified technique. A brief summary of the cases follow (16):

The first was an female nearly 7 years old who had a 2 year history of near daily headaches. The headaches were described as sharp and throbbing in the frontal and orbital regions and were without visual disturbances or prodromal symptoms. Following a chiropractic examination, adjustments were made to the upper cervical and lower thoracic regions during the initial visits with the ilium included on a subsequent visit. At

1½ months, headaches were reduced in intensity and frequency. Following that, she was pain-free, although there was a resumption of signs and symptoms following a fall and an involvement in a motor vehicle accident. After adjustments made following those traumas, she was again pain-free (16).

Case 2 was an almost 8-year-old male with classical migraine headaches. He complained of visual problems, nausea, and vomiting. Headaches could be set off by weather changes and food. His mother also had headaches. His birth was induced and forceps were used. He had seizures for a week after birth. Following a chiropractic examination, the occiput, lower cervical, and sacroiliac joint levels were adjusted. He was advised to avoid certain foods. After 1½ months, headaches were rare and migraines did not reoccur (16).

A third case was a near 8-year-old female with frontal headaches that sometimes disturbed sleep. The upper cervical and upper and midthoracic spine was adjusted. The pinnae of the left ear was also adjusted. Four months after initiation of care, she only had two instances of headaches (16).

A fourth case was a near 14-year-old male with migraine headaches which was medically diagnosed 5 years earlier. Auras were noted if the headaches occurred at mid-day. He received cervical and upper thoracic adjustments. Headache abated during the first two weeks. A fall while playing sports caused a resumption of headaches which again abated with adjustments (16).

The fifth case was a 15-year-old female with a 10 month history of severe generalized headaches that occurred several times each week. Pain relief drugs were prescribed. Adjustments were made in the upper cervical, upper thoracic, and lower lumbar spine. Two weeks after the initiation of care, headaches were of a low intensity and drugs were not required. Three months into care, headaches were rare and mild (16).

Cochran presented a case at the 1994 National Conference on Chiropractic and Pediatrics of a 10-year-old male with migraine headaches. He had headaches for three years. Adjustments were made in the cervical and thoracic spine using Thompson and diversified adjusting procedures. Two prodromal episodes were noted during the first month of care but these episodes did not result in a full migraine (17).

A chiropractor needs to look at other factors if headaches continue (assuming that there is not an underlying serious condition, such as aneurysm, tumor, infection, abnormal or vascular disorder) despite spinal adjustments. Diet (food allergies), temporomandibular joint dysfunction, poorly fitting shoes, stress, and eye strain are among many factors that may be involved.

There are numerous case reports and literature reviews on chiropractic care given to adults with headaches, including migraine headaches (10,18-20) (See also Chapter 1).

REFERENCES

1. Hewitt EG. Chiropractic care of a 13-year-old with headache and neck pain: a case report. Journal of the Canadian Chiropractic Association September 1994; 38(3):160-162.
2. Smith MS. Comprehensive evaluation and treatment of recurrent pediatric headache. Pediatric Annals September 1995; 24(9):450+.
3. Abu-Arefeh I, Russell G. Prevalence of headache and migraine in schoolchildren. British Medical Journal September 24, 1994; 309:765-769.
4. Singer HS. Migraine headaches in children. Pediatrics in Review March 1994; 15(3):94-101.
5. Sillanpää M. Prevalence of headache in prepuberty. Headache January 1983:10-14.
6. Sillanpää M. Changes in the prevalence of migraine and other headaches during the first seven school years. Headache January 1983:15-19.
7. Silberstein SD. Differential diagnosis of headache. Hospital Medicine January 1994; 30(1):49-60.
8. Mortimer MJ, et al. The prevalence of headache and migraine in atopic children: an epidemiological study in general practice. Headache September 1983:427-431.
9. Miller B, Maxwell JL, DeBoer KF. Chiropractic treatment of tension headache: a case report. Journal of the American Chiropractic Association 1984; 18(6):62-66.
10. Mindell JA, Andrasik F. Headache classification and factor analysis with a pediatric population. Headache February 1987; 27:96-101.
11. Maytal J, et al. Childhood onset cluster headaches. Headache June 1992; 32:275-279.
12. Bogduk N, et al. Cervical headache. Medical Journal of Australia September 2, 1985; 143:202+.
13. Vernon H. Spinal manipulation and headache of cervical origin. Manual Medicine 1991; 6(2):73-79.
14. Rothbart P. Unilateral headache with features of hemicrania continua and cervicogenic headache – a case report. Headache October 1992:459-460.
15. Lewit K. Manipulative therapy in rehabilitation of the locomotor system. 2nd ed. Oxford: Butterworth-Heinemann, Ltd. 1991. p.20.
16. Anderson-Peacock ES. Chiropractic care of children with headaches: five case reports. Journal of Clinical Chiropractic Pediatrics 1996; 1(1):18-27.
17. Cochran JA. Chiropractic treatment of childhood migraine headache: a case study. Proceedings of the National Conference on Chiropractic and Pediatrics 1994. pp.85-90. As abstracted by Masarsky CS. Headache and Torticollis (Research Review). ICA International Review of Chiropractic 1995; 51(1):45-47.
18. Grillo F. The differential diagnosis and therapy of headache. Annals of the Swiss Chiropractors Association 1961; 2:121-165.
19. Samms J. Chiropractic care of headache. Alternative and Complementary Therapies October 1994; 1(1):26-31.
20. Wright JS. Migraine: a statistical analysis of chiropractic treatment. J Chiro 1978; 12:563-567.

INFANTILE HYPOTONIA OR THE FLOPPY BABY

Infantile hypotonia or the "floppy baby" syndrome can be due to a variety of disorders. It is described below and was previously described in the chapter.

Lesions in the central nervous system cause some forms of hypotonia. Encephalopathy-caused hypotonia due to tonic cerebral palsy is usually associated with lesions in a normally formed brain often as a result of hypoxic-ischemic encephalopathy (1). Malformation of the brain may also cause atonia. Degenerative disorders of the brain, such as Tay-Sachs, may cause hypotonia (1). Cerebral palsy may also cause hypotonia (2).

Spinal cord lesions such as transection or maldevelopment may cause hypotonia (3). Anterior horn cell lesions such as Werdnig-Hoffman disease (acute infantile spinal muscular atrophy) and poliomyelitis produce hypotonia (3,4). Lesions in the peripheral nerves, myoneural junction, and in the muscles themselves may be a source of hypotonia. These include polyneuropathy, myesthesia gravis, myotonic dystrophy, and congenital muscular dystrophy (2-4).

Systemic disorders such as amino acid abnormalities, hypercalcemia, rickets, celiac disease, chronic diseases of the heart, kidneys, or liver, and congenital ligamentous laxity may also cause hypotonia (3,5). Chromosomal disorders such as Down syndrome may present with hypotonia (2). There is also a benign congenital form known as amyotonia congenita (3).

Because the "floppy baby syndrome" or hypotonia can be a result of any of a number of causes, a diagnostic work-up is difficult. The obstetrical history is very important in localizing the lesion (4). One of the first determinations is whether the lesion is in cerebral, spinal, or muscle/motor—upper and/or lower motor neuron involvement (2,6). Is it in the central or peripheral nervous system? The infant shows unusual postures, little resistance to passive movement of the joints, and increased range of motion. In an older infant, there are usually delays in motor milestones (7). The physical work-up includes tendon reflexes, palpation and strength test of the muscles, Babinski sign, and observation of cranial nerve function. Definitive diagnostic confirmation of the lesion site is usually by electrodiagnostic tests, imaging, biopsies, and lab work-up (1,4).

MEDICAL MANAGEMENT

Management depends upon the etiology of the condition. An extensive work-up may be required to differentiate and find the primary disorder causing it.

CHIROPRACTIC MANAGEMENT

It is difficult to ascertain the impact of the chiropractic adjustment on an infant suffering from infantile hypotonia. We are not aware of any case studies. Two of the authors have seen cases while doing volunteer work in Latin America but were unable to do follow-up on the cases nor conduct a proper work-up to determine the cause of the hypotonia. In one case, the head was carried in the anterior position, as in an AS occiput misalignment as described by C.S. Gonstead. Palpatory findings revealed fixation between the atlas and the occiput. It would be interesting to see if a course of chiropractic care would have an impact on some cases of infantile hypotonia.

REFERENCES

1. Netter FH. The CIBA collection of medical illustrations. volume 1: nervous system. Part: Neurologic and Neuromuscular Disorders. West Caldwell NJ: CIBA Pharmaceutical Co. 1986. pp. 15-16.
2. Swaiman KF. Pediatric neurology. St. Louis: C.V. Mosby Co. 1986. p.197.
3. Weiner HL, Urion DK, Levitt LP. Pediatric neurology of the house officer, 3rd ed. Baltimore: Williams & Wilkins. 1988. pp.11-17.
4. Crawford TO. Clinical evaluation of the floppy infant. Pediatric Annals June 1992; 21(6):348-352,354.
5. Paine RS. The future of the "floppy infant": a follow-up study of patients. Developmental Medicine and Childhood Neurology April 1963; 5(2):115-124.
6. Gilman S. The mechanism of cerebellar hypotonia. Brain 1969; 93(Part III):621-638.
7. Zellweger H. The floppy baby syndrome. Clinics in Developmental Medicine 1969; 31:1-107.

MENINGITIS

ASEPTIC MENINGITIS

The differentiation of aseptic meningitis from more potentially lethal illnesses is vitally important (See Chapter 16). Aseptic meningitis is inflammation of the meninges without culture of bacterial source. The incidence is about 11 to 27 per 100,000 population (1). It tends to occur in warm weather months (2,3). In children, it tends to occur to males between the age of 1 and 10 years (3). Neonate meningitis tends to be enteroviral origin rather than bacterial (3,4).

The most common source of aseptic meningitis is a viral agent (2). About 85% to 95% are associated with enteroviruses (echovirus, Coxsackie virus, and nonparalytical poliomyelitis),

mumps, herpes simplex type 2, lymphocytic choriomeningitis, and adenovirus (1,3). Arboviruses account for 5% and may cause encephalitis (3).

Viral meningitis may be a sequela of viral infections such as measles, rubella, or varicella; a sequela of bacterial meningitis, tuberculosis, or syphilis; or associated with other infections. It may also be associated with neoplasm, sinusitis, abscess, or meningeal disease (5).

Some vaccines can cause aseptic meningitis. The measles-mumps-rubella (MMR) and mumps vaccines have been implicated (3). Certain drugs, such as ibuprofen, are also suspected causes (3). It may also be caused by intrathecal injection (5).

Recovery is usually satisfactory but young infants may have neurological problems such as intellectual impairment or delayed speech (6). Studies have found subtle but significant deficits in receptive language processing. It was recommended that children who suffered enterovirus meningitis be carefully monitored in case there are deficits in language skills development that may require an increase in language stimulation (7).

CLINICAL FEATURES

The signs and symptoms of aseptic meningitis are similar to those of the bacterial form but tend to be less severe (2,8). It usually features acute onset fever, headache, nausea, and vomiting, sometimes preceded by several days of acute fever with general malaise and anorexia (3). Older children may present with myalgia, photophobia, and headache with only 50% presenting with nuchal rigidity (3). There are rarely neurological deficits or altered levels of consciousness (2). It is usually difficult to isolate the virus from CSF samples (8). Neutrophils tend to increase (8). Differential diagnosis is vitally important. In addition to the bacterial form, it must also be distinguished from its many forms and from many other disorders, such as poliomyelitis, mumps meningitis, arbovirus infection, leptospirosis, mononucleosis, sinusitis or mastoiditis, and as a secondary manifestation to neoplasm (1).

BACTERIAL MENINGITIS

Bacterial meningitis is a medical emergency and requires rapid treatment. It is in the interest of all to share responsibility for this case at an early stage. A high percentage die or have permanent neurological residuals.

The rate of frequency in children is 1 in 2,000 (2). The incidence is greatest during the first month (10 per 1000 live births) and falls significantly in the second month (4.5 per 1000) but peaks again in the six to eight months of age period (8 per 1000) (6). Of the 30,000 cases each year, 3,000 die and 6,000 to 12,000 have permanent neurological sequelae (2).

The bacterial organisms typically cultured from CSF of afflicted individuals tend to be, in 90% of cases, *Haemophilus influenzae, Salmonella pneumoniae, Escherichia coli, Neisseria meningitidis*, and Group B *Streptococcus. Streptococcus* seems to predominate (9). One retrospective study found that *E. coli* and *Listeria monocytogenes* predominated in the neonate (4).

The blood-brain barrier appears to be breached in the dural venous sinus system, above the cribriform plate, or in the choroid plexus. There is then infiltration into the subarachnoid space. In bacterial meningitis, the blood-brain permeability is

Table 13.26.   **Signs and Symptoms of Meningitis**

Age	Symptoms	Signs	
		Early	Late
0–3 months	Paradoxical irritability	Lethargy	Bulging fontanelle
	Altered sleep pattern	Irritability	
	Vomiting	Fever (±)	
	Lethargy		
4–24 months	Irritability	Fever	Nuchal rigidity
	Altered sleep pattern	Irritability	Decreased level of consciousness
	Lethargy		
>24 months	Headache	Fever	Brudzinski's sign★
	Stiff neck	Nuchal rigidity	Kernig's sign†
	Lethargy	Irritability	Decreased level of consciousness

★*Brudzinski's sign: Patient is supine. Examiner flexes the neck to approximate the chin to the chest. A positive sign is flexion of the knees. [LEFROCK]*
†*Kernig's sign: Patient is supine and is told to flex the knee and hip. The examiner attempts to extend the knee. A positive sign is marked irritation or pain. [LEFROCK]*
Adapted from Fleisher G, Ludwig S (ed). Textbook of Pediatric Emergency Medicine. Baltimore: Williams & Wilkins, 1988.

increased to proteins, ions, and other substances. The pathophysiology of bacterial meningitis includes cerebral edema which is aggravated by the release of antidiuretic hormone (ADH). Increased intracranial pressure may cause a wide variety of neurologic effects and may also lead to cerebral herniation. A vasculitis in the subarachnoid space may result in narrowing of the vessel lumina or thrombus formation potentially resulting in ischemia or infarct in the brain. CSF outflow may become limited as the subarachnoid space passageways to the dural sinuses may be limited (9).

CLINICAL FEATURES

Definitive clinical diagnosis of bacterial meningitis is difficult because of the variability and nonspecificity of presentation. This difficulty is particularly unfortunate because of the rapidly progressive and tragic nature of this disease.

The classical physical signs of bacterial meningitis are a history of high fever, stiff neck, severe headache, confusion and irritability, chills, petechiae and purpura (suggestive of meningococcal disease), and Brudzinski's and Kernig's signs (8,10). These tend to vary with the age of onset (See Table 13.26) (2). Brudzinski's and Kernig's signs are not always present (11).

A very young infant is difficult to diagnose. If there is a high fever at or greater than 38.5°C, meningitis is strongly under consideration until ruled out (2). Not all neonates will have a fever (4). A stiff neck may not be present in an infant. Lethargy is an important sign to pursue (12). Other signs in an infant are irritability, high pitched cry, cyanosis and lethargy (8). Occasionally, convulsion or seizures are presenting signs (2,8). Recently, researchers have found the cytokines, CSF interleukin-6 and tumor necrosis factor in the CSF of infants with meningitis and not in children without meningitis. Although CSF interleukin-6 has been found in many infants

with aseptic meningitis, the levels in bacterial meningitis were ten times greater. Many but not all infants with bacterial meningitis were found to have detectable levels of tumor necrosis factor in the CSF. None of the infants without meningitis nor those with aseptic meningitis showed any presence of tumor necrosis factor. The plasma levels of these two cytokines were not reliable or specific enough for differential diagnosis (13).

The definitive diagnostic sign is a positive culture from the CSF (2). Therefore, a lumbar puncture or cisternal tap is necessary. If CSF glucose levels are less that 23% of that of the serum level, CSF protein concentration is greater than 220 mg/dl, CSF white blood cell count is over 2000/mm^3, and PMN count is over 1180/mm^3, a diagnosis of bacterial meningitis is likely. CSF culturing and antigen assays round out the diagnosis (12). CAT scan rules out other lesions and is utilized if the fontanelles are closed and focal neurological signs are present (12).

MANAGEMENT

The typical medical intervention for bacterial meningitis is antibiotic therapy. The problems with antibiotic usage is the ability of the drug to pass through the blood-brain barrier, the bactericidal effect of abnormally acidic pH changes in the CSF, the means by which antibiotics are given, and the use of other drugs (9). If seizures are present, intervention with anticonvulsive drugs may be used. Steroids may be used to improve cerebral blood flow (12). Fluids are given in some cases of dehydration; in other cases, the intake of fluids is restricted as it may cause the abnormal release of antidiuretic hormone (ADH) which would contribute to cerebral edema (12). Monoclonal antibodies may also be given (9). Operative procedures may be used if an accessible brain abscess is present.

Attempts have been made to create vaccine against bacterial meningitis. Meningococcal vaccines were created by basing them on the polysaccharide capsule of the bacterium. The vaccine affords a temporary immunity and has not been effective in infants (15). A vaccine against Hemophilus influenzae has been more successful. It binds the capsule's polysaccharides to a protein carrier (15).

CHIROPRACTIC MANAGEMENT

Bacterial meningitis is usually an emergency situation, and rapid referral and intervention is appropriate and recommended. Based upon the following case, chiropractic intervention following referral may improve the outcome in some cases. Rubinstein, the author of the article, was contacted and upon arrival at the hospital, found a 10-month-old male in a coma who had been admitted suffering from bacterial meningitis. He was in an oxygen tent and was receiving IV feeding. The history included multiple birth defects and blindness and deafness, severe retardation, and abdominal contents which were located outside of the abdomen at birth. He also suffered from prenatal alcohol and cocaine syndrome. During the hospital stay, the infant required revival. The author noted that the head was in right lateral flexion and right rotation. A series of light thrusts were given (the author did not indicate whether thrusts were given to the skull or neck) with an A to P and left to right vector with the head in left lateral flexion and rotation. The child immediately began coughing and awakening. The following day, the child was fully conscious, was released from the intensive care unit, and has since recovered and been placed in a group home (16).

REFERENCES

1. Adams RD, Victor M. Principles of Neurology, 4th ed. New York: McGraw-Hill, Inc. 1989. p.599.
2. Fleisher G, Ludwig S, eds. "Textbook of Pediatric Emergency Medicine, 2nd ed. Baltimore: Williams & Wilkins. 1988. pp.420-426.
3. Maxson S, Jacobs RF. Viral meningitis. Postgraduate Medicine June 1993; 93(8): 153-66.
4. Shattuck KE, Chonmaitree T. The changing spectrum of neonatal meningitis over a fifteen-year period. Clinical Pediatrics March 1992; 31(3):130-136.
5. Berkow R. The Merck Manual of Diagnosis and Therapy, 14th ed. Rahway NJ: Merck & Co., Inc. 1982. pp. 1339-1346.
6. Powell KR. Meningitis. In: Hoekelman RA (ed). Primary Pediatric Care, (2nd ed). St. Louis, MO: Mosby Year Book. 1992. pp.1352-1359.
7. Baker RC, et al. Neurodevelopmental outcome of infants with viral meningitis in the first three months of life. Clinical Pediatrics June 1996; 35(6):295-301.
8. Weiner HL, Urion DK, Levitt LP. Pediatric neurology for the house officer, 3rd ed. Baltimore: Williams & Wilkins. 1988.
9. Tunkel AR, Wispelwey B, Scheld WM. Bacterial meningitis: recent advances in pathophysiology and treatment. Annals of Internal Medicine April 15, 1990; 112(8):610-623.
10. Pansky B, Allen DJ, Budd GC. Review of Neuroscience, 2nd ed. New York: Macmillan Publishing Co. 1988.
11. Moss RB, Sosulski R. Early meningitis. clinical pediatrics April 1991; 30(4):229-230.
12. Marks MI. Bacterial meningitis—an update. Clinical Pediatrics December 1991; 30(12):673-675.
13. Cytokine Measurements: A Marker for Meningitis. Emergency Medicine March 1996; 28(3):87.
14. Lefrock JL, Shapiro ED, Wenger J. Meningitis: find it early, treat it fast. Patient Care December 15, 1991; 25(20):133-136+.
15. Moore PS, Broom CV. Cerebrospinal meningitis epidemics. Scientific American November 1994; 271(5):38-45.
16. Rubinstein HM. Coma as a result of bacterial meningitis in the compromised child. Chiropractic Pediatrics 1994; 1(3):25-26.

MULTIPLE SCLEROSIS

Multiple sclerosis (MS) is uncommon in children—about 0.5% of MS cases (1-3)—and tends to occur after age 10 (4,5). It is a consideration in the differential diagnosis work-up for leukodystrophies (4).

MS is thought to be associated with an autoimmune process. A reduction in T5-cells has been found during acute MS episodes in both adults and children (6).

More females than males tend to be afflicted (5,6). The ratio ranges from 2:1 to 5:1—the adult ratio is 2:1 (6).

CLINICAL FEATURES

There have been no characteristic presenting symptoms or signs found, mainly because MS in childhood is rare (2,3). There can be one or more neurological changes with a gradual or sudden onset (1). The clinical presentation tends to be headaches, visual problems, and gait changes, but a variety of other symptoms may be present (2). Optic neuritis seems to be the most common presenting disorder (7,8). Abnormal neurological signs are present (5).

Currently, MRI seems to be the diagnostic modality of choice for visualizing MS (2,4,9).

REFERENCES

1. Gall JC, et al. Multiple sclerosis in children. Pediatrics 1958; 21(5):703-710.
2. Golden GS, Woody RC. The role of nuclear magnetic resonance imaging in the diagnosis of MS in childhood. Neurology 1987; 37(4):689-693.
3. Low NL, Carter S. Multiple sclerosis in children. Pediatrics 1956; 18(1):24-30.
4. Boutin B, et al. Multiple sclerosis in children: report of clinical and paraclinical features of 19 cases. Neuropediatrics 1988; 3(19):118-123.
5. Schneider RD, et al. Multiple sclerosis in early childhood. Clinical Pediatrics 1969; 8(2):115-118.
6. Steinlin MI, et al. Eye problems in children with multiple sclerosis. Pediatric Neurology 1995; 12(3):207-212.
7. Adams RD, Victor M. Principles of Neurology, 4th ed. San Francisco: McGraw-Hill, Inc. 1989. pp.755-768.
8. Sanders EACM, Bollen ELEM, van der Velde EA. Presenting signs and symptoms in multiple sclerosis. Acta Neurologica Scand 1986; 73(3):269-272.
9. Gebarski SS, et al. The initial diagnosis of multiple sclerosis: Clinical Impact of Magnetic Resonance Imaging. Annals of Neurology 1985; 17(5):469-474.

MUSCULAR DYSTROPHY

Many people's concept of muscular dystrophy is of tragically-disabled children being shamelessly paraded across the television screen in a pitch for research and medical care funding.

Muscular dystrophy (MD) is a progressive, degenerative skeletal muscle disorder without central or peripheral nervous system pathology. A family history of the disease is typical (1,2). There are several different forms of MD—Duchenne, Becker's, facioscapulohumeral, and limb-girdle, among others. There are other very rare types that seem to be isolated to certain families. A family history of MD is apparent in 59% of the cases (2).

Histologically, there is necrosis of the muscle fibers with signs of regeneration. These features are thought to be caused by the muscle cell membrane. A pseudohypertrophy of the muscle is due to the proliferation of collagen and fats cells between the muscle fibers (3).

CLINICAL FEATURES

The clinician must determine whether a child with muscle weakness has a congenital problem or an acquired problem. Is it a myopathy or another disorder which may cause muscle weakness?

In myopathy, there is usually a gradual onset of weakness. The child has difficulty climbing up stairs or running. Paresthesia is not present nor is bowel or bladder incontinence (4).

Weakness usually affects the proximal rather than distal limb muscles except in myotonic dystrophy. This differentiates it from neuropathies which tend to affect distal muscles (CSF proteins are normal in myopathies). Gower's sign occurs when hip and gluteal muscles are weak and the child must crawl up his legs with his hands when attempting to stand up from a lying down position. The flexor muscles are more affected than the extensors. Reflexes tend to be intact until the late stages. Sensation is normal. Muscle wasting may be present but not fasciculations (4).

Differentiating the type of muscular dystrophy is very difficult. Serum CK (creatinakinase) may be up to 400 times normal in Duchenne (5,6).

TYPES OF MUSCULAR DYSTROPHY

Duchenne or severe X-linked muscular dystrophy affects males and a rare female with Turner's syndrome or altered X chromosome (5). Duchenne's and Beck's MD is associated with a defect of a gene on the short arm of the X chromosome in the Xp21 band (3).

Onset is usually by age 4. Proximal muscles are affected symmetrically, usually in the pelvis and pectoral girdles. There is usually hypertrophy of the calf muscles. Muscle weakness is progressive. By age 10, many are unable to walk. There is cardiac involvement eventually. Death often occurs by the early twenties and is usually due to cardiac or respiratory failure. The incidence is 19-30 in 100,000 males. One third have no family history of it (5).

Symptoms of Duchenne MD include clumsiness, falls, waddling gait, and protruding abdomen. Walking may be delayed. Often the first sign is lack of briskness when walking. GI disturbances may be present as the muscles in the GI tract may be affected (5). There is intellectual impairment and problems in verbalization (3).

Becker or benign X-linked muscular dystrophy affects 3-6 of 100,000 males. The features are similar to Duchenne except muscle involvement is selective. Facial and cardiac muscles are usually not affected. Unlike Duchenne, onset is usually after age 5. Testing for serum CK level is not as definitive as dystrophin assay (normal amount but low molecular weight; in Duchenne, low amount and weight) (5).

They are often able to continue to walk into early adulthood. Intellectual impairment is usually not present. Cramps are common (3).

There are other rarer forms of muscular dystrophy. These include facioscapulohumeral, scapulohumeral, limb-girdle, myotonic, and congenital MD. There are also several forms associated with certain families.

MEDICAL TREATMENT

There are no medical treatments for muscular dystrophy except for symptomatic relief of some symptoms and genetic counseling (4). A procedure called myoblast transfer therapy has been tried on some individuals. This procedure involves injecting cultured muscle tissue from a volunteer into the muscles of a MD patient. At this point, the procedure has not worked.

Inactivity is known to be detrimental. Regular exercise is essential as progression is more rapid if the child is sedentary (5).

CHIROPRACTIC MANAGEMENT

Koren presents a case of a child with Duchenne muscular dystrophy who is in a program of chiropractic care along with 35 other children. The patient was diagnosed at age 6. All of the medical procedures, including myoblast transfer therapy have failed. When he presented at age 12 for chiropractic care, he had been in a wheelchair for three years. In addition to the loss of use of the lower extremities, he had lost upper body strength and was unable to lift a cup of water to his lips. After the first adjustment, he was able to raise a cup of water to his mouth. With further care, he has regained voluntary movement in his lower extremities. Other children with MD who are in this program have also shown improvement (7).

Bahan described two children with Duchenne muscular dystrophy. A 5-year-old diagnosed with Duchenne had not had further progression than difficulty getting up off of the floor. After a few months of chiropractic care using "Systemic Chiropractic" and seat wedges, he did not show further symptomatic progression and was able to get up off of the floor. The second case was a 7-year-old who had weakness, was falling constantly, and had a waddling gait. Within six months of initiating chiropractic care, falls became infrequent, coordination improved, he was less fatigued, and the size of the calves became smaller. He was less distracted in school and his educational performance improved. He was also able to do somersaults (8).

Sachey describes a case of a 9-year-old female as a illustration of the benefits of chiropractic for those afflicted with muscular dystrophy. This child was diagnosed with MD at age three (the type is not indicated). She went to numerous specialists and through a medical research program but the MD continued to progress. Upon presentation at the chiropractic office, she was unable to creep on hands and knees; movements were done with effort. She was unable to sit up straight. The child also drooled. Severe scolioses were noted. She was lightly adjusted in the sacroiliac, lumbar, and upper cervical areas by using light traction and a light thrust. After two months of chiropractic care, a letter written by the father noted that the progression of the condition ceased, she began to gain weight, she was able to creep, movements required less effort, drooling stopped, she sat straighter, body strengths and control improved. Therapeutic exercises were found to be an important adjunct to the adjustments (9).

REFERENCES

1. Adams RD, Victor M. Principles of neurology, 4th ed. San Francisco: McGraw-Hill, Inc. 1989. pp.1117-1132.
2. Aspegren DD. Voluntary muscular system. From: Lawrence DJ, ed. Fundamentals of Chiropractic Diagnosis and Management. Baltimore: Williams & Wilkins. 1991. pp.64-68.
3. Aicardi J. Diseases of the nervous system in childhood. clinics in developmental medicine 1992; 115/118:1172-1181.
4. Weiner HL, Urion DK, Levitt LP. Pediatric neurology for the house officer, 3rd ed. Baltimore: Williams & Wilkins. 1988.
5. Vickers J. LACC-sponsored chiropractic neurology course notes. Sunnyvale, Calif. February 9-10, 1991.
6. Chutkow JG. The work-up for muscular dystrophy. Hospital Medicine November 1993; 29(11):41-43+.
7. Koren T. Muscular dystrophy and chiropractic: the story of Eric Knapp. Chiropractic Pediatrics 1994; 1(1):18-20.
8. Bahan JR. The true power of "chiropractic working." American Chiropractor 1994; 16(5):48-52.
9. Sachey M. The chiropractic approach in treating progressive muscular dystrophy. Journal of the National Chiropractic Association 1952; 22(9):22-24, 71-72.

MYESTHESIA GRAVIS

Myesthesia gravis (MG) is a neuromuscular disorder affecting the postsynaptic acetylcholine receptors (1). The onset is typically insidious, but can be sudden (2).

The reported incidence ranges from 1-10/100,000 to 4-6/100,000 (3,4). Females are twice as likely to be affected as males, especially in early onset MG (3,5). If the mother has MG, one in seven live born children will have signs of MG. Those that survive will usually recovery fully within twelve weeks without later relapse (5).

CLINICAL FEATURES

The classical presentation is weakness and early fatigue of skeletal muscles (3). Ptosis and diplopia (double vision) are the most common symptoms. Dysphagia, dysarthria, and muscle weakness (especially the extra ocular muscles, triceps brachii, quadriceps femoris, and tongue) (5) may also be present. Use of the affected muscles exacerbates the symptoms. Life-threatening weakness of the respiratory muscles may occur (6). Remission and relapses may occur (5).

Tensilon or edrophonium test is conducted by injecting an anticholinesterase, edrophonium chloride. A positive test is the temporary return of normal muscle strength (2,3,5). If ptosis is present, the ice pack test may be used. Ice packs are applied to the affected eye until the area is cooled to below 20°C or to patient tolerance. A positive sign is return to normal strength which diminishes as the muscle warms (5). A simple screening is the repetitive action test in which the patient, by way of repetitive or sustained activity, fatigues the muscle. The MG patient fatigues sooner than a normal patient (3). Electromyography (EMG) is used to help confirm the diagnosis in some cases (6). Single fiber EMG appears to be becoming the definitive test for confirming MG (1). Muscle stretch/deep tendon reflexes are unaffected—an aid in differentiating it from Lambert-Eaton syndrome and multiple sclerosis (1). Other disorders to consider in the differential diagnosis are neurasthenia, botulism, intracranial mass, and progressive external ophthalmoplegia (1).

MEDICAL MANAGEMENT

Medical management falls in three categories: immunosuppression, elevating the safety factor for neuromuscular transmission, and avoiding factors that lower the neuromuscular transmission safety factor or risk respiratory distress (5). Treatment is by the use of cholinesterase inhibitors; in some cases, thymectomy, and in a few cases, corticosteroids (2,5). Cholinesterase inhibitors may cause further weakness (6).

CHIROPRACTIC MANAGEMENT

Araghi presented a case of a 2-year-old who acquired myesthesia gravis following an automobile accident. Presenting complaints were otitis media and ptosis of the right eye developing eight days post-trauma and lethargy, lower extremity weakness, bilateral toe-in, and moderate left head tilt. The diagnosis of myesthesia gravis had been confirmed prior to the chiropractic evaluation after a neurological evaluation which included a positive Tensilon test and positive EMG. After physical examination and x-ray studies were conducted, adjustments (Gonstead) procedures were made to S2, atlas, and later, the occiput. After five months of care, improvements were nearly 100% (7).

REFERENCES

1. Juhn MS. Myesthesia Gravis. Postgraduate Medicine 1993; 94(5):161-174.
2. Adams RD, Victor M. Principles of neurology, 4th ed. San Francisco: McGraw-Hill, Inc. 1989. pp.1150-1167.
3. Aspegren DD. Voluntary muscular system. From: Lawrence DJ,ed. Fundamentals of Chiropractic Diagnosis and Management. Baltimore: Williams & Wilkins. 1991. pp.68-70.
4. Drachman DB. The biology of myesthesia gravis. Annual Review of Neurosciences 1981; 4:195-225.
5. Vickers J. LACC-sponsored chiropractic neurology course notes. Sunnyvale, Calif. February 9-10, 1991.
6. Berkow R (ed). The Merck manual of diagnosis and therapy, 14th ed. Rahway NJ: Merck & Co, Inc. 1982. pp.1394-1396.
7. Araghi J. Juvenile myesthesia gravis: a case study in chiropractic management. Proceedings of the National Conference on Chiropractic and Pediatrics. Palm Springs CA. October 1993. pp.122-131.

NEUROTOXICITY / EXTRINSIC CAUSES OF ALTERED NEUROLOGICAL DEVELOPMENT

This has become an area of intense research and debate during the past several years with the lead paint disasters, Minamata mercury cases, Alar and other pesticide debates, among others. Many chemicals and metals have an effect on the developing nervous system of the child. They may have been introduced maternally or postnatally. The effect may be genetic, structural, functional, and/or behavioral. These substances include heavy metals, drugs, ethanol, foods and food additives. Environmental causes are believed to be the etiological factor in about 9% of the children born with malformations or impairments (1).

HEAVY METALS

Lead and mercury are well-known for their effect on the nervous system. Other metals have also been noted as having neurotoxic effects.

The typical sources of lead are paints and leaded gasoline. One study found impairment in cerebellar function in rats injected with lead acetate during the neonatal period (2). Effects were also noted in the visual cortex (2). Behavioral changes also appear to result from lead (2). Needleman found a six point lower mean IQ in children who were found to have a high lead content. Speech, language, behavior as rated by teachers, and attention measurements were also lower than in their low-lead controls (3). Fine motor function impairment was noted in high school students with lead exposure (3). Minor malformations were also found in infants with lead levels in the umbilical cord blood (3). The exact pathophysiological mechanism that lead has is not known, but it has been shown to affect enzymes and their activities, transfer RNA, and the development of the brain's endogenous opioid system (3). The U.S. Government has established 10 mg/dL as the toxic dose of lead. Seven percent of the children in the U.S. may have lead levels high enough to produce deficits (3). Fortunately, the use of leaded gasoline and paints has dropped considerably. Unfortunately, many old inner city housing projects and schools are known to still have lead painted walls.

Methyl mercury brought the developmental neurologic effects of heavy metal toxicity to the public. The tragic cases of the people in the Minamata region of Japan who suffer from severe disorders due to mercury poisoning have been well documented beginning in the 1950s. The damage is most profound in the cerebral cortex, the cerebellum, and the peripheral nerves. In acute and subacute cases, there is usually loss of peripheral sensation (hypesthesia), dysarthria, disturbed coordinated activity and gait, tremors, hearing impairment, and mental changes. Many also have Romberg's sign, hyperreflexia, and excessive salivation, among many other signs and symptoms. Congenital cases often had deformities as well (4).

SMOKING

Maternal smoking during the prenatal period has been found to have an effect on the growth on the child. A resultant increased risk of abnormal neurological and behavior problems has been found. Carbon monoxide, nicotine, and hydrogen cyanide are the three toxins found to have the highest concentration in smoking (5). Nicotine has a major effect on the autonomic ganglion cells acting with stimulus and depressive phases (5). Because it is highly soluble in lipids and water, it rapidly spreads throughout the body and readily crosses the placenta. Fetal concentrations have been found to exceed the maternal concentration and remain in fetal circulation longer. Nicotine causes vasoconstriction which reduces uteroplacental flow that is thought to cause fetal hypoxia (5). Carbon monoxide also crosses the placenta. Fetal carboxyhemoglobin levels have been found to be double the maternal with a half-life three times longer with a resultant chronic fetal hypoxia (7). Cyanide is thought to contribute to fetal growth retardation by depleting essential vitamins and amino acids (5).

Maternal smoking during pregnancy has been implicated in behavioral problems (6,7). Prenatal smoking has been implicated in hypertonicity and increased nervous system excitability at age one month, lower mental scores and altered auditory response at one and two years of age, and lower language and cognitive scores at three years of age (6). Children of mothers who quit smoking during pregnancy were found to perform better on cognitive scales than those of mothers who continued to smoke (8). Maternal smoking during the prenatal period was found to cause a two-fold increase in the risk of infantile febrile seizures (9).

DRUGS

Many drugs, such as anticonvulsants, chemotherapy drugs, and vitamin A, have been found to have neurodevelopmental effects (1).

Alcohol is probably the most abused maternally-ingested drug which causes neurological or behavioral changes to the offspring. Central nervous system manifestations that may occur include mental or motor retardation, hyperactivity, or tremulousness (10). The facial characteristics of fetal alcohol syndrome are well known (See Chapter 17). Recent studies appeared to have found a correlation between maternal prenatal alcohol consumption levels below those thought to cause fetal alcohol syndrome may cause in a decrease in cognitive and psychomotor skills (11).

Studies on maternal cocaine use have been on its fetal effects. Cocaine is known to have a vasoconstrictive effect which may affect the transfer of nutrients and oxygen to the fetus (12). Cocaine may also stimulate the fetal sympathetic nervous system leading to depletion of fetal nutrient stores (12). Brainstem auditory response has been found to be altered in infants with prenatal cocaine exposure (12). The effect on behavior requires more study but some alteration in behavior has been noted (12). SIDS was higher in prenatal cocaine exposed neonates, but not to the extent of those exposed prenatally to heroin or methadone at a level greater than those living in poverty alone (12). Postnatally, cocaine crosses over into breast milk. The postnatal effect is unknown (12).

Infants of mothers in a New York City methadone program for heroin addiction had a 5 to 10 times greater risk of SIDS than infants in the general population. Twenty-five percent of the infants who died during their first year of life died of SIDS compared to 10% of the infants in the general population. The infants in this study comparing drug users and controls found that those of drug-addicted mothers had a large number of abnormal neurological exams (13).

CHEMICALS

Many chemicals have been implicated in neurologic disorders or symptoms. Long term organophosphate exposure has been implicated. A case of hypertonicity in a neonate was thought to be due to organophosphate pesticide exposure (14). Vinyl chloride, PCBs, and other hydrocarbon-based substances have also been noted to have neurotoxic effects.

REFERENCES

1. Slikker W. Principles of developmental neurotoxicity. NeuroToxicity 1994; 15(1):11-16.
2. Kimmel CA. Critical periods of exposure and developmental effects of lead. In: Kacew S, Reasor MJ, eds. Toxicology and the Newborn. New York: Elsever, 1984. pp.217-236.

3. Needleman HL. The current status of childhood lead toxicity. Advances in Pediatrics 1993; 40:125-139.
4. Smith WE, Smith AM. Minamata. New York: Holt, Rinehart, and Winston. 1975. pp.180-192.
5. Nash JE, Persaud TVN. Embryopathic risks of cigarette smoking. experimental pathology 1988; 33(2):65-73.
6. Fried PA. Cigarettes and marijuana: are there measurable long-term neurobehavioral teratogenic effects. NeuroToxicology 1989; 10(3):577-584.
7. Olds DL, Henderson CR, Tatelbaum R. Intellectual impairment in children of women who smoke cigarettes during pregnancy. Pediatrics 1994; 93(2):221-227.
8. Sexton M, Fox NL, Hebel JR. Prenatal exposure to tobacco: III effects on cognitive functioning at age three. International Journal of Epidemiology 1990; 19(1):72-77.
9. Cassano PA, Koepsell TD, Farwell JR. Risk of febrile seizures in childhood in relation to prenatal maternal cigarette smoking and alcohol intake. American Journal of Epidemiology 1990; 132(3):462-473.
10. Fried PA. Alcohol and the newborn infant. In: Kacew S, Reasor MJ, eds. Toxicology and the Newborn. New York: Elsever. 1984: pp.85-100.
11. Larroque B, et al. Moderate prenatal alcohol exposure and psychomotor development at preschool age. American Journal of Public Health 1995; 85(12):1654-1661.
12. Frank DA, Bresnahan K, Zuckerman BS. Maternal cocaine use. Advances in Pediatrics 1993:65-99.
13. Rosen TS, Johnson HL. Drug-addicted mothers, their infants, and SIDS. Annals New York Academy of Sciences 1988; 533:203-210.
14. Wagner SL, Orwick DL. Chronic organophosphate exposure associated with transient hypertonicity in an infant. Pediatrics 1994; 94(1):94-97.

POLIOMYELITIS

Poliomyelitis was the dreaded disease in the 1920s and 1950s, and continues to be a problem in some countries. The vaccines for polio were developed in the 1950s, and mass inoculation programs were initiated (See Chapter 3). In the U.S., the primary cause of polio today is the oral, live cell vaccine.

Poliomyelitis is myelitis to the gray matter (1). Polio has been associated with a number of enteroviruses, particularly poliovirus types 1, 2, and 3 (2). The mode of entry is via the gastrointestinal system (2,3).

Polio is now categorized into abortive minor illnesses, nonparalytic illness, and paralytic illnesses (2,3). The site of lesion and the amount of destruction determines the manifestations. The worse form is bulbar poliomyelitis which affects the medulla oblongata.

For clinical purposes, paralytic poliomyelitis has been categorized into three types, bulbar, spinal and encephalitic (1). The spinal type is the most common while the encephalitic type is the least common (4).

Polio tends to occur in the summer and autumn in the temperate regions (2). Being associated with the gastrointestinal system, good sanitation and hygiene are important factors in reducing the incidence of this disease.

An interesting fact is that the diagnostic criteria for poliomyelitis was changed at the time of the introduction of the live-virus vaccine. The criteria for an epidemic was changed from 20 cases per 100,000 to 35 cases. The paralytic form originally required the stricken person demonstrating paralytic symptoms for 24 hours; this was extended to at least 60 days and at least two confirmations of residual paralysis during the course of illness. Aseptic meningitis was classified separately at that time as well. Many of those counted in the polio statistic prior to the introduction of the vaccine are now excluded. Obviously these changes would greatly alter the statistics on the effectiveness of the vaccine (5).

A 1952 chiropractic study of 300 polio cases from 1950 to 1951 found that 64% had injections or taken medication just prior to the onset of polio. Of these, more than one-half had received penicillin. It also found that 38% of the polio cases suffered from extreme fatigue prior to the onset of symptoms. Twenty percent had falls prior to the onset of polio (6).

The late sequelae or post-polio syndrome is becoming a problem of much concern as will be described below.

CLINICAL FEATURES

Its clinical presentation may include headaches, irritability, general malaise, fever, stiffness, muscular pain, paresis in the limbs, inability to roll over, stand, or walk, and respiratory and swallowing difficulty (4). Electrodiagnostic tests, such as nerve conduction tests and EMG, aid in the diagnosis (4).

The mortality rate of the paralytic form is from 5% to 25% (2).

MEDICAL MANAGEMENT

In the past, the enduring image of polio was the "iron lung." Those with bulbar poliomyelitis and compromised respiratory system required these huge chambers in order to survive.

There is little in the way of medical treatment except to make the patient as comfortable as possible. Mild analgesics and hot packs are given for muscle pain and meningeal irritation (1). The use of hot packs was loudly advocated by Sister Kenny and just as loudly denounced by the medical community who had little to offer. Splints are used for extremity paralysis (1). The problem with the use of splints and braces is, of course, disuse atrophy. Rest is very important, particularly in the acute phase (7). Proper body positioning is important to reduce the severity of deformities (7). Active and passive exercises are used but not to the point of fatigue (7). Electrotherapy may be used on the denervated muscles (7). If respiration is affected, then a respirator is necessary (1). The "iron lung" is still used with the remaining survivors of polio and some cervical cord injury cases (8). In some cases, surgery is used to correct deformities (7).

Medical treatment is primarily prophylactic via artificial immunization. There are two forms of polio vaccine—the injection administered Salk inactive or killed virus and the oral Sabin live attenuated virus. The Sabin vaccine is known to cause one case of paralytic poliomyelitis per three million doses (3) and is the primary cause of polio in the U.S. (5). The effectiveness of the vaccines is debatable as cases were dropping significantly prior to the arrival of the vaccines. The statistical measurement and diagnostic criteria also changed at the time of the introduction of the vaccines (5).

As an interesting sidenote, a few people hypothesize that early Salk and Sabin polio vaccines that were contaminated with the monkey virus, SV40, may be associated with the AIDS pandemic in Africa. This is a very controversial hypothesis with few adherents (9).

CHIROPRACTIC MANAGEMENT

A little known fact is that chiropractic protocol was being developed at the same time as the development of the vaccines. The protocol was developed from apparently successful chiropractic care of those afflicted. Robertson published a manual on the evaluation and chiropractic care of paralytic poliomyelitis (10). He is well known in chiropractic as the doctor who helped Winifred Gardella, a March of Dimes poster child, walk again. There was even a chiropractic polio clinic in Los Angeles, as well as a polio foundation put together by chiropractors.

A 1954 case report by Robertson described a patient who had a presenting history of three days of vomiting followed by difficulty swallowing, fever, severe headache, and exhaustion. The findings included a fever of 103.8°F, tenderness over the entire spine, neck stiffness, positive Brudzinski test, thick tenacious saliva, right arm and leg tenderness, slight facial paralysis, pharyngeal and esophageal paralysis, slight respiratory defect, and dyspnea. The patient refused to be hospitalized. The difficulty swallowing and right arm and leg pain persisted. After two weeks, the patient was able to eat solid food (initially fed intravenously and later liquid food). The paralysis and respiratory difficulty abated as well. The patient was refused an iron lung by local medical authorities because of his refusal to submit to their care. This patient responded positively to the chiropractic care of adjustments and heat packs (11) and, according to one of the authors of this chapter (PT), is reported by his brother to be active to this day without apparent ill effects, some 40 years later. Interestingly, another male of similar age in the same community was also stricken with bulbar poliomyelitis at nearly the same time. This individual was a dermatologist who followed the typical medical regimen at that time. He continued practicing but required the use of an iron lung until he died in the 1960s. Dr. Robertson stated that none of the cases of poliomyelitis under early chiropractic care experienced paralysis.

Another case in 1954 was described by Dr. Wilent, a chiropractor in Redwood City, California. The patient was a 24-year-old multiparous female who began noticing right leg soreness that progressed to an increasing body temperature, general malaise, cervical spine tenderness, and increasing right leg pain. The MD diagnosed a bladder infection and prescribed penicillin. The next day she felt better, but the following day, her temperature rose and she had neck pain and stiffness, headaches, and pain and loss of function of the right leg. The MD did a spinal tap and called in a polio specialist who gave drugs for pain and for sleeping. Dr. Wilent was consulted. He began a course of adjustments, hot packs, massage, and nutritional aid. She was adjusted hourly for 48 hours by a group of chiropractors working in shifts. During the first three hours, the temperature decreased and the headache, neck soreness, and leg pain abated. By the second day, she was responding well—temperature decreased and pain was reduced. Adjustments and hot pack frequency was reduced. On the fourth day, her temperature was normal, she felt "wonderful," and had a normal appetite (12).

Frame recommended giving chiropractic adjustments over the entire spine during the first three days of acute poliomyelitis. The goal is to improve circulation of CSF and blood as he noted that the inflammatory process blocks proper flow of fluids in the spinal cord creating congestion. Also noted is that the adjustments may stimulate the nerves to the paralyzed muscles. He also recommends avoiding overfatigue and removing refined foods and sweets from the diet (13).

According to a 1954 ICA study on chiropractic care of 300 cases of acute poliomyelitis, 86.7% had complete recovery, 11% were much improved, 1.31% were slightly improved, and 1% had no improvement. A National Foundation for Infantile Paralysis publication at the same time stated that 50% under medical care will recover completely, 25% will have slight paralysis, 17% will be permanently disabled, and 8% may die (14).

POST-POLIO SYNDROME (PPS)

Recently, people with varying degrees of recovery from polio have been experiencing a multitude of problems that are thought to be due to their previous episode of polio. Many, following the initial acute episode and recovery, were thought to be stable but recent findings have noted a number of effects occurring 30 to 40 years later (15). The most common symptoms are fatigue, pain, and muscle weakness, but symptoms such as dysphagia, muscle atrophy, muscle fasciculation, cold intolerance, dysphagia, dysphonia, sleep apnea, and dyspnea have been noted (15). Some have been found to have other disorders such as spinal stenosis that appeared to be causing their symptoms (16).

The diagnosis of post-polio syndrome is largely one of exclusion. If all other disorders that may cause similar symptoms have been ruled out, then the patient may be considered to have PPS.

EMG studies have found that action potentials of motor neurons to the muscles of those with PPS are not normal. Instead of the near simultaneous action potentials found in normal neural-muscle interactions, those with PPS have readings that are not synchronized and give a "jittery" reading (17).

Pathological studies of polio survivors dying of nonneurological causes tend to find signs of microglial, meningeal, or leukocyte infiltrates in the spinal cord sections studied (18).

In an Australian survey, 45% of those who sought chiropractic care for PPS found the care to be "very helpful" (15). It would be interesting to evaluate those who had gone through the intense chiropractic care described above and appeared to have recovered completely or near completely from acute poliomyelitis, find out their current state, and compare them to those survivors who underwent conventional medical care at the time of their acute poliomyelitis.

Whether to have a PPS patient engage in strength training is under debate. Some find that these patients lose strength after strenuous exercise but others found that a PPS patient benefits from strength exercise (19). From all appearances, it appears that an exercise program is recommended over inactivity. Programs emphasizing activities to maintain or enhance a patient's life activities are very important.

REFERENCES

1. Adams RD, Victor M. Principles of neurology, 4th ed. San Francisco: McGraw-Hill, Inc. 1989. pp.592-96, 726-27.
2. Nilsson AV. Chiropractic and poliomyelitis. Chirogram January 1954.

3. Berkow R. The Merck manual of diagnosis and therapy, 14th ed. Rahway NJ: Merck & Co., Inc. 1982. pp. 210-212.

4. Dean E, et al. Poliomyelitis. Part 1: an old problem revisited. Physiotherapy 1995; 81(1):17-22.

5. Miller NZ. Vaccines and natural health. Journal of Naturopathic Medicine 1994; 5(1):32-39.

6. Hilty J. A Recent survey shows the ratio between shots and poliomyelitis. Journal of the National Chiropractic Association 1952; 22(11):16.

7. Dean E, et al. Poliomyelitis. Part 2: revised principles of management. Physiotherapy January 1995; 81(1):22-28.

8. Markel H. The genesis of the iron lung. archives of pediatric and adolescent medicine 1994; 148(11):1174-1180.

9. Elswood BF, Stricker RB. Polio vaccines and the origin of AIDS. Medical Hypotheses 1994; 42(6):347-354.

10. Robertson L. Manual of acute and chronic poliomyelitis. Santa Cruz, CA: self-published. 1955.

11. Robertson L. Report of a case of successfully treated bulbar poliomyelitis. Chirogram January 1954.

12. Wilent EV. A case of poliomyelitis. In: Robertson L. Manual of Acute and Chronic Poliomyelitis. Self-published. 1955. pp.38-40.

13. Frame FD. Has the test tube fight against polio failed? Journal of the National Chiropractic Association 1959; 29(3):26, 66-69.

14. Bryan JE. No need to fear polio. ICA International Review of Chiropractic 1954; 13(12):3,31.

15. Westbrook MT. Clients' evaluation of chiropractic treatment for post polio syndrome. Journal of the Australian Chiropractors' Association 1990; 20(4):143-151.

16. La Ban MM, Sanitate SS, Taylor RS. Spinal stenosis presenting as 'The Postpolio Syndrome.' American Journal of Physical Medicine and Rehabilitation 1993; 72(6):390-394.

17. Dalakas MC, Bartfeld H, Kurland LT. Polio redux. The Sciences 1995; 35(4):30-35.

18. Kaminski HJ, et al. Pathological analysis of spinal cords from survivors of poliomyelitis. Annals New York Academy of Sciences 25 1995; 753: 390-393.

19. Spector SA, et al. Effect of strength training in patients with post-polio syndrome: a preliminary report. Annals of the New York Academy of Sciences 25 1995; 753:402-404.

RETT SYNDROME

Rett syndrome, first described in 1966 by the neurologist, Andreas Rett, is a progressive, neurodegenerative disorder affecting the young female (a few male cases have been reported) (1,2). It is considered to have a genetic basis, probably on an X-chromosome (3). The incidence in Europe is about 1:15,000 (3).

Rett syndrome does not became apparent until age six months to eighteen months—the infant appears to be normal up to that point (1). The child begins showing delays in or regression of intellectual development and motor skills. In later childhood to adulthood, mental retardation is in the profound range (1). Eighty percent of women with Rett syndrome are unable to walk (1). Sixty percent who had been able to walk, lose the ability (1). Those who do walk tend to have an ungainly wide-based, stiff-legged, unsteady gait (1). Seizures are not uncommon (4). Scoliosis is very common and often has rapid progression (3). Four clinical stages have been organized for classical Rett syndrome (3). The pathophysiology behind Rett Syndrome is unknown (1).

Alterations have been found in the brains of Rett victims. The substantia nigra has been found to be abnormal. Qualitatively, the number of neurons in the substantia nigra is normal but the neuron sizes are small, and the number of both the pigment cells and the amount of pigment in these cells is reduced. Substantia nigra abnormalities may be associated with some of the movement abnormalities. Abnormalities in the cerebral cortex, cerebellum, and other regions have been found (5).

CLINICAL FEATURES

The criteria developed for diagnosing Rett Syndrome includes an apparently normal prenatal and perinatal period and apparently normal psychomotor development during the first six months. Head growth decelerates between ages 5 months and 4 years. A loss of acquired purposeful hand skills is noted between ages 6 months and 30 months that appears to be associated with communications dysfunction and social withdrawal. There is the development of severely impaired expressive and receptive language, and the presence of apparent severe psychomotor retardation. Stereotypical hand movements are seen, such as hand wringing or squeezing, clapping or tapping, mouthing, and "washing" or rubbing automatisms, which appear after purposeful hand skills are lost. Gait apraxia and truncal apraxia or ataxia appear between ages 1 and 4 years.

When working up a case, there are supportive features, such as breathing dysfunction, EEG abnormalities, seizures, spasticity, scoliosis, growth retardation, and hypotrophic small feet. Exclusionary criteria include evidence of intrauterine growth retardation, organomegaly or other signs of storage disease, retinopathy or optic atrophy, microcephaly at birth, evidence of perinatally acquired brain damage, identifiable metabolic or other progressive neurological disorder, or acquired neurological disorders which resulted from severe infections or head trauma. Until age 4 or 5, the diagnosis is considered tentative (1,2).

MEDICAL MANAGEMENT

Some of the manifestations of Rett are treated medically. Those afflicted with Rett require constant care because of their inability to engage in most activities of daily living (1).

CHIROPRACTIC MANAGEMENT

One of the authors (STT) saw a 22-year-old female in Central America with characteristic features of Rett syndrome. The parents did not know the actual diagnosis so the diagnosis is tentative. The patient's physical appearance was of a young child about age 10. She walked poorly and required support, did not speak, held both hand in the air with a slight wringing motion, stuck her tongue out for long periods, and appeared conscious of the environment and others for brief moments at best. The head was carried in an anterior position. The manifestations apparently began at age 5 or so following a fall when she struck her head. Chiropractic adjustments were made to the sacrum and atlas over a two day period. Other observers commented that she seemed to become slightly more aware of her environment. It would be interesting to see the potential benefits that long-term chiropractic care of a Rett case would produce.

REFERENCES

1. Iyama CM. Rett syndrome. Advances in Pediatrics 1993; 40:217-237.

2. Woodyatt G, Ozanne A. Communication abilities and Rett syndrome. Journal of Autism and Developmental Disorders 1992; 22(2):155-173.

3. Hagberg B. Rett Syndrome: Clinical peculiarities and biological mysteries. Acta Paediatrica 1995; 84(9):971-976.

4. Morris J. Rett's syndrome: a case study. Journal of Neuroscience Nursing 1990; 22(5):285-293.
5. Bauman ML, Kemper TL, Arin DM. Pervasive neuroanatomic abnormalities of the brain in three cases of Rett's syndrome. Neurology 1995; 45(8):1581-1586.

REYE'S SYNDROME

Reye's or Reye-Johnson syndrome or hepatoencephalopathy is a disorder which usually occurs in children and adolescents (1). It is characterized by acute encephalopathy and visceral fatty infiltration (1,2) following viral infections (2,3). It has been associated with aspirin use in children (including adolescents) with viral infections such as influenza and varicella (See also Chapter 16). A downward trend in the number of cases has followed warnings against aspirin use by children with viral infections (2,4). The delay in delivering public warning of the association between aspirin and Reye's by the U.S. government is an interesting study in the influence of politics and economics on public health policy (5). Recently, the association of aspirin during viral infection and Reye's has been disputed. In one Australian study, 4 out of 42 confirmed cases of Reye's had taken aspirin while 12 had taken acetaminophen (5).

CLINICAL FEATURES

It typically begins with fever for several days, upper respiratory distress, nausea and profuse vomiting (1,2,3). The child may become disoriented or have delirium. Hyperventilation is a common feature (3). There can be rapid changes in mental status to extreme lethargy/stupor and coma (1,2). The comatose state may present with decorticate or decerebrate posture, seizures, hypotonicity, fixed and dilated pupils, and respiratory arrest (6). Signs of sympathetic overactivity and high level central nervous system dysfunction may be present (1). In later stages, seizures may be present along with cardiac or respiratory arrest (3). There is hypertonia and cranial nerve dysfunction (3).

The differential diagnostic mitochondria sign of Reye's from other metabolic encephalopathies is swollen and pleomorphic mitochondria from a liver biopsy (2). Lab findings include marked elevation of SGOT (serum glutamic oxaloacetic transaminase)/AST and slight elevation of serum ammonia (1).

MANAGEMENT

Medical treatment is aimed at altering the metabolic abnormalities by re-establishing homeostasis. This included rehydration, correcting hypoglycemia, reducing the elevated intracranial pressure, and controlling fever and seizures (1,2). Attempts are made to control the increased intracranial pressure that is usually present (6). The outcome is poor if there is early onset of seizures, profound hypoglycemia, and coma (1,2). Mortality runs from 20% in less severe cases to over 80% (6).

REFERENCES

1. Adams RD, Victor M. Principles of neurology, 4th ed. San Francisco: McGraw-Hill, Inc. 1989. p.855.
2. Glascow JFT, Moore R. Reye's syndrome 30 years on. British Medical Journal 1993; 307(6910):950-951,
3. Weiner HL, Urion DK, Levitt LP. Pediatric neurology for the house officer, 3rd ed. Baltimore: Williams & Wilkins. 1988. pp.177-181.
4. Soumerai SB, Ross-Degnan D, Kahn JS. Effects of professional and media warnings about the association between aspirin use in children and Reye's syndrome. Milbank Quarterly 1992; 70(1):155-182.
5. Orlowski JP, Campbell P, Goldstein S. Reye's syndrome: a case control study of medication use and associated viruses in australia. Cleveland Clinic Journal of Medicine 1990; 57(4):323-329.
6. Berkow R (ed). The Merck manual of diagnosis and therapy, 14th ed. Rahway NJ: Merck & Co, Inc. 1982. pp.1888-1890.

SEIZURES/EPILEPSY

A seizure is not necessarily epilepsy as it may be a single incident phenomena (1). A seizure is the result of abnormal cerebral electrical discharge (8). Epilepsy refers to recurrent, primary cerebral seizures of primary cerebral origin (2). Epileptic syndromes refers to a cluster of symptoms that commonly occur together (2). Seizures may also be classified as febrile or afebrile. Epilepsy and seizure are not synonyms.

Lipton and Rosenburg are studying the relationship of overstimulation of glutamate receptors in the occurrence of seizures (3).

"Kindling" occurs when repeated subthreshold electrical or chemical stimulation with no initial clinical effects leads progressively to more intense seizures with repeated stimulation. The result is generalized motor convulsions (4). This can happen in an otherwise normal cerebral cortex without an observable lesion (5). The kindling model is primarily a research model, although it is thought to be the mechanism in some forms of seizures (6).

CLASSIFYING SEIZURES AND EPILEPSY (2)

Changes in Terminology

Previous System	Current System
Focal or Jacksonian	Simple partial
Temporal lobe or psychomotor partial	Complex partial
Petit mal	Absence
Infantile spasms, akinetic, or minor motor	Myoclonic
Grand mal	Tonic-clonic

Clinical and EEG Classification of Seizures (23)

I. Seizures with a close association with EEG seizure discharges
   A. Focal clonic
   B. Myoclonic
   C. Tonic Clonic
   D. Apnea

II. Seizures with an inconsistent or no relationship to EEG seizure discharges
   A. Motor automatisms
   B. Generalized tonic
   C. Myoclonic

III. Infantile spasms

IV. EEG seizures without clinical seizures.

Classification of Epileptic Seizures (5)

1. Partial Seizures

a. Simple partial seizures
b. Complex partial seizures
c. Partial seizures progressing to secondary generalized seizures
2. Generalized Seizures
   a. Absence seizures
   b. Atypical absence seizures
   c. Myoclonic seizures
   d. Clonic seizures
   e. Tonic seizures
   f. Tonic-clonic seizures
   g. Atonic seizures
3. Unclassified seizures

Epileptic Syndromes in Children (2)
1. Primary generalized epilepsy
   a. Absence (petit mal)
   b. Myoclonic (grand mal)
2. Infantile spasms and hypsarrhythmia (West syndrome)
3. Aicardi syndrome
4. Lennox-Gastaut syndrome
5. Benign epilepsy of childhood with Rolandic spikes
6. Benign occipital epilepsy
7. Benign juvenile myoclonic epilepsy of Janz

FEBRILE SEIZURES

Febrile seizures affect 2% to 4% of children under age 5 making them the most common form of seizures in childhood (7,8). This form of seizure is caused by fever. When formulating a diagnosis, you must rule out intracranial infection, exogenous toxin or endotoxin, intracranial abnormalities causing the seizure, or idiopathic seizure disorder triggered by the febrile state (9). If the child is between ages 6 months and 5 years, is neurologically normal, and had a fever, the likelihood is a febrile seizure. In later childhood or adolescence, another cause needs to be investigated (9). Maturation of the brain and reduction in neuronal excitability diminishes the tendency for febrile seizures (10). With a high temperature fever, the likelihood that the seizure is fever induced is higher than that for a lower temperature fever. The latter requires more extensive investigation (10).

A high enough fever is known to cause seizures. The temperature levels varies with each individual and his/her state of health (9).

Febrile seizures and the initiation of epilepsy tend to occur most frequently between the ages of 4 months and 2 years (9). The reason is thought to be that the neuronal threshold of children in that age group is lower than in the newborn or those with a more mature cortex.

Children who have benign febrile seizures or rolandic epilepsy appear to be normal between episodes. Those with more serious forms of epilepsy often have some intellectual or neurologic deficits (8). After a febrile seizure, there is a 25% to 30% chance of a second febrile seizure (9). Risk factors also include the febrile seizure occurring during the first year or a family history of febrile seizures (9). There is 3% chance of children having afebrile seizures (8). Both single and multiple incidences of febrile seizures and febrile status epilepticus are not considered to be a cause of brain damage (9).

Electroencephalographs (EEG) were not found to be a predictor in the risk assessment for the recurrence of seizures. The rate of recurrence decreases with the child's age (11).

Phenobarbital is a commonly used medication for preventing recurrence of febrile seizures. Anticonvulsant medication has not been shown to prevent epilepsy or the rate of epilepsy (9). One study found that infants between age 8 to 36 months given phenobarbital following at least one febrile seizure had a mean IQ that was 8.4 points below the group taking a placebo (12).

AFEBRILE SEIZURES

Afebrile seizures must be differentiated from epilepsy. Epilepsy is two or more seizures without a precipitating cause (13).

There are two basic categories of seizures, generalized and partial. Generalized seizures involve both cerebral hemispheres. Partial seizures have focal involvement (14). Primary generalized seizures cause immediate involvement of both hemispheres and are subcategorized as absence, generalized tonic-clonic, myoclonic, and atonic. Secondary generalized seizures begin on one area of the brain before spreading to both hemispheres. Partial seizures are subdivided into complex or simple (14).

Generalized tonic-clonic seizures (previously called grand mal) are caused by discharges over a wide area of the cerebral hemispheres bilaterally. There is loss of consciousness, generalized tonic muscle stiffening, and extension of the body as a result of generalized muscle contractions. Tongue biting, salivation, frothing at the mouth, and urinary incontinence are not uncommon. There is a postictal state of limpness, obtundness, and unresponsiveness (15). Generalized tonic-clonic seizures may be the result of hyponatremia. These are often caused by water intoxication, commonly from using diluted formula. These seizures are often accompanied by respiratory insufficiency and hypothermia (16).

Lennox-Gestalt Syndrome is a severe form of seizure that is characterized by multiple, generalized, daily seizures and often results in injuries due to falls (17). During the episodes, there are tonic seizures which result in sudden, sustained contraction of muscle groups that may cause the person to fall (18). An episode begins and ends in an atypical absence seizure (18). Tonic seizures may occur during REM sleep (19). EEG is abnormal in the ictal and interictal periods (19). The onset usually occurs between the ages of 3 to 5 years. There is a slight male predominance (18).

Infantile spasms, West syndrome, or salaam episodes have an onset during the first year with the peak age of onset between three to seven months of age. There is a male predominance (18). Twenty-five percent of children with infantile spasms have tuberous sclerosis (18). During a seizure, there is typically dropping of the head, abduction of the shoulders, and flexion of the lower extremities. There may be a cry, pallor, flushing, grimacing, laughter, or nystagmus (18). The episodes tend to occur upon awakening, when drowsy, or when feeding (18). The prognosis is poor. There is a one in five mortality rate with 80% of the survivors suffering from mental retardation (18). Those who have remission often develop other forms of seizures (4). Colic must be differentiated from infantile spasms (20).

Simple partial seizures are of several types. Focal motor seizures involve the precentral gyrus or motor strip. It was previously known as Jacksonian seizures as tonic-clonic movements originate in one part of the body and spread, sometimes only on one side of the body. Autonomic seizures show autonomic changes, such as pallor, sweating, piloerection, and flushing (15).

Complex partial seizures are classified as focal seizures accompanied by changes in consciousness. There may be confusion. The temporal lobe is often involved. There may only be impaired consciousness or it may be accompanied by automatisms, masticatory movements, hallucinations (visual or olfactory), speech changes, affective or emotive symptoms, altered cognition, visceral sensations, or sensations of déjà vu (15).

In absence seizures, there is typically a brief staring spell. Muscle tone usually remains unchanged and any automatism is subtle. As hyperventilation for a few minutes may induce absence seizures, it is often used in a clinical setting to evaluate the effectiveness of the treatment (4). Absence seizures in children often diminish with age (8). Those with atypical absence seizures often have other forms of seizures (4).

Rolandic or benign partial epilepsy (also known as sylvian epilepsy or centrotemporal epilepsy) (18) typically occurs between ages 8 and 12 years and is self-limiting with remission usually around the ages of 9 to 12 years. It usually occurs at night (8,18). There is a male predominance (18). Typically, the child will awaken with twitching on one side of the face. Gurgling sounds may be made if the oropharyngeal muscles are involved. The ipsilateral upper extremity may be involved as well. The child will often remain conscious (18).

STATUS EPILEPTICUS

Status epilepticus (SE) refers to recurrent seizures without regaining consciousness (20,21). Status epilepticus is an emergency condition as death may ensue. There is a risk of asphyxiation. Control is more difficult and the risk of permanent sequelae increases with prolongation of an episode of status epilepticus (22).

The causes of SE can be divided into four categories: (22)

1. Idiopathic
2. Idiopathic with fever
3. Underlying acquired, developmental, or congenital disorder of the central nervous system
4. Acute central nervous system disorder

Most cases of SE occur in children with the average age being 3 years (22). In most cases, the first seizure is SE (22). Mortality is about 10% (22).

Febrile status epilepticus is a febrile seizure of more than 30 minutes duration (9). Approximately 25% of status epilepticus episodes have febrile origin (13,22).

The most common form of SE is generalized, convulsive seizures with loss of consciousness. Clonic status epilepticus is seen in infants and young children while tonic SE is more common in the adolescent. Myoclonic SE is seen in children and adolescents but is rare in the adult (22). Absence or partial SE is also seen in 10% of cases. These later two usually have a history of epilepsy (21).

In addition to neurological complications that may occur, there may be cardiac, respiratory, or renal failure because of the prolonged, repetitive contractions of the musculoskeletal system (22). Abnormalities at autopsy of the brains of infants who had suffered from SE tend to be more extensive than in the adult and tend to be unilateral (23). The primary histopathological damage is due to ischemia to the cells (23).

Incidence of subsequent seizures in children who do not have a history of prior seizures is 50% within two years or less (21). Of those who have an episode of febrile SE, 8% will develop afebrile seizures by the age of 20 years (21). For those without underlying neurological conditions, the risk of recurrence of SE is less than 5% (21).

FEATURES

A careful history is important to distinguish the form of the seizures and to differentiate it from other disorders. In the medical management of seizures and epilepsy, the correct diagnosis is very important as the wrong treatment could have a very negative effect. Most would have probably had a full work-up prior to presenting to your office so a diagnosis might have been made. But misdiagnoses are not uncommon or the pediatrician may have ignored subtle or not so subtle signs of seizures. Electroencephalograms (EEG) are used in the diagnosis of epilepsy but there are many false positives and false negatives. Video/EEG and 24 hour continuous monitoring have become helpful procedures in the work-up of some forms of seizures/epilepsy (2). Readings are taken in the waking and sleep states.

Not only is it important to distinguish the form of seizures or epilepsy, it must be differentiated from other conditions. Syncope, breath-holding, hypoglycemia, sleep disorders and vagal oversensitivity may be difficult to distinguish from seizures.

The history is vitally important in differential diagnosis. The following should be asked (2):

1. What time of day did it occur?
2. Was there a warning prior to the spell?
3. What was the first thing that happened to the child? (sudden fall, choking while feeding, etc.)
4. What were the abnormal motor activities?
5. What did the child's eyes do?
6. What did the child's mouth do? (lip smacking, chewing motions, unusual sounds, etc.)
7. Was the child's head turned one way or the other?

8. What were the child's extremities doing?

9. Was the child aware of his surroundings? (Did the child respond or recognize others)

10. Were there any strange vocalizing or activities? (Incoherent mumbling, aimless wandering, fiddling with clothing, etc.)

11. Was there loss of control of the bladder or bowel?

12. Did the child seem cold, hot, or clammy? (Was the seizure associated with hypoglycemia or fever?)

13. How long did the spell or episode last?

14. Was there a postictal period? (Generalized tonic-clonic seizures are followed by sleep while there are no postictal periods following myoclonic seizures)

Febrile seizures in a young child may also be associated with meningitis. There is controversy on the routine use of lumbar puncture in the first instance of febrile seizures. There is discussion on the age when all children with a first febrile seizure should have lumbar puncture. Some say that those under age six months having a first febrile seizure should have the procedure while others use a minimum age of between 18 months and 2 years (24).

MEDICAL MANAGEMENT

An interesting observation is made that conventional treatments for convulsions has a 30% to 80% success rate but is complicated by undesirable effects (14). Seizures are usually treated with drugs such as valproic acid and clonazepam. Blood tests are often necessary to check the serum levels of the drugs to minimize the risk of serious side effects (13). Drugs, such as Dilantin or carbamazepine, are sometimes used for rolandic seizures. Complex partial epilepsy and generalized tonic-clonic seizures are often treated with carbamazepine, phenytoin sodium (Dilantin), fosphenytoin, phenobarbitol, valproic acid, or divalproex sodium. Absence (petite mal) seizures are often treated with ethosuximide, valproic acid, or clonazepam. Myoclonic seizures are usually treated with valproic acid or clonazepam. Since 1993, four more drugs have been approved by the FDA: gabapentin, lamotrigine, felbamate, and topiramate. A fifth, vigabatrin, is used outside of the U.S. as are several other drugs (14).

There is some controversy on early drug intervention in cases of newly diagnosed tonic-clonic seizures in children. Because the anti-epileptic drugs have numerous side effects, the early use of drugs is important. One worry is that untreated tonic-clonic seizures will develop an uncontrolled, accelerating pattern of recurrent seizures. A 1988 retrospective study found that untreated tonic-clonic seizures tend to show an accelerating pattern with the intervals between seizures decreasing. In a 1992 2-year study using current patients, the opposite pattern was noted in a large number of untreated patients; even in those who had multiple episodes of seizures (25).

Febrile seizures are often treated with medication, such as phenobarbital, to prevent recurrence. It has been found that not only is it ineffective in preventing recurrence and is unsafe, but children in the treatment group were found to have a decrease of eight points in IQ (12).

One interesting treatment to prevent febrile seizures in infants suffering from a fever is to give them a source of N-3 polyunsaturated fatty acids, omega-3 fatty acids. The hypothesis is based on a possible mechanism of febrile convulsions that febrile seizures may occur due to a lowering of convulsion threshold in fever. Interleukin-1 is involved in mediating the febrile response. Interleukin-1 is carried to the CNS where it is involved in the synthesis of prostaglandins which contribute to the physiological actions involved in producing fever. N-3 polyunsaturated fatty acids reduce secretion of interleukin-1 (27).

Vagal stimulation has been tried in a group of children with medically intractable epilepsies. The vagal nerve stimulator is a devise that is implanted in a patient and is activated by holding a magnet against the battery. Of 12 patients, 5 had a greater than 90% reduction in the number of monthly seizures. Four were able to reduce antiepileptic drug usage (28). The implications relative to chiropractic care are obvious.

CHIROPRACTIC MANAGEMENT

Langley presents a case of a female child with epilepsy, as well as heart murmurs, hypoglycemia, nocturnal enuresis, and attention deficit disorder. This child had a difficult birth which resulted in the fracture of her mother's pelvis and an eventual caesarian section following five hours of labor and the administration of Demerol. The first seizure occurred eleven hours after birth. When the child presented at age eight for chiropractic evaluation, she had been evaluated by numerous medical specialists and had taken many drugs. She was experiencing ten to twelve seizures a day and was in a special education program. Six month after chiropractic adjustments to the upper cervical spine were initiated, enuresis had abated. After one year of care, the frequency of seizures have diminished to eight to ten per week and medication has been reduced. Medication was expected to cease a month after a neurological evaluation (29).

Goodman and Mosby wrote a case report on a 5-year-old white female with tonic, clonic, akinetic, and grand mal seizures. Mayo Clinic diagnosed Lennox-Gestalt syndrome. She was small at birth and had a breech birth. She had many episodes of viral infection and otitis media. She struck her head on the underside of a table at age 4 years, 8 months. She had a grand mal seizure within two hours of the injury and a second one during the first three weeks. When she presented at Mayo Clinic, seizures were occurring at a frequency of 10 to 30 per day. EEG showed abnormalities. Medications were given but most failed. Carbamazepine appeared to help the grand mal seizures, but she begin having drop seizures. When she presented, she was having 30 to 70 seizures a day and required protective gear to prevent injuries when falling. Communication skills were poor; neurological reflexes were hyperreflexive and asymmetrical. Cervical range of motion was restricted, and cervical paravertebral muscle spasms were noted. Chiropractic x-ray analysis showed upper cervical misalignment. Adjustments were given to the upper cervical spine daily for three days. At that time, post-x-rays showed a marked reduction in misalignment. Following the second and third adjustments, no seizures were noted for the rest of the day. Seventeen days following the last adjustment, she had nearly 100 seizures but on the 27th day, she did not have a seizure and seizures remained absent during the following four weeks. Speech was becoming normal and drug therapy was discontinued (30,31).

Young presented three cases of epilepsy who responded favorably to chiropractic care after long term medical care with little or no response. One case was a teenaged female who had seizures since a febrile condition at age 8 months that was accompanied by convulsions. She began receiving medications, such as Valium, Dilantin, Ritalin, Meciline, and Tegretol (carbamazepine). Her conditioned worsened over the years. She was tied to a chair in order to be fed and had difficulty walking. She was having four or five seizures daily when she was evaluated for chiropractic care. Over the course of chiropractic care, the frequency of seizures diminished and her medication was reduced. She also began showing academic excellence and began participating in sports. A second case was a 34-year-old female who had seizures since childhood in addition to chronic lower back pain. Medication controlled her seizures to a degree. She had an episode of status epilepticus. After beginning chiropractic care, seizures were controlled with the care, although she continued to take phenobarbitol and Dilantin. A third case was an elderly male who had upper extremity weakness and a history of seizures since age 14. The severity of seizures and auras reduced following the initiation of chiropractic care (32).

Gambino wrote of a 5-year-old male with seizures, hyperactivity, and clinical signs of autism. He was diagnosed as having idiopathic cerebral damage. He had been on Tegretol, Dilantin, and phenobarbitol. The mother placed an ad in the paper asking for help and a chiropractor answered her plea. The examination showed normal motor skills but minimal verbal skills. He was adjusted using Chiropractic Biophysics technique. Between the initiation of care in July 1992 until the paper was written in May 1995, he had three seizures. Prior to chiropractic care, he would have up to 55 seizures per month. His speech continued to be monosyllabic but improved and he is much calmer (33).

Hyman reported a 5-year-old male who suffered from petit mal or absence seizures (and lower extremity problems) that were noted at age 2 years. He would have a blank stare that would last 4-5 seconds at a frequency of 4-6 per hour. A pediatric neurologist prescribed Depakote following which the child began having involuntary movements of the head and upper extremities during the episodes, and the duration of the episodes increased to 8-10 seconds. The mother requested a change in prescriptions (to Zorantin) but, as the neurologist advised, the condition remained. The chiropractic examination noted segmental and global spinal and paraspinal abnormalities. Adjustments using Palmer Toggle Recoil and Thompson techniques were done in the upper cervical, mid-thoracic, and upper lumbar spine and sacroiliac joint. During the initial few visits, frequency of seizures had reduced from 4-6 per hour to 2-3 per two hours, and the duration and severity was reduced. After 2 months of care, he had one or no seizures of 2-4 seconds duration each day which were mild in intensity. He was able to cease taking the medication (34).

REFERENCES

1. Tharp BR. An overview of pediatric seizure disorders and epileptic syndromes. Epilepsia 1987; 28(Supplement 1):S36-S45.
2. Ferry PC, Banner W, Wolf RA. Seizure disorder in children. Philadelphia: J. B. Lippincott co. 1985.
3. Lipton SA, Rosenberg PA. Excitatory amino acids as a final common pathway for neurologic disorders. New England Journal of Medicine 1994; 330(9):613-622.
4. Epilepsy. Disease-A-Month 1996; 42(11):733-773.
5. Adams RD, Victor M. Principles of neurology, 4th ed. San Francisco: McGraw-Hill, Inc. 1989. pp.249-272.
6. Sadzot B. Epilepsy: a progressive disease? British Medical Journal 1997; 314(7078): 391.
7. Cassano PA, Koepsell TD, Farwell JR. Risk of febrile seizures in childhood in relation to prenatal maternal cigarette smoking and alcohol intake. American Journal of Epidemiology 1990; 132(3):462-473.
8. Fischer JH, French J, Leppik IE. Making the most of new seizure treatments. Patient Care 1996; 30(1):53+.
9. Freeman JM, Vining EPG. Decision making and the child with febrile seizures. Pediatrics in Review 1992; 13(8):298-304.
10. Mizrahi EM. Neonatal seizures: problems in diagnosis and classification. Epilepsia 1987; 28(Supplement 1):S46-S55.
11. Kuturec M, et al. Febrile seizures: is the EEG a useful predictor of reoccurrence. Clinical Pediatrics January 1997; 36(1):31-36.
12. Farwell JR, et al. Phenobarbital for febrile seizures—effects on intelligence and on seizure recurrence. New England Journal of Medicine 1990; 322(6):364-369.
13. Freeman JM, Vining EPG. Decision making and the child with afebrile seizures. Pediatrics in Review 1992; 13(8):305-310.
14. Hertz S, Gottesman M. New antiepileptic medications. Emergency Medicine 1997; 29(3):17-18+.
15. Netter FH. The CIBA collection of medical illustrations. volume 1: nervous system. Part: Neurologic and Neuromuscular Disorders. West Caldwell NJ: CIBA Pharmaceutical Co. 1986. pp. 15-16.
16. When are infant seizures caused by hyponatremia? Emergency Medicine 1996; 28(4):70.
17. Gomez MR, Klass DW. Epilepsies of infancy and childhood. Annals of Neurology 1983; 13:113-124.
18. Roddy SM, McBride MC. Seizure disorders. In: Hoekelman RA (ed). Primary Pediatric Care, 2nd ed. St. Louis: Mosby Year Book. 1992. pp.1481-1490.
19. Farrell K. Classifying epileptic syndromes: problems and a neurobiologic solution. Neurology 1993; 43(11; supplement 5):S8-S11.
20. Weiner HL, Urion DK, Levitt LP. Pediatric neurology for the house officer, 3rd ed. Baltimore: Williams & Wilkins. 1988. pp.33-61.
21. McBride MC. Status Epilepticus. Pediatrics in review October 1995; 16(10): 386-389.
22. Roberts MR, Eng-Bourquin J. Emergency Medical Clinics of North America 1995; 13(2):489-505.
23. Aicardi J, Chevrie JJ. Consequences of status epilepticus in infants and children. In: Elgado-Escueta AV, et al (eds). Status Epilepticus: Mechanisms of Brain Damage and Treatment. Advances in Neurology. Volume 34. New York: Raven Press. 1983. pp.115-125.
24. Moss RB, Sosulski R. Early meningitis. Clinical Pediatrics 1991; 30(4):229-230.
25. van Donselaar CA, et al. Clinical course of untreated tonic-clonic seizures in childhood: prospective, hospital based study. British Medical Journal 1997; 314(7078):401-404.
26. Freeman JM. Just say no! drugs and febrile seizures. Pediatrics 1990; 86(4):624.
27. Spirer Z, et al. Prevention of febrile seizures by dietary supplementation with N-3 polyunsaturated fatty acids. Medical Hypothesis 1994; 43(1):43-45.
28. Murphy JV, Hornig G, Schallert G. Left vagal nerve stimulation in children with refractory epilepsy. Archives of Neurology 1995; 52(9):886-889.
29. Langley C. Epileptic seizures, nocturnal enuresis, ADD. Chiropractic Pediatrics 1994; 1(1):22.
30. Goodman RJ, Mosby JS. Cessation of a seizure disorder: correction of the Atlas Subluxation Complex. Chiropractic: The Journal of Chiropractic Research and Clinical Investigation. 1990; 6(2):43-46.
31. Goodman R. Cessation of seizure disorder: correction of the Atlas Subluxation Complex. Proceedings of the National Conference on Chiropractic and Pediatrics. 1991. pp.46-56.

32. Young G. Chiropractic success in epileptic conditions. ACA Journal of Chiropractic 1982; 19(4):62-62.
33. Gambino DW. Brain injured child with seizures benefits from chiropractic care. Chiropractic Pediatrics Chiropractic Pediatrics 1995; 2(1):8-9.
34. Hyman CA. Chiropractic adjustments and the reduction of Petit Mal seizures in a five-year-old male: a case study. Journal of Clinical Chiropractic Pediatrics 1996; 1(1):28-32.

SLEEP DISORDERS

Sleep problems in children can be due to many causes. Twenty-five percent of all children and adolescents have some form of sleep disorder (1). These include nightmares and difficulty falling asleep.

Night terrors tend to occur within 30 minutes of falling asleep—during stage 3 or 4 of sleep (2). Persistence into adulthood is considered by some to be abnormal (2). Nightmares are common in both adults and children (2).

CHIROPRACTIC MANAGEMENT

Rome presented two cases of children with sleep disorders responding to chiropractic care. The first case is of a 12-month-old male whose mother stated that he slept poorly and when asleep, slept restlessly. While awake, he would be restless and irritable and would throw himself onto the floor. The medical doctor evaluated the infant but reported him as normal and gave a prescription for Panadol. Upon chiropractic evaluation, the physical examination was unremarkable but dysfunction was noted at C1/C2 and T8/T9. C1 appeared to be tender to palpation. C1 was gently adjusted. Following the adjustment, the baby slept for seven hours and was less restless for a few days. A little over a week later, the infant was adjusted again after some of the restless sleep reappeared. He was able to sleep well again. He was seen twice over a several week period a few months later; improved sleep patterns were noted after adjustments. When the child was 18-months-old, the mother stated that he had normal sleeping patterns and was less restless (3).

The second case is a 4-month-old male who slept poorly and fed poorly. After receiving an adjustment, he slept for 11 hours. Four months later, he was brought in after a few falls and he began sleeping poorly. Improved sleeping and feeding patterns returned after adjusting (3).

REFERENCES

1. Mindell JA et al. Pediatricians and sleep disorders: training and practice. Pediatrics 1994 94(2):194-200.
2. Adams RD, Victor M. Principles of neurology, 4th ed. San Francisco: McGraw-Hill, Inc. 1989. pp.311.
3. Rome PL. Case Report: The effect of a chiropractic spinal adjustment on toddler sleep pattern and behavior. Chiropractic Journal of Australia 1996; 26(1):11-14.

SPINAL CORD INJURIES

Severe spinal cord disorders may be due to trauma or disease. Approximately 10,000 spinal cord injuries were recorded in the U.S. in 1974 (1) (See also Chapter 19). One to ten percent of the spinal cord injuries are to children (2,3). Spinal stenosis, birth trauma, and achondroplasia may predispose a child to spinal cord injuries. Vehicular accidents, sports injuries (such as from diving), and violence are the most common causes of SCI (2). Disturbingly, of these, gunshot wounds and other violent injuries account for 19% of these cases in the preteen. In the African-American community, this level rises to 27%, making violence the second most common cause of SCI (2).

The cervical spine is the most common area to be injured followed by the thoracolumbar spine (3). The level of injury tends to be higher in the cervical spine in the child compared to the adult (2). C2 level was a common level injured in the preteen, C4 was commonly injured in the teen and C4-C5 in the adult (2). In the child, the head is relatively large and heavy compared to the level of development of the neck muscles, and the articulations. The cervical articular surfaces tend towards a horizontal orientation (3). Progressive deformity of the spine is a tendency in the young spine suffering injury. A sequela of cervical or thoracic spine injury is the development of scoliosis (4).

Five major directions of force that may cause sufficient trauma to the spine to affect the spinal cord include forward flexion, lateral flexion, rotation, axial compression, and overextension. Forward flexion injuries may cause wedge or teardrop fractures to the vertebral body. Coupled lateral flexion and rotation injuries may cause a unilaterally locked facet. Coupled forward flexion and rotation may tear ligaments, cause instability, and may cause dislocation. Axial compression may cause burst or Jefferson fractures. Overextension injuries may cause fractures of the neural arch and may also tear the anterior longitudinal ligament and injure the vertebral arteries (3).

Many chiropractors are aware of the work of Towbin, a pathologist. He studied the autopsies of newborns at birth or some time later. He found dural tears, spinal root avulsions, and lesions in the spinal cord and brain stem attributable to excessive longitudinal traction as done during forceful delivery of the infant. Hypoxia to neurological tissues may be the sequela. The neurological manifestations may be severe enough to cause "stillbirth" or cause neurological disorders, such as cerebral palsy or epilepsy. Some may cause very mild neurologic effects that are not attributed to the birth injury (5,6).

The spinal cord may be injured in many ways, including concussion, laceration, hematoma, and compression. The following are examples of forms of spinal cord injuries.

SPINAL CORD SHOCK

When there is sudden and complete severance of the spinal cord, one of the effects may be spinal shock. There will be loss of reflex function below the area of trauma and loss of autonomic reflexes. The areas of involvement depend upon the level of the lesion. The effects may last from weeks to months. On theory proposed on the cause of spinal shock is that the spinal motor neurons are kept in a continuous state of subliminal depolarization by the suprasegmental descending fiber system. This may be interrupted by trauma and result in the signs of spinal shock. Some think that the there may be alterations in neurotransmitters (7).

SPINAL CORD CONCUSSION

This is a blunt force to the spinal cord with a functional rather than neuropathological dysfunction. Usually function is restored in 1 to 2 days (3).

SPINAL CORD CONTUSION

This is a blunt injury to the spinal cord. There is neither continuous compression nor disruption of nerve tissue. There is incomplete recovery and central cord necrosis is common (3).

CENTRAL CORD SYNDROME

This is most commonly seen after a cervical hyperextension injury. A characteristic complaint is severe burning dysesthesia in the arms which is thought to be due to damage to the spinothalamic fibers, possibly at the point that they cross over in the anterior commissure. There may be upper limb weakness with preservation of the lower limbs. Pain and temperature may be lost in a cape-like distribution (1). Bilateral paralysis and loss of pain and temperature below the level of injury may be due to injury to the anterior spinal artery. Position sense and vibration (posterior column functions) would be spared in an anterior spinal artery injury.

BROWN-SEQUARD SYNDROME

This is a result of incomplete spinal cord injuries which leave the patient with neurologic deficits including ipsilateral loss of motor function, ipsilateral loss of vibration and position sense, and contralateral loss of pain and temperature sense (1).

CHIROPRACTIC MANAGEMENT

Schimp and Schimp reported a case of a 7-year-old male with a traumatically acquired hemiparesis due to being struck by an automobile. He was semicomatose when he arrived in the emergency room. Imaging studies of the head, neck, and spinal cord were negative. A hemiparesis was diagnosed and was thought to be due to a torqued brainstem. A week later, a chiropractic evaluation was done. The left arm was in a sustained position of internal rotation, flexion, and pronation. The left upper extremity muscles were graded as 3/5 and the left lower extremity muscles were graded at 4/5. The bicipital and patellar muscle stretch reflexes were 3+ (hyperreflexia) while clonus was noted on the ankle reflex. Bilateral Babinski sign was present. Nuchal rigidity was noted, and Kernig's and Brudzinski's tests were positive (meningeal irritation signs). Both the left superficial abdominal reflexes and the withdrawal responses were diminished on the left. He was noted to be restless, photophobic, and irritable. Gait was difficult due to left leg dysfunction and the left arm was nearly useless. Chiropractic analysis determined that there was cranial and upper cervical dysfunction. Toftness analysis and procedures were utilized. On the third day after the initiation of care, he was able to ascend stairs. On day five, upper extremity motor function began to return. After sixteen days, it was determined that upper extremity function was 90% and lower extremity was 70%. Sixty-one days post-accident, objective signs were negative and full restoration of function was demonstrated (8).

REFERENCES

1. Netter FH. The CIBA collection of medical illustrations. volume 1: nervous system. part II: neurological and neuromuscular disorders. West Caldwell NJ: CIB Pharmaceutical Co. 1986. pp.106-114.
2. Apple DF, et al. Spinal cord injury in youth. Clinical Pediatrics 1995; 34(2):90-95.
3. Rosman NP, Gilmore HE. Spinal cord injury. In: Swaiman KF (ed). Pediatric Neurology: Principles and Practice. St. Louis MO: C.V. Mosby Co. 1989. pp.735-743.
4. Babcock JL. "Spinal injuries in children." Pediatric Clinics of North America 1975; 22(2):487-500.
5. Towbin A. Spinal cord and brain stem injury at birth. Archives of Pathology 1964; 77:620-632.
6. Towbin A. Latent spinal cord and brain stem injury in newborn infants. Developmental Medicine and Childhood Neurology 1969; 11:54-68.
7. Adams RD, Victor M. Principles of neurology, 4th ed. San Francisco: McGraw-Hill, Inc. 1989. pp.718-722.
8. Schimp JA, Schimp DJ. The neuropathophysiology of traumatic hemiparesis and its association with dysfunctional upper cervical motion units: a case report. Chiropractic Technique 1992; 4(3):104-107.

SPINAL MUSCULAR ATROPHY

The characteristic feature of spinal muscular atrophies are the progressive degeneration of motor cells in the anterior horn of the spinal cord and may involve those in the motor nuclei of the brainstem as well (1). This group of disorders are the most common degenerative disorder of the CNS. They are also the second most common lethal genetic disorder of childhood (mucoviscidosis is the most common) (1). Onset can occur at any time from prenatal to adulthood (1). Motoneuron involvement may be diffuse or focal and affect certain muscle groups (1)

The best described and agreed upon type is SMA type I or Werdnig-Hoffman's disease. Werdnig-Hoffmann's disease or infantile progressive spinal muscular atrophy is a hereditary disease affecting the anterior horn cells of the spinal cord. Most cases are found at birth or within the first year of life (2). Progression is rapid (2). Those with early onset usually die before the first birthday (1). The infant will be alert, but hypotonic with a frog-leg posture. Deep tendon reflexes are absent and respiration is paradoxical. Fasciculations of the tongue is almost pathognomonic but are difficult to observe (3).

Hypotonia, muscle weakness, and delayed motor development are features which must also be distinguished from other disorders with similar manifestations (1). A key physical finding is intercostal muscle paralysis which causes a narrow chest and diaphragmatic breathing. There is constant retrognathism, a pulling back of the lower jaw. Deep tendon reflexes are not present. Other neurological signs, such are sensation and sphincter control, are intact and no pyramidal signs are present (1). EMG confirms the diagnosis of Werdnig-Hoffman (1).

REFERENCES

1. Aicardi J. Diseases of the nervous system in childhood. Clinics in Developmental Medicine 1992; 115/118:1095-1097.
2. Adams RD, Victor M. Principles of neurology, 4th ed. San Francisco: McGraw-Hill, Inc. 1989. pp.1146-1148.
3. Netter FH. The CIBA collection of medical illustrations. vol. 1: nervous system. part II: neurologic and neuromuscular disorders. West Caldwell, NJ: CIBA Pharmaceutical Co. 1986. p.16.

STROKE

Strokes can occur in childhood but are fortunately rare events. They can even occur in the prenatal or perinatal periods.

Childhood cerebrovascular disease may be ischemic (55%) or hemorrhagic (45%) (1). Acute nonvascular disease may cause focal neurological deficits (1). "Holes in the brain" are focal brain lesions of vascular and metabolic origin (1).

Strokes occur in 2.5 children per 100,000 population each year (1). Ischemic stroke rates are 0.63 per 100,000 (2). Strokes may be the result of vascular disease such as aneurysm or malformation, head trauma, maternal drug use, malignancies or the treatment for malignancies, metabolic disorders, infectious diseases, congenital heart disease, and vasculitis (1,2). Congenital heart disease is the most common cause of ischemic strokes (2). Fever or evidence of infection is present in about 50% of children presenting with cerebral infarction (2). Certain conditions appear to predispose the child to an increased likelihood of stroke recurrence. These conditions include sickle cell anemia, arteriovenous malformations, and metabolic disease (1).

The most common presenting sign of ischemic stroke is acute onset hemiparesis. It may be subtle with a presentation of asymmetrical use of the hands, a limp, or slight nasolabial fold asymmetry. Dysarthria may be present. Unlike adults, young children may have seizures at the time of the stroke. Headaches in older children are not uncommon. Fever is common.

In one study of perinatal strokes, 52% experienced seizures (2). Most achieved motor milestones at the expected times and I.Q.s tended to be in the normal range (3). MRI and CT scan are commonly used to localize the lesion.

REFERENCES

1. Pavlaki SG, Gould RJ, Zito JL. Stroke in children. Advances in Pediatrics 1991; 38:151-179.
2. Trescher WH. Ischemic stroke syndromes in childhood. Pediatric Annals 1992; 21(6):374-383.
3. Trauner DA, et al. Neurologic profiles of infants and children after perinatal strokes. Pediatric Neurology 1993; 9(5):383-386.

SUDDEN INFANT DEATH SYNDROME

Sudden Infant Death Syndrome, SIDS, crib death, or cot death is a tragic and perplexing dilemma. Despite the plethora of studies into the cause of SIDS, the cause (or causes) is still unknown.

SIDS is defined as the sudden death of an infant under one year of age. The cause of death remains unexplained after the performance of a complete postmortem investigation, which includes an autopsy, an examination of the scene of death, and a review of the case history. The diagnosis is one of excluding all other possibilities (1-4).

It is the leading cause of death between the age of 1 week and 1 year of age and accounts for 35% of the deaths (1,5,6). The incidence of SIDS in the United States, according to a 1988 report by the National Center for Health Statistics, was 1.4 per 1000 live births (3,7). World statistics range from 0.036 to 6.3 per 1000 live births (3). The peak incidence is between two and four months of age (1,6,8,9,10). Nearly all cases occur before six months of age (1). There is a preponderance of males (7,9). The incidence is greater in the autumn and winter months—60% to 65% (7,10). Poor socioeconomic conditions appears to be a risk factor as does low maternal age (8,9). Infant care practices related to culture may also be a factor (9).

Less than 10% of the infants are born before the thirty-sixth week of gestation but they account for 20% of the SIDS victims. One study found that nearly all of the term infants succumbing to SIDS do so by the thirty-second week postnatally but only 75% of the preterm have succumbed by this time. Preterm infants have a longer time frame during which they might become victims of SIDS (6). Both low gestational age and low birthweight seem to be factors (11).

The prone sleeping position is thought to be a risk factor. Most studies have found a correlation. In a few countries, advisories given to parents on the correlation between SIDS and prone sleeping position have appeared to have a positive effect on the reduction in the number of SIDS cases. Some studies have found a substantial reduction. A Norwegian study found the incidence in 1970 at 1.1/1000; 1989 at 2.0/1000; and 1990/91 rates to be 1.1/1000. In 1970, 7.4% of infants in the survey slept in the prone position at age three months; in 1989, 49.1% slept in the prone position; and in 1990, 26.8%; and in 1991, 28.3% slept in the prone position (12).

Prenatal maternal smoking appear to be a factor, possibly second only to the prone sleeping position. Chronic fetal hypoxia due to prenatal maternal smoking may cause growth retardation. Increased smoking has been found to be directly proportional to increased risk (9). There is evidence that exposure to passive smoke, be it the mother or others, may be a risk factor (4,13).

Another risk factor is drug use by the mother. Infants born to mothers who used drugs had a 5 to 10 times greater risk of SIDS that infants in the general population. SIDS claimed 25% of the infants dying in their first year who were born to mothers who are drug-addicts compared to 10% of infants in the general population (14).

Pathophysiological findings are very elusive in SIDS victims. In one study recording brainstem auditory evoked response of near-miss SIDS, 15% of these infants and their siblings were found to have abnormal studies suggesting possible delay of brainstem neural processing maturation (15). Also in near-miss infants under age three months, limb muscle tone abnormalities were found, particularly hypotonia of the shoulder musculature (16). Signs of chronic hypoxemia were noted in victims and near victims of SIDS (16) and increased respiratory rates were found in near victims compared to controls (17). Near victims tended to be less physically active, have more abnormal cries, be more exhausted and breathless after feeding, and react less intensely to external stimuli than their siblings (18). Siblings born after SIDS victims have a four to six fold greater risk of succumbing to SIDS compared to controls (9,18). Gilles, Bina, and Sotrel found atlanto-occipital instability in 10 of 11 SIDS victims and none in the controls

(19). A follow-up study by Schneier and Burns studied x-rays of SIDS victims. All films with atlas inversion into the foramen magnum were found in SIDS victims but not all SIDS victims had this (10). Towbin found evidence of birth-related spinal cord and brain stem injury. It may be possible that the brain stem injury from an excessively forceful birth could lead to respiratory compromise (20,21). The vagus nerve has significant control over respiration. One study found small myelinated vagus nerve fibers in SIDS victims. They suggested that the vagus nerve development in the SIDS victim is abnormal or delayed. That may cause respiratory compromise (22).

One hypothesis is that SIDS may be related to an infant dreaming of its previous fetal life. In fetal life, breathing is not necessary as the mother provides life support. It has been shown in sleep studies that the body's action corresponds with actions taken in lucid dreams. The authors hypothesize that lucid dreaming of fetal life causes a cessation of breathing. The authors feel that the prone position or tight wrapping in a blanket may mimic the environment in the womb and may initiate lucid dreams of fetal life. The suggestion is to reduce the resemblance of the infant's environment from that of the womb (23).

Another hypothesis concludes that there may be a relationship between SIDS and mitochondrial and thyroid function. The ability of the body to utilize oxygen would be affected, and the effect of the thyroid gland on ATP, which is necessary for the sodium/potassium pump, would affect thermogenesis. Reid found low selenium and iodine levels in the soil of two areas with the highest incidence of SIDS. Both are necessary for proper mitochondrial and thyroid function (24).

There is some speculation about the connection between the increased incidence of SIDS during autumn and winter months. Some feel that seasonal changes in melatonin levels may be involved (26).

There has been concern that bottle feeding is a factor in SIDS. Of 18 studies, 11 found an increased risk of SIDS with bottle feeding versus breast feeding. Many confounders have been found that could alter the findings, such as the sleeping position, maternal smoking, and length of gestation (11). Gilbert, et al. found an increased risk of SIDS with infants who only received bottle feeding but the increased risk diminished when confounders were factored out; although, some risk remained compared to infants who only received breast feeding (11).

One difficult area when determining the cause of inexplicable death is to distinguish death due to SIDS from that due to child abuse. An important part of the investigation is to rule out child abuse. Some errors have occurred where parents were accused of homicide but findings were inconclusive, and the parents had to suffer accusations in addition to their sorrow following the death of their child. On the other hand, a case is noted of a woman who had several children who suffered "SIDS" (3).

As can be surmised, the cause of and signs of SIDS are frustratingly unknown. Many tantalizing clues are being found in pathological and epidemiological studies. Abnormal factors such as gliosis in the brainstem regions, particularly those areas associated with respiration, abnormal retention of fetal hemoglobin, abnormal retention of periadrenal brown fat, increased levels of hepatic erythropoiesis, thymic petechiae, and signs of lung congestion may be present (4).

MEDICAL MANAGEMENT

The current recommendation is for the infant to sleep supine or on the side as sleeping prone appears to be a risk factor. Studies reported a 20% to 67% reduction in the incidence of SIDS following publication of the recommendation decrying the prone sleeping position in infants under age six months (4,7,26). In 1994, in spite of this recommendation, the Academy of Pediatrics found that many physicians and health care workers were not actively notifying parents of the connection between prone sleeping position and SIDS (27).

CHIROPRACTIC MANAGEMENT

Marion presented a case of a 6-week-old female infant who was found cyanotic by her mother. The mother revived her. The medical diagnosis was SIDS risk, and the mother was told that the infant had weak cervical musculature which could result in regurgitation and asphyxiation. On chiropractic evaluation, the infant was observed to have an aberrant flipping movement with the head and neck. An atlas subluxation and later a sacroiliac subluxation were found. After adjustments were made, the aberrant neck movements abated, and the mother stated that her infant was breathing and sleeping better (28,29).

REFERENCES

1. Beckwith JB. The sudden infant death syndrome. Rockville MD: U.S. Department of Health, Education, and Welfare. 1977.
2. Rammer L. Pathological definition. Acta Paediatrica 1993; 82(Supplement 389):15-16.
3. Reese RM. Fatal child abuse and sudden infant death syndrome: a critical diagnostic decision. Pediatrics 1993; 90:423-439.
4. Valdes-Dapena M. The postmortem examination. Pediatric Annals 1995; 24(7):365-372.
5. Elders JM. Reducing the risk of sudden infant death syndrome (from the surgeon general, U.S. Public Health Service). JAMA 1994; 272(21):1646.
6. Lipsky CL, et al. The timing of SIDS deaths in premature infants in an urban population. Clinical Pediatrics 1995; 34(8):410-414.0
7. Walsh S, Mortimer G. Unexplained stillbirths and sudden infant death syndrome. Medical Hypotheses 1995; 45(1):73-75
8. Banks BD, et al. Sudden infant death syndrome: a literature review with chiropractic implications. Journal of Manipulative and Physiological Therapeutics 1987; 10(5):246-252.
9. Dwyer T, Ponsonby A-L. SIDS epidemiology and incidence. Pediatric Annals 1995; 24(7):350-356.
10. Schneier M, Burns RE. Atlanto-occipital hypermobility in sudden infant death syndrome. Chiropractic: The Journal of Chiropractic Research and Clinical Investigation 1991; 7(2):33-38.
11. Gilbert RE, et al. Bottle feeding and the sudden infant death syndrome. British Medical Journal 1995; 310(6972):88-90.
12. Irgens LM, et al. Sleeping position and sudden infant death syndrome in Norway 1967-91. Archives of Disease in Childhood 1995; 72(6):478-482.
13. Klonoff-Cohen HS, et al. The effect of passive smoking and tobacco exposure through breast milk on sudden infant death syndrome. JAMA 1995; 273(10):795-798.
14. Rosen TS, Johnson HL. Drug-addicted mothers, their infants, and SIDS. Annals New York Academy of Sciences 1988; 533:89-95.
15. Petigrew AG, Rahilly PM. Brainstem auditory evoked responses in infants at risk of sudden infant death. Early Human Development 1985; 11(2):99-111.
16. Korobkin R, Guilleminault C. Neurologic abnormalities in near miss for sudden infant death syndrome infants. Pediatrics 1979; 64(3):369-374.
17. Williams A, Vawter G, Reid L. Increased muscularity of the pulmonary circulation in victims of sudden infant death syndrome. Pediatrics 1979; 63(1):18-23.

18. Hoppenbrouwers T, et al. Sudden infant death syndrome: sleep apnea and respiration in subsequent siblings. Pediatrics 1980; 66(2):205-214.
19. Gilles FH, Bina M, Sotrel A. Infantile Atlanto-occipital instability. American Journal of Diseases of Childhood. 1979; 133:30-37.
20. Kent C, Gentempo P. Sudden infant death syndrome and chiropractic. ICA International Review of Chiropractic 1992; 48(6):41-42.
21. Bussanich B. "SIDS: sudden infant death syndrome: some new ideas." The Digest of Chiropractic Economics 1982; 24-29.
22. Sachis PN, et al. The Vagus nerve and sudden infant death syndrome: a morphometric study. Journal of Pediatrics 1981; 98(2):278-280.
23. Christos GA, Christos JA. A possible explanation of sudden infant death syndrome (SIDS). Medical Hypotheses 1993; 41(3):245-246.
24. Reid GM. Sudden infant death syndrome (SIDS): oxygen utilization and energy production. Medical Hypotheses 1993; 40(6):364-366.
25. Douglas AS, Allan TM, Helms PJ. Seasonality and the sudden infant death syndrome during 1978-9 and 1991-3 in Australia and Britain. British Medical Journal 1996; 312(7043):1381-1383.
26. Guntheroth WG, Spiers PS. "Sleeping prone and the risk of sudden infant death syndrome." JAMA 1992; 267(17):2359-2362.
27. American Academy of Pediatrics. Infant sleep position and sudden infant death syndrome (SIDS) in the United States: Joint Commentary from the American Academy of Pediatrics and Selected Agencies of the Federal Government. Pediatrics 1994; 93(5):820.
28. Marion FB. SIDS, Chiropractic and you. Digest of Chiropractic Economics 1984; 27(2):89.
29. Marion FB. SIDS, Chiropractic and you. Today's Chiropractic 1984; 13(6):45.

TUMORS OF THE NERVOUS SYSTEM

BRAIN TUMORS

Brain or intracranial tumors are the second most common form of malignancy in children (leukemia is the most common) (1,2). The frequency rate of 2.4 per 100,000 is similar to that of acute lymphoblastic leukemia (3). About half occur above the tentorium and half in the posterior fossa (3). Unlike in adults, malignant tumors, glioblastomas and metastatic carcinoma, and benign tumors, meningiomas, acoustic neuromas, and pituitary tumors in children are uncommon (3). Medulloblastomas, ependymomas, and astrocytomas are the most common forms of pediatric intracranial tumors (1,4). The latter, astrocytomas, are the most common and represent more than 50% of intracranial tumors. Astrocytomas include cerebellar astrocytomas, high- and low-grade supratentorial astrocytomas, and brainstem gliomas (4).

Tumors tend to be supertentorial during the first six months of life (5). By the second year of life, the infratentorial region predominates (5).

The best survival rate is in children with cerebellar astrocytoma. The worst survival rate is with brainstem glioma (4).

CLINICAL FEATURES

The classical signs and symptoms of childhood brain tumors include frequent headaches which become progressively worse and are often accompanied by nausea or vomiting as well as other signs of increased, nonfocal intracranial pressure (3). Vomiting tends to occur in the early morning (5). A feature of increased intracranial pressure is papilledema but it may not be present if the fontanelles are open (5). Seizures, gait disturbances, and weakness may also be present (6).

The child's age and level of development, the tumor's location, as well as the degree of neurological integrity compromise, determines the signs and symptoms. The symptomatic course is usually progressive but can have regressions and exacerbations (4). Seventy-five to eighty percent of children with medulloblastoma are estimated to have the triad of headaches, nausea and emesis, and papilledema (7). Unsteadiness is a common sign of a posterior fossa tumor (5). Failure to thrive may indicate a tumor in the region of the hypothalamus (5).

In the exam, the eyes should be carefully observed as visual problems may accompany brain tumors. Sixth and third cranial nerves should be tested (6).

The diagnosis is usually confirmed by MRI or CT studies. If a tumor is suspected in the posterior fossa, MRI is more sensitive because of the particularities of the surrounding osseous structures (7).

The medical treatment is by surgery, radiation therapy, and/or chemotherapy. In low-grade gliomas, the 10-year survival rate following surgery is 80% for cerebral and 90% for cerebellar tumors (8). In high-grade malignant supertentorial gliomas, the five-year survival rate after medical intervention is 18% to 46% depending upon the treatments used (8). The five-year survival rate for medulloblastomas after intervention is 30% to 70%. Brainstem gliomas have a very poor prognosis. After complete surgical re-sectioning, the five-year progression-free survival rate for ependymomas is 60% to 80%.

SPINAL CORD TUMORS

Intraspinal tumors are rare in children (9). Of the primary tumors of the central nervous system found at Mayo Clinic, 15% were intraspinal (9). Spinal cord tumors are usually benign and their effects are usually due to compression of the cord as they expand. Tumors are often classified as intramedullary (within the substance of the cord) or extramedullary (outside of the spinal cord, e.g., vertebral body, epidural tissues, and meninges) (9). Nearly two-thirds of spinal cord tumors are benign (6).

The most common extramedullary tumors are neurofibromas and meningiomas. These constitute 55% of all intraspinal tumors (9). Neurofibromas tend to be found in the thoracic spine. Other extramedullary tumors include sarcomas, vascular tumors, chordomas, and epidermoid tumors (9).

Ependymomas and astrocytomas are the primary intramedullary tumors of the cord (9). Oligodendrogliomas are more rare. Other intramedullary tumors of the cord include lipomas, epidermoids, dermoid, hemangiomas, and metastatic carcinomas (9).

Metastatic intramedullary or extramedullary spinal cord tumors have been found to be more common than was once believed (9). In one study, nearly 10% of CNS metastatic tumors were found in the spinal cord.

CLINICAL FEATURES

Intraspinal tumors are often suspected when testing for a space-occupying mass in the spinal canal. Symptoms usually appear gradually. The main symptoms tend to be gait disturbances, weakness of the legs, clumsiness, pain, and loss of sphincter control (6). There may be severe back pain and spasm of the paravertebral muscles. Later stages include scoliosis and spastic weakness of the lower extremities (9). The clinical picture may be sensory-motor, radicular, or a syringomyelic syndrome (9).

Those with the signs of neurofibromatosis, e.g., café au lait spots, require further investigation as a spinal tumor may be present (6,10).

Scoliosis is seen associated with spinal cord tumors. It is important to give a good neurological examination when presented with a youth with scoliosis. An obvious exam procedure is checking for the Babinski sign or plantar reflex or similar signs (6).

REFERENCES

1. Friedberg SR. Tumors of the brain. CIBA-Geigy Clinical Symposia 1986; 38(4):1-32.
2. Posner JB. Brain tumor (editorial). CA—A Cancer Journal for Clinicians 1993; 43(5):261-262.
3. Albright AL. Pediatric brain tumors. CA—A Cancer Journal for Clinicians 1993; 43(5):272-288.
4. Cohen ME, Duffner PK. Tumors of the brain and spinal cord including leukemic involvement. In: Swaiman KF (ed). Pediatric Neurology: Principles and Practice. St. Louis: C. V. Mosby Co. 1989. pp.661-664.
5. Gordon GS, Wallace SJ, Neal JW. Intracranial tumours during the first two years of life: presenting features. Archives of Diseases in Childhood 1995; 73(4):345-347.
6. Sugar O. Tumors of the central nervous system in children. Pediatric Clinics of North America 1960; 7(3):689-701.
7. Newton HB. Primary brain tumors: review of etiology, diagnosis and treatment. American Family Physician 1994; 49(4):787-797.
8. Pollack IF. Brain tumors in children. New England Journal of Medicine 1994; 331(22):1500-1507.
9. Adams RD, Victor M. Priniciples of neurology, 4th ed. New York: McGraw-Hill, Inc. 1989. pp.742-746.
10. Netter FH. The CIBA collection of medical illustrations. volume 1: nervous system. Part: Neurologic and Neuromuscular Disorders. West Caldwell, NJ: CIBA Pharmaceutical Co. 1986. pp. 15-16.

GILLES DE LA TOURETTE SYNDROME

Gilles de la Tourette syndrome (TS) is a movement disorder that affects children. It can also be caused by antipsychotic drugs (1). The movie, "The Exorcist," showed an "early European treatment" for a cinematically exaggerated case of Tourette (2). Tics are the most notable feature of Tourette syndrome. There are both motor and verbal tics (1).

Earlier, TS was considered to be a psychiatric disorder but is now classified to be a neurological movement disorder (3).

Age of onset is about age 6-7 and ranges from 2 to 13 (2,4). One hundred thousand are thought to be afflicted in the U.S (2). Males are more commonly affected (3,5).

Fifty to sixty percent have attention-deficit hyperactivity disorder (ADHD) (6). Obsessive-compulsive disorder (OCD) or other behavioral disturbances may be present (4). A study by Como, et al. found that ADHD and OCD rarely appeared at a later date if not found on the initial evaluation (7).

Tourette syndrome remisses spontaneously in about 16% of the cases (2). There is some research indicating that the pathophysiology of Tourette may be associated with glutamate or glutamate-like toxins which may be affecting the basal ganglia (8).

CLINICAL FEATURES

Tics of the eye are a common initial symptom. Motor tics of the head, face, or neck are common presenting symptoms (2). Coprolalia (speaking profanity) may be an initial symptom. Coprolalia is common but often disappears (2). Motor tics are most common in the upper body, especially the head, face, and upper extremities (2). Common movements found to be difficult to engage in include touching, hitting, and jumping (2).

Differentiating must be made from Wilson's disease, Sydenham's chorea, and Bobble-head syndrome. Some manifestations of Wilson's disease not found in Tourette are hepatic involvement, Kayser-Fleischer corneal rings, changes in serum copper and ceruloplasmin (5). Sydenham's chorea is self-limiting (5). Bobble-head syndrome presents with rapid, rhythmic bobbing of the head and is associated with hydrocephalus (5).

MEDICAL MANAGEMENT

Drug therapy is the primary management in medical practice and is aimed at reducing tics or the associated disorders, such as ADHD, depression, or obsessive-compulsive disorder. Haloperidol has been a commonly used drug, but it has many side effects. Irreversible tardive dyskinesis is one of the hazards (9). Other short term side effects include sedation, lethargy, depression, pseudoparkinson's, akathisia (paces floor constantly) and dystonia (9). Clonidine and lithium are also used on some cases. Clonidine has been found to reduce motor or vocal tics in 50% of the children who received it. Side effects include sedation, excessive or reduced salivation, and diarrhea (5).

CHIROPRACTIC MANAGEMENT

Trotta presents a case of Tourette managed chiropractically over a three month period. This patient was a 31-year-old male who was diagnosed with Tourette at age four. He suffered from motor and vocal tics. He was unresponsive to drug therapy. He was found to have bilaterally diminished muscle stretch reflexes of the biceps brachii, triceps, and brachioradialis muscles. Foramen compression test was positive. Misalignments were found at atlas and C2 on x-ray. Adjustments were given in the upper cervical spine. During the course of care, the severity of symptoms diminished and reduced stress was noted in the Psychological Stress Audit Test (10, 11).

REFERENCES

1. Balduc HA. Neurologic system. In: Lawrence DJ,ed. Fundamentals of Chiropractic Diagnosis and Management. Baltimore: Williams & Wilkins. 1991. pp.80-81.
2. Shapiro AK, Shapiro E. Tourette syndrome: history and present status." In: Friedhoff AJ, Chase TN. Gilles de la Tourette Syndrome, Advances in Neurology, Volume 35. 1982. pp.17-23.
3. Hyde TM, Weinberger DR. Tourette's syndrome: a model neuropsychiatric disorder. JAMA 1995; 273(6):498-501.
4. Park S, et al. The early course of the Tourette's syndrome clinical spectrum. Neurology 1993; 43(9):1712-1715.
5. Greenberg DA, Aminoff MJ, Simon RP. Clinical neurology, 2nd ed. Norwalk, CT: Appleton & Lange. 1993. pp.226-227.
6. Leung AKC, et al. Attention-deficit hyperactivity disorder. Postgraduate Medicine 1994; 95(2):153-160.
7. Como PS, Cui L, Kurlan R. The early course of the Tourette's clinical spectrum. Neurology 1993; 43:1712-1715 (also reviewed in Literature Reviews: Neurology. Clinical Pediatrics 1994; 33(2):123.
8. Lipton SA, Rosenberg PA. Excitatory amino acids as a final common pathway for neurologic disorders. New England Journal of Medicine 1994; 330(9):613-622.
9. Borison RL, et al. New pharmacological approaches in the treatment of Tourette syndrome. In: Friedhoff AJ, Chase TN. Advances in Neurology, Volume 35: Gilles de la Tourette Syndrome. 1982. pp.377-382.
10. Trotta N. Chiropractic care in the management of an adult Tourette patient. Today's Chiropractic 1989; 18(4):90-92, 94
11. Trotta N. The response of an adult Tourette patient to life upper cervical adjustments. Chiropractic Research Journal 1989; 1(3):43-48.

APPENDIX 13.3

Selected Visceral Disorders

There are many reports of chronic or otherwise allopathically-unresolved visceral disorders which have resolved while the pediatric patient was under chiropractic care. Some visceral disorders have been previously described relative to possible neurological connections and the spinal segmental levels that may be associated with them. A few selected visceral disorders are described here.

For those chiropractors who wish to do outcome studies on the efficacy of chiropractic spinal adjustments on specific disorders, there are some basic criteria that must be met according to the established scientific and medical authorities. Obviously, you must research the disorder as completely as possible. You must find out the criteria used to determine the treatment efficacy used in researching treatments for that disorder. Documentation is a most important item, i.e., detailed history, complete examination, detailed notes on the care given, including any adjunctive care by yourself or others, and the visit-to-visit and overall response of the patient to the care. Long-term follow-up evaluation or contact with the patient or representatives of the patient must be done as well. Greater use of quality-of-life questionnaires is being made when determining the efficacy of the treatment being given. Objective findings are not enough, particularly if the treatment has a significant impact (positive, equivocal, or negative) on a person's life. This is of major importance in a child as they potentially have most of their life yet to live. Some disorders require special diagnostic studies pre and post care that may require other specialists to conduct because of the specialized diagnostic equipment used.

BRONCHIAL ASTHMA

Bronchial asthma has been defined as a condition of reversible airway obstruction of unknown etiology. One classification system is to classify it as exercise-induced, IgE-induced, intermittent, chronic, corticosteroid-dependent, and potentially fatal. There are variations on the classification such as whether it is seasonal or perennial. Another system of classification that has been devised divides the types into simple bronchoconstriction, bronchoconstriction and hypersecretion, and bronchiolar obstruction (1).

There is narrowing of the airways due to bronchospasm, edema, inflammation of the bronchial mucosa and the production of mucus (2). In response to localized hypoventilation, there is early hyperventilation. If the attack continues, there is further narrowing of the airways and fatigue of the musculature. This leads to arterial hypoxemia, increased pulmonary carbon dioxide levels, and respiratory acidosis. This can result in respiratory failure.

The neurological origins of asthma have been thought to be related to trophic disturbance of the respiratory sympathetic neuromeres (T2–T7) which causes sympathetic depletion or to facilitation of respiratory parasympathetic neuromeres (vagus nerve to C1) (2). When due to excessive parasympathetic effect, there is a disturbance in the cholinergic tone. Cholinergic tone is modulated by sympathetic adrenergic stimulation (anti-cholinergic effect) at the ganglion, in the airway, or both. Sympathetic neurotransmitters also inhibit secretions (immunological) by mast cells in the bronchial lining. Sympathetic (adrenergic effect) stimulation opens the airways and reduces edema and mucus secretion (3). In asthma, there is a hyperresponse to both cholinergic (parasympathetic) and alpha-adrenergic (sympathetic) neurotransmitters and a hyporesponse to beta-adrenergic (sympathetic) neurotransmitters) (3).

There has been an increase in the prevalence of asthma among U.S. children. Between 1982 and 1992, there was a 56.7% rise in newly diagnosed asthma cases in the U.S (4). One study found that there has been an almost 40% increase in the prevalence of childhood asthma between 1981 and 1988. The increase occurred among children ages 5 to 12 and adolescents but not in infants and young children under 5 (5). Of the 12 to 14 million cases of asthma in the U.S., more than four million are under the age of 18 (4).

A very disturbing trend is the increasing rates of mortality from asthma. Between 1979 and 1983-4, asthma death rates in the U.S. rose from 1.2 per 100,000 to 1.5 (6). There were nearly 5,000 deaths in the U.S. in 1992 compared to nearly 2,600 in 1979 (4). The increase in death rates among U.S. African-American was even greater (6). African-Americans account for 21% of the deaths due to asthma, although they make up 12% of the U.S. population (4,7). Other developed countries found similar increases as well. Some feel that it may be associated with the increased level of environmental pollutants. One U.S. study found increased rates of asthma mortality in areas with a greater density of medical specialists in allergy, asthma care, immunology, pediatrics, and emergency medicine (8). The use of a ß-agonist inhalant, fenoterol, has been implicated in some of the deaths (9-12). Increased use of the inhalants appears to be related to greater risk of fatal or near fatal asthma (7).

Aspirin and a few other NSAIDS have been found to induce asthmatic attacks in 10% to 20% of asthmatics. The ingestion of aspirin induces bronchospasm in these people (13). These studies were done on adults so the pediatric incidence is unknown.

A syndrome with signs similar to poliomyelitis has been seen in a few rare cases of those who are recovering from episodes of asthma. It has been reported that there may be permanent flaccid paralysis that may affect either the upper or lower extremities (14).

ANATOMY

An understanding of bronchial asthma depends upon an understanding of the anatomy from the trachea down to the terminals of the bronchioles. The outer trachea is composed of 16-20 connective tissue-covered cartilaginous rings. These crescent-shaped rings open posteriorly. The ends of the rings are attachment points for the trachealis muscle. This smooth muscle membrane contracts to narrow the tracheal lumen when coughing or upon forced expiration. Internally is a layer of nerves and mucus-secreting goblet cells in a connective tissue mesh. This layer has an epithelial lining which forms the inner wall of the lumen (15).

The bronchi branch left and right from the caudal aspect of the trachea to enter their respective lungs. These further subdivide into progressively smaller and more numerous bronchi up to ten orders of subdivision. The cartilage layer forms part of the structure of the bronchi, although, at the later divisions it exists as plates and then rods. These are joined together by smooth muscle and connective tissue network which contains nerves, blood vessels, and lymphatic vessels. The lumen is lined with ciliated epithelium (15).

The bronchioles form the eleventh and further orders of subdivision. Cartilage stops at this level. Elastic connective tissue and smooth muscle forms the walls of the bronchioles. Alveolar ducts branch off of the furthest sub-branches of the bronchioles. The alveolar ducts further subdivide into smooth muscle walled branches with outpockets called alveoli which have outpockets called air cells. Clusters of air cells are called alveolar sacs. The alveolar walls form a membrane where the transfer of gases occurs between the air passages and capillaries (15).

A surfactant material is synthesized and secreted in the alveolar wall. Macrophages involved in phagocytic action migrate up to the terminal bronchioles where they become embedded in the mucous coating and pushed upwards and outwards. The phagocytic action, sticky mucus, detoxification substances, and lymphatic drainage helps to filter and remove foreign matter from the respiratory tract (15).

The lungs and the tracheobronchial tree receive autonomic innervation. A variety of receptors send afferent impulses to the vagus nerve. Parasympathetic efferent impulses travel via the pulmonary plexuses and vagus nerve to the smooth muscles and glands causing muscle contraction, glandular secretion, and vasodilatation. Sympathetic efferent impulses pass from the sympathetic chain of the thoracic spine via the pulmonary plexuses to the lungs. This causes the opposite reaction compared to the parasympathetic supply, i.e., smooth muscle relaxation, inhibition of glandular secretion, and vasoconstriction (15).

In airway hyperresponsiveness, Th2 cytokines, a subclass of T helper cells, is thought to be involved. The exact mechanism does not appear to be established (16).

Exercise-induced Asthma

Physical exertion has been recognized as a cause of asthma or may aggravate an asthmatic condition. Up to 11% of world class athletes and 15% to 20% of the general population may be affected. Common symptoms include coughing, wheezing, chest tightness, and shortness of breath. This can occur during or following exercise. There are several theories on why exercise may induce asthmatic attacks. One theory is based upon the loss of water through the bronchial mucosa during exhalation which may cause bronchospasm and change the environment of the airway epithelium. Another is that the transfer of heat from the pulmonary vascular beds and rewarming after exercise leads to dilation and hyperemia of the bronchiolar vessels (17).

Medical Management

The treatment for asthma is to control it as there is no cure. The primary medical treatment is ß-agonist, corticosteroids, the-ophylline, cromolyn, and, in the case of IgE-induced asthma, allergen avoidance. Corticosteroids such as prednisone are a typical treatment for acute episodes. Inhalants are often used in early stages or for minor attacks.

New research has been looking at cytokine antagonists, anti-IgE antibodies, 5-lipoxygenase inhibitors, and phospho-diesterase isoform inhibitors, among others (16).

Chiropractic Management

There are several studies in the chiropractic literature on the effects of chiropractic care for those suffering from asthma (See also Chapter 1). The osteopathic literature implicates lesions in the midthoracic spine which cause a neurogenic reflex. Many chiropractors have seen asthmatic episodes abate after adjustments to the cervical or thoracic spine.

Vernon and Vernon note that spinal adjustments may benefit asthma sufferers because of the effect that adjustments/manipulation appear to have on the autonomic nervous system. In the field of neuroimmunomodulation, dysfunction in the musculoskeletal system may have an adverse effect on the immune system. They suggest a study comparing patients receiving chiropractic adjustments to those receiving drug therapy using peak flow meter and pulse oximeter measurements (18).

Arbiloff presented a case of a 7-year-old white male who was experiencing acute asthma. Ten months earlier he had an initial attack which was treated with bronchodilators and bed rest. Over the next several months, he had increasingly frequent and severe attacks. During the summer, attacks subsided but resumed in the fall. As an infant he had poor sleeping and eating habits. He had croup for five years from the age of one and one-half. In a lab work-up, blood values were within normal limits except an elevated eosinophil count, but Curschmann's spirals were found in the sputum. Chest x-rays were unremarkable. Adjustments were made in the upper thoracic spine using a posterior to anterior Meric double transverse thrust and rotatory adjustments to the cervical spine. Nutritional supplements were given as well. After the first adjustment, the difficulty in breathing and the wheezing ceased within two minutes post-adjustment and was followed by coughing with a large amount of thick, stringy, mucoid sputum being expectorated. He was adjusted three times a week for four months during which time he had two brief attacks, twice a week for 6 months during which he had six moderate intensity attacks, and once weekly for ten months during which he had three attacks (two during an upper respiratory infections and one after exposure to paint fumes) (19).

Mega gives two brief stories about asthmatics benefiting from chiropractic care in his article on the possible mechanism involved in asthma, particularly the neurological aspect. His introduction to chiropractic was his personal story of having asthma that did not respond to allopathic medical care. A chiropractor began adjusting him and encouraged him to change his diet. He was free of attacks until World War II. During the war, he began smoking and eating poorly and the asthma attacks resumed. After giving up smoking and changing his diet (he could not get adjusted), the attacks ceased. He mentions that he helped a medical doctor's son who had asthma (20).

In another article, Mega states that it is beneficial for asthma sufferers to remove toxic internal conditions. He states that asthmatics suffer from GI tract and liver dysfunction and, in many cases, pancreas dysfunction. He recommends removing acid producing foods, such as meat, eggs, and dairy products, and replacing them with vegetables and fruits. In some cases, the patient is put on three day orange or grapefruit juice fast or two days on distilled water. Adjustments are first given to the sacroiliac joints, then the lumbars, upper thoracic spine, and occiput. Breathing exercises are also given (21).

Jameson, et al. did a pilot study on the effects of chiropractic care on asthma. The measurements used included patient perception, forced vital capacity (FVC), forced expiratory volume in one second (FEV1), and maximum voluntary ventilation (MVV). Measurements were taken immediately prior to the care rendered and within five minutes postcare. Clinicians were 2 senior students and 15 patients aged 9 to 36 participated. Most of the patients were 28 or older. Four were less than 12-years-old. Most had mild to moderate cases of asthma. Seven treatments were given over a five week period. The care rendered included spinal adjustments, soft tissue work, mobilization, and home exercises. The study did not list the levels of the spine adjusted nor the type of adjustments given. Subjects were requested not to use bronchodilators during the four hours prior to receiving care. The trial was performed during an asthma "high risk" season. Subjectively, the subjects were satisfied with the care they received. One subject stopped taking medication and six others reduced their medication. The objective tests showed little overall change (22).

Nilsson and Christiansen did a retrospective study of 100 consecutive cases of patients with asthma from a private chiropractic practice. Seventy-nine of the cases had sufficient information to be included. Not all were children as the age range was 2–63 years old. The number of chiropractic treatments ranged from one to nine over an average period of one month. Those with the best improvement were the youngest patients. Those using the least amount of drugs, who were considered to be the least severe cases, responded the best (23).

Cohen described a case of an 8-year-old female suffering from severe asthma since age 2. The child was delivered in a breech presentation. She was a passenger in two automobile accidents which occurred at ages 6 and 7. The mother smoked during the pregnancy but apparently ceased, and the father still smoked but not in the presence of the child. The child was hospitalized regularly for asthma attacks and usually missed at least one day of school a week. As might be expected, the family was under significant stress because of the severity of her condition. She was prescribed Slobid, Alupent, and Ramtidine and also used three inhalants (Intal, Ventolin, and Azmacort). All medications were taken daily. She had previously been prescribed Prednisone and took Tylenol regularly for other complaints. The chiropractic evaluation found a right short leg, positive Derifield test, thoracolumbar scoliosis, and vertebral subluxation complexes in the upper cervical spine. She was examined three times a week for a month and, if indicated, adjusted. This was later reduced to twice weekly. The parents altered her diet by removing sugar, refined foods, and preservative-laden foods. During the course of care, the

pediatrician reduced the medication. At the time the report was written, the child no longer required drugs and for the past month, had not missed a day in school. It was reported that she had "steady improvement" (24).

Garde presented a case of a 5-year-old male with a history of respiratory problems. He was diagnosed with asthma and prescribed Beclovent and Ventolin inhalants which he used daily. Upon presentation for a chiropractic evaluation, his complaints included activity induced neck pain and stiffness, nasal passages closed by mucous, and an abnormal breathing pattern without diaphragmatic breathing. Based upon the history, examination, and x-ray findings, chiropractic care was commenced. Over a twelve month period, adjustments were made to the cervical, thoracic, and lumbar spine. Postural and breathing exercises were given. During the first six months of care, there were reductions in musculoskeletal abnormalities, his activities increased, use of the inhalers decreased, breathing improved, and mucous rarely blocked his nasal passageways. After a year of care, he ceased using the inhalers and did not have a recurrence of respiratory problems (25).

A study by Wiles and Diakow was based upon interviews of 241 chiropractors on how they care for asthmatic patients. Over 94% adjusted the patient. Other commonly used modalities included nutrition, soft tissue manipulation, exercise, psychotherapy, and electrotherapy. The primary area adjusted (almost 59%) was the T1 to T6 region. This is followed in descending order by the upper cervical spine (occiput to axis), lower thoracic spine (T7-T12), lower cervical spine (C3-C7), ribs, lumbars, and sacroiliac joints. The most common nutritional supplements were vitamin C and A. General dietary advice and avoidance of dietary triggers were made in many cases (2).

Bachman and Lantz describe a case of a nearly 3-year-old male with asthma and enuresis with a traumatic etiology. Metaproterenol syrup and Theodore Sprinkle were prescribed to control the asthma. A year later, an initial chiropractic work-up was done and chiropractic care was initiated. Over a 2-1/2 month period, 28 chiropractic adjustments were given using the Gonstead System protocols. T3, T12, and the second sacral segment were adjusted. After two weeks of care, asthmatic symptoms ceased. Two months later, asthma symptoms recurred along with nightly enuresis following a minor fall. Both symptoms ceased after three visits. A year later, the boy fell off of a horse and both symptoms reappeared. Chiropractic care was administered several months later with cessation of symptoms again. Over a year later, the child was evaluated, and no further symptomatic episodes since the last visit was noted. After beginning chiropractic care, asthma drugs were only used as needed (24).

Peet, et al. did a nine month study with 12 patients between the ages of 4 and 12 years old. Of these, eight completed the trial. Each patient had a medical diagnosis of asthma and was taking at least two drugs for the condition. Each was x-rayed and evaluated posturally with a Metrecom three-dimensional postural computer system. All were found to have abnormal findings. A peak flow meter was used to test lung capacity prior to the first adjustment and pre and post with subsequent adjustments. Mirror image maneuvers were also given to each patient as per the procedures of Chiropractic Biophysics technique. Over the course of care, seven of the eight completing the study were able to reduce or discontinue the use of drugs; lung capacity as measured with a peak flow meter increased, although, some decrease was noted after the tenth visit which was thought to be attributed to a rebound effect with decreased use of drugs. Post x-rays taken at the fifteenth visit showed an improvement in spinal alignment. At the end of the study, seven of the eight parents felt that chiropractic care reduced their child's need for asthma drugs. Four found that their children did not require drugs, and two found that their children did not required inhalers (27).

Burnier gives a brief mention of an 11-year-old male athlete with asthma who had been on theolair and alupent for the condition. A subluxation was determined to be at the C1 level. An adjustment was made at C1. After the first visit, the patient ceased taking medication. Six years after beginning chiropractic care, he had not had asthma nor required medication. Another 9-year-old male was mentioned. He suffered from chronic asthma and was taking Nasalcrom. After the first adjustment to the C1 vertebra, medication was not required and the patient had remained free of asthma at the time the article was written. Both reports were very brief with little information but those noted above (28).

Killinger described a 1949 case from the files of the B.J. Palmer Chiropractic Clinic. This case is an 18-year-old male who had been diagnosed with asthma two years prior to seeking chiropractic care. Attacks occurred daily, typically at night or in the early morning. The attacks began around the time that his neck was stepped on during a football game. Prior to that injury, he had a serious fall from a horse and had neck pain for several years. C1 was found to be misaligned and was adjusted using the Palmer Upper Cervical Specific or toggle-recoil technique. He received two adjustments during the first two weeks of care. Breathing improved and the severity and duration of attacks decreased. Over a five year period, he received care once a year and asthma symptoms had largely abated (29).

Case studies by Lines showed benefits from chiropractic adjustments and avoidance of substances that appeared to trigger asthmatic attacks. The patient or parent is instructed to keep a diary of foods and drinks ingested in the four hours prior to attacks for a seven day period. If foods and drinks do not appear to be the sole precipitators, exposure to other factors such as drugs, tobacco smoke, and physical activities are noted. Two of the three cases described were children, 5-year-old and 2-year-old females. Both had required hospitalization for the most severe attacks and took medication during attacks. Both were found to have foods that appeared to trigger the attacks. Common factors appeared to be milk, artificial colors, monosodium glutamate, and sulfur-based preservatives. These two children were adjusted and the offending foods removed. On 20+ months follow-ups, neither child had further attacks. He found that after a period of time the triggering substances did not have as significant an effect on the patient (30).

Beyeler and Hviid also wrote about the effects of chiropractic care on asthma and respiratory function (31,32).

Outcome Protocols

If chiropractors wish to do outcome studies (objective case reports) on the efficacy of chiropractic spinal adjustments for bronchial asthma, they should follow accepted protocols. Forced expiratory volume in one second (FEV1) and vital capacity are measured. Peak expiratory flow rate (PEFR) has also been used, although, FEV1 is thought to be a better tool. Another area that will probably be used more frequently in asthma studies are quality-of-life questionnaires. Quality-of-life studies are a fast growing area for studying the efficacy of different treatments in this era of managed care. There are many types of quality-of-life questionnaires used for asthma but most are better suited to adults. For children, there are the Childhood Asthma Questionnaires, Children's Asthma Symptom Checklist, and the Life Activities Questionnaire for Childhood Asthma (33).

REFERENCES

1. Tanizaki Y et al. Characteristics of airway responses in patients with bronchial asthma: evaluation of asthma classification systems based upon clinical symptoms. Arerugi: Japanese Journal of Allergology 1993; 42(2):123-130.
2. Wiles MR. Visceral disorders related to the spine. In: Gatterman MI. Chiropractic Management of Spine Related Disorders. Baltimore MD: Williams & Wilkins 1990. pp.391-393.
3. Kaliner M et al. Autonomic nervous system abnormalities and allergy. Annals of Internal Medicine 1982; 96(3):349-357.
4. Flieger K. Controlling Asthma. FDA Consumer 1996; 30(9):18-23.
5. Weitzman M, et al. Recent trends in the prevalence and severity of childhood asthma. JAMA 1992; 268(19):2673-2677.
6. Sly RM. Mortality from asthma. Journal of Allergy and Clinical Immunology 1988; 82(5, Part I):705-717.
7. Beausoleil JL, Weldon DP, McGeady SJ. Beta-2-Agonist metered dose inhaler overuse: psychological and demographic profiles. Pediatrics 1997; 99(1): 40-43.
8. Sly RM, O'Donnell R. Association of asthma mortality with medical specialist density. Annals of Allergy 1992; 68(4):340+.
9. Alberg AJ, Comstock GW. ß-Agonist use and death from asthma (Letters). JAMA 1994; 261(11):821.
10. Crane J, et al. Asthma deaths in New Zealand (Letters). British Medical Journal 1992; 304(6837):1307.
11. Pearce N, et al. Case-control study of prescribed fenoterol and death from asthma in New Zealand, 1977-81. Thorax 1990; 45(2):170-175.
12. Suissa S, Ernst P, Spitzer WO. ß-Agonist use and death from asthma (Letters). JAMA March 16, 1994; 261(11):821-822.
13. Park HS. Early and late onset asthmatic responses following lysine-aspirin inhalation in aspirin-sensitive asthmatic patients. Clinical and Experimental Allergy. 1995; 25(1):28-40.
14. Nihei K, Naitoh H, Ikeda K. Poliomyelitis-like syndrome following asthmatic attack (Hopkins syndrome). Pediatric Neurology 1987; 3(3):166-168.
15. Weiss EB. Bronchial asthma. CIBA Clinical Symposia 1975; 27(1 & 2).
16. Hall IP. The future of asthma. British Medical Journal 1997; 314(7073):45-49.
17. Storms WW, Joyner DM. Update on exercise-induced asthma. The Physician and Sportsmedicine 1997; 25(3):45-48+.
18. Vernon LF, Vernon GM. A scientific hypothesis for the efficacy of chiropractic manipulation of the pediatric asthmatic patient. Chiropractic Pediatrics 1995; 1(4):7-8.
19. Arbiloff B. Bronchial asthma: a case report. Journal of Clinical Chiropractic 1969; 2(4):40-42.
20. Mega JJ. Eliminating toxic conditions in the treatment of bronchial asthma. Journal of the National Chiropractic Association 1960; 30(1):11-12, 67-68.
21. Mega JJ. Bronchial asthma. American Chiropractor 1982 Jan/Feb: 26-27, 66.
22. Jamison JR, et al. Asthma in a chiropractic clinic: a pilot study. Journal of the Australian Chiropractors' Association 1986; 16(4):137-143.
23. Nilsson N, Christiansen B. Prognostic factors in bronchial asthma in chiropractic practice Journal of the Australian Chiropractors' Association 1988; 18(3):85-87.
24. Cohen E. Case history: an eight-year-old asthma patient. Today's Chiropractor 1988; 17(1):81, 122.
25. Garde R. Asthma & chiropractic. Chiropractic Pediatrics 1994; 1(3):9-16.
26. Bachman TR, Lantz CA. Management of pediatric asthma & enuresis with probable traumatic etiology. ICA International Review of Chiropractic 1995; 51(1):37-40.
27. Peet JB, Marko SK, Piekarczyk W. Chiropractic response in the pediatric patient with asthma: a pilot study. Chiropractic Pediatrics 1995; 1(4):9-13.

28. Burnier A. The side-effects of the chiropractic adjustment. Chiropractic Pediatrics 1995; 1(4):22-24.
29. Killinger LZ. Chiropractic care in the treatment of asthma. Palmer Journal of Research 1995; 2(3):74-77.
30. Lines DH. A wholistic approach to the treatment of bronchial asthma in a chiropractic practice. Chiropractic Journal of Australia 1993; 23(1):4-8.
31. Beyeler W. Experiences in the management of asthma. Swiss Annals 1965; 3:111-117.
32. Hviid C. A comparison of the effect of chiropractic treatment on respiratory function in patients with respiratory distress symptoms and patients without. Bulletin of the European Chiropractors Union 1978; 26(1):17-34.
33. McSweeny AJ, Creer TL. Health-related quality-of-life assessment in medical care. Disease-a-Month 1995; 61(1):37-40.

INFANTILE COLIC

Infantile colic is a frustrating problem of unknown etiology. It begins in early infancy and may persist for several months. Colic occurs in 20% to 39% of infants (1).

There are no fully accepted definitions of colic. It is not uncommon for the duration of daily crying to increase until the age of two months. The spells tend to occur during the evening hours (2). The characteristics of colic are paroxysms of crying, abdominal pain, and irritability (3). The crying tends to be incessant and leads to aerophagia, flatulence, and abdominal distention, although the infant eats well and has no problem gaining weight (3). A commonly used criteria for colic is the duration and frequency of crying in these infants who appear to be otherwise healthy and well-fed. One definition is at least three hours of crying per day at a frequency of at least three days a week over a period of at least three weeks (2,4). Another definition splits colic into two groups. There are those fitting the above criteria who are called Wessel's colic group and those with fewer crying days in the non-Wessel's colic group (2).

The physiological basis for colic has been difficult to ascertain. Studies to determine if there is excessive intestinal gas, allergic reaction, intestinal hypermotility, or digestive hormone imbalances have not been found a significant relationship (4). Maternal tension has also been studied but the correlation is poor (4,5). The presence of lactose in milk which leads to carbohydrate fermentation in the colon has been investigated in colicky infants but the results have been mixed (6). Higher levels of the intestinal hormone, motilin, have been studied as a cause but results have been mixed as well (6). Abnormal gall bladder function was found in more colicky infants than in the controls (7).

The potential problem is that a dysfunctional relationship could occur between infant and parent because of the frequent episodes of irritability and "fussiness." Physical abuse is a potential risk (4) (See Chapter 2). Retinal hemorrhage due to shaken baby syndrome should be investigated in suspected cases of child abuse, especially if the behavior of the parent(s) leads one to suspect it (5). Drug abuse, alcoholism, mental illness, and poor living conditions of the parent(s) or other caretaker are important considerations in the history of a child with excessive crying (8).

Other reasons for crying should be investigated as it may be secondary to an underlying disorder. In addition to child abuse, disorders, such as meningitis, otitis media, drug withdrawal, DTP vaccine reaction (See Chapter 3), and hyponatremia, among many others, should be under consideration (5).

Weissbluth and Weissbluth have been studying the relationship of infantile colic to the circannual rhythms. They reasoned that the crying spells usually occur in the evening hours. It tends to be in latitudes away from the equator (this factor may also be due to the few countries at the equatorial regions). The condition seems to begin at least one week after birth—in premature infants, it seems to begin one week after the expected birth date. During the first three months, the infant has not established its circadian rhythm (9-11).

MEDICAL MANAGEMENT

Typically, the parents are reassured that they are handling the child correctly and that the condition usually ceases shortly. Holding, rocking, or patting the infant may help. If the infant feeds quickly, a smaller nipple on the bottle should be tried. A pacifier or feeding in the upright position may help (3,12). A quiet environment or music or placing the infant in a warm bath and gently massaging the abdomen may be beneficial as well (5).

In a study by Colon, 30% of colicky infants from whom cow's milk was removed had a cessation of colic (6). Formula-fed infants have not been found to be more prone to colic than breast-fed infants (4).

In some cases, the colicky infant is given drugs. Some have been given a combination of dimenhydrinate (trade name Dramamine) and Donnatal (a combination of phenobarbital, hyoscyamine sulfate, atropine sulfate, scopolamine hydrobromide, and alcohol). These drugs contain anticholinergic and antimuscarinic agents, smooth muscle relaxants, and CNS depressants. Alcohol reduces lower esophageal sphincter tone which is associated with gastroesophageal reflux. These drugs appear to have caused instances of apparent life-threatening events (ALTE) in a few infants with cardiorespiratory control abnormalities or were otherwise at risk. The ALTE or apnea of infancy were characterized by choking, apnea, and cyanosis. In a study of eight infants under 14 weeks of age receiving the Dramamine/Donnatal combination for colic at the time of their ALTE, five were sleeping at the time of the episode while the remaining three were awake or feeding. Four required CPR, and the other half responded to stimulation (13).

Some colicky infants are given simethicone or methylpolysiloxane. It is used to treat the increased gastrointestinal gas that is thought be a factor in colic through its effect of altering the surface tension of gas bubbles. Simethicone is not absorbed by the GI tract. Results of its use have been questionable. In most trials, it has not been any more effective than placebo (12).

CHIROPRACTIC MANAGEMENT

The Danish Chiropractor's Association conducted a preliminary survey on the disorders of infants for which chiropractic consultations were sought and the outcome of the chiropractic care rendered. Seventy percent or 132 of 189 of the consultations were for infantile colic; average age was six weeks. The average number of treatments was two to three over an average one week time period. Fifty-four percent or 72 were cured, 37% or 48 were improved, and no change was noted in the remaining 12 or 9%. The improvement was considered to be associated with the care rather than spontaneous remission due to the age of the infants (14,15). A prospective cohort study which included 316 colicky infants by the same research group found most improved within the first two weeks. Most adjustments were made to the upper cervical spine (16).

A 9½ month old female was presented at a chiropractic office and was suffering from colic, irritability, and poor sleep. The history noted a difficult birth that resulted in caesarean section and an episode each of ear infection and the flu. The chiropractic evaluation showed postural deviations in the cervical spine and pelvis. Subluxations were found at C1 and T4-6. The orthopedic and neurological examinations were unremarkable. The lower cervical and mid-thoracic spine was adjusted manually while C1 and sacrum were adjusted with an instrument using Chiropractic Biophysics protocol. After the first adjustment, the child slept a full night and was happy. Adjustments were given over a three-week period with continued improvement in the sleep pattern, her personality, and in her posture. She was not seen for a three-week period, at the end of which some of the symptoms reappeared. Adjustments following continued her improvement in her sleep, personality, and postural problems. The colic had abated (17).

In the Gonstead System, a commonly found subluxation in an infant with colic is C2. The doctor holds the infant under the axillae and slowly tilts the child laterally left and right. The doctor watches the head position. If the head does not laterally flex on one side and C2 is palpated as abnormal, C2 is adjusted by a spinous process contact on that side in the sitting position with a primarily posterior to anterior line of drive. Subluxations could conceivably occur anywhere in the spine, necessitating a complete examination (18). Lawrence states that one should evaluate the T5 to T7 region (19).

Outcomes Protocol

Because of the nature of this condition, there are no objective tests for it. Parent diaries on the number of hours the infant cried each day is one means of recording. Another factor to remember is that it usually ceases spontaneously within a few weeks.

REFERENCES

1. Colon AR, DiPalma JS. Colic. American Family Physician 1989; 40(6):122-124.
2. Barr RC, et al. The crying of infants with colic: a controlled empirical description. Pediatrics 1992; 90(1):14-21.
3. Berkow R, ed. The Merck manual of diagnosis and therapy, 14th ed. Rahway, NJ: Merck & Co., Inc. 1982. pp.1852-1853.
4. Miller AR, Barr RG. Infantile colic: is it a gut issue? Pediatric Clinics of North America 1991; 38(6):1407-1423.
5. Nacey KA. Pediatric update: infant colic. Journal of Emergency Nursing 1993; 19(1):65-66.
6. Management of infantile colic. Drug & Therapeutics Bulletin. 1992; 30(4):15-16.
7. Klougart N, Nilsson N, Jacobson J. Infantile colic treated by chiropractors: a prospecive study of 316 cases. Journal of Manipulative and Physiological Therapeutics 1989; 12(4):281-288.
8. Singer JI. A fatal case of colic. Pediatric Emergency Care 1993:171-172.
9. Weissbluth L, Weissbluth M. The photo-biochemical basis of infant colic: pineal intracellular calcium concentrations controlled by light, Melatonin, and Serotonin. Medical Hypotheses 1993; 40(3):158-164.
10. Weissbluth M, Weissbluth L. Colic, sleep inertia, melatonin and circannual rhythms. Medical Hypotheses 1992; 3893):224-228.
11. Weissbluth M, Weissbluth L. Infant colic: the effect of serotonin and melatonin Circadian rhythms on the intestinal smooth muscle. Medical Hypotheses 1992; 39(2):164-167.
12. Metcalf TJ, et al. Simethicone in the treatment of infant colic: a randomized, placebo-controlled, multicenter trial. Pediatrics 1994; 94(1):29-34.
13. Hardoin RA, et al. Colic medication and apparent life-threatening events. Clinical Pediatrics 1991; 30(5):281-285.
14. Chapman-Smith DA. Infantile colic, medical tunnel vision and the art of chiropractic ACA Journal of Chiropractic 1989; 26(11):22-25.
15. Nilsson N. Infant colic and chiropractic. European Journal of Chiropractic 1985; 33(4):264-265.
16. Bronfort G. Is there a role for chiropractic management of infantile colic and chronic childhood asthma? Proceedings of the 1994 International Conference on Spinal Manipulation 1994. pp.131-133.
17. Krauss LL. Case study: birth trauma results in colic. Chiropractic Pediatrics 1995; 2(1):10-11.
18. Anrig CA. Chiropractic approaches to pregnancy and pediatric care. In: Plaugher G, ed. Textbook of Clinical Chiropractic. Baltimore, MD:Williams & Wilkins. 1993. pp.383-432.
19. Lawrence D. Fundamentals of chiropractic diagnosis and management. Baltimore: Williams & Wilkins. 1991.

INFECTIOUS DISORDERS

Infectious diseases have been a major feature of pediatric medical care. Much of the present medical intervention is prophylactic control through the use of vaccines. The goal of it is to establish artificial immunity to specific diseases. Vaccines have been developed or are being refined or developed for diphtheria, measles, rubella, mumps, tetanus, pertussis or whooping cough, hemophilus influenzae, chicken pox, and hepatitis (See Chapter 3). The effectiveness and the negative effects are both highly charged topics.

One area of concern is that artificial immunizations given to children do not confer lifetime immunity and increases the risk of more virulent adult forms of diseases than typically seen in childhood (1). Another concern is that subclinical vaccine-induced encephalitis may be more common than has been recognized and may be the cause of or a cause of many behavioral disorders, autoimmune diseases, SIDS, allergies, and other disorders that seem to be more common (2).

The DTP vaccine in particular seems to be quite problematic. No clinical trials have been conducted on children under one year of age to determine if it is safe or effective. The same dosage is given to a two month old and a four year old (3).

The MMR (measles, mumps, and rubella) vaccine appears to have many complications and questionable efficacy. A substantial number of those vaccinated have been found to be seronegative. The age of being afflicted with these diseases has been increasing. It is well known that those acquiring these condition at later ages have a higher risk of complications. The severity of these diseases may be increasing. In some studies, the incidence of people having these diseases is greater in those who were previously vaccinated (4).

A pilot study by Rose-Aymon et al. contacted chiropractic offices in Iowa and Illinois near Palmer College of Chiropractic. They were trying to determine if there was a relationship between the intensity of chiropractic care and the incidence of four infectious diseases—mumps, measles, rubella, and chickenpox. The study group was non-vaccinated children between the ages of 8 and 15. The results from this preliminary study was that children who had been under chiropractic care for at least one year and had at least seven visits a year had fewer incidences of these diseases than those with less frequent care (5).

The emerging field of psychoneuroimmunology has been finding that all cells of the body are able to receive specific neurochemicals. The immune cells have neurochemical receptors. Psychoneuroimmunology appears to be proving the importance of the nervous system in the function of the immune system as chiropractors have stated for many years.

REFERENCES

1. Miller NZ. Vaccine and natural health. Journal of Naturopathic Medicine 1994; 5(1):32-39.
2. Krieger DB. True value, effect of vaccinations questioned (Letters to Editor). APHA The Nation's Health 1995 September:2-3.
3. Coulter HL, Fisher BL. A shot in the dark. Garden City Park NY: Avery Publishing Group, Inc. 1991. p.13.
4. Lanfranchi RG. The facts and fallacies of measles, mumps and rubella. Journal of the American Chiropractic Association 1996; 33(2):69-75.
5. Rose-Aymon S et al. The relationship between intensity of chiropractic care and the incidence of childhood diseases. Journal of Chiropractic Research 1989; 5(3):70-77.

NOCTURNAL ENURESIS

Nocturnal enuresis is involuntary urination during sleep in the absence of a urological or neurological disorder (1). Two to three million children suffer from this disorder in the U.S (2). Ten to fifteen percent of 5-year-olds and 5% of 10-year-olds are afflicted (1,3).

The cause of nocturnal enuresis is unknown. Heredity seems to be a factor as enuretic patients are three to four times more likely to have a parent who was enuretic (4,5). Electroencephalograph abnormalities have also been found (5). Minor neurological dysfunctions, such as mild hypotonia, clumsiness, or mild dyskinesia are common (5). Nervous system dysfunction may affect bladder function and vasopressin release (4). Bladder size does not seem to be a factor (6).

Nocturnal enuresis tends to be self-limiting as it often resolves spontaneously (3). Unfortunately, there are many cases that persist.

The primary feature of nocturnal enuresis is accidental urination during sleep after the typical period of toilet training should have been accomplished. In its evaluation, neurogenic bladder and enuresis secondary to systemic disorders, such as diabetes, must be ruled out.

One important factor that is not usually mentioned is whether nocturnal enuresis is in some cases, a voluntary behavior. Evening fluid intake may also contribute to the problem.

ANATOMY

The urinary bladder is a reservoir with three orifices: one from each of the two ureters which carry urine from each kidney and one exit orifice to the urethra. The three orifices form the corners of the trigone of the bladder. The bladder wall has three layers: a serous layer which is the peritoneal covering, a triple layer detrusor muscle, and a mucous membrane (7).

The detrusor muscle surrounds the bladder, and its contraction is necessary for voiding. The sphincter muscle controls the outflow to the urethra by contracting to hold urine in or relaxing to void.

Unfortunately, the neurological control of the urinary bladder is somewhat vague. The urinary bladder appears to be controlled by the coordination of the somatic, sympathetic and parasympathetic systems. Parasympathetic preganglionic nerves from S2 to S4 cord levels form the pelvic splanchnic nerve and supply motor control to the bladder. The parasympathetic impulses contract the detrusor muscle and relax the sphincter muscle which allows urination to occur (8,19). Sympathetic fibers are from the T11 to L2 levels and are thought to be inhibitory to the bladder (9). The external sphincter is supplied by the pudendal nerve which arises from S2-S4 spinal nerves (10).

Afferent fibers accompany the efferent supply to the bladder. Afferent fibers that respond to distention of the bladder initially are received at the T12 to L2 dermatome levels and later to the S2 to S4 levels. These impulses ascend the spinothalamic and spinoreticular tracts. The sensation of bladder fullness, often conscious, is thought to be of sympathetic origin (11). Unconscious information from the bladder, e.g., unconscious sensations of bladder fullness so as to cause detrusor contraction, is thought to be via the parasympathetic supply (11). The somatic afferent fibers are thought to convey conscious sensation of urine flowing through the urethra via the pudendal nerve (11). Receptors thought to respond to pain as a result of overdistention form the vesical nerve plexus which is continuous with the inferior hypogastric plexus (9).

There are nerve axons and nerve cell bodies found in the bladder wall. These are neither cholinergic nor adrenergic, but some are peptidergic. The function of these nerves is unknown (11).

The neurologic control of micturition requires complex coordination of the nervous system and is still largely speculative, in particular, its supraspinal control (12).

MEDICAL MANAGEMENT

Behavior modification has been tried with mixed results. Dry bed training and an enuresis alarm in children over age 7 appears to be effective in about 70% of cases (4,5,13). Unfortunately, drugs with low effectiveness have been prescribed more frequently than the more effective behavior training with alarms (4).

Drug therapy usually consists of imipramine or desmopressin. Some have been able to remain dry during the course of treatment with desmopressin (DDAVP) intranasal spray (2,5). Prolonged effectiveness after the termination of treatment has been mixed (12% to 31%) (1,5,13-15), although some studies show greater effectiveness (16). It seems to be most useful on an occasional basis in social situations, such as sleeping away from home (5). Desmopressin is a synthetic analog of arginine vasopressin or antidiuretic hormone (ADH). The altered chemical structure of desmopressin from ADH emphasizes its antidiuretic tendencies and decreases its vasoconstriction or pressor activities (17). Its side effects appear to be uncommon and less than those of imipramine. The effects include hyponatremia, water intoxication, seizures, allergic reaction, and increased blood pressure (17,18).

Imipramine is a tricyclic antidepressant used in some cases of enuresis. The combination of imipramine and desmopressin is not recommended (19).

CHIROPRACTIC MANAGEMENT

There are many reports of the benefits of chiropractic care to reduce or resolve persistent or chronic cases of nocturnal enuresis. Unfortunately, most do not follow the recognized protocol for determining effectiveness or do not have long term follow-up so they fall in the category of "compelling." Most involve one or a handful of cases so are often considered to be anecdotal.

Blomerth describes a case of an 8-year-old male with primary nocturnal enuresis who wet the bed several days out of a week. This patient was receiving concurrent medical care for asthma. The mother checked the sheets on a daily basis. He was adjusted in the lumbar spine with follow-up four weeks later. At follow-up, the mother stated that the bedwetting had ceased. Two months later, he had two wet nights the previous week that appeared to begin after a fall off of a toboggan. The lumbar spine was adjusted with bedwetting ceasing. At one year follow-up, a recurrence was noted that ceased after two adjustments. At two years, another recurrence was noted that ceased after spinal adjustments. The child was not informed that the chiropractic care was for bedwetting as he had low back pain concurrently (20).

Bachman and Lantz describe a case of a 22-month-old male who received chiropractic care for asthma which ceased with care (The case is described in the section on bronchial asthma). After fall a couple of month later, asthma reappeared along with nightly enuresis. Both conditions ceased after three visits. Both recurred after another fall and again ceased after chiropractic care was administered. During a re-evaluation over one year later, it was reported that symptoms of neither had recurred (21).

Marko presents two cases. The first is a 9-year-old male who suffered from daily bedwetting for his whole life. During the first six months of receiving chiropractic adjustments, the day of receiving the adjustment and possibly the following day, he would be dry before being wet again. Changes in adjustments were made and he was adjusted diversified and with protocol of chiropractic biophysics. After one and one-half years of care, he is dry one-half to two-thirds of the time. The second is another 9-year-old male. After being seen by another chiropractor, he was dry some of the time. At this point he received diversified and chiropractic biophysics adjustments. After two to three months, he has been dry with occasional wet nights (22).

A case of an 8-year-old female with daily bed-wetting, in addition to epilepsy, heart murmurs, hypoglycemia, and attention deficit disorder is described by Langley. Adjustments were given in the upper cervical spine. After six months of chiropractic care, the bedwetting had resolved. After one year of care, it has apparently not returned (23).

A chiropractic study using appropriate protocol was conducted by LeBoeuf (24) who used senior chiropractic students as the clinicians rather than experienced chiropractors. This is not to cast aspersions on the skilled student clinicians, but as most people know, experience does make a difference and vertebral subluxations need to be carefully localized and very specific adjustments given. Knowing when to stop adjusting is

very important in these cases as adjusting beyond "correction" of the subluxation seems to coincide with resumption of bedwetting.

Forty-six children with nocturnal enuresis were studied at Palmer Institute of Research. At the end of the study, those receiving conventional manual adjustments had a mean frequency of wet nights of 7.6 nights per 2 weeks versus a sham treatment group with a mean of 9.1 wet nights per 2 weeks (25).

Wells, in 1939, stated that the chiropractor should look for subluxations at the L5 level, sacroiliac joints, and T11 to L2 region (26).

The chapter's authors have found that correction at the sacral segment or upper lumbar/lower thoracic spinal levels, but not limited to those levels, seems to have an effect on many pediatric patients suffering from nocturnal enuresis. It has been often been stated that sacral segments S2 or S3 may require adjustments but that is not always the case. If the sacral segment is involved, there should be a "v" appearance (posterior widening of the sacral segment rudimentary disc space between the involved segment and the superior segment, as well as palpable swelling and tenderness over the tubercle. If those findings are not seen, then you must search around. Sometimes we have found that the correction begins in the sacrum but then shifts to another area, such as the thoracolumbar region. "Overadjusting" the dysfunctioning vertebra may cause a resumption of symptoms; therefore, carefully following the patient's symptoms from visit to visit is necessary in order to prevent this. It is often helpful to find out if the child drinks before going to bed and, if so, cease or restrict it. Occasionally, you will find a child who simply likes to wet the bed.

OUTCOME PROTOCOLS

A detailed history is obviously important. If possible, a pre-care baseline observation of one month can confirm the severity. The parents can keep a diary noting whether each night was dry or wet. A common means of determining a successful outcome is 14 consecutive dry nights. Follow-up evaluations or queries should be made for at least two years. Dry for two years is considered a complete success (1).

REFERENCES

1. Alarm bells for enuresis. The Lancet 1991; 337(8740):523-524.
2. Toffler WL, Weingarten F. A new treatment of nocturnal enuresis (epitomes). Western Journal of Medicine 1991; 154(3):327.
3. Ghandi KK. Diagnosis and management of nocturnal enuresis. Current Opinions in Pediatrics 1994; 6(2):194-197.
4. Maizels M et al. Diagnosis and treatment for children who cannot control urination. Current Problems in Pediatrics 1993; 23(10):402-450.
5. Marcovito H. Treating bed wetting. British Journal of Medicine 1993; 306:536.
6. Watanabe H et al. Treatment system for nocturnal enuresis according to an original classification system. European Urology 1994; 25(1):43-50.
7. Warwick R, Williams Pl. Gray's Anatomy, 35th British ed. Philadelphia: W. B. Saunders Co. 1973. pp.1332-1333.
8. Darby SA. Neuroanatomy of the autonomic nervous system. In: Cramer GD, Darby SA (eds). Basic and Clinical Anatomy of the Spine, Spinal Cord, and ANS. St. Louis: Mosby-Year Book. 1995. pp.335-337.
9. Moore KL. Clinically Oriented Anatomy, 2nd ed. Baltimore: Williams & Wilkins. 1985. p.361.

10. Hanno PM, Wein AJ. A clinical manual of urology. Norwalk CT: Appleton-Century-Crofts. 1987. p.26.

11. Mathers LH. The peripheral nervous system: structure, function, and clinical correlations. Boston: Butterworth Publishers. 1985.

12. Brodal A. Neurological anatomy in relation to clinical medicine. New York: Oxford University Press. 1981.

13. Bradbury MG, Meadows SR. Combined treatment with enuresis alarm and desmopressin for nocturnal enuresis. Acta Paediatrica 1995; 84(9):1014-1018.

14. Donovan B. Treating bed wetting. British Medical Journal 1993; 306(6883):1003.

15. Moffatt ME, et al. Desmopressin acetate and nocturnal enuresis: how much do we know? Pediatrics 1993, 92(3):420-425.

16. Stenberg A, Lackgren G. Treatment with oral desmopressin in adolescents with primary nocturnal enuresis: efficacy and long-term effect. Clinical Pediatrics 1993; Special: 25-27.

17. Shulman LH, Miller JL, Rose LI. Desmopressin for diabetes insipidus, hemostatic disorders and enuresis. American Family Physician 1990; 42(4):1051-1057.

18. Hourihane J, Salisbury AJ. Use caution in prescribing desmopressin for nocturnal enuresis (Letters). British Medical Journal 1993; 306(6891):1545.

19. Hamed M, Mitchell H, Clow DJ. Hyponatremic convulsion associated with desmopressin and imipramine treatment. British Medical Journal 1993; 306(6886): 1169.

20. Blomerth PR. Functional nocturnal enuresis. Journal of Manipulative and Physiological Therapeutics 1994; 17(5):335-338.

21. Bachman TR, Lantz CA. Management of pediatric asthma & enuresis with probable traumatic etiology. ICA International Review of Chiropractic 1995; 51(1):37-40.

22. Marko RB. Bed-wetting: two case studies. Chiropractic Pediatrics 1994; 1(1):21-22.

23. Langley C. Epileptic seizures, nocturnal enuresis, ADD. Chiropractic Pediatrics 1994; 1(1):22.

24. LeBoeuf C, et al. Chiropractic care of children with nocturnal enuresis: a prospective outcome study. Journal of Manipulative and Physiological Therapeutics 1991; 14:110-115.

25. Reed W, et al. Chiropractic management of primary nocturnal enuresis. Journal of Manipulative and Physiological Therapeutics 1994; 17(5):596-600.

26. Wells BF. Enuresis and the spine. National College Journal of Chiropractic. 1939; 12(3):21-22.

OTITIS MEDIA

Otitis media now affects two-thirds of the children in the U.S. by the age of 2. It is the most common cause of hearing loss in children and is the most common diagnosis for a child under age 15 years visiting a medical office (1,2). About 17% of children have three or more episodes of acute otitis media during a six-month period (3). Between 1975 and 1990, there has been a 150% increase in the number of U.S. children diagnosed with OM (1).

The overall cost in the United States of otitis media is in the billions of dollars. There is not only the medical and surgical costs which is thought to be between $3 to $4 billion dollars (3), but also losses due to parents leaving work to care for their children as well as take them for medical care.

Otitis media may occur with or without infection. In many cases the middle ear fluid is sterile.

Ear pain can also be associated with pain referral from the sternocleidomastoideus (SCM) muscle. The SCM may refer pain to the external auditory canal. Pressure on trigger points should reproduce the pain pattern if the SCM is referring pain to the ear (4). The SCM is innervated by C2 and sometimes the C3 spinal nerve and the spinal portion of the spinal accessory nerve which arises from the upper cervical region. Upper cervical dysfunction may affect the SCM which may refer pain to the ear. A less than vigilant physician may be applying inappropriate treatments in these cases.

Breast feeding appears to have a preventive effect (5). This is logical since a healthy mother would be providing antibodies to her child through the milk.

Infectious complications are a risk with otitis media. Infectious complications include meningitis and mastoiditis, among others. The risk may be 1 in 10,000 (6). Another complication is hearing loss. This is usually a result of repeated infections.

MEDICAL MANAGEMENT

Drugs, such as antibiotics, steroids, and anti-histamines and/or decongestants, are commonly prescribed for OME (otitis media with effusion), either singly or in combination. The primary means of management of otitis media is antibiotic therapy. Drugs such as Amoxicillin, Ampicillin, and Cefaclor are commonly prescribed as are other antibiotics. Between 1977 and 1986, prescriptions for antibiotics for children under age 10 increased by 51% while their use in the general population declined (7). In 1986, 42% of all antibiotics prescribed to children were for otitis media (7). In studies of antibiotic-steroid combination drug therapy, antibiotics tended to slow resolution of OME (1).

A major issue today is the increase in the number of drug-resistant bacteria with the continued and indiscriminant use of antibiotics. In practice, cultures are not often taken of the middle ear fluid to determine if there is bacterial or viral involvement. Antibiotic therapy is often initiated merely by complaints of ear pain and the appearance of redness and distention of the tympanic membrane. A recent study by Dagan, et al. found a high failure rate or resistance to antibiotics by otitis media cases which cultured for Streptococcus pneumoniae (8).

Antibiotics are not without risks. Most adverse effects tend to be diarrhea or other GI tract problems or dermatological reactions. Some adverse reactions, though rare, can be quite serious (6).

Steroids such as prednisone and prednisolone are often used in otitis media (9).

When drugs fail, surgical procedures are often employed. Myringotomy with or without tympanostomy tubes is the usual surgical procedures done for OME. The efficacy of tympanostomy tubes is considered to be inappropriate or equivocal in most cases except if there is marked otoscopic findings, antibiotics have failed, and the condition has continued for 90 to 120 or more days (1).

Adenoidectomy or tonsillectomy singly or with myringotomy with or without tympanostomy tubes is not a recommended procedure for children under age 3 without pathology of the adenoids according to an AHCPR Panel consensus. It is considered a clinical option in children 4 and older with chronic bilateral OME, as one study has found that it reduces morbidity and recurrence of OME. In children under age 15, there is a 1 in 10,000 risk from general anesthesia. Significant postoperative bleeding is another risk. In Ontario, Canada, between 1968 and 1973, the mortality rate of combined adenoidectomy and tonsillectomy was 2 in 51,938. With the combined procedures, a 1992 study of operations between March 1987 and April 1990 found a rate of hemor-

Table 13.27. Adverse Effects of Antibiotic Medications Most Often Prescribed for Otitis Media in Children

Antibiotic	Adverse Reaction
Amoxicillin/Ampicillin	Diarrhea, usually mild and dose-related—20–30%
	Cutaneous allergic reaction—3–5%
	Rarely: hematologic, renal, hepatic effects
Amoxicillin/clavulanic acid	Diarrhea—9%
	Nausea and vomiting—4%
	Skin rashes/uticaria—3%
	Rarely: hematologic, renal, hepatic effects (mostly in adults)
Cefaclor	Diarrhea—2.5%
	Rarely: hematologic, central nervous system, renal, hepatic, dermatologic reactions; serum sickness (more common with cefaclor than with other antibiotics)
Cotrimoxazole	Skin rashes/uticaria—2%
	Nausea, vomiting, diarrhea
	Rarely: serious dermatologic reaction; hematologic, cardiovascular, central nervous system, endocrine, renal, hepatic, respiratory effects. Rare fatalities due to sulfonamides
Erythromycin	Gastrointestinal effects (dose related; 2–2.5% for ethylsuccinate or estolate salt administered to children)
	Subclinical elevations of liver function enzymes—5%
	Rarely: serious adverse effects reported for most organ systems
Sulfisoxazole	Gastrointestinal effects, uncommon—less than 1%
	Rarely: serious hematologic (e.g., blood dyscrasias), dermatologic (e.g., Stevens-Johnson syndrome), neurologic, allergic reactions—less than 0.1%

Modified from Agency for Health Care Policy and Research. Clinical Practice Guideline, #12: Otitis Media with Effusion in Young Children. Rockville, MD: U.S. Department of Health and Human Services, 1994; p. 50.

rhage of 0.49% (1). Tonsillectomy for OME is not recommended without signs of tonsillar pathology (1). In one study, reoccurrence rate of effusion following tympanostomy was 98% (10).

The direct and indirect cost of allopathic medical care of 2-year-olds was $1.09 billion. Average per patient cost of drug therapy was $406. Cost for myringotomy and tympanostomy tubes averaged $2,174—with adenoidectomy $3,433 (1).

CHIROPRACTIC MANAGEMENT

There are numerous case studies on children with otitis media who received chiropractic care and had positive results from cases resistant to allopathic medical care. Fallon presents a case of a 3-year-old male who had four previously diagnosed episodes of otitis media within the seven months before seeking chiropractic care. All episodes were treated with antibiotics by a pediatrician. The physical examination was normal except for bulging and swelling of the left tympanic membrane with loss of the light reflex. Chiropractic subluxation complexes were found at the occiput, C4, and T6. Lab work-up was normal except a slightly depressed

WBC level. He was seen five times over a nine day period. On the first day, the occiput was adjusted. On the second day, C4 and T6 were adjusted. On the fifth and ninth day, the occiput was adjusted. After the first adjustment, he had an overnight elevation of his temperature that returned to normal by morning. Tympanometric findings showed improvement with each visit and appeared to be normal by the ninth day (11).

Fysh briefly described two cases as an illustrative introduction to the presentation. The first case was a 22-month-old female with persistent otitis media for the previous eight months. One chiropractic treatment was given with the otitis clearing within 24 hours. On two week follow-up, no signs of otitis media was present. The second case is a 16-month-old male with otitis media for the previous five months. During the five month period, six trips were made to the emergency room for treatment. He had been on continuous antibiotic therapy during the time. One chiropractic treatment was given and the condition cleared up. The four week follow-up, showed no recurrence. Presumably, the "chiropractic treatments" were spinal adjustments and "clearing up" means symptomatic relief and negative tympanoscopic evaluation (12).

Burnier notes two male children, ages 6 and 9, who suffered from chronic ear infections for which antibiotics were given. C2, C3, T12/L1 subluxation were found on one child and occiput/C1and sacral subluxations on the other. Adjustments were given. Three years after beginning chiropractic care, no drugs were needed. No other information was given in these cases (13).

In a retrospective study of 46 children up to age 5 years had been seen in a chiropractic office and had complaints of ear infections or discomfort. Ninety-five episodes of ear infection/discomfort were noted among the 46 children. Of these 55% were male and 45% were female. Antibiotic use had been used by 62%. Multiple previous episodes were noted in 61%. Of the rest, 24% had one previous episode and 15% had no prior episodes. Forty percent were diagnosed with ear infections, the others were thought to have ear discomfort. Three had tympanostomy procedures. Chiropractic care consisted of the use of an Activator instrument as well as pelvic blocking (Sacro-Occipital Technique) and Applied Kinesiology. Outcome was based upon clinical signs and symptoms. Ninety-three percent were noted as improved (10).

The AHCPR Panel could not find randomized, controlled studies on the efficacy of chiropractic care or other nonallopathic procedures in the treatment of OME. They did recommend future studies since these types of therapy were inexpensive and without apparent notable risk of morbidity (1).

ALTERNATIVE MANAGEMENT

Nsouli found that 81 of 104 children with otitis media had allergies to food—one-third to milk and one-third to wheat. When the specific food was removed over a four month period, 70 of the children had improvement in the ear. When the 70 children were given the food back, the otitis media worsened (14). An ENT specialist placed children referred in for tympanostomy on a dairy product-free diet and found that three-fourths of the children did not require surgical intervention (7). Ramauro found a similar resolution by taking an infant with chronic ear infections off of dairy formula (6). Infant formula often contains sugars, particularly corn syrup. An infant may have a difficult time digesting it properly. If this is compounded by antibiotics which destroy the bowel flora, it could lead to problems such as diarrhea and ear infections (6).

The temporomandibular joint and altered bite is thought to be associated with some cases of otitis media.

Much lay information has been provided by Schmidt on otitis media through a book (15) and an article in a magazine (16).

OUTCOME MEASUREMENTS

Outcome studies for otitis media usually involve measurement systems, such as otoscopic evaluation, tympanometry, fluid culture studies, and/or pneumatic otoscopy. Outcome questionnaires that query parents are helpful as well.

REFERENCES

1. Agency for health care policy and research. Clinical Practice Guideline, #12: Otitis Media with Effusion in Young Children. Rockville MD: U.S. Department of Health and Human Services. 1994.
2. Bluestone CD. Otitis media with effusion in young children. Abstracts of Clinical Care Guidelines. 1994; 6(10):1-6.
3. Berman S. Otitis media in children. New England Journal of Medicine June 8, 1995; 332(23):1560-1565.
4. Travell J, Simons D. Myofascial pain and dysfunction: the trigger point manual. Baltimore: Williams & Wilkins. 1983.
5. Duncan B, et al. Exclusive breast-feeding for at least 4 months protects against Otitis media. Pediatrics 1993; 91(5):867-872.
6. Kohl M. Otitis media: treating an effect when you do not know the cause. Alternative & Complementary Therapies 1996; 2(2):68-70.
7. Schmidt MA. Otitis media in children. Journal of Naturopathic Medicine. 1994; 5(1):17-26.
8. Dagan R, et al. Impaired bacteriologic response to oral cephalosporins in acute Otitis media caused by pneumococci with intermediate resistance to penicillin. Pediatric Infectious Disease Journal 1996; 15:980-985. Abstracted in: Sadovsky R. Resistant Pneumococci and Acute Otitis Media (Tips from Other Journals). American Family Physician 1997; 55(4):1364.
9. Rosenfeld RM. New concepts for steroid use in Otitis media with effusion. Clinical Pediatrics 1992; 31(10):615-621.
10. Froehle RM. Ear Infection: A retrospective study examining improvement from chiropractic care and analyzing for influencing factors. Journal of Manipulative and Physiological Therapeutics 1996; 19(3):169-177.
11. Fallon J. Acute Otitis media in a 3-year-old: a case report. Chiropractic Pediatrics 1994; 2(2):1-3.
12. Fysh PN. Acute Otitis media in children: comparison of medical and chiropractic models of treatment. ICA Scientific Symposium. 1991.
13. Burnier A. The side-effects of the chiropractic adjustment. Chiropractic Pediatrics 1995; 1(4):22-24.
14. Nsouli TM, et al. Role of food allergy in serous Otitis media. Annals of Allergy 1994; 73(3):215-219.
15. Schmidt MA. Childhood ear infections. Berkeley CA:North Atlantic Books. 1990.
16. Schmidt MA. Ear infections in children. Mothering 1991 Spring:39-47.

14 Orthopedics

Peter N. Fysh

Orthopedic problems in children are common in general medicine, but are even more commonly encountered in the busy chiropractic clinic. Since the doctor of chiropractic's major area of expertise is the neuromusculoskeletal system, a child with symptoms of bone and/or joint pain might be brought to a chiropractor for evaluation. Although most adult orthopedic problems are straightforward in diagnosis, this is not always the case in the pediatric population. Pediatric spinal problems, particularly, require in-depth knowledge and experience for their accurate identification and management. Evaluation of pediatric problems requires a trained perception on the part of the doctor, in part because of communication difficulties, but also because of the young child's inability or reticence to demonstrate and perform tests appropriately. Examination of the child's movements during play and during relaxed walking and running is perhaps an ideal time to gather clinical data. Abnormalities of gait and posture are best evaluated without the child being made aware of the process, whereas ranges of joint motion can be estimated by visually examining the child's body movements before the physical examination.

Some of the most common pediatric problems confronting the chiropractor include conditions such as otitis media, asthma, tonsillitis, headache and enuresis; conditions that at first glance to the untrained may not appear to involve the neuromusculoskeletal system. The orthopedic conditions appearing in the pediatric "top ten" include mainly spine-related conditions, such as neck pain, low back pain, thoracic pain, scoliosis, and growing pains. As an introduction to understanding children's spinal problems, the doctor should have a good knowledge of the process of growth and development of the spine.

Development of the Spine

An understanding of the growth and development of the vertebral column is essential to the ability of the doctor of chiropractic in developing and modifying spinal evaluation and treatment plans to the needs of the pediatric patient.

At birth the length of the spinal column represents 40% of the total body height, the same percentage as in the adult. During embryonic development, the spine is shaped with a single primary anterior concave curve, which later changes to adapt to the human biped position. At birth, the secondary lordotic curves in the cervical and lumbar spinal regions are not fully developed. The cervical and lumbar lordoses continue to develop after birth. The cervical curve develops in response to the upright posture of the head at around 3 months and should be established by the time the infant can sit upright, at about 9 months. The lumbar curve develops in response to the child adopting the standing position and appears by the age of 12 months. The lumbar lordosis is well developed by the age of 18 months in response to walking, an activity that requires a postural shift so that the center of gravity can be maintained over the legs (1).

Spinal Growth

At birth the length of the vertebral column is approximately 24 cm. By the end of the adolescent growth phase this length will have increased to 70 cm. During the first year of life, the spine will increase in length by 12 cm and another 15 cm between the ages of 1 and 5 years. The first 5 years is the time of greatest spinal growth, even greater than that of the adolescent growth period.

From age 5 to 10 years the annual rate of spinal growth slows to 10 cm and increases again once puberty is reached. From 10 to 18 years, the spinal length increases by 20 cm in males and by 15 cm in females.

At around puberty, ossification centers appear for the vertebral secondary ring epiphyses and for the tips of the spinous and transverse processes. Ossification of the spine is finally completed at approximately 22–25 years of age. The lateral spinal radiograph at birth shows an anterior notch in the center of each spinal vertebrae, more prominent in the thoracic region, caused by the persistence of the intersegmental artery (2) (Fig. 14.1).

INTERVERTEBRAL DISC

The adjacent surfaces of each vertebrae are strongly connected to each other by fibrocartilaginous intervertebral discs. In the newborn and young infant, the intervertebral space appears greater than the actual height of the intervertebral disc due to the presence of the non-ossified part of the adjacent vertebral bodies. Although this might give the spine the appearance of weakness, in fact the connection of the vertebral body to the intervertebral disc is strong, such that in the case of vertebral

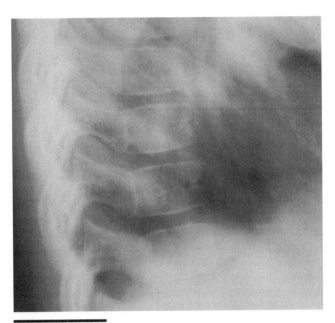

Figure 14.1.   Normal lateral radiograph of the thoracic spine demonstrating the radiolucency of the intersegmental artery.

fracture with displacement, there is no separation between the vertebral body and the intervertebral disc. As a result of this, the strength of the spine at birth is such that the bodies and the neural arches may be considered to be almost entirely ossified.

ATLAS

At birth, the anterior arch of atlas consists principally of fibrocartilage. The atlas vertebra has an anterior ossification center which usually appears by the end of the first year of life and is responsible for the development of the anterior arch and the greater portion of the lateral masses. Each neural arch has its own ossification center, present at birth, which is usually ossified by 6 to 12 months of age. The posterior arch of atlas is usually closed by the age of 3 years, but may occasionally remain ununited throughout life, as in spinal bifida occulta. The neural arches join with the anterior arch and fuse at about age 7 years. In the formative years, the anterior atlas would appear to derive much of its strength from the attachment of the transverse ligament to the odontoid process and from the odontoid process attaching to the anterior arch by ligamentous structures.

AXIS

The axis vertebra has four ossification centers at birth which are already partially ossified. The unossified sections are attached to each other by cartilaginous tissue. The synchondroses between the neural arches and the body fuse between 2 and 3 years of age and those between the body and odontoid process between the ages of 3 and 6 years. Occasionally the growth center may persist between the odontoid process and the axis body until about 11 years of age. This cartilaginous matrix is the homologue of the intervertebral disc. Traumatic disturbance of this growth center has been suggested as the cause of the development of an ossiculum odontoideum, or ununited odontoid process (3). The mechanism is proposed as an unrecognized injury to the C2 vertebra early in life, which causes pseudoarthrosis of the dens, disrupting the blood supply and resulting in progressive atrophy. The cephalad tip of the odontoid process at birth appears Y-shaped. The ossification center in the odontoid tip appears at about the age of 3 to 6 years and fusion is usually complete by about the age of 12 years. Failure of fusion of this secondary ossification center is known as an ossiculum terminale.

C3 TO C7

The bodies of the cervical vertebrae below the axis are almost fully ossified at birth. The neural arches close posteriorly at around age 2 to 3 years and anteriorly with the vertebral body at about age 3 to 6 years. The tips of the spinous processes and transverse processes appear by age 15 to 16 years and fuse to the rest of the processes by age 25 years. Ossification of the peripheral portion of the vertebral bodies takes place at around age 20 years. Hence the uncovertebral joints of von Luschka, i.e., lateral interbody joints, are not radiographically visible in the pediatric cervical spine.

CERVICAL RIBS

The anterior portion of the transverse process of the 7th cervical vertebra develops from a separate ossification center which usually fuses with the main ossification center around the age of 6 years. Failure of correct ossification of this section gives rise to the development of a cervical rib. The shaft of the cervical rib grows laterally and forward into the posterior triangle of the neck. In this area it may come into contact with the lower trunk of the brachial plexus affecting the C8 and T1 spinal nerves and the subclavian vessels, compressing these structures against a hypertonic anterior scalene muscle with resulting neurological and vascular symptoms (i.e., thoracic outlet syndrome).

THORACIC SPINE

The ossification of the thoracic spine is completed in the same pattern as that of the lower cervical spine, but closure of ossification centers generally occurs earlier than in the cervical spine. The ossification centers for the tips of the transverse and spinous processes appear at about 14 to 16 years of age and finally fuse with their more central structures around 25 years of age.

LUMBAR SPINE

Ossification of the lumbar spine is completed in the same pattern as that of the lower cervical spine, but closure of ossification centers generally occurs somewhat later. Similarly to the cervical spine, the ossification centers for the tips of the transverse and spinous processes appear at about 15 to 16 years of age and finally fuse with the main structure by about age 25 years.

Sacrum

At birth, the sacrum is mainly cartilaginous and represents typical vertebrae in that each segment ossifies independently. Fusion of one sacral segment to another does not commence until around puberty and the bodies of the sacral segments do not unite with one another until after the age of 20 years. The sacral discs may remain unossified until mid-life (4).

Coccyx

At birth the coccyx is made up of four rudimentary cartilaginous vertebrae. The ossification process starts after birth with the development of separate secondary ossification centers for each segment. Ossification centers develop at widely separated intervals from the first to the twentieth year of life. The coccygeal segments fuse with each other progressively up until about the age of 20 years. Late in life, the sacrum and coccyx may eventually fuse.

Growth of the Trunk

Although the spine grows at a steady rate after the first year of life, the trunk undergoes a period of rapid increase in height during the adolescent growth spurt at about 12 years of age in females and 14 years in males. This increase is most significant in the lower extremities and accounts for this rapid height increase combined with a relatively steadily lengthening spinal column (5).

Developmental Patterns and Anomalies

Crawling

Babies will usually be ready to crawl actively at about 9 to 10 months. Crawling is a natural protective reflex designed to prevent asphyxiation when the infant is lying face down. Delay in crawling may be an indication of orthopedic problems, such as congenital hip dislocation, or of neurological problems, such as cerebral palsy. However, the commencement of crawling is highly variable and parents should not be overly concerned if the child is a late starter. In one British study of infants who had not yet commenced to walk by the age of 18 months, 32 percent of the study group had an identifiable pathology to explain their late-walking (6).

The crawling action requires simultaneous use of opposite extremities, i.e., right arm with left leg, and vice versa, in a reciprocating motion. Because of the decussation of the outflow tracts from the brainstem to the spinal cord, the nerve impulses for motor activity in the extremities originate on the opposite sides of the brain, i.e., left brain controls right extremities and vice versa. Since crawling requires the simultaneous use of opposite extremities, each movement requires the use of both the right and left hemispheres of the brain. The act of crawling therefore is a complex action of neurological coordination. Studies of children who were categorized as "early walkers," i.e., those who crawled for a comparatively short period before commencing to walk, demonstrated lower performance scores on pre-schooler assessment tests support-

ing the importance of early cross-crawl patterning movements in the development of sensory and motor systems of the body and general motor skill development (7).

Baby Walkers

Baby walkers represent a cause of significant injury in the infant population. The use of walkers and other apparatus designed to prematurely assist infants to assume erect posture should be discouraged both as a potential cause of injuries including possible finger amputation. In a study of infants suffering trauma from the use of baby walkers, 88 percent of injuries were caused by a fall down stairs (8). A study using EMG demonstrated that the use of infant walkers alters the mechanics of locomotion inducing substantial mechanical errors in the walking process (9). Another study suggested that for some infants, the excessive use of babywalkers alters the pathway of normal locomotor development (10). One 1991 US survey found an estimated 27,804 injuries requiring treatment that resulted from the use of baby walkers, with most of the victims being under 2 years of age (11). A study of the mechanisms of walker-related injuries identified stairway falls (71%), tip-overs (21%), falls from a porch (3%), and burns (5%). Twenty-nine percent of the infants suffered significant injuries which included skull fractures, concussion, intra-cranial hemorrhage, cervical spine fracture and death (12). Baby walker-related injuries represent the third most common cause of injury in infants from 7 to 14 months and the use of such devices should be actively discouraged (13).

Walking

The age at which children commence walking can vary considerably. Typically, commencement of walking can occur at any time from 7 to 15 months. Parents of a "late walker" can be encouraged by the variability of the walking commencement date. The child's body has an innate understanding of the appropriate stage at which the bones, ligaments, joints, muscles and the nervous system are ready and coordinated to withstand the forces of erect stature. Encouraging children to walk prematurely may predispose them to increased stress on spinal musculo-skeletal structures, as well as to possible delay in developing neurological coordination. Several studies have hypothesized the importance of early crawling experience in the development of sensory and motor systems of the body and general motor skill development. One 1991 study which compared the performance of crawlers and non-crawlers on the Miller Assessment for Preschoolers showed non-crawlers to have lower average scores (14).

Initially the toddler walks on the fore foot or with a broad-based flat-footed gait with the hips held in slight flexion and no reciprocating arm swing. By the age of 2 years, most toddlers will have established an upright, heel-strike gait and will swing the arms. Abnormal walking patterns in young children are a source of much interest to the clinician.

A waddling gait may be an indicator of infantile coxa vara or of an undetected congenital hip dislocation, while abnormalities in position and placement of the feet may be due to congenital or acquired anomalies in the bones or joints of the lower extremities or pelvis. For example, medial or internal

(In) displacement of the ilium (the PSIS as the point of reference) joint with fixation may produce lateral rotation of the ipsilateral leg and foot. The converse is also true, where lateral sacro–iliac displacement with fixation may cause medial displacement of the ipsilateral leg and foot. Because sacro–iliac joint subluxation is frequently accompanied by a physiological short leg, frequent falls by a young infant while walking or running should be an indication to evaluate the position, alignment and length of the lower extremities.

Positional changes of the lower extremities should be evaluated to assess the likelihood of spontaneous correction or possible pathology. During the first year of life, rotational problems may present. At birth, the newborn infant's feet will usually turn inwards due to the typical position occupied in-utero. This internally rotated condition of the feet is called metatarsus adductus and usually resolves spontaneously by the end of the first year in 90% of infants (15). A most important step in examining an infant with metatarsus adductus is to check for congenital hip dysplasia, since CHD is more common in this group. Most cases of in-toeing resolve spontaneously by the end of the first year of life and require only observation on the part of the clinician. Torsional deformities of the lower extremity are covered in more detail later in this chapter.

Postural Abnormalities

Postural evaluation is an important component of the physical examination of the growing child. Evaluation of postural abnormalities should be made searching for evidence of underlying musculoskeletal or neurological problems. The following postural distortions may indicate an underlying problem: lateral head tilt, head rotation, unleveled shoulders, prominent scapulae, thoracic kyphosis, unleveled iliac crests, lumbar hyperlordosis or hypolordosis, internal or external rotation of an ilium, leg or foot and measured discrepancy of the length of the lower extremities.

Growth Rate

The velocity of growth in children varies with age, being particularly noticeable around the adolescent period. The average growth rate in children is around 4 to 6 cms each year, from 2 years of age until the commencement of the adolescent growth spurt. Once the adolescent growth spurt is reached, around age 11 to 12 in girls and 13 to 14 in boys, the rate of growth increases significantly to around 6 to 12 cm per year. The increase in growth during this period is almost entirely due to increase in length of the lower extremities and is not due to increased growth rate of the spinal column, which remains stable at around 2 cm per year. The adolescent growth spurt normally lasts around 2 years and completion of growth is normally achieved about 4 years after its start. The greater final height in males is reportedly due to a longer and more intense adolescent growth phase. The onset of the adolescent growth spurt can be reliably estimated by the stage of body development. In girls, the adolescent growth spurt precedes sexual maturation and is nearly complete by menarche, while in boys, it corresponds with the onset of testicular and penile enlargement.

Because the greatest risks of progressive spinal deformities have been identified as occurring during the rapid adolescent growth phase, it is important to have a reliable method of evaluating cessation of growth. Radiologic signs can be obtained from the wrist as an indication of growth completion. If the distal ulnar epiphysis is closed then growth can be considered to be almost complete. The most reliable estimate of completion of spinal growth is closure of the vertebral secondary ring epiphyses which usually occurs by the age of 17 to 18 years in girls and by 18 to 19 years of age in boys.

Normal rates of childhood growth have been extensively studied and are recorded in standard anthropometric charts. Length and weight percentiles for birth through 36 months are presented in Figure 14.2 (A–D). A slow rate of growth is of concern when the child's height is less than the third percentile for age, i.e., less than three standard deviations below the mean for that age. Growth rate should also be of concern when the child's height drops below a previously established growth curve as this may be an indication of an underlying pathology or metabolic problem.

Spinal Problems in Children

The diagnosis and treatment of spinal problems in children is a specialized task and should be undertaken with great care to ensure that a serious problem is not masquerading as a relatively minor complaint. Spinal problems in children can be difficult to diagnose. In infants, spinal problems may present simply with irritability, poor feeding and restlessness. Spinal pain can have many causes, such as birth trauma, trauma due to falls, motor vehicle accidents and child abuse, acquired torticollis, spondylolysis or spondylolisthesis, infections associated with meningitis, vertebral osteomyelitis or diskitis, and finally spinal pain can be due to juvenile rheumatoid arthritis. The causes of spinal pain therefore, include not only the ubiquitous vertebral subluxation, but also disease processes which directly attack the vertebrae and joint structures.

Symptoms of back and neck pain in children can sometimes be difficult to interpret due to difficulty in communicating effectively with young patients, but also because such symptoms do not always appear to be associated with or to specifically relate to spinal problems. As a child's age increases, so does their ability to communicate more effectively, thereby assisting the clinician in identifying the location and intensity of the symptoms and any associated activity which might have caused the problem. In evaluating the various spinal problems in children, one should be well aware that childhood back pain may be caused by a wide range of disorders. Whereas studies have shown that adult back pain most often has a non–pathological cause, back pain in children is more frequently associated with identifiable pathology (16). The spine in children is extremely flexible due to elasticity of the muscles, ligaments and intervertebral discs. Such increased elasticity provides for increased joint ranges of motion which allows for the extreme spinal positions associated with normal childhood activity.

Increased elasticity of spinal capsular ligaments, coupled with the falls and trauma of childhood, can predispose young children to vertebral subluxation (see Chapter 12). At around

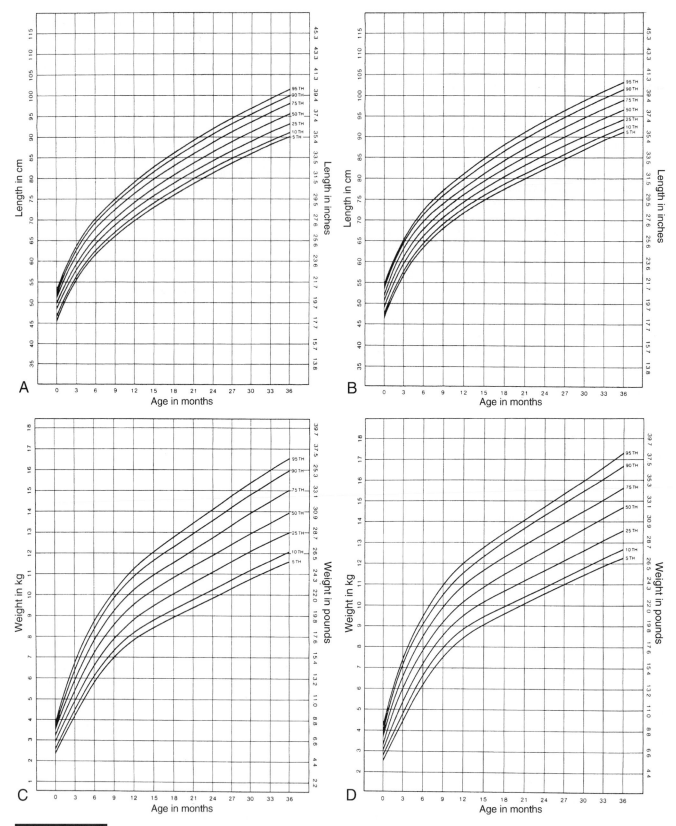

Figure 14.2. A. Length by age percentiles for girls aged birth-36 months. Reprinted with permission from Hamill PVV, Drizd TA, Johnson CL, et al. Physical growth: National Center for Health Statistics percentiles. Am J Clin Nutr 1979; 32:609. B. Length by age percentiles for boys aged birth-36 months. Reprinted with permission from Hamill PVV, Drizd TA, Johnson CL, et al. Physical growth: National Center for Health Statistics percentiles. Am J Clin Nutr 1979; 32:610. C. Weight by age per-

centiles for girls aged birth-36 months. Reprinted with permission from Hamill PVV, Drizd TA, Johnson CL, et al. Physical growth: National Center for Health Statistics percentiles. Am J Clin Nutr 1979; 32:611. D. Weight by age percentiles for boys aged birth-36 months. Reprinted with permission from Hamill PVV, Drizd TA, Johnson CL, et al. Physical growth: National Center for Health Statistics percentiles. Am J Clin Nutr 1979; 32:612.

the time of puberty, the spine gradually loses some of its elasticity and continues to lose flexibility as the teenage years progress.

During the adolescent phase, the developing spine is rapidly gaining strength through increasing bone density and progressive ossification, resulting in the closure of more epiphyseal growth centers. The adolescent patient will go through phases of rapid growth where height might increase by 6 inches in as many months. This rapid growth phase, known as the "adolescent growth spurt," is associated more with growth of the lower extremities than it is with growth of the spine. Growth of the spine remains fairly constant during adolescence, growing at about the same rate from the age of 5 years onwards. The adolescent phase is also a time when body structures are subjected to increasing trauma, through sporting activities, increasing body weight and increased velocity of movement. The effect of these changes can amplify any existing congenital or acquired spinal weaknesses, such as facet tropism, spondylolysis, spondylolisthesis or the results of previous spinal trauma. Spinal problems in children can be due to many causes and can be categorized by age group (Table 14.1).

Birth Trauma

The trauma of the normal birth process with its commonly applied rotation, lateral flexion and traction of the cervical spine has been identified as a possible cause of neurological trauma as well as vertebral misalignment with subluxation/fixation of the upper cervical spinal segments. Spinal problems associated with birth trauma can be associated with poor feeding, regurgitation, fussiness, tremors, and/or sleeping difficulties in the newborn infant. Atlas (C1) vertebral subluxation may be an etiological factor for a newborn infant who is difficult to feed, who spits-up consistently during and after each feeding, and who sleeps for only short periods of time. The problem with an infant who will only nurse from one breast and refuses or is difficult to feed on the opposite side can sometimes be corrected by restoring normal function to the involved cervical spinal segment(s).

Falls

It is not uncommon for infants to suffer trauma from falls encountered in negotiating their way through the developmental processes of the first two years of life. Such traumas may be due to rolling off a bed or changing table, crawling onto a stairway or to trauma associated with the monumental task of learning to walk. All of these examples can be common situations encountered in the infant's life which predispose the child to spinal problems and warrant regular spinal examinations. With increased mobility, growing children will encounter an even greater number of traumatic situations which may affect the spine, possibly resulting in back or neck pain or asymptomatic joint subluxation. At this stage of life, the spine is still undergoing secondary ossification, i.e. the vertebral structures are still comprised largely of cartilage which is being progressively ossified. Due to the presence of such an abundant mass of cartilage and to its relative flexibility, young children are less disposed to vertebral fractures. A further characteristic of the young spine is the comparative elasticity of the

Table 14.1. Causes of Back and Neck Pain by Age Group

Infants (0–2 yrs)

  Trauma/subluxation: falls, motor vehicle accidents, child abuse; congenital deformities

  Spinal cord malformation; tethering of the cord

  Spina bifida

  Klippel-Feil syndrome

  Malignancy; spinal cord tumor

  Birth trauma: rotation, lateral flexion or traction of neck

  Infection; vertebral osteomyelitis, diskitis

  Torticollis

Pre-school and grade-school years (3–10 yrs)

  Trauma/subluxation: falls, motor vehicle accidents, child abuse

  Infection; vertebral osteomyelitis, diskitis

  Spondylolysis, spondylolisthesis

  Tumor: leukemia

  Juvenile rheumatoid arthritis

  Torticollis

Adolescent years (11–19 yrs)

  Trauma/subluxation: sports injuries, overuse syndrome, motor vehicle accidents

  Poor posture

  Spondylolysis, spondylolisthesis

  Facet tropism (overuse syndrome)

  Scoliosis

  Ankylosing spondylitis

  Scheuermann's disease

  Infection; vertebral osteomyelitis, diskitis

  Tumors (benign): osteoid osteoma

  Tumors (malignant): osteoblastic sarcoma, Ewing's sarcoma

intervertebral ligament structures. While such increased elasticity provides a child with increased joint ranges of motion, it can also be the cause of vertebral subluxation, hypermobility or dislocation.

Motor Vehicle Injuries

Motor vehicle accidents frequently involve the entire family. However, it is not uncommon for infants and children involved in such incidents to go unchecked either medically or by a chiropractor simply because they have no overt symptoms, while the parents themselves receive an appropriate clinical evaluation. Because of the increased flexibility of an infant's spinal column, spinal trauma such as might be encountered in a motor vehicle accident is more likely to result in spinal cord injury, with associated neurological symptoms, than it is to result in severe damage to the motion segment soft tissues although this is extremely variable. It is important that every occupant involved in a motor vehicle accident, whether old or young, have a physical examination to check for the presence of such potential injuries. The potential must be recognized for a relatively minor stiff neck after an auto accident to be the precursor to long term spinal degeneration which eventually may destroy the alignment, biomechanics and integrity of joint structures, particularly in the cervical spine.

Motor vehicle occupant death rates for pediatric ages are extremely high. The highest death rate for infants is seen in cases where an unrestrained infant is riding on the lap of an adult. The reason for such a high mortality rate is because the child's effective weight is markedly increased during the deceleration phase of a collision, far exceeding the ability of the adult to hold on to the child. Further, the weight transfer of the adult during the collision may crush the infant against the interior of the vehicle. The highest death rate for motor vehicle injuries is in the adolescent population. Although teenagers travel fewer overall miles than adults, their lack of driving experience, coupled with driving speed and poor judgment has been identified as the likely cause of this increased mortality.

Children who are involved in auto accidents frequently suffer injuries without showing any overt symptoms. This fact is often overlooked after an auto accident, simply because the child does not complain of pain symptoms or because an infant or toddler is unable to communicate their symptoms to their parents. Symptoms such as irritability, lethargy, poor feeding, repeated squinting of the eyes, and restlessness may be the only evidence that a young infant has suffered injuries. In older children who are better able to communicate, symptoms may include fatigue, irritability, headache, or neck pain with or without restricted range of motion.

Injuries suffered by a child in an auto accident can be the cause of spinal problems which may not be evident for months or, in some cases, years after the incident. But worse than this, the children involved may have suffered significant spinal injuries which require immediate chiropractic attention, but which remain quite hidden due to the inability of children to communicate their symptoms. A thorough and careful parental consultation and pediatric evaluation of each child involved in an auto accident is essential to detect spinal problems that can have long-term consequences to the child's health.

The need for a detailed and thorough examination of the spine of all children involved in auto accidents is well documented in the pediatric literature. Because children have greater flexibility in their necks they are more likely to suffer spinal cord damage than they are to have fractures of the spinal vertebrae. This fact is due to the different rates of stretch between the spinal column, comprised of the vertebrae, muscles and ligaments, and the spinal cord which carries all important nerve impulses to and from the brain. The spinal column has been shown experimentally to have up to 5 cm (2

in) of stretch before vertebral or ligament damage occurs, whereas the spinal cord residing inside the spinal column has only a 1.25 cm (0.5 in) of stretch before rupture and hemorrhage can occur (16). As a result of this difference in the rate of stretch between these two structures, young children are more likely to suffer spinal cord and nerve damage than they are to fracture vertebrae or injure the ligament structures which hold the spinal vertebrae together. As a result of this potential for children to suffer spinal injuries without any apparent symptoms, it is important that all children involved in auto accidents, no matter how minor, should receive a detailed and thorough spinal examination to ensure that a proper differential diagnosis has been made. It should include a detailed and thorough examination of the child's nervous system to rule out any possible spinal cord damage. The neurological component of this examination requires evaluation of cranial and peripheral nerves, for both motor and sensory deficits. In very young infants, less than 6 months of age, evaluation of the primitive reflexes also will provide additional information on the status of the nervous system.

Parents ignoring the possibility of pediatric injury can lead either to short term effects on the child's health or to long term problems such as premature spinal degeneration, or both. The long term costs of ignoring the need for a child's spinal examination can be significant and may destine the child to a future of spinal pain, stiffness, spinal instability, headaches and other associated problems.

Child Abuse

Child abuse should be suspected in any infant presenting with injuries which do not correlate with the case history data (see Chapter 2). Injuries caused by abuse may sometimes be the result of the frustration of parents to control an infant's constant crying or other persistent symptom. Some infant habits may have a physical cause which can include early spinal trauma. All cases of non-accidental trauma must be recognized and reported by the attending primary care physician consistent with the laws of the particular jurisdiction. Child abuse incidents may be the cause of complaints of back and neck pain in children that a parent or guardian brings for treatment. In its simplest form, child abuse may be the cause of joint injuries or of recurrent headaches which have no other clinical explanation. More severe problems, such as fractures and joint dislocations, can be the result of increasingly violent trauma inflicted upon a child by a parent or guardian. Fractures are the most common result of child abuse in the toddler and skeletal x-rays are indicated in any case where suspicion of child abuse is present (17). Occasionally an x-ray finding of an old healed fracture site which does not correlate with the history, and for which detailed questioning cannot uncover the cause, may be evidence of previous or ongoing child abuse. Skeletal injuries can be dated so that the date of injury can be accurately estimated. The radiographic appearance of a healing bone after acute trauma follows the following predictable pattern; 0 to 5 days, radiolucent fracture line apparent, but no evidence of healing; 5 to 10 days, periosteal new bone formation evident; 10 to 14 days, soft callous formation; 14 to 21 days, hard callous formation (18).

Problems of the Neck and Cervical Spine

Children can present with an array of problems associated with the cervical spine. This section includes a discussion of problems such as torticollis, Klippel-Feil syndrome and developmental anomalies such as spina bifida, hemivertebra and odontoid anomalies. In addition to descriptions of these classic conditions, this chapter also includes discussion of other significant problems of the newborn cervical spine, as well as complaints of neck pain in children following involvement in an automobile accident, since this can be a significant cause of cervical spinal trauma (19).

Newborn infants can have subluxated spinal vertebrae. The upper cervical complex is an area of the spine which is frequently subjected to significant trauma during the birth process. Studies of newborn infants have identified the cervical spine and the atlanto-occipital junction as being the cause of a multiplicity of clinical findings affecting the newborn infant. Published studies have identified signs and symptoms of suboccipital strain/sprain in newborn infants and have highlighted the apparent clinical effectiveness of spinal adjustments in correcting the problem (20).

KISS Syndrome

Kinematic imbalances due to suboccipital strain, otherwise known as KISS syndrome, identify the pathogenic potential of the craniovertebral junction to produce a constellation of clinical findings. The most common clinical findings associated with KISS syndrome include restricted motion of the cervical spine, torticollis, scoliosis of the cervical spine, asymmetric paraspinal muscle development, delayed development of the femoral heads and acetabulae and asymmetrical or slow development of motor skills. Other findings include facial scoliosis, opisthotonus (retraction of the head and arching of the back, with infant unable to hold the head erect), deformities of the feet, restless sleep and poor feeding (20). The most common etiological factors causing suboccipital strain include intrauterine malposition of the fetus, the use of forceps or vacuum extraction during the birth process, prolonged labor and multiple fetuses. The incidence of these risk factors in affected infants varies significantly from the established normal birth statistics (20).

Correcting subluxation/fixations of the occipito-atlantal and the atlanto-axial joints of the cervical spine simplifies and shortens the course of the infant's problems and significantly reduces the need for physiotherapy. Indications for spinal adjustment in affected infants depend on first recognizing the clinical symptoms and then fitting them with the physical and radiological findings. Radiographic findings can be used to accurately evaluate the alignment of the atlanto-axial and occipito-atlantal joints as an aid in determining the most appropriate direction of adjustment, as well as to rule out the presence of any spinal deformities. Identification of suboccipital strain requires delicate digital palpation. Initial indications may be increased pain sensitivity of the suboccipital and upper cervical spinal regions and/or restricted movements of the head and neck. The atlas vertebra fixed on the right side relative to the occiput, has been reported in several studies to be the more frequent finding (20,21). Suboccipital strain can be managed effectively with specific adjustments of the cervical spine, usually only with a few treatments (20).

Torticollis

Torticollis is characterized most commonly by unilateral spasm or contracture of the sternocleidomastoid muscle (SCM). This condition is recognizable in a patient by the tilting of the head to one side while the chin is rotated away to the opposite side. Torticollis is generally classified as either congenital or acquired. The etiological factors include birth trauma, especially with breech birth and forceps delivery, spinal cord tumor, congenital spinal anomalies, such as hemivertebra in the cervical spine and subluxation of a cervical segment. Atlanto-axial rotatory subluxation is now a well recognized cause of childhood torticollis. Such rotatory displacements may occur spontaneously in-utero or be associated with trauma (22). Subluxations in other locations of the spine can also cause the torticollis or lateral head tilt presentation.

CONGENITAL TORTICOLLIS

Congenital torticollis, also known as congenital wryneck, may be present in the newborn infant or may appear within the first few weeks of life. The characteristic positional changes, caused by the SCM spasm, may be noted at birth or in some cases, may not be evident until the infant is 2 to 4 weeks of age. Congenital torticollis is commonly associated with hematoma and unilateral fibrotic contractures in the SCM, possibly caused by stretching trauma during the birth process or by the position of the head in-utero. If fibrotic contracture or a hematoma is the cause, then a mass, usually 1 to 3 cm in diameter, should be palpable in the involved SCM. If no mass can be palpated in the SCM, then x-rays of the cervical spine should be obtained to evaluate other possible causes of congenital torticollis. Congenital torticollis is frequently found in conjunction with congenital hip dysplasia and all newborns with congenital torticollis should be examined for this associated hip condition. Other causes of torticollis may include subluxation of the cervical or thoracic spine. Less commonly, vertebral dislocation, spinal cord tumor or osseous developmental anomalies associated with hemivertebra, Klippel-Feil syndrome and Sprengel's deformity may be the cause of congenital torticollis. Newborn infants with torticollis accompanied by a mass in the contracted SCM should undergo a treatment of chiropractic adjustments where indicated and passive stretching of the involved SCM. This protocol is nearly always successful if started prior to the age of one year. Newborns without a detectable mass in the SCM and without x-ray evidence of congenital anomalies of the cervical spine should be evaluated for subluxation in the cervical spine or mid to upper thoracic regions which, if present, should be treated by specific adjustment of the involved spinal motion segment(s).

ACQUIRED TORTICOLLIS

Acquired torticollis is a condition which is not present at birth but which has its onset at a later time, months or years after birth. Most cases of acquired torticollis in older children have sudden onset and may follow strenuous activity, mild trauma or sudden change in neck position. Significant spasm of the SCM can be identified and tenderness can be elicited in the belly of the muscle and in the area of the synovial articulations on the uninvolved side. X-rays will indicate a significant scoliosis in the cervical region, which may account for the tenderness and irritation of the ligamentous structures on the convex side of the spinal curve. Most medical pediatric textbooks now list the most common cause of acquired torticollis as rotational subluxation of the atlanto-axial complex.

Although the upper cervical spine can be involved in a sizable number of torticollis cases, it is important to examine the full spine carefully. Subluxations in the thoracic and lower cervical spine can also cause torticollis or lateral tilt presentations. If the patient's posture appears to be more of an antalgic lean due to a lower cervical/upper thoracic subluxation, the pain will be provoked on the side the patient leans away from when the doctor attempts to passively straighten the patient's neck and head. Where the torticollis is due to upper cervical subluxation, the spasmed SCM is painful on the ipsilateral side of tilt when the doctor attempts to passively straighten the patient's head and neck.

Other less common causes of acquired torticollis include intervertebral disc calcification, retropharyngeal infections, osteomyelitis of the cervical vertebrae, drug reactions, spinal tumors and atlanto-axial instability as seen in Morquio's and Down's syndromes. The use of radiographic studies and bone scans will usually be sufficient to identify any of the above causes of acquired torticollis.

Older children with acquired torticollis resulting from cervical or thoracic spine subluxation(s) usually respond quickly to care. A positive response is usually seen after the first adjustment, unless a great deal of chronicity is present. If needed, gentle manual traction to the contracted myofascial elements can be applied. In mild cases, torticollis and postural signs should be substantially resolved in the first week of care. The nature of the injury will determine the need for further care, to decrease the findings of subluxation and need for follow-up. Especially in colder climates, a soft collar worn during the initial few days of care may help to provide support and keep the neck muscles warm, although most cases can be managed without such appliances.

KLIPPEL-FEIL SYNDROME

The majority of cervical spine anomalies occur between the occiput and C2. Below the C2 level, developmental changes usually occur as multiple segmentation anomalies of which Klippel-Feil syndrome is an example (23). Klippel-Feil syndrome is a congenital spinal condition which is characterized by a short neck and limitation of head and neck movement. This rather characteristic picture is due to failure of segmentation of the developing cervical vertebrae with multiple block vertebrae being present. Clinically, the neck appears short and the hairline may appear low. Cervical ranges of motion are restricted and the neck may also be webbed. This webbing phenomenon is known as pterygium colli. Radiographs will reveal the underlying bony abnormality consisting of block vertebrae at multiple levels (see Chapter 8). Because of the presence of multiple block vertebrae, hypermobility may occur at the remaining intervertebral motion segments. Other anomalies which are frequently associated with Klippel-Feil syndrome include Sprengel's deformity, hearing impairment, and genitourinary, cardiopulmonary and nervous system anomalies.

ODONTOID ANOMALIES

Anomalies of the odontoid process of the C2 vertebra are well recognized in the radiological literature. The true incidence of anomalous defects in the C2 vertebra is unknown but certainly the prevalence is quite low. Disorders such as Klippel-Feil syndrome, Down's and Morquio's syndromes have a higher incidence of odontoid anomalies than can be identified in the general population (24). Anomalies of the odontoid process may include congenital agenesis or hypoplasia, ossiculum odontoideum and ossiculum terminale.

AGENESIS OR HYPOPLASIA

The odontoid process is formed from the first and second cervical somites. Failure of separation between the anterior arch of C1 and the odontoid process can lead to failure of formation or hypoplasia of the odontoid process. This condition can be associated with instability of the atlanto-axial region, and radiographic flexion/extension views should be obtained to evaluate for possible instability and orthopedic consultation and opinion should be sought. Spinal manipulation to this area, in the presence of instability, is contraindicated.

OS ODONTOIDEUM

Ossiculum odontoideum is considered to have either of two causes. Traditionally, os odontoideum was considered to be a congenital non-union of the dens at the neurocentral synchondrosis; however, more recently explanations suggest that the presence of an identifiable instability at the base of the dens is due to traumatic disturbance of the growth plate, giving the appearance of an un-united fracture (25). The atlas transverse ligament is usually intact with this condition, however symptoms due to cord compression or vertebral artery compromise may be present. Radiographic evidence of an os odontoideum in a young child is based on the finding of an odontoid process which is unstable relative to the base of the C2 vertebra. This is best identified on cervical flexion studies. Surgical stabilization of an unstable odontoid process should be provided as an option for the patient since further trauma may compromise the spinal cord and/or vascular structures in this region.

OS TERMINALE

Ossiculum terminale is a condition in which the tip of the odontoid fails to unite with the rest of the dens. Secondary ossification in this region is usually complete around the age of 12 years. Prior to this time, the odontoid tip may not be seen on plain film radiographs. In its place a V or Y shaped odontoid groove may be seen. Little clinical significance is attached to this anomaly and no instability is associated with its presence.

Problems of the Thoracic Spine and Trunk

Scoliosis

Few problems affect the thoracic spine and trunk in children, but those which do can represent serious disabilities which may significantly affect the child's future well-being. Possibly the most serious long-term disability of the thoracic spine and trunk which can afflict a child is scoliosis. Since scoliosis is a physical finding and does not represent a diagnosis, its etiology should be investigated in all cases and its classification established prior to commencing treatment (see Chapter 15). Scoliosis can be readily detected by postural evaluation and many cases of scoliosis are found during routine chiropractic physical examinations. Scoliosis screening is such an effective process for locating previously unidentified cases of scoliosis that screenings are becoming a regular occurrence in most schools.

Adolescent idiopathic scoliosis is the most common form of scoliosis and is a classification which is reserved for those scolioses which cannot be classified into any other appropriate category. The label idiopathic scoliosis may therefore be considered to be a diagnosis of exclusion. Adolescent idiopathic scoliosis has no associated spinal pain and therefore, any patient presenting with scoliosis who also complains of back pain should be carefully evaluated for an alternative cause. This type of scoliosis is more common in females and tends to progress more rapidly during an adolescent growth spurt.

Congenital scoliosis is associated with failure of appropriate formation of the spine during embryological development. It may be due to specific vertebral anomalies, such as hemivertebrae, or to failure of proper segmentation of the vertebral structures. Congenital scoliosis frequently presents concurrently with other developmental anomalies, such as genitourinary anomalies, cardiac anomalies and spinal cord tethering. The goal of any management program is to prevent the progression of the scoliosis. Classically, bracing has been the method of choice to prevent further progression of spinal curvatures associated with congenital scoliosis. Initial evaluation and progressive monitoring of congenital curvatures, especially small ones, is the appropriate course of action. Some congenital spinal curvatures can be non-progressive but this can only be determined by evaluation over a period of 6–12 months.

The detailed evaluation and management protocols for the child with scoliosis are delineated elsewhere in this text (see Chapter 15).

At this point, it is sufficient to point out that not all cases of scoliosis destine the child to a life of physical deformity. For each case of scoliosis, a careful and thorough evaluation must always be carried out to identify the type of scoliosis and regular follow-up evaluations must be made to assess the appropriateness and success of the selected program of scoliosis management.

Ankylosing Spondylitis

Ankylosing spondylitis (AS) is a chronic inflammatory condition of unknown etiology, primarily affecting the joints of the spine and pelvis. AS is classified as a sero-negative spondyloarthropathy. The sero-negative classification is defined as the absence of antinuclear antibodies and rheumatoid factor in the blood, however these patients are frequently HLA-B27 positive. The pathophysiology of AS involves chronic inflammation of the cartilage, ligaments and synovial linings of the joints. AS is a painful, progressive arthritic condition which occurs mainly in males between the ages of 18 and 30 years. AS is four times more common in males with the overall incidence being reported as being about 30 cases per 100,000 (26). The diagnosis of AS is frequently difficult because back pain is not always present early in the course of the disease. Characteristic clinical findings include night pain and morning stiffness in the hips and spine which is relieved by exercise. Exquisite tenderness and inflammation of the tendons, especially at the insertion of the Achilles and patella tendons has also been described as a common early clinical finding with AS (27).

Presenting symptoms may be low-back pain and stiffness, particularly around the sacro-iliac joints or lower extremity joint pain, characteristic of the arthritides. After initially involving the sacro-iliac joints, this disorder progresses further upward along the vertebral column to involve the lumbar, thoracic, and in some cases, the cervical spine. This disorder eventually results in bony ankylosis of the spinal joints with the inflammatory process eventually subsiding after about 10–15 years.

The best clinical diagnostic indicator has been suggested to be low-back pain and stiffness lasting for three months. Thoraco-lumbar pain has been shown to be a poor indicator for the diagnosis of AS (28). Upon examination, marked limitation of motion is usually encountered in the involved areas of the spine. Sacroiliac joint involvement can be identified by palpation and provocative stress testing. Involvement of the chest may produce restricted breathing capacity due to involvement of the costo-vertebral joints. Permanent stiffness of the involved joints usually results. The earliest radiographic changes involve a fuzziness of the sacro-iliac joints due to loss of cortical bone at the iliac margins of the sacroiliac joint. Destruction of the hyaline cartilage joint margins produces a joint outline which can no longer be clearly depicted thus producing a pseudo-widening of the joint space. As joint destruction progresses, discrete areas of destruction and sclerosis occur along the iliac margins of the joint leading to the classic "rosary bead" appearance. This is the stage where diagnosis of AS is usually made. Later x-ray changes may show complete obliteration of the sacro-iliac joint spaces with bony ankylosis of the lumbar, thoracic and occasionally of the cervical intervertebral joints.

Management of the patient with AS should involve activity rather than rest. Spinal adjustments may be used to maintain flexibility at the involved intervertebral motion segments. Spinal exercises have been shown to provide significant short-term improvements in spine and hip range of motion and should be instituted early in the course of treatment. In the longer term, spinal exercises have been shown to reduce the rate at which the loss of joint mobility occurs (29). Spinal exercises and adjustments should be instituted for the purpose of increasing joint range of motion, or at least to preserve what movement remains. The patient should be advised to sleep flat on the back, on a firm mattress, with a low pillow under the head and neck to prevent exacerbating the flexion deformity of the spine. The following five assessment criteria for accurately measuring progress in the treatment of AS have been identified: cervical rotation, tragus to wall distance, lateral flexion, modified Schober's and intermalleolar distance (30). These dimensions should be regularly monitored as a measure of the patient's progress.

Postural Kyphosis

The normal thoracic kyphotic curve should be present from birth. When evaluating the thoracic spine, palpation of the alignment of this curve should reveal a smooth kyphotic curve, devoid of flat spots, excessive ridges or lateral deviation. Individual vertebrae should be assessed for symmetry and conformity with the adjacent vertebral structures and for the presence of a slight springing motion. Tenderness to palpation can be an indicator for a more detailed examination of the involved area, the most common cause being vertebral subluxation at that level.

Postural kyphosis is an exaggerated kyphosis seen in the thoracic spine of adolescents which is essentially due to faulty posture. Occasionally this posture may be habitual and be seen in the patient's parents or role models. This posture can be helped with range of motion exercises and usually resolves with time and without excessive treatment.

Scheuermann's Disease

Scheuermann's disease is a disorder of unknown etiology which primarily affects the adolescent thoracic spine producing pain and cosmetic deformity. The average age at onset of Scheuermann's disease is between 13 and 17 years of age. Although the cause of this condition is unknown, recent studies have implicated spinal endplate fractures with bursting of the disc contents through the cartilage into the adjacent vertebral body as the likely etiological factor (31). Vertebral changes occur predominantly near the anterior margins where the greatest weight-thrust is borne. This causes defective growth of the affected part of the secondary ring epiphysis and the vertebral body becomes slightly wedge shaped. Several contiguous vertebrae are usually involved in the thoracic or upper lumbar regions. Symptoms include pain in the thoracic spine, easy fatigue and postural deformity. Postural changes can exhibit exaggerated mid-thoracic kyphosis, cervical and lumbar lordosis and anterior pelvic tilt. Radiographic findings demonstrate anterior vertebral body wedging, loss of disc height and irregularity of the vertebral endplates (see Chapter 8). Diagnosis is by history, clinical appearance and x-rays. Differential diagnosis should include tuberculosis of the spine, especially if the condition involves a single vertebra. The condition is self-limiting with the active stage lasting for about two years. Spinal adjustments in the involved regions may be used to reduce joint compression and to decrease associated joint symptoms. Scheuermann's disease predisposes to the later development of osteoarthritis.

Pectus Excavatum

Pectus excavatum, also known as "funnel chest," is a depression of the sternum which can be either developmental or second-

ary to severe obstructive airway disease. This condition is more common in boys and is usually not evident at birth, however the family history may reveal previous cases. The condition is mainly considered to be a cosmetic deformity, but may also be associated with mitral valve prolapse or Marfan's syndrome. The deformity may be corrected by surgical reconstruction of the involved muscles, usually at around 12 years of age.

Pectus Carinatum

Pectus carinatum is an outward protrusion of the sternum, also known as "pigeon breast." It is usually seen in association with children who have chronic respiratory disorders, such as asthma. Surgical correction is rarely undertaken.

Problems of the Lumbar Spine and Pelvis

Spondylolysis

Spondylolysis is a condition in which there is interruption of the bony integrity of the pars interarticularis. About 90% of spondylolysis cases involve the L5 vertebra. Recent reports have identified stress fracture as the likely cause of this condition (see Chapter 19). Radiographic examination of hundreds of fetal and newborn spines reveals no evidence of pars separation with the youngest recorded case of spondylolysis being in a four month old infant. Hence, this condition can be more correctly classified as an acquired rather than as a congenital disorder.

The most common cause of this condition is thought to be associated with athletic activities which involve hyperextension of the lumbar spine, such as diving, gymnastics, weightlifting and pole-vaulting. Wrestling and football have also been implicated by some authors in the etiology of this condition. Other authors point to the repetitive trauma associated with early attempts at walking as a possible cause. The most common stage for detection of this condition is after five years of age. Lower back pain can be a presenting symptom for spondylolysis if the traumatic event was a recent one. However, most commonly this condition is encountered incidentally without symptomatic evidence of back pain, suggesting ununited stress fracture as the more accurate diagnosis.

Spondylolisthesis

Spondylolisthesis is a condition in which there is anterior movement of a vertebra relative to the spinal structure immediately below, usually associated with an anomaly of the pars interarticularis. Spondylolisthesis may be due to any of the following three occurrences: a traumatic defect in the pars interarticularis, known as spondylolysis; congenital malformation, occurring as elongation of the articular processes; or degeneration of the posterior facet joints. Of these three etiologies, degeneration of the posterior facets is confined to adults and therefore not appropriate for discussion in this text. Elongation of the pars interarticularis, also known as dysplastic spondylolisthesis, is due to congenital weakness of the facet joints and intervertebral disc complex. The dysplastic form of spondylolisthesis is of concern due to the high incidence of nerve root compression symptoms encountered in affected patients. In such cases the intact lamina of L5 is pulled against the dural sac creating the compression symptoms. By far, the most common cause of spondylolisthesis in children is spondylolysis. In spondylolysis, loss of bony continuity occurs, as a result of fatigue fracture, between the superior and inferior articulating processes with the deficiency being bridged by fibrous tissue. If this fibrous tissue stretches or gives way, the consequent vertebral displacement may give rise to spondylolisthesis. In some patients the anterior movement of the affected vertebra can cause a spinal stenosis. The most common causes of separation of the pars interarticularis include early attempts at upright posture and sporting activities, especially those which involve repetitive hyperextension movements, such as gymnastics, or springboard diving which can involve hyperextension of the lumbar spine due to poor performance.

Spondylolisthesis is most often symptomless in children. Diagnosis is made most commonly from the lateral lumbar radiograph demonstrating the anterior vertebral slippage. Separation of the pars interarticularis may be readily observed on the oblique lumbar radiograph. The degree of spondylolisthesis is more likely to progress (e.g. from Myerding grade 1 to grade 2) during an adolescent growth spurt due to the relative weakness encountered in spinal structures at that time. For this reason children identified with this problem should be carefully supervised in sports which involve excessive axial loading of the spinal column, such as weight lifting and football, during that critical phase of growth. This is not to say that such sports are contraindicated during all of the adolescent period, but rather that restrictions may be reserved for those periods during which a characteristic rapid growth spurt is occurring. Patients with painful spondylolysis and without slippage may be treated conservatively with a soft lumbosacral corset to control their symptoms. Patients with a grade 1 spondylolisthesis may also be treated conservatively with anterior lumbar adjustments and bracing during the occurrence of pain symptoms. Children with a grade 2 slippage should be carefully evaluated and managed since a slippage of this magnitude in a child has a high probability of progression. Once the adolescent growth phase is completed, further slippage of a spondylolisthesis, with less than a Myerding grade 2 classification, is unlikely (32).

Facet Tropism

Facet tropism is a condition in which asymmetrical angulation exists between the facet joint facings of the left and right sides of the same intervertebral motion segment. This joint alignment predisposes to a reduction in the anterior-posterior osseous stabilization provided by the affected facet joint. The incidence of facet tropism is far more common than might be expected, being 50% at L5–S1 and slightly less at the L4–L5 level (33). The anomaly is thought to predispose to stretching and inflammation of the ligament capsule around the more sagittally aligned facet joint, resulting in the onset of lower back pain symptoms due to ligament sprain. One study showed that biomechanical instability exists on the side of the more oblique facet joint (34).

This condition has been associated with clinical symptoms of low back pain in athletic teenagers. Adolescents with facet tropism typically may complain of lower back pain which is exacerbated by sports participation, particularly those sports which involve sudden forceful hyperextension of the lumbar spine, such as volleyball, basketball and gymnastics. Subjects with tropism have a significantly higher prevalence of disc degeneration (35).

Facet tropism can generally be classified as an overuse syndrome associated with hyperextension of the lumbar spine. Clinically, radiographic examination is required to make this diagnosis, however, certain history and clinical findings make the presence of this condition more probable. Low back pain associated with facet tropism may frequently be identified in patients who are involved in activities which involve lumbar hyperextension. In the adolescent patient, sports such as volleyball and basketball can exacerbate this condition. Palpable tenderness which is confined to the area over a specific low lumbar intervertebral facet joint is a consistent finding in this condition.

An appropriate treatment protocol for facet tropism requires a combination of spinal adjustments at areas of subluxation and exercise. Since this condition is due to the existence of a hypermobile unstable facet joint, adjustments should be confined to those spinal joints which demonstrate fixation and not to the already hypermobile trophic facet. Adjust any subluxations which may decrease the compensatory hypermobility at the symptomatic facet joint. Management of this condition also requires a program of specific exercises to strengthen the supporting spinal musculature, specifically the abdominal and extensor lumbar muscles. It is important that any exercises which involve hyperextension of the lumbar spine beyond the neutral position be avoided as they tend to aggravate the patient's symptoms. Exercises to strengthen and stabilize the lumbar spine need to become part of the daily regimen for these patients. Temporary elimination of the offending activity until the symptoms are eliminated and an increased degree of abdominal strength is achieved is also recommended; temporary stabilization with a flexible back support may be required if symptoms persist.

Bilateral Sagittal Facets

Occasionally, a patient may have bilateral sagittal alignment of the lower lumbar intervertebral facet joints. This condition may be responsible for similar symptomatology to the unilateral condition of facet tropism and likewise, may potentially predispose the patient to accelerated intervertebral disc degeneration. Management of this condition requires a program similar to that previously recommended for facet tropism.

Congenital Anomalies of the Spine

Congenital spinal problems frequently have an associated physical deformity or present with neurological deficits. Progressive neurological loss which is evident when examining an infant may suggest a congenital lesion. Table 14.2 identifies the most common congenital anomalies associated with the spine.

Spinal cord malformation in an infant commonly results from tethering of the spinal cord, a condition in which thickening of the filum terminale prevents the normal ascent of

Table 14.2.	Congenital Anomalies of the Spine

Block vertebra

Butterfly vertebra

Hemi-vertebra

Agenesis of the dens

Cleft vertebra

Spina bifida occulta

Spina bifida vera

Persistent epiphysis

Facet tropism

Transitional vertebra

Lumbarization

Sacralization

Pseudo-arthrosis

the spinal cord from the sacral level at birth to the upper lumbar region (36). This condition may have associated cutaneous hemangiomas or tufts of hair in the lumbo-sacral region. Traction forces on the spinal cord during growth produces neurological loss. The diagnosis of spinal cord tethering may be confirmed by magnetic resonance imaging (MRI).

Spina Bifida

Spina bifida is a malformation of the spinal cord and vertebrae resulting in varying degrees of failure of closure of the spinal laminae. Spina bifida is the most common developmental defect of the central nervous system occurring most frequently in the lumbo-sacral region, usually at L5, in approximately 6% of the North American population (37) (see Chapter 8).

There are four classifications of spina bifida which can be identified as follows:

1. Spina bifida occulta (SBO), the most common type, has vertebral defect but usually no damage to the spinal cord and no external sac is visible
2. Meningocele (MC), in which an external sac, containing only meninges, bulges through the vertebral defect
3. Meningomyelocele (MMC), in which a bulging external sac containing neural tissue is present. Spinal cord damage is usually present in MMC
4. Encephalocele (EC), which is similar to meningomyelocele; however, the defect occurs over the skull instead of over the spine

Spina bifida occulta is frequently observed on routine lumbar spinal radiographs and is usually an incidental finding. Most cases of SBO are asymptomatic and the defect is small, less than ¼ inch gap between laminae. This condition does not present any problems with adjusting the spinal vertebrae;

however in rare cases, as the child grows there may be gradual development of cavus deformities of the feet and/or scoliosis as well as loss of bladder and bowel control. Symptomatic forms of SBO produce neurological deficit by tethering the spinal cord, resulting in symptoms early in childhood. Children with this condition have intact skin over the lesion but often have a cutaneous marker at the site, such as an hemangioma, a tuft of hair or dermal sinus.

In each form of spina bifida, the conus medullaris may be fixed in an abnormally caudal position, producing a progressive discrepancy between the length of the spine and the spinal cord as the child grows. This produces increased cord tension due to the inability of the cord to accommodate to spinal flexion and extension. Meningocele occasionally produces motor weakness or sphincter disturbance. Meningomyelocele may produce flaccid paralysis, loss of sensation and deformities of the legs. Children with MMC may have no voluntary function below the level of the lesion, while in cervical lesions there may be spasticity and hyperactive reflexes in the lower extremities.

In recent years, researchers have proposed that spina bifida is due to a folate deficiency in the mother early in the pregnancy. Since the neural tube closes at approximately the twenty-sixth day of gestation, deficiencies early in the pregnancy have been implicated (38). Further support for this theory comes from another study which identified a decreased incidence of spina bifida in infants born to mothers who were receiving vitamin supplementation prior to conception (39).

Neuromusculoskeletal Trauma

Neuromusculoskeletal trauma accounts for about 10 to 15% of injuries in children. The special characteristics of the osseous skeleton, with developing epiphyses, cartilaginous growth plates, relative elasticity of bones, and immature blood supply allow for a unique series of orthopedic problems and injuries.

The Limping Child

A child presenting with a limping gait must be suspected of having hip pathology as a primary concern. Since many pathologies of the hip region will cause a child to limp, a diagnosis of sprain/strain of the hip is an infrequent finding and should be rendered only after a careful and thorough evaluation of the patient. Disorders of the hip which may present with a painful limp can include Legg-Calvé-Perthes disease, slipped capital femoral epiphysis, joint infection (pyogenic/septic arthritis), infections of bone (osteomyelitis), acute lymphoblastic leukemia, transient synovitis, reactive arthritis and juvenile rheumatoid arthritis. Careful evaluation of the involved region should be carried out to rule out the above conditions before any alternative diagnosis is established.

Fractures

All injuries in which fracture is suspected should be evaluated by x-ray. Two opposing views are the minimum necessary to adequately assess such an injury. Frequently, comparison views of the opposite extremity or body part will be helpful in assessing problems which involve the epiphyseal growth plates. Children's fractures require careful description and identification, especially when communicating the initial clinical findings to an emergency room physician or other health care practitioner. Fractures should be described by identifying the exact location, the bone which is involved, the location in that bone where the fracture site is found, the fracture pattern (greenstick, etc.), the alignment and whether any surrounding soft tissues are affected (see Chapter 19).

Growth Plate Injuries

Cartilaginous growth plates are subject to frequent injury in children primarily because the epiphyses are not as strong as the surrounding bone. Trauma is more likely to cause epiphyseal separation than it is to cause fracture, especially when the trauma is close to a growth plate. Fractures which occur in the region of growth plates are likely to produce disruption of the surrounding vascular structures which may cause disturbance of longitudinal growth and subsequent avascular necrosis of the affected epiphysis.

Growth plate injuries should be assessed according to the Salter-Harris classification (Fig. 14.3). This classification provides an indication of the progressive risks for disturbance of growth. Care should be taken not to confuse a growth plate injury in a child with a torn ligament. An example would be to confuse a distal fibula physeal separation with a ligamentous sprain of the ankle. All suspected epiphyseal injuries should be referred to an orthopedist for evaluation and treatment.

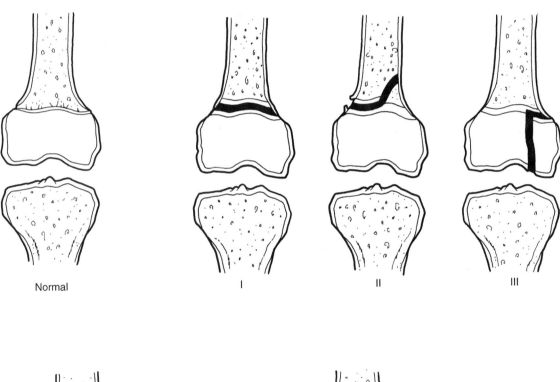

Normal   I   II   III

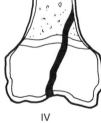   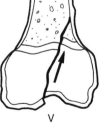

IV   V

Figure 14.3.   Salter-Harris classification of physeal injuries. The illustration shows normal, then, Type I. Isolated fracture through the growth plate (dark line). Type II. Fracture through the growth plate with separation of a corner of the metaphysis. Type III. The fracture extends along the growth plate and then moves towards the epiphysis. Type IV. Vertical oblique fracture extending through the metaphysis, growth plate and epiphysis. Type V. Compression deformity of the growth plate. The radiographs are usually initially interpreted as normal with this type of injury. Modified from Salter RB, Harris WR: Injuries involving the epiphyseal plate. J Bone Joint Surg 1963; 45A:587.

Clavicle Fracture

The clavicle is the first bone to calcify in-utero and is also the most common bone to be fractured during the birth process, especially with breech deliveries. Palpation of the clavicle should be performed for evidence of fracture when conducting a physical examination of any newborn infant. Fractures of the clavicle associated with the birth process are usually undisplaced, greenstick type fractures and can be identified by detecting a palpable "crunchiness" over the site of the fracture. The infant will usually display pseudoparalysis of the affected arm. Clavicle fracture in an infant usually does not require treatment, however bracing is an option to provide immobilization and increased comfort. The infant's parents should be made aware of the necessity to protect the clavicle from further injury by avoiding lifting the infant by the arms until union is complete, usually in about 2 to 3 weeks.

Forces sufficient to cause clavicle fracture may also cause other problems such as latent spinal injury, therefore a thorough spinal and neurological examination should be conducted on any child with a clavicle fracture.

Joint Sprains

Classification of sprains in pediatric joint injuries is based mainly on clinical findings. The assessment of a suspected joint sprain requires evaluation of the following clinical signs: pain on motion, tenderness to palpation, degree of swelling and the presence of joint instability. The following table provides a system of classifying joint sprains (Table 14.3).

Table 14.3.   Classification of Sprains

Grade 1

Degree of tearing: A small fraction of the ligamentous fibers is disrupted.

Clinical findings: Pain on motion, local tenderness, mild swelling.

Grade 2

Degree of tearing: Moderate tearing of ligamentous fibers is present.

Clinical findings: Pain on motion, more diffuse tenderness, moderate joint swelling, mild joint instability.

Grade 3

Degree of tearing: Complete disruption of ligamentous fibers.

Clinical findings: Severe pain on motion, marked tenderness, marked joint swelling, moderate joint instability.

Modified from Zitelli, BJ. Atlas of pediatric physical diagnosis. St. Louis: Mosby, 1987;19:16.

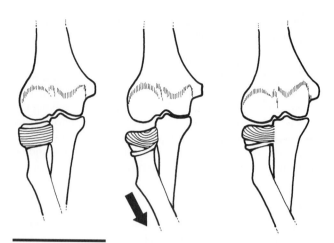

Figure 14.4.   The mechanism of radial head dislocation or subluxation. The annular ligament is partially torn when the arm is pulled. The radial head moves distally, and when the traction is discontinued, the ligament is carried into the joint. Modified from: Rang M. Children's fractures, (2nd ed.) Philadelphia: JB Lippincott Co, 1983:193.

Upper Extremity Evaluation

The elbow joint is an intrinsically stable joint. The wrist and finger flexors attach at the medial epicondyle while the extensors originate at the lateral epicondyle. Repetitive movements over a long period of time can result in apophysitis, i.e. pitcher's elbow at the medial epicondyle and tennis elbow at the lateral epicondyle. Treatment of these conditions generally involves specific evaluation and adjustment of the joints exhibiting restricted motion, followed by rest and cross-friction massage, and subsequent strengthening exercises. Pitching technique modification is also important in preventing recurrences.

Radial Head Dislocation (Pulled Elbow) (Nursemaid's Elbow)

Dislocation of the proximal head of the radius is an injury with frequent occurrence in toddlers. The radial head can be dislocated by sudden traction on the forearm causing the radial head to slip partly through the annular ligament, displacing and tearing the ligament. When the arm is released, the radial head traps the ligament between it and the capitulum (Fig. 14.4).

A typical scenario for this injury is when a child is forcibly pulled or lifted by the upward outstretched arm. The child with a pulled elbow will resist moving the arm due to pain, creating a condition of pseudoparalysis. The trapped annular ligament fibers can be reduced by placing the doctor's thumb over the dislocated radial head, applying gentle traction to the wrist with the other hand, while simultaneously applying full, quick supination of the forearm. A click is usually felt on reduction and a prompt return of function can be expected with correction. Immobilization is usually not required unless the problem is repetitive, in which case a posterior splint may be applied for several days.

Peripheral Nerve Trauma

Peripheral nerve trauma is most commonly seen in the newborn infant. The most common site of injury is at the brachial plexus and is due to lateral flexion of the neck during the process of delivery, resulting in a stretching injury to the brachial plexus. This type of injury is more common with shoulder dystocia (dislocation), breech delivery or forceps extraction. There are two major manifestations of peripheral nerve trauma, Erb's palsy and Klumpke's paralysis. Forces sufficient to cause either of these injuries may also be responsible for producing subluxation of the lower cervical spinal vertebrae. Specific adjustment of any subluxated vertebrae is indicated.

Erb's Palsy

Erb's palsy is a condition seen more commonly in newborn infants and presents with adduction, internal rotation and pronation of the arm, a position called the "waiter's tip" deformity. This injury involves the upper two nerve roots of the brachial plexus (C5 and C6). The injury is to the motor portion of the nervous system and sensation to the involved upper extremity is completely normal. Treatment consists of adjustments to subluxated levels (see Chapter 12) and passive range of motion to maintain mobility and prevent a frozen shoulder. Occasionally, ipsilateral paralysis of the diaphragm may be present due to involvement of the phrenic nerve.

Klumpke's Paralysis

Klumpke's paralysis has a similar mechanism of injury to Erb's palsy but in Klumpke's, the injury involves nerve roots to the seventh and eighth cervical nerves and usually also to the first thoracic nerve. This lower brachial plexus injury involves paralysis of the hand and is characterized by hyperextension of the metacarpophalangeal joints and wrist flexion. There is no associated sensory loss and treatment consists of passive range of motion to maintain mobility. Klumpke's paralysis may occasionally be associated with Horner's syndrome, characterized by ptosis, miosis and anhydrosis.

Sprengel's Deformity

Sprengel's deformity is a condition of unknown etiology in which one or both scapula are elevated and small. The anomaly represents a failure of the scapula, originally a cervical appendage, to descend to its normal thoracic position during in-utero development. In this condition, the scapular muscles are poorly developed or replaced by fibrous bands. Usually the scapula is smaller than normal and is medially rotated. Sprengel's deformity may be unilateral or bilateral, and the range of shoulder abduction is usually decreased to no more than 90 degrees of abduction, otherwise functional disability is slight. The child with this deformity usually cannot raise the arm completely on the affected side, since the rigidity of the scapula prevents its free rotation during abduction. Sprengel's deformity is occasionally seen associated with Klippel-Feil syndrome.

Lower Extremity Evaluation

Congenital Hip Dislocation and Congenital Hip Dysplasia

Congenital hip dislocation is a condition of spontaneous dislocation of one or both hips, occurring either before, during, or shortly after birth. Hip dislocation is most common in breech presentations and is seen about four to six times more often in female babies (40). The etiology is thought to be due to one of three main causes:

1. Ligament laxity around the hip joint due to either genetic joint laxity, or to hormonally induced ligament laxity, associated with the fetal uterus secreting the hormones relaxin and estrogen

2. Breech malposition where the sudden full extension of the hips may be the factor that precipitates dislocation, especially in the presence of ligament laxity

3. Defective development of the acetabulum

Developmental hip dysplasia represents a wide spectrum of hip problems ranging from mild instability to frank dislocation. Congenital hip dislocation is considered by most recent authors to be an inappropriate term since hip dislocation in the newborn can also occur after birth. The term congenital hip dysplasia (CHD) is preferred. The incidence if CHD can be influenced by hormonal, mechanical, environmental and genetic factors. CHD is not always detected at birth, with around 40% of the cases not being detected until later than the third month of life. In a case of unilateral dislocation, the involved extremity appears short and the inguinal creases will be asymmetrical. Clinical findings include limited abduction of the involved hip, which is a consistent finding in infants with dislocated hips. Assessment of the hip joints should be made using the Barlow, Ortolani or Galeazzi tests.

The Ortolani test consists of abduction of the flexed hips bilaterally (Fig. 14.5). Both hips should abduct to the point where they are flat against the examination table. If one hip will not abduct completely or if a palpable "clunk" is felt then hip dislocation should be suspected.

The Barlow test is performed by flexing and abducting the hip and then applying long axis traction or posterior pressure to the femur head (Fig. 14.6). Once again, the positive finding is a palpable "clunk."

Galeazzi's test compares the level of the knees after the baby is placed flat on the examination table with the hips and knees flexed. One hip protruding higher than the other is an indication of a dislocatable hip.

Radiographic examination will usually demonstrate proximal femoral displacement superior and laterally alongside a shallow acetabulum. The femoral head may not be visible due to delayed ossification associated with CHD. Radiographic findings will usually be diagnostic if:

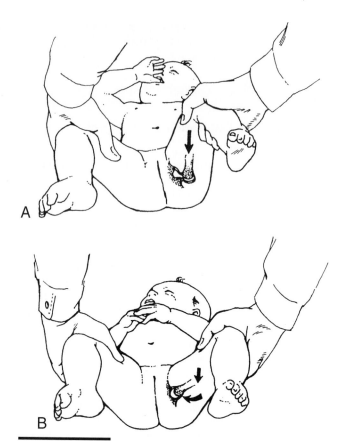

Figure 14.5. Procedure for the Ortolani maneuver for hip dislocation. A. Downward pressure further dislocates the hip. B. Medialward rotation of the hip will force the femoral head over the rim of the acetabulum, causing a "clunk." Modified from Graham JM. *Smith's recognizable patterns of human deformation,* (2nd ed.) Philadelphia: WB Saunders, 1988:25.

1. A disruption of Shenton's line (Fig. 14.7) is present.
2. The femoral head is located in the superior lateral quadrant (Hilgen-Reiner's method).
3. Skinner's angle is increased.

Positive Skinner's angle measurements are diagnostic if greater than 35 degrees in a newborn, greater than 27 degrees in pre-ambulatory stage, or greater than 25 degrees at the age of one year.

Early diagnosis of this condition simplifies the treatment process. The usual treatment involves fixing the hips in a position of flexion and abduction using a Pavlik harness for a period of at least 6 weeks. These methods will usually ensure a good prognosis (41). The therapeutic goal is to maintain the hips in contact with the acetabulum until sufficient growth and development has taken place to maintain stability. Cases of CHD which are not diagnosed at an early stage are usually predisposed to secondary degenerative changes and avascular necrosis which may cripple the child for their entire life (42).

Infantile Coxa Vara

The general term coxa vara includes any condition in which the neck-shaft angle of the femur is less than the normal angle of about 125 degrees, known as Mikulicz's angle (43). The neck-shaft angle is sometimes reduced to 90 degrees or less in this deformity which is aided mechanically by the stress of the body weight acting upon a femoral neck that is defective or abnormally soft and since this part of the femoral neck remains as unossified cartilage, it gradually bends during childhood. Bilateral presentation occurs in 30 to 50 percent of the cases detected (44). The diagnosis of coxa vara should be considered in any infant who walks with a painless waddling gait. The waddling gait is due to alteration in the femoral neck-shaft angle in which approximation of the origin and insertion of the gluteus medius muscle produces a characteristic Trendelenburg gait. Definitive diagnosis is by radiographic examination showing a reduced femoral neck-shaft angle. Treatment, if needed, can involve surgery to correct the deformity. Coxa vara can also occur after fracture of the trochanteric region with mal-union and with ununited fractures of the neck of the femur.

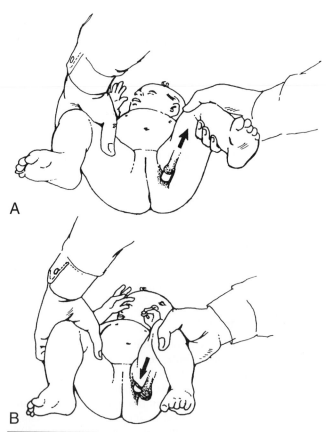

Figure 14.6. A. Barlow's test is performed by pulling on the femur causing distraction of the femur head. B. Passage of the femur over the rim yields a "clunk." Modified from Graham JM. *Smith's recognizable patterns of human deformation.* (2nd ed.) Philadelphia: WB Saunders, 1988:24.

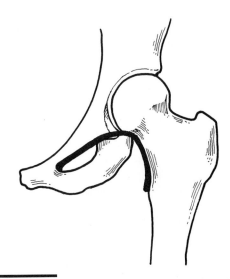

Figure 14.7. Shenton's line. The normal curvilinear line is present from the distal portion of the femoral neck to the inferior border of the superior pubic ramus. Disruption in this line occurs in hip dislocation.

Slipped Capital Femoral Epiphysis

Slipped capital femoral epiphysis (SCFE) is a condition of later childhood and adolescence in which the upper femoral epiphysis is displaced from its normal position on the femoral neck. The patient is usually adolescent and more frequently is a male who is obese or who is tall, thin and growing rapidly. The cause of the slippage is unknown but mechanical factors, such as pelvic asymmetry due to spinal or pelvic subluxation contributing to an uneven weight load distribution on the femur heads may be a contributing factor. Acute SCFE can result from shear forces applied to the area from severe trauma, motor vehicle accidents, child abuse, falls from heights or obstetric accidents. Hormonal factors have also been suspected. In about 10% of the cases, both hips are involved (45).

Most patients are chronic and present with a painful limp that occurred suddenly without identifiable cause. Patients with SCFE may also present with the only symptom being knee or groin pain. Examination of the hip will reveal restriction of internal rotation and a tendency to external rotation and flexion, a position which minimizes the discomfort. Flexion of the involved hip will exacerbate the symptoms. Definitive diagnosis can be made radiographically from the frog-leg view, which should always be included, since this condition may not be evident on an AP view (Fig. 14.8). Patients with SCFE should be referred for surgical consultation with the surgical objective being to pin the epiphysis in-situ to prevent further disruption to the vascular supply to the femoral head. The child should be non weight-bearing (e.g., provided crutches) after the entity has been identified. Complications with this condition include avascular necrosis, ankylosis and sequestration of the epiphysis.

Legg-Calvé-Perthes Disease (LCP)

Legg-Calvé-Perthes disease is an osteochondritis of unknown etiology which affects the epiphysis of the femoral head. It occurs in children usually in the age range 5 to 10 years and is more common in boys who are short in stature. The femoral head is temporarily softened and may become deformed. The condition, which usually affects only one hip, passes through the three classic pathological stages of condensation (avascularization), fragmentation (resorption) and regeneration (revascularization). The condition is self-limiting and progresses through the three stages in about 36 months.

The child with Legg-Calvé-Perthes usually presents with a limp of insidious onset and may complain of pain in the groin or knee. Because of the mild nature of the symptoms, many patients will have well-advanced disease by the time of presentation. Upon examination, restriction will be noted to all hip movements, but particularly on abduction and medial rotation (46). An internally rotated ilium may be noted and could be contributing to the groin pain symptoms.

Diagnosis is usually established by radiographic findings where the earliest changes show the shadow of a swollen joint capsule and widening of the joint space. The first osseous changes consist of widening of the epiphyseal plate, with widening of the femoral neck adjacent to the epiphyseal plate. Softening and flattening of the epiphysis may appear as a "jockey's cap" deformity. Eventually the texture of the bone

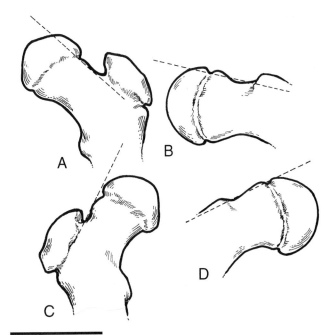

Figure 14.8. Analysis for slipped capital femoral epiphysis. For the AP projection "A" is normal, where the line superimposed on the superior femoral neck normally intersects a portion of the femoral head. In the frog-leg projection (B), the line should also intersect the femoral head. If it does not in either the AP projection (C) or in the frog-leg view (D), then a slipped capital femoral epiphysis is identified. Modified from Chung S. Diseases of the developing hip joint. Pediatr Clin North Am 1986; 33:1457.

returns to normal, but if flattening has occurred, the femoral head will be permanently deformed.

Treatment in the acute phase includes bedrest with containment of the femoral head deep within the acetabulum. A regular program of non-weight bearing leg abduction exercises may provide the best results for eliminating femoral head deformity. The most important factor in this management protocol is considered to be the maintenance of joint mobility which enhances synovium and cartilage nutrition. When joint pain and muscle spasms have subsided, use of crutches may be permitted; however the patient should be advised to avoid bearing any weight on the hip until the regeneration phase is completed. The primary goal of any treatment program for LCP is the reduction or elimination of degenerative joint disease later in life.

Transient Synovitis

Transient synovitis is a common cause of limping and hip pain in children. It is generally considered to be an acute inflammatory reaction in the acetabulum that follows an upper respiratory infection. The condition is self limiting and usually lasts about 10 days. It classically affects children between the ages of 3–8 years.

The patient usually walks with a limp and an antalgic gait. Hip pain is unilateral and some patients refuse to bear weight on the involved limb. Radiographic findings are usually normal. Before making a diagnosis of transient synovitis it is important to rule out slipped capital femoral epiphysis, Legg-Calvé-Perthes disease, pyogenic arthritis of the hip joint and osteomyelitis of the proximal femur.

Treatment involves bedrest to reduce weight-bearing in the acute phase. Patients with transient synovitis may respond to spinal adjustments to the lumbo-pelvic and sacroiliac region, especially if referred pain is involved.

Knee and Lower Extremity

A variety of painful conditions can affect the knee in the growing child. Most knee problems in children resolve without serious sequelae, however in managing knee problems it should be remembered that the knee is a frequent site of referred pain from hip pathology or from sacroiliac subluxation.

Acute Knee Injuries

Knee injuries in children are common and are usually associated with trauma, such as a falls or sporting injuries. The presence of hemarthrosis or the inability to walk after an injury suggests significant pathology. Ligamentous injuries in children are rare due to elasticity and flexibility of ligament fibers. The presence of epiphyses and the insertion of ligament fibers into epiphyseal cartilage is more likely to produce an avulsion fracture rather than to produce ligament damage.

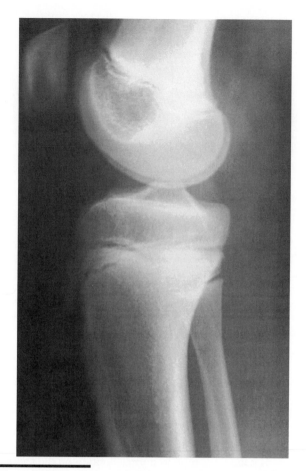

Figure 14.9. Osgood-Schlatter disease.

Osgood-Schlatter Disease

Osgood-Schlatter disease is a condition involving epiphysitis of the tibial tuberosity occurring most commonly in children between the ages of 10–14 years (47). The condition is characterized by pain at the tibial attachment of the patella tendon and localized swelling and tenderness is evident at the tibial tubercle. The proximal tibial tuberosity is generally tender to palpation and the knee will be otherwise normal on examination with the possible exception of mild limitation of flexion. This condition is most often seen in athletic children and is due to overuse of the quadriceps muscle group resulting in periostitis and/or avulsion of the patella ligament (quadriceps tendon). The most common mechanism of injury is forceful hyperextension of the knee joint producing associated micro-trauma to the fibers of the quadriceps muscle group. The resulting adhesions in the quadriceps muscle produce a tightening of the muscle, resulting in increased tension at the tendon insertion into the proximal tibial tuberosity.

Lateral radiographs of the knee may show fragmentation of the epiphysis of the tibial tubercle, but this finding alone without clinical findings of pain and swelling is insufficient evidence upon which to base a diagnosis (Fig. 14.9). Treatment consists of restoring the elasticity of the quadriceps muscles using cross-friction and longitudinal massage techniques, thereby reducing the ligament pressure being applied at the proximal tibial tuberosity. Compressive adjustment of the tuberosity can also be made. Stretching exercises involving forced knee flexion should be delayed until sufficient elasticity has been restored to the quadriceps muscles; otherwise it will tend to exacerbate the patient's condition. The use of a compressive strap around the knee may help with symptom relief, but generally does little to hasten recovery. The use of ice to control pain may also be appropriate. Ultrasound should not be used to treat this condition if the child has not yet reached skeletal maturity, as its use may have deleterious effects on the continued growth of epiphyses. Resumption of sporting activities can usually be achieved in 2–4 weeks.

Chondromalacia Patella

Chondromalacia patella is a painful condition of the knee caused by the cartilage on the under surface of the patella becoming roughened and fibrillated from repetitive microtrauma. The condition typically affects adolescent and young adult females. The mechanism of injury may include knee hyperextension, stress on the knee joint from ankle pronation, or pelvic subluxation and weakness of the vastus medialis muscle.

Clinical features include a deep aching pain behind the patella, which is exacerbated by climbing or descending stairs or by sitting with the knee flexed for extended periods, e.g., watching a movie. Often knee effusion is present and tenderness can be elicited upon palpating the underside of the patella or by displacing it to the lateral side. Fine crepitus may be present when mobilizing the patella. In more advanced chronic cases crepitus may be clearly audible during walking or when climbing or descending stairs. Radiographs typically show no abnormality.

Treatment includes identification and correction of the mechanical cause. Pronation can be corrected by fitting the patient with foot orthotics. Strengthening exercises for the vastus medialis muscle help to maintain centered patella tracking on the patella surface of the femur. An elastic support may help and the patient should restrict climbing activities until the problem is resolved. Surgery to correct this problem is rarely indicated at best; results are inconsistent.

Growing Pains

As many as 10–20% of children may complain of vague leg pain on a recurrent basis. The diagnosis commonly provided for these symptoms is "growing pains." However, the association of this problem with bone growth has been rejected by most authorities. The pains are usually unilateral, dull and non-specific and located deep within the lower extremity, most commonly in the thigh, knee or calf. Pains typically occur at night when the child is in bed and last 30 minutes to 1 hour. Systemic signs and symptoms are absent and x-ray findings and blood tests are normal. The leg pain symptoms are not present every night but frequently present after a day of intense physical activity. Differential diagnosis should include malignant and

benign bone tumors which can be ruled out on the basis of the duration and persistence of the symptoms. Case reports suggest that patients may respond to adjustment of the sacro-iliac joints, as the problem is thought to be associated with sacro-iliac subluxation producing referred knee pain to the ipsilateral extremity.

Leg Length Discrepancy

Leg length discrepancy is a common occurrence in children. Variation in the length of a child's legs may be anatomical, i.e., caused by variation in the length of the tibia or femur bilaterally; or it may be physiological, i.e., due to unilateral hypertonic muscle contraction associated with pelvic misalignment and/or subluxation/fixation of the lumbosacral or sacro-iliac joints. A study of patients with limb-length inequality showed significant asymmetry of lateral flexion of the spine together with the presence of a compensatory, non-progressive scoliosis (48).

Appropriate correction of leg-length inequality depends upon an accurate evaluation of its cause. Determination of leg-length inequality can be made radiographically or by measurement of the distance between appropriate body structures. Anatomical leg-length deficiency is present if the measurement from the anterior superior iliac spine to the medial malleolus differs from one side of the body to the other. Physiological leg-length discrepancy is present if the measurements from the umbilicus to the medial malleoli differ. Anatomical leg length discrepancy may be associated either with growth retardation or growth stimulation of the affected leg. Growth retardation can be associated with any of the following: congenital skeletal anomalies, infection around a joint or epiphysis, poliomyelitis, tumor or traumatic fracture which affects a growing epiphysis. Anatomical long-leg may be due to growth stimulation commonly due to diaphyseal or metaphyseal fracture of the femur or tibia in childhood.

Lower Extremity Development

Parental concern regarding the torsional and angular development of the lower extremities in children is a frequent occurrence in pediatric practice. The common valgus and varus deformities of the knees represent the normal development process of the lower extremities and will usually resolve with time and further growth. There are hereditary factors as well. According to Staheli (49) medial femoral torsion is frequently seen in the mother of the affected child (Fig. 14.10). A variety of positional deformities of the legs and feet are encountered in children. The distinction needs to be made between a pathologic and a functional cause. A joint which appears to be deformed will usually develop correctly if it can be put passively through a full range of motion. Alternatively, joints which exhibit restriction to passive movement should be evaluated further for possible pathologic causes, e.g. congenital anomalies of the tarsal bones, spasticity or misalignment/fixation of the tarsal bones. Painfully restricted movements of

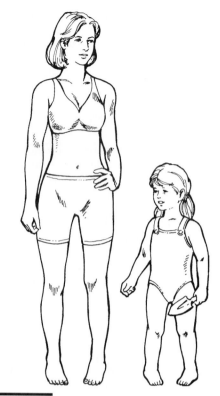

Figure 14.10. Medial femoral torsion can in some instances be hereditary. Modified from: Staheli LT. Torsional deformity. Pediatr Clinics North Am 1986; 33:1375.

the lower extremity joints may indicate joint infection or trauma and radiographic evaluation should be made to identify a possible etiology.

Genu Varus And Genu Valgus

Bowlegs and knock-knees generally represent normal variations in the developing limbs of children, although they may cause considerable anxiety in parents (Fig. 14.11). Most mild symmetric outward varus bowing deformities seen in toddlers represent normal lower extremity development and resolve spontaneously with growth, bone remodeling and time.

Due to the constraints of the uterus, children are often carried in a position in which the hips and knees are flexed and the feet and tibias are internally rotated with respect to the femurs. The medial capsule of the knee, especially the posterior oblique fibers, are contracted. When the child begins to learn to walk, these contractures are still present. As the child stands the tibia is internally rotated with respect to the femur (Fig. 14.12). For the child to walk straight, the femur must be externally rotated. The normally slight anterior curvature of the femur, when seen in profile, creates the bow legged appearance. This physiologic bowing can be corrected with manual pressure (Fig. 14.13). If after about 6 months of independent walking there is no apparent resolution of the genu varum and tightness of the posterior oblique fibers of the capsular ligament is present, then a parent can hasten the process by performing a passive rotation maneuver (Fig. 14.14). Wilkins (50) recommends performing the procedure at each diaper change.

Severe physiologic bowing of the lower extremities in children may be due to metabolic conditions, e.g., rickets (see Chapter 8), or to excessive ligamentous laxity or abnormal alignment of the feet.

A mild to moderate degree of genu valgus (knock-knees) is considered by most authors to be normal in children between the ages of 3 and 7 years. However, posterior sacral subluxation may be an associated entity, especially if the patient also

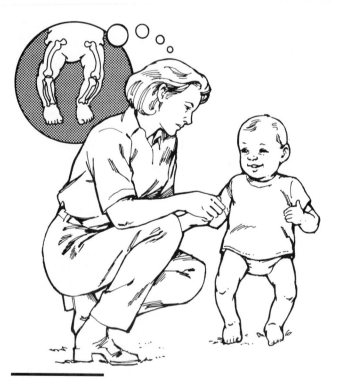

Figure 14.11. Parents may think that their child's bowlegs will persist although most resolve spontaneously. Modified from Wilkins KE. Bowlegs. Pediatr Clinics North Am 1986; 33:1430.

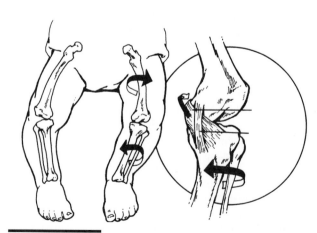

Figure 14.12. Physiologic bowing due to internal rotation of the tibia and external rotation of the femur. Modified from Wilkins KE. Bowlegs. Pediatr Clinics North Am 1986; 33:1431.

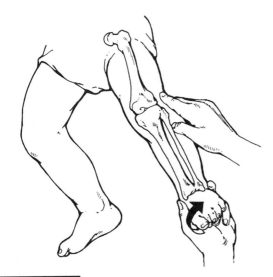

Figure 14.13.   Demonstration of correction of the bow-legged appearance by manually correcting the rotational positions. Modified from Wilkins KE. Bowlegs. Pediatr Clinics North Am 1986; 33:1432.

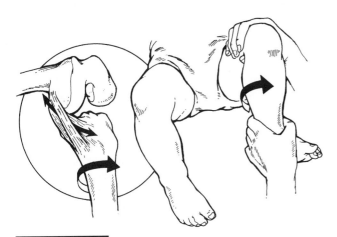

Figure 14.14.   Procedure for stretching the contracted posterior oblique fibers of the joint capsule by externally rotating the tibia with the knee flexed at 90°. Modified from Wilkins KE. Bowlegs. Pediatr Clinics North Am 1986; 33:1431.

demonstrates a bilateral "pigeon toe" deformity. This normal postural development of the lower extremities usually resolves by the age of 7 years. If deformities persist beyond this age then consideration should be given to the presence of pathologic causes.

In-Toeing

In-toeing, sometimes called "pigeon-toed" position, is defined as the turning of the feet toward the midline during walking. This positional characteristic may be due to one of three causes: in-turning of the foot, known as metatarsus adductus, inward tibial torsion, or inward femoral torsion. Subluxations which contribute to this condition may include

a base posterior sacrum (or posterior sacral segment) if the in-toeing is demonstrated bilaterally (Fig. 14.15) or an Ex ilium, if the in-toeing is unilateral (Fig. 14.16). The foot progression angle can be estimated by watching the child walk (Fig. 14.17).

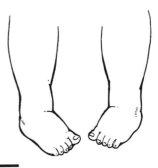

Figure 14.15.   Bilateral toe-in foot flare. Modified from Staheli LT. Torsional deformity. Pediatr Clinics North Am 1986; 33:1376.

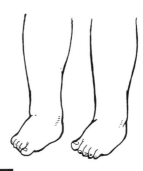

Figure 14.16.   Windswept appearance of unilateral toe-in. Modified from Staheli LT. Torsional deformity. Pediatr Clinics North Am 1986; 33:1376.

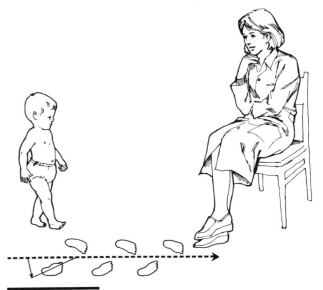

Figure 14.17.   Observation of in-toeing by estimate of the foot progression angle. Modified from Staheli LT. Torsional deformity. Pediatr Clinics North Am 1986; 33:1378.

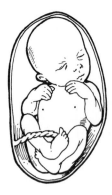

Figure 14.18. Intra-uterine constraint can cause various deformities of the feet, legs, hips, spine and cranium.

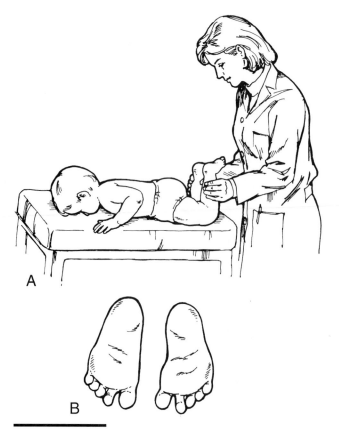

Figure 14.19. Plantar view of metatarsus adductus. Modified from Staheli LT. Torsional deformity. Pediatr Clinics North Am 1986; 33:1379.

METATARSUS ADDUCTUS

Metatarsus adductus probably results from intrauterine malpositioning (Fig. 14.18) and has a characteristic inward turn to the forefoot with the hind foot being in normal alignment. A curved lateral border to the foot is characteristic of this deformity, especially when viewed from the plantar surface (Fig. 14.19). The problem may be either unilateral or bilateral. Upon examination, the front of the feet are deviated medially but otherwise the feet appear normal in all other respects.

Evaluation of the feet for tarsal or metatarsal fixation subluxations is indicated. Spontaneous resolution occurs in approximately 85% of cases (47).

INWARD (MEDIAL) TIBIAL TORSION

Inward or medial tibial torsion is defined as excessive inward twisting of the tibia and is the most common cause of in-toeing in children under three years of age. Clinically, the hip, thigh and knee are normally aligned and the patella faces anteriorly but the lower leg and foot turn inward. The lateral malleolus will be seen to be positioned anteriorly to the medial malleolus, thus shifting the ankle mortise and foot to a medially oriented position. This deformity results in prominent in-toeing during walking, and may cause the child to trip frequently. Knee misalignment should be suspected, especially if there is a history of trauma or if palpable tenderness or edema are present over the knee joint of the affected lower extremity. Inward tibial torsion is considered to be a variation of normal limb development and corrects spontaneously with growth. Bracing is rarely indicated.

INWARD (MEDIAL) FEMORAL TORSION

Inward femoral torsion is the most common cause of in-toeing in children over three years of age and is caused by anteversion of the femoral neck relative to the knee. This condition usually resolves spontaneously in more than 95% of the cases with normal alignment by the age of 10 years (47). The child may sit in a "reverse tailor" position (Fig. 14.20) and this should be discouraged, since it exacerbates the medial femoral torsion.

Out-Toeing

Out-toeing may be caused by external, rotational contracture of the hip or by torsional variations in the femur and tibia (Fig. 14.21). Displacement and fixation of the innominate bone on the involved side may be implicated. Innominate fixation in an

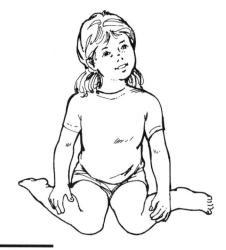

Figure 14.20. The typical sitting posture of a patient with inward or medial femoral torsion. Modified from Staheli LT. Torsional deformity. Pediatr Clinics North Am 1986; 33:1382.

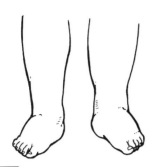

Figure 14.21. Out-toeing.

internally rotated position, i.e., the PSIS is more medially located, could be a contributing factor. It is rarely a functional problem and spontaneous correction is thought to be common. This condition may be caused by an internally rotated ilium and evaluation of pelvic joint mobility should be undertaken. Many toddlers will walk with an externally rotated gait when learning to walk (Fig. 14.22), as an aid to maintaining stability, but this posture should correct naturally by the age of 3 years. Upper cervical subluxation, especially the AS condyle (see Chapters 8 and 9) is sometimes associated with a bilateral toe-out foot flare.

Talipes Equinovarus

Talipes equinovarus, also known as clubfoot, has three anatomical components: equinus (plantar flexion) at the ankle, varus (inversion) at the heel and adduction and supination of the forefoot. Treatment for clubfoot depends on the etiology:

1. Congenital clubfoot which is the most common of the three categories is usually resistant to casting and requires surgery to correct the deformity.

2. Teratologic clubfoot is associated with other deformities, such as spina bifida (meningomyelocele), and typically requires surgery for correction.

3. Postural clubfoot which is due to intrauterine positioning resolves rapidly after birth, usually just with stretching.

Calcaneovalgus Foot

Calcaneovalgus deformity of the foot is a condition of intrauterine malpositioning in which the dorsum of the foot lies pressed up against the anterior tibia. This condition usually resolves rapidly after birth with simple stretching.

Pes Planus (Flat Feet)

All infants have flat feet for a year or two after they begin to stand. In this common condition, the longitudinal arch of the foot is reduced by the presence of a medial fat pad, so that while standing, the medial border of the foot contacts the ground (pronation). This fat pad usually disappears once weight-bearing stance is attained. The persistence of flat feet in children may be associated with generalized ligament laxity or muscle weakness. An appropriate evaluation for flat feet in

children is to examine the feet in both the standing and the supine positions. If the longitudinal arches are absent in the standing position but are present in the supine position, then the likely cause of the flat feet is ligament laxity. Generally, as the ligament laxity of childhood resolves, so do the flat feet. The use of arch supports and other orthoses in children with flat feet is not supported.

Sever's Disease (Calcaneal Apophysitis)

Sever's disease is due to chronic strain of the achilles tendon at the attachment to the calcaneal apophysis. The affected child is usually between the ages of 8 and 13 years and complains of pain behind the heel. A slight limp may be noticed and upon examination there is palpable tenderness over the lower posterior part of the tuberosity of the calcaneus. Radiographic appearance of fragmentation of the calcaneal apophysis is an insignificant finding since this may be present in children who do not have heel pain.

Treatment should include rest from sporting activities for several weeks, together with soft tissue therapy and stretching exercises to increase the elasticity of the calf muscles. Correction of the problem will usually be achieved in 2 to 4 weeks.

Infections of Bones and Joints

Osteomyelitis

Osteomyelitis is an infectious process which most commonly involves the long bones. The initial site of infection usually is

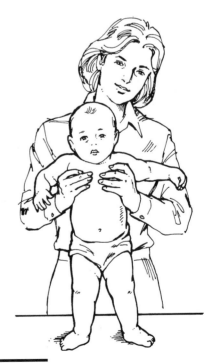

Figure 14.22. Normal out-toeing when a child begins to learn to walk. Modified from Staheli LT. Torsional deformity. Pediatr Clinics North Am 1986; 33:1381.

in the metaphyseal region, with the most common causative organism being Staphylococcus Aureus. Early signs of osteomyelitis include localized tenderness over the metaphysis of a long bone and pain on weight bearing, if the lower extremity is involved. Later, localized erythema, warmth, tenderness, swelling, fever and elevated pulse may be identified. Severe, constant throbbing pain over the end of the shaft of the affected bone, and limitation of joint motion can also be present.

No radiographic changes will be evident within the first 10 days of disease. Occasionally, expansion of the adjacent joint space will be noted but this is not due to infection of the joint but rather to sympathetic effusion. A joint tap of the proximate joint will usually be sterile unless the involved metaphysis lies within the capsule of that joint. Radiographic changes are only usually diagnostic after 10 to 14 days, at which time you should see spotty rarefaction of bone due to demineralization. This stage is followed shortly by periosteal new bone formation.

Early diagnosis of osteomyelitis can be made using a radionucleide bone scan (typically with radioisotope Technetium 99). The radionucleide bone scan will usually be positive as early as the first or second day of the infection. Early referral for antibiotic therapy is essential to save the affected bone and the prognosis is usually good if treatment is begun before radiographic changes are evident.

Pyogenic "Septic" Arthritis

Pyogenic arthritis is a condition in which joints can be infected by bacteria from one of the pyogenic groups, causing an acute inflammatory reaction within the joint tissues. The onset is usually acute with pain and swelling of the affected joint. There is systemic illness with malaise and fever. Typically there is acute joint infection of rapid development, but the infection may be sub-acute or even chronic. When pus is formed within the joint the condition is sometimes called suppurative arthritis. The most common causative organism is Staph. Aureus, except in a child under the age of 2 years when Hemophilus Influenzae is more common. Other causative organisms can include pneumococcus, gonococcus and meningococcus.

Organisms may reach the joint by any one of three routes — through the blood stream (hematogenous), through a penetrating wound, or by extension from an adjacent focus of osteomyelitis. This latter route is especially important when the metaphysis is wholly or partly located within the ligamentous joint capsule, as are the upper humeral metaphysis, the metaphysis at the elbow, and the upper and lower metaphysis of the femur.

SIGNS AND SYMPTOMS

In the young infant in the first year of life, early symptoms can include poor feeding, irritability, and low or normal temperature. Later, as the infection destroys more of the joint there may be pseudo-paralysis of the involved joint and the overlying tissues may become swollen, tender and warm. In older children, early signs include fever, malaise and refusal to walk. The child may complain of severe pain and myospasm and joint splinting may be evident. Pyogenic arthritis must be differentiated from acute infections near the joint, especially acute osteomyelitis.

Definitive diagnosis is by aspiration and culture of fluid from the infected joint. The rapid onset of symptoms, fever, leucocytosis and the presence of pathogenic organisms in the aspirated joint fluid are important diagnostic features. Earliest radiographic changes include distention of the joint capsule. Subsequent changes include narrowing of the cartilage space, erosion of the subchondral bone, irregularity and fuzziness of the bone surfaces, bone destruction and diffuse osteoporosis.

Early referral for a joint tap and antibiotic therapy is essential to save the affected joint from destruction. Prognosis depends on the speed with which treatment is commenced and the outcome can vary from complete resolution with normal function, to total destruction of the joint with fibrous or bony ankylosis.

Spinal Infections

Infections of the spine can be associated with meningitis or diskitis. A patient with back pain accompanied by fever must be considered to have spinal infection until proven otherwise.

Meningitis

Meningitis is a condition in which inflammation of the spinal meninges occurs, usually due to infection with staph aureus bacteria. Ninety percent of cases occur in children between 1 month and 5 years of age, with the first year of life being the period of greatest risk. Signs of meningitis in a young infant can include subtle signs of a tense or bulging anterior fontanel, fever, irritability, disinterest in feeding, drowsiness and vomiting. In older infants and young children, some of the characteristic signs of headache, nuchal rigidity, extension of the head and neck (opisthotonus) and positive Brudzinski's or Kernig's signs may be present. Brudzinski's sign is elicited in the supine position by flexing the patient's chin to the chest and observing involuntary flexing of the hips. Untreated meningitis is usually rapidly fatal, and delay in treatment greatly increases the chance of death or permanent sequellae, thus early diagnosis and treatment is essential.

Diskitis

Diskitis is a condition in which infection of the intervertebral disk occurs mainly in the lumbar spines of young children. Infants and young children with this condition may refuse to walk or stand. Symptoms may include mild fever and localized back pain. Early diagnosis of diskitis may be made by bone scan. As with osteomyelitis, roentgenographic changes may not be present for several weeks.

Pediatric Neoplasms

Pediatric neoplasms can frequently present a challenge to the doctor attending to a young child with bone or joint pain. Pediatric neoplasms need to be considered together with orthopedic and infectious conditions when considering the possible causes of a child's symptoms.

Leukemia

Acute lymphoblastic leukemia is the most common form of cancer in the pediatric age group, representing almost 40% of this entire group of disorders. The highest incidence is in children between the ages of 2 and 5 years of age. Acute lymphoblastic leukemia is associated with a malignant proliferation of immature white blood cells.

The child with leukemia usually has a significant history of illness over the preceding months. The presenting symptoms may be confined to bone pain and/or joint pain which is caused by leukemic cells invading the periosteum and joint capsules. Upon examination the child will usually be anemic with malaise and fever. The anemia is due to the bone marrow gradually being replaced by leukemic cells.

Diagnosis is confirmed by running a complete blood count. Red blood cell count and hemoglobin levels will usually be low with white cells being either elevated, normal or depressed. Thrombocytopenia is the most consistent finding with leukemia and is responsible for the purpuric hemorrhages and easy bruising seen in these children. Anemia is generally normochromic, normocytic and uric acid and LDH levels will usually be elevated. Radiographs may sometimes show fuzzy white bands in the metaphyseal area of the affected bones, a finding which is not due to leukemic cells but rather is due to disordered bone growth. Management of acute lymphoblastic leukemia requires referral to an oncologist.

Hodgkin's Disease

Hodgkin's disease is usually seen in patients in their mid to late teens or in young adults. The disease begins in the lymphoid tissue and is characterized by the presence of Reed-Sternberg cells (abnormal monocytes). Symptoms may include anorexia, weight loss in excess of 10% of body weight, malaise and fever, fatigue, night sweats and pain on ingestion of alcohol. The diagnosis of Hodgkin's disease should be suspected in any patient with painless, asymptomatic lymphadenopathy, most commonly in the cervical region, but other regions such as the axilla, supraclavicular and inguinal areas may also be affected. The disease may progress through four stages with the prognosis being a 90% cure rate if found before stage III:

Stage I. Involvement of one lymph node region only.

Stage II. Involvement of two or more lymph node regions unilaterally.

Stage III. Involvement of lymph nodes on both sides of diaphragm.

Stage IV. Extralymphatic organ involvement.

Nephroblastoma (Wilm's Tumor)

The nephroblastoma is a solid tumor which develops within the renal parenchyma and enlarges with distortion and invasion of adjacent renal tissue. The diagnosis should be suspected in any patient with the finding of a non-tender abdominal mass, who also complains of flank pain. Treatment is by surgical excision.

Neuroblastoma

Neuroblastoma is a tumor arising from cells in the sympathetic ganglia and adrenal medulla. It is the third most frequent pediatric neoplasm with the highest incidence being found at 2 years of age. Symptoms generally include failure to thrive, anorexia, black eyes, fever, diarrhea, hypertension, pallor, irritability, and masses. Diagnosis may be made from plain film radiographs with the finding of multiple destructive lesions of bone and a "moth-eaten" appearance seen throughout all bones. Appropriate management includes referral to an oncologist.

Retinoblastoma

Retinoblastoma is the most common malignant tumor of the eye found in the pediatric age group. Its occurrence, however, is rare and it is often inherited, with the children of survivors having a 50% chance of developing the problem. Retinoblastoma mainly occurs in the first few years of life and diagnosis should be suspected in any child with a missing red reflex and the finding of a whitish, gray mass on ophthalmological examination. Treatment is by radiation and cauterization of the tumor.

Bone Tumors

Characteristically, the pain associated with bone tumors is persistent and of increasing severity. Any child who complains of localized bone pain should be x-rayed to rule out tumor as a possible cause. Radiographic examination will usually help make the diagnosis.

Primary Malignant Bone Tumors

The two most common primary malignant bone tumors are osteogenic sarcoma and the Ewing's tumor.

OSTEOGENIC SARCOMA

Osteogenic sarcoma arises most frequently in the metaphysis of long bones, such as the femur or tibia. The initial complaint is often pain over the affected bone. As the tumor progresses there may be symptoms of swelling, tenderness and heat. Radiographic examination reveals evidence of bone destruction and periosteal new bone formation, with an "onion skin" or "sunburst" appearance. The tumor often metastasizes to other bones or to the lungs and radiographs should be obtained to identify possible metastasis. The definitive diagnosis is made by biopsy. Treatment is initially with chemotherapy for up to one year to control metastasis together with or later followed by amputation of the affected bone with sufficient margin to ensure complete removal of the tumor. This tumor has been known to follow irradiation and is sometimes seen in patients who have been treated for retinoblastoma.

EWING'S SARCOMA

Ewing's sarcoma may occur in any bone. It most frequently involves the long bones such as the femur and tibia and occasionally flat bones such as the scapula. Metastasis can occur to the lungs and to other bones. Initial findings include localized pain in the affected bone with swelling, tenderness and heat. Later, the patient may develop fever. On plain film radiographs, Ewing's sarcoma resembles an abscess and is characterized by bone destruction and soft tissue mass. Treatment currently consists of radiation and chemotherapy.

Benign Bone Tumors

Benign tumors are more likely to be painless, however there are two notable exceptions, osteoid osteoma and benign osteoblastoma.

OSTEOID OSTEOMA

Osteoid osteoma may typically affect long bones and/or vertebrae. A patient with osteoid osteoma will usually complain of pain which is characteristically worse at night and relieved by aspirin. Diagnosis is by plain film radiography or bone scan with the finding of a small radiolucent nidus surrounded by a sclerotic border.

BENIGN OSTEOBLASTOMA

Benign osteoblastoma is similar to the osteoid osteoma except that the radiolucent lesion is larger than an osteoid osteoma and the surrounding bone is less sclerotic.

Pediatric Arthritides

Arthritis

Clinically, arthritis is characterized by pain and restriction of movement at a joint, arising spontaneously. In superficial joints these features are usually accompanied by obvious swelling and thickening. Table 14.4 identifies the clinical manifestations of arthritis.

Juvenile Rheumatoid Arthritis (JRA)

Juvenile rheumatoid arthritis is the most common form of arthritis in children. JRA has several forms of onset each with its own characteristic set of symptoms. The diagnosis of JRA is a diagnosis of exclusion, i.e., the diagnosis is only made after all other possible conditions have been ruled out. The conditions which should commonly be considered and excluded prior to making a diagnosis of JRA are listed in Table 14.5.

Table 14.4.   Clinical Manifestations of Arthritis

Joint swelling

Joint pain at rest

Joint pain on palpation

Joint pain on motion

Heat

Redness

Loss of motion

Table 14.5.   Differential Diagnosis of Juvenile Rheumatoid Arthritis

Rheumatic diseases
  Acute rheumatic fever
  Systemic lupus erythematosus
Infectious diseases
  Pyogenic arthritis
  Transient synovitis
  Osteomyelitis
Malignancies
  Leukemia
  Neuroblastoma
  Hodgkin's lymphoma
Orthopedic disorders
  Spinal subluxation
  Legg-Calvé-Perthes
  Osgood Schlatter
  Kohler's
  Fractures (battered child syndrome)
  Joint injuries
  Chondromalacia patella syndrome
Reactive arthritis

Reactive Arthritis

Reactive arthritis is characterized by sterile joint effusion occurring 10–14 days after a bacterial infection of the gastrointestinal tract by Salmonella, Shigella or Yersinia Enterocolitica. The presence of HLA-B27 in patients with reactive arthritis suggests a genetic predisposition.

Juvenile Rheumatoid Arthritis (JRA)

Juvenile rheumatoid arthritis is a chronic deforming arthritis of unknown etiology, affecting children under 16 years. The onset of the disease has two peaks, one between the ages of 2 and 5 years and a second peak between the ages of 9 and 12 years. The female to male ratio is about 2:1. JRA differs from adult rheumatoid arthritis in the following ways:

1. Systemic features such as high fever, pericarditis, uveitis and rash are common.

2. Blood tests for rheumatoid factor are usually negative.

3. The child is less likely to complain of joint pain than the adult.

4. Remission is frequently characteristic.

The diagnosis of JRA demands chronicity and joint swelling must be present for a period of at least 6 weeks before a diagnosis of JRA can be made. An attack of JRA can frequently be preceded by physical or emotional trauma suggesting a diverse neuroimmunological etiology. Osteopathic physicians (51) have recommended manipulative treatment in patients with JRA. Treatment is directed at reducing swelling and increasing range of motion of the affected articulations. These physicians do not recommend high velocity manipulation in patients with inflamed or unstable joints; soft tissue and muscle energy techniques can be applied. Mobilization techniques that pump the affected joint are believed to be capable of reducing immune complexes and inflammatory mediators within the joint through lymphatic drainage (51).

ACUTE SYSTEMIC (STILL'S DISEASE)

In some children, systemic symptoms are the first manifestation of JRA. In the acute systemic form of JRA, typically fever will spike with daily or twice daily elevations of temperature to 103 to 104 degrees. The child may appear quite ill during the period of elevated temperature and surprisingly well when the temperature falls. A characteristic salmon-pink maculo-papular rash often accompanies the fever. This rash is migratory and generally non-pruritic. Other symptoms can include myalgia, lymphadenopathy, hepatosplenomegaly and pericarditis. Joint manifestations may not be present, but when they do occur the patient's symptoms usually follow a similar course to that of the polyarticular form of JRA.

POLYARTICULAR ARTHRITIS

With polyarticular JRA, joint tenderness and soft tissue swelling is present in both large and small joints. The pattern of joint involvement is usually symmetrical with hip, knee, ankle, elbow and small joints of the hands being involved. Cervical spine involvement may occur with stiffness or acute pain and occasionally torticollis. The temperomandibular joint (TMJ) may be involved in this type of JRA with symptoms which can include difficulty in opening the mouth, jaw stiffness and occasionally shortening of the mandible (micrognathia).

PAUCIARTICULAR (OLIGOARTICULAR) OR MONOARTICULAR

The most common type of arthritis to affect the spine in children is the pauciarticular type of JRA, identified as type II. The large joints such as the knees, ankles and wrists are usually involved in an asymmetric pattern. There is usually considerable swelling of the involved joints. At onset, only one joint may be involved, but the symptoms can migrate later to involve other joints. The affected child may limp, especially in the morning. Involved joints may be warm and tender but there is usually no erythema of the overlying skin evident. In pauciarticular JRA, boys around 8 years of age are most commonly affected, initially in the hips, knees and ankles. Later involvement may affect the sacro-iliac joints and the lumbar and thoracic vertebrae. The presenting complaint is usually lower back pain with accompanying hip and thigh pain. A family history of anky-

losing spondylitis may be helpful in diagnosing this condition, but is not pathognomonic. This problem can be the precursor to the more classic ankylosing spondylitis which presents some years later. Iridocyclitis (uveitis) is a common complication of this type of JRA and since blindness is common with uveitis, referral to an ophthalmologist for evaluation and treatment is essential.

Sports Injuries

Spinal Injuries and Associated Sports

FOOTBALL

Football is the most common sport for "collision injuries" in American children. About half of the sporting injuries to high school and college students are the result of tackling in football. In the US, in one 12 month period (1975-76), 13 fatalities occurred from football, while only four fatalities occurred from other sporting activities (52). The most common injuries occurring from football involve the head and neck. Cervical spine injuries are the greatest cause of long term disability and therefore represent the most serious type of injury suffered with injuries to the neck usually being the result of inappropriate tackling procedures. The problem with head tackling is that inexperienced players, just before a head tackle, will tend to flex the neck prior to impact, producing the potential for axial loading of the spine resulting in vertebral fractures. Severe flexion injuries may also result in fracture or dislocation of the spine. One survey of collision injuries in football revealed that of 40 spinal injuries suffered, 39 were in players under the age of 20 years (53). Thirty five of these players were quadriplegic upon admission and of whom six recovered some degree of ambulatory function.

Lateral flexion injuries to the neck which involve traction injury to the brachial plexus are less serious but are the more common type of football injuries. This type of injury, known as a "burner" involves a sudden shooting or burning pain down the arm. Later the player usually has difficulty in moving the arm, but this quickly resolves leaving just a dull aching sensation in the extremity. Players injured in this way should not be allowed to continue to play in that game and a detailed examination should be conducted. Any young player who suffers a "burner" should be examined also for underlying congenital anomalies of the cervical spine.

WATER SPORTS AND DIVING

A common sports related injury to the cervical spine is that associated with diving. Diving into shallow water and hitting the head on the bottom or on a submerged object is the most common cause of this type of neck injury. Most such injuries involve cervical spine fracture and/or spinal cord damage. Studies have shown that the velocity of the body at entry into the water is not significantly dissipated until the diver reaches a depth of 10-12 feet. Diving technique has been shown to have a significant impact on the incidence of injury.

Experienced divers will use their hands to precede the entry of the body into the water. This technique significantly protects the head upon entry. Inexperienced divers, with no particular technique, tend to leave their head unprotected, leading to a higher incidence of injuries. Studies of low back injuries, particularly of spondylolysis, have demonstrated a significant incidence of this type of injury in inexperienced divers. The cause of the associated fracture to the pars interarticularis appears to be poor diving technique. In particular, hyperextension of divers' legs at the point of entry to the water causes the lumbar spine to hyperextend resulting in compression of the pars interarticularis with resulting fracture.

GYMNASTICS AND TRAMPOLINE INJURIES

Gymnastics, and especially trampoline programs, have come under considerable criticism in the literature for the high incidence of cervical and lumbar spine injuries encountered (54). The incidence of such injuries was of great concern prior to the publication of a policy statement in 1977 by the American Academy of Pediatrics. Subsequent banning of trampoline programs took place in most schools and the incidence of cervical spine injuries diminished. The recommendations for the use of trampolines in gymnastics programs state in part... "highly trained personnel who have been instructed in all aspects of trampoline safety must be present when the apparatus is used" and "...maneuvers, especially somersault, should be attempted only by those qualified to become skilled performers."

SKIING

Spinal injuries related to skiing are primarily associated with injuries to the cervical spine. The high incidence of collisions where the head hits an object has been cited as the major cause of these injuries. Injuries typically involve anterior-posterior movements of the head with associated hyperextension/hyperflexion rebound injuries.

WEIGHT-LIFTING

Spinal injury due to weight lifting is a common occurrence, especially in adolescence. Hyperextension facet syndromes are the most common injuries associated with weight-lifting in this age group while injuries such as vertebral endplate fractures can occur without significant pain. Scheuermann's disease of the lumbar spine is also common in teenage weight-lifters. The mechanism of injury is hyperextension and the pathophysiology is associated with repeated stress to the apophyseal ring of the vertebral body producing a herniation of the nuclear material anteriorly into the apophyseal defect. The problem usually resolves with rest.

Spondylolysis and spondylolisthesis can be aggravated by weight-lifting during the adolescent period. It is thought that lumbar hyperextension, associated with squats, is the mechanism of injury, particularly during the adolescent growth spurt, when spinal structures are characteristically weak. The rule is to discourage squats and power-lifting in adolescents during the growth-spurt period.

REFERENCES

1. Warwick R, Williams P, eds. Gray's Anatomy, 35th edition, Longman, Edinburgh, 1973:248.
2. Warwick R, Williams P, eds. Gray's Anatomy, 35th edition, Longman, Edinburgh, 1973:245.
3. Ogden J. Development and maturation of the neuromusculoskeletal system. In: Lovell and Winters, eds: Pediatric Orthopedics. Philadelphia: J.B. Lippincott, 1990.
4. Warwick R, Williams P, eds. Gray's Anatomy, 35th edition, Longman, Edinburgh, 1973:246.
5. Anderson M, Hwang SC, Green WT. Growth of the trunk in normal boys and girls during the second decade of life. J Bone Joint Surg 1965; 47A:1554.
6. Chapelais JD, Macfarlane JA. A review of 404 "late walkers". Arch Dis Child 1984; 59:512-6.
7. McEwan MH, Dihoff RE, Brosvic GM. Early infant crawling experience is reflected in later motor skill development. Percept Motor Skills 1991; 72:75-9.
8. Rieder M, Schwartz C, Newman J. Patterns of walker use and walker injury. Pediatrics 1986; 78:488-93.
9. Kauffman IB, Ridenour M. Influence of an infant walker on onset and quality of walking pattern of locomotion. Percept Motor Skills 1977; 45:1323-9.
10. Crouchman M. The effects of babywalkers on early locomotor development. Dev Med Child Neurol 1986; 28:757-61.
11. Trinkoff A, Parkes PL. Prevention strategies for infant walker-related injuries. Public Health Rep 1993; 108:784-8.
12. Chiaviello CT, Christoph RA, Bond GR. Infant walker-related injuries: a prospective study of severity and incidence. Pediatrics 1994; 93:974-6.
13. Mayr J, et al. Baby walkers-an underestimated hazard for our children. Eur J Pediatr 1994; 153:531-4.
14. McEwan MH, Dihoff RE, Brosvic GM. Early infant crawling experience is reflected in later motor skill development. Percept Motor Skills 1991; 72:75-9.
15. Grundy PF, Roberts CJ. Does unequal leg length cause back pain? A case-control study. Lancet 1984; (8397):256-8.
16. Sponseller PD. Bone, joint and muscle problems. In Oski FA, ed. Principles and practice of pediatrics. Philadelphia: J.B. Lippincott, 1994.
17. Wissow L. Child Maltreatment. In: Oski FA, ed. Principles and practice of pediatrics. Philadelphia: JB Lippincott, 1994.
18. Sty JR, et al. Diagnostic imaging of infants and children. Maryland: Aspen, 1992:246.
19. Rachesky I, et al: Clinical prediction of cervical spine injuries in children. Am J Dis Child 1987; 141:196-201.
20. Biedermann H. Kinematic imbalances due to suboccipital strain in newborns. J Manual Med 1992; 6:151-156.
21. Jirout J. Roentgenologische Bewegungsdiagnostik der Halswirbelsaule. Sittgart: Fischer, 1990.
22. Burkus JK, Deponte RJ. Chronic atlantoaxial rotatory fixation correction by cervical traction, manipulation and bracing. J Pediatr Orthop 1986; 6:631-5.
23. Dolan KD. Developmental abnormalities of the cervical spine below the axis. Radiol Clin North Am 1977; 15:167-75.
24. Hensinger R, Fielding J. The cervical spine. In: Morrissey RT, ed. Pediatric orthopedics. Philadelphia: J.B. Lippincott, 1990.
25. Ogden JA. Development and maturation of the neuromusculoskeletal system. In: Morrissey RT, ed. Pediatric Orthopedics. Philadelphia: J.B. Lippincott, 1990.
26. White JI. Back pain in the pediatric patient. In: Spine: State of the Art Reviews 1990; 4 (1).
27. Ross EP, Malleson P. Spondyloarthropathies in childhood. Pediatr Clin North Am 1986; 33:1079-96.
28. Rigby AS, Wood PH. Observations on diagnostic criteria for ankylosing spondylitis. Clin Exp Rheumatol 1993; 11: 5-12.
29. Ytterberg SR, et al. Exercise in arthritis. Clin Rheumatol 1994; 8:161-89.
30. Jenkinson TR. et al. Defining spinal mobility in ankylosing spondylitis. J. Rheumatol 1994; 21:1694-8.
31. Alexander CJ. Scheuermann's disease: A traumatic spondylodystrophy? Skel Radiol 1977; 1:209.
32. Winter RB. Spinal problems in pediatric orthopedics. In: Morrissey RT, ed. Pediatric orthopedics. Philadelphia: J.B. Lippincott, 1990:693.
33. Murtagh FR, et al. The role and incidence of facet tropism in lumbar spine degenerative disc disease. J Spinal Dis 1991; 4:86-9.
34. Cyron BM, Hutton WC. Articular tropism and stability of the lumbar spine. Spine 1980; 5:168-72.
35. Noren R, et al. The role of facet joint tropism and facet angle in disc degeneration. Spine 1991; 16:530-2.
36. Ment LR, Fishman MA. Neuroembryology. In: Oski FA, ed. Principles and practice of pediatrics, 2nd ed. Philadelphia: J.B. Lippincott, 1994:342.
37. Scoles PV. Pediatric orthopedics in clinical practice, 2nd ed. Chicago: Yearbook Med Publishers, 1991:265.
38. Yates JW, Ferguson-Smith, MA. Is disordered folate metabolism the basis for the genetic predisposition to neural tube defects? Clin. Genet 1987; 31:279.
39. Seller MJ, Nevin NC. Periconceptional vitamin supplementation and the prevention of neural tube defects in south-east England and north Ireland. J Med Genet 1984; 21:325.
40. Carter CO, Wilkinson JA. Genetic environmental factors in the etiology of congenital dislocation of the hip. Clin Orthop 1964; 33:119.

41. Grill F, et al. The Pavilk harness in the treatment of the congenitally dislocating hip. J Pediatr Orthop 1988; 8:1.
42. Pavlik A. Stirrups as an aid in the treatment of congenital dysplasias of the hip in children. J Pediatr Orthop 1989; 9:157.
43. Guebert G, et al. Congenital anomalies and normal skeletal variants. In: Yochum T, Rowe L, eds. Essentials of skeletel radiology. Baltimore: Williams & Wilkins, 1987:128.
44. Kehl DK, et al. Developmental coxa vara. Orthop Trans 1993; 7:475.
45. Behrman RE, ed. Nelson textbook of pediatrics. 14th ed. Philadelphia: WB Saunders, 1992:1710.
46. Weinstein, SL. Legg-Calve-Perthes disease. In: Morrissey RT, ed. Pediatric Orthopedics, Lippincott, Philadelphia, 1990;2(23):868.

47. Staheli, LT. The lower limb. In: Morrissey RT, ed. Pediatric orthopedics. Philadelphia: J.B. Lippincott, 1990:763.
48. Papaioannou T. Stokes I, Kenwright J. Scoliosis associated with limb-length inequality. J Bone Joint Surg 1990; 64A:59-62.
49. Staheli LT. Torsional deformity. Pediatr Clinics North Am 1986; 33:1373-1383.
50. Wilkins KE. Bowlegs. Pediatr Clinics North Am 1986; 33:1429-1438.
51. Pertusi RM, Rubin BR, Blackwell D. Juvenile rheumatoid arthritis. J Am Osteopath Assoc 1996; 96:298-301.
52. Cantu RC. Head and spine injuries in the young athlete. Clin Sports Med 1988; 7:459-472.
53. Alley RH. Head and neck injuries in high school football. JAMA 1964; 188:418-422.
54. Zimmerman HM. Accident experience with trampolines. Res Q 1956; 27:452.

15 Scoliosis

Raymond R. Brodeur, Gregory Plaugher, Richard A. Elbert, and Charles A. Lantz

Scoliosis is defined as an appreciable lateral deviation of the spine. It can affect patients of all age groups with complications varying from cosmetic deformity to severe cardiac and pulmonary compression and death. When viewed from the frontal plane, and assuming relative anatomical and loading symmetry, the ideal shape is a straight spinal column; however, anatomists more than 200 years ago described everyone as having a slight scoliosis (1). Most children are not posturally symmetrical, with most having a slight right scoliosis and slight right rib hump. In a recent study, only 2 of 265 children were symmetrical, with most of the children having a short left leg, a left lumbar hump and a right thoracic rib hump (2). Since true symmetry is rare, the clinician needs to consider the point at which spinal asymmetry is a concern to the patient and the parents.

Currently, the Scoliosis Research Society defines scoliosis to be a lateral deviation of the spine of greater than 10°. This may be adequate for the orthopedic surgeon, who has no treatment modality to recommend until a curve exceeds 20°. However, the chiropractor is likely to assume that any lateral deviation is of concern and should be treated as soon as possible. Recent reports have used 5° as the minimum degree of curvature as an inclusion criterion for the presence of scoliosis (3,4).

In this chapter, we will discuss the current state of knowledge regarding scoliosis diagnosis and patient treatment, concentrating on progressive adolescent scoliosis, the type that is of most concern to clinicians and patients alike.

Scoliosis Identification and Measurement

The apex of a scoliosis is at the vertebra having the largest lateral deviation from the mid-line of the spine when viewed on an AP radiograph. A scoliotic curve is named according to the location of the apex of the curve. For example, a scoliosis is a thoracic curve if the apex is in the thoracic spine.

The curve is either a "right" or "left" scoliosis as defined by the convexity. A right scoliosis is convex to the right and a right thoracic scoliosis indicates that the apex of the curve is in the thoracic spine and that the curve is convex to the right. If the apex is in a transitional area, the curve is classified as transitional. For example, if the apex is between T11 to L1, then the curve is called a thoraco-lumbar scoliosis.

Cobb Angle

Cobb (5) first defined his method for measuring scoliosis in 1948. His method is well known to many clinicians and remains the primary measurement tool for analyzing scoliosis, in spite of many attempts to develop improvements.

The end-vertebrae of the curve are those having the greatest angulation towards the apex of the curvature. Lines are drawn parallel to the superior endplate of the cephalic end-vertebra and the inferior endplate of the caudal end-vertebra. The angle between these two lines is the Cobb angle (Fig. 15.1).

The Cobb angle has been shown to have a high measurement error, with repeated measure standard deviations of between 2° to 3° for the same examiner measuring the same film (6) and has been reported to be as large as 4° for multiple examiners (7). In addition to technical variabilities in the measurement, the Cobb angle does not provide any description of the three-dimensional aspects of scoliosis and has been shown to under-estimate the actual severity of the curve (7). However, in spite of these short comings, it is likely to remain the primary method for measuring scoliosis curves for the foreseeable future.

Other Measurements of Scoliotic Curves

The Cobb angle is independent of the number of vertebrae involved in a scoliosis and provides only a limited description of the true shape of a scoliotic spine. Voutsinas and MacEwen (8) have suggested additional measurements for describing spinal curves. It is possible for two curves to have the same Cobb angle, as shown in Figure 15.2, but the distance of the apex of the curve from the long-axis of the spine may vary significantly, as depicted. The ratio of the width of the curve to the length of the curve is a descriptor that requires further investigation (6).

Many methods have been proposed for describing scoliotic curves. Moire topography (9) and other photographic methods have been proposed to describe the trunk topography (10).

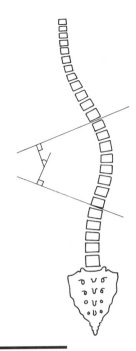

Figure 15.1. Cobb angle measurement.

However, it is difficult to determine underlying skeletal changes from surface features and thus these approaches are still experimental as well as controversial. More recently, CT scans have been used to more thoroughly describe scoliotic curves (11). Three-dimensional methods using stereo or bi-planar radiography have also been proposed for describing scoliotic shapes (7). With the increasing use of computers, the means for describing the full three-dimensional aspect of the scoliotic curve will be easier for the clinician (12). At the present time, the above measurement tools are either too controversial or too experimental to be used by most clinicians.

Torso Balance

Ideally, when viewing a full spine standing AP or PA radiograph, a line connecting T1 to S1 should be vertical. The extent to which there is some deviation in this line is graded as the torso balance (13). A vertical line is drawn from S1 to the top of the radiograph. The horizontal distance from T1 to the vertical line is used to describe the torso balance grade (Fig. 15.3). A grade 1 corresponds to less than 1.5 cm from T1 to the vertical line passing through the mid-line of the sacrum. Grade 2 corresponds to a distance between 1.6–3.0 cm, grade 3 from between 3.1–5.0 cm and grade 4 if the distance from T1 to the sacral mid-line is greater than 5 cm.

Vertebral Rotation

Nash and Moe (14) suggested measuring relative vertebral rotation based on the distance between the pedicles. Normally the pedicles are symmetrical relative to the spinous process and are oval in shape. The pedicles shift toward the concave side of the scoliosis (the spinous points toward the concavity). The amount of rotation is graded from 0 to 4 and the grade for the

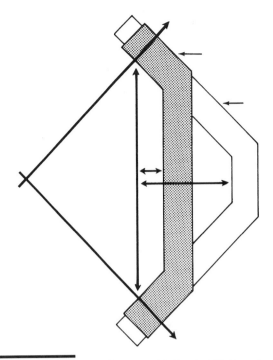

Figure 15.2. Two spinal curves with identical Cobb angles are represented (a and b). Although both curvatures are quite different in terms of magnitude, using Cobb's angle as the sole criterion for assessment leads to identical measurements. The differences in the two curves can be more accurately assessed by scrutinizing the ratio between the length (L) and their respective widths (W and W1). Modified from Voutsinas, MacEwen GD. Sagittal profiles of the spine. Clin Orthop 1986; 210:236.

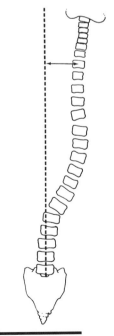

Figure 15.3. Torso balance.

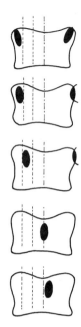

Figure 15.4. Vertebral rotation using the method of Nash and Moe. Modified from McAlister WH, Shackelford MGD. Measurement of spinal curvatures. Radiol Clin North Am 1975; 13:119.

patient is defined by the most rotated vertebra, which is usually at the apex. The vertebral body is divided into segments as shown in Figure 15.4. No rotation corresponds to a grade 0; grade 1 is the rotation of the pedicle into the first segment, at a grade 2, the pedicle is in the second segment; with a grade 3, the pedicle is at the mid-line of the vertebra; and grade 4 occurs when the pedicle crosses the mid-line of the vertebra. The pedicle position can also be used to estimate the number of degrees of vertebral rotation (13,14) as shown in Figure 15.4. Pedicle rotation is described as a percentage of the position on the vertebral body, with each percentage point corresponding to one degree. For example, if the pedicle is at 25% of the body, it corresponds to a rotation of 25°.

The vertebra with the most rotation occurs at the apex of a structural scoliosis. However, the relative rotation is smallest at the apex and largest at the junction of the structural curve with the upper and lower compensatory curves (15). Thus, although the total amount of rotation is largest at the apical vertebra, it is a result of the summing of rotations from the vertebrae above and below the apex. The vertebra at the apex has very little rotation relative to the vertebra above and below. When assessing the relative rotations at an individual motion segment, as is the case when determining a listing for a specific adjustment, it is important to carefully compare the relative pedicle sizes with the neighboring levels.

Vertebral Wedging

In moderate to severe scoliosis, the vertebrae often become wedge-shaped when viewed on AP or PA radiographs. Wedging may also occur as a result of a congenital anomaly. If the vertebral body height decreases laterally by less than

1/6, it is considered grade 1 wedging (13). A decrease in vertebral height of between 1/6 to 1/3 the contralateral height is considered grade 2 wedging; 1/3 to 1/2 is grade 3 wedging, and a difference in left-right vertebral height of more than ½ the contralateral height is considered grade 4 wedging (Fig. 15.5).

Wedging of vertebrae may develop as a result of unequal loading on the vertebral endplates (i.e., Heuter-Volkmann Law) (16). Some structural curves may begin without initial osseous deformity, but start with changes in the viscoelastic elements instead (e.g., in discs, muscles, etc.). Any treatment would likely be optimally effective if it could alter the initial soft tissue deformity rather than attempting to change the secondary osseous changes that have occurred.

Classifications for Scoliosis

Structural and Non-Structural Scoliosis

There are many different causes for scoliosis, but the vast majority are considered to be idiopathic in origin. Table 15.1 is a summary of scoliosis classifications originally described by Winter (17) and modified by Plaugher and Lopes (18). Essentially, scoliosis can be divided into structural curves and nonstructural or functional curves. A structural scoliosis will not straighten when the patient flexes during forward bending, while functional curves will reduce or disappear on forward bending and lateral bending to the side of the convexity.

A functional scoliosis is caused by factors external to the spine. A short leg or a pelvic asymmetry are common causes. Lateral flexion subluxations can occur (Fig. 15.6). In some cases, structural scoliosis may begin as functional curves. If such asymmetries occur at a young age, it has been proposed that the stresses on the vertebral growth plates may be sufficient to cause bone remodeling and thereby creating a structural curve (18).

Curve Patterns

Structural curves are classified into commonly occurring patterns (13):

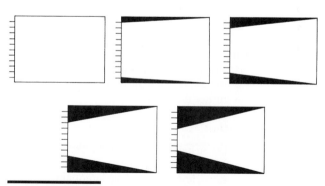

Figure 15.5. Vertebral body wedging. Modified from McAlister WH, Shackelford MGD. Measurement of spinal curvatures. Radiol Clin North Am 1975; 13:120.

Table 15.1.   Classifications of Structural and Functional Scoliosis

Structural Scoliosis	Functional Scoliosis
I. Idiopathic	I. Postural scoliosis
A. Infantile (0–3 years)	II. Hysterical scoliosis
1. Resolving	III. Nerve root irritation
2. Progressive	A. Herniation of the intervertebral disc
B. Juvenile (3–10 years)	B. Disk block subluxation
C. Adolescent (>10 years)	C. Tumors
II. Neuromuscular	IV. Segmental
A. Neuropathic	V. Inflammatory
1. Upper motor neuron lesion	VI. Leg length inequality
2. Lower motor neuron lesion	VII. Hip joint muscle contractures
3. Dysautonomia	
B. Myopathic	
III. Congenital	
A. Failure of formation	
B. Failure of segmentation	
IV. Neurofibromatosis	
V. Mesenchymal disorders	
VI. Rheumatoid disease	
VII. Trauma	
VIII. Extraspinal contractures	
IX. Osteochondrodystrophies	
X. Infection of bone	
XI. Metabolic disorders	
XII. Related to lumbosacral joint	
XIII. Tumors	

1. Cervicothoracic
2. Thoracic
3. Thoracolumbar
4. Lumbar

Double structural curves:

1. Double thoracic
2. Combined thoracic and lumbar
3. Combined thoracic and thoracolumbar

Right thoracic structural curves are far more common than left thoracic curves and extend from about T5 to T11 with the apex near T8. In fact, the right thoracic pattern is so common that if the opposite (left thoracic scoliosis) is found, then further

examination of the patient is warranted. Patients with syringomyelia or Arnold–Chiari type 1 malformation have a greater likelihood of having a left convex thoracic scoliosis (19,20). In a review of more than 1600 scoliosis cases, Coonrad et al. (21), identified only 27 left thoracic curve patterns. Of these 27 cases, 9 had a neurologic etiology.

With the right thoracic structural curve, there is usually a compensatory lumbar curve that is often confused with a double structural curve. The difference is that the compensatory lumbar curve is functional and can be completely reduced with flexion or lateral flexion whereas the thoracic curve cannot. Patients with a large thoracic structural curve have more severe cardiorespiratory distress and statistics show that they die earlier (22,23).

The thoracolumbar curve extends from about T8 to L3 with the apex near T11. These curves are less likely to have any associated compensatory curves and the center of gravity of the

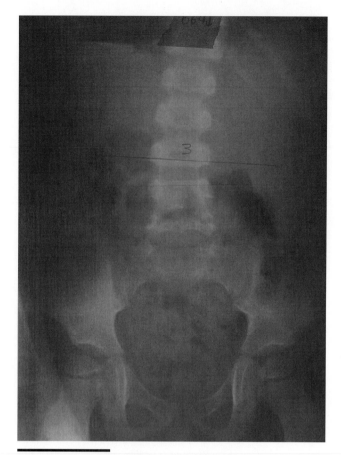

Figure 15.6.   Lateral flexion subluxation of L3.

head is often displaced slightly lateral to the mid-line of the pelvis. Patients with thoracolumbar curves suffer from fewer cardiopulmonary problems; however, curve progression in adulthood is more likely (24).

The structural lumbar curves range from about T12 to L4 with the apex near L3. This curve is most often convex to the left and usually has a pelvic obliquity associated with it, giving the appearance of a short leg on the side of the concavity. A thoracic compensatory curve is commonly found, but the thoracic curve is mild by comparison. These patients often suffer from arthritic changes in the lumbar spine later in life. Lateralisthesis at the apex of the curve is a late sequelae of annular injury. Lumbar curves are less likely to progress than other types (24).

The most common double structural curve is the combined thoracic and lumbar. As the name implies, both curves are structural, that is, neither curve will disappear on forward flexion or lateral bending. Generally, they have a right thoracic and a left lumbar curve. Patients with combined thoracic and lumbar curves are more likely to maintain torso balance and to have less cosmetic deformity. However, they usually have a smaller torso height due to the increased curvature as well as more arthritic changes and pain in the lumbar spine in later life (24).

Infantile

Infantile scoliosis is defined as that occurring during the first three years. It is more common in males (3:2 ratio) and the curve is most often in the thoracic spine and is usually convex to the left. This condition is rare in North America. Positioning of a baby in its crib may play a role in the development of this type of scoliosis, but this does not explain why it is more common with males (25). The condition has been highly correlated with low birth weight, prematurity, mental retardation, and delayed muscle development. Although most cases resolve on their own (74–97%), progressive curves become very severe and disabling.

The difference in the left and right rib-vertebral angle can be used to indicate the probability of progression for infantile scoliosis (Fig. 15.7). Mehta (26) and others (27) have reported that rib-vertebra angle (RVA) differences greater than 20° are more likely to progress. Also, if the RVA is less than 68° at the apex, then progression is also likely.

Juvenile

Juvenile scoliosis is defined as that occurring after three years and before the onset of puberty. It occurs more often with females and most cases begin before the age of ten. There are many who argue that adolescent idiopathic scoliosis (AIS) cases are simply cases of juvenile scoliosis that went undetected. The current trend in scoliosis screenings is to try to detect the onset of scoliosis before puberty begins (15,18,28). Juvenile curves are most likely to progress and must be monitored radiologically at a minimum of 3–6 month intervals. Curves that show no sign of progression after follow-up can be monitored less frequently with radiographs. Individual patients with objective signs of subluxation (e.g., tenderness, motion restriction) may require more frequent clinical examinations and treatment (e.g., chiropractic).

Juvenile patients must be monitored throughout adolescence since curve progression is most likely to occur during this growth period. Severe spinal deformity results if progressive curves are left untreated.

Adolescent

Adolescent idiopathic scoliosis (AIS) takes place at any time between puberty and adulthood. It is the most common type of idiopathic scoliosis. Since it occurs at a time when physical appearance is most important to an individual, progressive

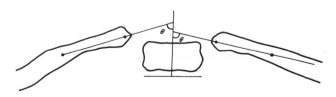

Figure 15.7.   Coronal plane view of Mehta's rib-vertebra angle measurement.

cases can leave physical as well as emotional scars. For curves of less than 20° the female to male ratio is 1:1, but for curves greater than 20° the occurrence is much higher for females (up to 5.4:1) (29).

Progression of a scoliotic curve varies greatly between individuals. For the most part, adolescent curves are not progressive. It is estimated that only one to six per thousand will ever require treatment for scoliosis (29–32) . However, because we can only know in retrospect which curves progress, deciding which cases need monitoring is a challenge. All authorities agree that monitoring is most important during the rapid growth phase of puberty. However, there is a great variability in the growth rate as well as the onset of growth. The sections below will describe the natural history of AIS and the many variables that have been shown to affect curve progression.

NATURAL HISTORY OF ADOLESCENT SCOLIOSIS

Present screening procedures are based on a limited knowledge of the natural history of adolescent scoliosis. The early symptomatic stage shows slight postural asymmetry as well as a rib hump on forward flexion. However, the point at which the lateral deviation requires referral for diagnosis and treatment is not well defined (30,33–38).

The cause of progressive spinal scoliosis is far from being understood but our knowledge of its clinical course is improving. Dickson (15,34) has reported that progressive idiopathic scoliosis has a characteristic loss of the normal thoracic kyphosis at the area of the apex of the scoliosis. This loss of kyphosis is often a local thoracic lordosis. The loss of thoracic kyphosis in the presence of progressive spinal scoliosis is supported by Willner (39) and Somerville (40). Willner reports a consistent loss of the thoracic kyphosis in children with scoliosis compared with a normal population. Somerville hypothesized that progressive scoliosis consists of a local lordosis, rotation, and lateral flexion of the vertebrae involved. In studies involving clinical, cadaveric, biomechanical and radiological investigations of the pathogenesis of progressive spinal scoliosis, Dickson and co-workers have concluded that there is always the presence of a local lordosis at the level of the apex of the scoliosis (15,41–43).

Investigations into the normal spinal development of children reveals a constant decrease of the thoracic kyphosis from the age of 8 to 12 years. After the 12th year the angle of the kyphosis begins to increase again (44). Dickson (41) has proposed that this normal loss of kyphosis in combination with the rapid growth spurt of adolescence may be a primary consideration in the cause of progressive scoliosis. When the thoracic kyphosis is at its minimum in girls, they are at their peak growth velocity; whereas with boys their peak growth velocity does not occur for another two years. This may be why girls are more prone to suffer from progressive scoliosis than boys. In a study by Archer and Dickson (45), girls with adolescent progressive scoliosis did not differ from girls with pelvic tilt scoliosis or normal girls in growth velocity. However, there was an increase in standing height among the girls with progressive scoliosis. They propose that the increase in height was due to the uncoiling of the spine as the thoracic kyphosis decreased and that the scoliosis progression was accelerated by the loss of the thoracic kyphosis. Girls with progressive scoliosis have been reported to reach menarche sooner, are taller than their peers when initially diagnosed with scoliosis, and have an earlier pubertal growth spurt (46).

Another consideration is the height to width (slenderness) ratio of adolescent vertebrae. In females, vertebral body height increases by 50% during adolescent growth, but vertebral body width only increases 15%. Males have wider vertebrae during their adolescent growth period and, in addition, their thoracic kyphosis is at or near its maximum (47).

EPIDEMIOLOGY

The prevalence of scoliosis (proportion of the population affected at a given time period) as reported by various screening programs, varies over a range, from 0.29–14.4% (34,48–53). This range is due primarily to the criteria for referral (51,53). The prevalence for scoliosis treatments has a much smaller range of one to six per thousand children screened (51,53). This indicates there is a need for improvement in the current screening methods. The small range of variation for treatment indicates that there is more agreement on when to treat scoliosis than on agreement on when to refer.

The incidence of scoliosis (rate of new cases) is difficult to determine since many studies claiming to be incidence studies are in fact prevalence studies (51). However, the following facts have been reported: Male to female ratio at screening vary from 1:1 to 1:3.2 (48,50–52); for small curves (6°–10°), the ratio is 1:1 (52); for larger curves (over 20°), the ratio is 1:5.4. Rogala (52) concluded that scoliosis was equally prevalent in both sexes but that larger curves are predominant in females, possibly due to hormonal and familial influences. Others also report a familial tendency for scoliosis (31,50,52) (See case study).

CASE REPORT
Two Brothers

Christopher

The first brother is a 14-year-old Filipino male with a history of "allergies," consisting of a runny nose, sneezing, itching of the chest and eyes and watering of the eyes. The child's only recorded trauma was a fall he sustained while riding a bicycle approximately 6 years before presentation.

CLINICAL AND RADIOLOGIC FINDINGS

The clinical signs of subluxation such as fixation dysfunction, edema, tenderness, and skin temperature differentials are present at the L5 segment, the right sacroiliac joint, L1, and C7-T1. The initial or pre-AP full spine radiograph demonstrates an 11° thoracolumbar scoliosis (Fig. 15.8A). The lateral full spine (in two exposures) shows a retrolisthesis at L5 and hyperextension of the upper lumbar spine (Fig. 15.8B). The thoracic kyphosis appears reduced and the cervical spine has a straight posture with anterior carriage of the head.

TREATMENT AND FOLLOW-UP

Short lever arm specific contact manual adjustments (i.e., Gonstead), were primarily directed at L5, the sacrum, L1 and C7. A total of 50 visits over approximately five months were made before comparative x-rays were obtained. The AP view shows a reduction of the scoliosis to approximately 4° (Fig. 15.8C). The lateral radiograph demonstrates a slight reduction in the retrolisthesis of L5 (Fig. 15.8D). The cervical lordosis is improved in the lower region of the neck but persists in a kyphotic posture at the segments above. There is less anterior carriage of the head.

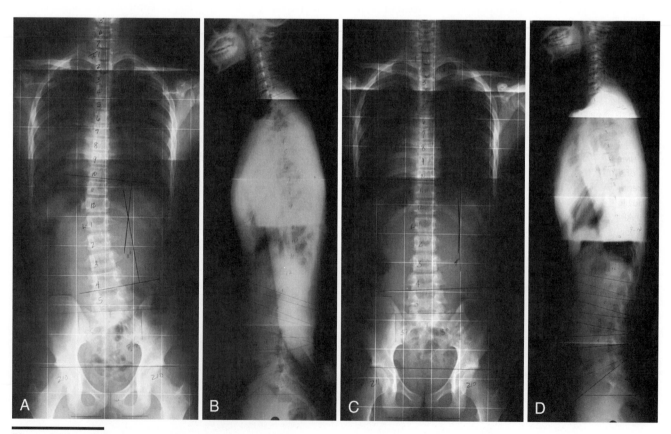

Figure 15.8.   A. Pretreatment AP radiograph. An eleven degree lumbar scoliosis is present. B. Pretreatment lateral radiograph. C. Comparative AP radiograph after 5 months. D. Comparative lateral radiograph after 5 months.

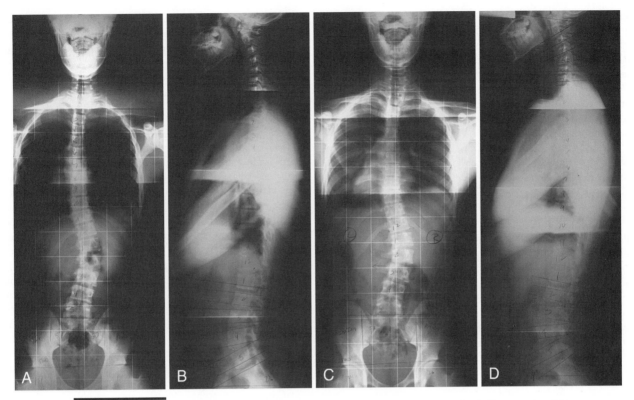

Figure 15.9. A. Pretreatment AP radiograph. B. Pretreatment lateral radiograph. C. Comparative AP radiograph after 6 months. D. Comparative lateral radiograph after 6 months.

Charles

This 16-year-old male is the older brother of the child described in the earlier case report. His symptoms are mostly neuromusculoskeletal in nature, including low back and upper lumbar pain.

CLINICAL AND RADIOLOGIC FINDINGS
Signs of subluxation, including motion restriction, skin temperature differentials, edema, and tenderness were present at L5 and at various levels (e.g., T12, L1, L2) of the thoracolumbar junction. The initial AP radiograph demonstrates a moderate thoracolumbar scoliosis of approximately 30° (Fig. 15.9A). The lateral radiograph shows a hypolordotic upper lumbar spine, a hypokyphotic/lordotic thoracic spine and a kyphotic cervical spine (Fig. 15.9B). Anterior carriage of the head is present.

TREATMENT AND FOLLOW-UP
Short lever arm specific contact manual adjustments (i.e., Gonstead), were primarily directed at L5 and at the apex of the scoliosis. Approximately 50 visits were made over about a 6-month period. Follow-up radiographs were obtained. The comparative AP view shows a nearly identical magnitude of the thoracolumbar scoliosis (i.e., approx. 30°) (Fig. 15.9C). The comparative lateral findings (Fig. 15.9D) are virtually identical to the initial radiograph (see Fig. 15.9B).

Physical Findings of Progressive Scoliosis

The progressive curve is most often in the thoracic spine where there is either a local lordosis or a loss of the thoracic kyphosis at the apex, when viewed from the true lateral of the apical vertebra as opposed to the lateral view of the patient (41–43). In addition, there is usually a decrease in the lumbar lordosis. The clinician should be alert to the presence of subluxations in the lumbar spine or pelvis that might cause hypolordosis of the lumbar spine (54).

Studies on spinal posture during puberty indicate there is a loss of thoracic kyphosis during the growth spurt (44). The patient is generally taller than her peers and her pelvis also appears taller than normal (28,45). This may be due to the loss in the lumbar lordosis, increasing the pelvic height on radiographs (44,45).

The patient has less thoraco/lumbar range of motion (ROM) on flexion/extension as well as lateral flexion and rotation. The loss of ROM is highly correlated with the degree of curvature. Patients with more than a 35° Cobb angle have an average of an 8° loss in forward flexion, a 7° loss in right rotation, a 9° loss in left rotation, and an 8° loss in both right and left lateral flexion when compared to patients with a Cobb angle of less than 25° (55).

An examination of the patient's x-ray will show that, in the thoracic spine, a functional scoliosis has an associated spinous rotation to the convex side (i.e., the spinous rotates right for a right convex functional scoliosis). With a structural scoliosis, the spinous processes of the thoracic spine rotate to the concavity (spinous rotates left with a right convex structural scoliosis) (56,57).

Hand Dominance

For small angles, there is a significant correlation to hand dominance. However, this is not true for large angles. In a study of 14 subjects with over a 20° left convex curve, ten were right handed, two were left handed and two others were ambidextrous (58). As discussed earlier, the clinician should examine the patient for other neurological conditions if a left scoliosis is found. A high incidence of neurological diseases such as syringomyelia or Arnold-Chiari type 1 malformation have been associated with left convex scoliosis (21).

Back Pain

When compared with adolescents in general, the incidence of back pain is not significantly larger for adolescent scoliotic patients; however, adult scoliotic patients have been reported to have a higher incidence of back pain (59).

Surgery and Back Pain

The conventional theory is that the more vertebrae fused during a scoliosis surgery, the greater the risk of future back pain (60). Paonessa and Engler (61) found that 92% of patients fused from L3 or caudally had suffered from at least one episode of severe low back pain during the past two years. They also found that patients having a lumbar lordosis greater than 30° suffered from fewer and less severe episodes of low back pain. They recommended that spinal fusions allow motion below L2 if possible or contouring the fusion so that a lordosis of at least 30° is maintained. However, in a recent cohort study, Poitras et al. (60) investigated the prevalence and nature of back pain for patients who had Harrington rod surgery for adolescent idiopathic scoliosis. They found that 73% of subjects had back pain in the last year, but found no correlation with the level of lumbar fusion. Poitras et al. found a slight increase in the incidence of back pain if more lumbar vertebra were fused (69% for L1, 88% for S1) but this increase was not statistically significant. Furthermore, they could not show any relationship between the degree of scoliosis correction and back pain. In a related study, Mayo et al. (62) showed that adult scoliosis patients (including those that had Harrington rod surgery when first diagnosed with AIS) had a greater incidence of back pain compared with the general adult population (73% versus 56%).

Grubb et al. studied adults having both scoliosis and back pain. They reported that spinal fusion resulted in a reduction of pain by 80% and that the patients had improved walking and sitting tolerances (63).

Cosmetic Deformity

In a recent survey (3,60,62,64) scoliosis patients were reported to have a poor body image as well as more visits to their physician and more sick days than the general population. In addition, the effect on social life may be important; it has been reported that 76% of females having scoliosis did not marry (22). However, despite a poor body image, scoliosis patients do have a positive perception of themselves as a whole and are capable of coping with their affliction (4). One might expect that scoliosis patients who were treated using surgery would have a poorer self image than those treated with braces. Paonessa and Engler (61) reported that 79% of Harrington rod surgery patients were satisfied with their appearance post surgery. Patients who received thoracoplasty for the reduction of rib hump reported higher satisfaction with their postoperative appearance than patients who underwent fusion without thoracoplasty (65). This may be a significant finding since conventional surgery has been shown to decrease the Cobb angle as well as the lateral deviation from the spinal axis (mid-sagittal plane), although it does not correct the axial rotation of the vertebra (66).

The reaction of others is probably the principal factor in forming a self image for those afflicted with scoliosis. This is probably even more important to adolescents, especially girls. Theologis et al. (67) described a cosmetic index whereby others quantified the cosmetic deformity caused by scoliosis. They found that the slight reduction in rib hump when treated with bracing did not significantly change the cosmetic index. However, for those who underwent Harrington instrumentation, all parameters characterized within the index improved.

Scoliosis Screening

The U.S. Preventive Services Task Force reports that "there is insufficient evidence to recommend for or against routine screening of asymptomatic adolescents for idiopathic scoliosis" (68), mainly as a result of the lack of evidence indicating that early detection results in better patient outcomes. However, at this point in time several states require all children to undergo screening for scoliosis. The current objective of screening is early detection including the referral and monitoring of positive cases. The greatest worry is over-referral of healthy children who may then be exposed to unnecessary radiographs and mental stress. When screening, the examiner must keep in mind that the incidence of scoliosis over 5° is about 4.5% and for curves over 20° the incidence is between one and five individuals per thousand cases.

A study of current screening methods reveals questionable validity, with a sensitivity of 26%, specificity of 98% and false positives of 75% (33). This large degree of error is unacceptable and there is a need to further evaluate the validity of current scoliosis screening. Burwell (35) emphasized the need to define "normal" before screening for abnormal can be performed and Dickson (34) stressed the need for understanding the clinical course of the disease.

Other studies indicate there is a problem with over-referral and hence the over-exposure of children to unnecessary x-ray. Leaver (30) states that screening programs can lead to 10% of 11 to 15 year old children being referred for x-ray when only one in five of those referred would have a scoliosis and of those, only one in ten would require treatment (i.e. bracing or surgery). Burwell (35) describes the forward bending test (visual inspection for scoliosis followed by forward bending for the presence of a rib hump) as being highly sensitive, but having too many false positives. When using this procedure, between 1.9% and 15% of the children are referred for x-ray, but only 2-3 per thousand are treated. Howell (36) concludes that educational methods for screeners must be improved and that the criteria for referral need to be better established.

Vercauteren et al. (2) studied the normal variations in symmetry of children aged 7 to 18. The study was designed to determine the ranges of physiological normal values for a child's posture. The left-right measurement discrepancies were quite common in the children; shoulder height: 1.0 cm; scapular height: 1.0 cm; iliac crest height: 1.0 cm; rib hump on forward flexion: 0.8 cm.

The primary purpose of any screening program is to detect the existence of a particular disease or condition. Screening tests are not meant to be diagnostic, but they must sort out the person who may have the disease or condition from those who probably do not. A properly designed screening program requires that the epidemiology and the natural history be well understood (30,37). Epidemiology provides the information that allows society as a whole to determine if the cost of screening programs are economically feasible (30). The natural history allows early diagnosis through understanding the early symptomatic stages of a disease (37). In addition, a thorough understanding of the natural history may aid in treatment as well as in measuring the effect of treatments. Unfortunately, the natural history of scoliosis is not very well understood. There has been a great increase in our understanding of progressive idiopathic scoliosis and ongoing studies will add to our knowledge base.

In order for a screening program to be successful, Cochrane and Holland (38) state that it must be simple to administer, acceptable to the subjects, sensitive (give a positive finding when the subject has a scoliosis) and specific (give a negative finding when the subject does not have the disease). In addition, the cost of the program to the community must be compared with the cost of the problem if there was not an early detection. Very little information is available on screening cost; however, in a recent U.S. Preventive Services Task Force policy statement, the cost of screening was reported to range between \$.41 to \$2.31 per child and the average cost of treatment of confirmed cases ranged between \$3500–\$3900 per case (68).

Screening Procedure

Children should be screened at or before 10 years of age. The screening procedure must involve inspection of the entire back from the cervicals to the pelvis.

1. Children should be wearing shorts or swimming suits, females should wear a two-piece swim suit. Gowns exposing the back are not acceptable since gowns hide postural attitudes.

2. Inspect for lateral spinal deviation, pelvic asymmetry and/or shoulder asymmetry.

3. Adams test (forward flexion) differentiates structural from functional scoliosis. The back should be inspected in at least three forward bending positions. The patient holds his/her hands together while bending forward so that they hang in the mid-line of the body:
   a. Bending forward at about 45°, the thoracic spine is examined for rib-hump
   b. Bending forward a few degrees further, the thoraco-lumbar spine is examined
   c. Bending full forward to examine the lumbar region
   d. Any trunk rotation (rib-hump or lumbar-hump) should be measured using an inclinometer (also called a scoliometer) or the difference between left and right should be measured in mm
   e. Trunk rotations (thoracic or lumbar) greater than 7° as measured by an inclinometer or rib humps greater than 11 mm should be referred for x-ray (69,70)

4. The side bending test further differentiates a structural from a functional scoliosis. Functional curves disappear during lateral flexion to the side of convexity, while structural curves remain.

Screening Effectiveness

Torell et al. (71) described the effectiveness of a Swedish screening and treatment program over a ten year period. The number of patients detected below the age of 20 years and having a scoliosis of 20° or greater tripled during the first four years of the program, and reached a plateau after the sixth year. Between the sixth and tenth year, the incidence of scoliosis of 20° or greater was 0.4%. The mean referral age of the patients dropped from 15 to 13 years by the end of the 10-year period reported on by the study. In addition, the Cobb angle of the average scoliosis referral decreased from an average of 46° to 28°. The average Cobb angle of the ten worst cases for each year also decreased from 63° to 46°.

Screening Thermography

Cooke et al. (72) studied the use of thermography (infrared) for the detection of scoliosis. One hundred fifty-four children were included in the study. Twenty-nine subjects had previously been identified through clinical examination and radiography for the presence of scoliosis (mean=27° SD=12°). A second group of 125 individuals had no history of scoliosis and were asymptomatic. All subjects underwent full spine radiological examinations and thermography. Assessment of thermograms selected at random from these two subject pools showed that thermography had a sensitivity of 98.2% and a specificity of 91.0% when compared to the gold standard of radiography. The authors conclude that thermographic examination is a noninvasive and simple means for screening adolescents for scoliosis and recommended it for further prospective large-scale investigations.

Clinical Examination

Posture

When a patient is referred because of a suspected scoliosis, a thorough examination of the posture of the patient is required. The patient's entire back area including the shoulders must be exposed in order to determine the presence of any asymmetries or spine humps. It is important to compare postural findings with full spine radiographs as well as functional testing. The most common causes of functional scoliosis are leg length differences due to a true anatomical short leg, pelvic asymmetry, or foot pronation. Muscle spasm and pain can also cause a functional scoliosis.

If a scoliosis is obvious with a postural examination, then it must be determined if the curve is structural or functional. The Adam's test (forward flexion) should be performed, as described above. The curve will disappear on flexion if it is functional. If the curve does not disappear, it is common for the torso to rotate during flexion, giving the appearance of a rib hump or lumbar hump. The extent of rib or lumbar humping should be measured with an inclinometer; the left-right difference in the hump can be measured in mm. As stated earlier, trunk rotations (rib or lumbar humps) of 7° or more indicate the need for a radiographic examination (69). Rib and lumbar humps having a left-right difference of 11 mm or more also indicate the need for a radiographic examination (70). A lateral flexion test should also be performed. If the curve disappears on lateral flexion to the side of convexity, then the curve is functional.

The clinician should further examine the patient if the scoliosis is a left thoracic scoliosis. As mentioned earlier, a left thoracic curve has a greater likelihood of occurring in patients with syringomyelia or Arnold-Chiari type 1 malformation. In addition, cafe-au-lait spots may be indicative of neurofibromatosis. A patch of hair over the lumbosacral region may indicate diastematomyelia. Ehlers-Danlos syndrome is associated with abnormal scarring and extreme elasticity of the skin.

Additional spinal examination procedures that are usually performed are covered in Chapter 11.

Radiography

If it is determined that radiographs are necessary, then a minimum of two radiographs must be taken: (a) full spine AP (or PA) and (b) full spine lateral (see Chapter 8). The PA radiograph is preferred since it provides better protection of breast and/or reproductive tissue from radiation exposure (73). If adequate prepatient shielding is available, then the AP view is preferred because the patient can be positioned closer to the bucky without head or cervical spine rotation. In addition, the use of rare-earth gradient screens, three-phase or high frequency generators, gonadal shielding, and a high density grid all reduce the radiation exposure to the patient (74).

A full view of the spine from the ischial tuberosities to the top of the cervical spine is the ideal exposure. This allows an examination of the pelvis and femur heads as well as the location of the head relative to the pelvis. Complete visibility of the ischial crest is also important since the degree of apophyseal fusion is a key method for determining skeletal age (Risser's sign; this method is described in more detail in the next section).

The PA radiograph gives a slightly larger distortion of the spine due to the fact that the spine to film distance is increased. The distortion is greater for those vertebrae furthest from the central ray. Thus, the clinician must be consistent if comparisons are to be made. The cervical spine is sometimes distorted so that it gives the appearance of a pillar view in some PA films. Positioning of the patient is crucial as is the anatomical location of the central ray. The slightest change in radiographic protocol can change the Cobb angle by several degrees.

On the AP (or PA) radiograph, the rotation of the spinous process should be examined in the area of the scoliotic curve. If the spinous rotation is due to a functional lateral flexion of the spine (i.e., leg length inequality, hemivertebrae or pelvic asymmetry), then the spinous process rotates to the contralateral side (i.e., spinous rotates right for a right functional scoliosis). With a structural scoliosis, the spinous process rotates to the concavity (spinous rotates left with a right scoliosis).

Barge (75) recommends that a sacral base radiograph be used to determine any asymmetry in the sacrum or L5 since the standard AP (or PA) full spine view does not usually provide an adequate view of these structures. Barge reports that 29% of scoliosis patients have a level sacral base, 32% have a low right and 39% a low left sacral base. In the early stages of scoliosis, Dickson et al. (76) recommend close examination of the sacrum. In a study of over 1700 children, Dickson et al. found 2.5% having a scoliosis of greater than 10°. Of these, 21% (0.53% of the total group) were due to sacral tilt. None of the children having scoliosis due to sacral tilt had any progression in the scoliosis (76).

It is also recommended that a recumbent radiograph be ordered, with the patient laterally flexing to the side of the convexity, in an effort to reduce the curve as much as possible. This provides insight on the flexibility of the curve as well as information on the effect gravity has on the curve. The more a curve corrects on the recumbent radiograph, the less the curve will progress (77).

Most chiropractic clinics do not have the ability to perform a recumbent radiograph. As an alternative, lateral flexion radiographs are recommended to determine the flexibility of the curve and examine potential sites for spinal adjustments (18). Motion segments that have a loss of normal motion should be examined closely to determine if the fixation is due to soft tissue or caused by anatomical changes in the vertebra.

Recently, Beauchamp et al. (78) reported that the Cobb angle has a diurnal variation of about 5°. They recommend that follow-up radiographs be performed at the same time of day as the initial x-ray. It has long been known that the intervertebral disc has a diurnal variation in height, so it should not be surprising that the Cobb angle may vary as well. Gravitational forces on the disc would not be as uniform in scoliotic patients, causing changes in disc height through the day in such a way as to affect the Cobb angle.

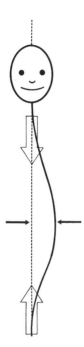

Figure 15.10. Loads and torque acting on the apical vertebra when the spine is offset laterally. Modified from Schultz AB. The use of mathematical models for studies of scoliosis biomechanics. Spine 1991; 16:1212.

Predicting Scoliosis Progression

The most important factor for predicting curve progression is the Cobb angle of the patient. In terms of the mechanics of the spine, it is not surprising that a large curve is more likely to progress than a small curve. Figure 15.10 shows the loads and torque acting on the apical vertebra for a scoliotic spine. The larger the Cobb angle, the larger the torque acting on the apical vertebra, and thus the greater likelihood for progression.

However, existing angle is not the only factor in scoliosis progression; age and the extent of rib-cage deformity are also factors that have been shown to play a role in affecting progression. If the Cobb angle is large (more than 20°) and the patient is of a young skeletal age, then the chances of progression are very high. Because skeletal age has been shown to be a very important factor in progression, the next few paragraphs summarize different methods for determining skeletal age.

Risser's method (79) is one of the easier procedures for determining skeletal maturity. With age, the iliac crest epiphyseal plate closes from the caudad end towards the cephalic end of the ilium (Fig. 15.11). This progression moves from the anterior towards the posterior portion of the ilium.

The crest is divided into four quadrants and the location of epiphyseal excursion is graded as follows:

Grade 1 = 25% excursion

Grade 2 = 50% excursion

Grade 3 = 75% excursion

Grade 4 = 100% excursion

Grade 5 = Full excursion and complete fusion

For example, a patient with a Risser's sign of 1 is more likely to have a scoliosis progress since the skeleton is relatively immature and the patient's growth rate is likely to be rapid in the near future.

Radiographs of the wrist are the classic means of identifying skeletal age (80). However, this requires additional radiation exposure at a time when it can be most harmful to developing tissue. In addition, it has been shown that there is an increase in spinal height after skeletal maturity has been achieved (as measured by wrist radiography). That is, the spinal column continues to grow after skeletal maturity. For girls, the sitting height increases an average of 6.9 mm 1 year after skeletal maturity and 14.2 mm 3 years after maturity. For boys, the increase is even more dramatic, averaging 13.5 mm 1 year after maturity and 16.2 mm 2 years after maturity (81). Examining the epiphyseal plates of the vertebral bodies to confirm skeletal maturity is not a reliable means of verifying maturity since the true epiphysis is not visible on radiographs. The radiographically obvious ring apophyses are the result of traction on the vertebra from the anulus of the disc (81).

Tanner (82) provides a series of methods for estimating the current stage of puberty using breast development for females, genital development for males and pubic hair development for both sexes as key factors (see Chapter 18).

Izumi (83) has proposed the use of alkaline phosphatase as a biochemical means of determining skeletal maturity and the potential for growth. The advantage to this method is that it does not require additional radiographs. In general, if alkaline phosphatase were greater than 25U, the subject is experiencing the highest growth rate, while subjects with less than 10U have completed bone growth (Table 15.2).

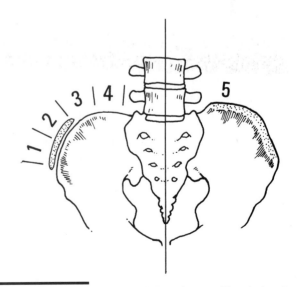

Figure 15.11. Risser's Sign. A Risser's sign of 2 is depicted on the left and a Risser's sign of 5 on the right.

Table 15.2.   Alkaline Phosphatase Level and Skeletal Maturity

Group	Average Alk-Phos (U)	Average Age (years)	Average Months after Menarche	Average Growth Velocity (cm per year)	Avg. Risser's Sign
I	>25.0	12.4 [1.3]	3.4 [10.8]	4.1 [2.1]	1.6 [1.8]
II	20–25	13.2 [1.3]	4.5 [13.0]	3.5 [1.8]	2.5 [1.8]
III	15–20	13.9 [1.1]	9.9 [10.3]	1.7 [1.6]	3.5 [1.5]
IV	10–15	14.4 [1.2]	21.3 [12.2]	1.3 [1.2]	4.2 [0.9]
V	<10	14.7 [1.0]	24.7 [11.1]	0.5 [0.6]	4.7 [0.5]

The greatest growth velocity occurs during the periods of highest alkaline phosphates levels. (Values in [ ] indicate the standard deviation). Adapted from Izumi, 1993.

For girls, the AIS curves are more likely to cease progression by Risser's sign 4 while boys with AIS have a substantial rate of progression up to Risser's sign 5 (84,85). Thus, for boys, there is a greater chance of progression right up to the end of their skeletal development (85) whereas for girls progression is less likely after Risser's sign has reached stage 4. This is probably due to the dramatic growth of the spine seen in boys even after the rest of the skeleton has matured (76).

Predicting the progression of a scoliotic curve is difficult at best. The results of the aforementioned discussion can be summarized in the curve progression chart shown in Figure 15.12 (86). Given the current Cobb angle, Risser's sign and the chronological age, the incidence of scoliosis progression can be estimated. Unfortunately, there is very little reliability in predicting the progression of small angles (less than 20°); thus, the smallest angle shown is 20°.

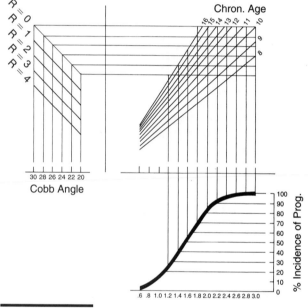

Figure 15.12. Curve progression chart. Follow the child's Cobb angle through their age to determine the likelihood for progression. Modified from Lonstein JE, Carlson JM. The prediction of curve progression in untreated idiopathic scoliosis during growth. J Bone Joint Surg 1984; 66A:1061.

Case Management

Infantile Scoliosis

Current information indicates that nutrition is one of the more important factors for infantile scoliosis. Thus questioning the parents regarding the infant's diet as well as the mother's diet (if the child is being breast-fed) is an important aspect to consider. Signs of neurological problems as well as any compromise of cardiovascular function should also be investigated. If the rib-vertebra angle difference (see Fig. 15.7) is greater than 20°, the curve is more likely to progress and the chiropractor needs to monitor the infant closely and should refer for an orthopedic evaluation. Most cases resolve on their own, but often with significant cosmetic deformity (25). Chiropractic adjustment of normal or hypermobile joints is contraindicated. Short lever adjustments of hypomobile joints are best approached from the convexity of the curve (18).

Adult Scoliosis

If the curve is less than 30°, the chance of progression is minimal and increases greater than 10° after skeletal maturity are rare (87,88). For the adult, the function of the spine is of

primary importance, with the cosmetic curve reduction a secondary concern. Correcting leg-length inequalities and/or sacral base deformation can reduce lumbar scoliosis, but usually does not completely eliminate the curve. Once skeletal maturity is reached, there is little that can be done to reduce a scoliosis. Curves of 50° or greater are more likely to progress and surgery is likely to be the only means of arresting the progression and reducing the deformity. Curves of 80° often interfere with cardiopulmonary function.

The chiropractor needs to investigate short leg and pelvic asymmetries as a means of reducing a lumbar scoliosis. Adult lumbar curves of up to 35° have been reported to be reduced to near zero once limb and pelvis inequalities have been corrected (89). Adults with lumbar scoliosis have more low back pain, with women having more cases of lumbar scoliosis as well as more back pain than men (90). However, pelvic asymmetries have only affected the lumbar spine, with no evidence indicating that the thoracic spine is affected. Large primary thoracic curves are not likely to respond to leveling sacral asymmetries (89). In addition, in the case of structural curves, the shape of the vertebral bodies are permanently deformed and no amount of therapy will reduce such a deformation (91).

The chiropractor also plays an important role in maintaining function of the scoliotic spine. Patients with scoliosis have more back pain than those without scoliosis (62). In addition, the stresses on the scoliotic spine are greater than those on the normal spine. The chiropractor must recognize the importance of back pain and other neurological dysfunction associated with scoliosis as well as the cosmetic or quality of life concerns the patient may have (92).

Juvenile and Adolescent Idiopathic Progressive Scoliosis

The treatment of any malady requires knowledge of the cause and mechanisms of the disease. There are many theories about the cause of progressive idiopathic scoliosis, all having some evidence to support their tenets but none explain all aspects of the disease. Epidemiologic studies show that progressive scoliosis has a familial tendency and is speculated to be a dominant sex-linked (X-chromosome) disease. About 25% of scoliotic patients have a family history of the disease with relatives of female patients more frequently affected than the relatives of male patients (93). See the case studies presented in Figures 15.9 and 15.10. If both parents have scoliosis, the chances of the children having scoliosis increase to 40% (94). However, the fundamental cause of progressive scoliosis still remains elusive.

LEG LENGTH INEQUALITY AND SCOLIOSIS

Limb length inequality and pelvic asymmetry affect the mechanics of the lumbar spine and generate lumbar scoliosis. Leveling of the sacrum has been shown to reduce the lumbar curve to residual levels of between 4° to 8° (78,89,90,95). In some patients, sacral leveling can cause a reversal in the curve (89). The effect of limb length inequality has been shown to be completely compensated for in the lumbar spine for adults; however, the effect on children is not known (89). Plaugher and Lopes (18) suggest that stresses on the thoracic vertebra due to limb-length inequalities may lead to permanent changes in vertebral architecture, setting the stage for structural scoliosis.

NEUROPHYSIOLOGICAL AND NEUROMUSCULAR CONSIDERATIONS

Sectioning of the dorsal (sensory) roots of spinal nerves has been shown to cause scoliosis in laboratory animals (96,97). Post-mortem examination of the spinal columns of scoliotic patients reveals that there is damage to the dorsal root ganglia (98,99). This factor may lead to an imbalance in the paraspinal musculature, causing a scoliosis. The convex side of the scoliosis is always on the side of damage to the dorsal nerve or dorsal nerve root ganglia. In animal models, the chances of scoliosis occurring increases with the number of dorsal nerve roots cut as well as the location of the nerve roots. Pincott and coworkers (100) researched nerve sectioning on cynomolgus monkeys and found that sectioning the L1 dorsal nerve root had the greatest chance of causing a scoliosis. In summary, proprioceptive loss to certain muscles can generate a scoliosis; however, it must be pointed out that surgeries that lead to scoliosis in animals do not necessarily mean that the same mechanisms are responsible for generating scoliosis in humans.

Yamada and Yamamoto suggest that impairment of the postural regulation between brainstem centers and proprioceptive input could be a factor in idiopathic scoliosis (101). They found that about half of the patients with idiopathic scoliosis demonstrated abnormal occulo-vestibular reflexes, indicating dysfunction of the brainstem. In addition, they reported a positive correlation between brainstem dysfunction and curve progression. Although similar reports have been made (102) Sahlstrand and Lidstrom found no difference between progressive and non-progressive scoliosis patients with regard to stabilometry, electronystomography (ENG) and electroencephalography (EEG) studies (103). However, there were only ten subjects having progressive curves in Sahlstrand and Lidstrom's study, none having any indication of occulo-vestibular dysfunction. Yamada and Yamamoto reported that only 48 of 86 scoliotic cases revealed abnormal function. This indicates that there is a need for further work in this area.

Kennelly and Stokes have shown that the lumbar multifidus muscle cross-sectional area is smaller on the side of the concavity in primary thoracic curve scoliosis. For lumbar curves, the multifidus cross-sectional area was smaller on the side of the convexity (104). Electromyography (EMG) studies have shown that there is increased muscle activity on the convex side of the curve (105). This is true whether the curve is located in the thoracic or lumbar spine. Since there is more activity on the side of the convexity, it has been proposed that the muscles have been weakened, with more fibers firing to maintain a given force to balance the spine (106). This is supported by histological studies showing that the proportion of type I fibers and the capillary density of the muscle is higher on the convex side of scoliosis patients. This indicates that there is a histological change in the muscle due to chronic fatigue (107,108).

It is hypothesized that small muscles play a role of kinesiological monitors and larger muscles are more important as force generators. In the spine, muscles that cross one vertebral level have approximately six times the spindle density of muscles that cross two vertebral levels. Muscles that cross three to five levels (multifidus) have the same spindle density as those crossing six to eight levels (semispinalis). Although muscles like the rotatores and other small muscles of the back can generate forces, it is highly unlikely that they can generate forces that can cause even small intervertebral movements (109).

BIOMECHANICS

There have been several biomechanical models developed in an effort to understand the mechanical causes of scoliosis, as well as to predict the results of surgery. In general, these models have provided insight into the mechanics of scoliosis but have not been successful in predicting the full three-dimensional structural changes involved in scoliosis. Early models of spinal geometry and muscle lines of action have shown that mild scoliotic curves can be generated and corrected with muscle force alone (110,111). However, these models could not generate the full three-dimensional shape of the spine as seen in progressive scoliosis.

Models of Harrington instrumentation have been used to predict the upper and lower boundary of the forces needed to provide correction, as well as the forces that will lead to failure of the appliance post-surgically. As the distraction on the spine increases, the angle of the scoliosis decreases, but if the distraction forces are too large, the danger of hook breakout from the bone increases. As a result, the forces on the rod are often measured during surgery to insure maximum correction and to reduce the chance of failure due to hook breakout (112).

Dickson and co-workers have developed a model for progressive scoliosis that combines vertebral rotation with lateral flexion. They have generated progressive scoliosis in rabbits by forcing a local lordosis in the thoracic spine and forcing a slight lateral flexion. Under these circumstances, progressive scoliosis results, with both the lateral flexion and vertebral rotation progressing (15,42,113). In these animal studies, the apex of the scoliosis is always at the most lordotic vertebra, supporting the theory that scoliosis requires both a local lordosis as well as an initial lateral flexion before progression can take place. Dickson and co-workers have also described radiological, histological, and morphometrical data supporting a basic sequence of mechanical attributes that are consistently seen with scoliosis and have consistently been shown to generate scoliosis in animal studies. Morphometric studies of osteological specimens and radiologic studies of patients with progressive structural scoliosis have a local lordosis at the apex of the scoliotic curve. On standard lateral radiographs (i.e., mid-line of the patient) the same area of the spine appears kyphotic, and often appears hyper-kyphotic. Radiologic studies of the true lateral (i.e., the patient is positioned so that the true lateral view of the apical vertebra can be seen on the radiograph) reveal that a local lordosis always exists at the apex (40–42,113).

The biomechanical model proposed by Somerville, Dickson and others is illustrated in Figure 15.13. A small local thoracic lordosis and slight lateral deviation (convexity to the right) predisposes the spine to the development of progressive thoracic scoliosis. Flexion and/or compression (as occurs with gravity) of the thoracic spine results in the rotation of the spinous processes toward the concavity (40–42,113). In spite of the success of animal models, a computer model of this mechanism did not produce the desired effect of lateral flexion and rotation (114). However, this may only be an indication of weakness within the computer model. Two independently developed mechanical models did obtain the same results found with scoliosis: a local lordosis within a kyphotic section, combined with slight lateral flexion, produced further lateral flexion and rotation when the model was flexed forward (40,115). Further research on the precise mechanisms involving the generation of a scoliosis are needed.

MORPHOMETRIC CHANGES TO THE VERTEBRAL BODY

An examination of the vertebral body of scoliosis patients and cadavers shows that the change in shape of the body is usually not uniform. Approximately 95% of the vertebral bodies have a non-uniform distribution of the deformation (Fig. 15.14). The vertebral endplates are normal except at the area closest to the concavity (91). This indicates that there is extremely high stress acting at the growth cartilage, inhibiting vertebral body growth and contributing to the progression of the curve.

Morphometrical examination of vertebrae from human specimens having structural scoliosis show very consistent patterns. The concave pedicle is thinner than the convex pedicle and the vertebral body is asymmetrical with bone growth radiating toward the concavity (Fig. 15.15).

The data in Table 15.3 summarizes the changes in radiographic appearance of the apical vertebra (as well as two vertebra above and below the apex) as a function of Cobb angle. Vertebral wedging, disc height and the rib-vertebra angle are given as a function of Cobb angle. As the Cobb angle increases, vertebral wedging and disc wedging both increase (116). The rib vertebra angle also increases with increasing Cobb angles, but the left-right difference is greatest two levels above the apex, while the rib-vertebra angles are nearly equal at the level of the apex.

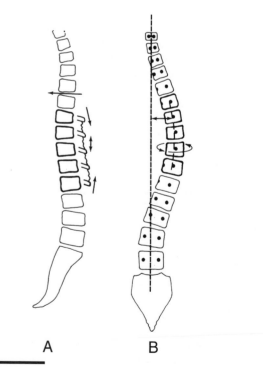

Figure 15.13. Local lordosis (A) combined with slight lateral flexion can cause progressive scoliosis (B) in animal models. Modified from Dickson RA, Lawton JO, Archer IA, Butt WP. The pathogenesis of idiopathic scoliosis: biplanar spinal asymmetry. J Bone Joint Surg 1984; 66B:9.

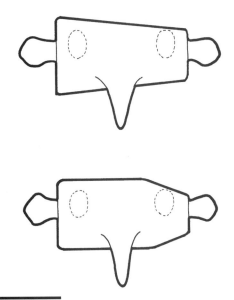

Figure 15.14. Uniform and non-uniform shapes of vertebral bodies in scoliotic curves. A. Uniform deformation (5% of scoliotic vertebrae). B. Nonuniform deformation (95% of scoliotic vertebrae. Modified from Perdriolle R, Becchetti S, Vidal J, Lopez P. Mechanical process and growth cartilages: essential factors in the progression of scoliosis. Spine 1993; 18:343.

The changes in the morphology of scoliotic joints have been well documented (117). It has been proposed by Kennelly and Stokes (99) that such joint abnormalities can lead to reduced muscle activity. Abnormal joint morphologies have been shown to reduce muscle activity via reflex inhibition, even if pain is not present (118). Such reflex inhibition of the muscle may result in weakness and instability of the joint, leading to further damage to the joint. This assumes pre-existing changes in the joint leading to changes in muscle function, but once established, such a mechanism could be a factor in the progression of scoliosis.

TREATMENT CONSIDERATIONS FOR PROGRESSIVE SCOLIOSIS

Of all the treatments for scoliosis, only surgery has been shown to consistently reduce scoliotic curves. Early in this century, medicine had created a "health crisis" of sorts concerning those afflicted with scoliosis (119,120). This attitude continues today (121). Patients are sometimes led to believe that scoliosis is generally a life-threatening condition (23,122). Because scoliosis is often associated with severely debilitating disorders such as polio, Marfan's syndrome, neurofibromatosis, and muscular dystrophy (123), the crisis position (121) was used as justification for invasive procedures to correct the deformity, culminating today in an array of "spinal instrumentation" ranging from Harrington rods (124) to halo traction devices (125). By the 1950s, orthopedists were prone to exaggerate the risks associated with scoliosis and to carry out surgical fusions of the spine which were often unnecessary (126). Recent

research, however, has questioned the basis of surgical intervention (127,128). When curves progress beyond 60–90°, pulmonary function is compromised, even in the absence of other comorbid factors, and cardiac impingement can interfere with circulatory function. In such cases, surgery is the only viable alternative.

Although most scoliotic curves do not progress, those that do begin as slight curves and it has been brought forth that functional curves are the precursors to the structural deformities (129). This simple observation is at the heart of current trends in conservative management (130).

If the patient's scoliosis can be managed before it has an opportunity to undergo significant progression, the chances of therapeutic success are believed to be greatly enhanced (131,132). The conventional medical approach is to wait until a curve reaches 20° before intervening therapeutically. Withholding treatment until significant progression occurs biases the clinical outcome towards the negative; at some unknown critical degree of progression, surgical intervention is the only reasonable alternative (133). With a shift among clinicians towards early detection and early conservative treatment, the

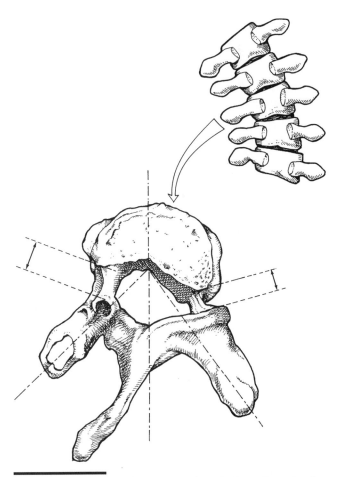

Figure 15.15. The deformity in scoliosis is three dimensional. Transverse plane view of a scoliotic vertebra. Modified from White AA, Panjabi MM. Clinical biomechanics of the spine, 2nd ed. Philadelphia: JB Lippincott, 1990.

Table 15.3. **Vertebral Angle, Disc Angle and Rib-Vertebra Angle for the Apical Vertebra and Two Vertebra Above and Below the Apex**

Cobb Category Angle Range Average Angle	Group I 0°–3° 2.1°	Group II 4°–7° 5.7°	Group III 8°–15° 11.1°	Group IV 16°–30°+ 22.9°
Vertebral wedge angle (deg.)				
2 levels above	−0.1	0.1	0.9	1.7
1 level above	0.4	1.4	1.6	3.6
Apical vertebra	0.2	1.4	1.6	4.2
1 level below	0.3	0.9	1.6	2.6
2 levels below	0.3	0.3	0.8	0.9
Disc height (mm) (convex side minus concave side)				
2 levels above	>0.01	0.11	0.51	1.02
1 level above	0.07	0.06	0.91	1.33
Apical vertebra	0.04	0.68	0.79	1.75
1 level below	−0.08	0.22	0.73	1.00
2 levels below	0.11	0.15	−0.32	0.30
Rib-vertebra angle (deg.) (convex angle minus concave angle)				
2 levels above	1.7	−2.3	−9.8	−15.2
1 level above	0.2	0.4	−5.6	−8.1
Apical vertebra	−0.8	1.5	−3.6	−1.5
1 level below	−0.1	3.2	1.7	3.9
2 levels below	−1.3	2.7	2.8	4.9

incidence of patients "requiring" surgery has substantially decreased (134–136). This has been accompanied by a three-fold increase in the numbers of patients being treated for scoliosis, since curves of much smaller magnitude are now being managed. These changes in therapy approaches have developed despite the absence of any medical intervention program until curves reach a magnitude of approximately 25°. Due to the increased numbers of children diagnosed with scoliosis, the percentage of those with progressive curves will decrease for purely statistical reasons (130).

The issue of mild curve (i.e., <20°) management deserves particular attention in any conservative treatment program. Positive treatment of mild curves is usually rejected by medical/surgical dogma which demands a "wait and see" approach (137). The fallacy of this approach is obvious on even modest scrutiny. If curves are more likely to progress as they become more severe, then simply waiting until they become more severe to initiate treatment assures that a certain amount of progression will inevitably occur (130). Part of the problem current therapists face is that medicine offers no viable treatment options, short of the application of braces. Chiropractic, in contrast, offers treatment alternatives which could

be applied during the "observation" period of mild scoliotic curve management (130).

There are essentially two factors that handicap conservative treatment for progressive scoliosis. The first is the visco-elastic deformation of normal healthy tissue under abnormal physiological loading conditions. The second is the permanent change in tissue as a result of growth inhibition from abnormal stresses. A single chiropractic adjustment cannot lengthen a ligament that has shrunk due to contractures occurring over a period of months or years. Any conservative treatment must take place before there are significant changes in the architecture of the spinal column. In the following paragraphs, we provide a summary of conservative treatments and the evidence available on the efficacies of these treatments.

BRACING

Braces are designed to apply traction and lateral forces to the spine to decrease the compression and to force a lateral correction. Traction in a brace system has minimal effect on correcting scoliotic curves (138), and current braces are designed to maximize the lateral force. However, current bracing techniques can exaggerate the thoracic lordosis and to have minimal effect on vertebral rotation (139).

The effectiveness of bracing as a treatment for scoliosis is being questioned and the debate is currently very vigorous. Focarile et al. (140) could not determine any difference in the progression rates between bracing and not bracing patients. Approximately 29% of the patients receiving brace treatment progress while only 15% of those not receiving brace treatment progress (140). Goldberg et al. (141) examined the effectiveness of brace treatment on girls with Risser's sign 0 and Cobb angles between 15–35°. They found no statistical difference in curve progression between bracing and non-bracing and concluded that bracing has no effect on the natural history of scoliosis. In addition, they concluded that their results remove the ethical problem associated with studying the natural history of scoliosis where the only treatment permitted to a control group is surgery.

Associated with the question of brace effectiveness is the compliance of the patient. A poor self image created by the need to wear an unattractive brace can reduce the willingness of the patient to cooperate and thus reduce any effect the brace may have (142). As few as 15% of patients have been reported to have high compliance and, in general, patients wear the brace only 65% of the recommended 23 hours/day (143).

ELECTRICAL MUSCLE STIMULATION

Biomechanical models of the spine have been used to predict the muscle groups that would best correct a scoliosis (111,144). Muscle stimulation over a prolonged period, such as at night while the patient sleeps, was expected to reverse the effect of stresses on the spine and paraspinal tissue during daily activity. Muscle stimulation as a treatment for scoliosis had very promising initial results (145); however, follow–up studies did not show any significant changes in curvature (146). In addition, electrical muscle stimulation can produce an uncomfortable sensation that disturbs sleep and irritates the skin (147).

EXERCISE

Exercise has not been shown to affect scoliosis curvature (68); however, exercise is an important aspect to spinal health in general. Swimming or any exercise that minimizes the stresses on the spine are best for the scoliotic patient. Specific therapies can be given for strengthening weak paraspinal musculature and for stretching the chronically contracted fascia and muscles. The chiropractor must be aware of any existing hypermobile spinal motion segments and educate the patient about avoiding stretching or exercises that stress those spinal levels.

CHIROPRACTIC ADJUSTMENTS AND OTHER TREATMENT CONSIDERATIONS

The EMG and histological findings indicate that the muscles on the convex side of the curve are reacting to increased loads required to maintain postural stability. As a result, muscle activity increases and histological changes occur to reduce the inevitable fatigue of fast twitch fibers by increasing the number of slow twitch fibers.

The morphologic and radiographic studies indicate that the change in vertebral body shape is dramatic, leading to the permanent deformation of the vertebrae. In addition, there is a local lordosis that appears at the apex of the scoliosis, if viewed from the true lateral of the apical vertebra. Thus, with an established structural curve there is little hope that chiropractic adjustments could have an effect on the curve shape. However, for the developing curve, it may be that chiropractic care could make the difference between progression and stabilization or even reversal of small curves.

Leg length differences and pelvic asymmetry can generate a lumbar scoliosis (75,89). Slight structural changes in the spine may cause asymmetrical loading resulting in changes in vertebral body shape. If these changes are large enough, they may result in setting the stage for progressive scoliosis (18).

The chiropractor can examine the child for obvious structural problems and correct them as necessary to maintain a symmetrical spinal column. In addition, examination of intervertebral motion for hypomobility is especially important for the thoracic spine. In light of animal studies and morphological examinations, the existence of flexion fixations and/or the presence of a local thoracic lordosis may be early signs of progressive scoliosis (15,41,42,113).

No definitive studies exist on the efficacy of specific contact short lever-arm chiropractic adjustments in the reduction of scoliosis. Case reports have documented positive changes in the magnitude of scoliosis in adults (95,148,149) as well as juveniles and adolescents (18,75,150,151). Another report cites improvement (152) in 84% of a group of approximately 1000 chiropractic patients undergoing treatment for scoliosis; total correction in 6.8%, "significant" correction in 35.6%, and small correction in 41.2%. In 16.4% of patients, the curves either progressed or were unchanged. While this report appears promising, this must be tempered by the fact that there were no inclusion criteria presented and quantitative aspects of the study were severely lacking; no indication of the range of curves, the mean Cobb angle or the magnitude of change. Cohort studies as well as more rigorous experimental designs such as the randomized controlled trial will need to be performed before the true measure of chiropractic's efficacy and effectiveness on scoliosis can be determined.

ADJUSTIVE MANAGEMENT

The specific short lever arm adjustment is designed to restore function at a dysfunctional motion segment. In addition, both the intersegmental as well as the global posture of the spine may be affected. Since scoliosis is a global postural problem, finding the causes of the curvature is often difficult but important.

The most caudal portion of the curve may be the genesis of the scoliosis. Lateral flexion malpositions can cause a scoliosis. These malpositions could be due to disc, or disc and posterior joint trauma. It is especially important to accurately detect this type of misalignment, often in the lumbosacral region in the younger child (e.g., with an AP radiograph). If left undetected or mismanaged, the lateral flexion misalignment may lead to permanent osseous remodeling. The lateral radiograph is used to complete the diagnostic inquiry and determine if retrolisthesis or anterolisthesis of the segment is present.

The apex of the curvature is another likely site for subluxation. The long lever arm at this area allows a large lateralward bending moment to be created at the spine due to the force of gravity.

If it is determined that the apex is freely moveable, then adjustments are contraindicated. Mobile and hypermobile FSUs are contraindicated for any adjustive intervention. Intersegmental spinal mobility can be more accurately evaluated with stress plain film analysis as opposed to motion palpation.

It is important to approach all adjustments from the convexity of the curve, to reduce the likelihood of increasing the lateralward deviation. Generally, this is also likely the best approach for reducing the curvature. Pretensioning in side posture is also helpful when the clinician is attempting to reduce a lumbar scoliosis.

Disturbances in the vestibular apparatus has been associated with scoliosis patients (153). Also, dysfunction in proprioception has been documented (154). Whether these findings are a cause of the scoliosis or simply an effect of the disorder is unknown. Lewit (155) has hypothesized that mechanical dysfunction in the upper cervical spine may have an influence on the curve or its genesis. Biedermann (156) has proposed that upper cervical subluxation (i.e., KISS syndrome) (see Chapter 8) can create postural scolioses as a result of compensation to the upper cervical lesion. As with any patient, the doctor should examine all segments of the spinal column, pelvis and cranium for signs (e.g., edema, tenderness) of subluxation, since the lesion can occur at any level.

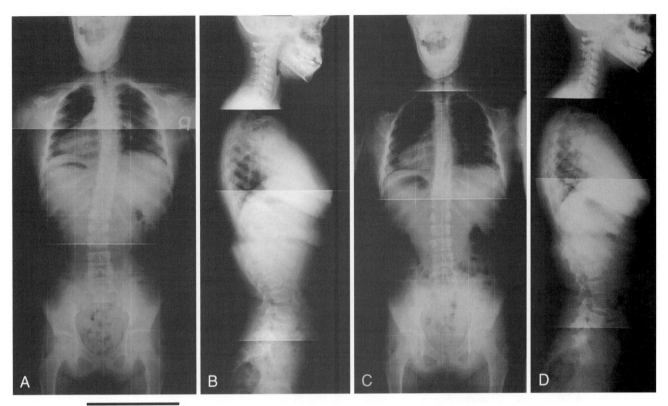

Figure 15.16. A. Pretreatment AP radiograph. B. Pretreatment lateral radiograph. C. Comparative AP radiograph after 10 weeks. D. Comparative lateral radiograph after 10 weeks.

C A S E   R E P O R T
11-year-old Caucasian Female

*T*his 11-year-old female patient has low back pain and "leg pains." Her legs have hurt since she was born. As a baby, the intensity of the pain would cause the child to scream at night. By the age of 11, the pains were nearly constant. She usually takes Tylenol at least twice each week. Prolonged standing appears to aggravate the leg pain. Other symptoms this patient has include neck pain with referral to both upper extremities, and headaches, which occur usually 3-4 days each week. The headache is frontal. The child also reports that her stomach hurts from time to time, usually on one occasion in a given week. The patient's past history included recurrent otitis media. The patient's birth history revealed that labor had been induced and hard labor occurred for about eight hours before the attending physician had discovered that the baby's right arm and leg had wrapped around her head. She was then delivered by caesarean section.

CLINICAL FINDINGS
Right-handed dynamometer readings were as follows: L: 40,35,38; R:40,42,35. The left biceps and left achilles deep tendon reflexes were diminished (+1). Foraminal compression tests were negative and shoulder depression was positive on both sides. Cervical ranges

of motion were 60° flexion; 80° extension; 90° left rotation; 60° right rotation; 50° left lateral flexion; and 55° right lateral flexion. Thoraco-lumbar range of motion findings were 95° flexion; 20° extension; 20° left lateral flexion; and 35° right lateral flexion. Romberg's was negative and there was a positive Trendelenburg sign on the left. The following orthopedic tests were positive: Lasegues and Braggards (right), double leg raise and leg lowering, FABERE (left), Bechterew (bilateral). There was a positive Deerfield on the right and a positive Soto-Hall.

Observation showed the patient to have a high right shoulder and right ilium. Static palpation disclosed bilateral trapezium muscle hypertonicity. Tenderness, edema, fixation dysfunction and skin temperature differentials were present at L5, T3, T7, and the right SI joint.

RADIOLOGIC FINDINGS
The initial AP radiograph demonstrates a low femur on the left of 3 mm (Fig. 15.16A). Lumbarization of the sacrum is present. An approximately 10° thoraco-lumbar scoliosis is present. There is head rotation to the left (+Θ Y). L5 is listed as PRS-m (-Z,+Θ Y, -Θ Z; mamillary process as contact point). The lateral borders of the sacrum from S2 measured 53 right and 49 left, indicating little if any sacral rotation. Analysis of the pelvis demonstrates external rotation of the PSIS on the left (-Θ Y). The seventh cervical spinous is rotated to the right (+Θ Y).

The lateral full spine (in two exposures) shows a posterior widening of the rudimentary disc space between S3 and S4 (Fig. 15.16B).

Lumbarization is present at S1. Hyperextension and slight retrolisthesis of L5 is visible. The cervical spine is mildly lordotic from C7 through C4 but then changes to a kyphotic posture at the upper cervical segments. The head is forward flexed on C1.

TREATMENT AND FOLLOW-UP

The treatment frequency proposed was daily care for 2 weeks, 3 times per week for 7 weeks, twice per week for 7 weeks and once per week for 7 weeks. Twenty visits were completed during the first month of care. At the first seven visits the S3 sacral segment was adjusted (listed as posterior). The L5 subluxation was then adjusted on three occasions followed once by the sacrum. After 2 weeks, L5 and T6 were adjusted (3X), L5, T6 and C7 (4X) and L5, T6 and T1 (1X). A brief clinical examination (e.g., skin temperature instrumentation, static and motion palpation) was performed at each visit to monitor the patient and determine the location for the adjustment(s). The radiographs were used to determine the direction for the adjustment following an assessment of the motion segment level through the clinical examination procedures. The patient made gradual improvement during the first month of care.

After two adjustments to the third sacral segment, decreased edema was noted. The lumbar spinal muscles also became less hypertonic and she began sleeping better. The legs became less painful, after the first adjustment to L5.

A progress examination was performed 5 weeks after initiation of treatment. The patient reported subjectively that the leg pains were improved. Mild low back pain was still present. Right handed dynamometer readings were Left: 40,35,35 and Right: 35,35,30. Braggards was positive on the left. The Deerfield test showed positive on the left. FABERE of the hip was still positive on the left. All other previously positive orthopedic findings were normal. All deep tendon reflexes were normal. Foramina compression was positive on the right and shoulder depression was also still positive on the right.

Cervical ranges of motion overall gradually increased with the most marked improvement for right head rotation which was normalized.

Thoraco-lumbar range of motion was increased to 40° for extension but pain was also present. Left and right lateral flexion increased to 50° to each side. Mild pain was still present at the extreme of end-range. The left sacroiliac joint was still tender to palpation. Mild hypertonicity of the lumbar spinal muscles and the trapezium was also noted. The patient had two exacerbations during the first phase of treatment in which she fell while roller skating during the first week of care and was hit on the head during an outing with the Girl Scouts in the fifth week. Following the progress examination, the patient was then scheduled for a treatment frequency of 3 times per week for one week and then 2 visits per week for five weeks.

During the next 5 weeks of care, the patient was seen on 13 occasions. Progressively, L5,T6 and T1 were adjusted four times, L5, T6 and C7 on two visits, and L5, T6 and C6 on one occasion. The sacrum, T8 and C7 were adjusted two times. L5 and C7 were predominately adjusted during the ninth and tenth weeks of care. Follow-up radiographs were obtained after 10 weeks of care.

The comparative AP (Fig. 15.16C) shows a decrease in the magnitude of both the thoracic and lumbar portions of the scoliosis (compare with Fig. 15.16A). The comparative lateral full spine radiograph (Fig. 15.16D) shows a slight decrease in the retrolisthesis of L5. The head is in a more forward looking direction but this is mainly accomplished by the extension occurring at C1-C2 (compare with Fig. 15.16B).

During the next 9 months, the patient was seen a total of nine times and she was mostly asymptomatic during this time period; objective signs of subluxation continued, e.g., restrictions in intersegmental range of motion. L5, T6 and C7 were the most frequently adjusted segments during this time period. No further follow-up is available on this patient.

CASE REPORTS
Cohort Study Participants

*T*he following five case scenarios are derived from an ongoing cohort study by one of the authors (CAL). The study includes approximately 40 participants. All subjects received chiropractic care over an approximately 1-year period. Care consisted primarily of manually delivered specific contact short lever arm adjustments. Adjustments were full spine and were usually delivered at the apex of any scoliosis and at the base of the curvature. In addition, adjustments to the sacroiliac articulation(s) were performed in most cases. Cervical adjustments were performed when indicated. The precise location for the delivery of the adjustment was determined

through a combination of x-ray findings and palpatory indications of fixation dysfunction. Adjustments of the lumbar spine in the side posture position were performed with the spine in a pre-stressed position before the introduction of the thrust. Patients were seen at a frequency of two to three visits per week for the entire 1-year duration of the study. The following cases are presented to show some of the varying types of responses to chiropractic care in adolescent patients with scoliosis.

Case No. 1

This patient is a 13-year-old female. The initial radiograph discloses a lumbar and thoracic scoliosis (Fig. 15.17A). The comparative (after 12 months) radiograph shows no sign of progression or remission of the magnitude of the curvature (Fig. 15.17B).

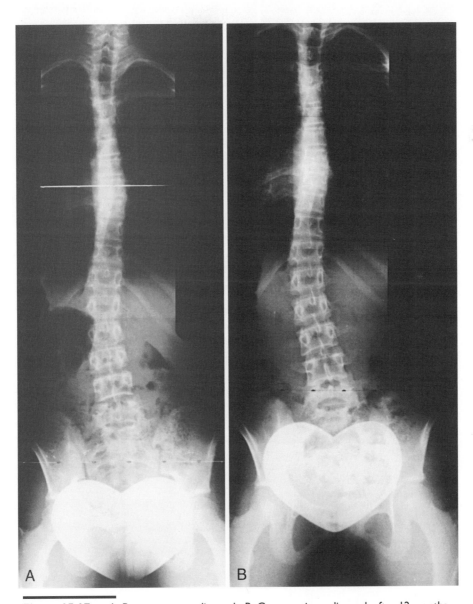

Figure 15.17.   A. Pretreatment radiograph. B. Comparative radiograph after 12 months.

Case No. 2

This patient is an 11-year-old female. The pre-treatment radiograph demonstrates a mild lumbar and thoracic scoliosis (Fig. 15.18A). The comparative (after 7 months) radiograph shows that the scoliosis has progressed in both the lumbar and thoracic regions (Fig. 15.18B).

Case No. 3

This patient is a 14-year-old female. A moderate lumbar and thoracic scoliosis is evident on the pretreatment radiograph (Fig. 15.19A).

The comparative (after 12 months) radiograph shows little progression in the scoliosis (Fig. 15.19B).

Case No. 4

This patient is an 11-year-old male. The initial radiograph discloses a mild lumbar scoliosis (Fig. 15.20A). The comparative (after 12 months radiograph) shows minimal change in the curvature (Fig. 15.20B). The lumbar portion appears to have increased slightly while the thoracic portion is somewhat reduced.

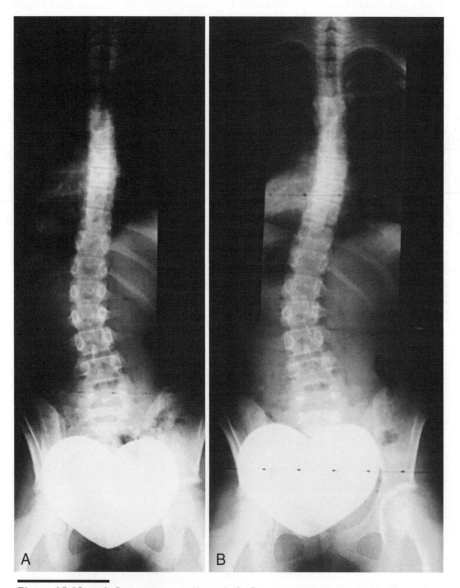

Figure 15.18.   A. Pretreatment radiograph. B. Comparative radiograph after 7 months.

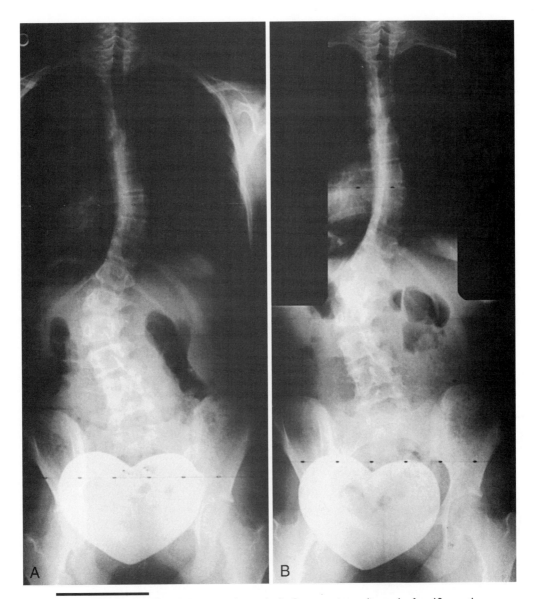

Figure 15.19. A. Pretreatment radiograph. B. Comparative radiograph after 12 months.

Case No. 5

This patient is an 11-year-old male. The pretreatment radiograph shows a mild thoracic scoliosis with the convexity to the left (Fig. 15.21A). The comparative (after 12 months) radiograph shows that the configuration of the curvature has markedly changed. The thoracic convexity is now to the right (Fig. 15.21B).

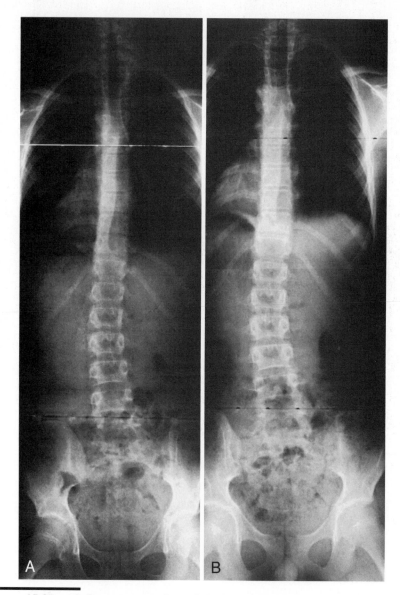

Figure 15.20.   A. Pretreatment radiograph. B. Comparative radiograph after 12 months.

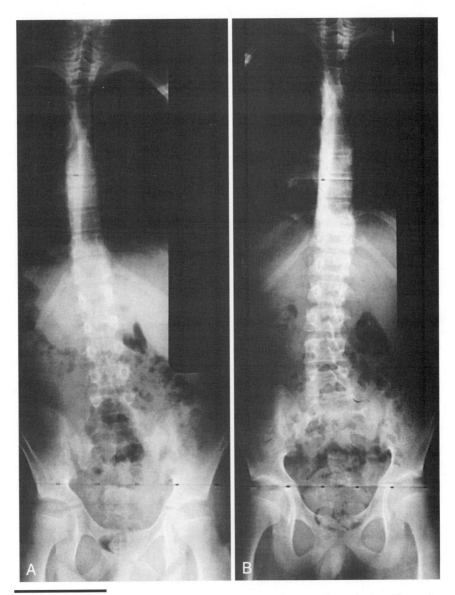

Figure 15.21.   A. Pretreatment radiograph. B. Comparative radiograph after 12 months.

Terminology

One of the major hindrances with scoliosis research has been the confusion created by authors using the same word but with different interpretations of the terminology. The Scoliosis Research Society has developed a glossary of terms to create a common language for the researcher as well as for the clinician with an interest in scoliosis.

GLOSSARY

adolescent scoliosis. spinal curvature presenting at or about the onset of puberty and before maturity.

adult scoliosis. spinal curvature existing after skeletal maturity.

apical vertebra. most axially rotated vertebra in a curve; the most deviated vertebra from the vertical axis of the patient.

cafe-au-lait spots. light brown irregular areas of skin pigmentation. If sufficient in number and having smooth margins, they are suggestive of neurofibromatosis.

congenital scoliosis. scoliosis due to congenital anomalous vertebral development.

curve measurement. Cobb's method: select the upper and lower end vertebrae with the steepest inclination towards the concavity of the curve. Erect perpendiculars to lines drawn through the endplates of the end vertebrae (see definition for end vertebra given below). If the endplates are poorly visualized or anomalous, then draw a line which bisects the centers of the pedicles.

double major scoliosis. scoliosis with two structural curves.

end vertebra. 1. The most cephalad vertebra of a curve, whose superior surface tilts maximally towards the concavity of the curve. 2. The most caudal vertebra whose inferior surface tilts maximally towards the concavity of the curve.

fractional curve. compensatory curve that is incomplete because it returns to the erect. Its only horizontal vertebra is its caudad or cephalad one.

full curve. curve in which the only horizontal vertebra is at its apex.

gibbus. sharply angular kyphotic deformation.

hyperkyphosis. sagittal alignment of the thoracic spine in which there is more than the normal amount of kyphosis.

hypokyphosis. sagittal alignment of the thoracic spine in which there is less than the normal amount of kyphosis.

hysterical scoliosis. nonstructural deformity of the spine that develops as a manifestation of a conversion reaction.

idiopathic scoliosis. structural spinal curve for which there is no known cause.

iliac epiphysis, iliac apophysis. The epiphysis along the wing of an ilium.

inclinometer. instrument used to measure the angle of thoracic inclination or rib hump.

infantile scoliosis. spinal curvature which is developing during the first three years of life.

juvenile scoliosis. spinal curvature which is developing between the skeletal age of three and the onset of puberty.

kypos. change in alignment of a segment of the spine in the sagittal plane that increases the posterior convex angulation; an abnormal kyphosis.

kyphoscoliosis. spine with a scoliosis and a true hyperkyphosis. A rotatory deformity with only apparent kyphosis should not be described by this term.

lordoscoliosis. scoliosis associated with an abnormal anterior angulation in the sagittal plane.

major curve. term used to designate the largest structural curve.

minor curve. term used to describe the smallest curve. This curve is always more flexible than the major curve.

nonstructural curve. curve that has no structural component and that corrects or overcorrects on recumbent or standing lateral bending radiographs.

pelvic obliquity. deviation of the pelvis from the horizontal in the frontal plane. Fixed pelvic obliquities can be attributable to contractures either above or below the pelvis. Functional obliquity can be caused by leg length inequality.

primary curve. first or earliest of several curves to appear, if identifiable.

rotational prominence. in the forward bending position, the thoracic prominence on one side is usually due to vertebra axial rotation causing rib prominence. In the lumbar spine, the prominence is usually due to axial rotation of the lumbar vertebrae.

skeletal age, bone age. age obtained by comparing an AP radiograph of the left hand and wrist with the standards of Gruelich and Pyle Atlas.

structural curve. segment of the spine with a lateral curvature that lacks normal flexibility.

vertebral ring apophysis. most reliable index of vertebral immaturity, seen best in lateral radiographs or in the lumbar region in AP lateral bending radiographs.

REFERENCES

1. Sabatier. Traite complete d'anatomie. Paris, 1777 (Cited by Farkas A. Physiological scoliosis. J Bone Joint Surg 1941; 23:607-627.
2. Vercauteren M, Van Beneden M, Verplaetse R, Croene, Uyttendaele D, Verdonk R. Trunk asymmetries in a Belgian school population. Spine 1982; 7:555-562.
3. Goldberg MS, Mayo NE, Poitras B, Scott S, Hanley J. The Ste-Justine adolescent idiopathic scoliosis cohort study. Part I: Description of the study. Spine 1994; 19:1551-1561.
4. Plaugher G, Cremata EE, Phillips RB. A retrospective consecutive case analysis of pretreatment and comparative static radiological parameters following chiropractic adjustments. J Manipulative Physiol Ther 1990; 13:498-506.
5. Cobb JR: Outline for the study of scoliosis. In Instructional Course Lectures, The American Academy of Orthopaedic Surgeons, 1948; 5:261-275.
6. Nordwall A. Studies in idiopathic scoliosis relevant to etiology, conservative and operative treatment. Acta Orthop Scand (Suppl) 1973; 1-178.
7. Jeffries BF, Tarlton M, De Smet AA, Dwyer SJ, Brower AC. Computerized measurement and analysis of scoliosis. Radiology 1980; 134:381-385.
8. Voutsinas SA, MacEwen GD. Sagittal profiles of the spine. Clin Orthop 1986; 210:235-242.
9. Willner S. Moire topography for the diagnosis and documentation of scoliosis. Acta Orthop Scand 1979; 50:295-302.
10. Ischida A, Suzuki S, Imai S, Mori Y. Scoliosis evaluation utilizing truncal cross-sections. Med Biol Eng Comput 1982; 20:181-186.
11. Ho EKW, Chan FL, Hsu LCS, Leong JCY: New methods of measuring vertebral rotation from computed tomographic scans. Spine 1993; 18:1173-1177.
12. Hierholzer E, Luxmann G. Three-dimensional shape analysis of the scoliotic spine using invariant shape parameters. J Biomech 1982; 15:583-598.
13. McAlister WH, Shackelford MG. Measurement of spinal curvatures. Radiol Clin North Am 1975; 13:113-121.
14. Nash CL, Moe JH. A study of vertebral rotation. J Bone Joint Surg 1969; 51A:223-229.
15. Dickson RA, Lawton JO, Archer IA, Butt WP. The pathogenesis of idiopathic scoliosis. J Bone Joint Surg 1984; 66B:8-15.
16. White AA, Panjabi MM. Clinical biomechanics of the spine, 2nd ed. Philadelphia: JB Lippincott, 1990.
17. Winter RB. Classification and terminology. In: Moe JH, Bradford D, Lonstein J, Ogilvie J, Winter RB, eds. Moe's textbook of scoliosis and other spinal deformities. 2nd ed. Philadelphia: WB Saunders Co, 1987.
18. Plaugher G, Lopes MA. Scoliosis. In: Plaugher G, ed. Textbook of Clinical Chiropractic: a specific biomechanical approach Baltimore: Williams & Wilkins, 1993:266-278.
19. McGuire DJ, Keppler L, Kotagal S, Akbarnia BA. Scoliosis associated with type I Arnold-Chiari malformations. Orthop Trans 1987; 11:122-127.
20. Arai S, Ohtsuka Y, Moriua H, Kitahara H, Minamia S. Scoliosis associated with syringomyelia. Spine 1993; 18:1591-1592.
21. Coonrad R, Richardson WH, Oakes WJ. Left thoracic curves can be different. Orthop Trans 1985; 9:126-127.
22. Nilsonne U, Lundgren KD. Long term prognosis in idiopathic scoliosis. Acta Orthop Scand 1968; 39:456-465.
23. Nachemson A. A long term follow-up study of non-treated scoliosis. Acta Orthop Scand 1968; 39:466-476.
24. Keim H. The adolescent spine. New York, NY: Springer-Verlag, 1982.
25. McMaster MJ. Infantile idiopathic scoliosis: Can it be prevented? J Bone Joint Surg 1983; 65B:612-617.
26. Mehta MH. The rib-vertebrae angle in the early diagnosis between resolving and progressive infantile scoliosis. J Bone Joint Surg 1972; 54B:230-243.
27. Kristmundsdottir F, Burwell RG, James JI. The rib-vertebra angles on the convexity and concavity of the spinal curve in infantile idiopathic scoliosis. Clin Orthop 1985; 201:205-209.
28. Hagglund G, Karlberg J, Willner S. Growth in girls with adolescent idiopathic scoliosis. Spine 1991; 16:108-111.
29. Rogala EJ, Drummond DS, Gurr J. Scoliosis: Incidence and natural history. J Bone Joint Surg 1978; 60A:173-176.
30. Leaver JM, Alvik A, Warren MD. Prescriptive screening for adolescent idiopathic scoliosis: A review of the evidence. Intl J Epidemiol 1982; 11:101-111.
31. Belstead JS, Edgar MA. Early detection of scoliosis. Br Med J 1978; 2:937-938.
32. Lonstein JE. Screening for spinal deformities in Minnesota schools. Clin Orthop 1977; 126:33-42.

33. Wynne EJ. Scoliosis: To screen or not to screen. Canadian J Public Health 1984; 75:277-280.
34. Dickson RA. Scoliosis in the community. Br Med J 1983; 286:615-618.
35. Burwell RG, James NJ, Johnson F, Webb JK, Wilson YG. Standardized trunk asymmetry scores. J Bone Joint Surg 1983; 65B: 452-463.
36. Howell JM. Problems in scoliosis screening. Canadian J Public Health 1978; 69:293-296.
37. Whitby LG. Screening for disease: Definitions and criteria. Lancet 1974:819-821.
38. Cochrane AL, Holland WW. Validation of screening procedures. Br Med Bull 1971; 27:3-8.
39. Willner S. Spinal pantograph: A non-invasive technique for describing kyphosis and lordosis in the thoracolumbar spine. Acta Orthop. Scand 1981; 52:525-529.
40. Somerville EW. Rotational lordosis: The development of the single curve. J Bone Joint Surg 1952; 34B:421-427.
41. Dickson RA, Lawton JO, Archer WP, Berkin CR, Bliss P, Womervill EW, Jobbins B. Bi-planar asymmetry: The pathogenesis of idiopathic scoliosis. J Bone Joint Surg 1984; 66B:143-144.
42. Deacon P, Flood BM, Dickson RA. Idiopathic scoliosis in three-dimensions: A radiographic and morphometric analysis. J Bone Joint Surg 1984; 66B:509-512.
43. Dickson RA, Lawton JO, Archer IA, Butt WP, Jobbins B. Combined median and coronal plane asymmetry: The essential lesion of progressive idiopathic scoliosis. J Bone Joint Surg 1983; 65B:368.
44. Willner S, Johnson B. Thoracic kyphosis and lumbar lordosis during the growth period in children. Acta Paediatr Scand 1983; 72:873-878.
45. Archer IA, Dickson RA. Stature and idiopathic scoliosis: A prospective study. J Bone Joint Surg 1985; 67B:185-188.
46. Goldberg CJ, Dowling FE, Fogarty EE. Adolescent idiopathic scoliosis: Early menarche, normal growth. Spine 1993; 18:529-535.
47. Veldhuizen AG, Bass P, Webb PJ. Observation on the growth of the adolescent spine. J Bone Joint Surg 1986; 68B:724-728.
48. Daruwalla JS, Balasubramaniam P, Chay SO, Rajan U, Lee HP. Idiopathic scoliosis: Prevalence and ethnic distribution in Singapore school children. J Bone Joint Surg 1985; 67B:182-184.
49. Brooks HL. Current incidence of scoliosis in California. In: Zorba PA, Siegler D (eds), Scoliosis, London, Academic Press, 1980:7-12.
50. Brooks HL, Azen SP, Gerberg E, Brooks R, Chan L. Scoliosis: A prospective epidemiological study. J Bone Joint Surg 1975; 57A:968-971.
51. Leaver JM, Alvik A, Warren MD. Prescriptive screening for adolescent idiopathic scoliosis: A review of the evidence. Intl J Epidemiol 1982; 11:101-111.
52. Rogala EJ, Drummond DS, Gurr J. Scoliosis: Incidence and natural history. A prospective epidemiological study. J Bone Joint Surg 1978; 60A:173-176.
53. Kane WJ. Scoliosis prevalence: A call for a statement of terms. Clin Orthop 1977; 126:43-46.
54. Walters PJ. Pelvis. In: Plaugher G, ed. Textbook of clinical chiropractic: a specific biomechanical approach. Baltimore: Williams & Wilkins, 1993:150-189.
55. Poussa M, Mellin G. Spinal mobility and posture in adolescent idiopathic scoliosis at three stages of curve magnitude. Spine 1992; 17:757-760.
56. White AA. Kinematics of the normal spine as related to scoliosis. J Biomech 1971; 4:405.
57. Lovett RW. The mechanism of the normal spine and its relation to scoliosis. Boston Med Surg J 1905; 153:349.
58. Goldberg C, Dowling FE. Handedness and scoliosis convexity: a reappraisal. Spine 1990; 15:61-64.
59. Kostiuk JP, Bentivoglio J. The incidence of low back pain in adult scoliosis. Spine 1981; 6:268-273.
60. Poitras B, Mayo NE, Goldberg MS, Scott S, Hanley J. The Ste-Justine adolescent idiopathic scoliosis cohort study. Part IV: Surgical correction and back pain. Spine 1994; 19:1582-1588.
61. Paonessa KJ, Engler GL. Back pain and disability after Harrington rod fusion to the lumbar spine for scoliosis. Spine 1992; 17(8S):S249-S253.
62. Mayo NE, Goldberg MS, Poitras B, Scott S, Hanley J. The Ste-Justine adolescent idiopathic scoliosis cohort study. Part III: Back pain. Spine 1994; 19:1573-1581.
63. Grubb SA, Lipscomb HJ, Suh PB. Results of surgical treatment of painful adult scoliosis. Spine 1994; 19:1619-1627.
64. Goldberg MS, Mayo NE, Poitras B, Scott S, Hanley J. The Ste-Justine adolescent idiopathic scoliosis cohort study. Part II: Perception of health, self and body image, and participation in physical activities. Spine 1994; 19:1562-1572.
65. Geissele AE, Ogilvie JW, Cohen M, Bradford DS. Thoracoplasty for the treatment of rib prominence in thoracic scoliosis. Spine 1994; 19:1636-1642.
66. Stokes IAF, Ronchetti PJ, Aronsson DD. Changes in shape of the adolescent idiopathic scoliosis curve after surgical correction. Spine 1994; 19:1032:1038.
67. Theologis TN, Jefferson RJ, Simpson AHRW, Turner-Smith AR, Fairbank JCT. Quantifying the cosmetic defect of adolescent idiopathic scoliosis. Spine 1993; 18:909-912.
68. U.S. Preventive Services Task Force Policy Statement. Screening for adolescent idiopathic scoliosis. JAMA 1993; 269:2664-2672.
69. Bunnell WP. Outcome of spinal screening. Spine 1993; 18:1572-1580.
70. Duval-Beaupere G. Rib hump and supine angle as prognostic factors for mild scoliosis. Spine 1992; 17:103-107.
71. Torrel G, Nordwall A, Nachemson A. The changing pattern of scoliosis treatment due to effective screening. J Bone Joint Surg 1981; 63A:337-341.
72. Cooke ED, Carter LM, Pilcher MF. Identifying scoliosis in the adolescent with thermography: a preliminary study. Clin Orthop 1980; 148:172-176.
73. Ardran GM, Coates R, Dickson RA, Dixon-Brown A, Harding FM. Assessment of scoliosis in children: low dose radiographic technique. Br J Radiol 1980; 53:146-147.
74. Smet AA, Fritz SL, Asher MA. A method for minimizing the radiation exposure from scoliosis radiographs. J Bone Joint Surg 1981; 63A:156-158.
75. Barge FE. Scoliosis: Identifiable causes detection and correction. Bawden Brothers, Inc. Davenport, Iowa, 1988.
76. Dickson RA, Stamper P, Sharp AM, Harker P. School screening for scoliosis: cohort study of clinical course. Br Med J 1980; 281:265-267.
77. Duval-Beaupere G, Lespargot A, Grossiord A. Flexibility of scoliosis; what does it mean? Is the terminology appropriate? Spine 1985; 10:428-432.
78. Beauchamp M, Labelle H, Grimard G, et al. Diurnal variation of Cobb angle measurement in adolescent idiopathic scoliosis. Spine 1993; 18:1581-1583.
79. Risser JC. The iliac apophysis: An invaluable sign in the management of scoliosis. Clin Orthop 1958; 11:111-119.
80. Tanner JM, Whitehouse RH, Cameron N, et al. Assessment of skeletal maturity and prediction of adult height. (TW2 method). 2nd edition, London, Academic Press, 1983.
81. Howell FR, Mahood JK, Dickson RA. Growth beyond skeletal maturity. Spine 1992; 17:437-440.
82. Tanner JM. Growth at adolescence, 2nd edition. Oxford, England: Blackwell Scientific, 1962.
83. Izumi Y. Alkaline phosphates as a biochemical maturity index in female adolescence. Spine 1993; 18:2257-2260.
84. Terver S, Kleinman R, Bleck EE. Growth landmarks and the evolution of scoliosis: a review of pertinent studies on their usefulness. Develop Med Child Neurol 1980; 22:675-684.
85. Karol LA, Johnston CE, Browne RH, Madison M. Progression of the curve in boys who have idiopathic scoliosis. J Bone Joint Surg 1993; 75A:1804-1810.
86. Lonstein JE, Carlson JM. The prediction of curve progression in untreated idiopathic scoliosis during growth. J Bone Joint Surg 1984; 66A:1061-1071.
87. Collis DK, Ponsetti IV. Long-term follow-up of patients with idiopathic scoliosis not treated surgically. J Bone Joint Surg 1969; 51A:425-444.
88. Scott MM, Piggot H. A short-term follow-up of patients with mild scoliosis. J Bone Joint Surg 1981; 63B:523-525.
89. Papaioannou T, Stokes I, Kenwright J. Scoliosis associated with limb-length inequality. J Bone Joint Surg 1982; 64A:59-62.
90. Perennou D, Marcelli C, Herisson C, Simon L. Adult lumbar scoliosis: Epidemiologic aspects in a low back pain population. Spine 1994; 19:123-128.
91. Perdriolle R, Becchetti S, Vidal J, Lopez P. Mechanical process and growth cartilage: Essential factors in the progression of scoliosis. Spine 1993; 18:343-349.
92. Diakow PRP. Pain: A forgotten aspect of idiopathic scoliosis. J Can Chiro Assoc 1983; 27:11-15.
93. Wynne-Davies R. Familial (idiopathic) scoliosis. A family survey. J Bone Joint Surg 1968; 50B:24.
94. Czeizel A, Bellyei A, Barta O, Magda J, Molnar L. Genetics of adolescent idiopathic scoliosis. J Med Genet 1978; 15:424-427.
95. Mawhiney RB. Clinical report: reduction of minor lumbar scoliosis in a 57-year-old female. Chiropractic: J Chiropractic Res Clin Invest 1989; 2:48-51.
96. Liszka O. Spinal cord mechanisms leading to scoliosis in animal experiments. Acta Med Pol 1961; 45-63.
97. MacEwen GD. Experimental scoliosis. Clin Orthop 1973; 93:69-74.
98. Lloyd-Roberts GC, Pincott JR, McMeniman P, Bayley IJL, Kendall B. Progression in idiopathic scoliosis: a preliminary report of a possible mechanism. J Bone Joint Surg 1978; 60B:451-460.
99. Pincott JR. Observations on the afferent nervous system in idiopathic scoliosis. In: Zorab PA, Siegler D, eds. Scoliosis, New York, Academic Press, 1980:45-59.
100. Pincott JR, Davies JS, Taffs LF. Scoliosis caused by section of dorsal spine nerve roots. J Bone Joint Surg 1984; 66B:27-29.
101. Yamamoto H, Tani T, MacEwen GD, Herman R. An evaluation of brainstem function as a prognostication of early idiopathic scoliosis. J Pediatr Orthop 1982; 2:521-527.
102. Sahlstrand T, Peterson B. A study of labyrinthine function in patients with adolescent idiopathic scoliosis. Acta Orthop Scand 1979; 50:759.
103. Sahlstrand T, Lidstrom J. Equilibrium factors as predictors of the prognosis in adolescent idiopathic scoliosis. Clin Orthop 1980; 232-236.
104. Kennelly KP, Stokes MJ. Pattern of asymmetry of paraspinal muscle size in adolescent idiopathic scoliosis examined by real-time ultrasound imaging. Spine 1993; 18:913-917.
105. Reuber M, Schultz A, McNeill T, Spencer D. Trunk muscle myoelectric activities in idiopathic scoliosis. Spine 1983; 8:447-456.
106. Zuk T. The role of spinal and abdominal muscles in the pathogenesis of scoliosis. J Bone Joint Surg 1962; 44B:102-105.
107. Green RJL. Histochemistry and ultrastructure of paraspinal muscles in idiopathic scoliosis and control subjects. Med Lab Sci 1988; 16:171-176.
108. Zetterberg C, Aniansson A, Grimby G. Morphology of the paravertebral muscles in adolescent idiopathic scoliosis. Spine 1983; 8:457-461.
109. Peterson BW, Richmond FJ. Control of head movement. Oxford University Press, NY, 1988.

110. Schultz AB, LaRocca H, Galante JO, Andriacchi TP. A study of geometrical relationships in scoliotic spines. J Biomech 1972; 5:409-420.

111. Schultz AB, Haderspeck K, Takashima S. Correction of scoliosis by muscle stimulation: Biomechanical analyses. Spine 1981; 6:468-476.

112. Schultz AB, Hirsch C. Mechanical analysis of Harrington rod correction of idiopathic scoliosis. J Bone Joint Surg 1973; 55A:983-992.

113. Smith RM, Pool RD, Butt WP, Dickson RA. The transverse plane deformity of structural scoliosis. Spine 1991; 16:1126-1129.

114. Stokes IA, Gardner-Morse M. Analysis of the interaction between vertebral lateral deviation and axial rotation in scoliosis. J Biomech 1991; 24:753-759.

115. Pope MH, Stokes IAF, Moreland M. The biomechanics of scoliosis. CRC Critical Reviews in Biomedical Engineering, 11:157-188.

116. Xiong B, Sevastik JA, Hedlund R, Sevastik B. Radiographic changes at the coronal plane in early scoliosis. Spine 1994; 19:159-164.

117. Enneking WF, Harrington P. Pathological changes in scoliosis. J Bone Joint Surg 1969; 51A:165-184.

118. Shakespeare DT, Stokes M, Sherman KP, Young A. Reflex inhibition of the quadriceps after meniscectomy: lack of association with pain. Clin Physiol 1985; 5:137-144.

119. Kane WJ. Scoliosis prevalence: a call for a statement of terms. Clin Orthop 1977; 126:43-46.

120. Risser JC. Scoliosis: past and present. J Bone Joint Surg 1964; 46A:167-199.

121. Lenox Hill Hospital. Health Tip Sheet: scoliosis. Lenox Hill Hospital. Health Education Center, 1080 Lexington Avenue, New York, NY 10021.

122. Hildebrandt RW. Science, medicine and chiropractic theory. J Manipulative Physiol Ther 1986; 9:181-182.

123. Keim HA. Scoliosis. CIBA clinical symposia. 1978; 30:1-30.

124. Bjerkreim I. Operative treatment of scoliosis with the Harrington instrumentation technique. Acta Orthop Scand 1976; 47:397-402.

125. Dewald RL, Ray RD. Skeletal traction for the treatment of severe scoliosis. The University of Illinois halo-loop apparatus. J Bone Joint Surg 1970; 52A:233-238.

126. Ponseti IV, Friedman B. Prognosis in idiopathic scoliosis. J Bone Joint Surg 1950; 32A:381-395.

127. Tolo VT. Progression in scoliosis. A 360 degree change in 75 years. Spine 1983; 8:373-377.

128. Ziporyn T. Scoliosis now subject of numerous questions. JAMA 1985; 254:3009-3019.

129. Faraday JA. Current principles in the nonoperative management of structural adolescent idiopathic scoliosis. Phys Ther 1983; 63:512-523.

130. Lantz CA. Conservative management of scoliosis. Chiropractic 1995; 9:100-107.

131. Blount WP. Editorial: the virtue of early treatment of idiopathic scoliosis. J Bone Joint Surg 1981; 63A:335-336.

132. McCarthy RE. Prevention of the complications of scoliosis by early detection. Clin Orthop 1987; 222:73-78.

133. Lloyd-Roberts GC, Pincott JR, McMeniman P, Bayley IJL, Kendall B. Progression in idiopathic scoliosis. A preliminary report of a possible mechanism. J Bone Joint Surg 1978; 60B:451-460.

134. Lonstein JE, Bjoklund S, Wanninger MH, Nelson RP. Voluntary school screening for scoliosis in Minnesota. J Bone Joint Surg 1982; 64A:481-488.

135. Madigan RR, Wallace SL. What's new in scoliosis? J Tenn Med Assoc 1983; (May):292-297.

136. Torell G, Nordwall A, Nachemson A. The changing pattern of scoliosis treatment due to effective screening. J Bone Joint Surg 1981; 63A:337-341.

137. Bunnell WP. Treatment of idiopathic scoliosis. Orthop Clin North Am 1979; 10:813-827.

138. Andriacchi TP, Schultz A, Belytschko T, DeWald R. Milwaukee brace correction of idiopathic scoliosis: A biomechanical analysis and a retrospective study. J Bone Joint Surg 1976; 58A: 806.

139. Labelle H, Dansereau J, Poitras B. Evaluation of the 3-D effect of the Boston brace. Presented at the annual Scientific Meeting of the Pediatric Orthopaedic Society of North America, 1991:35.

140. Focarile FA, Bonaldi A, Giarolo MA, et al. Effectiveness of non-surgical treatment for idiopathic scoliosis. Overview of available evidence. Spine 1992; 16:395-401.

141. Goldberg DJ, Dowling FE, Hall JE, Emans JB. A statistical comparison between natural history of idiopathic scoliosis and brace treatment in skeletally immature adolescent girls. Spine 1993; 18:902-908.

142. Fallstrom K , Cochran T, Nachemson A. Long-term effects on personality development in patients with adolescent idiopathic scoliosis: influence of type of treatment. Spine 1986; 11:756-758.

143. DiRaimondo CV, Green NE. Brace-wear compliance in patients with adolescent idiopathic scoliosis. J Pediatr Orthop 1988; 8:143-146.

144. Yettram AL, Jackman MJ. Equilibrium analysis for the forces in the human spinal column and its musculature. Spine 1980; 5:402-411.

145. Axelgard J, Brown JC. Lateral surface stimulation for the treatment of progressive idiopathic scoliosis. Spine 1983; 8:242-260.

146. Sullivan JA, Davidson R, Renslaw TS, et al. Further evaluation of the scolitron treatment of idiopathic adolescent scoliosis. Spine 1986; 11:903-906.

147. Francis EE. Lateral electrical surface stimulation treatment for scoliosis. Pediatr Nurs 1987; 13:157-160.

148. Sallahian CA. Reduction of a scoliosis in an adult male utilizing specific chiropractic spinal manipulation: a case report. Chiropractic: J Chiropractic Res Clin Invest 1991; 7:42-45.

149. Mawhiney RB. Chiropractic proof in scoliosis care. Dig Chiro Econ 1984; (Mar/Apr):65-70.

150. Aspergren DD, Cox JM. Correction of progressive idiopathic scoliosis utilizing neuromuscular stimulation and manipulation: a case report. J Manipulative Physiol Ther 1987; 10:147-156.

151. Bosler J. Scoliosis cured by manipulation of the neck. Med J Aust 1979; 1:3,95.

152. Betge G. Scoliosis correction. Euro J Chiro 1985; 33:71-91.

153. Byrd JA. Equilibrium dysfunction and sensitivity to vibration in scoliosis. Clin Orthop 1988; 229:114-119.

154. Barrack RL, Whitecloud TS, Burke SW, Cook SD, Harding AF. Proprioception in idiopathic scoliosis. Spine 1984; 9:681-685.

155. Lewit K. Manipulative therapy in rehabilitation of the motor system. Boston: Butterworths, 1985.

156. Biedermann H. Kinematic imbalances due to suboccipital strain in newborns. J Manual Med 1992; 6:151-156.

16 The Febrile Child

Shahinaz E. Soliman, Gregory Plaugher, and Joel Alcantara

One of the most common pediatric clinical presentations is that of the febrile child. In an office-based study by Hoekelman et al. (1), 10.5% of 1068 children, ages 3 to 24 months, had temperatures >38.2° C. Fever comprises approximately 30% of the principal complaints brought to a pediatrician (2). Twenty percent of pediatric emergency room visits (3) and approximately ⅔ of all children in the United States will be evaluated by a health care provider for an acute febrile illness during the first two years of life (4). To practitioners and parents alike, it is an alarming and anxiety-provoking issue. The purpose of this chapter is to examine the issues involved in the evaluation and management of the febrile child and the causes of fever in children.

Control of Body Temperature

Body temperature regulation is based on an equilibrium between heat production and heat loss. Heat production depends on the basal metabolic rate, which varies with physical activity, thyroxine level and catecholamine levels. On the other hand heat loss is mediated through evaporation, conduction and convection. The control of heat production and heat loss is maintained by the thermoregulatory center in the hypothalamus. The hypothalamus regulates the normal body temperature by receiving inputs from two main sources; the first source is the peripheral thermoreceptors. The second source is the temperature of blood perfusing the hypothalamus itself. When the body temperature rises and the hypothalamus receives input from the above two sources it responds by vasodilatation, sweating and shivering (also a mechanism of pyrogenesis).

Pathophysiology of Fever

Toxins, infectious agents, or antigen-antibody complexes from many different sources, known as exogenous pyrogens, produce fever in humans by initiating the production of a protein, endogenous pyrogen, from phagocytic leukocytes (5). This protein interacts with specialized receptors in the anterior hypothalamus, leading to the production of prostaglandins, monoamines and probably cyclic adenosine monophosphate (5). Thus, the body thermostat is set to a higher level and the patient becomes feverish. The primary pyrogen responsible for

fever is interleukin-1 (6). This endogenous pyrogen is not stored in the phagocytic leukocytes and takes from 1 to several hours to be synthesized. When fever takes place, the body responds by vasodilatation temporarily raising the skin temperature allowing heat loss through the skin to the cooler environment. On the other hand, sweating promotes heat loss via evaporation and at the same time the subject feels warm and seeks a colder atmosphere (7).

The Role of Fever

There is an increasingly large body of evidence that appears to support the positive role fever places on the host defenses (8). The fever improves the body's ability to fight infection by increasing leukocyte mobility, increasing leukocyte bacteriocidal activity, enchancing the interferon effect, and T-cell proliferation and decreasing available trace metals for the pathogenic infection. In animals, the inability to mount a febrile response in the presence of infection is highly associated with increased mortality.

Fever is associated with the release of endogenous pyrogens, leading to the activation of T cells which presumably enhances the host defenses (9). Elderly or debilitated patients often have little or no fever and this factor is considered to be a poor diagnostic sign. However, Petersdorf states that there is no reason to believe that fever accelerates phagocytosis, antibody formation or other defense mechanisms (9).

Fever Defined

Normal body temperature varies diurnally with the high temperature occurring in the early evening and low temperature in the early morning. Depending on which authority is consulted (5,8,9), there is a discrepancy as to what is considered normal and abnormal temperature. Normal rectal temperature can range between 96.8° and 98.6° F (36° and 37° C); however, on rare occasions it may be as low as 95.5° F (35.3° C) or as high as 100.4° F (38° C) (8). For this discussion, in the appropriately clothed child, a rectal temperature more than 38.0° C (100.4° F) will be defined as fever. Oral and axillary temperatures are usually 0.6° C (1° F) and 1.1° C (2° F) lower than rectal, respectively (5). Infrared tympanic membrane thermometry appears to be a reliable method for measuring body temperature, although in children less than three months of age the reliability of this method has been questioned. Because even a low grade fever in this age group can be serious, it is prudent to rely on rectal temperatures in this population of patients (5).

Pediatric and emergency medicine residency directors were surveyed and defined fever as greater than 38° C and 38.1° C, respectively (10).

General Considerations

A complex dilemma for any primary health care provider is to determine the mechanism, clinical relevance, and case management of fever in a child. Within the field of medicine there remains a lack of consensus with regard to the treatment of the febrile child (5,8,9).

Infections of the gastrointestinal tracts or the respiratory system account for the majority of fevers in all age groups. Most of these infections are viral in origin (e.g., influenza virus, parainfluenza virus, respiratory syncytial virus, adenovirus, rhinovirus, rotavirus, entero virus) they are generally self-limiting and children recover without specific therapy (8,11).

The challenge for the chiropractic clinician is to determine which children have uncomplicated fevers of viral origin versus those that may be caused by a serious bacterial infection (e.g., meningitis) which requires prompt referral to an emergency room. As an increasing number of parents choose a chiropractor as their primary health care provider for their children, the challenge of managing the patient with fever will increase in complexity. Co-management (MD and DC) of patients, especially when some uncertainty exits with regard to the diagnosis, is in the best interest of all. In this chapter the authors will discuss the different clinical presentations of a febrile child, causes of fever in children and the possible avenues for case management.

The challenge for the medical physician is to adequately treat children with serious bacterial infections while not overtreating the vast majority of children who have a viral infection (11).

History

Careful attention to the patient's case history and physical examination will provide the most important clues as to the diagnosis as well as the overall toxicity of the child and thus the urgency of the situation (e.g. will an emergency room referral be required?). The doctor should query the onset and duration of the fever, the degree of temperature (if taken by the parent), any medications given (including antipyretics), associated signs and symptoms or behavioral changes, and the presence of any similar patterns in siblings or playmates (8).

The physician should also inquire about the child's past medical history such as recurrent febrile illnesses (8), chronic illness or drug regimens that may compromise the defenses of the host, such as malignancy, sickle cell disease, dysplasia or immunosuppression (8,11). The Rochester criteria (12) are used to identify those infants unlikely to have a serious bacterial infection. In addition to the observation that the infant appears generally well, seven historical criteria are used to identify those infants at low risk:

1. Born at term (at least 37 weeks gestation)
2. Did not receive prenatal antimicrobial therapy
3. Was not treated for unexplained hyperbilirubinemia
4. Had not received and is not receiving antimicrobial agents
5. Had not been previously hospitalized
6. Had no chronic or underlying illness
7. Was not hospitalized longer than mother

The Rochester criteria also includes information derived from the physical and laboratory examinations. Infants at low risk are those that have:

1. No evidence of skin, soft tissue, bone, joint or ear infection
2. Laboratory values:
   a. Peripheral blood WBC count 5.0 to 15.0×10^9 cells/L (5000 to 15,000/mm^3)
   b. Absolute band form count less than or equal to 1.5×10^9 cells/L (less than or equal to 15000/mm^3)
   c. Less than or equal to 10 WBC per high power field ($\times$40) on microscopic examination of a spun urine sediment
   d. Less than or equal to 5 WBC per high power field ($\times$40) on microscopic examination of a stool smear (only for infants with diarrhea)

Questions that should be included in the history include:

1. Foreign travel
2. Animal exposure (e.g., leptospirosis)
3. Drug intake
4. Vaccination history (see Chapters 3 and 7).
5. Skin rashes (onset, pattern, distribution)
6. Any skin changes
7. Magnitude and pattern of temperature
8. Any difficulty in breathing
9. Cough expectoration
10. Seizures (number, duration)
11. Level of consciousness
12. Earache present
13. Any difficulty in swallowing
14. Any bleeding tendency
15. Any pallor changes
16. Any loss of weight or failure to thrive
17. Trauma (e.g., falls, MVA, etc.)
18. Any nasal discharge
19. Swollen gums

20. Diarrhea
21. Constipation
22. Any abdominal cramps
23. Red eye(s), or eye swelling
24. Any blurring of vision
25. Difficulty in micturation
26. Any change in color of urine
27. Cough
28. Headache
29. Neck rigidity and/or pain
30. Food ingestion within the last 48 hours
31. Abnormal gait/crawling
32. Any difficulty in movement
33. Swelling/edema (anywhere on the body, including joints)
34. Pain (e.g., muscle aches, bone pain, pain of any kind)
35. Family history (e.g., diabetes insipidus, familial Mediterranean fever)

Chiropractic Management

Once a chiropractor has been presented with a febrile child, he/she must address two main considerations. First, what is the source of the fever and second, what is the best management approach for the patient.

Clinically, the chiropractic and osteopathic communities have observed the effect of spinal adjustments and its apparent influence on immune system function in a variety of disorders (13-15). The chiropractor is now challenged to determine when correcting the vertebral subluxation and its impact on the immune system is sufficient or when a referral to the pediatrician or emergency physician for further evaluation and treatment is necessary. Referral for evaluation and treatment does not exclude the continuation of chiropractic care where indicated. Provided that no contraindications exist (i.e., joint laxity as in SLE), an adjustment should be administered when signs of subluxation exist regardless of the patient's concurrent disease state. Chiropractic care falls under the rubric of overall supportive care in the case management of most patients with fever.

In deciding upon the appropriate course of management of the acutely febrile child, the following examination procedure is recommended (16,17). After a complete history (see above discussion), the vital signs of the child should be examined, followed by a thorough physical and spinal examination (see Chapters 7 and 9) (Fig. 16.1).

Vitals

TEMPERATURE

For the young infant, the rectal temperature is measured. Place the infant in the prone position and with the infant's buttocks spread, a well-lubricated thermometer is inserted slowly through the anal sphincter to approximately one inch.

PULSE

Determine the pulse by auscultation of the heart. The average heart rate of a newborn ranges from 120–140 beats per minute. Wide fluctuations may occur to as fast as 190 during crying to 90 during sleep.

RESPIRATORY RATE

Both the respiratory rate and respiratory effort should be carefully assessed. The respiratory rate varies between 30 and 50 per minute and should be observed for 1–2 minutes due to periods of apnea and periodic breathing, especially among pre-term infants. Look for grunting respirations and chest retractions, which are signs of respiratory distress.

BLOOD PRESSURE

Blood pressure may be difficult to assess in a child, especially for infants under six months of age. In such cases, the flush method may be used. The arm is elevated while an uninflated cuff is applied. The arm is then "milked" from the fingers to the elbow so that blanching of the skin occurs. The cuff is inflated to just beyond the estimated blood pressure. The arm is then placed by the patient's side and the cuff pressure is allowed to fall slowly. A sudden flush of skin color occurs at a pressure level slightly lower than the true systolic pressure. In this method, the systolic blood pressure of a one day old child is about 50 mm/Hg and by the second week of life, it is 80 mm/Hg. By the end of the first year, it is 95 mm/Hg.

Physical Examination

In the course of the physical examination, the following body systems should be scrutinized for abnormal findings (16). We refer the reader to the chapter on physical diagnosis for a more complete discussion on the subject. Keep in mind that the physical exam findings should be correlated with the signs and symptoms of the various non-infectious and infectious causes of fever as discussed.

EYES, EARS, NOSE, AND THROAT

Conditions with this area that are accompanied by fever may be, for example, teething with an accompanying runny nose and dribbling. Herpes simplex ulcerations on the tongue and mucous membranes, aphthous ulcers, gingivitis, tonsillitis and pharyngitis can also cause a fever. There may be otitis media, cervical adenitis, retropharyngeal abscess, or rheumatic fever.

RESPIRATORY SYSTEM

With respect to this system, one must be aware of respiratory tract infections. In addition to fever, one must observe for the presence of cough and chills, signs of respiratory distress such as flared nostrils, tachypnea, and retraction of the supraclavicular, intercostal and subcostal areas. Upon auscultation, observe for the presence of crackles and wheezes over the affected lobe. Chest radiography should be considered when there is evidence of lung consolidation. The spine is also scrutinized on the AP chest/thoracic radiograph (see Chapter 8).

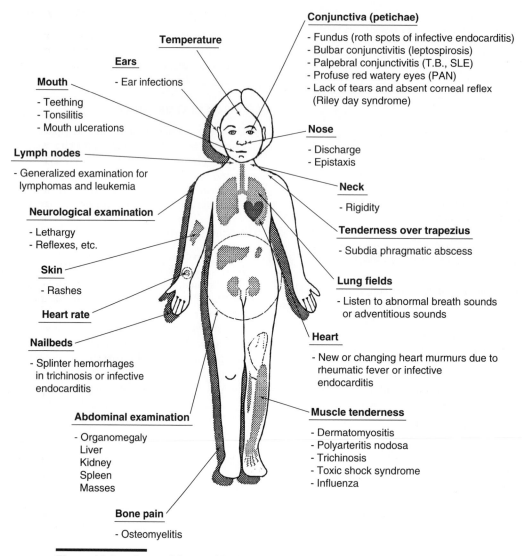

Temperature

Ears
- Ear infections

Mouth
- Teething
- Tonsilitis
- Mouth ulcerations

Lymph nodes
- Generalized examination for lymphomas and leukemia

Neurological examination
- Lethargy
- Reflexes, etc.

Skin
- Rashes

Heart rate

Nailbeds
- Splinter hemorrhages in trichinosis or infective endocarditis

Abdominal examination
- Organomegaly
  Liver
  Kidney
  Spleen
  Masses

Bone pain
- Osteomyelitis

Conjunctiva (petichae)
- Fundus (roth spots of infective endocarditis)
- Bulbar conjunctivitis (leptospirosis)
- Palpebral conjunctivitis (T.B., SLE)
- Profuse red watery eyes (PAN)
- Lack of tears and absent corneal reflex (Riley day syndrome)

Nose
- Discharge
- Epistaxis

Neck
- Rigidity

Tenderness over trapezius
- Subdia phragmatic abscess

Lung fields
- Listen to abnormal breath sounds or adventitious sounds

Heart
- New or changing heart murmurs due to rheumatic fever or infective endocarditis

Muscle tenderness
- Dermatomyositis
- Polyarteritis nodosa
- Trichinosis
- Toxic shock syndrome
- Influenza

Figure 16.1. Some of the possible physical examination findings in the febrile child.

GASTROINTESTINAL SYSTEM

In the case of gastrointestinal involvement there may be, in addition to fever, abdominal cramping, nausea, vomiting and diarrhea. One must discern for food poisoning, acute appendicitis, and peritonitis. In those cases, laboratory tests are helpful.

INTEGUMENTARY SYSTEM

One must be aware of dermatological manifestations that are accompanied by fever. These involve, for example, viral infections resulting in measles, mumps, and chicken pox.

NERVOUS SYSTEM

With respect to this system, one must be aware of certain conditions which require emergency care. These include subdural hematoma due to trauma (see Chapter 2), encephalitis, and meningitis (see Chapter 13). With respect to screening for infants that are at low risk for serious bacterial infection,

we remind the reader to review the characteristics of the toxic child, particularly lethargy. Figure 16.1 depicts an overview of some of the physical examination findings in an acutely febrile child.

The findings from the history and physical examination of the child should assist in determining when/if the patient may need to be referred for additional care. The authors propose the following criteria for referral:

1. The infant is younger than 2 months and the child's temperature exceeds 38° C.

2. The fever persists for several days at 40–40.5° C.

3. There is a positive Kernig's or Brudzinski's sign.

4. The child has febrile seizures that last longer than 15 minutes.

5. There is an acute airway obstruction (e.g., acute epiglottitis, retropharyngeal abscess). There may be stridor,

drooling, retractions, and maintenance of the head and neck in the "sniffing position" (the neck is slightly flexed, and the head is slightly extended on the neck and held quite still).

6. Cardiorespiratory compromise (e.g., severe pneumonia, pericarditis) including dyspnea, cyanosis or pallor, tachypnea, tachycardia and hypotension.

Laboratory and Radiographic Examinations

Most fevers are self-limiting and resolve in a few days requiring very little in terms of sophisticated diagnostic tests or specific therapy. Supportive measures are indicated. In cases of persistent fever it is important to realize that more detailed examinations will be required to arrive at an accurate diagnosis. Laboratory examination can begin with urinalysis and/or culture. Hematology will also need to be considered including a full blood count, erythrocyte sedimentation rate and any cultures. Radiological examination of the chest and/or any area that may have sustained a trauma may be needed. In addition to the general types of examinations described above, specific tests such as a bone marrow biopsy (e.g., leukemia, lymphoma) and the Mantoux test for the detection of tuberculosis may be required for the differential diagnosis.

Medical Management

Medical management of febrile infants and children is commonly based on the 1993 guidelines by Baraff et al. (18). In this study, an expert panel of individuals in pediatrics, infectious diseases or emergency medicine examined the scientific literature to develop guidelines for the care of infants and children from birth to 36 months of age with fever without a known source. For brevity of discussion of the guidelines, the definition of low-risk febrile infants and toxic appearing infants and children must first be presented.

DEFINITION OF LOW-RISK FEBRILE INFANTS

The criteria for low-risk febrile infants includes: previously healthy, absence of a focal bacterial infection upon physical examination and negative results on laboratory screening. Negative laboratory screening is defined as white blood cell (WBC) count of 5,000-15,000 per cubic millimeters, less than 1,500 bands per cubic millimeters, normal urinalysis and if diarrhea is present, less than 5 WBCs/ high power field (hpf) in the stool.

Toxic Appearing Infants and Children

Toxic appearing is defined as a clinical picture consistent with the sepsis syndrome. This is characterized by lethargy, signs of poor perfusion or marked hypoventilation, hyperventilation or cyanosis. Lethargy is further defined as a level of consciousness characterized by poor or absent eye contact or failure of the child to recognize parents or failure to interact with persons or objects in the environment.

Medical Management Options By Age Group

The medical management options for a febrile child are dependent and categorized according to age: infants less than 28 days old, 28 to 90 days old and 3 to 36 months of age.

INFANTS <28 DAYS OLD

There are two management options for infants in this category. All febrile infants should have a sepsis evaluation and be hospitalized for parenteral antibiotics while waiting for the laboratory results. The sepsis evaluation includes cerebrospinal fluid (for cells, glucose and protein), blood (complete blood cell and differential count) and urinalysis.

The second option for low risk infants is hospitalization, sepsis evaluation and careful observation without parenteral antibiotics.

INFANTS 28 TO 90 DAYS OLD

The management of infants in this category are further delineated based on those children that are low-risk or non-low-risk.

LOW-RISK INFANTS

There are two management options for infants in this category; outpatient management with blood and urine cultures and an intramuscular injection of ceftriaxone; or outpatient observation without antibiotic therapy.

NON–LOW-RISK INFANTS

The management option for infants in this category is sepsis evaluation and hospitalization for parenteral antibiotics while waiting for the laboratory results.

CHILDREN 3 TO 36 MONTHS OLD

For previously healthy children in this category, the management options involve the following:

a. Child appears toxic: admit for hospitalization and perform sepsis workup and administer parenteral antibiotics.

b. The child does not appear toxic and does not have a fever greater than or equal to 39° C. Outpatient observation without antibiotic therapy or diagnostic tests. Acetaminophen is recommended at 15 mg/kg per dose every 4 hr for fever. The child is returned to the hospital if the fever persists for longer than 48 hr or the child's clinical condition deteriorates.

c. The child does not appear toxic but has a fever greater than or equal to 39° C. For the child in this category, the following management considerations are recommended. Urinalysis for males <6 months of age and females <2 yr of age. Stool culture for those with blood and mucus in their stool or greater than /equal to 5 WBCs/hpf in the stool. A chest radiograph is recommended if the patient presents with dyspnea, tachypnea, rales, or decreased breath sounds. A blood culture is recommended for all with antibiotic therapy as well as acetaminophen at 15 mg/kg per dose every 4 hr for fever. A follow-up is recommended in 24–48 hours. If the blood culture is positive, admit for sepsis evaluation and parenteral antibiotics. If the urinalysis is positive, the patient is admitted if they are febrile or ill-appearing. If the child is afebrile and well, outpatient management with antibiotics is the treatment recommended.

Parental Considerations

The association of fever with serious illness may lead parents to "fever phobia" (19) and overreaction resulting in mismanagement or unnecessary visits to the doctor. This mismanagement is not without its consequences as indicated by concerns regarding aspirin poisoning (20) and acetaminophen overdosage (21). In addition to management considerations discussed above, the following should be brought to the parents' attention (22):

- While fever may signal the need for a doctor's attention, the fever itself is rarely harmful and is a sign that the child is fighting the disease.

- Place more emphasis on changes in the child's behavior than the thermometer readings.

- Prior to taking the temperature, the mercury thermometer should be shaken to below 35° C.

- Children younger than 5 years of age should have their temperature taken rectally. The thermometer should be well lubricated, inserted into the rectum carefully and approximately 1 inch and placed for 2-3 minutes.

- Children older than 5 years of age should have their temperature taken orally. The thermometer should be placed under the child's tongue with prior instructions to purse the lips around the thermometer, not to bite down and to breathe through the nose.

- If the child's temperature is 38–39° C, the medical recommendation is to give him/her acetaminophen in the recommended dosage, ensure plenty of fluid intake, do not overheat by clothing or blankets and reassess his/her temperature and every 4 hours.

- If the child's temperature is greater than 39° C, the medical treatment recommendation is acetaminophen as above. After one hour, if the fever persists, sit him/her in a tub of lukewarm water and sponge-bath him/her for a half-hour, even if he/she shivers or cries; if the fever persists four hours after giving acetaminophen, continue giving it at 4-hour intervals and continue observing the child.

- The child should be referred to a medical physician if the child has a fever and if any of the following apply:
  a. The child is younger than 3 months.
  b. The child's fever exceeds 38° C for more than 24 hours (and is unresponsive to conservative measures).
  c. The child's face, arms, and legs are twitching.
  d. The child is irritable or drowsy even without medication.
  e. The child complains of belly ache, ear ache, or pain on micturition.
  f. The child is vomiting, suffering from diarrhea, wheezing or has difficult breathing.

Febrile Seizures

The febrile seizure occurs usually between the ages of 6 months and 5 years. The seizure (tonic-clonic response) is preceded by a quick onset of increased body temperature. The fever range is typically between 38° C and 41° C. The seizures may last up to 15 minutes and normally only one seizure occurs. It should be noted that 1–2% of these seizures may go beyond 15 minutes. This duration is extremely dangerous for the child and warrants immediate emergency care. Seizures that go beyond 60 minutes may cause severe brain damage as a result of hypoxia.

Fever of Unknown Origin (FUO)

Fever of unknown origin is defined as a persistent fever of 101° F (38° C) or more for more than three weeks without underlying obvious disorder or etiology after an inpatient evaluation (23). DiNubile (24) notes that another type of FUO, an acute form, which arises more frequently in children. He proposes that this entity be called an acute fever of unknown origin and cautions against using antibiotic therapy in most stable immunocompetent patients.

Case Management

The most optimum treatment strategy for a child presenting with fever of unknown origin remains a controversy. The child who presents with fever may be at risk for a serious bacterial infection and may develop serious complications as meningitis or pneumonia. Therefore, the treatment of a child who presents with fever of unknown origin typically consists of hospitalization, empiric antibiotic treatment and further diagnostic testing (25). However, other clinicians disagree with the above treatment option and elect a more selective "conservative" approach such as outpatient management with or without antibiotics but with close observation (26). The treatment option is dependent on the risk of complications from serious infection traded off against the risks and costs of hospitalization, unnecessary antibiotics and laboratory testing. Certain studies clearly indicate that a strictly defined low-risk group of febrile infants can be cared for at home safely and effectively without the administration of antibiotics, but this form of management should be used only after a complete laboratory evaluation for sepsis and after clinical assessment of the infant by an experienced clinician (27). On the other hand, numerous studies evaluating the role of laboratory tests and clinical judgment in identifying children at risk for serious complications have shown that as many as 23–50% of serious cases are not identified by such methods (18, 28, 29, 30, 31). If risk factors are not present and the fever appears to be viral in origin, extensive diagnostic testing (e.g., hematology) is not needed unless the fever becomes persistent or escalates to an unsafe level.

Although the identification of a specific diagnosis is sometimes difficult, even for the most seasoned clinician, it is important to always attempt to identify those children at risk for a serious bacterial infection (e.g., meningitis). For the treating clinician, the Rochester Criteria as outlined above should be considered. Jaskiewicz et al. (12) performed a prospective study on 1057 eligible infants to test the hypothesis that infants unlikely to have serious bacterial infections can be accurately identified by the low risk criteria of the Rochester Criteria. They found that among well appearing febrile infants, the Rochester Criteria may be applied to determine infants unlikely to have serious bacterial infection. The child should be brought in for emergency care if he is (1) lethargic, has a seizure, or a stiff neck, (2) the child is three months old and has a fever greater than or equal to 38°C or (3) the parent is anxious (32). Infectious causes of fever include those from viral, bacterial, protozoan, or rickettsial sources. These infectious agents are most likely to cause a disease process in the immunocompromised patient. Noninfectious causes of fever include various drugs, trauma (spinal or otherwise), teething, dehydration, heat stroke, poisoning, neoplastic disorders (e.g., lymphomas, leukemia, neuroblastoma, reticulum cell sarcoma, Wilm's tumor), inflammatory disorders (e.g., regional enteritis, ulcerative colitis), endocrine disorders (e.g., hyperthyroidism, virilizing adrenal hyperplasia), infantile cortical hyperostosis (Caffey's disease), allergies, central nervous system fever (i.e., altered thermostat), and collagen vascular disorders (e.g., polyarteritis nodosa, polymyositis, Kawasaki disease, Stevens Johnson syndrome, systemic lupus erthythematosis) (7, 33–36).

Noninfectious Causes of Fever

TRAUMA

Physical trauma can cause a child to develop a fever. There should be a history of trauma. The overlying skin may show bruises or swelling. This may be accompanied by underlying pain or bone fracture. It is important to notify child protection services if child abuse is suspected (see Chapter 2). The physical trauma (e.g., subluxation, fracture) is treated according to the specifics of the case (see Chapter 10).

TEETHING

Normal childhood teething can cause fever. The patient may have swollen and tender gums. There may also be manifestations of gastroenteritis such as vomiting and/or diarrhea. The resistance of the child may be lowered leading to recurrent or persistent viral or bacterial infections. The mother can have difficulty during feeding of the child and anorexia may develop.

DEHYDRATION

Dehydration, due to common factors such as poor fluid intake or exercise, can also result from gastroenteritis. Signs and symptoms of dehydration include fever, loss of skin turgor, thirst, reduced urinary output, soft sunken eyes, fontanelle (if present) depression, prominent skull sutures, increased pulse rate, diminished pulse volume, dry mouth, diminished tearing, lethargy, orthostatic hypotension in older children and cool pale skin. Laboratory findings include elevated hematocrit value, diminished renal functions and electrolyte imbalances (Na+ and K+). Treatment is rehydration therapy with correction of the electrolyte imbalance.

DRUG FEVER

The fever is usually persistent in this syndrome. Essentials for diagnosis include a history of drug intake, which may be accompanied by skin eruptions. Common drugs that can lead to this reaction are aspirin, penicillin and sulfonamides. Reactions to a single injection, e.g., depot penicillin, can last for months. Treatment is through discontinuance of the offending drug. Symptomatic treatments are usually very effective.

REGIONAL ENTERITIS

Regional enteritis is an acute inflammation of the lining of the intestine accompanied by fever, vomiting and diarrhea. Treatment is supportive and includes fluid replacement.

NEOPLASTIC DISORDERS

HODGKIN LYMPHOMA

This disease is more common in older children (i.e., adolescent age). Lymphadenopathy (firm, rubbery, non-tender) often involving the cervical nodes may be present. Hepatomegaly can occur with or without splenomegaly. The fever is intermittent (Pel-Epstein). There may also be night sweats, fatigue, weight loss, and generalized pruritus. Pain is present at the site of the nodes upon ingesting alcohol.

The blood laboratory may reveal anemia, leucocytosis or leucopenia, thrombocytosis, or thrombocytopenia. Eosinophilia may be present. Serum alkaline phosphatase levels, SGPT, SGOT (hepatic involvement) should be checked.

A Gallium scan can show the site of involvement. Lymph node biopsy will establish the diagnosis. Bone marrow biopsy and CT scans may also be used to establish the diagnosis/ prognosis. Laparotomy and splenectomy are often performed. Chest x-ray may show parenchymal or mediastinal nodal disease. Lymphangiography shows "foamy" filling defects in enlarged nodes.

Complications include susceptibility to herpes zoster and fungal infections. Treatment can lead to acute toxicity (e.g., nausea, vomiting, anorexia, alopecia, bone marrow suppression, radiation disease, pneumonitis and an increased incidence of second malignant tumors such as acute myelogenous leukemia, which is a fatal complication.

Due to the splenectomy, there is increased susceptibility to infection especially pneumococcal pneumonia. Medical treatment is combined chemo-radiotherapy according to the stage of Hodgkin lymphoma.

NON-HODGKIN LYMPHOMA

Non-Hodgkin lymphoma afflicts more boys than girls. It is also more common in the lymphoid structures of the intestinal tract, usually in the ileocecal area. Involvement of the central nervous system produces symptoms due to cord compression or increased intracranial tension

Laboratory findings are similar to Hodgkin lymphoma except that the "routine" laparotomy and splenectomy are not done. Lumbar puncture with cytologic examination of the CSF needs to be done on all patients. Medical treatment is with combined chemo-radiotherapy.

CLINICAL STAGING OF HODGKIN LYMPHOMA

Stage I disease is confined to one group of nodes. In stage II disease findings are present in more than one group of nodes but is limited to one side of the diaphragm. Stage III disease involves nodes on both sides of the diaphragm with splenomegaly. In stage IV there is hematogenous spread to the liver, bone marrow, lungs, etc.

LEUKEMIA

Symptoms and Signs. Acute lymphoblastic leukemia is the most common form of leukemia. Other types include acute non lymphoblastic leukemia and chronic myelocytic leukemia.

There is an increased incidence in children with Down's Syndrome or in rare familial diseases as ataxia telangiectasia, Bloom's syndrome, Fanconi's anemia, Kleinfelter's Syndrome and neurofibromatosis. The Epstein Barr virus is implicated in Burkitt's leukemia, lymphoma. In the early stages of leukemia, fever may be present. Other symptoms include headache, pallor, fatigue, irritability and palpitation. Anemia is present. The patient easily bruises and epistaxis or gum bleeding may be present. Increased susceptibility to infections may develop leading to toxemia and septicemia. Bone and sternal tenderness and nuchal rigidity are musculoskeletal signs in later stages. Blurring of vision from increased intracranial tension can develop.

Laboratory findings include anemia (normochromic, normocytic), thrombocytopenia, and leucocytosis with neutropenia or even leucopenia. Lymphocytosis may be present with or without blast cells in the peripheral blood. Bone marrow biopsy will show the replacement of the normal marrow with malignant cells.

Metabolic abnormalities include hyperuricemia, renal failure and increased lactic acid dehydrogenase (LDH).

The chest x-ray is used to evaluate for a mediastinal mass or hilar adenopathy and for pulmonary infiltrations suggestive of infection. Ultrasound may be used to assess splenomegaly or renal enlargement suggestive of leukemic infiltration.

Patient Management. The optimal medical drug therapy is not yet known and still investigational. Most often chemotherapy and radiotherapy are combined. Bone marrow transplantation is the treatment of choice.

NEUROBLASTOMA

Neuroblastomas are of neural crest origin and may arise anywhere along the sympathetic ganglion chain or in the adrenal medulla. It is the most common tumor in children less than one year of age in the United States.

Symptoms and Signs. Fifty percent of patients present with manifestations of metastasis. Any of the following may be present: abdominal mass, weight loss, anemia, failure to thrive, abdominal pain and distention, fever, bone ache, diarrhea, hypertension in 25% of cases, Horner's syndrome (ptosis, meiosis, enophthalmos, heterochromia of iris), orbital ecchymosis, dysphagia, paraplegia, cauda equina syndrome, flushing, sweating irritability and cerebellar ataxia.

CT scan or MRI of the chest, neck, abdomen or pelvis (depending on location of the tumor) is required for diagnosis. Laboratory findings may show anemia and thrombocytopenia. Chest x-ray, bone marrow aspiration, and renal function tests are additional diagnostic tools.

The staging of neuroblastoma presented is that of Evans:

I. Confined to single organ, completely resected
II. Extends beyond organ of origin but does not cross midline
III. Extends across midline
IV. Distant metastasis
V. Infants under one year with metastasis to liver, skin or bone marrow sparing cortical bone.

Patient Management. Treatment is according to the stage of the disease and can be in the form of surgical resection, chemotherapy, radiotherapy and bone marrow transplantation.

WILM'S TUMOR

Wilm's tumor is an embryonal renal neoplasm containing blastoma, stromal or epithelial cell types usually affecting children under five years of age.

Symptoms and Signs. Most patients are asymptomatic. If symptoms develop, they take the form of fever and abdominal pain. There may be a palpable upper abdominal mass. Other signs include cardiac murmurs, hepatosplenomegaly, ascites, prominent abdominal wall veins, varicocele, gonadal metastasis, and rarely signs of an acute abdomen with free intraperitoneal rupture.

In addition to anemia (low CBC), urine analysis may reveal hematuria. The chest x-ray and abdominal scout views may reveal calcifications. Additional imaging includes the CT scan and contrast studies of the chest and abdomen. Biopsy is also used.

Patient Management. Treatment usually is with chemotherapy and radiotherapy. Other supportive measures are recommended.

CAFFEY'S SYNDROME (INFANTILE CORTICAL HYPEROSTOSIS)

This is a benign disease of unknown cause occurring before 6 months of age. Fever is a symptom. Non-suppurative, tender, painful, swellings that can involve any bone in the body and are frequently widespread develop. The mandible and clavicle are affected in 50% of cases. The ulna, humerus and ribs may be affected as well. The disease is limited to the shafts of bones and does not involve subcutaneous tissues or joints. It is self limiting but may persist for weeks or months. Laboratory findings include anemia, leukocytosis, and high ESR and serum alkaline phosphatase. Radiographs show the lesions.

POLYARTERITIS NODOSA

Polyarteritis nodosa is a collagen-vascular disorder. A vasculitis of medium sized arteries with fibrinoid degeneration in the media extending to the intima and adventitia leads to aneurysmal dilation of the vessels and thrombus formation with organ infarctions in addition to fibrosis of the vessels. There is no known cause but immunological involvement is suspected.

SYMPTOMS AND SIGNS

The clinical picture includes fever, weakness, weight loss, malaise, myalgia, livido reticularis, headache, and abdominal pain. The following may be present in multisystem involvement; musculoskeletal: myalgia, migratory arthralgia and arthritis; skin: purpura, urticaria, subcutaneous hemorrhages, polymorphic rashes, subcutaneous nodules, Raynaud phenomena; gastrointestinal: recurrent and severe pain, hepatomegaly nausea, vomiting and bleeding; lung: hilar adenopathy, patchy infiltrates, reticular or nodular lesions, often fleeting; renal: hypertension, hematuria, proteinuria, progressive renal failure; CNS: seizures, confusion, headaches; peripheral nervous system: monomuritis multiplex; cardiac: pericarditis, congestive heart failure associated with hypertension and/or myocardial infarction; and genitourinary: usually asymptomatic but may have testicular, epididymal, ovarian pain.

A CBC may reveal neutrophilia, eosinophilia (rare), and anemia. Elevated ESR, hypergammaglobulinemia may be present. Biopsy of involved vessels can be made (very specific test).

PATIENT MANAGEMENT

Treatment is supportive. The patient should decrease salt in the diet if the condition is associated by hypertension. Medical interventions include prednisone and cyclophosphamide. Plasmapheresis may also be added.

DERMATOMYOSITIS (POLYMYOSITIS)

This is a systemic connective tissue disease characterized by inflammatory and degenerative changes in muscles sometimes accompanied by a characteristic skin rash. It is of unknown etiology. Cell mediated autoimmunity viruses may be a possible participating factor.

SYMPTOMS AND SIGNS

The clinical picture includes difficulty when arising from sitting or lying positions, difficulty kneeling, difficulty climbing stairs, difficulty raising arms, joint pain/swelling, dysphagia, buttock pain, respiratory impairment, symmetrical proximal muscle weakness, decreased deep tendon reflexes, muscle swelling, stiffness and, induration, rash over the face (eyelids, nasolabial folds), upper chest and dorsal hands, and periorbital edema.

Laboratory findings may show increased creatinine phosphokinase (CPK), increased aldolase, increased SGOT, increased LDH, myoglobinuria, increased ESR, positive rheumatoid factor (less than 50% of patients), leukocytosis, anemia, hyperglobulinemia and increased creatinine.

PATIENT MANAGEMENT

Supportive measures (e.g. nutrition, psychological counseling, chiropractic care, etc.) should be instituted. Medical treatment is with prednisone or azathioprine or methotrexate.

KAWASAKI'S DISEASE (MUCOCUTANEOUS LYMPH NODE SYNDROME)

The clinical features of this disease are erythema of the conjunctivae and mucous membranes, a maculopapular rash with subsequent desquamation, and dominant lymphadenopathy of the anterior cervical chain. Fever may be present as well. Bilateral conjunctival injection, truncal rashes, palmar erythema, and non-pitting edema of the hands and feet may be present. There is firm skin overlying the lesion and desquamation takes place 2-3 weeks after the onset of the disease beginning in the extremities and progressing centrally. There may an injected pharynx, dry fissured lips and a strawberry tongue.

SYMPTOMS AND SIGNS

The following are relatively common findings: cervical lymphadenopathy, pneumonia, diarrhea, arthralgia, arthritis, photophobia, tympanitis, meatitis, meningitis and carditis. Less common features may include severe abdominal pain, hydropic gall bladder, cardiac tamponade, congestive heart failure, pericarditis, myocarditis, coronary artery thrombosis, aneurysm of the cardiovascular system, febrile convulsions, pleural effusions, tonsilar exudate, encephalopathy, jaundice and renal abnormalities.

Leucocytosis, anemia (mild), thrombocytosis and an increased ESR may be present. Urinalysis may reveal phoria or proteinuria. The CSF may reveal an increase in the number of cells. There may either be normal or elevated serum immunoglobulin and complement levels. Liver involvement is indicated by elevated transaminase activity. The electrocardiogram may show changes.

PATIENT MANAGEMENT

No scientifically proven treatment has been established. In addition to supportive measures, symptomatic treatment to improve the clinical features, e.g., aspirin for fever, or treatment of underlying congestive heart failure may be needed.

STEVENS JOHNSON SYNDROME

Stevens Johnson syndrome is characterized by conjunctivitis, stomatitis and balanitis. The skin lesions vary from small papules to extensive bullae. The oral cavity is involved in 50%

of cases. The lips are often covered with hemorrhagic exudate. Erythematous plaques on the mucosa may develop into vesicles or bullae that subsequently rupture forming shallow erosions covered by a pseudomembrane. These lesions may become infected secondarily. The etiology is unknown but may be secondary to a drug reaction or follow upper respiratory tract infection.

Treatment of mild illness is with local mouth wash and antihistamines. In severe illness systemic corticosteroids are often used.

SYSTEMIC LUPUS ERYTHEMATOSUS (SLE)

The following symptoms and signs can occur in SLE: fever, arthritis, myalgias, skin lesions, malar (butterfly) rash, oral ulcers, anorexia, malaise, eye pain and/or redness, chest pain and/or shortness of breath, pallor, nausea, vomiting, diarrhea, muscle tenderness, aching and stiffness, headaches and visual problems, and psychosis/delirium.

Laboratory tests show a positive antinuclear antibody (ANA) and/or an anti-double standard DNA (dsDNA), and/or Anti-Sm, and/or false positive VDRL, and/or positive LE preparation. These tests have either a high sensitivity (ANA, false positive VDRL) or specificity (anti dsDNA, anti Sm and LE preparation) and are included as American Rheumatology Association (ARA) criteria for the diagnosis of SLE along with the clinical features. Other laboratory findings and positive tests may include an increased ESR, anemia, leukopenia, lymphopenia, abnormal urinary sediment, proteinuria, increased prothrombin time, hypoalbuminuria, positive anti cardiolipin, thrombocytopenia, increased serum creatinine, positive coombs test, complement levels (Cryoglobulins, Raji cell test, Clq precipitins), coagulation studies (lupus anticoagulant), biopsy of skin, kidney and peripheral nerves, cerebral angiography, chest x-ray, MRI, and an echocardiogram.

Adjustments or manipulation is contraindicated at joints exhibiting signs of laxity/hypermobility. Medical treatment consists of steroidal treatment for skin lesions; minor arthritis is treated with NSAIDS and severe disease with immunosuppressants.

Infectious Causes of Fever

Infectious causes of fever include influenza, mumps, measles and other viral agents and bacterial organisms (33–36).

INFLUENZA

Influenza is caused by a virus droplet infection in a susceptible host.

SYMPTOMS AND SIGNS

An abrupt onset of high fever may be accompanied by toxic appearing manifestations. This upper respiratory tract illness is in the form of a runny nose, cough and difficulty in breathing. In infants it may be associated with the croup syndrome.

Pharyngeal or nasal secretion can be examined with fluorescent labeled antibody for rapid identification of influenza virus. Serum antibody obtained early and late in the course of infection can be of value in retrospective diagnosis. Radiographic findings reveal extensive bronchial pneumonia or simply hyperaeration.

REYE'S SYNDROME AND OTHER COMPLICATIONS

Reye's syndrome is an encephalopathy with fatty degeneration of the viscera that occurs in children receiving aspirin (salicylates) during acute influenza infections. Clinically it can be suspected when an upper respiratory tract infection is followed by excessive vomiting and convulsions; later on it may be further complicated by liver dysfunction and hypoglycemia. It is absolutely contraindicated in all children (including adolescents) to ingest aspirin during an influenza infection.

Influenza may progress in rare cases (susceptible individuals) to pneumonia, croup, cardiac arrest, emphysema, pneumothorax and Reye's syndrome.

PATIENT MANAGEMENT

Supportive measures include proper hydration, nutrition and rest. Supplements that support immune function include vitamins A, C, E, and zinc. Chiropractic care is indicated at sites of subluxation. Certain herbs (e.g., echinacea) may be helpful.

Medical referral is required in severe cases where the airway needs to be supported. Tracheotomy may be needed. If respiratory or cardiovascular complications develop, these are treated medically.

PARAINFLUENZA VIRAL INFECTION

The etiology of parainfluenza (type 30 viral infection) is also by droplet infection but is more common in infants one year of age (33–36). The symptoms and signs are similar to that of regular influenza but is more commonly associated with croup and hoarseness of the voice. Patient management is the same as in viral influenza infections.

MUMPS

The etiology of mumps is infection by the mumps virus in a susceptible individual. Thirty to forty percent of those infected have no symptoms (33–36). The incubation period is two to three weeks and symptomatic individuals develop a mild upper respiratory tract illness prior to the onset of parotitis. Infection can also take the form of orchitis or oophoritis, meningoencephalitis, and pancreatitis. Other glands that can become infected include the thyroid (thyroiditis) and the mammary and Bartholin's glands.

PAROTITIS

A high fever and headache may accompany the infection. Other symptoms and signs include a bilateral or unilateral painful swelling of the parotid gland. Lymphedema of the face may occur and makes the parotid swelling indistinct. Obliteration of the angle of the mandible may be present or upward and lateral displacement of the earlobe. There may be a reddened and pointed opening of Stensen's duct. The lateral and anterior aspects of the neck may be swollen due to the involvement of submaxillary and sublingual salivary glands.

MENINGOENCEPHALITIS

The mumps virus is the most common cause of aseptic meningitis in children. Aseptic meningitis may occur with or without parotitis. Clinically it is characterized by fever, headache, nuchal rigidity and gastrointestinal symptoms (e.g., nausea and vomiting). Central nervous system irritability and convulsions are uncommon. Recovery is usually spontaneous within three to ten days usually without complications.

Very rarely the complications can be in the form of deafness, post infectious encephalitis syndrome, myelitis, facial neuritis and myocarditis.

PANCREATITIS

A high fever, chills and prostration is accompanied by moderate abdominal pain, nausea, and persistent vomiting in this form of mumps infection. This disease could be complicated by diabetes mellitus in some children.

ORCHITIS OR OOPHORITIS

These forms are more often seen in post pubertal individuals. There is usually a sudden onset of fever, chills and systemic manifestations. Males will have testicular pain and swelling. Females will complain of low abdominal pain and tenderness. The symptoms usually subside in 3–14 days. Sterility is very uncommon because the infection in the majority of cases is unilateral.

OTHER GLANDULAR INVOLVEMENT

Thyroiditis, inflammation of the mammary gland and Bartholin's gland can also occur rarely. Other complications can include nephritis (rare), unilateral nerve deafness, optic neuritis, dacryoadenitis, uveokeratitis, scleritis, central retinal vein thrombosis, arthritis and post mumps thrombophlebitis.

LABORATORY

An elevated serum amylase level is present in 75% of cases during the acute attack. Normal levels are achieved again after two to three weeks. The cerebrospinal fluid may show pleocytosis with lymphocytosis (often 500–1000 cells/uL) and is associated with elevated levels of proteins in the CSF and normal levels of glucose.

The mumps virus can be isolated from the following body secretions: saliva, urine or the cerebrospinal fluid.

A four-fold rise in serum antibody titer is diagnostic. Serum should be collected as early as possible in the clinical course and again in two weeks.

PATIENT MANAGEMENT

Mumps is usually a self-limited infection, recovery is spontaneous and complete immunity is life long. Supportive measures include adequate rest, a nutritious diet and chiropractic care where indicated.

MEASLES (RUBEOLA)

Measles is a highly contagious disease usually affecting susceptible preschool children. The infection is airborne (droplet infection) and the incubation period is 9–14 days (33–36).

SYMPTOMS AND SIGNS

The prodromal period is manifested clinically by fever, conjunctivitis, photophobia, coryza and cough. Koplik's spots, small white specks on a red base on buccal mucosa appear one or two days before the rash and are pathognomonic of measles. In some cases the spots may be absent. Occasionally Koplik's spots can be seen on the nasal mucosa also.

The rash begins near the hairline as faint macules and papules which rapidly progress to involve the face, trunk and arms. When the rash appears on the lower extremities it begins to fade on the face and then gradually disappears over the period of three to six days. The lesions begin as discrete macules and papules that gradually coalesce involving larger areas of the skin. Fine desquamation may accompany healing.

The coryzal symptoms reach their peak during the first four to five days and persist throughout the illness. The cough is more at night and is barking and harsh.

The look of a child suffering from measles is in the form of a red-eyed patient with puffy eye lids and a swollen nasal bridge, a distressed apathetic look, copious nasal secretions and violent harsh cough. The illness lasts for 9–10 days.

The laboratory will show leucopenia (1500–3000/uL) and lymphocytosis. If bacterial superinfection occurs, abrupt leukocytosis may be evident. A four-fold rise in serum antibody can be demonstrated in paired sera.

Radiographic findings may show patchy pneumonic infiltrates or the typical hilar pneumonia pattern. Overinflation of the lungs may occur as well. In the presence of bacterial pneumonia, the x-ray reveals lobar or lobular consolidation.

PATIENT MANAGEMENT

Measles is generally a self-limited disease lasting for 7–10 days. However, complications include upper and lower respiratory tract secondary bacterial infections, occurring in 5–15% of cases (e.g. otitis media, pneumonia, sinusitis, mastoiditis, cervical adenitis and tonsillopharyngitis). CNS complications may take the form of encephalitis occurring in 1:1000 during the acute attack or subacute sclerosing panencephalitis, a rare degenerative disease occurring years after infection. Multiple sclerosis and Jakob-Creutzfeldt disease occurs also in a latent period due to slow measles viral infections. Hemorrhagic measles, with bleeding in gastrointestinal tract, mucous membranes and CNS accompanied by fever and toxicity, is a fulminant type of measles and can occur.

Other complications include thrombocytopenia, diarrhea, acute appendicitis, and vomiting. These are rare in the United States. Conjunctivitis, corneal ulcers, optic nerve damage are also rare complications. Myocarditis and cardiac failure can occur but are also rare. Nephrosis, asthma and eczema may exacerbate during measles infection. Measles can also exacerbate tuberculosis. Measles during pregnancy may result in stillbirth, abortion or premature delivery.

In addition to supportive measures cited previously, there may need to be maintenance of clear nasal passages. Reduction of fever may be required in some cases. If secondary bacterial complications develop, they should be specifically diagnosed and treated where indicated.

RESPIRATORY SYNCYTIAL VIRUS (RSV) DISEASE

Respiratory syncytial virus (RSV) disease is caused by droplet infection in a susceptible host. It is spread by hand contact between hospitalized infants and hospital staff and leads to nosocomial infections with RSV (33–36).

SYMPTOMS AND SIGNS

Fever is very common. There may be a history of upper respiratory tract illness which progressed to lower respiratory tract disease. Non specific symptoms include rhinitis, nasal stuffiness and bronchitis.

Bronchiolitis is caused by RSV in 70% of cases. Dyspnea and severe respiratory distress is associated with nasal and pharyngeal secretions. Fine rales and marked expiratory wheezes are heard by auscultating the chest. There is usually a high fever. Overworking of the accessory muscles of respiration and severe respiratory effort is usually quite evident.

Bronchial pneumonia from RSV infection is associated with dyspnea and tachypnea. Rales may or may not be present. A small proportion of sudden infant deaths may be due to overwhelming RSV infection, especially in very young infants.

Fluorescent antibody identification of RSV can be made in nasal or pharyngeal secretions. A four-fold antibody rise is seen in paired sera. Radiographic findings may reveal generalized hyperaeration and the level of the diaphragm may be depressed. Diminished respiratory excursion is seen on fluoroscopy.

PATIENT MANAGEMENT

In addition to supportive measures (proper hydration, nutrition, etc.), bronchiolitis may require maintenance of an airway and oxygenation, which may save the child's life.

Ribavirin is an antiviral agent prescribed in severe conditions and is particularly useful in treating children with underlying diseases in whom RSV infection could cause serious morbidity or death. The dose is 6 g in 300 ml of water delivered by a special aerosol apparatus for 12–18 hours each day, usually for 3–8 days.

HERPANGINA

Herpangina (coxsackie A virus types 2,6,8 & 10 infection) tends to occur in epidemics during the summer in temperate climates. The spread is enhanced by over crowding and poor hygiene. The incubation period is two to ten days (33–36).

SYMPTOMS AND SIGNS

The clinical manifestations include fever (prominent particularly in the young), dysphagia, anorexia, and vomiting. Tiny vesicles which rapidly ulcerate on the anterior fauces and elsewhere in the posterior pharynx can occur. The ulcers are often arranged linearly on the anterior fauces (diagnostic).

Convulsions are common early in the course of fever. Parotitis or vaginal ulcerations may occur but recovery is usually complete. If needed, the virus can be isolated from a throat swab or stool specimens.

PATIENT MANAGEMENT

The disease is self-limiting within 2–6 weeks. Only symptomatic/supportive therapy is required.

PARALYTIC POLIOMYELITIS

Paralytic poliomyelitis occurs in susceptible individuals by droplet infection from a case or a carrier through a fecal-oral route. The incubation period is 7–10 days (33–36).

SYMPTOMS AND SIGNS

Fever is accompanied by headache, lassitude, nausea, vomiting, neck rigidity, and stiffness of the back.

There are variable degrees of CNS depression or excitability, followed by pain and tenderness of the affected muscles. Acute lower motor neuron paralysis can occur which is purely motor with no sensory changes. It is asymmetrical with a spotty distribution.

Involvement of the spinal cord segments and the brain stem may lead to respiratory muscle paralysis and cranial nerve involvement with palatal facial and laryngeal paralysis. Severe involvement may lead to irregular respirations, apnea, and peripheral vascular collapse.

Further complications include respiratory arrest, hypertension, static pneumonia, decubitus ulcers, renal calculi, and disuse atrophy of the affected muscles.

The polio virus may be persistent in the stools for 6–8 weeks after the primary infection so it can be isolated from the stools during this period. Isolation of the virus can also be made from the throat. There may be an increased titer of serum antibody. CSF findings are those of aseptic meningitis, with early mild pleocytosis with poly-morpho nuclear leucocytosis. Later, lymphocytosis will be evident. There may be a raised protein concentration during the paralytic stage in the second or third week of illness.

PATIENT MANAGEMENT

Complete bed rest is essential. Chiropractic care is provided where indicated. Heat packs (the Kenny method) reduces spasm and tenderness and helps early rehabilitation.

An endotracheal or transtracheal tube may be required to maintain a clear airway. Use of oxygen, assisted ventilation and a humid respirator may also be necessary.

PLEURODYNIA

Pleurodynia, also known as epidemic myalgia and Bomholm disease, is caused by a Coxsackie B viral infection in a susceptible host.

SYMPTOMS AND SIGNS

In addition to headache, other prodromal symptoms include malaise, anorexia, headache and muscle aches. Severe unilateral chest pain may be present that frequently is paroxysmal and pleuritic and therefore is aggravated by movement. The pain is severe and the patient usually describes it as being a crushing pain. Abdominal pain, hiccups, vomiting, diarrhea and a stiff neck can also occur. Physical examination may reveal limitation of respiratory excursions, muscle tenderness, normal breath sounds and ipsilateral pleural friction rub in about 25% of cases. Mild to moderate nuchal rigidity may be present. The illness may last as long as a week, but light variable complications are uncommon and include aseptic meningitis, orchitis, pericarditis and pneumonia. The virus can be isolated from the stools or with a throat swab.

PATIENT MANAGEMENT

Supportive measures include splinting of the chest, analgesics, rest, proper nutrition/hydration, chiropractic care, etc.

GENERALIZED NEONATAL INFECTION

The etiology for this common viral infection is by the Coxsackie B3 and B4 viruses invading a susceptible host. It is more common in sick infants who are in nurseries or recently discharged and is also more common if the mother has a history of an upper respiratory tract infection prior to delivery (33–36).

SYMPTOMS AND SIGNS

The clinical picture includes a sudden onset of fever. Symptoms of gastro-intestinal disturbance occur 1-2 days preceding the major illness. Manifestations of acute heart failure develop; cyanosis, tachycardia and increasing size of liver and heart are all observed. Pneumonia can occur in addition with clinical manifestations of cough, dyspnea and vomiting. The condition may progress rapidly to death in about 50% of cases.

The ECG may reveal myocardial damage. Cardiomegaly may be evident on a chest x-ray. The virus can be isolated from feces in very severe conditions. Serologic confirmation is possible in surviving infants.

PATIENT MANAGEMENT

The complications include encephalitis, pancreatitis, focal hepatitis and myositis. Lines of management include intensive supporting measures: oxygenation support of ventilation and circulation and treatment of heart failure.

ISOLATED MYOCARDITIS AND PANCARDITIS

The etiology is infection by the Coxsackie B virus in a susceptible host.

SYMPTOMS AND SIGNS

The clinical picture varies from very mild to fulminant cases and simulates all other cases of myocarditis and pericarditis. The virus can be isolated from stools and pericardial fluid (33–36).

PATIENT MANAGEMENT

Case management is similar to that of generalized neonatal infections (see above) but if there are manifestations of pericardial effusion, the fluid should be aspirated.

ACUTE LYMPHONODULAR PHARYNGITIS

Acute lymphonodular pharyngitis caused by an infection of the Coxcakie A virus (Type 10) in a susceptible host.

SYMPTOMS AND SIGNS

The clinical picture shows a papular, white or light yellow lesions of the uvula, anterior pillars and pharynx. A sore throat is accompanied by headache and fever. The illness lasts from 1–2 weeks. There are no vesicles.

PATIENT MANAGEMENT

Complications are uncommon. Symptomatic treatment and general immune supportive measures (proper rest, nutrition, chiropractic care) are options.

VESICULAR EXANTHEM

Vesicular exanthem, otherwise known as hand, foot, mouth disease is caused by an infection of the Coxsackie A Virus (Types 5, 10,16) in a susceptible individual.

SYMPTOMS AND SIGNS

Vesicular Exanthem involves the oral mucosa, tongue, interdigital and digital surfaces of both upper and lower extremities. Non-vesicular forms may occur. Diagnosis can be made by virologic isolation and serology (33–36).

PATIENT MANAGEMENT

Treatment is symptomatic and supportive (see above).

HERPES SIMPLEX

Herpes simplex Type I viral infection leads to lesions in the oral cavity, central nervous system and skin, while herpes simplex Type II leads to genital lesions and most cases of congenital herpes viral infections (33–36).

HERPETIC GINGIVOSTOMATITIS

The clinical picture is that of fever, irritability, pain in the mouth and throat, dysphagia, lassitude, and disinterest in surroundings.

Shallow, yellow ulcers of the buccal mucosa occur, mainly in the gingival, tonsillar and pharyngeal mucosae and are frequently accompanied by crusting of the lips. A half open mouth with drooling and foul breath odor are present. Palpation reveals cervical lymphadenopathy. The disease typically lasts 7–14 days.

HERPETIC VULVOVAGINITIS OR URETHRITIS

Similar ulcerations as in cases of gingivostomatis occur in the vulva and vagina. They are accompanied by painful micturation and inguinal lymphadenopathy.

RECURRENT HERPETIC LESIONS

Sensory manifestations of the symptomatic infection vary from vague discomfort to neurologic pain. Erythematous papules on the mucocutaneous junction of the lips can occur. Vesicles, pustules and crusting can occur on top of papules. Regional lymphadenopathy and lymphadenitis may occur and the lesions tend to occur in groups.

HERPETIC KERATOCONJUCTIVITIS

Acute herpetic corneal infection is usually accompanied by conjunctival inflammation. Cloudiness and corneal ulcerations may accompany the condition. Stromal edema, hypopyon or rupture of the globe can complicate the condition leading to blindness.

HERPETIC ENCEPHALITIS

Herpetic encephalitis may be in the form of aseptic meningitis, cranial nerve pulsics and cortical symptoms. The condition can be further complicated by coma or convulsions and death occurring in the second to third week of the illness.

NEONATAL HERPETIC INFECTION

Neonatal herpetic infections should be suspected if there is a history of recent herpes virus infection in either parent before delivery. The illness may be present at birth or it may appear during the first week of life with generalized vesiculation of the skin and either a high or low temperature. Jaundice, hepatosplenomegaly, dyspnea, heart failure, hemorrhage, and CNS manifestations can all occur. Death can occur following 2 to 4 days of illness. Mild neonatal infections are not associated with CNS involvement. A congenital anomaly syndrome is associated with early intrauterine infection, (e.g. microcephaly, mental retardation, intracranial calcification, microphthahnia, retinal dysplasia, chorioretinitis).

ECZEMA HERPETICUM

Kaposi varicelliform eruption (eczema herpeticum) can be accompanied by fever, prostration, vesicular lesions and eczema. It is frequently fulminant and fatal especially when large areas of the skin are involved.

The cerebrospinal fluid will reveal pleocytosis. The virus can be recovered from vesicular lesions, skin and corneal scrapings, throat swabs, blood, and cerebrospinal fluid. A four-fold or greater rise in serum antibody is detectable from patients with primary infections.

Lines of management for corneal infections include topical agents; 1% trifuluidin or 3% acyclovir or 3% vidarabine or 0.1% idoxuridine.

HERPETIC LESIONS IN SKIN OR MUCOSA

Oral acyclovir is used. Topical antiviral agents can be used except for topical acyclovir which is not effective.

ENCEPHALITIS

Systemic acyclovir (drug of choice) or vidarabine can be used to treat the infection. General measures include the maintenance of fluid intake, topical anesthetics for painful lesions, analgesics and Vitamin B_{12} injections.

VARICELLA (CHICKEN POX) AND HERPES ZOSTER (SHINGLES)

The diseases are transmitted from person to person and are caused by the varicella virus. Chicken pox is highly contagious. On the other hand, herpes zoster is sporadic and less infectious. The incubation period is 10–20 days. The illness is usually preceded by manifestations simulating the common cold with rhinitis for 1–3 days before the eruptions occur.

Chicken pox has an abrupt onset. A rash that appears in crops with faint erythematous macules, rapidly develops into papules and vesicles. The vesicles are thin walled and superficial on the skin (dewdrop on a red base). The rash is heaviest on the trunk and spreads to the extremities. Lesions in all stages can be seen at one time without bacterial infections. The crusts fall off in one to three weeks leaving no scars. Hemorrhagic lesions occur and are associated with thrombocytopenia particularly in children with leukemia. Bullous and gangrenous forms occur in very severe conditions. Systemic manifestations are usually absent or mild. Shallow mucosal ulceration may also be present which, if involving the posterior pharynx or esophagus, will cause difficult and painful swallowing.

Herpes zoster occurs in older age groups. It is usually unilateral and limited to one or more adjacent dermatomes. Common sites are the thoracic and lumbar spine, cervical roots, and the ophthalmic division of the trigeminal nerve. Maculopapules appear in closed patches, rapidly vesicular and they frequently coalesce. They follow the dermal distribution of the nerve root and often end abruptly at the mid line of the body. Concomitant or preceding pain may be very severe. The disease is uncommon in children as are complications. Complications can include secondary bacterial infections, abscesses, lymphangitis, septicemia, osteomyelitis, pneumonia (very rare), hepatitis, fatal hypoglycemia, optic neuritis, orchitis and transverse myelitis. Complications are more common in newborns and/or immunosuppressed children due to malignancies or the intake of medications.

Laboratory tests may show leucocytosis neutrophilia. Vesicular scrapings will reveal inclusion bodies of the eosinophilic intranuclear type (cowdry type A). The chest x-ray may reveal diffuse nodular pneumonia and emphysema in varicella pneumonia.

PATIENT MANAGEMENT

Symptomatic treatment includes maintaining fluid intake, control of itching, antipyretics where indicated (avoid high doses of aspirin) and the treatment of complications.

MURRAY VALLEY ENCEPHALITIS

This is also called Australian X disease or encephalitis. It is a severe encephalitis with a high mortality rate. It occurs in the Murray Valley of Australia. The disease is the most severe in children and is characterized by fever, headache, malaise, drowsiness or convulsions, and nuchal rigidity. Extensive brain damage is the most severe complication. The virus is of the genus Flavivirus (37).

DENGUE

Dengue is caused by group B arboviruses which are transmitted between an arthropod (e.g., tick) and non-human vertebrates (33–36). Humans are affected as a secondary host. The disease is more common in preschool children or during early school years.

SYMPTOMS AND SIGNS

There may be a sudden onset of fever, severe headache and/or retro-ocular pain. There is also severe pain in the extremities and back (thus it is known as the break bone fever). Examination may show lymphadenopathy and a maculopapular or petechial hemorrhagic rash. The course of the disease shows period of remissions and exacerbations. CNS symptoms and pneumonic symptoms may be present. Shock and peripheral vascular collapse may lead to death in the first week of illness.

Laboratory diagnosis shows leucopenia, thrombocytopenia, a prolonged bleeding time, and maturation arrest of mega karyocytes. The virus may be isolated from the blood.

PATIENT MANAGEMENT

Supportive measures for shock may be needed. Blood replacement of severe hemorrhage and in very severe cases corticosteroids are indicated. Antipyretics and analgesics are used in uncomplicated cases.

YELLOW FEVER

Yellow fever is caused by an infection of the arbovirus (33–36). The mode of infection is similar to dengue fever. The incubation period is between 3 and 7 days.

SYMPTOMS AND SIGNS

The clinical manifestations follow three phases. In the first, there is an abrupt onset of fever, headache, lassitude, nausea and vomiting, and muscle aches. The second phase is a short period of remission. The final phase is severely toxic. A high fever, bradycardia (Faget's sign), severe jaundice, and gastrointestinal hemorrhage progress to shock and death. It may also be fulminant without a remission period. The disease can be abortive with mild clinical manifestations.

Laboratory diagnosis shows leucopenia, proteinuria, azotemia, hyperbilirubinaemia, and elevated BUN. Liver function tests may show abnormalities. The virus can be isolated from the blood.

PATIENT MANAGEMENT

Symptomatic and supportive treatment includes fluid and blood replacement, antipyretics and support of peripheral circulation.

RUBELLA (GERMAN OR 3-DAY MEASLES)

This infection is from the rubivirus through a droplet infection from a patient infected by the virus. The incubation period is 14-20 days (33–36).

SYMPTOMS AND SIGNS

The clinical manifestations may be mild, varying from asymptomatic to only associated with lymphadenopathy. In adolescents the prodroma may be associated with mild respiratory constitutional symptoms and lymphadenopathy. In children these prodromal manifestations are absent.

Suboccipital and post-auricular lymphadenopathy typically precedes the rash. The rash appears about the face as a pinkish, discrete macular eruption and rapidly spreads to the trunk and proximal extremities. Within 2 days the rash disappears from the face and trunk to involve the distal extremities. Thereafter the rash rapidly disappears and rarely desquamates. The rash may be the first sign of rubella. Fever and constitutional symptoms are usually very mild. Only in infants is the fever and the rash very severe. Other clinical features may include purpura or petechiae, and arthritis.

Laboratory tests may show leukopenia and thrombocytopenia. Isolation of the virus can be made 2 weeks before the onset of the rash and as late as 2 weeks after the onset, from throat specimens and urine analysis. The virus can be also isolated from the blood prior to the rash. Fecal specimens may also yield the virus. An increase in rubella antibody titer may be detected in paired sera collected 2 or more weeks apart.

PATIENT MANAGEMENT

Rubella is always a self limited uncomplicated disease. Encephalitis is uncommon.

Rubella is a teratogenic virus that can lead to severe fetal malformation if the mother becomes infected during the first trimester of pregnancy. Because of this, therapeutic abortion is often recommended.

No specific therapy for rubella is available. Symptomatic treatment is provided for the constitutional symptoms.

ROSEOLA INFANTUM (EXANTHEM SUBITUM)

No specific virus has been isolated in this disease. The clinical picture begins with three days of sustained high fever. Convulsions may occur. A discrete pink rash which is evanescent appears as the fever decreases. The rash is often generalized and may coalesce. There may be edema of the eyelids. It can be complicated by encephalitis. Leukocytosis or leucopenia may be present. Roseola infantum is a benign self-limiting disease that does not need specific treatment; only symptomatic/supportive treatment is required (33–36).

INFECTIOUS MONONUCLEOSIS

The etiology of this disease is infection by the Epstein Barr virus in a susceptible host. The clinical picture may include fever, sore throat, exudative tonsillitis, malaise, generalized lymphadenopathy, splenomegaly, headache, jaundice, epistaxis, abdominal pain and a morbilliform or maculopapular rash (33–36).

Complications can take the form of hepatitis, encephalitis, meningitis, polyradiculoneuritis, pneumonitis, carditis or Burkitt's lymphoma.

Laboratory diagnosis may reveal leucocytosis between 10,000–20,000/uL. Normal WBC count may be present or even leucopenia. Atypical lymphocytes in the peripheral blood may range from 50 to 90%. A normal Hb, hematocrit value and platelet count are usually found. Rarely thrombocytopenia and autoimmune hemolytic anemia may be present.

The screening test for mononucleosis is the Monospot test. Serology: the Paul Bennell test is positive in a titer above 1:112. Antibody to viral capsid antigen (VCA) rises to titers in excess of 1:160 during the acute phase of the disease. Specific IgM antibody is detectable in 97% of acute infections. Antibody to EB nuclear antigen (EBNA) appears only after several weeks of infection. Case management is symptomatic/supportive (see above).

ACQUIRED IMMUNODEFICIENCY SYNDROME

Although some controversy exists (38,39), and the degree of biological susceptibility does vary, the infective agent in AIDS is HIV. The mode of infection is by blood transfusion, Factor VIII concentrate transfusion, or through infected parents.

Essentials to the diagnosis of this syndrome include the presence of lymphadenopathy, hepatosplenomegaly, high IgG levels, failure to thrive, recurrent infections, lymphopenia and unresolved pneumonia (33–36).

Treatment is symptomatic and supportive. Symptomatic improvement following IgG replacement has been reported.

INFANT BOTULISM

The etiology of infant botulism is infection of a nonresistant host through the ingestion of spores from contaminated honey, light or dark corn syrup, or from unknown sources (33–36). The clinical presentation varies between mild and fulminant cases.

SYMPTOMS AND SIGNS

Symptoms can include generalized weakness and lethargy that takes place over one to four days. There may be constipation, drooping of the eyelids, slow and incomplete feeding, or a week feeble cry.

There may be a sluggish pupillary reflex, generalized hypotonia, or ptosis of the eyelids. Autonomic nervous system dysfunction (e.g., flushing, bradycardia or tachycardia) can occur. There may also be a sluggish gag reflex. Paralysis can progress to respiratory arrest. Complications with this infection can include aspiration pneumonia, necrotizing enterocolitis, otitis media, urinary tract infections, misplaced endotracheal tubes, or death.

PATIENT MANAGEMENT

Laboratory investigations can include electromyography, which may reveal BSAP (brief, small, abundant potentials). The feces should be tested for c. botulinum spores and botulinal toxins. Hospitalization is recommended with monitoring of respiratory and cardiac activity and gavage feeding (the mother's breast milk with its immune components can and should be used if possible). Antibiotics should only be used to treat secondary infections. Trimethoprim sulfamethoxazole (Bactrim) is the drug of choice for secondary infections in patients with botulism.

Frequent emptying of the urinary bladder by Crede's method should be used to minimize the risk of urinary tract infections. Close contact with other infants should be avoided for 3 months or until excretion of the organisms has ended.

BRUCELLOSIS

The etiology of Brucellosis is infection in a compromised host by the organism Brucella, transmitted through infected animals such as dogs, cattle, swine, and goats (33–36). The transmission is either by direct contact or when humans ingest the infected animal's secretions in milk or cheese.

SYMPTOMS AND SIGNS

The patient may have a non-specific fever (septic-sustained or low grade). In chronic stages, the patient can present with an undulant fever where normal periods alternate with febrile episodes. The patient may have chills, malaise, weakness, body aches, sweating and lethargy.

Complications of brucellosis include spondylitis, suppurative arthritis, subacute endocarditis, meningitis, encephalitis, and chronicity.

PATIENT MANAGEMENT

Organisms can be recovered from the blood, urine and cerebrospinal fluid early in the course of the disease. Agglutination test using serial dilutions of patient serum and Babortus antigen, with an agglutination titer of 1:160 or greater is diagnostic of the infection.

Bed rest, nutritional support, and spinal examination/adjustment are indicated as part of comprehensive approach to patient management. Medical management can include the drainage of abscesses. Tetracycline is the drug of choice given by mouth in standard doses for 3–4 weeks. In cases of severe illness or relapse, the treatment is augmented by intramuscular administration of streptomycin 15–30 mg/kg/day. This daily dose of streptomycin should be divided into two equal doses and given every 12 hours. Steroids may be necessary at the onset of therapy to reduce the risk of herxheimer reaction. This disease is preventable by avoiding animal contact and the ingestion of unpasteurized dairy products.

PSITTACOSIS

The etiology of this infection is by the organism chlamydia psitta in a compromised host. Chlamydial infection is contracted by humans from infected birds, primarily through inhalation (33–36).

SYMPTOMS AND SIGNS

The incubation time for the organism is 7–14 days. The fever rises steadily. Chills, headache, pneumonia, malaise, and/or nausea can all be a part of the clinical picture.

PATIENT MANAGEMENT

If pneumonia is present, then a chest x-ray may reveal extensive interstitial infiltrations. Serological studies can reveal a four-fold rise of specific antibodies. Isolation of the infective agent is done with a tissue culture. In addition to supportive measures, medical management includes the administration of tetracycline either orally or parenterally for 21 days.

CHLAMYDIA PNEUMONIA

The usual etiology of chlamydial pneumonia is infection of a susceptible infant by c. trachomatous in an infected birth canal. This type of infection is an important differential for the infant during the first six months of life. Ten to twenty percent of infants born through an infected genital tract will develop chlamydial pneumonia (33–36).

Symptoms and Signs. There is usually an insidious onset of tachypnea and coughing, often in paroxysms. The infant is typically afebrile.

Patient Management. Eosinophilia with more than 400 cells/mm^3 is common in this type of pneumonia The chest x-ray will reveal an interstitial type of pneumonia with over inflation. Culturing of chlamydia can be done from the nasopharynx. Anti-chlamydial antibody levels can be assessed. The medical management of this condition is with erythromycin for 2–3 weeks. Maternal and paternal infections, if present, should also be treated.

NEWBORN INCLUSION CONJUNCTIVITIS

The etiology of newborn inclusion conjunctivitis is through infection by chlamydia in an infected birth canal (33–36).

Symptoms and Signs. An acute purulent conjunctivitis is identified in the newborn. The incidence is 10–80 cases per thousand live births. The incubation period is between 5 and 12 days. A watery discharge from the eyes becomes gradually more purulent and the eyelids become more swollen. Lymphoid follicles and membranous conjunctivitis can develop and persist for weeks or months.

Patient Management. Conjunctival cultures can be done on blood and chocolate agar media. Medical management consists of topical conjunctival treatment with sulfonamides, tetracycline or erythromycin. Oral erythromycin, at 40–50 mg/kg/day, is prescribed for two weeks. Conjunctivitis can be prevented by instilling erythromycin ointment at birth as the legally mandated prophylaxis against gonococcal and chlamydial conjunctivitis.

CHOLERA

The organism that causes cholera is vibrio cholerae. The incubation period varies between 6 hours and 5 days. The manifestations of cholera vary from asymptomatic infection or mild gastroenteritis to profuse watery diarrhea, usually in a malnourished and compromised host (33–36).

SYMPTOMS AND SIGNS

The onset of symptoms usually begins with mild abdominal discomfort and anorexia. This is followed by the appearance of brownish feces in the liquid stool. As the diarrhea becomes more severe, the stool takes on a pale gray color, and loses its odor, except for a faint fishy smell; it contains mucus flecks ("rice water stool"). Vomiting may occur after the onset of diarrhea. A normal or subnormal temperature is usually present although a low grade fever is occasionally seen.

The complications of cholera include severe dehydration, hypovolemic shock, hypoglycemia, convulsions, loss of consciousness, hypokalemia, renal failure, and death.

PATIENT MANAGEMENT

Examination of the stools is made with dark field or phase microscopy. Active motile vibrio organisms are seen in large numbers of choleric stool. A rectal swab and stool culture is made.

Replacement of fluid and electrolyte losses is the first priority. Intravenous rehydration or oral rehydration, if the condition permits, is of extreme importance. The rehydration therapy should contain 2.0 to 2.5 percent glucose, 70–90 m Eq/L sodium and 20 m Eq/L potassium from 40–75 mL/Kg, depending on the estimated deficit and should be administered every four hours. Following rehydration an oral maintenance solution should be given. The maintenance solution contains 2–2.5% glucose, 40–60 m Eq/L sodium and 20 m Eq/L potassium. The administrated volume of the maintenance solution should not exceed 150 ml/kg /24 hours. If additional fluid is needed, water, breast milk, or low solute fluid can be given.

Complications such as electrolyte imbalance and renal failure are treated. Antibiotic treatment is of secondary importance. Tetracycline 30 mg/kg/day if given every 6 hours for 2–3 days will shorten the clinical course, reduce the volume requirement for rehydration and decrease the period of bacterial excretion. Cholera is also sensitive to trimethoprim-sulfamethoxazole, amino glycosides, chloramphenicol, and furazildone.

DIPHTHERIA

Diphtheria is caused by an infection in a compromised host by the corynebacterium diphtheria organism. The most common form is that of nasal diphtheria and is usually seen in infants and young children. A profuse, grayish mucoid nasal discharge is present. After a few days, when the membrane begins sloughing, there is often blood in the discharge. This is the mildest form of diphtheria (33–36).

Other mucous membrane and skin diphtheria can occur on rare occasions. The primary sites of infection are the mucous membrane of the eye, vagina or ear. Ulcerating lesions with exudate or pseudomembrane forms occur. The lesions are self limiting in most occasions without any toxicity.

Toxic Manifestations of Diphtheria

Toxic myocarditis, which may lead to severe dysrhythmia that can be life threatening, can occur on rare occasions. Toxic nephropathy and renal failure may also occur. Isolated peripheral nerve palsies and the muscles in the peripharyngeal area are commonly affected early in the course of the disease. Paralysis of the extraocular muscles, diaphragm and muscles supplied by peripheral nerves can occur between the second and sixth week (33–36).

Patient Management

A complete blood count may reveal leukocytosis in the peripheral blood. Thrombocytopenia and disseminated intravascular coagulopathy are rare. There may be a mild anemia. The CSF examination will reveal albuminocytologic dissociation and urine examination may show albuminuria cells and casts. Isolation of the organism from the local lesions can be made.

The medical management consists of administering diphtheria antitoxin, intravenously, as soon as possible after performing a sensitivity test. The sensitivity test is obtained by installing a 1:10 dilution into the conjunctival sac or performing an intradermal test dose with a 1:100 dilution of the antiserum. If the patient has an immediate reaction, a desensitization procedure is done. The dose of antitoxin varies according to the severity of the condition. If the diphtheria is diagnosed to be nasal, pharyngeal or laryngeal, or diagnosed in less than 48 hours, then the antitoxin dose should be 20,000–40,000 U. If the diphtheria is severe (e.g., bull neck diphtheria or diagnosed after 48 hours of the onset), the antitoxin dose should be 80,000–100,000 U. In cases of laryngopharyngeal diphtheria, 40,000–60,000 U of the antitoxin is administered. Asymptomatic susceptible contacts should receive 5,000–10,000 U of the antitoxin.

BACTERIAL MENINGITIS

The etiology of bacterial meningitis is usually infection with hemophilus influenza encapsulated type B; the most common cause of bacterial meningitis in the U.S. The infection is transmitted by respiratory droplets (33–36).

Symptoms and Signs

This disease is more common in children under 2 years old, between 4 and 24 months of age, but can also occur in older children and adults. The clinical picture is nonspecific early in the course of the disease in the form of temperature instability (hypothermia or hyperthermia), respiratory distress, feeding difficulties, irritability, lethargy, apnea, abdominal distention, vomiting, diarrhea, hepatosplenomegaly, jaundice, petechiae and seizures. A bulging fontanelle is a late sign of meningitis in neonates. Kernig's and Brudzinski's signs are rare in the neonate.

Complications of bacterial meningitis include death in 40–50% of cases. Auditory impairment is the most common lasting deficit. Subdural effusions can develop in one third of patients. Disseminated intravascular coagulopathy is another complication.

Patient Management

Medical management includes blood cultures, a spinal tap, Gram stained CSF smears, Latex particle agglutination (LPA) and countercurrent immuno-electrophoresis (CIE). Detection of antibodies in the CSF is usually rapid and specific. The patient's Hb level should be monitored because anemia is a frequent finding in Hemophilus influenza infection.

Intravenous chloramphenicol and ampicillin is a recommended therapy and should be initiated intravenously followed by oral administration of ampicillin at a dose of 200–400 mg/kg given every 4–6 hours for 7 to 21 days. Precautions should be taken with chloramphenicol therapy for its possible side effects. In cases of bacterial resistance, ampicillin cefuroxime 200–400 mg/kg every 6–8 hours can be given for 7 to 21 days. The patient is also treated for any electrolyte imbalance. Anticoagulant therapy is used if disseminated intravascular coagulopathy develops. Anticonvulsants are administrated if necessary. Medical recommendations for prevention of H. influenza meningitis is by chemoprophylaxis and immunization (See also Chapter 3).

BACTEREMIA

This blood infection is also due to H. Influenza type B. The clinical picture includes a high fever with no other focus of infection. It is common in children younger than two years of age. Nonspecific symptoms include fever, myalgia, irritability or vomiting (33–36).

Patient Management

The medical management includes blood culture and other investigations similar to bacterial meningitis. The case management is also similar to that of bacterial meningitis.

PNEUMONIA

Pneumonia generally occurs in children less than six years of age. The infective agent is usually H. influenza. It is also clinically indistinguishable from other types of bacterial pneumonia. Pleural effusion, empyema and pericarditis are common complications of H. influenza pneumonia (33–36).

Patient Management

A chest x-ray may reveal segmental, subsegmental or lobar pneumonia patterns. Blood cultures are important for the diagnosis, and antigen detection in the blood or urine may be of some diagnostic assistance. The management of the patient is as in the case of bacterial meningitis.

EPIGLOTTIS

The etiology of infection of the epiglottis and supraglottic tissues is due to H. influenza type B in susceptible host. It is more common in older children 2 to 7 years of age (33–36).

SYMPTOMS AND SIGNS

There is usually an acute onset of the disease, with high fever, sore throat, dysphagia and lethargy. This is usually followed by accumulation of secretions in the oropharyngeal region which can lead to respiratory distress in the form of tachypnea, stridor and cyanosis. This condition may be associated by H. influenza B bacteremia. Usually the epiglottis is examined directly in the operating room to secure the airway with an endotracheal tube.

PATIENT MANAGEMENT

A blood culture is performed. An endotracheal tube may be needed to secure the airway. Antibiotics, similar to the treatment in bacterial meningitis, should be given for 10–14 days even after the clinical cure of epiglottitis.

CELLULITIS

Cellulitis is an H. Influenza type B infection of the skin. Facial cellulitis is an uncommon development in children during the initial year of life (33–36).

SYMPTOMS AND SIGNS

The disease is characterized by raised, warm, tender and indurated areas of skin with a bluish-red hue. It is more common over the cheek, but it may also appear on the extremities. The child appears to be toxic with a high fever. The complications include high fever, orbital and periorbital cellulitis meningitis.

PATIENT MANAGEMENT

A blood culture is obtained. The patient management is similar to that of bacterial meningitis.

SEPTIC ARTHRITIS (OSTEOMYELITIS)

H. Influenza type B infection is the leading cause of septic arthritis in children under two years of age. It affects large joints and may cause contiguous osteomyelitis in the knees, ankles, hips or elbows (33–36).

SYMPTOMS AND SIGNS

The clinical picture starts with an upper respiratory tract infection which is followed later by pain in the involved joint and the child appears toxic with fever.

PATIENT MANAGEMENT

A culture of joint fluid and blood can be made. There may be antibodies in the blood or urine. The medical management includes the administration of antibiotics for at least 10–14 days and longer if osteomyelitis is suspected. Draining the joint through repeated needle aspiration or open drainage is often useful.

LYME DISEASE

The etiology of lyme disease is through an infection by a spirochete through a bite which spreads through a variety of different ticks. The incubation period is 3–20 days after the tick bite (33–36).

SYMPTOMS AND SIGNS

There are intermittent symptoms in the form of a unique skin lesion which begins as a macule or papule followed by progressive expansion of an erythematous ring over approximately seven days. The ring typically reaches 15 cm in diameter and has red borders and central clearing. Sometimes the central area is indurated, discolored or even necrotic. The lesions most often appear on the thigh, groin or axilla and they may be itchy or painful. Approximately half of the patients will develop multiple, smaller, annular secondary lesions and some will have recurrent lesions. Symptoms resembling those of flu or aseptic meningitis usually appear with the skin lesions. These symptoms often include headache, stiff neck, myalgia, arthralgia, malaise, fatigue, lethargy and lymphadenopathy. High grade fever is present in only about half of the patients and is usually low grade among adults.

After a few weeks or months, the second stage of the disease begins. Neurologic and cardiac manifestations in the form of headache, neck pain and stiffness can occur. Ten percent of patients will develop frank meningitis which may be recurrent with cranial or peripheral radiculopathies and cardiac manifestations in the form of myocarditis and dysrhythmia.

In the final stage of the disease which occurs weeks to years after stage 2, arthritis is the primary feature. The arthritis is monarticular or oligoarticular and affects the large joints. It takes place in the form of intermittent attacks of joint swelling and pain that lasts weeks to months in a given year. Less commonly the arthritis is migratory which can be complicated by chronic destructive joint changes.

PATIENT MANAGEMENT

There may be an elevated ESR, IgM and aspartate transaminases. Patients with neurologic manifestations or arthritis often possess the B-cell alloantigen, DR2. Medical management includes the administration of antibiotics against the etiologic spirochete. Penicillin, in a dose of 50 mg/kg/day is probably the agent of choice. Tetracycline, in a dose of 250 mg/kg/day is the alternative for older children while erythromycin in a dose of 30 mg/kg/day is the alternative for younger children. The therapy should last 10–20 days and be guided by the patient's clinical response.

LEPTOSPIROSIS

This infection is the by the organism leptospira interrogans (icterohemorrhagic sero group from swine and the canicola sero group from cattle and dogs). The incubation period ranges between 2–20 days (33–36).

SYMPTOMS AND SIGNS

There is usually a sudden onset of fever, headache, myalgia and gastrointestinal disturbances such as abdominal pain, nausea and vomiting. Physical examination may reveal conjunctivitis, pharyngeal infection, lymphadenopathy, hepatosplenomegaly, macular exanthematous and icterus.

The fever ends by lysis and the patient may remain asymptomatic and comfortable for 1–3 days until the start of a second phase of the disease which in most patients is asymptomatic. In those who have symptoms in the second phase, the clinical manifestations will be in the form of meningitis and low grade fever. Ten percent of patients develop a severe form of the disease characterized by prolonged fever, azotemia, hemorrhage, vascular collapse and altered states of consciousness.

Complications of this disease can include thrombocytopenia, renal failure, acute calculus cholecystitis, hydrops of the gall bladder, cholangitis pancreatitis and peripheral gangrene.

PATIENT MANAGEMENT

During the first phase leptospiras may be detected in the patients blood by culture or inoculation of guinea pigs or mice. One can determine the specific IgM using the DOT. ELISA method which is the most accurate and least expensive.

During the second phase, examination of the CSF shows features characteristic of aseptic meningitis with mononuclear pleocytosis usually not exceeding 500 cells/mm^3, a normal glucose level and an elevated protein concentration. There is no leptospira in the blood in this phase but the urine will reveal leptospiruria. The efficiency of antimicrobial treatment is still controversial. The only antimicrobial treatment that should be given for children younger than the age of 12 is penicillin.

MENINGOCOCCAL INFECTIONS

These infections occur when meningococci is transmitted from person to person by droplet infection. Incubation period in a susceptible host is 3–4 days during which the organism multiplies in the nasopharynx (33–36).

SYMPTOMS AND SIGNS

There is usually a fever, rash and meningitis. Typical petechiae or larger purpuric lesions are found usually on the chest, upper arms and axillae. In the fulminant form of the disease, meningitis may be absent, but signs and symptoms of septic shock often heralded by spreading hemorrhagic rash, can progress rapidly and lead to death within hours. Rarely a chronic form of meningococcemia occurs that produces intermittent fever, chills, joint pains and petechial or maculopapular eruptions that persist for several days, over months. With recurring episodes, there is gradual clinical deterioration and enlargement of the spleen, endocarditis, meningitis or death may supervene at any time.

PATIENT MANAGEMENT

The laboratory diagnosis includes CIE, ELISA or LPA, all based on detecting specific bacterial antigen in serum, spinal fluid or urine. C. reactive protein or CSF lactate concentration can be used to differentiate between viral and bacterial meningitis. Culture of the meningococci in the blood is performed.

Penicillin is the drug of choice in medical management. If the patient is allergic to penicillin, chloramphenicol or cefotaxime can be used. Treatment should be given by EV route and continued for at least seven days. Respiratory isolation during the first 24 hours of antimicrobial therapy is recommended. Vital signs, especially blood pressure should be monitored if hypotension develops. If present, an immediate effort should be made to maintain the blood volume.

PLAGUE

Yersinia (Pasteurella pestis) is the infective agent in plague. It is transmitted from rats to humans by the flea, mostly xenopsylla cheopis, or by wild rodents. In the pneumonic form of the disease, it can be transmitted directly from person to person through the air (33–36).

SYMPTOMS AND SIGNS

The incubation period is between 1–10 days. The clinical manifestations of plague are divided into two types: bubonic and pneumonic.

Bubonic Plague. A sudden fever of 40° C or more, is accompanied by shaking, chills. The fever peaks during the first 24 hours and then continues at slightly lower levels for 3 to 4 days with occasional morning remissions. This may be followed by a second steep rise. If no complications develop, the fever will decline once again after the seventh or tenth day of the illness. A sudden drop of body temperature to normal or subnormal body temperature always precedes death.

Tender lymph nodes can be felt corresponding to the lymph channels draining the anatomic area of the bite. The skin overlying the enlarged bubonic lymph nodes is erythematous. These lymph nodes vary from one to several centimeters in diameter. As the fever continues, other manifestations in the form of malaise, headache, photophobia, abdominal pain, nausea, vomiting, diarrhea, restless, myalgia, weakness and often convulsions occur. The buboes increase in size during this time and become fluctuant and the overlying skin becomes hemorrhagic. The buboes may be reabsorbed slowly with clinical recovery or they may rupture. Occasionally the condition may become chronic with the formulation of ulcers and draining fistulas.

Pneumonic Plague. Pneumonic plague is quickly fatal. It is characterized by alveolar hemorrhages and massive pulmonary edema. The majority of untreated patients die within a few hours.

PATIENT MANAGEMENT

In bubonic plague, profound leukocytosis of more than 40,000 leukocytes/mm^3 is detected. In the pneumonic form, leukopenia or leukocytosis may be found with various proportions of young and immature polymorphonuclear leukocytes. Blood culture, sputum smears or aspiratal from the buboes will reveal the typical gram negative organisms. Agglutination tests can be performed.

Immediate therapy consists of isolating for 12 hours. The discharges should be handled with rubber gloves and a patient with pulmonary involvement should wear face masks. Also, careful attention must be paid to waste disposal because feces may be contaminated. Treatment for shock, seizures, fever and fluid loss is begun. For mild to moderate cases, tetracycline should be given orally in a dose of 40–50 mg/kg/day after a loading dose of 30 mg/kg. After 24 to 48 hours the dose can be reduced to 25 to 30 mg/kg/day. If intravenous therapy is desirable, tetracycline at a loading dose of 10 mg/kg is followed by 15 mg/kg/day. Oral therapy should be substituted as soon as possible for fear of hepatic and renal toxicity. For severe cases with sepsis or pneumonia, streptomycin should be used cautiously at a dose of 20–30 mg/kg/day given intramuscularly into three equal doses for 5 days. Tetracycline should be given at an oral dose of 30 mg/kg/day divided into four equal doses for an additional 5 days. Treatment is generally continued 1 week after the body temperature returns to normal. Chloramphenicol can be given at a dosage of 50 mg/kg/day in four divided doses.

RAT BITE FEVER

The infectious agent in rat bite fever is streptobacillus moniformis (in the U.S.) and by spirillum minus (in Japan) which occurs after the bite of a rodent, usually a rat (33–36).

SYMPTOMS AND SIGNS

The clinical picture in S. Moniformis consists of fever and chills, headache, myalgia and weakness. The incubation period is 7–10 days. There may be maculopapular eruption-arthralgia and polyarthritis. The lesions heal without suppuration.

In S. Minus (Sodoku), the incubation period is 1–3 weeks. Erythema, induration and tenderness of the wound develops. Lymphadenitis, intermittent fever, rash and chills are part of the clinical picture. The rash occurs with the febrile period and disappears between them. The disease runs a relapsing course and the fever subsides in the course of several weeks.

PATIENT MANAGEMENT

Culture of the organism is made with the blood. The medical management consists of moderate doses of aqueous procaine penicillin for 7–10 days.

RELAPSING FEVER

The etiology of relapsing fever is an infection by the borrelia recurrentis organism which is transmitted by lice and ticks. The incubation period is 7–10 days (33–36).

SYMPTOMS AND SIGNS

The disease begins abruptly with a very high fever, prostration, headache, myalgia and arthralgia. Diarrhea, cough and chest pain develops. Splenomegaly is common and hepatomegaly and jaundice may also occur. Each episode lasts for 3–6 days with a symptom free period for 5–10 days between each episode. Without treatment the mortality rate is about 40%.

PATIENT MANAGEMENT

The laboratory diagnosis should demonstrate borrelia in a blood smear. Borrelia can be also found in the urine or CSF when the CNS is involved. The medical management consists of standard oral doses of tetracycline or chloramphenicol for 5–10 days. It is important to caution that Herxheimer's reaction (fever), chills, fall in the blood pressure, and leucopenia can occur with treatment as a result of the release of large number of endotoxin from the killed borrelia.

SALMONELLA INFECTION

The infective agent is the salmonella organism transmitted by ingestion of contaminated food (e.g. chicken) or water. The highest frequency of infection is at the age of 2–4 months. The median age of infection is 14 years (33–36).

SYMPTOMS AND SIGNS

Gastroenteritis develops with diarrhea after an incubation period of 8–72 hours followed by dysentery and cramping abdominal pain. A high fever begins within the initial day of onset and lasts for more than 48 hours. The clinical picture can include headache, chills, anorexia, nausea, vomiting and malaise. The symptoms are usually present for seven days; rarely they may persist for 2 weeks.

Complications: can include dehydration, metabolic acidosis, hypovolemic shock, bacteremia, prolonged secretory diarrhea (more evident in infants than older children), and failure to thrive after the acute infection.

Bacteremia. This is more common in newborns and infants less than 3 months old. Also predisposed are those with immune deficiency (e.g., due to malnutrition, malignancy or previous antimicrobial and cortico steroid therapy). Symptoms are usually indistinguishable from acute gastroenteritis. The patient appears acutely toxic with a high fever.

Focal Infections. Local focal infections can occur after salmonella gastroenteritis. CNS involvement can consist of brain abscess and meningitis. Respiratory tract involvement includes pneumonia, lung abscess and pleuritis. Cardiovascular involvement manifests in endocarditis, pericarditis and mycotic aneurysms. Hepatic involvement occurs with liver abscess. Reticuloendothelial involvement manifests as splenic abscess and mesenteric lymphadenitis. In the musculoskeletal system, osteomyelitis or arthritis develops. The urinary tract can be affected with renal abscess and cystitis. Patients with sickle cell anemia are predisposed to salmonella osteomyelitis.

Enteric Fever. This is a fever that starts insidiously and gradually increases over the initial week to as high as 40° C. Relative bradycardia disproportionate to the temperature elevation is a unique feature; headache, chills anorexia and malaise are also present. Initially diarrhea may be present, but later, constipation will be the prominent feature. Diffuse abdominal tenderness, hepatomegaly and splenomegaly may be present.

The complications may include intestinal perforation, peritonitis, septic shock, and focal infections. Decreased bowel sounds indicates paralytic ileus. Discrete palpable erythematous lesions known as Rose spots can appear on the trunk during the second week and the fever usually ends by lysis at the end of 3 weeks.

PATIENT MANAGEMENT

Medical evaluation includes stool cultures and CSF culture, especially in infants less than three months old. Serial blood cultures should be obtained if the first culture is negative because of the intermittent occurrence of low inoculum bacteremia. Urine can be cultured. Biopsy may be positive in the spleen, liver or mesenteric lymph nodes. In epidemiological studies, serological tests can be helpful in the diagnosis (e.g., Widal's test).

Uncomplicated salmonella gastroenteritis requires no antimicrobial therapy, however gastroenteritis in infants less than 3 months old requires antimicrobial treatment. Enteric fever requires antibacterial treatment. Any complications are treated. The types of antimicrobial therapy given in cases of enteric fever are Ampicillin 50–150 mg/kg/day IM or IV divided every 6 hours, Chloramphenicol 50–75 mg/kg/day PO or IV divided every 6 hours, or trimethoprim-sulfamethaxote 5–10 mg TMP/25–50 mg SMZ/kg/day PO or IV divided every 8–12 hours. The therapy may range from as little as 10 days for uncomplicated septicemia to at least 3 weeks for meningitis and 3 months or more for osteomyelitis.

SHIGELLOSIS

Shigellosis infection arises in a susceptible host through the ingestion of contaminated food or water by the shigella organism, which can survive in buffered food stuffs (e.g., milk and grains). Direct person to person spread by contaminated fingers or through indirect vectors is also common. The incubation period is 1–7 days (33–36).

SYMPTOMS AND SIGNS

The clinical features begin with a high fever (40° C) that usually disappears within 72 hours. Generalized malaise and crampy abdominal pain are often present. An uncomplicated generalized seizure may occur. Diarrhea is present, and may recur within seven days, or proceed to dysentery, tenesmus, fecal urgency, diffuse abdominal pain and prostration.

On examination, the abdomen is often diffusely tender, usually without rebound tenderness and the pain is intense in the lower quadrants. There may be hyperactive bowel sounds. An atonic portion of the rectum may be prolapsed. Proctoscopy may reveal friable, ecdemic, hyperemic mucosa, areas of severe erythema with focal ulcerations covered by exudate.

Complications are common in debilitated children or infants and can include chronic enteropathy with persistent

diarrhea, dehydration and weight loss. The compromised child may also develop secondary hypochromic anemia, bacteremia, or suppurative focal infections

PATIENT MANAGEMENT

Investigations include a stool culture. There may also be an increased portion of immature granulocytes known as band forms, seen in the peripheral blood. Since shigelaemia can occur in malnourished infants, blood culture and lumbar puncture are highly recommended for that group of patients. Determination of shigella-specific serum antibodies is useful in characterizing the incidence and prevalence of epidemic infections.

Management includes oral or parenteral fluids as indicated by the clinical condition of the patient. Shigellosis is a self limiting disease and antibiotic treatment is only indicated to reduce the duration of fever, diarrhea and to reduce the public health risk associated with shigella carriage. The antimicrobial treatment may be in the form of ampicillin, administrated orally 50–150 mg/kg/day, divided every 6 hours for 5 days. In the case of resistance to ampicillin, trimethoprim-sulfamethoxazole 5–10 mg TMP 25–50 mg SM2/kg/day divided every 8–12 hours can be used.

ENTERIC ESCHERICHIA COLI

E. coli infection is through the ingestion of contaminated food such as dairy products, meats (e.g., undercooked hamburgers) and uncooked vegetables. In underdeveloped countries the main mode of transmission is by ingestion of contaminated water. Direct person to person contact is another mode of transmission. The incubation period is less than 24 hours (33–36).

SYMPTOMS AND SIGNS

Clinical features include sudden onset of explosive diarrhea, rapid dehydration, metabolic acidosis, and systemic hypotension. Associated symptoms include fever, vomiting, loss of appetite and systemic toxicity, lethargy and abdominal distention. This clinical manifestation in the United States is in the form of mild non-specific diarrhea which occurs after an incubation period of 6–24 hours. Watery, liquid large volume stools without blood or mucus are passed 3–10 times per day, usually for a total of 2–5 days. The patient can be afebrile or the fever can be as high as 40° C, usually within the first 2 days. Malaise, abdominal pain, anorexia and vomiting can occur as well. Enteroinvasive escherichia coli infection can produce mild dysentery with high fever. The disease is self limiting and ends in less than 1 week although stools may be abnormal for several weeks.

PATIENT MANAGEMENT

The main proof of escherichia coli invasiveness is a positive sereny test but the procedure is time consuming, expensive and not widely available. E. coli infection is usually a self-limiting disorder. Thus, the main lines of treatment are appropriate replacement of electrolytes and water, either by water or parenteral fluids. Nutritional support is needed with proper amounts of proteins, fats and carbohydrates. Antibacterial therapy for diarrhea genic escherichia coli is controversial. Prophylactic treatment is through proper sanitation and cooking. In rare cases death can occur.

STAPHYLOCOCCAL COLONIZATION AND DISEASE

Infection by staphylococcus aureus in the newborn is by contaminating the newborn nares or umbilicus from nursery personnel or attendants. Older infants and children can be infected by staph aureus when they have altered host resistance. Gastroenteritis can be caused by ingestion of food contaminated with a strain of staph aureus (33–36).

SYMPTOMS AND SIGNS

This infection is more common in newborns and infants with altered host resistance. In the newborn it appears as Staphylococcal scalded skin syndrome. This syndrome affects mainly the skin although the primary site of infection can be distant from the skin (e.g., in the conjunctiva or at the site of a circumcision). The patient is generally afebrile. Clinical features also include impetigo, septicemia, osteomyelitis, pneumonia, localized boils and meningitis.

In older infants and children, the clinical features can include septicemia, staphylococcal pneumonia, endocarditis, enterocolitis, meningitis, brain abscesses, furunculosis, osteomyelitis, cellulitis, bullous impetigo, exfoliative dermatitis, skin rash and toxic shock syndrome.

If the disease is acquired through surgical incision, abrasion or insect bite, it is characterized by the sudden onset of fever, diarrhea shock, hyperemia of the mucous membranes and a diffuse macular erythematous rash followed by desquamation of the hands and feet. Fluid loss and shock are a common cause of death in this disorder.

Enteric Infection. The incubation period is 3–8 hours for enteric infections. There is usually sudden onset of vomiting and diarrhea. The disease is self limiting and symptoms usually drop abruptly within 24 hours. The most severe form of staphylococcal infection is staphylococcal enterocolitis which is usually complicated by fluid loss and shock.

PATIENT MANAGEMENT

Examination begins with a stool culture to identify an enteric infection. Minor skin infections require no treatment. Abscesses should be drained. If the infection occurred in infants and was caused by staph aureus strain, bactericidal drugs should be used (e.g., benzylpenicillin). For hospital strains infection, B-lactamase resistant penicillin is the drug of choice. If the patient is allergic to penicillin, a first generation cephalosporin erythromycin should be used. Cancomycin or oral treatment is not recommended because of the unpredictable absorption. Enteric infection by staphylococci is usually self limiting and does not need antimicrobial therapy. The main line of treatment in this case is to correct the water and electrolyte imbalance.

STREPTOCOCCAL INFECTIONS

Group A B. hemolytic streptococci infections are transmitted through the air with salivary droplets. Nasal discharge is another mode of transmission and skin to skin transmissions also occur if skin infections are present (33–36).

SYMPTOMS AND SIGNS

The clinical features vary from mild to severe. Pharyngitis is present. In severe cases, the child suffers with a high fever (102.5° F), malaise, headache and severe pain on swallowing. Vomiting and abdominal pain may be prominent early symptoms. Nasal discharge, hoarseness, cough and diarrhea may occur. On examination the pharyngeal tissues may appear beefy red with edema of the uvula. A confluent grayish exudate on the tonsils is usually present. Tiny doughnut-shaped hemorrhages on the soft palate can be present. The patient usually has enlarged and tender anterior cervical lymph glands. Skin petechia and scarlatina form rash may occur. In mild conditions the clinical findings are less characteristic.

PATIENT MANAGEMENT

Laboratory investigations consist of blood agar throat culture from a swab. Rapid screening for streptococci can be done from throat swab with antigen agglutination kits. Leukocytosis may be present. The conventional medical treatment consists of penicillin for a 10 day course. If the patient is allergic to penicillin, erythromycin should be given.

SCARLET FEVER

Scarlet fever is streptococcal infection of the upper respiratory tract with a characteristic rash. The rash appears within 24–48 hours after the onset of symptoms (33–36).

SYMPTOMS AND SIGNS

In addition to fever, the characteristic rash often begins around the neck and spreads over the trunk and extremities. It is a diffuse, finely papular, erythematous eruption which blanches on pressure. The rash is often more intense along the creases of the elbows, axillae and groin. The skin has a goose dimple appearance and feels rough to the touch. Transverse red streaks in skin folds of the abdomen, antecubital spaces and axillae "Pasha's Line" may also be present. The face is usually spared with circumoral pallor. After 3–4 days the rash begins to fade with desquamation of the skin. Similar clinical manifestations as in streptococcal pharyngitis are present.

On examination, punctate erythematous lesions on the palate may be evident. The tongue is coated and the papillae are swollen. After desquamation, the reddened papillae are prominent, giving the tongue a strawberry appearance.

ERYSIPELAS

Erysipelas is a rare type of streptococcal skin infection in infants and children, characterized by swollen, red, very tender superficial skin blebs. This can be accompanied by reddish streaks of lymphangitis that project out of the margins of the lesions. A septic fever and other signs of infections may also be present. The complications include cervical adenitis, mastoiditis, otitis media, sinusitis, metastatic infection, (e.g., in the meninges, bones or joints), glomerulonephritis, and rheumatic fever (33–36).

PATIENT MANAGEMENT

Clinical laboratory cultures will show leukocytosis > 15,000. Streptococci may be cultured from exudate or from non-involved sites. ASO, streptozyme anti DNAase may be helpful in the diagnosis. Medical treatment consists of penicillin for at least 10 days at 20–50 mg/kg/day.

RHEUMATIC FEVER

This disorder is a fever that follows a streptococcal infection of the throat. It is variably associated with acute migratory polyarthritis (37).

SYMPTOMS AND SIGNS

According to the Jones criteria, the clinical manifestations of rheumatic fever are classified into major and minor manifestations (33–36). Major manifestations may include:

1. Pancarditis, affecting the three cardiac layers
2. Murmurs
3. Cardiomegaly
4. Pericarditis
5. Congestive heart failure
6. Polyarthritis, mainly in the large joints, migratory in nature, with redness, tenderness and swelling of the affected joints
7. Chorea, which is more common in females. It occurs in the form of sudden aimless irregular movements of the extremities that increases with excitement and laughing, disappearing during sleep. This condition is usually associated with emotional instability of the child.
8. Erythema marginatum; evanescent, pink erythematous macules with a clear center and serpiginous outline. The rash is transient, migratory and non-pruritic. It blanches with pressure and is found primarily on the trunk and proximal extremities.
9. Subcutaneous nodules; painless, small (0.5–1 cm) swellings over body prominences, over the extensor tendons of the hands, feet, elbows, scalp, scapulae and vertebrae.

Minor manifestations may include:

1. History of previous rheumatic fever
2. Arthralgia
3. Fever
4. Increased ESR, C reactive protein, and WBC count
5. Prolonged P-R and Q-T intervals on EC

Two major manifestations or one major and two minor manifestations with recent evidence of streptococcal infection indicates a high probability of rheumatic fever. However failure to meet the Jones criteria does not exclude rheumatic fever. Additional findings in rheumatic fever may include abdominal pain, epistaxis, facial tics and facial grimace.

PATIENT MANAGEMENT

Laboratory findings may demonstrate an elevated ESR and C. reactive protein. A prolonged P-R interval may be present. Studies of serum antibodies against the organism are the most reliable proof of infection. The most commonly used titer is antistreptolysino titer (ASO). Titers of at least 333 units in children and 250 units in adults are considered elevated.

The medical management consists of 1.2 million U of benzathine penicillin G as a single intramuscular injection, or 600,000 U of procaine penicillin G given as a daily injection for 10 days. Erythromycin 1g orally for 10 days may be substituted for penicillin in patients allergic to penicillin. Prophylaxis against recurrent rheumatic fever should be reinstituted immediately. 1.2 million U of benzathine penicillin G is given as a monthly injection, or 200,000 U of penicillin given orally twice each day or 1 g sulfadiazine given orally once each day. The prophylactic treatment should be given until adolescence and should start again if the patient is re-exposed to streptococcal infection. Salicylates and steroids are useful in controlling the clinical manifestations of acute rheumatic fever. Prednisone in a dose of 1–2 mg/kg/day is given in cases complicated by carditis. In other cases where carditis is absent, salicylates are preferred. Acetyl salicylic acid is recommended in a dose of 70–100 mg/kg/day. The minimum period of treatment of acute rheumatic fever is 6 weeks. Gradual withdrawal of salicylates or steroids is recommended to be over a period of 4–6 weeks. If rebound occurs, full therapy has to be reinstituted for an additional 4–6 weeks. Chorea may require treatment with haloperidol. Supportive measures are indicated.

TULAREMIA

The etiology of tularemia is infection by francisella tularensis which follows bites by ticks, fleas, mites, and contact with infected animals (e.g., rabbits, sheep, cats). Other causes are by contact with infected carcasses which can penetrate unbroken skin or by ingestion. The incubation period averages between 3 and 4 days (33–36).

SYMPTOMS AND SIGNS

The picture varies between low-grade fever with regional lymphadenopathy to fulminant fatal infections. Nearly all cases have fever, chills, fatigue and malaise.

Ulceroglandular tularemia is characterized by a non healing ulcer and regional adenopathy. A glandular form has localized lymphadenopathy without ulceration. The typhoidal type is characterized by fulminating septicemia with pleuropulmonary involvement. The oropharyngeal form has an exudative and/or membranous pharyngitis with cervical adenopathy and the oculoglandular is characterized by purulent conjunctivitis, and periauricular and cervical adenopathy.

PATIENT MANAGEMENT

Laboratory investigations will show a four-fold rise in antibody titer; an elevated ESR; delayed growth on specific media or blood culture; and normal WBC count but increased percentage of polymorphonuclear neutrophils. Lymph node aspiration can be performed. The medical treatment consists of streptomycin 30–40 mg/kg IM per day divided b.i.d. for 7–14 days. Alternative medications include gentamycin, chloramphenicol, tetracycline, and coxycyclin.

TUBERCULOSIS

Tuberculosis is a specific disease caused by the infection of mycobacterium T.B. by droplet infection in a susceptible host. To a lesser extent infection can occur through the ingestion of milk contaminated by the bovine type of mycobacterium T.B. The main predisposing factor of infection is the degree of immuno-suppression. The incubation period is 2–10 weeks following the initial infection (33–36).

SYMPTOMS AND SIGNS

The clinical feature of primary pulmonary tuberculosis is persistent low-grade fever of about 102° F, lasting 2–3 weeks. There may be weight loss, fatigue, irritability and malaise. Some patients are asymptomatic. The disease may progress to bronchopneumonia or lobar pneumonia, which are characterized by cough, high fever, night sweats and hemoptysis. The signs are usually in the form of rales, dullness and diminished breath sounds. If there is endobronchial involvement, the cough becomes brassy and paroxysmal and wheezes can be heard over the chest. Pleural effusion may complicate primary pulmonary tuberculosis but it is less common in children under 6 years; it is usually unilateral; and clinically it may vary from mild illness with malaise, cough, fever and weight loss to illness with acute onset of chills and pleuritic pain. In can be complicated in severe conditions by respiratory distress. Physical examination usually reveals dullness to percussion and a lack of breath sounds.

Chronic pulmonary tuberculosis is more common during adolescent life as a result of reactivation of the primary type or due to re-infection. Clinically it is characterized by dyspnea, malaise, cough and fever. As the disease advances the amount of sputum increases. Hemoptysis may occur and the patient may appear to be chronically ill with weight loss.

Hematogenous tuberculosis (military T.B.) may complicate primary tuberculosis or chronic tuberculosis and is due to invasion of the blood stream by tuberculous bacilli. The clinical picture is usually in the form of anorexia, weight loss, and low grade fever. Although the child may appear acutely ill, there are few respiratory signs and symptoms. Respiratory distress and cyanosis may complicate the conditions or hepatosplenomegaly, lymphadenopathy, choroidal tuberculosis, and meningitis.

Extrapulmonary tuberculosis includes T.B. meningitis—skeletal tuberculosis of the spine or other joints. Infections can also occur in the urinary tract, in superficial lymph nodes, in the skin, eyes, middle ear or mastoid cells. The heart can be affected (i.e., pericarditis), and infection can arise in the abdominal lymph nodes, the spleen, liver, tonsils, adenoids, and buccal mucosa.

PATIENT MANAGEMENT

Laboratory investigation includes the tuberculin test. It is a purified protein derivative (PPD); the mantoux skin test method is 5 units intermediate strength 0.1cc volar forearm. An intradermal wheal should be read at 48-72 hours. Greater than 10 mm is positive (>5 mm in HIV positive patient).

Nonspecific laboratory includes anemia and sterile pyuria. Lumbar puncture is performed if meningitis is suspected. Bone marrow biopsy and liver biopsy may be used for a culture. Fluorescent staining and DNA probes can be used for a rapid diagnosis. Ziehl Neelsen or auramine rhodamine stain of the sputum, gastric aspartate, broncho alveolar lavage fluids, peritoneal fluids, bone marrow aspirates, or cerebro-spinal fluid can be made.

Chest x-rays may show infiltrate with or without effusion with primary disease. Cavitary lesions and upper lobe disease with hilar adenopathy is common in primary infection of children.

The medical management is with the drug Isoniazid, orally 10–20 mg/kg (maximum 300 mg as a daily dose), or twice weekly 20–40 mg/kg. Rifampin can be given orally daily in a dose of 10–20 mg/kg (maximum 600 mg) or twice weekly at 10–20 mg/kg (maximum 600 mg). Pyrazinamide at 20–30 mg/kg (maximum 2 g) is another alternative as is streptomycin, daily IM 20–40 mg/kg (maximum 2 g) or twice weekly IM 25–30 mg/kg. Other drugs include ethambutol used only if the patient is old enough to cooperate for visual acuity tests.

REFERENCES

1. Hoekelman R, Lewin EB, Shapira MB, Sutherland SA. Potential bacteremia in pediatric practice. Am J Dis Child 1979;133:1017-1019.
2. Van der Jagt EW. Fever. In Hoekelman R, ed. Primary pediatric care. St. Louis:Mosby, 1992:923-928.
3. Henretig FM. Fever. In: Flesher GR, Ludwig S, eds. Textbook of pediatric emergency medicine, 3rd ed. Baltimore:Williams & Wilkins, 1993:202-209.
4. Powell KR. Fever without localizing signs in infants and children. In: Rudolph AM, Hoffman JIE, Rudolph CD. Rudolph's pediatrics, 20th ed. Stamford, CT: Appleton & Lange, 1996:521-526.
5. Henretig FM. Fever. In: Flesher GR, Ludwig S, eds. Textbook of pediatric emergency medicine, 3rd. ed. Baltimore: Williams & Wilkins, 1993:202-209.
6. Grossman M. Fever. In: Rudolph AM, Hoffman JIE, Rudolph CD. Rudolph's pediatrics, 20th ed. Stamford, CT: Appleton & Lange, 1996:521.
7. Schwartz, Charney, Curry, Ludwig, eds. Principles and Practice of Clinical Pediatrics. 1987; 394.
8. Van der Jagt EW. Fever. In: Hoekelman R, ed. Primary pediatric care, 2nd ed. St. Louis: Mosby, 1992:923-928.
9. Petersdorf R. Chills and fever. In Petersdorf R, et al., eds. Harrison's principles of internal medicine. 10th ed. New York: McGraw-Hill 1983;57-65
10. Baraff LJ. Management of the febrile child: a survey of pediatric and emergency medicine residency directors. Pediatr Infect Dis J 1991;10:795-800.
11. Powell KR. Fever without localizing signs in infants and children. In: Rudolph AM, Hoffman JIE, Rudolph CD. Rudolph's pediatrics, 20th ed. Stamford, CT: Appleton & Lange, 1996:521-526.
12. Jakiewicz JA, McCarthy CA, Richardson AC, White KC, Fisher DJ, Dagan R, Powell KR, Febrile Collaborative Study Group. Febrile infants at low risk for serious bacterial infection - an appraisal of the Rochester Criteria and implications for management. Pediatrics 1994;94:390-396.
13. Allen JM. The effects of chiropractic on the immune system: a review of the literature. Chiro J Aust 1993; 23:132-135.
14. Purse FM. Manipulative therapy of upper respiratory infections in children. J Am Osteopath Assoc 1966; 65:964-972.

15. Kline CA. Osteopathic manipulative therapy, antibiotics and supportive therapy in respiratory infections in children: a comparative study. J Am Osteopath Assoc 1965; 65:278-281.

16. Davies NJ. Chiropractic management of the acute febrile paediatric patient. J Austral Chiro Assoc 1987;17:126-130.

17. Swartz MH. Textbook of Physical Diagnosis, 2nd ed. Philadelphia: W.B. Saunders, 1994.

18. Baraff LJ, Bass JA, Fleischer GR, Klein JO, McCracken GH, Powell KR, Schriger DL. Practice guidelines for the management of infants and children 0 to 36 months of age with fever without source. Pediatrics 1993;92:1-12.

19. Schmitt BD. Fever phobia. Am J Dis Child 1980;134:176-181.

20. Done AK. Aspirin overdosage:Incidence, diagnosis and management. Pediatrics 1978;62(supp):890-897.

21. Weiss CF. Acetaminophen:Potential pediatric hazard. Pediatrics 1973;52:883.

22. Atkins HA. Febrile kids and overheated parents. Emergency Medicine 1993; Feb 15:125-129.

23. Petersdorf RG, Beeson PB. Fever of unexplained origin. Medicine 1961; 40: 1-30.

24. DiNubile MJ. Acute fevers of unknown origin: a plea for restraint. Arch Intern Med 1993; 153:2525-2526.

25. Long S. Approach to the febrile patient with no obvious focus of infection. Pediatr Rev 1984;5:305-315.

26. Baker MD, Bell LM, Avner JR. Outpatient management without antibiotics of fever in selected infants. New Engl J Med 1993; 329:1437-41.

27. McCarthy C, Powell K, Jaskiewics J, et.al. Outpatient management of selected infants younger than two months of age evaluated for possible sepsis. Pediatr Infect Dis 1990;9:153-175.

28. Timmermans DRM, Sprij AJ, De Bel CE. The discrepancy between daily practice and the policy of a decision-analytic model. Medical Decision Making 1996;16; 357-366.

29. Saladino R, riskson M, Levy N, et.al. Utility of serum interleukin-6 for diagnosis of invasive bacterial disease in children. Ann Emerg Med 1992;21:1413-1416.

30. McCarthy PL, Lembo RM, Baron MA, Fink HD, Cicchetti DV. Predictive value of abnormal physical examination findings in ill-appearing and well appearing febrile children. Pediatrics 1985;76:167-171.

31. McCarthy PL, Sharpe MR, Spiesel SZ, et.al. Observation scales to identify serious illness in febrile children. Pediatrics 1982;70:802-809.

32. Atkins HA, ed. Overcoming fever phobia. Emergency Medicine 1993; Apr 30:51-52.

33. Kempe, Silver, O'Brien, Fulginiti (eds). Current pediatric diagnosis and treatment, 9th Ed. Lange, 1987.

34. Dambro MR, ed. 1996 Griffith's 5 minute consult. Baltimore: Williams & Wilkins, 1996.

35. Braunwald E, et al., eds. Harrison's principles of internal medicine, 12th ed. New York: McGraw Hill, 1991.

36. Rudolph A, ed. Pediatrics. Nineteenth Edition. Norwalk, CT: Appleton & Lange, 1991.

37. Stedman's medical dictionary, 25th ed., Baltimore: Williams & Wilkins, 1990.

38. J Clin Invest 1997; T cells

39. Caulfield CR, Goldberg B. The anarchist AIDS medical formulary: a guide to guerrilla immunology. Berkeley: North Atlantic Books, 1993.

17 The Challenged Child

Cheryl E. Goble

This chapter is designed to assist the doctor of chiropractic in the care and management of the challenged child. In today's society, children who are physically or mentally challenged are accepted and therefore appear to be more prevalent. The health care provider must be prepared to aid in the treatment of these children. One of the most significant necessities of this assistance is to participate as part of the child's health care team. Services from therapists, teachers, optometrists, nutritionists, psychologists, medical physicians and social workers are many times essential to the total well-being of the patient; and therefore, the doctor of chiropractic must be cooperative with these providers.

The following chapter will review the clinical history, chiropractic evaluation, and chiropractic treatment of the challenged child. The author will address four specific disorders as to the chiropractic diagnosis, management and prognosis of these cases: cerebral palsy, Down syndrome, attention deficit hyperactivity disorder, and fetal alcohol syndrome.

History

The clinical history of the child is of utmost importance; adequate time must be made available with the child and parents or caretaker of the child to properly evaluate the child's past and present history. The environment of the office should be one of comfort and accessibility. It is suggested the child have appropriate toys, such as puzzles, puppets, or drawing tools to occupy his/her time during the evaluation period.

The first element of the assessment is the child's birth. Information should be compiled regarding the type of delivery. Complications of pregnancy or birth trauma are more frequent in cases of the handicapped child than in the histories of other children (1). Because a number of childhood disabilities are caused by abnormalities of pregnancy and labor, a history of gestation and delivery should be obtained (2). Prenatal and intranatal complications arouse the suspicion of central nervous system damage (3).

The child's development, including physical, mental and emotional abilities, should be assessed. Accomplishment of skills in gross and fine motor function, along with social skills, are significant in the child's overall developmental representation. Oftentimes the parent or caretaker is unable to adequately detail the progress of these developmental milestones. Table 17.1 provides guidelines regarding normal skills (4). The parent or caretaker can provide information regarding the child's academic progress and social behavior, as well as the child's ability to adapt in a normal everyday lifestyle. Many times, the child's capabilities and limitations can be observed during the evaluation period in the office.

In review of the general health of the child, a chronological order of symptoms, signs and treatment should be analyzed. The category of general health should include immunizations, medications, diagnostic test, injuries, surgical procedures, medical treatment and hospitalizations (3). Social behavior can be easily observed, and with adequate inquiry, one can determine the activity capabilities, temperament, sleeping habits, eating patterns, discipline problems and interactive skills. The doctor can gain a vast amount of knowledge about the child by having the child, parent or caretaker give a description of a "typical day" for the child. As with all patients, the clinical history provides a wealth of cumulative information in which the doctor can use to determine an accurate diagnosis, treatment plan and prognosis for the patient.

Examination

As with any patient, cooperation is essential in obtaining accurate findings. The patient should be in a comfortable and appropriate position for examination. A flexible approach to the child is necessary; initial evaluation should begin with general observation of the child and his/her capabilities. Throughout the evaluation, the doctor should be aware of the developmental stage of the child (5) (Table 17.1). A significant amount of information can be collated about the neuromuscular system, alertness, behavior, and parent-child interaction by observing the child in spontaneous activities (6). The neurological examination begins with observation; special attention is given to the child's gait, motor function, and postural deviances. The doctor must take advantage of opportunities provided by the patient (4). Should the patient be confined to a wheelchair, the doctor must make adaptations to properly evaluate the child in this position (Figs. 17.1, 17.2). If the child is able to sit on his/her own, the cervical chair is an appropriate tool to be used for the evaluation.

One component of the chiropractic evaluation is the use of a hand held temperature differential instrument (7–9). If the

697

Table 17.1. **Screening Protocol for Developmental Delay**

Age: 3 mo.

Gross motor: Supports weight on forearms

Fine motor: Opens hands spontaneously

Social skills: Smiles appropriately

Language: Coos, laughs

Age: 6 mo.

Gross motor: Sits

Fine motor: Momentarily transfers objects

Social skills: Shows like and dislike

Language: Babbles

Age: 9 mo.

Gross motor: Pulls to stand

Fine motor: Grasps (Pincer)

Social skills: Plays patty cake & peek-a-boo

Language: Imitates sound

Age: 12 mo.

Gross motor: Walks with one hand held

Fine motor: Releases object on command

Social skills: Comes when called

Language: Speaks one to two meaningful words

Age: 18 mo.

Gross motor: Walks upstairs with assistance

Fine motor: Feeds from a spoon

Social skills: Mimics actions of others

Language: Speaks at least six words

Age: 24 mo.

Gross motor: Runs

Fine motor: Builds a tower of six blocks

Social skills: Plays with others

Language: Speaks two- to three-word sentences

patient is able to sit, the instrument can be used in a normal glide pattern. If unable to sit, the child may be more comfortable in a prone position for this portion of the examination.

When evaluating the child for evidence of vertebral subluxation, motion and static palpation of the spine and paraspinal areas for tenderness, edematous areas, hypertonicity or hypotonicity of musculature reveals potential levels of vertebral subluxation (10). Intersegmental motion palpation of the spine from occiput to the sacrum (including sacroiliac articulations) provides useful clinical information regarding the biomechanical function or lack of normal function of the joint (10).

To appropriately evaluate the child, plain film radiography is a fundamental way of determining if chiropractic treatment will be appropriate (11). Spinal alignment derived from a specific radiographic marking system can add to the analysis of the child regarding the application of a specific chiropractic adjustment. To appropriately evaluate the child, full spine radiographs taken anterior to posterior (AP) in a single exposure and also a lateral projection taken in two exposures are recommended (12), provided the patient can be adequately positioned. In certain disorders covered in this chapter, additional views may be recommended to properly assess the biomechanics of the spine.

In summary, the chiropractic evaluation and examination of the challenged child requires patience on the part of all parties involved. Many times, the examination may require more than one office visit depending on the child's physical status, emotional and mental capabilities, as well as the child's level of cooperation during this important portion of the child's care.

Common Disorders

The following section is a collation of the most commonly seen challenged-child disorders in this author's practice. A chiro-

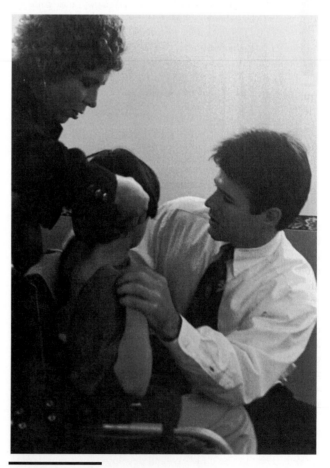

Figure 17.1. Assessment of upper cervical mobility in Y-axis rotation in a patient with cerebral palsy.

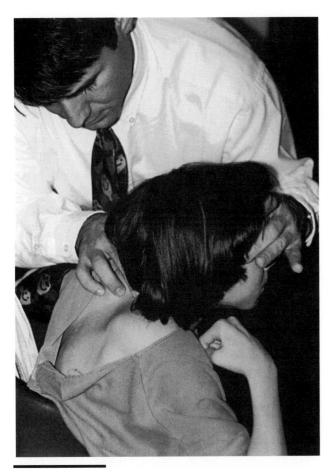

Figure 17.2.   Motion palpation of the lower cervical spine in a patient with cerebral palsy.

practic approach to each disorder is presented as well as information regarding prognosis, where applicable.

Cerebral Palsy

In the United States, approximately 300,000 individuals manifest this central motor deficit. This syndrome is described as a nonprogressive motor disorder resulting from gestational or perinatal CNS damage and characterized by an impairment of voluntary movement (13). In this category of neurologic defect there is evidence of a major disturbance of motor function. Numerous causes of cerebral palsy have been investigated; these include physical trauma to the brain at birth (4), complications of pregnancy which include placental complications, abnormalities or presentation (face, brow, and transverse), breech delivery, prolapse of the umbilical cord, and fetal growth retardation, although most term growth-retarded infants develop normally (14,15). For low birth weight infants born by breech delivery, the cerebral palsy rate reached almost 5% in a study performed at the National Institute of Neurological and Communicative Disorders (14). Risk factors include child abuse, prematurity, encephalopathy or seizures in the perinatal period, interventricular hemorrhage in the perinatal period, in-utero infections, postnatal meningitis or encephalitis, and hypoxic ischemia (16).

Intrapartum fetal asphyxia has been implicated as a cause of cerebral palsy, although most cases of cerebral palsy occur in persons without evidence of birth asphyxia or other intrapartum events (17–20). Based on formalized review processes the U.S. Preventive Services Task Force has not recommended that routine electronic fetal monitoring for low risk women in labor be used (21). The Task Force also concluded that there was insufficient evidence to recommend for or against intrapartum electronic fetal monitoring for high-risk pregnant women.

CLINICAL SIGNS AND SYMPTOMS

Cerebral palsy can be grouped into four main categories: spastic, athetoid, ataxic, and mixed forms. Spastic syndromes are most common, representing approximately 70% of the cases (13). The spastic form of cerebral palsy is characterized by stiff, awkward movements of the affected limbs, muscular hypertonicity, increased deep tendon reflexes, "scissors gait" and toe-walking of the lower extremities. There may be stiffness and incoordination of the hands and arms evident in spastic quadriplegia. This form accounts for 30% of cerebral palsy cases, and these children are generally markedly retarded and nonambulatory (22). Children with spastic hemiplegia or paraplegia frequently have normal intelligence and a good prognosis for social independence (13). Movements of the extremities are slow, writhing and involuntary. Emotional tension seems to cause an increase in the motions with a disappearance of the motions during sleep. Ataxic cerebral palsy is commonly associated with sclerotic lesions of the cerebellum (22). These patients have difficulty with rapidity of fine movement, weakness, incoordination and a wide based gait. The fourth category of cerebral palsy is the mixed form. These are classified most often as spasticity and athetosis; less often, ataxia and athetosis (13).

RADIOLOGIC EVALUATION

In addition to the full spine AP and lateral views, a flexion view of the cervical region is beneficial in determining the potential vertebral subluxation. It is often difficult to radiograph these children and technological assistance is of utmost importance. Due to the patient's condition multiple levels of malalignment will usually be present. It is of utmost importance to evaluate the mobility of any motion segment determined to need an adjustment and all adjustments should be administered in ways that promote improved posture of the spine at both the segmental and global level.

A subluxation is often detected in the upper cervical region in the patient with cerebral palsy, either as an effect of the disorder or preceding it, most commonly the antero-superior (AS) condyle (23). The integrity of the position of the occiput in relationship to the atlas is noted on the neutral lateral, flexion and AP cervical views. When the condyle slips anterior and superior, the space between the posterior arch of the atlas and the occiput is diminished. The space will remain closed even when the cervical spine is in flexion (24).

Abnormalities of the brain, identifiable with CT and/or MRI include cysts, cerebral atrophy, calcification, tumors, malformation and stroke (16).

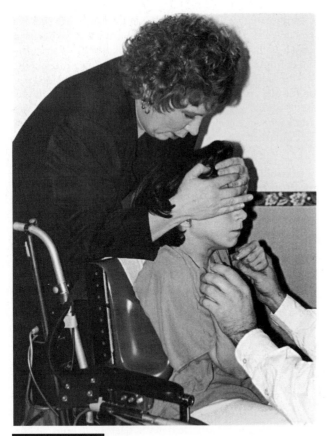

Figure 17.3. Adjustment of an AS condyle subluxation in a patient with cerebral palsy.

SUBLUXATION CONSIDERATIONS

The vertebral subluxation complex can be determined by visual inspection, motion and static palpation, and instrumentation. The correlation of these findings, along with radiographic studies are optimal in the location and correction of the vertebral subluxation. Special attention should be directed to the upper cervical region; many times the child will present with a "starward gaze" in their head presentation. This could be indicative of an AS condyle misalignment. Careful analyzing of this region, along with the entire spine (including the cranium and pelvis) can produce the specific level of the vertebral subluxation. In correlating the objective findings along with the radiological findings, a specific listing can be determined, thus assisting in a specific correction (Figs. 17.3–17.6).

After analyzing the cerebral palsy child and determining the area of subluxation, a specific adjustment is necessary. The adjusting thrust should be gentle, as well as specific due to the spasticity in many of these children. The thrust should also be of a high velocity, low amplitude character.

Cranial and pelvic structures should be checked carefully for subluxation and addressed accordingly. The removal of neurological stresses that may be present can promote a more normal functioning of the nervous system, resulting in improved general resistance.

PROGNOSIS

The child with cerebral palsy has many special needs. In caring for these children, special time should be appropriated for not only evaluation and adjusting, but for communication with their caretakers. In this author's experience many parents have noted a more positive attitude, relaxation, improved sleep patterns, better coordination and stronger resistance to stresses. These observations should be systematically evaluated for evidence of efficacy.

Spinal contractures will increase during growth, resulting in scoliosis. This factor will require careful scrutiny by the attending chiropractor. The general course for most patients is to improve in function with time (16).

General follow-up is important in patients with cerebral palsy by the appropriate health care provider. Specific areas to be addressed during the child's growth are the development of contractures, epilepsy, learning disabilities, strabismus, hearing loss, and mental retardation (16).

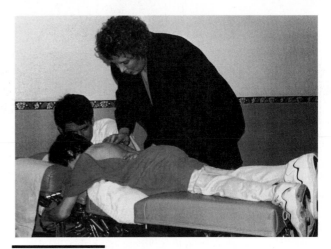

Figure 17.4. Demonstration of a vertebral count in the prone position.

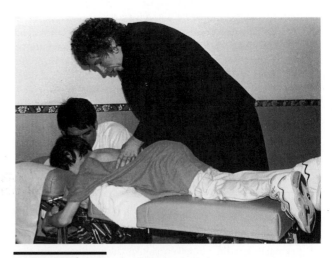

Figure 17.5. Thoracic adjustment in the prone position on the hi-lo table with a double-thumb contact.

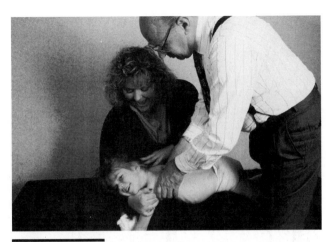

Figure 17.6. Prone thoracic adjustment using an assistant/ parent in a patient with cerebral palsy.

Down Syndrome

John Langdon Down was the first to publish a study on children with exaggerated mongoloid facial features, mental retardation, and hypotonia (25). These manifestations, along with other recognizable appearances constitute what is called Down syndrome. Down syndrome is caused by trisomy of chromosome 21 or translocation of parts of this chromosome (22). It is the most common chromosome abnormality and occurs in all races with equal frequency (26).

Ninety percent of patients have the extra chromosome 21 in all cells. Translocation of the chromosome occurs in 5% of cases usually to number 13 or 15. For these cases one half are new and the other half is from a parental carrier. Another 5% of cases have been termed Mosaic because two or more cell populations are found, usually trisomy with normal cells. The clinical manifestations in these patients are usually more mild (26).

Population-based surveillance programs have reported a Down syndrome birth prevalence of 0.9/1,000 live births. The incidence of Down syndrome is higher than the birth prevalence, however, since many fetuses are spontaneously aborted, some are recognized in utero and electively aborted, and some cases are not recognized at birth.

Affected children are characterized by physical abnormalities that include congenital heart defects and other dysmorphisms, and varying degrees of mental and growth retardation. Although there are therapies for some of the specific malformations associated with Down syndrome, there are no proven therapies available for the cognitive deficits. Life expectancy for infants born with Down syndrome is substantially lower than that of the general population. Based on 1988 cross-sectional data, the lifetime economic costs of Down syndrome have been estimated to be $410,000 per case (27).

The risk for Down syndrome and certain other chromosome anomalies increases substantially with advancing maternal age. At age 20 the risk for Down syndrome is approximately 1/2000, at age 35 it increases to 1/200, 1/100 at age 37, and 1/20 at age 45 (26).

Parents carrying chromosome-21 rearrangements are also at an increased risk of Down syndrome pregnancies, with the risk being much higher if the mother carries the rearrangement than if the father does. Also at higher risk are those who have previously had an affected pregnancy, independent of advancing maternal age and chromosome rearrangements (27).

SCREENING FOR DOWN SYNDROME

Prenatal diagnostic testing is accurate and reliable for detecting Down syndrome, but it is associated with a procedure-related fetal loss (i.e., death) of about 0.5% for second-trimester amniocentesis and 1.0–1.5% for chorionic villus sampling (CVS), and a measurable risk of transverse fetal limb deficiency after CVS. The currently accepted medical practice of routinely offering amniocentesis or CVS for prenatal diagnosis to pregnant women ages 35 and older or otherwise at high risk is based on the mother's increased risk of having a fetus with a chromosome abnormality balanced against the risk of fetal loss associated with these procedures and therefore includes an element of judgment (27). It can be predicted from available data (i.e., odds of Down syndrome during the second trimester) that a program offering amniocentesis to all pregnant women at age 35 has the potential of exposing 200–300 normal fetuses to this procedure for every case detected (27–28). With an estimated procedure-related fetal loss rate of 0.5%, a normal fetus would be lost by amniocentesis for every one to two chromosome anomalies detected in such women. For CVS, the number of normal fetuses lost per case detected would be higher, and for first-trimester amniocentesis, it may be higher still. The older the maternal age, the more favorable is the ratio of affected fetuses to fetal loss. Most women who request such testing and receive a diagnosis of a Down syndrome pregnancy choose to abort the pregnancy, resulting in a measurable reduction in Down syndrome births (27).

For those for whom Down screening is an option, identification and selective abortion of Down syndrome pregnancies raise important ethical concerns, a full discussion of which is beyond the scope of this chapter. These concerns include the implicit message that Down syndrome is an undesirable state, the interpretation of induced abortions in eugenic terms by some persons, and societal and economic pressures that may stigmatize families with a Down syndrome member. Attitudes held by both physicians and by society towards individuals with Down syndrome have changed over time, and various Down syndrome associations now offer support for families and individuals with Down syndrome, promote their participation in society, and seek respect for them (29–30). These issues highlight the importance of offering screening and prenatal diagnosis of Down syndrome in a value-sensitive fashion with emphasis on reliable information about Down syndrome itself as well as about the potential risks and benefits of screening procedures (27).

The United States Preventive Services Task Force has recommended the offering of amniocentesis or chorionic villus sampling for chromosome studies for pregnant women ages 35 and older and to those at high risk of Down syndrome for other reasons (e.g., previous affected pregnancy, known carriage of a chromosome rearrangement associated with

Down syndrome). The Task Force also recommends the offering of screening for Down syndrome by serum multiple-marker testing for all low-risk pregnant women, and as an alternative to amniocentesis and CVS for high risk women. This testing should be offered only to women who are seen for prenatal care in locations that have adequate counseling and follow-up services (27).

CLINICAL SIGNS AND SYMPTOMS

Many of the signs of Down syndrome can be recognized in the neonatal period. The child may present with a combination of any of the following. The sill tends to be small and round with flattening of the occiput. The ears are small and dysplastic (31). The eyes slant slightly upward and outward owing to the presence of a medial epicanthal fold and gray-white specks of depigmentation are seen in the iris (i.e., Brushfield's spots) (22). The nose appears to be flattened with no apparent bridge. Features of the mouth include corners turned down, highly arched palate and the tongue is usually enlarged and protruding. The hands are short and broad with single transverse palmar crease. The fingers are often short and curved inward (22). The neck exhibits loose skin posteriorly and the pelvis is dysplastic (31). Congenital defects, usually cardiac, are found in come cases.

RADIOLOGIC EVALUATION

The reported incidence of atlantoaxial instability in Down varies from 15% up to 50% (32). This instability is due to the absence of the transverse ligament of the atlas. It is imperative that radiographs, especially of the cervical region, are taken to determine the atlanto-dental interval (ADI). The normal ADI distance is 2 to 5 mm on a lateral cervical radiograph. Any distance greater that 5 mm is indicative of atlanto-axial ligament instability (33). The views to be taken must include a neutral lateral view, full cervical flexion and extension views of the cervical spine. It is also recommended that weightbearing full spine AP and lateral radiographs be taken to assess other biomechanical abnormalities or spinal anomalies.

SUBLUXATION CONSIDERATIONS

Neurological examinations should include the evaluation of muscle tone, gait disturbances, deep tendon reflexes and Babinski's sign. Most infants with Down syndrome exhibit subluxations of the atlas, axis or occiput most frequently, with cranial base faults being the next most common area of involvement (31). In several cases there has been evidence of lumbosacral subluxations, therefore, this area of the spine cannot be overlooked. Many of these children exhibit poor muscle tone and hyperlaxity of the musculature, so the adjusting thrust should be gentle with a low force and depth but high velocity.

PROGNOSIS

Clum (34) suggests that chiropractic care be investigated as an alternative to traditional allopathic care in the care of the Down syndrome patient. The conservative method of chiropractic care is one way of improving the quality of life for Down children. This author has observed positive changes in Down syndrome patients undergoing chiropractic care including more calmness and an increase in patience, as well as increased abilities in walking and running, along with general coordination improvement. Correction of the subluxation can only create more normal function of an already challenged system. It is important that both medical clinicians and as well as researchers consider the role of chiropractic in the health of the Down syndrome patient.

Complications in patients with Down syndrome include congenital heart disease in the form of endocardial cushion defect or ventricular septal defects occurring in 50% of patients. Bowel obstruction from intestinal fistulas or anomalies occurs in 10% of cases. Hyper or hypothyroidism is present in 5–8% of patients and Hirschsprung's disease occurs in 3% (26).

The natural history of Down syndrome is as follows. Approximately one-third of cases develop normally during their first year of life, the other two-thirds being mildly delayed. After the age of one, the child's development slows with language and cognition being moderately delayed. The patient's long-term outcome and longevity is dependent primarily on the presence or absence of congenital heart disease. Premature aging occurs and most individuals die at 50–60 years. After the age of 35 one-third of patients have clinical Alzheimer's disease (26).

Some adult individuals can work in protected situations. A small percentage of individuals can function largely independently. Most adults can care for their personal needs and although they are retarded (IQ = 40–45), they are usually very personable and cooperative. A small percentage of patients are nonverbal and some individuals have autistic features (26).

Attention Deficit Hyperactivity Disorder

As early as March 1902, Dr. George Still spoke before the Royal College of Physicians in London regarding children "who seemed to him restless, passionate, and apt to get into trouble." Still's lecture is often billed as the first recorded discussion of hyperactivity (35). The term "attention deficit disorder" is defined as developmentally inappropriate inattention and impulsivity, with or without hyperactivity (13). ADD or ADHD may be known as the single most prevalent childhood behavioral problem today. ADD is many times linked with learning disabilities or disorders. Researchers agree that ADHD is estimated to occur in 5–10% of school age children with incidence four to six times greater in boys than girls (4).

CLINICAL SIGNS AND SYMPTOMS

The primary signs of ADD with or without hyperactivity are a child's display of inattention or impulsivity. ADD with hyperactivity is noted when the signs of overactivity are obvious (13). According to recent guidelines for attention deficit hyperactivity disorder, the problem must be noticed before the age of seven and must persist for at least 6 months (36). The following criteria are used by parents, teachers, and health care providers to adequately recognize this disorder:

1. Fidgets with hands or feet or squirms in seat (restlessness)
2. Has difficulty remaining seated when required to do so
3. Is easily distracted by extraneous stimuli
4. Has difficulty waiting turn in games or group situations
5. Often blurts out answers before the question has been completed
6. Has difficulty sustaining attention in tasks or play activities
7. Often shifts from one uncompleted activity to another
8. Has difficulty playing quietly
9. Often talks excessively
10. Often interrupts or intrudes on others
11. Often does not seem to listen to what is being said to him or her
12. Often loses items that are necessary for tasks or activities without considering possible consequences

One must realize that many of these signs are subjective and rely on a particular person's judgment. A study performed by two Canadian researchers, Cohen and Minde (35), found that most of the children who had been diagnosed with ADHD had altogether different psychological problems or else seemed to be suffering poor nutrition or too little sleep; only 0.8% were categorized as hyperactive after a more rigorous screening. Many times motor incoordination, neurologic immaturity and minimal brain dysfunction are noted. Some problems may have their origin in prenatal or postnatal birth trauma (37). In some studies of ADHD, there is evidence that diminished activity of the brain neurotransmitter dopamine may exist and that this neurotransmitter abnormality may contribute to the pathophysiology of this syndrome (38). Others have implicated food allergies, diet and the indiscriminate use of antibiotics in contributing to this syndrome in children (39).

SUBLUXATION CONSIDERATIONS

As with any chiropractic patient, the entire spine should be analyzed for potential vertebral subluxations; however, the doctor should devote special attention to the upper cervical region (i.e., C0 to C3) in these cases (23). There is a correlation between upper cervical adjustments and apparent improvement in mental function (40). Giesen et al. (41), in a time-series investigation noted that hyperactivity and other impairments of patients responded well to chiropractic care. Studies showing microtrauma of brain stem tissues and suboccipital structures, usually as a result of birth trauma, resulting in abnormal motor development (42,43) reveal the necessity for specific evaluation and correction of vertebral subluxation in the child exhibiting ADD or ADHD.

PROGNOSIS

No definitive studies exist on the effects of chiropractic care either in the short or long term on individuals with ADHD. The natural history of the disorder suggests that the overt restlessness tends to diminish in adolescence, but that impulsiveness and emotional liability usually persist (44). Large-scale follow-up studies of ADHD have confirmed a less favorable outcome of hyperactive children compared to control groups, although many hyperactive persons do well (44). When aggressiveness is a feature of the disorder, it usually persists and appears also to be related to the development of early onset alcoholism (45,46).

ADHD tends to last through school years and on into adulthood. The disorder becomes easier to control with increasing age (47). Although Ritalin (methylphenidate) is the universal medical panacea for ADHD, its widespread prescription by medical physicians is very controversial (48). Parents should make use of conservative measures first in the child diagnosed with ADHD, including chiropractic (38,40), nutritional (39) and psychosocial or behavioral factors (35).

Fetal Alcohol Syndrome

Fetal alcohol syndrome (FAS) is seen in babies born to mothers who consume alcohol during their pregnancy. Even moderate maternal alcohol consumption (2–3 ounces of hard liquor per day) may produce fetal alcohol effects (49). Maternal alcohol abuse is thought to be the most common cause of mental retardation (49). Infants born to chronic alcoholic mothers not only exhibit signs of mental retardation, but also prenatal and postnatal growth deficiency and other malformations.

Alcohol problems are common in the primary care setting, but they often go undetected by clinicians (50). Although imperfect, asking patients direct questions about the quantity, frequency, and pattern of their drinking is an important way to identify those who are most likely to experience problems due to alcohol. Questions about tolerance to the effects of alcohol may circumvent denial among pregnant women and heavy drinkers. The CAGE (Table 17.2) and other brief screening instruments are useful supplements to the standard patient history, but they may be less sensitive for early problems and hazardous drinking. The AUDIT (Table 17.3) may detect a broader range of current drinking problems, but its performance in the primary care setting needs further evaluation. Although laboratory tests such as GGT are not sufficiently

---

Table 17.2.   Four-question CAGE Instrument (Popular Screening Tool in the Primary Care Setting)

C: "Have you ever felt you ought to Cut down on drinking?"

A: "Have people Annoyed you by criticizing your drinking?"

G: "Have you ever felt bad or Guilty about your drinking?"

E: "Have you ever had a drink first thing in the morning to steady your nerves or get rid of a hangover (Eye opener)?"

sensitive or specific for routine screening, they may be useful in selected high-risk patients to confirm clinical suspicion or to motivate changes in drinking. Neither questionnaires nor laboratory tests should be considered diagnostic of problem drinking without more detailed evaluation (50).

The U.S. Preventive Services Task Force (50) has recommended the following clinical interventions for primary care physicians. Screening to detect problem drinking and hazardous drinking is recommended for all adult and adolescent patients. Screening should involve a careful history of alcohol use and/or the use of standardized screening questionnaires. Patients should be asked to describe the quantity, frequency, and other characteristics of their use of wine, beer, and liquor, including frequency of intoxication and tolerance to the effects of alcohol. One drink is defined as 12 ounces of beer, a 5-ounce glass of wine, or one 1.5 fluid ounces of distilled spirits. Brief questionnaires such as the CAGE or AUDIT may help clinicians assess the likelihood of problem drinking or hazardous drinking. Responses suggestive of problem drinking should be confirmed with more extensive discussions with the patient (and family members where indicated) about patterns of use, problems related to drinking, and symptoms of alcohol dependence (51). Routine measurement of biochemical markers, such as serum GGT (y-glutamyl transferase), are not recommended for screening purposes. Discussions with adolescents should be approached with discretion to establish a trusting relationship and to respect the patient's concerns about the confidentiality of disclosed information.

All pregnant women should be screened for evidence of problem drinking or risk drinking (two drinks per day or binge drinking). Including questions about tolerance to alcohol may improve detection of at-risk women. All pregnant women and

Table 17.3. AUDIT Structured Interview

Question	Score				
	0	1	2	3	4
How often do you have a drink containing alcohol?	Never	Monthly or less	2–4 times/mo	2–3 times/wk	4 or more times/wk
How many drinks do you have on a typical day when you are drinking?	None	1 or 2	3 or 4	5 or 6	7–9*
How often do you have six or more drinks on one occasion?	Never	Less than monthly	Monthly	Weekly	Daily or almost daily
How often during the last year have you found that you were unable to stop drinking once you had started?	Never	Less than monthly	Monthly	Weekly	Daily or almost daily
How often last year have you failed to do what was normally expected from you because of drinking?	Never	Less than monthly	Monthly	Weekly	Daily or almost daily
How often during the last year have you needed a first drink in the morning to get yourself going after a heavy drinking session?	Never	Less than monthly	Monthly	Weekly	Daily or almost daily
How often during the last year have you had a feeling of guilt or remorse after drinking?	Never	Less than monthly	Monthly	Weekly	Daily or almost daily
How often during the last year have you been unable to remember what happened the night before because you had been drinking?	Never	Less than monthly	Monthly	Weekly	Daily or almost daily
Have you or someone else been injured as a result of your drinking?	Never	Yes, but not in last year (2 points)		Yes, during the last year (4 points)	
Has a relative, doctor, or other health worker been concerned about your drinking or suggested you cut down?	Never	Yes, but not in last year (2 points)		Yes, during the last year (4 points)	

A score greater than 8 (out of 41) is suggestive of problem drinking and indicates a need for more in-depth assessment. Cut-off of 10 points recommended by some to provide greater specificity. ★5 points if response is 10 or more drinks on a typical day. Reprinted with permission from the U.S. Preventive Services Task Force. Guide to clinical preventive services, 2nd ed. Baltimore: Williams & Wilkins, 1996:577.

women contemplating pregnancy should be informed of the harmful effects of alcohol on the fetus and advised to limit or cease drinking. Although there is insufficient evidence to prove or disprove harms from occasional, light drinking during pregnancy, abstinence from alcohol can be recommended on other grounds: possible risk from even low-level exposure to alcohol, lack of harm from abstaining, and prevailing expert opinion. Women who smoke should be advised that the risk of low birth weight is greatest for mothers who both smoke and drink (50).

Patients with evidence of alcohol dependence should be referred, where possible, to appropriate clinical specialists or community programs specialized in the treatment of alcohol dependence. Patients with evidence of alcohol abuse or hazardous drinking should be offered brief advice and counseling. Counseling should involve feedback of the evidence of a drinking problem, discussion of the role of alcohol in current health or psychosocial problems, direct advice to reduce consumption, and plan for regular follow-up. Problems related to alcohol, such as physical symptoms, behavioral or mood problems, or difficulties at work or home, should be monitored to determine whether further interventions are needed. There is no single definition of "hazardous" drinking in asymptomatic persons, but successful intervention trials have generally defined five drinks per day in men, three drinks per day in women, or frequent intoxication to identify persons at risk. Several U.S. organizations have suggested lower limits for "safe" drinking: two drinks per day in men and one drink per day in women (52). All persons who drink alcohol should be informed of the dangers of driving or other potentially dangerous activities after drinking. The use of alcohol should be discouraged in persons younger than the legal age for drinking, although the effectiveness of alcohol abstinence messages in the primary care setting is uncertain (50).

CLINICAL SIGNS AND SYMPTOMS

The infant who is subjected to maternal alcohol abuse should be observed carefully within 72 hours after delivery. Clinical signs include irritability, vomiting, diarrhea, sweating and convulsions. Newborns rarely die from withdrawal, but long-term effects have not been studied (13).

SUBLUXATION CONSIDERATIONS

As with any newborn, it is optimum if the Fetal Alcohol Syndrome child can be evaluated as soon after birth as possible. This author has observed that these children often exhibit primary subluxations in the upper cervical region. The author has also observed that FAS patients under chiropractic care appear to have an improved quality of rest, restoration of normal muscle tone and remission of digestive disturbances. These observations should be systematically evaluated by clinicians and scientists in order to determine the relative efficacy of different treatment strategies.

Summary

In summary, the needs of the challenged child are great. It takes a team of caring individuals to work together for the good of

Table 17.4. Organizations and Clinics for Children with Special Needs

Kentuckiana Children's Center
P.O. Box 16039
Louisville, KY 40256-0039
502-366-4658

Oklahaven Children's Chiropractic Center
4500 N Meridian Ave.
Oklahoma City, Oklahoma 73112-2404
405-948-8807

Resources for Children with Special Needs, Inc.
212-677-4650

National Parent Resource Center, Federation for
    Children with Special Needs
617-482-2915

Administration on Children, Youth and Families, Dept.
    of Health and Human Resources
202-205-8348

Local or State Chapters of United Way

Crippled Children Services (State regulated)
National Number
800-772-1213

Special Olympics International
202-628-3660

United States Organization for Disabled Athletes
516-484-3701

National Wheelchair Athletic Association
719-574-1150

National Down Syndrome Congress
1-800-232-NDSC
listserv@vm1.nodak.edu

United Cerebral Palsy Associations
7 Penn Plaza, Suite 804
New York, NY 10001
1-800-USA-1UCP

the child. Clinically, doctors of chiropractic are working as a part of this team to assist the child in achieving optimal function. As part of the responsibility, one must sometimes assist the parents in seeking organizations designed to aid in the child's special needs. Table 17.4 includes a list of organizations that may be beneficial for the parents of a challenged child (37,53).

REFERENCES

1. Nelson K, Ellenberg J. Obstetric complications as risk factors for cerebral palsy or seizure disorders. JAMA 1984; 1843–1848.
2. Swaiman KF, Wright FS. The practice of pediatric neurology, 2nd ed. St. Louis: CV Mosby Co., 1982.
3. Molnar GE. A developmental perspective for the rehabilitation of children with physical disabilities. Pediatric Annual 1988; 17:766.
4. Behrmann E. Textbook of pediatrics, 14th ed. Philadelphia: WB Saunders Co., 1992.

5. Illingworth RS. Development of the infant and young child: normal and abnormal. New York: Churchill Livingstone, 1987.

6. Brown SB. Neurologic examination during the first 2 years of life. St. Louis: CV Mosby Co., 1982.

7. Plaugher G. Skin temperature assessment for neuromusculoskeletal abnormalities of the spinal column. J Manipulative Physiol Ther 1992; 15:365–381.

8. Plaugher G, Lopes MA, Melch PE, Cremata EE. The inter- and intraexaminer reliability of a paraspinal skin temperature differential instrument. J Manipulative Physiol Ther 1991; 14:361–367.

9. Ebrall PS, Iggo A, Hobson P, Farrant G. Preliminary report: the thermal characteristics of spinal levels identified as having differential temperature by contact thermocouple measurement (Nervo Scope). Chiro J Australia 1994; 24:139–146.

10. Lopes MA, Plaugher G, Walters PJ, Cremata EE. Spinal examination. In Plaugher G, ed. Textbook of clinical chiropractic: a specific biomechanical approach. Baltimore: Williams and Wilkins, 1993;73–111.

11. Plaugher G. The role of plain film radiography in chiropractic clinical practice. Chiropractic Journal of Australia 1992; 22:153–161.

12. Rowe SH, Ray SG, Jakubowski AM, Picardi PJ. Plain film radiography in chiropractic. In: Plaugher G, ed. Textbook of clinical chiropractic: a specific biomechanical approach. Baltimore: Williams and Wilkins, 1993;112–149.

13. Holvey D. The Merck manual. Merck & Co., Inc. 1972.

14. Nelson K, Ellenber J. Obstetric complications as risk factors for cerebral palsy or seizure disorders. JAMA 1983:1843–1848.

15. Goldenberg RL, Davis RO, Nelson KG. Intrauterine growth retardation. In: Merkatz IR, Thompson JE, eds. New perspectives on prenatal care. New York: Elsevier, 1990;461–478.

16. Russman BS. Cerebral palsy. In: Dambro MR, ed. Griffith's 5 minute clinical consult. Baltimore: Williams & Wilkins, 1996;188–189.

17. Freeman JM, Nelson KB. Intrapartum asphyxia and cerebral palsy. Pediatrics 1988; 82:240–249.

18. Nelson KB, Ellenberg JH. Antecedents of cerebral palsy. Multivariate analysis of risk. N Engl J Med 1986; 315:81–86.

19. Shy KK, Larson EB, Luthy DA. Evaluating a new technology: the effectiveness of electronic fetal heart rate monitoring. Annu Rev Public Health 1987; 8:165–190.

20. Goodlin RC, Haesslein HC. When is it fetal distress? Am J Obstet Gynecol 1977; 128:440–445.

21. U.S. Preventive Services Task Force. Guide to clinical preventive services, 2nd ed. Baltimore: Williams & Wilkins, 1996;433–442.

22. Jeffers J, Scott E. Principles of internal medicine. 11th ed. McGraw-Hill, Inc: 1987.

23. Anrig CA. Chiropractic approaches to pregnancy and pediatric care. In: Plaugher G, ed. Textbook of clinical chiropractic: a specific biomechanical approach. Baltimore: Williams and Wilkins, 1993:383–432.

24. Cox D. The condyle subluxation in Infants. Intl Rev Chiro 1991; Mar/Apr:23–29.

25. LaFrancis M. A chiropractic perspective on atlantoaxial instability in Down's syndrome. J Manipulative Physiol Ther 1990; 13:157–159.

26. Benke PJ. Down's syndrome. In: Dambro MR, ed. Griffith's 5 minute clinical consult. Baltimore: Williams & Wilkins, 1996:324–325.

27. U.S. Preventive Services Task Force. Guide to clinical preventive services, 2nd ed. Baltimore: Williams & Wilkins, 1996:449–465.

28. Palomaki GE, Haddow JE. Maternal serum alpha-fetoprotein, age, and Down syndrome risk. Am J Obstet Gynecol 1987; 156:460–463.

29. Haslam R, Milner R. The physician and Down syndrome: are attitudes changing? J Child Neurol 1992; 7:304–310.

30. Inglese C. Is the cultural approach towards Down's syndrome people changing? Am J Med Genet 1990; 7:322–323.

31. McMullen M. Handicapped infants and chiropractic care. Int'l Rev Chiro 1990; July/Aug: 32–35.

32. Haldeman S. Modern developments in the principles and practice of chiropractic. New York: Appleton-Century-Crofts, 1986;369.

33. Yochum TR, Rowe LJ. Essentials of skeletal radiology. Baltimore: Williams & Wilkins, 1987.

34. Clum GW. Atlantoaxial subluxation in Down's syndrome. Today's Chiropractic 1985 May/Jun:33–36.

35. Kohn A. Suffer the restless children. Atlantic Monthly 1989 Nov:90–100.

36. Gundersen K. The misunderstood child. April 1989:1–3.

37. Gordon S, Dickman I. Learning disabilities-a family affair. Public Affairs Committee, Inc. April 1983.

38. Webster L. The hyperactive child and chiropractic. Today's Chiropractic. 73–74.

39. Crook WG. Help for the hyperactive child. Jackson, Tennessee: Professional Books, 1991.

40. Thomas MD, Wood J. Upper cervical adjustments may improve mental function. J Manual Med 1992; 7:215–216.

41. Giesen M, Center D, Leach R. An evaluation of chiropractic manipulation as a treatment of hyperactivity in children. J Manipulative Physiol Ther 1989; 12: 353–363.

42. Biedermann H. Kinematic imbalances due to suboccipital strain in newborns. J Manual Med. 1992: 6:151–156.

43. Gottlieb M. Neglected spinal cord, brain stem and musculoskeletal injuries stemming from birth trauma. J Manipulative Physiol Ther 1993; 16:537–543.

44. Kinsbourne M. Disorders of mental development. In: Menkes JH. Textbook of child neurology, 5th ed. Baltimore: Williams & Wilkins, 1995:924–964.

45. Kellam SG, Ensminger ME, Simon MB. Mental health in first grade and teenage drug, alcohol, and cigarette use. Drug Alcohol Depend 1980; 5:273–304.

46. Tarter RE, Alterman AI, Edwards KL. Vulnerability to alcoholism in men: a behavior-genetic perspective. J Stud on Alcohol 1985; 46:329–356.

47. Novak LL. Attention deficit hyperactivity disorder. In: Dambro MR, ed. Griffith's 5 minute clinical consult. Baltimore: Williams & Wilkins, 1996:108–109.

48. Hancock L. Mother's little helper. Newsweek 1996; March 18:51–56.

49. Moore K. The developing human. Philadelphia: WB Saunders, 1988.

50. U.S. Preventive Services Task Force. Guide to clinical preventive services, 2nd ed. Baltimore: Williams & Wilkins, 1996:567–582.

51. American Psychiatric Association. Diagnostic and statistical manual of mental disorders, 4th ed. Washington, D.C.: American Psychiatric Association, 1994.

52. Bradley KA, Donovan DM, Larson EB. How much is too much? Advising patients about safe levels of alcohol consumption. Arch Intern Med 1993; 153:2734–2740.

53. Faust-Baron R. Exceptional families-meeting the medical needs of children with physical disabilities, 1993; Nov:115–126.

18 Care of the Adolescent

Phillip S. Ebrall

*A*s adults, we may recall our adolescence as a time of optimism, idealism, and potential (1). Sadly, today more than ever, adolescence is also a time of stress and social conflict (2), with some youth finding the structure they seek for their lives in the shopping malls of suburbia (3). On the one hand, adolescence is a time when the individual faces many potential health care problems, and on the other, it is the ideal time for preventive care (1). Adolescent medicine has existed as a discipline for about 35 years; today it is growing, with a developing number of professional organizations for those interested in providing health services to this group (4,5).

Adolescent health care makes front page news (6) but has not, until now, seriously drawn the interest of the chiropractic profession. The medical profession is coming to grips with its responsibilities to provide specialized health care for the adolescent population (7–9) and the Society for Adolescent Medicine (8) has identified the five key issues:

1. Quality of health care for adolescents
2. Research
3. Health services for adolescents
4. Communications among health professionals caring for adolescents
5. Training of individuals providing care to adolescents

These five issues are equally applicable to chiropractors, even though it is accepted that the precedence for providing health care to the adolescent has been within orthodox medicine, particularly with pediatricians (9).

Adolescent Care: Beyond Pediatrics

The increasing responsibility demonstrated by the chiropractic profession for developing a specialized pediatric knowledge base from the chiropractic perspective (10), in addition to conducting continuing education and postgraduate programs evolved from the accepted, broad-scope pediatric knowledge base (11), cannot be taken as automatically conferring those particular abilities demanded for the provision of competent "adolescent" care.

Adolescents have needs and problems sufficiently distinguishable to warrant consideration as a distinct group for health care provision (12), consequently the differences between the adolescent patient and the pediatric patient are many. Pediatrics has its own complexities but they can broadly be considered as congenital, developmental, or transitional related to the commencement of schooling. Pediatrics can therefore be considered the speciality of the neonate, the preschooler and of childhood, ranging up to the onset of puberty at which time the greatest musculoskeletal and psychosocial developments are unleashed. Development within adolescence is complicated by the major social adjustments associated with sexuality and the expanded transition to life outside the family orbit.

With the pediatric patient, the parent or guardian is more often the historian and the doctor–patient relationship exists largely within the patient's existing frame of reference, the family. The adolescent period sees progression to the patient being the historian and coming to take responsibility for his/her own health. Not that this happens easily. The response of adolescents suggests that the health professions are failing in their efforts to specifically reach them (13). Not only was consultation time seen as inadequate, but medical practitioners were felt to be hard to approach and impersonal. Among the suggestions and strategies to remedy this problem is mention of the requirement for greater awareness of youth needs, and greater availability of doctors for young people (13).

Adolescence is the time for the greatest growth and change of the musculoskeletal system, and the more doctors of chiropractic who accept the unique challenges associated with the provision of quality, competent and relevant adolescent health care, the greater will be the enrichment of our society. By taking up the stimulating challenge of providing specialized musculoskeletal care during this period, chiropractors can make two unique contributions to a young life: first, the relief of pain through the correction of musculoskeletal dysfunction; and second, the provision of a corrected structural foundation to allow a more normal adult life.

The World Health Organization has identified two approaches necessary to effectively deliver complete health care to adolescents, namely "curative" and "preventive (14)." Traditionally the curative care for adolescents is delivered by remote professional figures who are specialists in mainly medical areas. Chiropractors already have a reputation of being easily approachable primary contact practitioners (15–17), and are in a unique position to develop a practice style of curative musculoskeletal care with which adolescents can feel comfortable.

The curative approach is problem oriented. The chiropractor's ability to gain ready access to an adolescent population must be supported by clinical competency in not only the wide spectrum of musculoskeletal disorders encountered in adolescence, but also with the extremely wide range of psychosocial issues which are integral to adolescent care. The preventive approach is designed to address the needs of adolescents and involves a wide selection of qualified paramedics with an emphasis on the psychosocial aspects. There is a very broad scope here for chiropractors to implement preventive strategies related to neuromusculoskeletal health.

Age of Adolescence

Adolescence is accepted as commencing around the time of puberty, in the second decade of life. Accordingly, 10 years is considered a demarcation for entry into adolescence (18), although 12 may be a more convenient age with regard to age and school grouping (19). The point at which adolescence ends, however, is not as clearly defined. Traditionally it has been 21 years, with the proviso that in special cases, such as chronic disease, care may continue past 21 (9,20); however, contemporary thinking is that the end point of "adolescence," or, as it is becoming to be known more generically, "youth" (21), is more realistically about age 25 years (22), the time when the "late adolescent" period blends into young adulthood. There are two arguments in favor of the 25th birthday being considered as the more appropriate end point to adolescence, namely:

1. While adolescence is a period of physical growth, including the "growth spurt" of high peak annual height velocity (23,24), growth actually concludes with the fusion of the secondary ossification centers of the spine by about the twenty-fifth year (24–27), notwithstanding that the spurt occurs earlier in females than males (28).

2. Adolescence is a period of psychosocial growth and central nervous system maturation, with the development of formal operational thinking (4). In recognition of this, the statistical measurement of young people is grouped as 15–19 and 20–24 years. The former statistical grouping excludes late adolescents; the latter includes them (19). These psychosocial considerations support the view that adolescence is a cultural phenomenon as an inevitable by-product of adult, Western civilization (29).

From the chiropractic perspective of the neuromusculoskeletal system, the most appropriate age range for "adolescence" is therefore 10 to 24 years, and on this basis the typical adolescent population in Western countries represents about one quarter of the total national population. Within a three kilometer radius of the clinics in an Australian study the proportion ranged from 23.4% in the rural/urban fringe up to 29.4% in an outer metropolitan suburb (30).

The clear implication is that a chiropractic practice can reasonably expect to have adolescents as patients, and specific reports of the usage of chiropractors by adolescents are now becoming available (31,32). They suggest attendance by adolescents for new visits can range up to 29% of all new patient visits, thereby approaching their proportional representation in the population at large (between 24% and 29%); however, for return visits the rate is only about half of what could be expected, at about 12%.

Of greater concern however was the adolescent participation rate in chiropractic management under the provisions of workmen's compensation. In the Australian studies, adolescents aged in their early 20s had double the national average participation rate (18% compared to 9%). The implications are obvious; musculoskeletal injury in general and low back injury in particular represent the lion's share of work related, compensable injury in the U.S. (33). The majority of this musculoskeletal injury is amenable to chiropractic management (34), a fact no longer overlooked by health economists who continue to demonstrate the significant cost effectiveness of the chiropractic management of low-back pain (35). Add to this the various preventive strategies used within chiropractic practice, such as the "Back School" (36) and preemployment assessment (37), and chiropractors can be seen as holding a preeminent position for the provision of care for the adolescent.

Growth and Development in Adolescence

Adolescence is a journey through physiologic, cognitive, and psychologic stages, an integral aspect of which is the development of the adolescent as a sexual being. A successful journey through adolescence will result in the successful development of the individual's sexuality, and subsequently largely determine his/her nature as an adult.

Western society places unreasonable pressure on adolescents which is reflected in difficulty with finding their roles as sexual beings. Television and take-away videos provide easy and non-stop access to distorted sexual attitudes and activity. Many youth have faced the horror of child sexual and verbal abuse, and all are affected by the quality (good or bad) of the sexuality education we, as adult society, give them. The comprehension of adolescent sexuality is not easy, even for health care workers. It is a physioanatomic, biologic, psychosocial, moral, and ethical phenomenon, existing as a continuum (instead of an endpoint), within a community which itself is grappling with constantly changing stressors and varying standards of sexuality.

The sexuality issues of the adolescent begin in childhood. Those youth who lived with a childhood of abuse, neglect, parental divorce, family chaos or other negative experiences have less than the ideal template for the development of their adolescent sexuality. Parental attitudes towards clinically normal sexual development are vitally important to the overall development of the emerging individual.

Regardless of one's chosen scope of chiropractic practice, an understanding of adolescent sexuality is vital for the establishment of an adequate professional relationship with the adolescent as a patient. Should your scope of practice be broad enough to include the room to work with issues of adolescent sexuality then further study and membership of appropriate professional bodies is essential. On a day-to-day basis, the chiropractor needs to understand that the adolescent patient is neither a child nor an adult, therefore management strategies which are otherwise effective in one's practice may singularly fail for the adolescent patient. Further, adolescence is a journey in itself and not just a whistle-stop one passes through while progressing from the cradle to the grave. As such, it has a myriad of nuances which interact to varying degrees at varying times. Fortunately for the practitioner, however, the journey through adolescence can largely be considered in three stages.

Stages of Adolescence

Adolescence can be viewed in terms of early, mid and late, each with its own characteristics and problems. Traditionally the early stage is 10 to 14 years, middle 14 to 18, and late 18 to 21 or 22, with a crossover phase into adulthood and growth completion between 21 and 24 years. The stages are only guidelines, however, and it is important to always remember that all patients have the right to present in the stage of development in which they find themselves at the time. On the basis of there being some sort of mean range within which developmental landmarks generally occur, it can be said that some teenagers have precocious development while others are delayed, but remember the term "delayed" is only a label, and one must be cautious before thinking about whether or not to apply it.

Each stage has its own characteristics for growth, cognition, psychosocial self, family relationships, peer group relationships, sexuality and chronological age range. They are listed in Table 18.1. There are further stages that can add to one's concept of adolescence, such as those of Kolberg, Freud, Sears, Havighurst, Kinsey, Lidz, and Gillian, Miller and Chodorow; these can be explored at one's discretion and leisure.

EARLY ADOLESCENCE

The chronological age range is 10 to 14 years. Sexual function will occur before biologic maturation, and generally the concepts of sexuality are initiated in the youth's mind by the events of puberty. The body increases in height and weight as growth accelerates, and the secondary sexual characteristics appear. The time lapse between childhood and adulthood stages is from 2 to 4 and perhaps 5 years.

Growth is initiated by the hypothalamus through stimulation of the anterior pituitary, and is controlled by various hormones. The amount of sex steroids produced by the body slowly increases from about age 6 years. Puberty commences with the triggering of gonadotropin releasing hormone (Gn-RH). It is believed that this system is controlled by a highly sensitive, negative feedback system which inhibits the synthesis of effective levels of Gn-RH earlier in life. As age increases, it is thought the sensitivity of the negative feedback mechanism decreases, and the hormones reach endocrinologically effective levels. The critical weight hypothesis of Frisch-Revelle (38) suggests that the decreasing sensitivity is related to a statistically significant correlation between menarche and the achievement of a critical body weight of 47.8 kg. The hypothesis has been modified to relate more to a ratio between body fat, total body water, and lean mass (22) and remains a useful clinical indicator.

The biologic changes are categorized by Tanner, with genital maturity ratings that range from 1 to 5 (Tables 18.2, 18.3). They apply to the secondary sexual characteristics of the male and the female, and allow a "staging" of the individual's biologic development (Figs. 18.1, 18.2). Although not used in day-to-day chiropractic practice, they do form an important part of the patient record for complaints such as delayed menarche (primary amenorrhea) or short stature. As Tanner staging should only be performed by a chiropractor in the presence of a chaperone of the same sex as the patient or in the presence of the patient's parent or guardian, it is often easier to use the "self-reporting" method, in which the patient is asked to identify which of a series of Tanner drawings most closely resembles himself/herself. This method has been found to be reasonably reliable (39), has also been recommended by other chiropractic authors (40), and is much more practical for use outside the office; for example when conducting pre-participation examinations for a sporting organization.

Adolescent growth, these times of tremendous biological change, occurs at different chronological ages in males and females. Female puberty is heralded by thelarche (the budding of the breast) at about age 11 (range 8 to 15), Tanner stage 2. Puberty starts 1.5 to 2 years later in the male and takes nearly twice as long to complete. Menarche occurs approximately 2.5 years after the onset of puberty or during stage 4, at which stage the female has attained 90 to 95% of her adult height.

In males, the first observable change is testis enlargement, beginning at 11.6 years of age (range 10 to 14.8). The male growth spurt usually begins at stage 3, peaks during stage 4, and is all but complete by stage 5; however, some males will continue to grow up to 2 cm more in height over the ensuing 5 years. Another characteristic of importance to manual practitioners is the period of male puberty, which sees rapid muscle growth, the "strength spurt," at the end of stage 4.

Linear growth follows these early changes in sexual characteristics, with an initial increase in the length of the long bones which causes a rise in the body's center of gravity. This is followed by growth of the spine which reestablishes equilibrium in the ratio of upper to lower body segments. This is the "growth spurt" of Tanner, or the period of peak height velocity, which in females commonly starts in Tanner stage 2, reaches a peak midway between stages 3 and 4, and ends at stage 5. In males, the peak height velocity occurs later, during genital stage 4. During the growth spurt the "average" female will grow at a peak velocity of 8 cm per year, and the "average" male at 10 cm per year, adding as much as 20 cm to his height. Similar dimensional increases occur in every body system apart from the lymphatic, in which total tissue volume decreases.

Because youth have such a varying time of entry to puberty, any comparison between individuals is best made on the basis of Tanner staging. We therefore have chronological age, Tanner stage, cognitive level and psychosocial development as aspects to consider when talking about adolescents. It is essential to understand these relationships, together with their standard deviations, to correctly evaluate normal and problematic growth states such as delayed puberty, short stature, or delayed menarche.

Piaget has described the cognitive stages of development, which reach the concrete operational stage between 7 and 11 years. The adolescent will generally be making the entry into adolescence and puberty from the concrete stage, however the stage may last until well into adolescence. Concrete thought is limited to considering things and specific situations in existential terms, with no ability to extract general principles from one experience and apply them to a wholly new experience.

A feature of the concrete operational stage of interest to chiropractors is the monosyllabic nature of responses to questioning. There should be some ability with understanding the concepts of symmetric relationships and serializations,

Table 18.1.   Characteristics of Early, Mid, and Late Adolescence

Characteristics	Early Adolescence	Mid Adolescence	Late Adolescence
Growth	Secondary sexual characteristics have begun to appear Growth rapidly accelerating; reaches peak velocity	Secondary sexual characteristics well advanced Growth decelerating; stature reaches 95% of adult height	Physically mature; statural and reproductive growth virtually complete
Cognition	Concrete thought dominant Existential orientation Cannot perceive long-range implications of current decisions and acts	Rapidly gaining competence in abstract thought Capable of perceiving future implications of current acts and decisions but variably applied Reverts to concrete operations under stress	Established abstract thought processes Future oriented Capable of perceiving and acting on long-range options
Psychosocial Self	Preoccupation with rapid body change Former body image disrupted	Reestablishes body image as growth decelerates and stabilizes Preoccupation with fantasy and idealism in exploring expanded cognition and future options Development of a sense of omnipotence and invincibility	Emancipation completed Intellectual and functional identity established May experience "crisis of 21" when facing societal demands for autonomy
Family	Defining independence–dependence boundaries No major conflicts over parental control	Major conflicts over control Struggle for emancipation	Transposition of child–parent dependency relationship to the adult–adult model
Peer Group	Seeks peer affiliation to counter instability generated by rapid change Compares own normality and acceptance with same sex/age mates	Strong need for identification to affirm self-image Looks to peer group to define behavioral code during emancipation process	Recedes in importance in favor of individual friendships
Sexuality	Self-exploration and evaluation Limited dating Limited intimacy	Multiple plural relationships Heightened sexual activity Testing ability to attract opposite sex and parameters of masculinity or femininity Preoccupation with romantic fantasy	Forms stable relationships Capable of mutuality and reciprocity in caring for another rather than former narcissistic orientation Plans for future in thinking of marriage, family Intimacy involves commitment rather than exploration and romanticism
Age Range	Initiates between ages 11 and 13 and merges with mid-adolescence at 14 to 15 years	Begins around 14 to 15 years and blends into late adolescence about age 17	Approximately 17 to 21 years; upper end particularly variable; dependent on cultural, economic, and educational factors

Table 18.2.   **Male Secondary Sexual Characteristics**

Stage	Pubic Hair	Penis	Testes
1	None	Preadolescent	Preadolescent
2	Scanty, long, slightly pigmented	Slight enlargement	Enlarged scrotum, pink, texture changed
3	Darker, begins to curl, small amount	Longer	Larger
4	Resembles adult type, but less in quantity; coarse, curly	Larger, glans and breadth increase size	Larger, scrotum darker
5	Adult distribution, spread to medial thighs	Adult	Adult

Table 18.3.   **Female Secondary Sexual Characteristics**

Stage	Pubic Hair	Breasts
1	Preadolescent	Preadolescent
2	Sparse, slightly pigmented, straight, at medial border of labia	Breast and papilla elevated as small mound, areola diameter increased
3	Darker, beginning to curl, increased amount	Breast and areola enlarged, without contour separation
4	Coarse, curly, abundant, but amount less than in adult	Areola and papilla form secondary mound
5	Adult feminine triangle, spread to medial surface of the thighs	Mature, nipple projects, areola part of general breast contour

untouchable. Accordingly they do not perceive the risks that attend risk-taking behavior because they feel they are "special" and essentially "untouchable" by any future danger. This magical thinking can extend well into late adolescence (to include about 30% of late adolescents) and even adulthood, as evidenced by the number of adults who take drugs, smoke, drive irresponsibly and abuse alcohol. Generally the adolescent progresses to formal operational thinking by mid adolescence.

The psychosocial self of adolescence is dominated by the rapid physiologic growth changes of puberty with its various aches and musculoskeletal pains. These can lead to a hypochondriacal phase until the changes become more familiar. The family relationship lessens with a commensurate strengthening of the peer group relationship. As the teenager starts to move away from the parent he/she forms stronger friendships and bonds with peers, the new source of one's own sense of self-worth. This is a time of strong comparison with one's peers, and friendships tend to be of the same gender, with some possible homosexual experimentation.

MID ADOLESCENCE

The chronological age range is 14 to 18 years and the formal operational thinking patterns are now developing. This abstract thinking permits the conceptualization of possibilities beyond past and present experiences. The emerging phase is attended by a preoccupation with fantasy and ideas which develop into a strong ability to comprehend logic which can be used in profound arguments to counter parental direction. Any guidance given by health care workers needs to be extremely clearly presented with fully explained rules or recommendations, especially with preventive health strategies.

These youth are balancing the newfound power of formal operational thinking with the emergence of needs for independence. They lack the level of experience needed to avoid errors in judgment, especially when "magical thinking" remains, but they can achieve independence and make career and lifestyle choices while their personal value system emerges. Formal thought may not be applied at all times; some simple situations may not need it, while some other occasions may overwhelm the person who then reverts to irrational thought.

although this ability can be expected to vary greatly between adolescents. Concrete thinkers may well be interested in the physical aspects of their bodies but may be unable to express themselves clearly and in detail. Questionnaires can be useful at this stage to identify the key points of a health history. Teaching aids are also of great benefit to extend the patient's knowledge and understanding. The thinking of the concrete adolescent is very much in the present, with a resultant difficulty to think in futuristic terms.

The implication for clinical practice is that therapeutic recommendations need to be accompanied by evidence of an immediate benefit. For example, "sex is OK" because "it feels good right now"; the risk of pregnancy and delivery is 9 months in the future and is not comprehensible. The future cannot be appreciated except as a direct projection of clearly visible, current operations. The difficulty of counseling around inappropriate behavior is compounded by the concept of "magical thinking," in which the adolescent feels he or she is

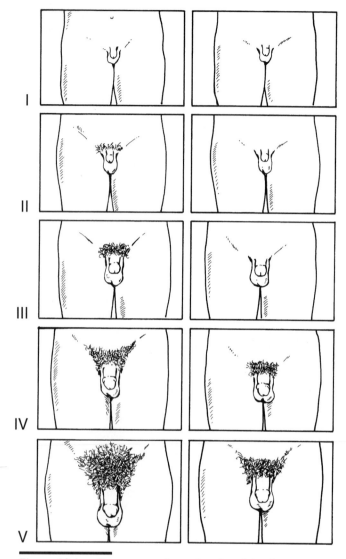

Figure 18.1. Tanner stages for male pubertal development. Modified from Strasburger VC, Brown RT. Adolescent medicine, a practical guide. Boston: Little, Brown & Co., 1991:3.

The psychosocial self shows a stronger reliance on peers with an acquisition of greater independence and emancipation from the parents. The kind of youth with which one associates reflects one's sense of self worth. Individuals with undesirable peer group associations, such as those with drug taking habits, seem more prone to depression at this stage. While self confident youth generally associate with similarly self confident youth, parents and health care workers should be aware of the futility of attempting to force certain relationships onto the adolescent.

Heterosexual experimentation is inevitable and parental attitudes become critical. A youth who is rebelling against authority may demonstrate such rebellion sexually. Coital activity is common with the resultant high rates of pregnancy, abortion and STDs, which in turn can further complicate parent-adolescent relationships. The developing emancipation and heterosexual experimentation strengthens the cognitive abilities. Various adults may serve as role models (good or bad), and youth often turn to other adults for counselling in addition to or instead of their parents. It is at this time that your influence as a chiropractor is significant, especially as questions of a moral, ethical and religious nature are often asked. The difficulties experienced vary greatly. Some adolescents may pass through this stage with little upheaval, while others may turn to drug experimentation and exhibit transient school dysfunction, moodiness and irritability. This is a relevant time to consider the appropriate type of counselling should it be indicated.

LATE ADOLESCENCE

The chronological age range is from 18 years to the end of skeletal growth, between 21 and 24 years. By the 25th birthday, all secondary ossification centers should be fused and growth should be complete. The adolescent will exhibit sound formal operational thinking with strong cognitive skills, and can be considered as an adult, with both the independence and experience needed to reduce errors in judgment. There is some final physiologic fine tuning, such as regulation of menstruation and male muscular development. The male growth spurt should be all but complete by Tanner stage 5, however it must be appreciated that some males will continue to grow up to 2 cm more in the ensuing 5 years. Another characteristic of importance to chiropractors is the period in males which sees rapid muscle growth, the "strength spurt," at the end of stage 4.

The psychosocial self will by now be resolving the issues of emancipation and the youth-parent relationship, which should be more adult-adult in nature, and more comfortable. Ideally, a young pre-adult emerges, a person who likes him or her self as a male or female and has come to grips with important issues of human sexuality. The body image will be secure and the gender role established, two keys to potential success in late adolescence and adulthood. Any necessary corrections to the musculoskeletal system from the chiropractor's viewpoint will have been made and the entry into adulthood should be based on a firm, pain-free, fully functional structural foundation. Those youth who still experience difficulty in this stage may also experience considerable anxiety or depression and care must be taken to distinguish between genuine physical need for adjustive treatment, and a perceived demand based on retaining the patient in a "comfort zone." The rest of this transitional period involves the acquisition of adult lifestyles and habits, and one or several of a variety of sexual orientations will be adopted. This is also the time for establishment of vocational skills and of training to meet the complexities of modern society.

Youth Oriented Practice

Adolescence is the bridging period between childhood naivete and adult experience. As such it is reasonable to treat adolescent patients with an understanding based on their individual psychologic and physiologic development, taking care to develop a doctor-patient relationship built on mutual trust and respect. The process of physical change that occurs during adolescence is a cause of increased self consciousness, self awareness and self centeredness. On the one hand the adolescent is striving to gain independence, while on the other he or she may be in need of your support and understanding, not just as a chiropractor but also as a person.

The joy of working with adolescent patients comes from their capacity to warmly return the effort you put into your relationship with them. If you are a caring chiropractor, and exhibit empathy, you will be rewarded with countless opportunities to improve the quality of life of your adolescent patients through (i) the short term benefits of the relief of musculoskeletal pain, and (ii) the long term benefit of the provision of a healthy body and mind as a springboard into

adult life. The doctor's attitude needs to encompass both the concepts of the appropriate treatment program for the immediate presenting complaint, and of a tailored preventive health care program based on your long term advice and guidance.

Bennett, a leading adolescent medicine physician, has identified seven important steps to promote a successful doctor/patient interview (41). These steps, and their application in the chiropractic office, are:

1. *See the patient alone, at least for part of the interview.*

Start the initial interview with the parent present by all means if patient (usually in the 10 to 16 age group) attends with their parent, but then excuse the parent at the point where you wish to establish your one-on-one relationship with the patient. Doing this will avoid the appearance of you being aligned with the parents and will invite a more mature and

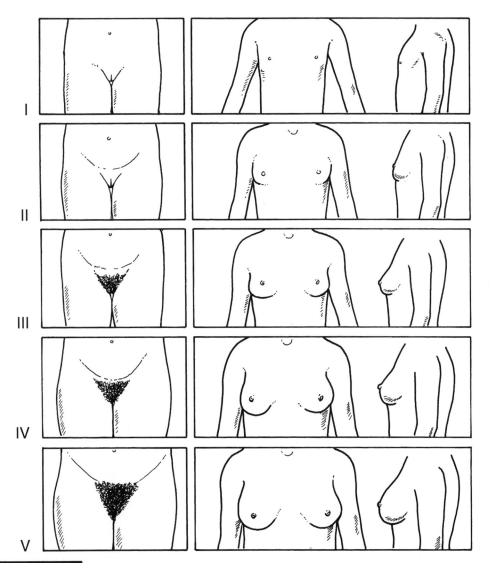

Figure 18.2.   Tanner stages for female pubertal development. Modified from Strasburger VC, Brown RT. Adolescent medicine, a practical guide. Boston: Little, Brown & Co., 1991:4.

responsible response within this doctor/patient relationship. Before relaying any information to the parent, ask your patient for permission to do so. Use your judgment and perhaps ask the patient if he or she agrees with you "filling (the parent) in on the basic details" ... this will let you retain an area of confidentiality with the patient and will strengthen the parental cooperation with your proposed treatment plan.

2. *Define the basis of confidentiality.*

Your adolescent patients must feel they can trust you, especially in personal areas which to them may be highly sensitive. Exceptions are, of course, proposed self destructive or dangerous behavior, however you can also lay a ground rule with your patients when alone with them that "if any problems come up which are too big for the both of us," you will help form a team with the appropriate professional (maybe a clinical psychologist) and maybe a parent to work it through together. This signals a comfort zone to your patients and shares the decision making responsibilities without disempowering or "controlling" them.

It is important for all parties to know that the history you have taken and will continue to take when alone with the patient is confidential between you and the patient and will only be shared with parent(s) or guardian(s) with the patient's permission. In practical terms this arrangement works well, usually because the patient has willingly attended with the assistance of the parent who is keen to help their child grow to greater independence, however there are no predictable answers for the rare case where, subsequent to a breakdown in communication between the younger adolescent and the parent, the parent may insist on exercising what they see as their right to know the contents of their child's history and treatment file.

As a guide, the issues at play are the age of the patient (whether they are legally a minor), the social standing and emancipation of the patient (whether they have left home and can demonstrate independence), and the agreement reached between all parties at your initial interview. You may elect to have the parent sign a "consent to treatment" clause on the patient's history and have that clause include statements of confidentiality. You may elect to operate "a family history" with no recorded confidential matters, or you may elect to tough it out fully on the side of the adolescent. Legal opinion will vary widely, not only between but also within jurisdictions.

From a pragmatic point of view, such disputes tend to happen as the adolescent is attempting to assert independence and while in some jurisdictions the "age of consent" may be literally enforced, issues of patient confidentiality tend to revolve around the level of independence and intellectual cognizance of the patient.

3. *Respond openly to the adolescent's initial reactions.*

If your patient has not been to a chiropractor before, his/her expectation of the experience will be based on any previous interaction with the medical profession. You can defuse hostility by commenting on the patient's apparent and expected discomfort. Don't handle this lightly or with humor. At all times be "matter of fact" and fully professional, but demonstrate your awareness of what the patient is feeling and act in a manner which allows them to place his/her confidence in you.

It is a good idea to "talk through" all that you do, from the simple scoliosis screen to the complex neurological evaluation. The assessment of sexual development can be an acute embarrassment to both you and the patient. A very effective method in the chiropractic office, as previously mentioned, is to show the patient a set of sketches of the Tanner staging (breast contour and pubic hair development for females, and testicular size, penis size and pubic hair development for males), asking the patient to indicate which sketch they feel most accurately looks like them at this time. Be sure to include sketches of both circumcised and uncircumcised penises.

This approach allow you to gently work with any "taboo" or fear of sexual matters and development, and to open a conversation in which the patient may raise any questions with you. As with all inquiry about personal matters your approach must be open-ended. Such questions are best phrased "most young men I see wonder whether their penis is like other people's..." or "most young ladies I see wonder whether their breasts are the right shape..."; "what do you think about yours?" or "how often do you or your friends wonder about that?" Again, it is vital to be non-judgmental and to demonstrate genuine empathy with this very special human being who is putting trust in you.

4. *Clarify the reasons for the consultation.*

From the adolescent patients' point of view their care is largely "symptom care" (curative) and it is very important for you to explain why you may be conducting adjunctive assessments of areas which they may not relate to the presenting complaint. The patient may also be in your office against his or her will because a parent (perhaps a patient of yours) has brought them to you "to fix their headache and bad temper." Be alert for signs of this and make the effort to establish a reason for the consultation that the patient accepts and understands.

If you detect a problem that the patient is reluctant to confront with you, then the open-ended questioning style can be used to invite a response. Again, you may say "I see many patients of your age who worry about being ... too heavy or too light.../...too short or too tall .../...whether smoking is really bad ..." and so on. Two-way conversations, in a discussive manner, with complete honesty in your responses, are a very effective method of communication with adolescents.

5. *Be a good listener.*

The conversation must be "two-way," meaning you are expected to listen. In fact, the art of adolescent health care may be summarized by saying "hear what your patient is telling you." Listen, listen, then listen. Adolescents frequently convey their concerns in an indirect style of conversation. Listen for the subtle nuances which may tell you what the patient is really trying to say, but don't try and listen for cues to generate an automatic response from you. Neuro-linguistic programming has no place in adolescent health care. Converse and listen with honesty and integrity.

6. *Allocate ample time.*

The examination and treatment of the adolescent can not be rushed. The real investment you make in adolescent health is your time and your availability; now and then you may actually adjust! The chiropractic office which wants to earn its place in the overall network providing adolescent health care needs to be an office where the adolescent comes first. Late afternoons, early evenings and Saturdays are good times to have your office open for adolescents. On week-days, consider structuring the hours at the end of the day as "adolescent only" hours, with music in your office to match, but be sure to retain a high level of professionalism in the dress of yourself and your staff. The adolescent patient expects to see professional figures, not confused grownups attempting to dress like kids. Also, make sure your office works in an open and relaxed manner to reflect a well planned schedule which has ample time allocation for each individual patient.

The greatest honor your adolescent patient can give you is to bring a friend with them to watch their treatment session with you, or perhaps because the friend may have a similar problem to that of your patient. You need to have enough time within the patient visit framework to accommodate the friend and their problem. This is not to suggest you should treat the friend at this time, rather, this situation can be viewed as being an ideal patient and future patient education session. At 12 or more patients an hour and with the waiting room full, you won't have the time and your young patient will know it.

7. *Answer questions simply and honestly, and particularly in a nonjudgmental manner.*

Adolescents, especially when in a group situation such as a basic health class you may be teaching for your local high school, have a great talent for asking questions from left field. Any hesitation or embarrassment you may feel will be picked up by their sixth sense. Always answer as best you know how, at all times showing genuine respect for their concerns and point of view. Above all, if you don't know an answer, say so! Offer to find out about an issue and report back next visit.

Outreach Activity

Care of the adolescent is not limited to your chiropractic office, nor is it limited to the simple "fee for service" paradigm. Chiropractors, as primary health care providers (42), have the potential to provide a wide range of community services, many of which may be focused on the particular needs of early and mid adolescents. Some of these services may include acting as the physician at your local high school, providing a service at no cost to the school community but one which places you in the forefront as a gatekeeper for adolescent health concerns in your community.

You may offer your professional services as a team physician for a particular sporting club in your community and extend your duties to the junior ranks as well as the senior players you are paid to look after. On the other hand, you may again work with your local high school by offering to conduct an annual "pre-participation" sports examination. There is no reason why you could not offer this service free to your local high school and set an example in community participation and interaction. The format and content of such examinations are beyond the scope of this chapter, however you can obtain relevant information from your professional association and detailed formats from the literature (43,44).

A number of chiropractic communities are also extending their services at no cost to the socially disadvantaged, through "Hands on Health" clinics and other such services aligned with welfare agencies. Within this system you will be working with homeless youth, dysfunctional youth, and at times, detainees. It is imperative that you have a high level of competence with the essential components and substance of adolescent health care in order to be able to adapt your assessment and intervention to what will, at times, be a practice environment essentially incompatible with the generally accepted patient management strategies, the absence of which places a greater responsibility on you as a practitioner.

The Initial Visit

There are several scenarios within which you will conduct your initial consultation with an adolescent patient, not withstanding any outreach activity you may be undertaking. The most likely scenarios are where the parent who is a patient of yours brings their son or daughter to you for either a "check-up" or for your opinion on a particular problem, in which case the patient will generally be in early or mid adolescence, and secondly, where a patient in the late adolescent stage will seek your services on their own volition. Depending on the nature of your practice, you may also receive adolescent patients on referral from other primary health care practitioners, or on self-referral through the new patient being a friend of an adolescent patient of yours. The following recommendations for the conduct of the initial visit are intended for the scenario where the patient attends with a parent or guardian.

The aim of the initial visit is twofold: firstly you need to establish the framework in which the patient is operating, the health status which they carry from childhood, the things which worry them and which they think you can do something about, and other concerns which they don't see as being any of your business; and secondly the patient needs to establish how he or she sees you and your clinic, and to work out what it means to him or her. Only the most optimistic practitioner would think they will practitioner will subtly gather a little more "historical" information on each subsequent visit, realizing they are establishing a long term "doctor-patient" relationship which has the potential to span many years.

Introduction to the Clinic

The normal administrative matters for new patients of your clinic should be conducted for the adolescent patient, including the taking of demographic information and determining the terms of payment. There is no reason why the fee for an adolescent consultation should be any different to the normal office fees; however, more time will be spent with the adolescent patient, especially on the initial visit, than with an adult. A separate file should be established in the name of the patient and it should indicate the name by which the patient prefers to be called. It is inappropriate for any person other than the doctor to seek to elicit any health-related or psychosocial information from the patient prior to the consultation.

The adolescent should be advised at this stage that he or she may be required to expose parts of the body for examination by the doctor, and to simultaneously inform him or her that a gown and a private room in which to change will be provided.

This should apply to male patients as well as to females, and the patient should be instructed to keep underwear on. It is beneficial for clinic reception staff and chiropractic assistants to be trained by the doctor to have an understanding that a "guidance-cooperation" relationship is appropriate and effective for most early to mid stage adolescents, while a "mutual participation" relationship is more suited for some middle and most late-stage adolescents.

Consent

All patients are required to give informed consent before you commence your examination, treatment and management. Additionally, a consent from the parent(s) or legal guardian(s) of the patient, on behalf of the patient, is required where the patient may be either viewed as a minor in the jurisdiction of practice, or be deemed incompetent to give informed consent due to being intellectually challenged. The issue of consent is not new to the chiropractic literature (45–48) and it has been termed the "search for protection" (49). The literature contains examples of appropriate consent forms and their rationale (45,49–51) and the consent form used in the author's practice and in the chiropractic teaching clinics of Royal Melbourne Institute of Technology (RMIT) is reproduced as Figure 18.3. It is the responsibility of the doctor to be familiar with the laws as they relate to the age of consent in the jurisdiction in which the practice is conducted, and to ensure the appropriate documentation is completed and placed in the patient's file.

The issue of "minor consent" has been blurred over recent years with the emergence of the unofficial concept of the "mature minor doctrine," which broadly holds that minors who can demonstrate emancipation in some form may accept responsibility for seeking and consenting to their treatment. In this case it is "emancipation" which becomes the pivotal term, the interpretation of which varies from jurisdiction to jurisdiction. Again, it is the practitioner's responsibility to come to an understanding of the situation as it may apply in his or her practice, always remembering s/he has the right to not accept a patient for treatment in certain circumstances.

History

It is common practice for chiropractors to require new patients to fill out a "tick the box" type of questionnaire, which purports to gather historical and contemporary health information. The validity of these self-reporting instruments has yet to be demonstrated and they are generally unsuited for the adolescent patient who may not only be an unreliable historian, but also may not have the required level of literacy to understand the questions and specific terms used. It is preferable to gather all information in the framework of the face to face, doctor-patient interview.

Although open-ended questions are likely to lead to appropriate areas for discussion, there are some advantages in gaining the screening history through a closed question and answer session. This can commence with the parent present to ensure the childhood history is accurate, and then continue when alone with the patient to record current information. The total history taking process will be a combination of direct questioning, open-ended questioning, and observation. Sexual experiences and drug use (including alcohol and tobacco) should be sensitively explored, and the screening history should also include an assessment of the patient's level of functioning, obtained from gaining knowledge about his or her family relationships, peer relationships, special interests, hobbies and skills, school and career performance, and goals. Be alert for unresolved learning disability and emotional conflicts. An effective way to establish the framework in which the patient is operating is to use the mnemonic HEADSS (41,52) as a guide for the screening history:

H = home
E = education, employment
A = activities, ambition, anxieties
D = drugs, depression
S = sexuality, self esteem
S = stress, suicide

Open-ended questioning in a conversational style within each of these areas will quickly build a medicosocial and psychosocial picture of your patient and establish a two-way rapport which you can build on as you return to explore certain areas in detail during the full history taking process.

Your history can then include such straightforward questions as "why are you coming to see me today?" and then "what other problems do you think you have that I can help you with?" Remember the basic concept of avoiding questions which can be answered with "yes" or "no"; for example, it is preferable to say, "Some young men think they have cancer because they are always tired. How much does tiredness worry you?," than to ask "Do you think you have cancer?" Another way to phrase general questions is to say, "Some young people are really bothered by dizzy spells and stomach aches; how often do these things worry you?"

The parent or guardian can be present during these conversations; however, you must ensure the patient is given every opportunity to express his or her own answer to your questions. It is sometimes difficult to stop a parent from answering on behalf of the patient, particularly if you are experienced with treating children and babies. There is wisdom in carefully arranging the seating in your office to place yourself behind your desk, the patient diagonally across from you at the end of the desk, and the parent out of the eye-line between you and your patient, perhaps using the desk as a barrier. This method allows you to maintain direct and close eye contact with the patient as you gather your history, and requires the physical effort of moving your body to acknowledge or address the parent.

This seating configuration can easily become functionally triangular at your instigation as you reach the section of the history which details the health status the patient has carried from childhood. The parent will be more reliable in providing confirmation and dates of the gestation and birth process, childhood illnesses such as hepatitis, rheumatic fever and tuberculosis, immunizations, allergies and any hospitalization.

RMIT
The Chiropractic Unit

> Please read the information on this form carefully before you sign. Please ask us if you need help to understand any part of this form, or if you want anything explained further.

Patient consent form

I, _____ being the parent or legal guardian of
    Print given name (s) and family name

_____ hereby consent to this person receiving
    Patient given name (s) and family name

examination, x ray, and treatment in this clinic. _____
                                            Signature   Date

Chiropractors, medical practitioners and other registered practitioners using manual therapy treatments for patients with neck problems are required to explain there have been rare cases of injury to the arteries of the neck following treatment of the cervical spine. This occurrence has been known to cause stroke, sometimes with serious neurological (nervous system) changes. The chances of this happening are extremely remote, approximately 1 per one million treatments. Several manual tests will be performed on you to help identify if you may be susceptible to this risk. If you have any questions about this please do not hesitate to speak with the Head of Clinic or the duty clinician.

I have read, or have had read to me and explained to my satisfaction, the above statements and I understand what they say. I accept the risk mentioned, and hereby consent to treatment for myself or for the above minor under my care.

Signed:
    _____   _____
            Signature   Print given name (s) and family name

of: Dated: _____
    _____   _____
            Number / Street   Suburb / Town

Witnessed by: _____
                  Signature   Print given name (s) and family name   Date

---

I understand that this clinic is a teaching clinic of RMIT and hereby give permission for the information contained within this file to be used within the approved protocols of The Chiropractic Unit of RMIT for research and teaching purposes on the condition that no information which may identify the patient as an individual will be published, and with the understanding that I may revoke this permission at any time without prejudicing due care and treatment.

Signed: _____
         Signature   Print given name (s) and family name   Date

---

I accept financial responsibility for my treatment in this clinic, or for the treatment of the above minor under my care, and agree to pay the fees which have been explained to me at the time service is rendered unless I have made prior arrangement with the Head of Clinic.

Signed: _____
         Signature   Print given name (s) and family name   Date

Figure 18.3.   Consent form appropriate for use with adolescent patients. Reproduced with permission from the author and RMIT, Melbourne.

The parent may also be more forthright about any current medication, and recent medical, dental, visual and hearing check-ups.

At the end of this stage it is appropriate to say to the parent, "You have certainly given me a good idea of where we are up to but I would now like to examine (patient name) further and determine what treatment we might need to arrange. This could take a while so you might like to have a coffee in the waiting room and we'll ask you to come back in when we're done." Once the parent is excused you can repeat your contract of confidentiality with the patient and commence the physical examination, interspersing it with conversation designed to help you build a complete history.

When you have completed your history, physical and chiropractic examinations, you can then explain the situation to the patient in terms they will understand, bearing in mind the operational state appropriate to their age and status. You should ensure your patient understands what you are saying and extend every opportunity for them to ask any questions and settle any fears. It is also paramount that you reach an agreement at this point on what you are about to share with the parent and what stays as part of the confidential file. When you have agreed on this it is appropriate for you to invite the parent or guardian back into the room, at which stage you will present a summary of your findings and outline your plan of management.

It is important at this point that you stick to the plan you have developed with the patient and that you do not spring any surprises. In fact, it is sometimes effective as a reinforcement to have the patient explain the findings to the parent. It is then appropriate to outline the exact treatment you propose, to ensure your consent form covers this, and then to invite the parent to stay in the room while you treat the patient. You will find this to be a most rewarding experience, especially if the parent is a patient of yours, as you have established a common bond for the patient and their parent. You will find the parent may bring the patient in the future (if transport is needed) but that the parent has no particular interest in sitting in on further treatments. Eventually the patient will become old enough to drive themselves but might still pay with one of "mom's checks."

Common Neuromusculoskeletal Disorders

The presenting complaint of adolescents attending chiropractors has been found to most often be "back pain," shared about equally between "low back pain" and "mid back," "thoracic pain," or "general spinal pain" (32). In that study pain descriptors relating to the upper quadrant (head, neck, shoulder, arm) were given in almost half (48.75%) of patient visits. Further, most return visits included a complaint of upper quadrant pain, and while most new visits were specifically for low back pain, there was about an equal distribution between complaints of the upper quadrant and of the lower quadrant (32).

It would seem there is no predominant musculoskeletal condition in adolescence which drives presentation to chiropractors, although typically there will be a complaint of headache, and/or neck and shoulder pain, and/or low back pain. Multiple presenting complaints are to be expected in that they may well represent the "constellation of symptoms" that has recently been identified as being associated with persisting pain (53). Chiropractors can also expect a number of visceral-type conditions to be given as the presenting complaint by adolescents (32), however most will have a causal relationship with neuromusculoskeletal conditions and be within the management scope of chiropractic practice.

A number of musculoskeletal conditions which may surface during adolescence have been previously identified and are listed here as Table 18.4 (30). It is beyond the scope of this chapter to provide detailed etiological, diagnostic and management information on each entity, however it is appropriate to consider several important and common presentations.

Adolescent Spine

The adolescent disk is more prone to herniation than older, adult disks. After the third decade of life, the nucleus of the disk is not sufficiently fluid to be expressed through an annular fissure under most normal circumstances. For older disks to herniate, the nucleus needs to undergo autolysis and relative liquefaction, whereas the adolescent nucleus is fluid (54).

Weak points in the cartilage plates at the former notochordal track are identified as the sites of origin for Schmorl's nodes in adolescence (55,56). Taylor also identifies potential tracks along the remnants of the vascular canals which run between the ring apophysis and centrum of the developing adolescent vertebra. It is along these channels that nuclear material may herniate through the cartilage plates into the anterior vertebral spongiosa or out under the anterior longitudinal ligament (55,56).

During adolescence the sexual dimorphism of the spine becomes clearer. The female spine grows more rapidly in height while the male spine grows more rapidly in transverse diameter up to about age 13. After 13 years the growth in vertebral height is greater in males, together with the greater growth rate in vertebral girth. The female spine thus becomes more slender, less stable and less resistant to bending forces than the male spine (55–57), a finding confirmed by Veldhuizen, Baas and Webb (58). The lumbar disk height of adolescent females is similar to that of adolescent males, but the endplate length is considerably shorter, another factor to explain the greater flexibility of adolescent females (59,60).

Posture

Adolescence is perhaps the last period in which beneficial corrections can be made to postural habits. The reeducation of posture revolves around passive and active exercises. Contracted musculature can be treated with soft tissue techniques after Bates, which involves passive stretching combined with gentle, specific trigger point work (61).

The motor strength of postural muscle groups can be enhanced by specific daily exercises designed to match the improving motor performance of various muscle groups (62). It is also important to correct any pelvic inclination in the

Table 18.4.   **Musculoskeletal Considerations in Adolescence**

Spinal:	Scheuermann's disease (spinal osteochondrosis)
	adolescent disk syndrome
	subluxogenic pain
	postural scoliosis
	idiopathic scoliosis
	tuberculosis of the spine
	sprain/strain syndromes
	prolapsed intervertebral disks
	Schmorl's nodes
	ankylosing spondylitis
	pyogenic osteitis
	coccydynia
	spinal stenosis
	sickle cell disease
	diskitis
	disk space calcification
	sacroiliac pyoarthritis
	spinal epidural abscess
	juvenile rheumatoid arthritis
	spondylolysis
	spondylolisthesis
	neoplasia (vertebral column and intraspinal)
	transverse myelitis
	classic (juvenile) myaesthenia gravis
	Bertolotti's syndrome
Systemic:	ataxia
	fatigue, lassitude
	hypotonia
	Lyme disease
	periarticular-onset juvenile rheumatoid arthritis
	psoriatic arthritis
	inflammatory bowel disease
	acne fulminans
	systemic lupus erythematosus
	syncope–vasodepressor
	micturition
	orthostatic
	tussive
	psychological
	vertigo—cervicogenic
	tall stature disorders—familial
	Marfan's syndrome
	Klinefelter's syndrome
	stress related enuresis
Chest:	costochrondritis
	osteomyelitis
	slipping rib syndrome
	lower cervical/upper thoracic nerve root compromise
	pectus excavatum
	pectus carinatum
	congenitally absent pectoral muscles
Shoulder:	recurrent dislocation
	acromioclavicular dislocation
	sternoclavicular dislocation
	staphylococcal osteitis
	uncommon infections—tuberculosis and gonococcal arthritis
	Sprengel's deformity
	scapula exostosis
Elbow:	epicondylitis
	post-trauma myositis ossificans
Wrist:	extensor tenosynovitis

Hand:	trigger finger/thumb
Cervical:	Klippel Feil syndrome
	subluxogenic pain
	non-traumatic torticollis
Head:	headache—vascular, non-migraine
	vascular, migraine
	cluster
	tension
	cranial inflammation
	ear/eye/sinus disorders
	traction, tumor
	traction, abscess
	intracranial hemorrhage
	pseudo tumor cerebri
	psychogenic
Foot:	March fracture
	Freiberg's disease
	pes cavus, verruca pedis
	tarsal coalition
	early hallux rigidus
	bunion
	hallux valgus
	nail problems
	cuneiform exostosis
	peroneal flat foot
	calcaneal exostosis
	bursitis
	Sever's disease of late onset
	fifth metatarsal head exostosis
	fifth metatarsal base exostosis
Ankle:	osteochondritis tali
	tendo calcaneus
	footballer's ankle
Leg:	tibial stress fracture
	osteoid osteoma
	osteoblastoma
	osteosarcoma
	Ewing's sarcoma
	Brodie's abscess
	anterior compartment syndrome
	shin splints
	Blount's disease of late onset
Knee:	osteochondritis dissecans
	Osgood-Schlatter's disease
	longitudinal meniscus tears
	first incidents of patella dislocation
	chondromalacia patellae
	fat pad injury
	popliteal cyst
Hip:	infective arthritis
	slipped femoral capital epiphysis
	ankylosing spondylitis
	Reiter's syndrome
	pelvic inflammatory disease
	osteoid osteoma
	osteo-arthritis secondary to Perthes'
	undetected congenital dislocation of the hip
	undetected Legg-Calve-Perthes disease
	benign limb pain (muscle overuse)

sagittal plane with exercise. A reduction in pelvic tilt will be reflected by a decrease in other spinal curves with a concomitant improvement in posture and gait (63).

Scoliosis

Estimates of the incidence of scoliosis among adolescents vary widely. Some medical authors who have reviewed the studies suggest about 3% to 4% of all adolescent females are affected and that 15% of these instances are serious enough to warrant aggressive intervention (64). Others suggest a prevalence in school screenings ranging between 0.3% to 15.3% with a prevalence for larger curves of between 1% and 3% (65,66).

As a specialty subject in itself, with numerous current developments and proposals regarding etiology and treatment, scoliosis is deserving of more attention than can be given in a chapter of this nature (see Chapter 15). A comprehensive approach to scoliosis for chiropractors has been published by Souza (40), from which the algorithm in Figure 18.4 is taken. Given the comparatively low incidence of scoliosis which progresses to require surgical intervention, and given that serious congenital scoliosis is likely to have been identified in your adolescent patient prior to his or her visit to your office, it is appropriate to summarize an approach for chiropractors to scoliosis as follows:

1. Screen every adolescent patient through the Adams test, using a "scoliometer" style device to quantify rib-hump.
2. Identify contributing factors, including biomechanical, environmental, familial, and congenital.
3. Where clinically indicated, obtain appropriate radiographs and quantify the scoliotic curvature.
4. Clearly date all relevant findings in the patient's file.
5. Treat to normalize spinal segmental mobility, muscle balance, and postural alignment and assess and treat other presenting complaints within your normal clinical framework.
6. Manage and monitor the patient.

A word of caution is required regarding the use of computerized electrogoniometry to attempt to quantify spinal curvatures. Whilst definitive evidence is not yet published, it should be recognized by the clinician that any such non-invasive measurement is subject to considerable clinical variation, including the temporal variation of the patient, which, in some cases, may exceed the size of the dimension one is attempting to quantify (67,68).

Headaches

Headache activity in adolescents is of a frequency to be of concern. King and Sharpley (69) studied 900 Australian youth aged 10 to 18, and reported only 36.8% as never experiencing a headache. Some 4.6% indicated that they experienced headache almost all the time, 24.8% every few days or once a week, and 33.7% every 2–3 weeks or once a month (69). Almost a third of respondents affirmed their headaches to be a problem, and more than three-quarters considered it was

difficult to concentrate in class or on their homework during a headache (69). When the frequency categories were collapsed into high frequency (once a week) and low frequency (once every 2–3 weeks and below), girls report significantly more headaches than boys (69).

Linet et al. (70) report that 6.9% of males and 15% of females aged 18–23 had consulted a physician within the preceding 12 months because of headache, while 4.4% (male) and 1.2% (female) had consulted a chiropractor. Within this age grouping, 56.8% (males) and 78.3% (females) reported their most recent headache as occurring within the previous 4 weeks (70). The incidence is similar in the 12–17 age grouping, being 55.9% (male) and 73.6% (female) (70).

Headaches in adolescents are more common than recognized (71) and there is a specific opportunity for chiropractors to develop and demonstrate further expertise with the problem.

Dysmenorrhea

Primary dysmenorrhea is painful menstruation which develops within a few years of menarche in the absence of any organic pelvic disease. A Finnish study reported an incidence of 48% among 12-year-old girls, increasing to 79% at age 18 (72), and a Melbourne study of 427 female adolescents (age: 10–12) reported an incidence of 82.1% for dysmenorrhea (73). Further, 19.3% of girls missed school or classes because of the pain, and another 24% limited their activities for the same reason (73). Dysmenorrhea was reported by one third of the Melbourne girls as occurring with their first period, while two thirds reported the onset as being within the first 16 months of menstruating (73). Interestingly, while a higher incidence was found in overweight girls, the underweight girls suffered from more severe pain (73).

Posture was considered an etiological factor as early as 1943 (74), so chiropractic treatment is considered beneficial for patients with dysmenorrhea (75, 76). Liebl and Butler describe one case in which a patient with dysmenorrhea realized fewer episodes of pain as well as lower pain ratings during the treatment phase (77). Dysmenorrhea is a prevalent problem in adolescence and represents a leading cause of recurrent school absenteeism (78). As such it warrants close attention by chiropractic clinicians, not just for the identification and correction of subluxation, but also for nutritional counselling, given the presence of elevated prostaglandins (E2 and F2a) (79,80).

Low-Back Pain

The published evidence demonstrates that adolescent low-back pain, particularly in males, is a serious public health problem (81,82). One study has found the point prevalence of adolescent low-back pain (ALBP) to be 16.7% , with a sample prevalence of 57%, suggesting that nearly two out of three adolescent males experience an episode of LBP in their lifetime (82). Given that the lifetime occurrence of LBP is typically estimated at 80% (83), it is valuable to learn that this figure may be approached within an adolescent population, i.e., in a population before it enters the work force. This fact alone raises implications with respect to the efforts of reducing work-

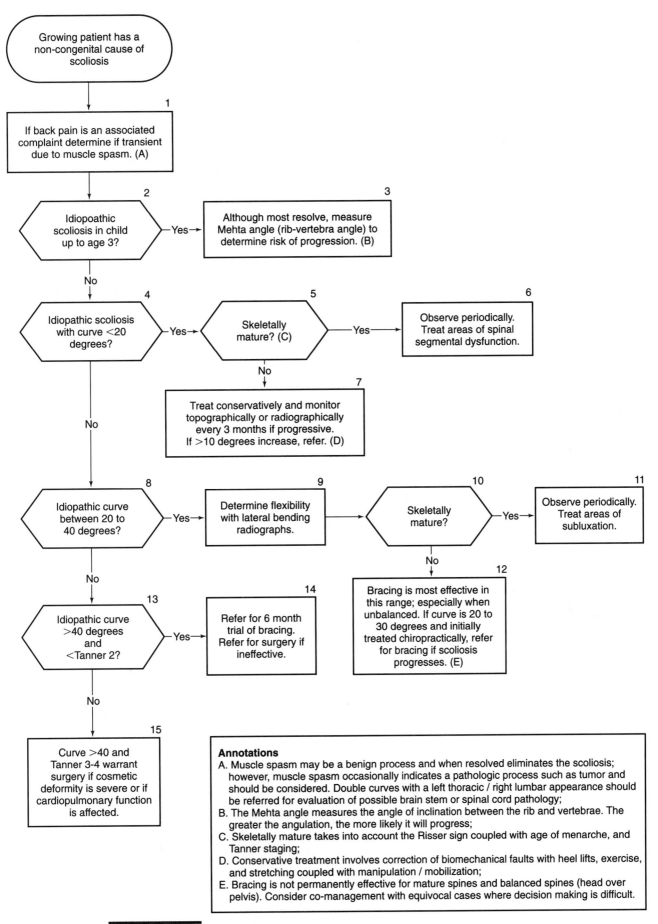

Figure 18.4. Decision making with scoliosis management-algorithm for idiopathic scoliosis.
From Souza TA. Top Clin Chiro 1994; 1:75.

related LBP, and suggests non-traumatic, occupational LBP may result more from an aggravation of preexisting (adolescent) dysfunction than from an unsafe or unsuitable work environment.

The clinical characteristics and correlates of ALBP have been reported to a small extent, and include the finding of Mierau and Cassidy of a high degree of association between sacroiliac dysfunction and LBP (84). Salminen found a subgroup with recurrent LBP having a different spinal mobility pattern as well as decreased trunk muscle strength (85). The typical sufferer of ALBP reports chronic LBP experienced up to a few days at a time, several times a month (82).

Interestingly, several anthropometric characteristics have been identified as having an association with ALBP (86), and it is suspected the association may be causative. The anthropometric picture associated with ALBP is one in which the upper body segment is increased, as indicated by an increased sitting height and increased upper body length (S4 to vertex), resulting in the ratio of the upper body segment to the lower body segment being closer to unity (1:1). In other words, the risk factor is not just being taller, it seems to be a comparatively longer upper body segment. This matter is still being actively researched by the author (87,88).

The practical application of this knowledge is that LBP is a clinical entity of some commonality and concern to chiropractic practice. The clinician must be very thorough with the diagnostic procedures to rule out disk protrusion, limbic fractures and other pathologies, and be aware that, to be complete, any management program must include rehabilitative and strengthening exercises for the low back, with an awareness that some adolescents may be more prone to mechanical LBP than others.

Sports Injuries

The sport which causes the most injuries is American football, followed by gymnastics; while the most severe injuries happen on the track and in basketball. Sprains and strains account for 57% of all injuries (89). The most common adolescent sporting injury in soccer is reported as ankle sprain (90). It is essential for the chiropractor to be competent with both the initial and the subsequent management of such injuries, and particularly when acting as a team physician, to be fully versed in the application of cryotherapy.

The safest and most effective method of applying cryotherapy is to use "wet ice" in the form of about 500 g of broken ice cubes placed within a single layer of cloth, such as a light cotton or linen towel, and then wetted with water to the point where the pack is slowly dripping (91). This pack can then be molded to closely fit the injured body part, and applied without fear of creating an ice burn, given that the temperature of wet-ice (using normal water) is always greater than the freezing point.

The most appropriate application cycle of a wet-ice pack has been found through research to be "10 minutes on, 10 minutes off, then 10 minutes on again" (91). This will provide a reduction of the temperature of the injured body part to the therapeutic range of less than 20°C for over 60 minutes. In the case of acute injury, cryotherapy can be repeated after about

two hours from the first application. During the sub-acute stage a twice-daily application is generally appropriate. It is imperative that any team member who suffers an injury requiring cryotherapy be not allowed to return to the field after ice has been applied, as the subsequent risk of more serious injury to cold soft tissues is very high, due to their increased tensile nature.

More than 70% of running injuries involve the knee or leg. Females report more leg injuries while males report more knee injuries, and over two thirds of all injuries result from a training error (92). Traditional teaching is that disruption of the ligaments about the knee is a rare injury in younger adolescents because the ligaments are stronger than the adjacent growth plates and that injuries that tear adult ligaments will produce epiphyseal disruption in an immature skeleton (93). Further, it is shown that there is an entity of knee pain in adolescence associated with segmental spinal dysfunction, and that such pain may be relieved by a specific treatment programme which includes spinal manipulation (94).

The current concept is that ligamentous injuries, although uncommon in the skeletally immature patient, can be found either in isolation or in association with physeal injury (95). A high level of competence with differential diagnosis of such injuries about the knee is particularly important as the prompt recognition and management of such ligamentous injuries in the adolescent is essential if good recovery is to be made by the patient.

Comprehensive diagnostic and management information regarding the spectrum of sporting injuries is available in text form (96) as well as in paper form throughout the literature. It is expected that a chiropractor who wished to practice in the area of sports medicine would seek membership of the International Federation of Sports Chiropractic (FICCS) (97), the world governing body for sports chiropractic, and gain additional educational qualification through either a Masters program in Sports Chiropractic, offered by university based chiropractic programs (98,99), or a post graduate program from a private chiropractic college (100).

Health Maintenance in Adolescence

Although adolescents have many real and significant health problems, they are not regarded as prolific users of the health care system, especially for counselling on health related matters (12,13,101). A major problem with implementing health care strategies for adolescents is gaining access to them as individuals (3,13,19,101–105). A chiropractor is well placed within the community to provide preventative as well as curative care to adolescents. Some of the more common matters which arise as health maintenance issues in adolescence are alphabetically described below.

Asthma

Management of the asthmatic patient centers around an established "management plan" (106). Even within the limitations of any such plan which may include a pharmacological component, the chiropractor has an important role to play with respect to musculoskeletal health, as with the patient retaining mobility of the thoracic musculoskeletal structures. All medical management plans require the identification and avoidance of trigger and aggravating factors, a written action plan by the patient to facilitate rapid medical intervention when indicated by serial peak expiratory flow readings, plus specific patient education and regular review.

Within the wholistic, neuromusculoskeletal chiropractic paradigm the opportunities are very much broader (107). No matter which particular empirical model (108,109) the chiropractor elects to follow, it must be remembered that the responsibility of the chiropractor as a primary health care practitioner is not only to adjust in accord with a chosen model, but to ensure the patient has a defined, understood and agreed action plan, and has appropriate access for pharmacological assistance when indicated.

Lines (107) has argued the suitability of the "clinical ecology" model in the management of bronchial asthma, a model which contends that many causes of ill-health lie within the environment of the sick person. In addition to the known precipitants which include allergens, infection, exercise, air pollution, food additives, occupational exposures and psychosocial factors, other substances known to trigger asthma attacks in susceptible individuals include aspirin, beta-blockers, NSAIDS, and monosodium glutamate. Added to this list are suspected precipitants such as cow's milk, preservatives, artificial colors and flavors, and some cereal grains (107). The inclusion of the clinical ecology approach in chiropractic practice would seem to be an appropriate method of broadening and indeed strengthening the chiropractor's role in the management of asthma (107).

Breast Self Examination

There is some controversy as to whether it is appropriate for adolescent females to be taught breast self examination (BSE), on the basis of the low incidence of breast cancer in this age group. It is generally recommended that as a preventative measure, patients should be questioned from the age of 25 years to determine whether they fall into a high-risk group (identified by the presence of familial breast cancer and/or the presence of a lump, swelling, or pain in the breast, or bleeding or discharge from a nipple) and that BSE instruction should commence from about age 40 (110).

However, an essential characteristic of primary health care practice is the provision of "self-help" skills to patients (111), and this includes the skills of BSE for the late adolescent female. Logic suggests that if the accepted preventative measures are enacted from about age 25, then some form of basic instruction should be given before then so the patient has a knowledge base from which she can give an informed response. It seems fitting for even the mid-stage adolescent to be taught how to explore her body and become familiar with its cyclical changes, and it is appropriate to ensure all female patients beyond adolescence have the knowledge and skills to conduct BSE. Whether they choose to do so remains their prerogative; however, at some future stage, one can be fairly sure the skill will become an essential part of the patient's personal health care strategy.

There is a variety of brochures available from public agencies which are suitable for distribution in the chiropractic clinic. The contemporary approach to BSE is to palpate vertically in parallel lines over the breast tissue, starting from the sternum and moving laterally in finger width increments to conclude with the axillary tail of breast tissue and axillary lymph nodes, while lying supine with a small pillow under the shoulder on the side of the breast being examined, and with the homolateral hand placed under the head.

It is important to emphasize to the patient that she is "not looking for cancer"; instead she is getting to know her body and at some stage when there may be a variation from the familiar, she will be able to detect it early and describe it to the appropriate practitioner. It is important to also ensure the patient understands the components of observation, effected by standing undressed in front of a mirror and leaning forward with the hands on the hips, and of individual nipple inspection, including gentle distraction and squeezing to determine whether there is any discharge.

Chronic Fatigue Syndrome

The challenge of chronic fatigue syndrome (CFS) to the chiropractor is the establishment of the diagnosis without resorting to a battery of serological and other laboratory tests (112). The criteria for diagnosis have been identified (Table 18.5) (113), as have the differential diagnoses (Table 18.6). Alternate terms for CFS include "yuppie flu," "post viral fatigue syndrome," "chronic mononucleosis syndrome," and "systemic immunodeficient Epstein-Barr virus syndrome," (114) and although chiropractic adjustment may afford some relief for patients with CFS (114, 115), it is not seen as a "cure." As with homeopathic intervention (116), the successful management of idiopathic CFS would seem to warrant the inclusion of a balanced diet with nutritional support, and stress management.

Key aspects of the history of an adolescent with a complaint of fatigue include onset, severity, duration, aggravating and relieving factors, exercise tolerance with respect to the patient's peers, the level of physical activity, adequacy of sleep, recent weight gain or loss, dietary review, medication review, depression (as with sadness, concentration or declining school performance, and depression secondary to the stress of peer or parental conflict), and exposure to contagious disease (117). In addition to the history, it is wise to determine any avenue of secondary gain to the patient; however, this may take several consultations and a broader knowledge of the family environment.

The physical exam is used to rule out systemic causes, with particular attention being paid to the cardiovascular system. Most congenital cardiac conditions are diagnosed before adolescence; however, the clinician must be alert for undetected conditions. Murmurs that indicate a need for referral and subsequent evaluation of an organic cause include those in an adolescent with a history of chest pain, syncope, shortness of breath, or exertional dyspnea; a diastolic, pansystolic or continuous murmur; a murmur of intensity greater than grade 3; a murmur associated with abnormal splitting of S2; and a systolic ejection murmur with maximal intensity in the aortic

Table 18.5.   Diagnostic Criteria for Chronic Fatigue Syndrome

Required

Both major criteria plus 8 minor criteria
or
Both major criteria plus 6 minor criteria *and* 2 physical criteria

Major Criteria

Persistent fatigue for at least 6 months, not relieved by bed rest, causing at least a 50% impairment in daily activity

Absence of other medical conditions that would explain the fatigue

Minor Criteria (present for at least 6 months)

Fever (37.5°-38.6°C orally)
Sore throat
Cervical or axillary adenopathy
Unexplained general weakness
Myalgias
Headaches
Migratory arthralgias
Neuropsychiatric symptoms (e.g., inability to concentrate, depression, confusion)
Sleep disturbance

Physical Criteria

Documented fever
Nonexudative pharyngitis
Palpable or tender anterior or posterior cervical or axillary nodes

---

area (118). Chronic pulmonary, cardiac or liver disease may be suggested by digital clubbing, and a tachycardia may indicate the use of illicit drugs.

According to Cavanaugh (117), pallor may be associated with iron-deficiency anemia or chronic inflammation. Anorexia nervosa may give a yellowish cast to the skin due to an elevation in serum carotene. Jaundice suggests hepatitis or increased red cell destruction. Other skin abnormalities may indicate SLE or JRA. Iritis, uveitis, stomatitis, glossitis or gingivitis may indicate inflammatory bowel disease, while hyperpigmentation of the gums suggests Addison's disease. Joint tenderness or restricted motion may indicate a collagen vascular disorder or inflammatory bowel disease, while bone pain and/or tenderness on direct palpation is suggestive of malignancy or a benign lesion.

Cavanaugh (117) also points to the value of determining the patient's strength to differentiate disorders with an associated muscle weakness from other causes of fatigue. Muscle weakness only late in the day, or after physical activity, may suggest myasthenia gravis, in which case the patient should also be examined for ptosis, weakness of the extraocular muscles, and dysphagia (117).

The tired patient with cervical lymphadenopathy, fever and sore throat is indicative of infectious mononucleosis (IM), one of the most common infectious diseases of adolescence and most commonly associated with Epstein-Barr virus (EBV). Cytomegalovirus (CMV) is more commonly found in those older than 25 years of age. Other considerations include toxoplasmosis, hepatitis A and adenovirus. The typical viral prodrome of headache, chills, sweating, loss of appetite and inability to concentrate is accompanied by a fever with afternoon and evening peaks of 100°F to 103°F. There may be whitish tonsillar exudate and other pains, such as shoulder or abdominal, from associated adenopathy. Other clinical signs include periorbital edema and soft palate petechiae. IM secondary to EBV and CMV is a not a differential diagnosis of CFS, given it is not a chronic clinical presentation, but it does need to be clearly differentiated within all adolescent patients who present with fatigue. The acute phase of IM generally subsides spontaneously after 2 to 4 weeks but may be followed by a variable period of ill defined fatigue. The management is symptomatic with advice to avoid physical activity and sport which may threaten injury to the spleen should it be enlarged.

Contraception

As with BSE, it is more the right of the patient than the comfort or convenience of the practitioner which should be considered in relation to the issues surrounding contraception during adolescence. It is a responsibility of every primary health care practitioner to be a source of accurate information and advice for their adolescent patients in this matter.

Contraceptive methods fall into two groups; either they require prescription and/or fitting (oral contraceptive, diaphragm, inter uterine devices, cervical cap) and as such fall outside the scope of chiropractic practice, or they are non

Table 18.6.   Differential Diagnoses for Chronic Fatigue Syndrome

Extremely common	Depression
	Pregnancy
	Stress related disorders: anxiety, hyperventilation syndrome, school avoidance, psychosomatic disorder
Common	Eating disorders
	Rapid or excessive change in weight
	Excessive physical activity
	Allergic tension fatigue syndrome
	Anemia: dysfunctional uterine bleeding, nutritional
Uncommon	Cardiomyopathy or congestive heart failure
	Asthma
	Hyperthyroidism or hypothyroidism
	Connective tissue disease
	Inflammatory bowel disease
	Leukemia or lymphoma
	AIDS
	Hepatitis
	Myasthenia gravis
	Obstructive sleep apnea

prescriptive (condoms, vaginal spermicides, contraceptive sponge, douching, coitus interruptus, natural family planning). Of this latter group, perhaps the most effective method for a sexually active adolescent is the condom; it is easily available, inexpensive, has no side effects (apart from a rare allergic reaction to latex), may contribute to a reduced risk of cervical cancer, protects well against pregnancy, and protects almost completely against sexually transmitted diseases (119).

Apart from contraception, the benefits of condom usage include a lower rate of transmission of Chlamydia trachomatis, Neisseria gonorrhea, herpes virus and human papilloma virus; however, only latex condoms offer protection against cytomegalovirus, hepatitis B virus, and human immunodeficiency virus (120,121).

As condoms become more freely available in the community, there will be a greater compliance with their usage by adolescents; however, the availability of condoms should not be seen as an encouragement of sexual activity. While the adolescent care provider is not a moralist, he or she has the obligation as a primary health care practitioner to provide the level of support deemed to be in the best interest of the patient. Where an adolescent declares a decision for abstinence, this must be supported, especially as abstinence is indeed the most effective way to prevent both pregnancy and sexually transmitted diseases.

On the other hand, when the need for prevention and protection is identified, the responsibility becomes one of supporting the patient as he or she moves towards self sufficiency in these matters. When natural family planning is appropriate, perhaps for married youth with religious conviction, it is a responsibility to know where to refer the couple for ongoing counseling, advice and assistance. When oral contraception is sought, the most qualified person to provide the advice and to determine the better type of pill, is the prescribing practitioner. In summary, for matters of contraception, it is the chiropractor's duty, as a primary health care provider, to ensure the patient receives the best level of most appropriate care from all members of the health care team, including the chiropractor.

Growth Disorders

Variations in the time of onset of puberty, the duration of puberty, and the overall stature of the individual are considered as being disorders of growth. Generally, concerns are raised when puberty is delayed beyond the general limit of commencement in males of 13.2 years, or appears to be unduly lengthy, beyond the normal completion within 4 or 5 years of commencement.

The management of growth disorders would seem to lie outside the chiropractic scope of practice, however it is essential for every practitioner working with adolescents to be aware of the key clinical information which are required to identify the patient who may benefit from referral, to competently effect the referral, and then to retain an informed role in the co-management of the patient.

About 50% of short stature is nonpathologic (familial, idiopathic, or constitutional delay), however this assumption cannot be made without an investigation to rule out pathologic short stature which includes intrinsic causes (such as osteo-

chondrodystrophy, or chromosomal abnormalities), nutritional deprivation, psychosocial deprivation, and disease-related short stature.

Serial height measurement is the most important diagnostic tool in firstly the identification, and secondly the evaluation and management of short stature (122,123). Short stature is considered when the patient's height falls below two standard deviations (SD) from the mean. The benefit of serial height measurement is that it can show whether the short stature is a normal variant (a long history of being less than 2 SD below the mean) or acquired (a move towards 2 SD below the mean from a growth curve previously within 2 SD of the mean). It is essential that the growth chart which you choose to use is one which bears relevance to the population in which you practice, the most obvious distinctions being between American Caucasians and American blacks. Additional clinical information may be gained from bone age as determined by radiographs of the wrists and knees, and by accurate Tanner staging.

For intervention to have any effect, there must be potential for growth; it is important for the early adolescent's record to include a growth chart from the first visit. Concerns regarding short stature must be addressed promptly, and, when known to not be acquired secondary to nutritional deprivation, generally require referral to a pediatric endocrinologist.

Menstrual Disorders

The role of the chiropractor within primary health care practice is to gather the clinical information relating to complaints of menstrual disorders and then make a determination between the continuation of monitoring within the chiropractic management paradigm, or referral to a pediatric or adolescent gynecologist.

In Western societies, menarche occurs from 1 to 5 (average 22) years after the onset of puberty, at a mean age of 12.2 years. Although this is between Tanner stages 3 and 4, some 15% of females achieve menarche after reaching stage 5 (124). Although primary amenorrhea correctly describes the situation in which menstrual flow has never occurred, a preferred term is delayed menarche. The preferred term for secondary amenorrhea is postmenarchal amenorrhea, and is when menses ceases after at least three menstrual flows in a 3 to 6 month time frame (125).

Delayed menarche is evaluated with reference to the onset of puberty. If puberty has not commenced (absence of breast budding) by 13.2 (some authors say 13) years, the patient should be referred to an endocrinologist for evaluation. If puberty is present but no menses has occurred within 4 years of the onset of puberty, then referral is indicated to an adolescent gynecologist for investigation of anatomic, obstructive defects. Complaints of postmenarchal amenorrhea require that pregnancy be ruled out, and if so, then referral for assessment of the hypothalamic-pituitary-ovarian axis (22,125–127).

Complaints of dysfunctional uterine bleeding (DUB) include oligomenorrhea, hypomenorrhea, polymenorrhea, hypermenorrhea, menometrorrhagia, and breakthrough bleeding. They all require appropriate referral by the chiropractor as the investigation will most likely include a gynecological examination which lies outside the general scope of chiropractic practice.

Nutrition

Diet, fitness, and health are closely interlinked concerns of adolescents (128). Any provision of advice must be tempered by a knowledge of the living environment of the patient. For example, school students may not be able to obtain fresh food through their school canteen, or may be subjected to traditional gender stereotyping in the school's approach to teaching home economics and cooking, or indeed may be taking a cooking class which teaches a curriculum devoid of healthy food prepared in a healthy manner.

Most young people are aware of the link between diet and health, and, notwithstanding any stated attempt to achieve a balanced diet, seem to be lazy about food choices, responsive to fast-food advertising, and not generally motivated to make the effort to achieve a reasonably nutritious balance. In late adolescence there is the risk of the negative cycle of unemployment, low income, inadequate diet, and poorer health (128).

The role of the chiropractor is to promote and reinforce the concepts of healthy eating. This can be achieved in a front line manner by making appropriate leaflets available in the waiting room, and by conducting "healthy eating" classes for schools and community groups. On the more intimate doctor/patient level, the concept of a "health contract" may be introduced, based on the work and recommendations of Jamison (129).

A beneficial chart to have in your clinic is Jamison's "Nutritional well-being: A self assessment tool" (Fig. 18.5). The power of this instrument lies in its subliminal proactive message: the patient is led to assess his or her current diet and set a two stage goal for improvement. The same chart has been used successfully by the author in his work with socially disadvantaged adolescents, in which case the column headings "current/intended/achieved" become "never/sometimes/always," and the instrument serves as a cross sectional survey of nutritional habit. A discussion of the findings from such a survey with the study group then opens the way to negotiate individual health contracts, referring to the original instrument to address and discuss the nutritional reasoning underlying each line item and to set a time period for achievement.

Pap Smear

In contrast to BSE, the use of the Papanicolaou smear test is appropriate for all women who have been sexually active and who have not had a hysterectomy (130). It is a preventative intervention thought to reduce the incidence and mortality from invasive cervical cancer through the early detection of cancer of the uterine cervix.

Given that the conduct of this test is not a component of chiropractic practice, the role of the chiropractor becomes one of screening all female patients to counsel on the advisability of the test and to arrange appropriate referral where needed. With adolescent females, it is preferable to couch the questioning in a discussive, open-ended manner; however, discretion must be used with respect to you making an initial judgment that the patient may be sexually active.

When consulting with an 18-year-old patient for example, you could say, "One of the important things a woman can do is look after her personal health. Having a pap smear is one way to do that. Have you had a pap smear yet?" If the answer is in the affirmative you can deduce the patient has a certain level of awareness and thus take a supportive role to reaffirm her actions. If the answer is in the negative, you may then say, "A smear is a good thing to have when you start having sexual intercourse," and then, depending on your interpretation of the patient, either, "Is there something here you'd like to talk about or would you like me to refer you for a smear test?" or "When you are ready we can talk about it more and I'll give you further information."

Skin Cancer

Chiropractors hold a unique place in the primary health care model due to the nature of their practice providing frequent opportunity for thorough observation of the patient's skin, especially on the back where it is difficult for the patient to self-assess. The fourth most common cancer in white Australians is malignant melanoma, and all patients should be considered to be at risk. In other countries (such as Canada), the risk group has been reduced to outdoor workers and those in contact with polycyclic aromatic hydrocarbons (131).

The history taken by the chiropractor should include the question, "Have you had any recent change, such as an increase in number, size or thickness, or any change in shape or color, or any itchiness or bleeding from any mole or freckle on your skin?" An affirmative response will obviously lead to a more detailed history and examination, while a negative response should be kept open until confirmed by your examination. Early identification of suspicious lesions, followed by prompt intervention, is an effective preventative health strategy.

Testicular Self Examination

Testicular cancer is rare in adolescents but remains the most common malignancy in men aged between 18 and 30 years (132,133). When other scrotal concerns of adolescence are considered, there is strong reason for every adolescent male to be taught the principles of testicular self examination (TSE). The philosophy of BSE applies to TSE, namely the patient is not being taught to look for cancer; he is being helped to become familiar with his body, its parts, and their function.

The best time for TSE is during a shower or in bed when the patient is warm and relaxed. The technique is to use both hands to gently roll each testicle between the thumb and fingers. The epididymis is located as an irregular, sausage shaped structure at the back of the testicle. While both hands support the scrotum, the size and weight of each testicle is noted. The patient is instructed to become familiar with the various irregularities of the contents of the scrotum, including points of tenderness and firmness. The objective is to detect any change early, and to be able to describe it to an appropriate practitioner who will examine and comment.

The patient needs to be told that the most common cause of irregularities in the scrotum are congenital or caused by infection. The whole objective of TSE (as with BSE) is empowerment of the individual. The patient is helped to

Nutritional Well-Being: A Self-Assessment Tool

There is evidence to suggest that diet influences health. Many of the nutritional recommendations for good health proposed by health authorities can be achieved by implementing the dietary suggestions listed in the following nutritional index.

Complete the following quiz noting your CURRENT score on all items listed in the first column. Identify those items which you intend to alter and commit yourself to a time (INTENDED) at which you anticipate having achieved the desired eating pattern. Perform continual self-monitoring (ACHIEVED). Score 1 point for every true statement.

	CURRENT	INTENDED	ACHIEVED
I eat fresh fruit or raw vegetables twice or more daily.			
I eat two or more servings of vegetables each day.			
I eat nuts, legumes, fish, or chicken without the skin each day.			
I eat nuts, legumes, fish, or chicken in preference to red meat.			
I eat yellow/orange and cruciferous vegetables each day.			
I eat from a calcium source, e.g., lowfat milk or yogurt, sardines, sesame seeds, etc. each day.			
I eat liquid vegetable oils in preference to animal fats or solidified vegetable oils.			
I avoid excess salt.			
I eat wholegrain/wholemeal products in preference to refined products.			
I limit my sugar intake.			
I limit my fat intake.			
I limit my alcohol intake.			
I avoid charred, barbecued food.			
I avoid cured or smoked food.			
I maintain my ideal bodyweight.*			
NUTRITIONAL HEALTH INDEX			

To maintain an ideal body weight ingest 15 kcal for every pound of ideal body weight; to lose weight ingest 10 kcal for every pound of desired body weight; to gain weight ingest 20 kcal for every pound of desired body weight.

Figure 18.5. Self assessment instrument for nutritional well-being. From Jamison JR. Health promotion for chiropractic practice. Gaithersburg: Aspen, 1991:54.

become very familiar with a part of his body which is all too frequently hidden, yet paradoxically, can give rise to a rapid robber of life.

All scrotal complaints raised by the patient require prompt referral, and where testicular torsion is suspected (acute onset of testicular/scrotal pain, mostly with scrotal edema and erythema, and with nausea and vomiting in about 50% of cases), it must be considered a surgical emergency as infarction occurs within 5 to 6 hours. Other presentations requiring prompt referral for diagnosis and management include acute epididymitis, orchitis, varicoceles and hematoceles.

Other Matters

There is a range of other matters the management of which, while intimately related to adolescent health, may not be most appropriate for inclusion within typical chiropractic practice. Such matters include alcohol abuse, destructive behavior (risk taking), drug experimentation or abuse, pregnancy and related issues such as abortion and adoption, sexual orientation, sexually transmitted diseases, and trauma from motor vehicle accidents.

The chiropractor who elects to begin the journey of developing a practice oriented towards the adolescent patient would wisely seek out the existing groups and professionals in his or her community and start to establish a network of interactive support, not just for the practice, but most importantly, for the patient. The care of the adolescent is attended by new and greater responsibilities, and these should be met through continuing education, postgraduate study, and interactive community participation.

REFERENCES

1. Nelms BC. Adolescent health care - the need is great. J Paediatric Health Care 1987;1(2): 59.
2. Eckersley R. Casualties of change: social and economic issues affecting youth. Bull Nat Clearinghouse Youth Studies 1988;7(4): 3–8.
3. Thomas L. Adolescent health. Alabama Med 1988;57(9): 41–2.
4. McAnarney ER. Adolescent medicine: growth of a discipline. Pediatrics 1988; 82(2): 270–2.
5. Campbell D. From the editor: Community education. Aust Assoc Adolescent Health National Newsletter 1990;1: 3.
6. Gross J. Afraid and hurt, young turn to clinics. The New York Times 1992 Jan 28: 1.
7. Bennett D. Preface. In Bennett D and Williams M, eds. New universals, adolescent health in a time of change. Curtin, Brolga Press. 1988: vii.
8. Jenkins RR. Reassessing our leadership role for the health of adolescents. J Adol Health Care 1989;10: 435–7.
9. Sanders Jr. JM. Health care delivery to adolescents and young adults by pediatricians. Pediatrics 1988;82(3)Pt2: 516–7.
10. Anrig-Howe CA. Chiropractic approaches to pregnancy and pediatric care. In: Plaugher G, ed. Textbook of clinical chiropractic: a specific biomechanical approach. Baltimore: Williams and Wilkins, 1993: 383–432.
11. Master of Applied Science in Clinical Practice (Chiropractic Paediatrics). Course information handbook. The Chiropractic Unit, Faculty of Biomedical and Health Sciences, RMIT, Melbourne, 1994.
12. Wheeler MJ. Adolescents and health care. Nursing: the add on journal 1981;1(24): 1028–30.
13. Youth Policy Development Council. Health for Youth Final Report. Health Promotion Unit. Victoria. Health Department, 1987.
14. Friedman HL. World Health Organization initiatives in adolescent health and some future directions. In: Bennett D and Williams M, eds. New Universals, Adolescent Health in a Time of Change. Curtin: Brolga Press, 1988: 72–5.
15. Coulehan JL. Chiropractic and the clinical art. Soc Sci Med 1985;21(4): 383–90.
16. Wardwell WI. The Connecticut survey of public attitudes toward chiropractic. Proceedings of 1989 International Conference on Spinal Manipulation. Arlington: FCER 1989: 230–5.
17. Jamison JR. Chiropractic's functional integration into conventional health care: some implications. J Manipulative Physiol Ther 1987;10: 5–10.
18. Hofmann AD, Greydanus DE. Adolescent Medicine. 2nd ed. Norwalk: Appleton and Lange, 1989: xi–xiii.
19. Coulter ID. The chiropractic patient: A social profile. J Canadian Chiropr Assoc 1985;29: 25–8.
20. Council on Child and Adolescent Health. Academy of Pediatrics. Age limits of pediatrics. Pediatrics 1988;81: 736.
21. Australian Health Ministers' Advisory Council Working Party on Child and Youth Health. Draft National Policy on Child and Youth Health. Canberra. Australian Government Publishing Service 1994: 1.
22. Garn SM. Physical growth and development. In: Friedman SB, ed. Comprehensive adolescent health care. St. Louis: Quality Medical Publishing, Inc. 1992:18–23.
23. Brunader RA, Moore DC. Evaluation of the child with growth retardation. Am Fam Physician 1987;35(2): 165–76.
24. Lowrey GH. Growth and development of children. 7th ed. Chicago. Year Book Medical Pub Inc 1979: 207–99.
25. Bullough PG, Boachie-Adjei O. Atlas of spinal diseases. New York. Gower Publishing 1988.
26. Moore KL. Before we are born. Toronto: WB Saunders, 1983.
27. Taylor JR, Twomey LT. Vertebral column development and its relation to adult pathology. Aust J Physiotherapy 1985;31: 83–8.
28. Taylor JR, Twomey LT. Sexual dimorphism in human vertebral body shape. J Anat 1984;138: 281–6.
29. Strasburger VC, Brown RT. Adolescent medicine, a practical guide. Boston: Little, Brown and Company, 1991: 400.
30. Ebrall PS. Adolescent health care: chiropractic's investment in the future. Chiro J Aust 1991;21: 13–9.
31. Ebrall PS. Adolescent attendance at chiropractic clinic. A pilot study. Unpublished minor thesis. School of Chiropractic and Osteopathy. Melbourne: Phillip Institute of Technology, 1990.
32. Ebrall PS. A description of 320 visits to chiropractors by Australian adolescents. Chiro J Aust 1993; 24: 4–8.
33. Burton CV, Cassidy JD. Economics, epidemiology and risk factors. In Kirkaldy-Willis WH, Burton CV, eds. Managing low-back pain, 3rd ed. New York: Churchill Livingston 1992: 1–6.
34. DeCoster LD, Ebrall PS. A description of WorkCare claims where chiropractors wrote the initiating certificate: Victoria 1990/91. Chiropr J Austral 1993; 23:33–7.
35. Manga P, Angus D. The effectiveness and cost effectiveness of chiropractic management of low-back pain. Ottawa. Pran Manga and Associates, University of Ottawa. 1993.
36. Dutro CL, Wheeler L. Back school and chiropractic practice. J Manipulative Physiol Ther 1986;9: 209–12.
37. Ebrall PS. Pre-employment musculoskeletal assessment: the imperative for outcome studies. Chiro J Austral 1992; 22: 9–14.
38. Johnson RL. Adolescent growth and development. In: Hofmann AD, Greydanus DE. Adolescent Medicine, 2nd ed. Norwalk: Appleton and Lange, 1989:9–15.
39. Kreipe RE, Gewanter HL. Physical screening for participation in sports. Paediatrics 1985;75:1076–80.
40. Souza TA. Decision making with scoliosis management. Top Clin Chiro 1994;1(3): 39–54.
41. Bennett DL. The approach to the adolescent patient. Aust Fam Physician. 1988:17(May): 345–6.
42. Ebrall PS. Commentary: Chiropractic and the cul de sac complex. Chiropr J Aust 1994; 24: 106–12.
43. Bar-Or O, Lombardo JA, Rowland TW. The pre-participation sports exam. Patient Care 1988;Oct 30: 75–102.
44. Fields KB, Delaney M. Focusing the pre-participation sports examination. J Fam Pract 1990;30: 304–12.
45. Sweaney JA. Informed consent: A practitioner's viewpoint. J Aust Chiropractors' Assoc 1984;14: 57–8.
46. Jamison JR. Beyond informed consent: Competent practitioner-patient communication. J Aust Chiropractors' Assoc 1984;14: 62–4.
47. Harrison JD. Informed consent, as a growing obligation. ICA Int Rev Chiropr 1990;Nov/Dec: 23–7.
48. Bolton SP. "Informed consent" and all that jazz. Chiropr J Aust 1993;23: 141–2.
49. Campbell L, Ladenheim CJ, Sherman R, Sportelli L. Informed consent: a search for protection. Top Clin Chiro 1994;1(3): 55–63.
50. Chapman-Smith D. Cervical manipulation and vertebral artery injury. In: Chapman-Smith D, ed. The Chiropractic Report 1994;8(3): 1–6.
51. Appendix E. Top Clin Chiro 1994;1(3): 77–80.
52. Goldenring JM, Cohen E. Getting into adolescent heads. Contemp Pediatr 1988; 5:75.
53. Klapow JC, Slater MA, Patterson TL, et al. An empirical evaluation of multidimensional clinical outcome in chronic low back pain patients. Pain 1993: 107–18.
54. Twomey L, Taylor JR. Structural and mechanical disc changes with age. J Man Med 1990;5: 58–61.
55. Taylor JT. The development and adult structure of lumbar intervertebral discs. J Man Med 1990;5: 43–7.
56. Taylor JR, Twomey LT. Vertebral column development and its relation to adult pathology. Aust J Physiotherapy 1985;31(3): 83–8.
57. Taylor JR, Twomey LT. Sexual dimorphism in human vertebral body shape. J Anat 1984;138(2):281–6.
58. Veldhuizen AG, Baas P, Webb PJ. Observations on the growth of the adolescent spine. J Bone Joint Surgery 1986;68-B(5): 724–8.
59. Twomey L, Taylor JR. Structural and mechanical disc changes with age. J Man Med 1990;5: 58–61.
60. Bradford DS, Hensinger RN. Development of the vertebral column. In: The pediatric spine. Thieme. New York 1985: 9–14.
61. Bates T, Myofascial pain. In Green M, Haggerty R, eds. Ambulatory Pediatrics II. WB Saunders. Philadelphia 1977: 147–8.
62. Beunen GP, Malina RM, Van't Hof MA, et al. Adolescent growth and motor performance. Illinois. Human Kinetic Books 1988.
63. Keim HA. The adolescent spine. New York. Grune and Stratton 1976; 23–6.
64. Greydanus DE, Hofmann AD. The musculoskeletal system. In: Hofmann AD, Greydanus DE. Adolescent medicine, 2nd ed. Norwalk: Appleton and Lange, 1989: 203–30.
65. Strasburger VC, Brown RT. Adolescent medicine, a practical guide. Boston: Little, Brown and Company, 1991:95–105.
66. Macy NJ. Orthopaedics. In: Friedman SB, ed. Comprehensive adolescent health care. St Louis: Quality Medical Publishing, Inc., 1992:1116–9.
67. Ebrall PS, Alevaki H, Cust S, Roberts NJ. An estimation of the measurement error of the Metrecom for computation of sagittal spinal angles. J Chiropr Technique 1993; 5:104–6.
68. Ebrall PS, Alevaki H, Cust SL, Roberts NJ. Preliminary report: Evidence of temporal variation in the values of three sagittal spinal angles. In: Minter W, ed. Proceedings of the National Conference, Chiropractors' Association Australia, 1993 Oct 22–24. Sydney: Chiropractors' Association of Australia 1993:81.
69. King NJ, Sharpley CF. Headache activity in children and adolescents. J Pediatr Child Health 1990; 26: 50–4.
70. Linet MS, Stewart WF, Celentano DD, et al. An epidemiologic study of headache among adolescents and young adults. JAMA 1989;261(15):2211–6.
71. Rothner AD. Headaches in children and adolescents. Postgrad Med 1987;81: 223–9.

72. Teperi J, Rimpela M. Menstrual pain, health and behaviour in girls. Soc Sci Med 1989; 29:163–9.

73. Verbowski G, Matthews M, Tucker C. The incidence of primary dysmenorrhoea in 427 adolescent girls in years 10–12 in one Melbourne school. J NZ Reg Osteopaths 1991: 24–7.

74. Adams TW. Painful menstruation with a special reference to posture as an etiologic factor. Pac Med Surg 1943; 42:88–98.

75. Arnould-Frochet S. Investigation of the effect of chiropractic adjustments on a specific gynecological problem: dysmenorrhoea. Bull Eur Chiro Union 1977; 25(1):17.

76. Wiles M. Gynaecology and obstetrics in chiropractic. J Canadian Chiro Assoc 1980; 24:163–6.

77. Liebl NA, Butler LM. A chiropractic approach to the treatment of dysmenorrhoea. J Manipulative Physiol Ther 1990;13: 101–6.

78. Alvin PE, Litt IF. Current status of the etiology and management of dysmenorrhoea in adolescence. Pediatrics 1982; 70: 516–25.

79. Strasburger VC, Brown RT. Adolescent medicine, a practical guide. Boston. Little, Brown and Company 1991:238.

80. Jamison JR. The management of rheumatoid arthritis: considerations for chiropractic practice. Chiropr J Aust 1994; 24: 83–90.

81. Olsen TL, Anderson RL, Dearwater SR, et al. The epidemiology of low back pain in an adolescent population. Am J Public Health 1992; 82:606–8.

82. Ebrall PS. The epidemiology of male adolescent low-back pain in a north suburban population of Melbourne, Australia. J Manipulative Physiol Ther 1994;17:447–53.

83. Goertz MN. Prognostic indicators of acute low-back pain. Spine 1990; 15: 1307–10.

84. Mierau D, Cassidy JD, Yong-Hing K. Low-back pain and straight leg raising in children and adolescents. Spine 1989;14: 526–8.

85. Salminen JJ, Maki P, Oksanen A, Pentti J. Spinal mobility and trunk muscle strength in 15-year-old schoolchildren with and without low-back pain. Spine 1992;17: 405–11.

86. Ebrall PS. Some anthropometric dimensions of male adolescents with idiopathic low back pain. J Manipulative Physiol Ther 1994; 17:296–301.

87. Ebrall PS. Adolescent musculoskeletal health. In: Seater SR, Callahan DL, eds. Proceedings of the 1994 International Conference on Spinal Manipulation 1994, June 10–11, Palm Springs, CA. Arlington. Foundation for Chiropractic Education and Research 1994:134–5.

88. Ebrall PS. Low-back pain and relevant anthropometric dimensions in male adolescent Australian Aborigines. J Manipulative Physiol Ther (in press).

89. McLain LG, Reynolds S. Sports injuries in a high school. Pediatrics 1989; 84(3): 446–50.

90. Editorial. Soccer injuries and physical maturity. Am Fam Physician 1989; 39(2): 312–5.

91. Ebrall PS, Bales G, Frost B. An improved clinical protocol for ankle cryotherapy. J Man Med 1992; 6:161–5.

92. Paty JG, Swafford D. Adolescent running injuries. J Adol Health Care 1984;5: 87–90.

93. Kannus P, Jarvinen M. Knee ligament injuries in adolescents. J Bone Joint Surg 1988;70-B(5): 772–6.

94. Sweeting RC, Crocker B. Anterior knee pain and spinal dysfunction in adolescence. J Man Med 1989;4: 65–8.

95. Sullivan JA. Ligamentous injuries of the knee in children. Clin Ortho 1990; 255:44–50.

96. Schafer RC. Chiropractic management of sports and recreational injuries. Baltimore: Williams and Wilkins, 1982.

97. Press SD, ed. The role of chiropractic in athletic injuries and sports science, a position paper. Stirling Western Australia. International Federation of Sports Chiropractic, 1989.

98. Master of Applied Science in Clinical Practice (Sports Chiropractic). Course information handbook. The Chiropractic Unit, Faculty of Biomedical and Health Sciences, RMIT, Melbourne, 1994.

99. Master program in sports chiropractic. Course information handbook. The Centre for Chiropractic, Macquarie University, Sydney, 1994.

100. International Sports Injuries Video Series. Course information folder. Northwestern College of Chiropractic. Bloomington, 1994.

101. Joffe A, Radius S, Gall M. Health counselling for adolescents: What they want, what they get, and who gives it. Pediatrics 1988; 82(3):481–5.

102. Bennett DL. Adolescent health care in the 1980s. In: Bennett DL, ed. Problems of adolescents at work and at play. Sydney: Australian Association for Adolescent Health 1985:47–51.

103. Patrick K. Student health: Medical care within institutions of higher education. JAMA 1988; 260(22): 3301–5.

104. Nyiendo J, Haldeman S. A prospective study of 2,000 patients attending a chiropractic college teaching clinic. Medical Care 1987; 25(6): 516–27.

105. Phillips RB. A survey of Utah chiropractic patients. Am Chiropr Assoc J Chiropr 1981; 15: S113–34.

106. Woolcock A, Rubinfeld AR, Seale JP, et al. Asthma management plan, 1989. Med J Aust 1989;151: 650–3.

107. Lines DH. A wholistic approach to the treatment of bronchial asthma in a chiropractic practice. Chiropr J Aust 1993; 23:4–8.

108. Plaugher G, Lopes MA, Konlande JE, et al. Spinal management for the patient with a visceral concomitant. In: Plaugher G, ed. Textbook of clinical chiropractic: a specific biomechanical approach. Baltimore: Williams & Wilkins, 1993:369–70.

109. Wiles MR. Visceral disorders related to the spine. In: Gatterman M. Chiropractic management of spine related disorders. Baltimore: Williams & Wilkins, 1990: 379–96.

110. Couch MHA, ed. Health assessment for adults. North Ryde: Commerce Clearing House Inc, 1989: 23–7.

111. WHO and UNICEF. Alma Ata 1978, primary health care, a report of the international conference on primary health care at Alma Ata. Geneva. WHO, 1978.

112. Strasburger VC, Brown RT. Adolescent medicine, a practical guide. Boston. Little, Brown and Company 1991:71.

113. Holmes GP, Kaplan JE, Gantz NM, et al. Chronic fatigue syndrome: a working case definition. Ann Intern Med 1988;108: 387–389.

114. Gerow G, Poierier MB, Alt R. Chronic fatigue syndrome. J Manipulative Physiol Ther 1992;15:529–35.

115. Farinelli E. Effective treatment for chronic fatigue syndrome: case studies of 70 patients. Am Chiropr 1988;Nov:58–61.

116. King FJ. Homeopathic management of chronic fatigue syndrome. Dig Chiropr Economics 1992; July/Aug: 40–3.

117. Cavanaugh Jr RM. Evaluating adolescents with fatigue. Am Fam Physician 1987;Mar: 163–8.

118. Goldfield N, Neinstein L, Wohlgelernter D. Cardiovascular evaluation of adolescents and young adults. Postgrad Med 1986; 79:111–9.

119. Shearin RB, Cope JU. Contraception. In: Hofmann AD, Greydanus DE, eds. Adolescent Medicine. 2nd ed. Norwalk. Appleton and Lange, 1989:383–401.

120. Strasburger VC, Brown RT. Adolescent medicine, a practical guide. Boston: Little, Brown and Company 1991:212–8.

121. Neinstein L. Overview of sexually transmitted disease in adolescents. In: Bennett D and Williams M, eds. New Universals, Adolescent Health in a Time of Change. Curtin: Brolga Press 1988:117–21.

122. Cervantes CD, Abdenur J, Lifshitz F. Growth disorders. In: Friedman SB ed. Comprehensive adolescent health care. St Louis: Quality Medical Publishing Inc. 1992:175–86.

123. Strasburger VC, Brown RT. Adolescent medicine, a practical guide. Boston: Little, Brown and Company 1991:14–27.

124. Brookman RR. Menstrual and pelvic disorders. In: Hofmann AD, Greydanus DE, eds. Adolescent medicine, 2nd ed. Norwalk: Appleton and Lange 1989:371–382.

125. Strasburger VC, Brown RT. Adolescent medicine, a practical guide. Boston: Little, Brown and Company 1991:248–65.

126. Sanfilippo JS, Hertweck SP. Menstruation. In: Friedman SB, ed. Comprehensive adolescent health care. St Louis: Quality Medical Publishing, Inc 1992:917–46.

127. Howard CP. Endocrinology of puberty. In: Hofmann AD, Greydanus DE. Adolescent Medicine, 2nd ed. Norwalk: Appleton and Lange, 1989:17–20.

128. Crooks ML, ed. Health for youth. Youth Policy Development Council, Health Department Victoria. Melbourne, Health Department Victoria, 1988:43–4.

129. Jamison JR. Health promotion for chiropractic practice. Gaithersburg: Aspen, 1991.

130. Couch MHA, ed. Health assessment for adults. North Ryde: Commerce Clearing House Inc 1989:51–3.

131. Couch MHA, ed. Health assessment for adults. North Ryde: Commerce Clearing House Inc 1989:89–91.

132. Raghaven D. Towards the earlier diagnosis of testicular cancer. Aust Fam Physician 1990; 19:865–72.

133. Raghaven D. Cancer of the testis - diagnosis. Patient Management 1990; August:57–61.

SUGGESTED READINGS

Friedman SB. Comprehensive adolescent health care. St Louis. Quality Medical Publishing, Inc 1992.

Hofmann AD, Greydanus DE. Adolescent medicine, 2nd ed. Norwalk: Appleton & Lange, 1989.

Strasburger VC, Brown RT. Adolescent medicine, a practical guide. Boston: Little, Brown and Company, 1991.

19 Adolescent Patients with Acute Spinal Fractures

Gregory Plaugher, David J. Rowe, David L. Cichy, Cheryl E. Goble, Richard A. Elbert, Christopher R. Hart, J. Larry Troxell, and Peter Thibodeau

*A*lthough contemporary chiropractic authors have devoted considerable time in their writings to the discussion of acute traumatic disorders of the spinal column (1–3), the subject of chiropractic management of patients with spinal fractures and dislocations has not been presented. This may be a reflection of the relatively specialized nature of the endeavor and/or the lack of scientific substantiation for these treatments in the literature. It is important for the reader of this chapter to keep in mind the seriousness of evaluating and/or treating any patient who has suffered a trauma, especially one capable of causing a fracture or spinal dislocation. It is also the authors' intent to provide as much detail as possible about this specialized area of chiropractic, while also acknowledging the fact that not all clinicians will necessarily participate in this area of practice. It should go without saying that practice procedures for an individual patient cannot be gleaned from a textbook or single writing (e.g., case report) but arise from interactions and consultations with others more experienced with careful attention paid to the nuances of the individual case.

The chiropractic scientific literature consists primarily of individual case reports or multiple case series of both successes and failures in the area of fracture management. The orthopedic, neurosurgical and medical management literature also consists of both uncontrolled reports and non-randomized comparisons of different customary (medical or surgical) procedures.

The relatively few case reports of the chiropractic management of spinal fractures or dislocations involve inappropriate diagnosis of the lesion with subsequent manipulation. Manipulation either did not resolve the patient's complaints or aggravated the condition, necessitating eventual medical or surgical treatment (4,5), or, there was directed referral of the patient for surgical intervention (6). Rowe (7) was the first author to report in a thorough manner the successful chiropractic management of both acute, subacute and chronic patients with spinal fractures and dislocations. Ironic as it may seem, many of the case reports presented by Rowe were initially misdiagnosed by medical doctors. Less than appropriate practice occurs in both the medical and chiropractic professions (see Missed Fractures).

Rowe (7) has presented the biomechanical factors associated with spinal and pelvic fractures and dislocations, leaving the reader with a preliminary introduction to the topic. In this chapter we will present more detail on the specific chiropractic management of patients with spinal fractures and dislocations. The case studies are also presented in as much relevant detail as possible in order for the student and doctor to gain an appreciation for the nuances of this specialized form of chiropractic practice. Future comparison of chiropractic, medical or surgical methods in combination or as sole treatments in specific patient populations will begin to attempt to sort out the most efficacious treatment.

Patient Population

Chiropractic pediatrics encompasses the care of children from birth through adolescence. Adolescence is defined as beginning with puberty and ending with completed growth and maturity (8). The cessation of skeletal growth is between the ages of 18 and 25 (9). The case studies presented in this chapter comprise adolescents and all injuries were a result of severe trauma.

Several of the cases presented in this chapter were a result of automobile injuries (See Chapter 14). There are also two water sports injuries. These two populations of children, automobile passengers and individuals engaged in recreation or sports, constitute the majority of adolescent injuries. For younger children (e.g., younger than 8 yr), falls comprise the majority of precipitating events.

Etiology

The group presented in this chapter represents the major kinds of trauma commonly encountered in adolescents. Injuries during this time can lead to lifetime deformities. Many such injuries may be missed on initial presentation because the radiographs are either incorrectly interpreted, improperly exposed or positioned, or not obtained at all. Since skeletal growth is not complete, deformity at this stage can progress as the bones continue to grow. At times there can also be growth that tends to mitigate the effects of the injury.

As can be seen from the types of acute spinal disorders presented here, the type of injury is mostly dependent on the mechanism of trauma and the amount of force involved rather than on any spinal biomechanical function substantially different from the adult. Although it is more common in the child, there can be severe neurological injury without fracture or dislocation at any age (10).

The cervical spine attains functions that are similar to the adult after approximately 8 years of age (11). In the case of the adolescent, cervical injuries, including fractures and dislocations, occur predominantly in the mid and lower cervical spine. In infants and toddlers, the general patterns of injury to the neck seem to favor the upper cervical region, with injuries such as occipital subluxations and dislocations, fractures of the dens and atlanto-axial rotatory fixation being typical examples (11).

McGrory et al. (12) reviewed the records of 143 patients admitted to the Mayo clinic between 1950 and 1991. All patients had sustained injuries to the cervical spine. The injuries included fractures, dislocations or subluxations, and fractures with subluxation or dislocation. There was a clear demarcation of injuries sustained by two separate age groups. Children younger than 11 years of age had fewer injuries as a group. This group also had more injuries to the upper cervical spine and most of the trauma was a result of falls. There was also a higher rate of mortality in children younger than 11 years of age. Children between the ages of 11 and 15 years were more often injured through sports and recreational activities. This group had injuries more often to the lower cervical spine. There was also a higher male to female ratio in this sample and the pattern of injury was similar to that seen in adults (12). The age- and sex-adjusted incidence of cervical spine fractures and dislocations is 7.41 per 100,000 population per year (12).

Chiropractic Literature

There is scant literature on the topic of chiropractic management of spinal fractures and dislocations (7,13,14). The literature detailing successful chiropractic management practices is contained in uncontrolled case reports that are fraught with confounding variables lessening both their interpretability and generalizability.

Guebert and Thompson (6) present a burst-compression fracture of the lumbar spine that was initially diagnosed by a chiropractor, but subsequently referred to an orthopedist

who performed Harrington rod surgery. The patient was neurologically intact at the initial presentation.

Clements, et al. (15) report on fractures of the thoracolumbar spine in three adults. The cases were managed by either bracing, rest, physical therapy, mobilization, or massage. Clements et al. (15) advise that manipulation should be applied in these types of cases only above and below the site of the fracture. The authors of this chapter suggest an entirely alternate approach. If subluxation findings are present, then the fracture site, at times, will need to be adjusted (see Fracture-Subluxation and Dislocation-Subluxation).

Haldeman and Rubinstein (5) have brought attention to the factors involved in patients undergoing spinal manipulation who have compression fractures. The authors noted that of the 89 cases referred to their offices involving malpractice litigation, four cases directly implicated chiropractic adjustments as the cause of the spinal compression fracture. There was no cause-effect relationship demonstrated by Haldeman and Rubinstein in their report for precipitation of a spinal compression fracture following manipulation (16). Iatrogenesis is probably more prevalent within the medical profession when long-term use of steroid treatments leads to bone demineralization. Their widespread use runs contrary to the lack of good evidence that these drugs are efficacious for the seemingly endless varieties of disorders for which they are prescribed (16).

Nykoliation et al. (4), reviewed three cases of cervical spine fractures and dislocations that were missed during examinations performed by chiropractors. Cervical manipulation was subsequently performed without positive results. The patients eventually underwent spinal surgery. Nykoliation et al. (4) advise that manipulation of a patient with this disorder is contraindicated. While it is true that an improper diagnosis prior to an adjustment would contraindicate the procedure, it is the authors' clinical experience that properly performed specific adjustive procedures applied at segmental levels where there is not reproduction of the mechanism of injury are not contraindicated. However, delaying surgical intervention when the neurological condition (see Chapter 13) of the patient continues to decline while under chiropractic care is not appropriate (7).

Chiropractors in Trauma Centers

The authors are aware of several instances where chiropractors have adjusted patients with severe subluxations and fractures in the hospital. One such patient is the case study of a burst fracture of T7, presented later. Ideally, there should be more cooperation between chiropractors who specialize in this area of patient management with the nursing staff, emergency room physicians and orthopedists or neurologists involved with the case. The patient can only benefit from such open communication and interdisciplinary case management. For too long, absence of avenues of communication between doctors has been to the detriment to the patient.

Duke and Spreadbury (17) lament about surgeons and anesthesiologists overcoming their dread of making things worse in attempting closed reductions of lesions with manipulation. They advise performing the manipulation while the patient is under anesthesia. Duke and Spreadbury (17) present a case involving a bilateral facet dislocation of C5 on C6. A spondylolisthesis was present at the involved level. Closed manipulation resulted in good alignment. At nine days follow-up there had been some forward slippage of the motion segment due to the rupture of the various ligamentous elements. Chiropractors could fill an important role in trauma cases where highly skilled hands are necessary. The authors recommend more cooperation between skilled chiropractors and medical doctors in cases of acute spinal trauma.

Manipulation under Anesthesia

The subject of spinal manipulation of patients while they are under conscious sedation, not with complicating factors (e.g., fracture), has a limited but growing following of advocates within the chiropractic profession. None of these advocates has described protocols for the pediatric population with or without complicating factors such as fracture. In neurologically stable patients, especially those seen on an outpatient basis, the subject of the role of manipulation under anesthesia deserves some mention here.

It is the authors' opinion that in order to properly adjust patients who present with spinal fractures or dislocations, it is necessary that the patient be fully conscious and understand the nature of the treatment. The patient's cooperation during both the assessment and adjustment process is essential. It is necessary that the treating doctor be in full oral communication with the patient. Certain aspects of the adjustive process, such as preload thrust and the use of reflexive contraction of surrounding musculature (discussed later) as an indicator of the point of motion segment tension, are impossible to properly determine if the patient is sedated. The chiropractor must always be able to assess the patient's tolerance to the adjustment through constant communication. Any procedure, such as conscious sedation or general anesthesia, that restricts the ability of the patient to interface with the doctor during the adjustment is contraindicated.

Chiropractic Scope and Standards of Practice

The scope of chiropractic practice varies from state to state in the U.S. and in all jurisdictions throughout the world. In some U.S. states the issue of patients being adjusted when fractures are present is often not addressed.

Research on which to base standards of practice is sorely lacking for professionals who treat patients with spinal injuries. Chiropractic benefits cannot be discounted due only to the lack of currently available evidence, when scientifically validated alternatives do not exist in many circumstances. The first axiom of the doctor must be to above all do no harm (Primum Non Nocere).

Neither surgical techniques nor conservative medical management with collars, bracing, and exercise has been subjected to valid scientific scrutiny. In the absence of evidence to the contrary, any attempt by governing bodies to limit therapies without adequate trial runs counter to the patient's right to choose.

Informed consent should be obtained from all patients (or a suitable guardian) with a specific explanation of the patient's current condition and options for management.

Denying patients access to chiropractic services may lead to increased lifetime spinal distortions, scoliosis and other disorders linked to the axial locomotor system. Doctors unfamiliar with the management of these disorders should consult with others more experienced in this field. Complex lesions are better evaluated with advanced imaging.

Surgery is an invasive procedure, the effects of which are irreversible. Since there is evidence that delaying certain surgical procedures when there is no neurological deterioration does not result in a more unfavorable prognosis, conservative procedures, including chiropractic, should be applied initially.

It is unfortunate, but some chiropractic patients are likely treated in the absence of proper identification of a spinal fracture. Neural arch fractures and compression injuries are the most likely fractures that are missed without the proper imaging examination, although missed cervical spine dislocations have been reported (4).

Frequency of Injuries in Chiropractic Practice

Winterstein (18), in his review of stable acute compression fractures, mostly in older women with signs of osteoporosis, has described a role for chiropractic intervention in these patients. He advises light adjusting/mobilization above and below the fracture site. He also acknowledges that there is some controversy in this area of chiropractic management. In Winterstein's article, it was reported that up to 9% of patients presenting to a chiropractic clinic may have compression fractures.

There has been no systematic study of the frequency of patients with spinal fractures and dislocations presenting for chiropractic evaluation. The greater the trauma (e.g., sports, auto accidents) encountered by the patients in the practice will determine how frequent these injuries occur. If radiographs are not customarily obtained both old and sometimes acute injuries can go unnoticed (See Missed Fractures). Due to misdiagnosis, many of these lesions may remain hidden and be treated both inadvertently and inappropriately.

Chiropractic Education

The chiropractic management of spinal fractures and dislocations has received little attention in chiropractic colleges. The authors are aware of only one current post graduate education program that teaches management procedures in this area (19), although the subject has likely been presented in other venues in the past.

The subject is currently taught at two chiropractic colleges, but the content is usually dependent on the particular clinical experience of the practitioner teaching the course. Some of this material may be presented in trauma management courses during the student's final year at chiropractic college, if it is presented at all. Unfortunately, this unevenness in instruction has led to some graduates not having sufficient education to recognize that limited expert consultation is available in some regions of the country and patients with these conditions deserve to be evaluated and possibly treated by some chiropractors. Practitioner fear may also be present due to generalized confusion regarding scope of practice (it may not be legal in one state but it may be in another) and reimbursement issues, as well as simple ignorance about handling the acute trauma patient. It is advised that individuals with less experience handling these injuries work closely with at least one other chiropractor with more experience in the area of interest.

Society Costs for Spinal Cord Injury

Cervical spinal cord injuries are a major cause of death and disability in the U.S. Injuries from motor vehicle accidents result in 500 to 650 quadriplegics per year (20). The approximate cost to society for each new cervical spinal cord injury in the U.S. each year is $400,000 (21). Approximately 10–11,000 new cases of spinal cord injury (from all causes) occur each year, costing more than $4 billion annually (21,22).

Cotler et al. (23) studied the medical and economic impact of closed cervical spine dislocations. Patients that had initial nonoperative treatment, but later needed to undergo surgery, had higher overall costs. The nonoperative group's mean hospital charges per case was $61,351.14. The operative group's mean charge per case was $42,944.00.

These costs are similar per case to that seen by Roye et al. (24) in a survey of 71 cervical spine fracture patients admitted to a medical center over a 2 year period. Twenty-two patients had neurological injuries. Six patients died in the intensive care unit. The average hospital stay for survivors was 45 days. The average hospital charges were $50,370.00.

Prevention of Spinal Fractures and Dislocations

Reath et al. (25) studied the injury prevalence and costs of restrained versus unrestrained motor vehicle crash victims. Hospitalization following a crash was more frequently required for unrestrained victims.

Mandatory seatbelt laws have increased seatbelt usage two to four-fold in New York. This has resulted in reduced serious and fatal casualties and insurance claims (26).

Since children are often passengers in the rear seat of a vehicle, they are more vulnerable to a Chance fracture, due to the presence of lap seat belts. All seats in a vehicle should have as a minimum, both lap and shoulder restraining devices. Lap seat belts, in addition to causing another type of spinal injury (i.e., Chance Fracture), can also cause severe trauma to the abdominal organs (27).

When improperly used, any restraint may accentuate the trauma (27–29). Wang et al. (27) present a case of a 2-year-old patient that was involved in a car accident while sitting in the front seat on her mother's lap, face to face with a three-point harness wrapped around both individuals (27). The 2-year-old did not lose consciousness following the accident and there were no visible lesions. Five hours later the patient began projectile vomiting. Computerized tomography of the abdomen disclosed a fractured left pedicle of L2. Part of the jejunum was interposed between the left kidney and the vertebral body of L2. The patient was then transferred to another hospital. A plain film taken of the abdomen disclosed the fracture of the left pedicle. An upper GI series demonstrated obstruction of the proximal jejunum at the level of the spinal fracture. Resection and end-to-end anastomosis of the perforated segment of jejunum was performed. The patient was discharged from the hospital 20 days later in stable condition.

The greater availability of airbags should also help to prevent some injuries. Safety harnesses over both shoulders (in order to avoid the roll-out phenomenon), similar to that seen in racing cars, may also be an alternative for automobile manufacturers to consider (7).

Scher (30,31) advises that individuals engaged in contact sports, such as rugby, undergo a limited radiographic examination (lateral cervical radiograph) prior to participation in these activities. Analysis can then be made for congenitally small spinal canals and congenital fusions that may predispose the individual to neurological injury should he/she receive trauma to the cervical spine.

Surgical and Nonoperative Methods

There is ample evidence that many types of fractures and fracture-dislocations can be managed through non-operative methods (32–34) such as bracing and bed rest. It is of concern to some researchers in the arena of fracture care that there is a lack of long-term follow-up studies on patients undergoing fusion surgery. In the case of thoracolumbar fractures and fracture-dislocations, fusion surgery for a fracture at one vertebra will require stabilization instrumentation for five to seven vertebral levels (32). There is literature that suggests that occupational limitation may also result from surgical fusion procedures (32,35).

Hanley and Eskay (36) reviewed the records of 57 patients who suffered fractures and fracture-dislocations of the thoracic spine that presented for medical evaluation over a ten year period. They found in no case was there a patient with a complete neurological deficit that exhibited improvement following surgical stabilization. In a review of tetraplegic cases by Burke and Berryman (37), no patient with a complete lesion made a satisfactory recovery following either closed medical manipulation under anesthesia, traction, or surgical reduction with fusion. In a study of 18 patients who had lower thoracic and lumbar fractures combined with neurological deficits, only nine showed some neurological improvement (38). The patients had an average 1.125 Frankel's Grade improvement.

Jacobs et al. (39) compared the results of surgical treatment with laminectomy and Harrington rods vs. bed rest accompanied with bracing. The laminectomy group fared much worse as has been confirmed in other studies. No patients that were Frankel A, improved. Jacob's et al. (39) remark about the presence of an alignment abnormality of the spine that was usually present causing the neurological injury may be of interest to chiropractors. If such a deformity was not present, then a burst fracture with resultant fracture pieces encroaching upon the spinal canal was assumed.

Traction and closed reduction methods vs. surgery were compared in a survey of 68 patients over a 12 year period by Hadley, et al. (40). The patients ranged in age from 14 to 63 years. Neither group showed a difference in neurological outcome due to treatment, but when there was a difference in the timing of the reduction, patients undergoing early reduction had better neurological improvement.

Remarkably, research continues into which method of surgical fusion is necessary. This therapeutic approach is based mostly upon enlarging and immobilizing the spinal canal when there is no correlation between the amount of canal decompression, the initial canal compromise or the nature of the neurologic lesion, and neurological recovery (41). Small groups of patients have been retrospectively evaluated with widely different lesions, no randomization, and without blinding of assessments or control groups for comparison. From these types of studies broad statements are made regarding the efficacy and appropriateness of different surgical procedures (42). Only through well conducted randomized studies can differentiation be made between the myriad of therapies currently available. Conservative methods, including specific spinal adjustments and bracing, need to be compared in trials, both by themselves and with surgical procedures. Further research will only yield more benefits to patients suffering with these afflictions.

Although hypotheses abound, some surgeons acknowledge that there is no proof for their methods (43). This situation is probably a sign of the dearth of scientifically valid medical research in general (44). Of particular note is a tendency for surgeons studying the issue to focus on outcomes in terms of surgical constructs, rather than on patient oriented functional measures (45).

The authors stress the need for comparison research between chiropractic, medical and surgical methods. Combined approaches also may prove to be of some benefit, especially when severe neurological injury has occurred. The rehabilitative physical therapists need also to work more closely within an interdisciplinary setting.

The contradictions between the medical and chiropractic approaches to spine trauma is illustrated by a report from Jacobs et al. (39). They stress that when the patient is moved into a position of extension, direct pressure at the fracture site is always avoided. This advice is contrary to that provided by chiropractors familiar with fracture management. The fracture site is often where the majority of high or low velocity load(s) or thrust(s) would be applied. This is especially true with flexion trauma when there is a tendency for this injury to cause the motion segment to be translated posteriorward. In these cases posterior to anteriorly directed forces will help to diminish the tendency towards progressive flexion deformity.

Frankel's Grading (42):

Frankel A indicates no sensory or motor function below the level of the injury.

Frankel B indicates sensory sparing but no distal motor function.

Frankel C indicates that there is lower extremity motor function present, but it is functionally useless.

Frankel D indicates that there is functionally useful motor sparing.

Frankel E indicates normal sensory and motor function although hyperreflexia may be present.

Surgery should be questioned as a general panacea due to the lack of good evidence demonstrating its efficacy, but particularly, when there is incomplete neurologic injury or no neurologic deficits (32). Gaines and Humphreys (32) advise orthopedists to manage fractures that do not have large neurologic deficits non-operatively for two to four months. If canal decompression is needed after this time period, then surgery can be performed (46), preferably at only one level. Similarly, Bohlman, et al. (47) report on 45 patients who had spinal surgery after an average of 4.5 years following the initial trauma. These patients had continued pain or paralysis that had not responded to conservative measures (not including chiropractic). Surgery in these patients resulted in favorable outcomes (e.g., reduced pain) despite the delay in treatment.

In the case of traumatic spinal cord injury with paraplegia, certain medical methods are necessary to prevent the development of chronic instability, spinal deformity, and complications from other body systems affected by the injury (48). Complications following spinal cord injury include bowel and bladder dysfunction and other organ system trauma, pulmonary emboli, etc.

Donovan and Dwyer (48) state that indications for surgery that are not controversial include correction for an unacceptable deformity or instability. They advise medical (bracing, rest, observation) management and not surgical treatments for most cases of traumatic paraplegia.

Place, et al. (49) studied the impact of surgical stabilization on initial rehabilitation and complications in patients with traumatic paraplegia. One hundred thirteen patients' records in the retrospective analysis were reviewed. Each patient had a minimum of five years of follow-up. The review demonstrated that patients who received surgical stabilization versus those who were treated nonoperatively showed a statistically significant increase in complications. Neurologic recovery was also not significantly altered through surgical intervention.

Vlach and Bayer (50) studied laminectomy surgery in patients with fractures of the thoracolumbar spine. The majority of patients undergoing laminectomy had a more severe kyphotic deformity when compared to a conservatively treated group. The kyphotic deformity in the surgical patients was also more frequently progressive.

Burke and Berryman (37) advise the use of gentle closed manipulation under anesthesia to reduce dislocations of the cervical spine. In a report covering a seven year period of 425 patients with spinal column injury and neurological lesions, cervical spine dislocations were discovered in 76 individuals. Closed gentle manipulation to reduce the dislocation combined with mild skeletal traction resulted in a good result in most patients. But traction applied to certain kinds of patients where ligamentous sprain and rupture are present will complicate the injury. Overdistraction can cause further dislocation and/or movement of fracture or disk fragments (Fig. 19.1).

Surgery should be reserved for those patients exhibiting continued or deteriorating neurological instability (37). The advice of Knight et al. (33) is particularly poignant, "Physicians who care for patients with traumatic spinal deformities should resists the temptation to be technicians and not apply metal to every fracture seen."

Biomechanics of Bone

Cook, et al. (51) studied the association of bone mineral density and pediatric fractures. They concluded that reduced bone density is unlikely to play a significant role in acute traumatic pediatric fractures. Chan, et al. (52) also concluded that pediatric fractures are a result of the particular activities the child engages in, rather than any intrinsic bony susceptibility.

In the case of cancellous bone, as collapse occurs there may or may not be a loss in compressive strength (53). Since the vast majority of compression fractures do not result in a loss of compressive strength, instability should not be assumed from isolated compressive deformity alone. The biomechanical properties of spongy bone are depicted in Figure 19.2.

Major Injuring Vector

Throughout this chapter the authors will refer to the major injuring vector or MIV in each fracture or dislocation case. This terminology reflects the primary force causing the presenting injury. It is helpful to understand the biomechanics of injury in order that the treatment procedures (e.g. the adjustment or advice on preferred patient postures) do not reproduce the mechanisms of injury. It is often the case that the adjustive intervention should be directed in a line of drive precisely opposite that of the major injuring vector or opposite the "net effect" of the MIV.

Spinal Stability

White and Panjabi (53), define spinal stability as that situation in which a spine placed under normal physiological load is able to resist further positional deformation, neurological damage and irritation. It is important for the chiropractor to understand the biomechanics of stable and unstable injuries. Each clinical scenario will mandate different approaches to treatment, affect the prognosis of the patient, and will help delineate those cases that may require more aggressive stabilization procedures (e.g., bracing and surgery).

Three Column Model of Spinal Stability

Denis (54,55) has put forth the three column concept of spinal stability. He divides the spine into three columns; anterior, posterior and middle. Through a review of biomechanical studies Denis determined that instability would not occur if only posterior ligamentous structures were damaged. He found that instability occurred only when there was disruption of the middle column combined with posterior column damage. Denis was the first to recognize the independent importance of the middle column. Denis (55) suggests that spinal instability can only occur when there is damage to two of the three columns, one of which has to be the middle column. Dislocations usually result in disruption of all three columns.

Ferguson and Allen (56) have concurred with Denis on the inadequacy of two-column model descriptions of spinal injury. However, they prefer the term elements over columns since the tissues involved do not resemble columns in terms of their anatomy and do not behave as columns in the biomechanical sense (57). Ferguson and Allen's description of the three elements or columns differs slightly from the Denis model in that the anterior column consists of the anterior longitudinal ligament (ALL), the anterior two-thirds of the vertebral body, and the anterior two-thirds of the intervertebral disc. The middle element consists of the posterior one-third of the vertebral body and intervertebral disk as well as the posterior longitudinal ligament. The posterior element comprises the posterior bony complex (pedicles, lamia, articular processes, and spinous process) and the posterior ligamentous complex (57). The slight difference in this description from the Denis model is that the latter divided the anterior column from the middle at the midpoint of the intervertebral disc. The three element model is depicted in Figure 19.3 (57).

James et al. (58) further refine the Denis model by presenting a unique situation that is a clear example of a two column injury that does not involve the middle column but does produce instability. The example is a burst fracture that compresses the anterior column and causes distraction injury to the posterior column.

In this chapter, the authors will classify fractures or dislocations as unstable if any two of the three columns or elements are damaged to the degree that they could potentially lead to further mechanical deformity or to increased neurological damage or irritation when placed under normal physiological loading (7).

The Fourth Column

The rib cage is an integral biomechanical component to the spinal column. There are several important mechanical functions of the rib cage, including (53,59):

1. To stiffen and strengthen the spine. Resistance to displacement is provided by two mechanisms:
   a. The costovertebral joint provides additional ligamentous structures and attachments which contribute to spinal stiffness and strength. Mobility is also reduced.

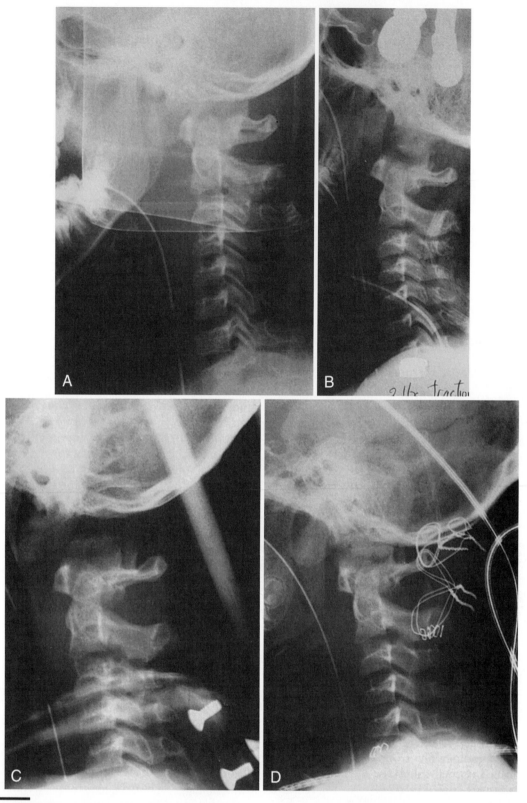

Figure 19.1. A 6-yr-old child was involved in a motor vehicle accident. He received prompt resuscitation at the scene of the accident and was quickly transferred to a local emergency room. A. The child was intubated because of respiratory distress. A lateral cervical spine x-ray film appeared to show distraction and anterior displacement of the occiput on the atlas. B. The child was immediately placed in skull tongs and 5 lb of traction applied. A lateral x-ray film showed worsening of the occipito-atlanto-axial separation. Weight was sequentially removed, but even at 1 lb, pathological separation persisted. C. The child was then placed in a halo body jacket. This x-ray film shows that during the application of the halo body jacket the vertical and anterior separation worsened. D. The child was then taken to the operating room where an occiput to C2 fusion was carried out. This fusion was ultimately successful, but the child remained a ventilator-dependent quadriplegic. Reproduced with permission from MacEwen GD, Kasser JR, Heinrich SD, eds. Pediatric fractures. Baltimore: Williams & Wilkins, 1993:226.

b. An increased moment of inertia of the thoracic spine. Moment of inertia is a measure of the distribution of a material about its centroid. This distribution determines the strength in bending and torsion. The addition of the rib cage to the thoracic spine effectively increases its cross sectional area and mass. The increased moment of inertia stiffens the spine when it is subjected to lateral bending and axial torsion. The added stiffness of the spine provided by the rib cage has been well described by Andriacchi et al. (59,60) (Fig. 19.4). It is evident that the results of sternum removal have as devastating an effect as removal of the entire rib cage.

2. To add energy absorbing capacity to the spine structure during trauma.

3. To serve as a protective barrier against lateral or anterior impacts.

For the thoracic spine, fractures in this area can also involve the sternal–rib complex. A proposed fourth column to the Denis three column spinal model has been made by Berg (61). Two cases are presented, one managed conservatively, and one surgical, with combined sternal and spine fractures. Berg (61) notes that overriding, displaced sternal fracture is a marker for a severe flexion-distraction thoracic spine injury with a propensity for instability and further deformity.

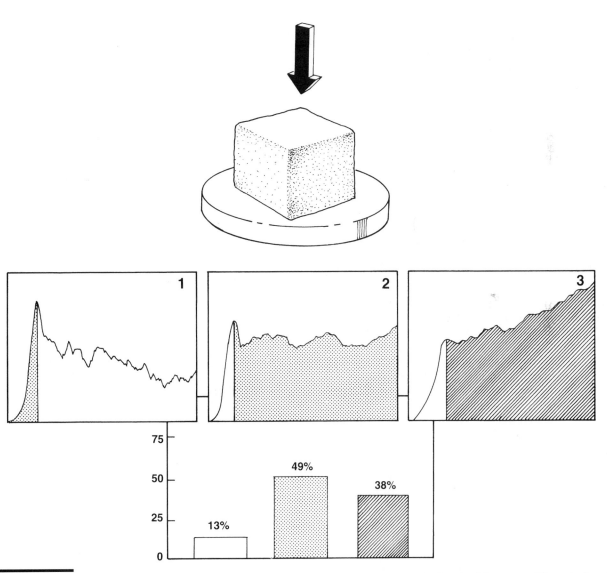

Figure 19.2.   Cancellous bone failure patterns from compression injury. There are three types of load-deformation curves presented. Type 1 demonstrates decreasing strength after the maximum load is reached. Type 2 maintains its strength and type 3, increases in strength after the failure point. The majority of the samples in this study had type 2 curves. Modified from White AA, Panjabi MM. Clinical biomechanics of the spine. 2nd ed. Philadelphia: J.B. Lippincott Co., 1990:36.

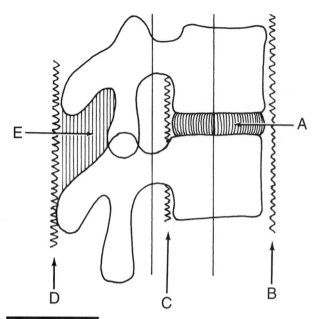

Figure 19.3. Three element model of spinal stability. The anterior column is composed of the anterior portion of the disc (A) and the anterior longitudinal ligament (B). The middle column includes the posterior disc and the posterior longitudinal ligament (C). The posterior column is comprised of the supraspinous (D) and interspinous (E) ligaments. Modified from Kaye JJ, Nance EP. Thoracic and lumbar spine trauma. Radiologic Clinics North Am 1990; 28:362.

Etiology of Fractures, Dislocations and Subluxations

Birth Injuries and Neonatal Deaths

The spinal cord can undergo tremendous traction forces during acceleration–deceleration and distraction types of injuries. This is due to the fact that the cord can only deform approximately 10% of its original length (62). Flexible behavior transforms to stiff resistance when an attempt is made to deform the cord further (62). The spinal column, in contrast, can stretch much more due to the elasticity of the spinal ligaments and disc. As such, the mechanical properties of the joints may be preserved (few signs of subluxation and no signs of fracture or dislocation) with pronounced trauma to the spinal cord and/or nerve roots.

Towbin (63) performed autopsies of infants during the neonatal period. They were cases of crib death now called sudden infant death syndrome or SIDS. A total of eight infants were autopsied and in seven there was spinal epidural hematomas (63). The brain stem resides in the cervical cranial junction and disruption in this area can have a major impact on the breathing centers. Excessive torsion of the upper cervical spine may also cause compression or stretch to spinal cord in the upper cervical region. It is fortunate that now U.S. pediatricians are recommending that infants be placed on their back for sleeping. Other countries and chiropractors for many years

have recommended this practice. Foreign countries correlate reduced incidence of SIDS with this practice. It is acknowledged that there are also other factors involved with SIDS, such as second-hand smoke. The supine position avoids the increased rotation of the upper neck, which is necessary for proper respiration while in the prone position.

There is good evidence that some birthing methods involve excessive rotation and lateral flexion of the head and neck. The use of forceps, and the difficulties encountered with breech deliveries, can lead to spinal column or cord injury (64,65). Severe hyperextension of the cervical spine during child birth can also cause cord injury or death (66).

Shulman et al. (67) has reported on the rare complication of transection of the spinal cord during cephalic delivery. The authors note that mild injury appears to be very frequent. An injury less than cord transection or dislocation may have sufficient force to cause spinal subluxation.

A cross species presentation of the possible trauma that can be involved in some birthing practices has been presented by Agerholm et al. (68). They confined their analysis to the incidence of vertebral fractures in newborn calves. A major problem in the cattle industry is the high frequency of stillborn calves and calves dying during their neonatal period. In a study

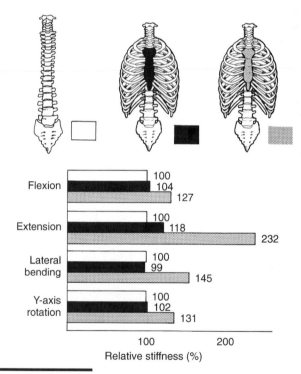

Figure 19.4. Relative stiffness of a ligamentous spine (white), removal of the sternum (black), and intact spine and rib cage (shaded). Notice that the ligamentous spine behaves similarly to a spine and rib cage that has the sternum removed. Modified from White AA, Panjabi MM. Clinical biomechanics of the spine. 2nd ed. Philadelphia: J.B. Lippincott Co., 1990:59. Based on data from Andriacchi TP, Schultz AB, Belytschko TB, Galante JO. A model for studies of mechanical interactions between the human spine and rib cage. J Biomech 1974; 7:497-507.

of 100 cases involving still birth, death during the neonatal period, or a locomotor disturbance, it was discovered that approximately 7% had sustained vertebral fractures. Anatomical, radiographic and microbiological techniques were used to analyze the calves. Of interest was the determination that manually applied traction forces during delivery appeared to be a contributing factor to the injuries. Most fractures were epiphyseal separations in nature and confined to the thoracolumbar junction.

Motor Vehicle Accidents

Motor vehicle accidents are a cause of many of the spinal cord injuries in adolescents and the precipitating etiology in the majority of the case studies presented in this chapter (See Chapter 16). As in the case of adults, many of these injuries are preventable with the use of proper safety belts and other devices (e.g. air bags). Unfortunately, the unrestrained head and cervical spine may encounter high acceleration/deceleration forces despite the proper use of lap and shoulder restraint belts.

Recreational and Sports Injuries

Reid and Saboe (69) reviewed 1,447 spine fractures over a seven year period. Two hundred and two (n=145) were related to sports or recreation. Of these, nearly half (42%) were associated with paralysis. The high incidence of catastrophic injury is second only to motor vehicle accidents. Approximately 25% of these injuries were caused by the following activities: snowmobiling (10%), snowskiing (5%), tobogganing (5%), and ice hockey (3%) (See Chapter 4).

Physical Abuse

Spine and spinal cord trauma may possibly be present in the battered child syndrome (70) (See Chapter 2). Violent shaking can produce a cervical lesion much like that seen in a whiplash-type of injury. Uncomplicated vertebral fractures can also be asymptomatic (70), leading to avoidance in x-raying the spine.

Ahmann et al. (71) present two cases of spinal cord infarction due to physical trauma. One patient, a 4 yr-old girl, fell when she was pushed out of a swing by another child. The other patient, a 22 month old boy, was cuffed (a blow with the palm of the hand) at the jaw and face and fell to the floor. The first child died 48 days following the trauma and the other died six months later following respiratory arrest. The pattern of infarction was thought to be related to spasm of the distal branches of the central sulcal arteries in a terminal arterial bed (71).

The number of new cases of nonaccidental head injury does not appear to be reducing despite public information campaigns (69). Child abuse does not occur within any one racial, religious or political group, nor is it confined to the socially disadvantaged. Physical abuse remains a major concern as a preventable cause of death and disability in childhood (72).

It is important for clinicians to be alert to the signs that may indicate physical abuse and/or central nervous system injury. The cardinal findings include (73) (See Chapter 2):

1. An uncertain history or one that seems to be at odds with the physical findings;
2. New onset of seizures in association with retinal hemorrhages (74); and
3. Intradural surface hemorrhages on the CT scan or MRI.
4. Infants with the above signs may have suffered a nonaccidental injury.

Fracture Subluxation

The major types of injuries encountered by the spine include fractures, dislocations or subluxations (75), and fractures with subluxation or dislocation (12). Fracture at one spinal level combined with injury (e.g. subluxation) at neighboring or distant motion segments can lead to an overall complex biomechanical disorder.

A fracture-subluxation is present when signs of subluxation (75) or the vertebral subluxation complex (75) (See Chapter 12) are also present at the fracture site (i.e., the involved motion segment). The presence of a spinal fracture alone does not necessarily indicate that a subluxation is present at the involved level. A systematic examination of the area will bring forth information necessary in making the proper determination.

In instances of severe trauma or when the index of suspicion for a spinal fracture or dislocation is very high, the practitioner must always keep in mind that a complete subluxation examination (e.g. motion palpation) prior to the radiologic examination may not be possible to be performed.

Static Palpation

Probably one of the more prevalent findings that should be weighed heavily with the multi-parameter examination is the presence of a soft edematous area over the spinous process. Palpation with the pads of the finger tips should be used to determine the presence of edema.

The examination for tenderness should be performed by palpating with the tip of the finger or thumb slightly underneath the involved spinous process. Repetitive comparisons of tenderness of spinal levels above, at, and below the fracture site should be performed. The patient should be in a slightly flexed posture to aid the examination. The presence of tenderness should be weighed heavily in the multiparameter examination for signs of subluxation.

Skin Temperature Instrumentation

Skin temperature instrumentation (76,77) may or may not demonstrate positive findings. In cases of acute trauma the presence of generalized skin inflammation due to marked trauma in the area may not provide the examiner with specific readings at one spinal level as is commonly found in patients with less severe injuries. The absence of instrumentation findings does not necessarily rule out the presence of subluxation at the involved level.

Motion Palpation

Patient assisted motion palpation of the fracture site will generally provide little information beyond assessing the patient's functional capabilities before receiving a specific adjustment in a slightly stressed position. However, due to the acute nature of the lesion and the presence of prominent inflammation and pain, the patient can generally not tolerate the adjustment in anything more than predominantly neutral spinal postural positions. For this reason, motion palpation is of little use in providing clinically useful information in these cases. The fact that moderate spinal movements may either reproduce the mechanism of injury or otherwise aggravate the site of the fracture or dislocation, illustrates why this procedure should not be performed prior to a thorough radiological examination.

Plain Film Radiography

Plain film radiographic examination is essential in the evaluation of trauma to the pediatric patient (See Chapter 8). Although marked radiographic findings may not be present, especially in the younger age groups (< 8 yrs), in cases of trauma to the spinal column, it does not contraindicate the need for the examination.

In addition to specialized sectional radiographic projections such as obliques and pillar views, the examination should include an antero-posterior full spine radiograph. The single exposure AP full-spine radiograph, either on a 14 × 36 or 14 × 17 film, with appropriate collimation and shielding, is necessary in order to accurately determine the vertebral count (See Chapter 8). An opposing lateral projection should also be obtained. When the full spine is imaged, it is possible to get even penetration with selective prepatent filtration. This results in less radiation exposure when compared to multiple sectional views. During sectional radiography of the full spine, there is necessary overlap in the lower thoracic/upper lumbar area and at the cervicothoracic junction (See Chapter 8).

Although the plain film is sensitive for identifying lesions such as compression or burst fractures when they occur, it does not accurately depict the actual transient injury that occurs during impact (78). During burst injuries of the cervical spine, there is significant recovery of axial height after impact (78).

Motion x-ray studies, when appropriately used, can be helpful in the evaluation of the stability status of an injury.

Accuracy of Count

The doctor will need to be able to palpate the exact location of the subluxation and/or fracture in order to insure that the thrust is delivered at the exact vertebra intended. The lateral full-spine radiograph or spot lateral of the cervicothoracic junction taken in either the swimmer's or a direct lateral position, is essential in assessing the site of subluxation, fracture or dislocation, since these injuries occur with frequency at

these levels. The AP radiograph, obtained with one exposure, is the most accurate method for determining the exact count of cervical, thoracic and lumbar vertebrae.

Missed Fractures

As is shown in several of the cases presented in this chapter, some of the fractures were missed following initial plain film interpretation by medical sources. The exact incidence of missed fractures when only spine injury is present is currently unknown. Delays in diagnosing spinal fractures when other (sometimes more life-threatening) injuries are present occur within 3.2% to 16.7% of the population (79). Keenen et al.'s (79) review demonstrated that non-contiguous spinal fractures were present in 52 cases (6.4%). A mean delay of 53 days in diagnosing the injury has been reported by others who have investigated trauma patients (80).

Even such severe injuries as bilateral facet dislocations of the cervical spine may go unnoticed, especially when other significant injuries are present (81). This may occur more commonly in patients with larger central spinal canals, since there is more room for the cord to maneuver (81).

Both inadequate radiographs as well as poor interpretation skills are culprits in the misdiagnosis of fractures. In addition to improper radiographic factors, a late diagnosis may be due to an incomplete clinical assessment of symptoms that may initially appear to be have less significance to the physician unfamiliar with the complexity and seriousness of spinal disorders (82). Simple compression fractures of the vertebral bodies, endplate and epiphyseal fractures, and spondylolisthesis are probably overlooked quite often due to insufficient radiological examinations. Radiological findings occur frequently in children participating in athletics.

Nykoliation et al. (4), reviewed three cases of cervical spine fractures and dislocations that were missed during examinations (both clinical and radiologic) performed by chiropractors. Cervical manipulation was subsequently performed without positive results. The patients eventually underwent spinal surgery.

Upon initial radiological assessment some fractures may remain occult if displacement is minimal or a callus has yet to be formed. Follow-up radiographs are needed, especially in patients unresponsive to care or when a suspicion of fracture or other injury remains.

The chiropractor needs to be aware of spinal lesions in order that the adjustive thrust is directed exactly opposite to the mechanism of injury. Future research in this area is necessary in order to provide incidences of radiographic trauma findings in varying pediatric populations.

Advanced Imaging

Plain films are the primary diagnostic test to be used in the case of cervical spine injuries and should direct further diagnostic investigations (57,83). Computerized tomographic scans are helpful in the evaluation of patients who have sustained blunt and other types of trauma (84,85). If an adequately positioned and exposed plain film of the cervical spine is normal, it is unlikely that a CT examination will reveal a fracture. However, should a fracture be evident on the plain film, the CT may disclose additional fractures (e.g., pedicle) of the involved segment or at neighboring levels (84,86). Complex motion tomographic studies (TOMOS) may be superior in some instances to conventional CT scans in detecting injuries of the upper cervical spine involving the atlanto-occipital motion segment (87).

CT scans can be deficient in imaging fractures that are parallel to the axial plane. Without intrathecal enhancement, the spinal cord is poorly visualized with CT (88). Since MRI is superior to CT in imaging neurological structures, the intervertebral disc and major ligaments, it should be the imaging modality of choice following plain films (89). Its use is limited in many instances due to the lack of facilities in some countries and certain regions of the U.S. In some cases, computerized tomography (with more widespread availability and lower cost) or a bone scan (to diagnose the age of the fracture) may be the more appropriate imaging choice following plain films.

Bone scans (called scintigrams) are recommended when the age of the fracture is important to the management or prognosis of the patient. Insidious development of back pain and the suspicion of bone pathology may warrant a bone scan examination (90). Bone scans can image signs of fracture and other bony pathological processes, helpful in arriving at a differential diagnosis, but usually plain films, CT, or MRI are needed to fully evaluate the patient.

Hildingsson et al. (91), studied the sensitivity of the bone scan for detecting spinal fractures in the multiply injured patient in a series of 20 patients with a total of 38 fractures. A negative bone scan was insufficient in detecting all spinal fractures. Therefore, a negative test does not exclude the possibility that a spinal fracture may be present.

Adjustment of the Acute Fracture-Subluxation

Very few general recommendations can be made regarding the adjustment of spinal fractures exhibiting signs of subluxation. However, in the case of a spinal fracture, it is considered very rare for the motion segment exhibiting signs of subluxation to be the articulation above the fracture site. It is far more likely that the fracture itself will be the site of subluxation, or a more caudal vertebra, either subjacent to the fracture site or from one to several segments inferior to it.

Adjustment of the Dislocation-Subluxation

Although each case needs to be evaluated independently, some general considerations for the mid and lower cervical area appear to emerge. In general, the segment below the site of dislocation will need to be adjusted in the case of a dislocation directly above. The motion segment that the doctor is usually trying to influence is the articulation below the dislocation site. No attempt is made in this instance to realign the dislocated vertebra.

In the case of perched facets undergoing fusion, or dislocation combined with fracture pieces into the IVFs or central canal, then dislocation reduction is ill-advised. The case study

presented in this chapter involves a perched facet with fracture that was not reduced prior to the cervical adjustment.

Cervical Collars

A patient with an acute or healing noncomplicated, neurologically stable fracture of the cervical spine should be advised to wear a soft cervical collar for the first few weeks post injury. More complex lesions, such as dislocations and odontoid fractures, may require a more rigid orthosis such as the Philadelphia collar. The duration of usage will vary greatly and should generally not exceed six to eight weeks because muscular atrophy may ensue. The collar should especially be worn if the patient is operating or riding in an automobile or engaging in an activity where the cervical spine may be moved in rapid fashion or otherwise put at risk. The collar should also be worn when the patient sleeps. If the patient is irritated by the appliance or its usage causes an increase in symptom, then it should be used on a limited basis or perhaps not worn at all.

Contraindications for Adjustments of Spinal Fractures and Dislocations

Full fracture through the lamina or neural arch would contraindicate a thrust in a direction which could potentially aggravate the fracture site and result in further displacement of the fracture pieces or cause further dislocation. Adjacent levels to a neural arch fracture can be safely adjusted providing attention is paid to stabilizing surrounding areas during the thrust. It is preferred, in some cases where there is great potential for migration of fracture pieces to a further encroaching position, to wait a few days to weeks prior to the administration of a high velocity/low amplitude thrust. This also may be true, in some instances, for adjusting patients who might have fractures adjacent to or at the site of the subluxation. Each case needs to be evaluated individually prior to making any determination.

In neurologically deteriorating patients, consideration needs to be given to the possibility of complicating the site of the lesion with a high velocity thrust. In these cases, a low velocity preloading force can help to determine the patient's tolerance for a more vigorous procedure.

In the pediatric patient with acute lymphoblastic leukemia, 23% to 59% will present with back pain (92,95). In this disorder, spontaneous compression fractures of the thoracic spine are relatively common. Only adjustive techniques with extremely light force should be applied. The possibility of a fracture occurring spontaneously, independent of an adjustive procedure, is very high. The common occurrence of spinal fracture in these patients should be brought to the attention of the parent and child. Prednisone treatment of the leukemia (usually over a long period of time) or the disease process itself could be responsible for the fracture. In a 9 yr-old patient with back pain and compression fractures presented by Oliveri et al. (94), long term follow-up following calcitonin, calcium and Vitamin D treatment demonstrated remission of symptoms. After 2 years, there was restoration of height of one vertebral body. Most segments had a "bone within a bone" sign.

A thrust of too great a magnitude is contraindicated. It is often necessary to apply a thrust with very low velocity and in a high amplitude manner. This is true of acute burst fractures of the thoracic spine in which the doctor is attempting to push the segment from posterior to anterior. The ligaments will hold the pieces together and there may be approximation of the fracture pieces. An audible noise will generally be heard during this maneuver. Sustained pressure should be applied in lieu of a thrust.

The thrust can be of a high velocity/low amplitude nature provided there is not marked separation of the fracture pieces or severe encroachment of the spinal canal. In every instance, the doctor needs to apply a preloading force in order to assess the patient's tolerance for the procedure. Failure to do this would contraindicate an adjustment.

Analysis of MIV

The patient history or any superficial lacerations or bruises, will assist the doctor in determining the MIV for the injury. The static radiograph should be used to identify the area of the bone fractured. It also assists in making the determination of the major injuring vector by the direction of the osseous failure. High quality plain films of good detail should always be obtained prior to the initiation of treatment.

Analysis of Static Position

Once the doctor has determined that the site of fracture also presents signs of subluxation, static radiographic analysis of the segmental position of the vertebra should be performed (See Chapter 8). Vertebral rotation, posteriority and lateral flexion malposition are all common findings in fracture patients since most injuries involve multiple and or combined force directions. The complex coupling motions of the spinal column in normal individuals will also lead to multiaxis directions of static malalignment.

Analysis of Active and Passive End-Range Position

In almost every case, the adjustment of a fracture subluxation or dislocation subluxation should be made with the patient in a neutral position. Typically, many chiropractic adjustments are performed with the spinal column moved toward its passive end-range in one or more planes. This type of end-range positioning is contraindicated in patients with acute trauma. All positions of the patient should be constantly monitored for any change in the patient's symptom status.

Contact Point

The contact should generally be light in order to minimize patient discomfort. In some cases a brief cold application, such as ice, will provide the skin with an analgesic, making contacting the vertebra less painful. The contact point should be very specific and take into account the nature of the fracture site. The doctor needs to consider the overall stability of the spinal column and which areas are affected. The Denis spinal model will provide the practitioner with a generalized basis for the stability of the motion segment. The thrust should be made in the opposite direction of the major injuring vector. The contact point and tissue pull should be in line with and in the direction of the adjusting force. In most cases the contact point should be much lighter than a typical case, not involving a fracture or dislocation.

Preload

A noncomplicated spinal adjustment usually involves preloading the motion segment prior to the administration of a high velocity low amplitude thrust. The preloading of the joint will help to determine if a high velocity thrust may be contraindicated. In the case of a spinal fracture or dislocation, this preload must be necessarily of short duration and of very minimal force. The spinous process is usually contacted and a gentle push is applied in the exact line of drive that would be used for the high velocity thrust. If the preloading force does not cause an increase in symptomatology, this finding can then be used as a positive indicator for the application of additional loads, more pronounced preload or a high velocity thrust.

Preloading forces can be applied in succession, with each loading followed by a careful assessment of the patient's response to the loading. In some cases, the preloading force can substitute for a high velocity thrust intervention during the first few treatments, especially in cases of severe trauma.

Thrust

The "line of drive" of the thrust has to be considered with respect to the *exact* location of the fracture site(s). Each injury represents a different set of forces involved and each patient must be evaluated as an individual. The reader should note that the mechanism of correction for a unilateral or bilateral neural arch fracture would differ greatly from a simple compression of the vertebral body.

Should the doctor decide that a high velocity thrust adjustment can be performed, the segment can be preloaded slightly until there is a detectable slight reflexive spasm of the surrounding musculature. Then, the preload force should be reduced slightly until the splinting of the musculature is ceased. At this level of preload, the high velocity thrust can usually be administered. High velocity thrusts should always be of extremely shallow depth, in order to gauge the patient's response to the intervention before more vigorous adjustments are applied.

Introduction to Case Presentations

The subject of spinal fracture and dislocation management is very serious. It is imperative for all practitioners to be aware of the parameters used in the evaluation and treatment of the individual case. The intention of this chapter is not to lead the reader into believing that every chiropractor should treat these cases in his/her practice. It is important for the reader to understand that the management practices employed in each case evolved over many years and has been passed on to less experienced practitioners through expert consultation.

It is the intention of the authors that these practices be documented in writing, thus expanding one's awareness of management practices in this area beyond isolated consultation. However, there are no two spinal trauma cases that are alike. Life presents a myriad of different mechanisms of injury that are combined with unique genetic and environmental factors affecting the skeletal structure in complex ways. The case studies presented are examples of appropriate management by extremely skilled practitioners familiar with fracture and dislocation management. The cases should not be construed as "cook book" instruction for someone unfamiliar with this area of clinical care.

In some practices, close to 10% of patients may present with spinal fractures (7). Although more common in the geriatric populations, injuries in younger individuals do occur as evidenced by the source material for this chapter. It should be of considerable interest to the reader that all of the patients presented here had acute spinal injuries. Whether or not the reader ever decides to add fracture treatment to his/her armamentarium of practice skills is an individual choice. The authors want to be clear that these cases do present to outpatient chiropractic facilities and that we would be negligent as educators if this information was left hidden to the profession.

The practice of fracture management is not a process to be taken lightly. The approach necessitates careful scrutiny, is often very time consuming, and carries added risks beyond less complex spinal injuries. When and if a fractured segment is adjusted, it is done so only after extensive clinical testing to ensure proper management.

During the actual moment of a spinal adjustment at a fractured site, there is an extremely heightened state of awareness that is difficult to describe, other than to say that the doctor may experience a change in his or her perspective of practicing chiropractic. Adjusting spinal fractures is not for the squeamish.

The reader is encouraged to seek out others engaged in this area of clinical care if he or she desires specific information on an individual case. The chapter should not be used as a "guide to management."

Burst Fracture of C7

INTRODUCTION

This 19-yr-old male presented himself for chiropractic consultation the day before following a motor vehicle accident. He had no prior history of any accident or injury. The patient was referred to the clinic by another patient. The patient stated that on 6-7-94, at approximately 2:30 p.m. he was sitting as the front middle passenger in a tow truck with a car in-tow. A third vehicle rear-ended the car in-tow and tow truck at approximately 45 m.p.h. causing the car in-tow to be totaled. The towed vehicle launched into the cab of the tow truck, primarily damaging the top portion of the cab. The patient was not wearing a seatbelt. The other two occupants were also injured but neither sustained a fracture. The patient was transported by rescue to a hospital emergency room where he was examined and radiographs of the cervical spine were performed. The patient was provided a diagnosis of cervical strain, given a soft cervical collar, and released. The patient

then presented for chiropractic evaluation. The chiropractor requested that the patient sign a release of records form so that he could obtain the hospital radiographs. The patient did so, and returned on the morning of 6-8-94.

CLINICAL BIOMECHANICS

The burst fracture is produced through a compressive (-Y) force to the head, leading to failure in a mid or lower cervical vertebra. The compressive force above pushes the nucleus through the endplate, bursting the vertebral body at right angles to the MIV. The vertebral body "bursts" apart into fracture fragments (7).

Fragments are often times driven posteriorward, damaging the posterior longitudinal ligament and compressing the anterior portion of the spinal cord. A classic anterior spinal syndrome may ensue, causing immediate and complete motor paralysis, and cutaneous sensory nerve loss of pain and temperature below the level of nerve damage. Bilateral vibration and position sense are often left unaffected (7).

The lateral radiograph demonstrates flattening of the comminuted vertebral body centrally. Anterior and posterior displacement of fragments can be visualized but do not necessarily give a clear indication of spinal stability (7,21).

The AP radiograph often demonstrates a vertical fracture line in the body of the vertebra. This radiographic sign is usually present in the burst fracture and absent in the simple compression fracture, making it useful as a differentiating factor (96).

The burst fracture is often missed, due to its tendency to reposition to a more normal shape and position following the injury. This is due to the centering effect of the ligaments of the motion segment. The centering effect of the ligaments is thought to assist reorientation of the fracture fragments during the adjustment (Personal communication: Dr. W. Alex Cox). Experimental evidence suggests that the reorientation of fracture pieces for thoracolumbar burst fractures is most likely due to the strong attachment of the annulus fibrosis rather than the effect of the posterior longitudinal ligament (97).

This natural repositioning effect following burst fractures may leave the practitioner uncertain as to the level of neurological deficit if the radiograph shows no alterations (53). The CT scan is the best method of determining the level of comminution and fracture (96). Due to the fact that the burst fracture involves the anterior and middle or posterior columns, it is always biomechanically and often neurologically unstable.

In a survey of cases with cervical spine trauma investigated with MRI, it was discovered that when a fracture was present combined with an acute disc herniation, it was the disc below the level of the fracture that was usually involved (89).

EXAMINATION

The patient complained of right-sided severe neck pain that extended across the superior fibers of the right trapezius. Initial static palpation revealed severe interstitial edema over the lower cervical area and moderate edema in the mid thoracic region. Palpation of the cervical and thoracic spinous processes demonstrated a progressive increase in tenderness that peaked at the lower cervical and midthoracic motion segments.

Temposcope (76,77,98) findings showed changes in skin temperature symmetry at C7-T1 and T5-T6.

Radiological Assessments

The hospital films were reviewed by the chiropractor. The radiological impression at this time was a burst/superior endplate compression fracture of C7. The patient was unaware of any fracture since the hospital's report was negative. The chiropractor had radiographs of the full-spine performed (AP and right lateral) (Fig. 19.5A, B). An additional left lateral cervical radiograph (Fig. 19.5C) was also obtained to determine if any differences were detectable between this radiograph and the right lateral portion of the full-spine view. To further evaluate the nature of the fracture, obliques of the cervical spine (unremarkable) and pillar views were also obtained (Fig. 19.5D,E). Additional radiographic analysis disclosed seven cervical vertebrae with an acute burst fracture of C7 with an increase in the anterior/posterior boundaries of the vertebral body. Eleven thoracic and five lumbar vertebrae were present. The full spine radiograph was helpful in determining an accurate vertebra count since this patient had eleven thoracic vertebrae. Bilateral cervical ribs were present at C7. At the C6 vertebra, the segment directly above the site of the burst fracture, there appeared to be some slight depression of the anterior-inferior aspect of the vertebral body. There is also some slight decrease of the C6-C7 disc space height, possibly as a result of the recent trauma. The full spine radiographs revealed the multiple intersegmental and global postural static malalignments (e.g., positional dyskinesia) (98-100). The biomechanical analysis of the radiographs was performed following additional physical examination procedures.

The patient reported to the doctor that a hospital doctor released him after x-rays and examinations, not informing him that any pathology was present on the x-rays taken at the hospital.

Clinical Assessments

All vital signs were normal. The patient is 5 feet 7 inches in height and weighs 149 lbs. As a result of the C7 burst fracture, no cervical compression tests were performed as these reproduce the mechanism of injury. Active range of motion of the cervical was markedly limited. The patient was unable to extend or left lateral flex his neck. Flexion, right lateral flexion, and right and left rotation were severely restricted. When the patient initiated all neck movements, they were performed very slowly and in a guarded fashion. Thoracic range of motion showed only slight reduction in global ranges of motion.

A tuning fork applied to the C7 spinous process provoked pain. The left biceps reflex was absent and all other reflexes were within normal limits. Soto-Hall's test was positive although the patient's head was never put into forced flexion because any attempt at cervical flexion caused an increase in lower cervical pain. Single trial right-handed dynamometer readings were 110 lbs right and 100 lbs. left.

DIAGNOSIS

Based on the primary findings of edema, palpable spinous process tenderness, skin temperature asymmetry and motion restriction at C7-T1 and T5-T6 it was determined that these levels were to be adjusted utilizing short lever arm articular procedures. A subluxation was diagnosed at T5-T6 and a fracture-subluxation at C7-T1. Although the patient presented with films from the hospital, the patient was first examined clinically to determine where the primary sites of subluxation were. The x-ray was used to further assess how these areas were to be adjusted and not to diagnose the level of subluxation.

TREATMENT

The radiographs were used to further evaluate how C7 and T5 were to be adjusted. Line analysis (101,102) (See Chapter 8) is used to more precisely ascertain the spatial orientations of the motion segment. The adjustment is directed three-dimensionally opposite the patient's presenting configuration and towards the primary center of motion for the segment.

The patient was provided the results of all examinations and fully informed of his condition. He consented to receiving chiropractic care. On 6-8-94, T5 was adjusted on the hi-lo table. The segment was listed as "P" (-Z) and was adjusted from posterior to anterior using a spinous process and soft-pisiform contact points.

On 6-10-94, T5 was adjusted again and C7 was given a preload force to see if there was any increase in symptomatology, locally or peripherally. On 6-15-94, T5 was adjusted and C7 was adjusted as PR-inf-sp (-Z, -θX, +θY, spinous process contact). The thrust was primarily directed posterior to anterior, through the plane lines of the zygapophyseal joints and the anterior-posterior plane of the disc. The patient was adjusted in the seated position. The neck was maintained in a neutral position during the adjustment with no lateral flexion of the spine. The patient's spinous process was contacted with the distal, palmar, lateral aspect of the index finger (Fig. 19.5F). When the high velocity, low amplitude thrust was made, a slight audible was detected consistent with facet joint coaptation. After the adjustment, the patient was able to slightly extend his neck and he stated that although his neck had been painful, he thought the adjustment felt "very good."

It is of interest that the hospital's review of the radiographs failed to identify the burst fracture of C7. A review of these films, as well as the additional radiographs ordered by the chiropractor (i.e., AP and lateral full spine, left lateral, obliques and pillar views) by a second medical radiologist, disclosed the burst fracture of C7, but was termed a compression fracture in the medical radiologist's report.

FOLLOW-UP

Between 6-15-94 and 7-22-94, the patient was adjusted on 10 occasions. He was adjusted on 14 occasions from 7-25-94 through 12-5-94. At each visit both T5 and C7 were adjusted, with the exception of 6-24-94. The patient was also adjusted at T5 on 6-8-94, the day following the accident. The cervical

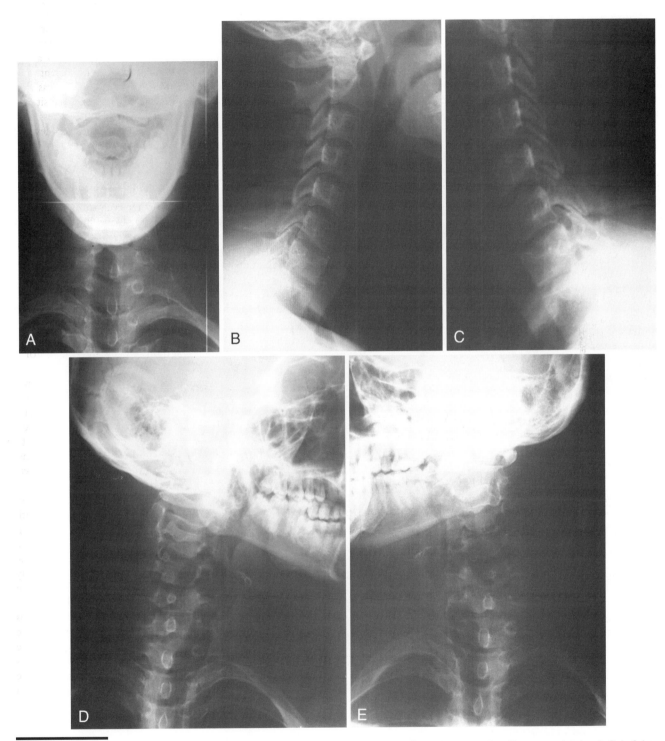

Figure 19.5. A. AP radiograph demonstrating a slight widening in the interpedicular distance at C7. B. Right lateral radiograph. There is compression of the superior endplate at C7 with an increased anterior-posterior distance at that level. C. Left lateral radiograph with similar findings as B. D. Right pillar view. E. Left pillar view.

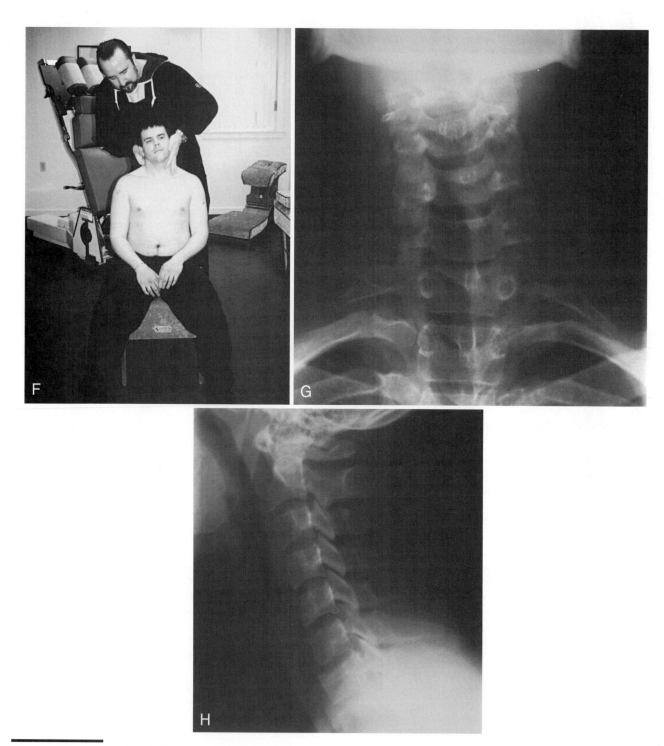

Figure 19.5—(*continued*).   F. Demonstration of the seated patient positioning for the C7 adjustment. The thorax restraining strap is not pictured. Also present in the photo are the hi-lo, pelvic bench and knee-chest adjusting tables. G. AP comparative radiograph. H. Lateral comparative radiograph.

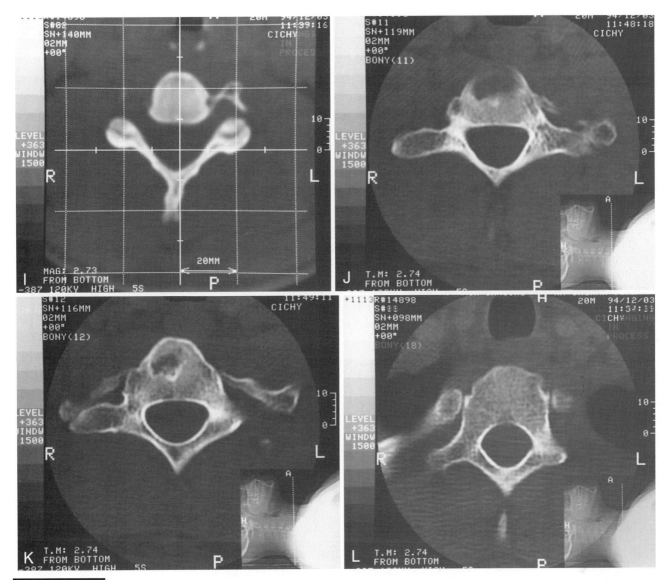

Figure 19.5—*(continued)*.   I. CT scan (six months post-injury) at the level of C6 demonstrating no sign of fracture. J. CT scan (six months post-injury) at the superior endplate portion of C7 demonstrating a radiolucency in the centrum of C7. The margins of the fracture are corticated and smooth and there is no sign of a burst fracture with separation of fracture fragments. K. CT scan (six months post-injury) at the middle of C7 demonstrating alteration in the shape of the anterior aspect of the vertebral body (compare to Figure 19.5I of C6). No sign of persistent burst injury is detectable. L. CT scan (six months post-injury) through the inferior portion of C7 demonstrates no sign of separation of fracture fragments and that proper healing had taken place.

spine was not adjusted on this date, not because of any inherent contraindication, but rather, additional radiographic analysis was needed before an accurate determination of the patient's condition could be made. The patient continued to do well during the course of treatment and was relatively asymptomatic after about three months of care.

Follow-up radiographs were obtained on 12-3-94 approximately 6 months post-injury consisting of full spine AP and lateral projections (Fig. 19.5G, H). They revealed that the C7 fracture had properly healed and that the patient's cervical lordosis has been maintained.

CT scans, obtained approximately six months post injury demonstrated that proper healing had taken place (Fig. 19.5I to L).

Unilateral Fracture-Dislocation of C6

INTRODUCTION

This 19-yr-old male suffered a fracture dislocation to the cervical spine while diving head first into a shallow portion of the ocean. The patient was driven to a hospital for examination.

CLINICAL BIOMECHANICS

The direction of injury in a unilateral interfacetal dislocation is flexion coupled with rotation (37,96,103) (Fig. 19.6). The dislocation occurs at only one zygapophyseal joint and leaves the injured inferior articular surface resting in the intervertebral foramen of the vertebra below. The nondislocated zygapophyseal joint usually subluxates with the inferior articulating process of the involved vertebra moving cephalad to the superior articulating process of the subjacent segment. There may be a concomitant articular pillar fracture.

In 1963, Beatson (104) described the concomitant injuries to the ligamentous elements for cervical dislocations. For a unilateral dislocation, the posterior ligaments are torn along with the capsular ligament on the side of dislocation, but there is usually sparing of the longitudinal ligaments and the disc (Fig. 19.7A,B). Bilateral dislocations invariably have some associated disc involvement. With the advent of specialized imaging such as MRI it has been discovered that disc herniation can occur in both bilateral and unilateral dislocations. It has been reported that approximately 60% of facet dislocation cases will show evidence of disc herniation on MRI (105).

The lateral cervical radiograph will give several indications of this condition. The body of the dislocated vertebra will be misaligned anteriorly on the body of the vertebra below, although usually not as far as in bilateral dislocations. There is also a disruption in the alignment of the facets which often exhibit a "bow tie" or "bat wing" appearance on the lateral radiograph (7,103,106).

CT scans of the patient should be obtained in order to determine the extent of injury to the neural canal and associated neural arch fractures. Stress films are indicated if no neurological deficits are increased during active motion. The flexion radiograph is important in gauging the stability of the motion segment. If the segment translates more than 3.5 mm

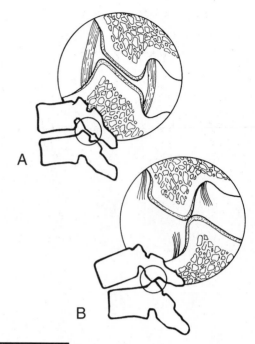

Figure 19.7.   A. Normal motion segment. Modified from White AA, Panjabi MM. Clinical biomechanics of the spine. 2nd ed. Philadelphia: J.B. Lippincott Co., 1990:226. B. Demonstration of the perched and dislocated facet joint with capsular ligament rupture. Modified from White AA, Panjabi MM. Clinical biomechanics of the spine. 2nd ed. Philadelphia: J.B. Lippincott Co., 1990:226.

(FFD = 72 in.) or has a disc space angle at the motion segment in question that is 11 degrees greater than the neighboring motion segment, then instability is present (53).

EXAMINATION

While the patient was in the hospital, CT scans and plain films of the cervical spine were obtained (Fig. 19.8A-G). The CT scan clearly shows a displaced fracture of the vertebral body of C6 with a hairline fracture of the pedicle. The transverse process is also fractured.

The patient's chief complaint was moderate neck pain and numbness of the right upper arm and hand. The patient was placed in a Philadelphia collar and surgery was recommended. The patient then elected to travel out of state to seek chiropractic treatment.

Twenty days following the initial trauma, the patient presented to an outpatient chiropractic facility with complaints of neck pain and numbness of the right arm and hand.

CLINICAL ASSESSMENTS

The patient presented with a Philadelphia collar and exhibited very guarded movements. He described a numbness sensation of the right forearm corresponding to the C7 dermatome. There were no alterations in deep tendon reflexes.

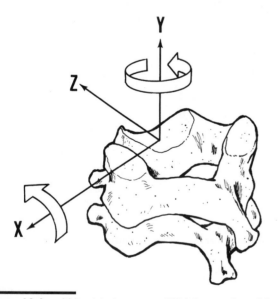

Figure 19.6.   Major injuring vector (MIV) for a unilateral facet dislocation.

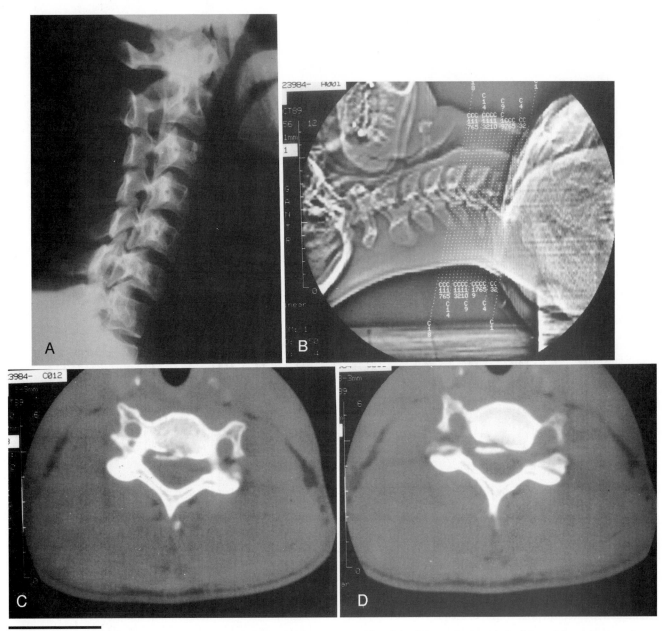

Figure 19.8.   A. Lateral radiograph of the cervical spine demonstrating unilateral facet dislocation at C6. The hospital radiograph was obtained immediately following the injury on 10-11-89. B. Scout view for the CT scan. Slices C12, C11, C10, C7 and C6 are pictured in Figure 19.8C-G. C. Slice C12 through the middle of the C6 vertebral level. Avulsion of the right posterior vertebral body is noted. D. Slice C11 through the lower C6 vertebral level. The fracture line is more extensive than in the previous slice.

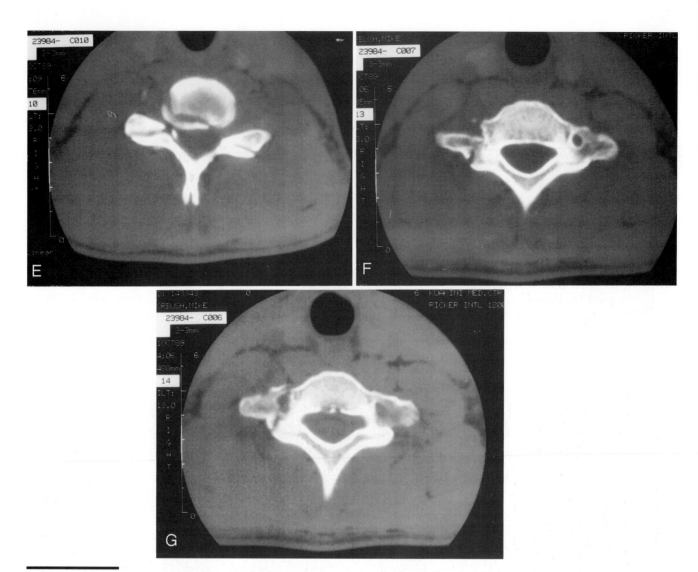

Figure 19.8—(continued). E. Slice C10 through the C6 inferior vertebral endplate. Avulsion of the right posterolateral vertebral body is noted. There is a small displaced vertebral fracture fragment near the right lateral recess. Asymmetrical facet align-ment is noted. F. Slice C7 through the C7 vertebral level demon-strating fracture of the right transverse process. G. Slice C6 through the C7 vertebral level demonstrating fracture and mild displacement of the right transverse process.

Dynamometer evaluations revealed weakness of grip strength on the right dominant hand side (Right: 52/62/62; Left: 75/78/85). Range of motion examination of the cervical spine demonstrated the following:

Flexion: 49/75

Extension: 48/60

Right Lateral Flexion: 26/45

Left lateral Flexion: 34/45

Right Rotation: 62/80

Left Rotation: 40/80

Skin temperature instrumentation findings (i.e., right left differentials) (76,77) were present at C6, C7, T5, and L5.

Moderate edema was noted at C6, C7, T1 and T5. This edema gradually decreased while the patient was under chiropractic care.

Tenderness was most pronounced at C6, C7, T1 and T5. These segments also exhibited reductions in range of motion during palpatory examinations.

RADIOLOGICAL ASSESSMENTS

Additional full spine radiographs were obtained in addition to the films taken at the hospital. Radiological examination disclosed the fracture dislocation of the C6 vertebra (Fig. 19.9 A, B). The right inferior articulating process of C6 had dislocated anteriorly to the right superior articulating process of C7. Slight hyperextension of C7 on T1 was also present.

DIAGNOSIS

A unilateral fracture-dislocation of C6 with subluxation of C7-T1 and T5-T6, L5-S1 and the sacrum was diagnosed.

TREATMENT

The patient was adjusted on the first visit as a C7 PR (-Z,+θY) using a spinous process contact with the patient in the prone position. A succession of *very* light thrusts were applied with a gradually increased force in order to gauge whether the patient's symptoms were worsened with the procedure. During the first adjustment, no audible was obtained with the adjustment. On subsequent visits, audibles were detected with progressively more movement of the C7 vertebra. At no time did the patient's symptoms increase following an adjustment. After five adjustments in the prone position over an approximate three week period, the patient began to receive the cervical adjustment in the seated position.

Beginning with the second visit, the fifth thoracic vertebra was adjusted as a PRS (-Z,+θY,-θZ) in the prone position, using a single hand contact.

The patient was provided a Philadelphia collar at the hospital. He continued to wear the device for two months while under chiropractic care. During the latter part of this time period, the patient only wore the collar at night. It is generally advised in fracture cases for the patient to wear a collar for at least eight weeks or until adequate healing has occurred. Beatson (104) has advised in those patients having suffered dislocations of the cervical spine, that a cervical collar is unnecessary. In the case presented here, the dislocation was combined with a fracture.

FOLLOW-UP

Follow-up radiographic examinations one month later were obtained in order to determine the alignment of the motion segment and to further gauge the stability of the motion segment (Fig. 19.10 A to D). The radiographs demonstrate no progressive instability at C6-C7.

On 10-30-89, after one adjustment and three days, pin wheel tests of the upper extremity showed barely detectable differences in sensation which was a considerable improvement

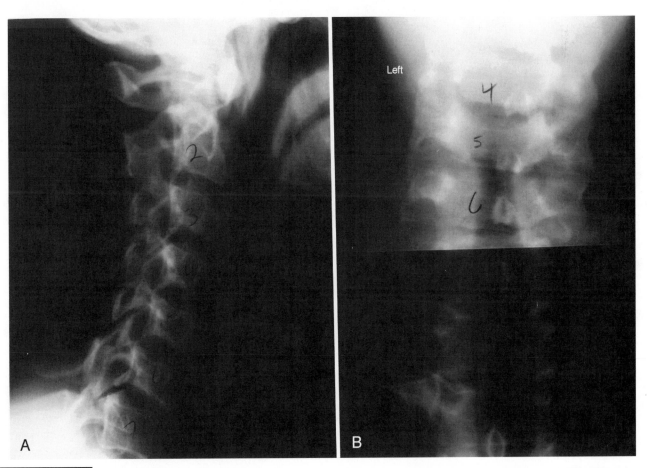

Figure 19.9. A. Lateral cervical projection with the central ray positioned at T1 taken 20 days following injury. Unilateral facet joint dislocation of C6 is noted. B. AP portion of the full spine radiograph 20 days post-injury. Notice the inferior- ward tipping of C6 on the right side indicative of the right inferior articular process of C6 moving up and over the right superior articular process of C7.

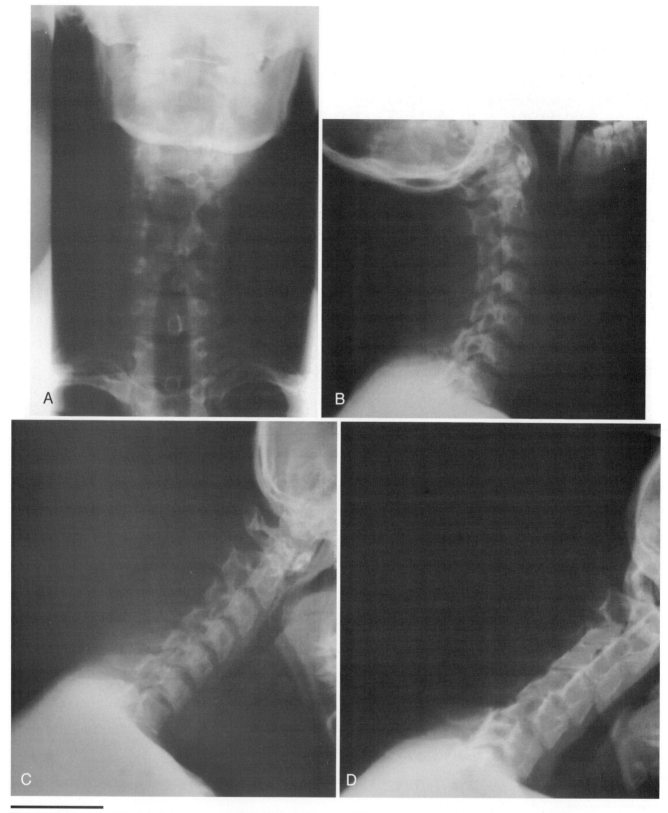

Figure 19.10.   A. AP radiograph after 1 month of chiropractic treatment and approximately 7 weeks post-injury. B. Extension radiograph 7 weeks post-injury and after 1 month of chiropractic care. C. Partial flexion of the cervical spine 7 weeks post-injury. Slight anterolisthesis of C6 is present. D. Full flexion of the cervical spine 7 weeks post-injury. Slight anterolisthesis of C6 is present.

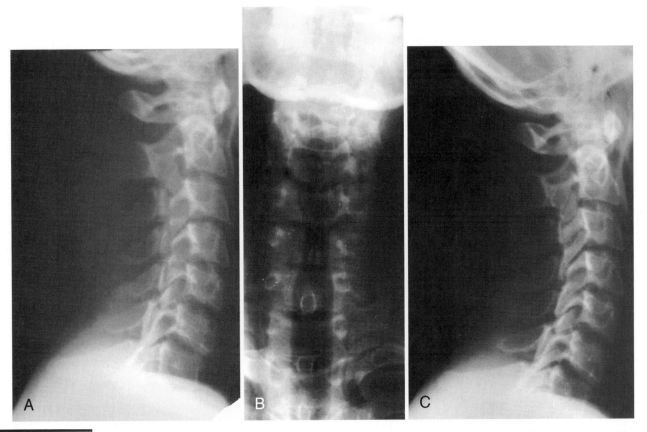

Figure 19.11.   A. Follow-up lateral radiograph on 6-24-91, approximately 20 months post-injury. B. Follow-up AP radiograph at approximately 25 months post-injury. C. Follow-up lateral radiograph at approximately 25 months post-injury.

from just three days earlier. The patient had ceased taking pain medication (i.e., Motrin 800 mg., Tylenol, Codeine) on this date as well. All reflexes of the upper extremities were normal. All reflexes remained normal over the five year period of treatment. If there had been any deterioration in the patient's neurological status over this period, then this information would have been used to alter the nature of the treatment that the patient was receiving.

On 7-16-90 dynamometer readings of grip strength were obtained. They were as follows: Right Dominant: 77/78/79; Left: 88/81/81.

As of 9-28-94, approximately 5 years following the accident, the patient has received 43 adjustments. The patient was seen intensively at first and then only intermittently during the last two years. There was no predetermined treatment plan of visits provided for this patient. Care was scheduled as the doctor felt necessary based on the objective findings of skin temperature instrumentation, as well as motion and static palpation findings. The patient's symptomatology also played a role in the timing of visits. The patient has had intermittent soreness of the mid back, low back and neck over the course of five years. There has been no hand numbness. Most of the discomfort follows physically stressful activities. The patient water skis, surfs and plays basketball.

Follow-up static radiological examinations did not demonstrate any progressive deformity. The neutral and flexion/extensions radiographs are presented in Figure 19.11A–C. The static films indicate no change in the position of the right zygapophyseal articulation. It is most likely that a natural fusion has occurred at the involved zygapophyseal joint with healing through a bony bridge or fibrous tissue (37).

DISCUSSION

Late diagnosis commonly occurs in cases of cervical spine fracture-dislocations. The lesion may be diagnosed as much as two weeks following the initial trauma (107,108). This problem of late diagnosis occurs due to three factors (103):

1. Inadequate radiographic technique with failure to visualize the cervicothoracic junction;
2. The presence of associated injuries to other areas of the body that leads concern away from the cervical spine, and;
3. Lack of marked symptoms. Patients often have no neurologic deficits or only an isolated radiculopathy that may be overlooked during a cursory examination.

Continued presence of a dislocation following treatment does not necessarily mean there is instability (109,110). Manipulative reduction of dislocations by osteopathic clinicians has been reported (37,109). Mahale et al. (111) studied 16 patients who deteriorated neurologically following reduction of cervical spine dislocations. They advise not reducing these lesions with traction, manipulation, or surgery since additional trauma to the vertebral arteries, ligaments, or the edematous spinal cord could result. In the case report presented here, the adjustment was rendered at the level of the subluxation (i.e., C7–T1) and no attempt was made to reduce the dislocated zygapophyseal joint.

Spinal cord compression and nerve root compression symptoms have been found to not only improve without reduction but to also persist following reduction (107).

In a review of 36 patients treated over a ten year period, Beyer et al. (103) found that there was virtually no statistical difference in treatment outcomes in patients treated with discectomy, reduction and fusion when compared to patients treated non-operatively with halo-traction and collars. None of these treatments have been compared to the natural history of the disorder or to alternative treatments such as chiropractic (7) or other non-surgical methods (111). In the review by Beyer et al. (103) it was also discovered that segmental dysfunction (i.e. hypermobility) adjacent to the dislocation site can develop due to the altered biomechanics (i.e. fixation dysfunction) in the area. Adjustments delivered at surrounding segments exhibiting motion restriction would likely minimize compensatory hypermobility at adjacent levels. This is especially true for subluxation present in the upper thoracic spine since compensatory hypermobility will necessarily occur in the middle cervical spine, a relatively common site for fractures and dislocations.

Traction applied to patients with dislocations has been reported to cause neurological injury (112). This usually occurs because of the presence of disc material displaced posteriorly. When the segment is brought posteriorly, back into alignment, the disc material may then compress the spinal cord. The anterior displacement associated with a unilateral dislocation does not usually interfere with the contents of the spinal canal unless gross instability is present. If reduction is achieved, but there is disc material present or a congenitally narrow spinal canal, then cord compression may ensue (112). Disc injury is very common during fracture-dislocation injuries necessitating their prompt evaluation with CT or MRI (113).

Hadley (114) found that when lesions such as facet dislocations were combined with a fracture, then restabilization occurred more often. This subgroup of an analysis of 68 patients had a natural fusion rate of 97% without surgery.

The vertebral artery is prone to injury from cervical spine trauma because of its intimate relationship to the bony structures of the spine (115). Flexion distraction injuries resulting in unilateral facet dislocations may lead to occlusion of the vertebral artery (115,116). Occlusion of the artery is less likely to produce a risk than the more dangerous arterial dissection or pseudoaneurysm formation (115). In a study of 12 consecutive patients admitted to a hospital,

there was a bilateral dislocation present in seven patients and a unilateral dislocation in the remainder. Of the five patients with a unilateral dislocation, four (80%) had occlusion of the vertebral artery. In the sample of seven patients with a bilateral dislocation, five (71.4%) patients had vertebral artery occlusion. The occlusions did not necessarily always occur at the site of the dislocation but also above and below the level of dislocation. In patients with unilateral occlusion of the artery, neurological findings may not be significant unless the other artery is compromised. Approximately 15% of patients have hypoplasia of one vertebral artery (116).

Willis et al. (115) reviewed 26 consecutive patients who sustained cervical spine trauma resulting in fractures and dislocations. Nearly one half of the patients sustained significant vertebral artery injury confirmed with preoperative vertebral arteriography. A thorough search for neurological symptoms must be made by the doctor of chiropractic managing a patient with a cervical spine dislocation. Although symptoms of vertebral artery occlusion are very often transient and do not necessitate treatment, if neurological symptoms are present above the level of the dislocation, then angiography is indicated. However, due to the small but finite risk of vertebral angiography, diagnostic modalities such as MRI (117) and duplex sonography (118) should be considered first. Small, but potentially harmful intimal tears can be better imaged through angiography. Angiography should definitely be considered where there are comminuted fractures of the foramen transversarium (115). In the case presented here the dislocation was at C6. Since the vertebral artery enters the foramen transversarium at C6, there is more mobility of the artery at this level. This may explain the lower incidence of vertebral artery occlusion in patients with dislocations at this level (116).

Cotler et al. (23) studied the medical and economic impact of closed cervical spine dislocations. There were 25 males and 10 females with an average age of 35.3 years (range, 12–75 years). Medical care consisted of traction for an extended period of time, combined with bracing. Surgery patients usually had a shorter duration of traction followed by fusion. Of interest is that all of the patients in the sample had immediate reduction of the dislocation attempted. In contrast, the case study presented here did not have reduction attempted. One should wonder what the natural history would be in dislocations without fractures, if they were kept in a dislocated position. In the study by Cotler et al. (23) patients that had initial nonoperative treatment but later needed to undergo surgery had higher overall costs. The nonoperative group's mean hospital charges per case was $61,351.14. The operative group's mean charge per case was $42,944.00.

Continued clinical research in the area of conservative management of cervical spine dislocations is needed. Comparison clinical trials with randomized or matched groups undergoing control (natural history), chiropractic (adjustments, bracing, rest, etc.), and orthopedic treatments (bracing, surgery, etc.) should begin to answer some questions and provide others.

Compression Fracture of C5 with Spondylolysis and Spondylolisthesis of L5

INTRODUCTION

This 16-yr-old male was involved in a motor vehicle accident involving three automobiles in which he was thrown through the windshield. He was not wearing a seatbelt. The patient suffered multiple injuries including a compression fracture of C5. The patient also presented with a spondylolysis and spondylolisthesis of L5.

CLINICAL BIOMECHANICS

COMPRESSION FRACTURE

The MIV for the wedge fracture is forced hyperflexion ($+\theta X$) of the spine creating a compression on the anterior or anterolateral portion of the vertebral body. Most (2/3) wedge fractures occur at the fifth, sixth and seventh cervical segments (96). Supportive soft tissues are usually spared and no major ruptures occur to either the anterior longitudinal ligament, the disc structures, or the posterior ligamentous elements. The simple wedge compression fracture is a relatively stable injury because only the anterior column is affected (7).

The cervical wedge fracture is best seen on the lateral radiograph. The vertebral body is usually compressed anteri-

orly and the anterior vertebral body height measurement is generally at least 3 mm (based on an FFD of 72 in.) less than that of the posterior.

Prevertebral edema and hemorrhage can increase the retropharyngeal interspace (96). The measurement taken from the anterior margin of the vertebral bodies of the upper and mid cervical vertebrae to the posterior aspect of the tracheal air shadow should not exceed 40% of the anterior to posterior measurement of C4. An increase in this measurement suggests anterior vertebral trauma (Fig. 19.12). The normally radiolucent fat stripe which runs within the prevertebral soft tissue may be locally displaced at the level of the trauma (7,106).

The wedge fracture often shows a disruption in the normal smooth and regular contour of the vertebral body at the point of cortex break. The best view for visualizing a compression fracture is the lateral radiograph. The AP view does not typically give a clear indication of the injury since no fracture line can be visualized. Once a fracture has been identified, the doctor should search for concomitant injuries. If the attending physician is unfamiliar with potential fracture variants, then films should be interpreted by a chiropractic or medical radiologist.

Seizure attacks can lead to fracture of the cervical spine in rare cases. This accounts for approximately 2.5% of all hospitalized "non-traumatic" fractures of the spine (119). It is generally not contraindicated to use the fracture segment as a contact vertebra for an adjustment. If an adjustment is indicated, it can be performed in the prone or seated position using the spinous process as the short lever arm.

SPONDYLOLYSIS AND SPONDYLOLISTHESIS

Definition. Spondylolytic defects of the pars interarticularis are acquired lesions of the neural arch and can occur anywhere in the spine. Although they are also common in the cervical spine, spondylolytic defects occur most often at the lower lumbar levels. We will use the following definitions in this discussion:

Spondylolysis: a uni- or bilateral defect in the neural arch of the vertebra (120), which often occurs in conjunction with spondylolisthesis.

Spondylolisthesis: forward slipping of a vertebra in relation to the vertebra below. This forward displacement can happen in any area of the spine, but occurs most frequently at L5. It is graded I–IV according to Meyerding. There are five classifications of spondylolisthesis depending on the degree of slippage (121):

1. Isthmic spondylolisthesis: Break in the pars interarticularis, or an elongation without separation;
2. Degenerative spondylolisthesis: Degenerative erosion of the facet joints;
3. Congenital spondylolisthesis: Inadequate development of the posterior elements;
4. Posttraumatic: Fracture of the bony hook other than the pars;
5. Pathological: Generalized or local bone disease.

Anterolisthesis: Like spondylolisthesis, anterolisthesis has forward vertebral body slippage, but does not necessarily imply a break in the neural arch of the involved vertebra.

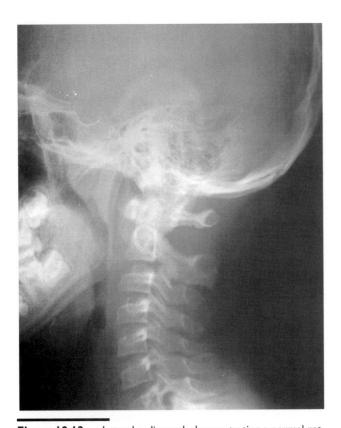

Figure 19.12.   Lateral radiograph demonstrating a normal retropharyngeal interspace.

Sacro-horizontal angle: the angle between a line parallel to the upper endplate of the sacrum and the horizontal plane on lateral views obtained in the standing, neutral position (122).

Etiology. Although defects in the pars interarticularis of lumbar vertebrae have been recognized for many years, the precise etiology of the defect remains unclear. There are four plausible explanations of the origin of this defect.

Although no longer widely accepted, spondylolysis was once regarded as a congenital failure of fusion of two growth centers (123). There is no evidence however that lysis of the pars is congenital, since autopsies of stillborns and fetuses have never shown the defect (124).

More generally accepted is the view that this defect is of a mechanical origin. It is considered a stress fracture, but may be a fatigue fracture with an underlying hereditary diathesis, such as a thin isthmus (124). Some pars interarticularis are exaggeratedly long and thin, creating anterolisthesis with or without spondylolysis (125,126). An intact but elongated pars interarticularis is seen in about a third of symptomatic children and adolescents with spondylolisthesis. This condition is known as dysplastic spondylolisthesis, lumbosacral subluxation, or isthmic Subtype B spondylolysis (121). If the defect is ultimately of mechanical origin, then the amount and distribution of cortical bone within the pars interarticularis must be important (127).

In some cases spondylolysis may be caused by acute trauma, although the strength and stiffness of the neural arch tends to preclude this in favor of multiple mechanical fatigues as the usual mode of failure (127). The stiffness is important because the neural arch has been shown to bend away from the vertebral body when a force acts on the inferior articular facets (127). This flexibility makes a fracture due to a single trauma difficult (127). Hence spondylolysis should be attributed to repeated loading causing a stress fracture in the pars interarticularis.

Demographics. The incidence of spondylolysis in the general population varies from 4% to 6%. Spondylolysis is never present at birth, and is uncommon before age 5 (128–130). This lesion usually occurs between the ages of 5 and 7 years (121). The majority of lesions are thought to occur before the end of the adolescent period (131). Progression to spondylolisthesis usually occurs before the age of 20 (132).

Although spondylolysis is not considered congenital, there is an increased incidence of the defect among families (133,134) and certain racial groups (135,136). For example, the prevalence of this defect reaches an extreme of 52.6% in Eskimos north of the Yukon (137). This suggests that there are some genetic factors which may predispose an individual to develop the defect (127).

With respect to anatomical level, findings suggest that 86% of pars defects (spondylolysis) occur at L5 (120,137,138). Spondylolysis is most common at the fifth lumbar vertebra because its position creates a mechanical disadvantage due to the increased anteriorward shear forces (127).

Predisposing Factors. As we have seen above, spondylolysis is not considered to be a congenital defect, although there are several factors which are believed to predispose to the stress fracture. These four factors are:

1. Anatomical Structures: The stiffness of the neural arch suggests that mechanical failure is caused by repeated loading, rather than a single trauma (127,139,140);

2. Biomechanical Misalignments/Motion and Position: There is an increased risk for fatigue failure of the neural arch by overload in flexion, forced rotation, and unbalanced shear forces (140). An increased sacro-horizontal angle may predispose to spondylolysis, because the load on the pars interarticularis in the lower lumbar vertebrae increases with an increasing inclination of the upper endplate of the sacrum (122);

3. Age: Young people are more likely to develop spondylolysis since they frequently engage in strenuous activities at a time when their intervertebral discs may be less resistant to shear and their neural arch has not reached its maximum strength (139);

4. Activity Type: Mechanical fatigue can occur during prolonged periods of strenuous or unaccustomed activity (127). Such activities produce repetitive cyclic stress across the pars interarticularis. Over time a fatigue fracture may develop (127). There is an increased incidence of spondylolysis among athletes, supporting the concept of overload as a cause of the defect (122). Sward (122) found that athletes had a larger sacro-horizontal angle than non-athletes, especially among football players. Further, the sacro-horizontal angle was larger in athletes with spondylolysis as compared with those without, predisposing them to a pars defect.

Symptoms. Most cases of spondylolysis are asymptomatic in the early stages (131,133). Symptomatic subjects often have low back pain, usually in adulthood, sometimes after a low back strain injury (123). There is often decreased activity associated with symptomatic stages of spondylolysis (141). For instance, subjects will be unable to bend or lift with normal agility. Athletes (e.g., gymnasts, football players), are usually forced to refrain from engaging in sports.

Screening. Because there is an increase of spondylolysis among athletes, screening of subjects prior to participation in impact athletics is necessary. As a result of the screening, risk factors can be evaluated. A decision can then be made to either refrain from participation or to correct the biomechanical predisposition (e.g., reduction of the sacral base angle). Screening for adolescent scoliosis and general pediatric examinations are two methods for ensuring pre-athletic evaluation.

Clinical Chiropractic. Only when a spondylolisthesis exhibits signs of subluxation and symptomatology is care considered necessary. The authors operationally define a subluxation for this discussion as a misaligned joint that is fixated, edematous, and causing neurological irritation or interference which will affect the normal neurological transmission to the end organ or end tissue. Assuming signs of subluxation and symptomatology are present, diagnosis and treatments of spondylolisthesis should be conducted in the following manner:

Postural Examination. Postural analysis from the lateral perspective can give indications of increased sacro-horizontal angle which may predispose the patient to spondylolisthesis.

Though not present in all cases, there may be a noticeable posterior protrusion of the sacral base causing a triangular appearance below the level of the fifth lumbar. This is best viewed from the posterior to anterior. If a spondylolisthesis is present, the L5 spinous process may appear posterior upon visual examination due to elongation. This is known as a step defect. The elongation is thought to predispose the pars interarticularis to traumatic separation (142).

Skin Temperature Instrumentation. Asymmetrical skin temperature findings (termed readings or breaks) may be present at the level of disc involvement in cases of both cervical and lumbar spondylolisthesis.

Static Palpation. During static palpation the L5 spinous process may be more prominent than in a spine without a spondylolisthesis. Again, this may be due to an elongated spinous process. Especially in acute cases, there will be palpable edema in the area of disc involvement, and the sacral base will be more prominent to touch. The first sacral tubercle is often more tender to the touch than the fifth lumbar spinous. If there is severe hyperextension at the L5-S1 motion segment, the SI tubercle may be underneath the L5 spinous process and not readily palpable.

Motion Palpation. Movement examination of the patient with a potential spondylolisthesis is best performed in the seated position. During motion palpation the anterior glide of the sacral base may palpate more rigidly.

Orthopedic and Neurological Testing. Selective orthopedic tests should be performed in the case of the patient presenting with low back pain or lower extremity symptoms. If the injury is not severe, many of these tests are relatively insensitive for detecting abnormalities. The absence of positive orthopedic findings does not rule out the presence of injury. Subtle signs of sprain injury can be detected through other subluxation examination procedures. Neurological testing of sensation, reflexes and strength should be performed.

Radiography. The doctor should attempt to differentially diagnose a spondylolisthesis from a retrolisthesis of L5 and the base posterior sacrum (100). The lateral film is used for determining posteriority of the sacral base. The margins of the bodies of the fifth lumbar and sacrum may be assessed for retrolisthesis or posteriority, or lines may be drawn along the anterior and posterior borders (George's line) to compare the positioning of the vertebral bodies. The lateral lumbar film only shows whether the vertebrae has slipped anterior or posterior in relation to the adjacent vertebrae. Therefore, the determination of a spondylolysis must be made upon examination of oblique lumbar projections. Once a break in the pars interarticularis has been identified, the lateral film is used to establish the grading of the spondylolisthesis in relation to the vertebra below (its foundation vertebra) according to Meyerding.

Adjustive Procedures. Evidence of a subluxation must exist before adjustments are made. Adjustments cannot be made on the basis of misalignments alone. Though total realignment is rarely accomplished, in order to re-establish a more normal function and alignment between the posterior sacral base and the fifth lumbar, the sacrum is adjusted underneath the fifth lumbar.

Adjusting the fourth lumbar or the segment above the involved segment is generally not indicated when there is a spondylolisthesis of the fifth lumbar because the risk of increasing lumbosacral misalignment is too great.

The doctor's contact point for the adjustment is the pisiform, and the segmental contact point is the S1 or S2 tubercle. The S1 tubercle is the preferred contact point due to its proximity to the L5 disc. However, there is often marked hyperextension of the L5-S1 motion segment. This factor, in combination with an often elongated L5 spinous process, makes the S1 tubercle not readily palpable, necessitating an S2 contact.

The table of choice for achieving proper correction with the greatest patient comfort is the pelvic bench with the patient in the side posture position. The line of drive is P-A and S-I through the disc plane line, unlike that for correction of a base posterior subluxation which is P-A and I-S.

The second table of choice for achieving proper correction with greatest patient comfort (when adjusting is difficult on the pelvic bench in the side posture position) is the knee chest table. The line of drive is P-A and S-I. The third table of choice is the Zenith Hi-Lo with the patient prone. For grade III and grade IV spondylolistheses the abdominal section is locked to keep the lumbar spine from moving anterior during the thrust.

Contraindicated Adjustments for Spondylolisthesis. Adjusting through the abdominal wall in order to correct the anterolisthesis is never indicated due to the delicate nature of the soft tissue organs beneath (e.g., abdominal aorta, small and large intestines, and bladder). In addition, it is impossible to obtain a specific contact point on the involved segment.

DIFFERENTIAL DIAGNOSIS OF THE NORMAL L5-S1 DISC, POSTERIOR FIFTH LUMBAR, BASE POSTERIOR SACRUM, AND SPONDYLOLISTHESIS

The technique for analysis is to scribe lines on the endplates of each of the involved vertebrae and note the configuration presented. With practice, simple visual assessment of the disc space of the motion segment will suffice for interpretation.

Normal L5-S1 Disc Space. For the normal L5-S1 disc space, especially in the younger child, the endplates of L5 and sacral base will have a parallel configuration (Fig. 19.13). Some very slight decrease in the posterior portion of the disc space when compared to the anterior section should also be considered normal, especially when there is absence of any clinical findings suggestive of subluxation (e.g., tenderness, edema, fixation, etc.).

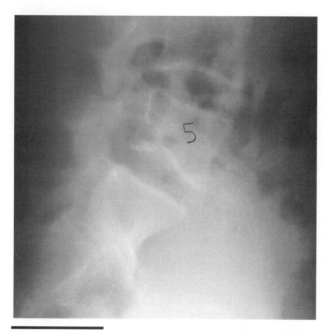

Figure 19.13.   Radiographic presentation of a relatively normal L5-S1 disc space. Nuclear endplate invagination is present.

Retrolisthesis of L5. In this presentation the endplate lines will diverge anteriorly. There is usually a break in George's line, with L5 subluxed posteriorly to the sacral base. With increasing hyperextension of the motion segment, there is usually a progressive decrease in the amount of posteriorward translation visualized (Fig. 19.14). Tenderness will be increased upon pressing the L5 spinous process cephalad, compared to the S1 tubercle.

Base Posterior Sacrum. The base posterior sacrum will essentially appear either the same as a normal disc (i.e., endplate lines parallel), or with the disc space widened at its posterior aspect (Fig. 19.15). Both subjective and objective signs are used to distinguish it as a subluxation. With this subluxation tenderness will be greater when pressing the S1 tubercle posterior to anterior and caudal when compared to pressing the L5 spinous process cephalad. In addition, motion examination will demonstrate restriction in nutation of the sacral base.

Spondylolisthesis. A spondylolisthesis of L5 can present as any of the following configurations: parallel endplate lines, a disc widened in the anterior and narrow at its posterior aspect, or a disc widened at the posterior (Fig. 19.16A–C). In most nonacute presentations the disc space will be more widened at its anterior aspect. Symptomatology related to a spondylolisthesis can vary from none to great. In order for a spondylolisthesis to occur in the pediatric patient, there must be either a break or an elongation of the pars interarticularis, or other congenital anomaly combined with an anterior slippage of the involved segment when compared to the segments above and

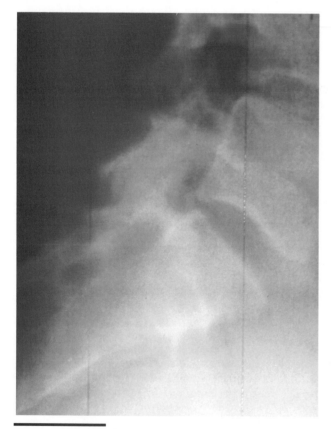

Figure 19.14.   Radiographic presentation of a retrolisthesis of L5.

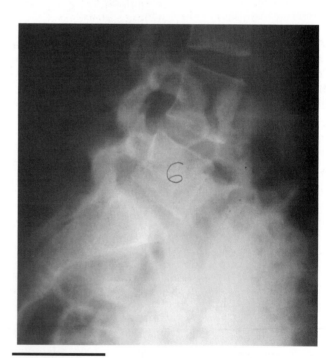

Figure 19.15.   Radiographic presentation of a base posterior sacrum. The L5-S1 endplate lines are parallel. This finding must be correlated with the palpatory or stress-x-ray assessment in order to differentiate the finding from a normal disc space.

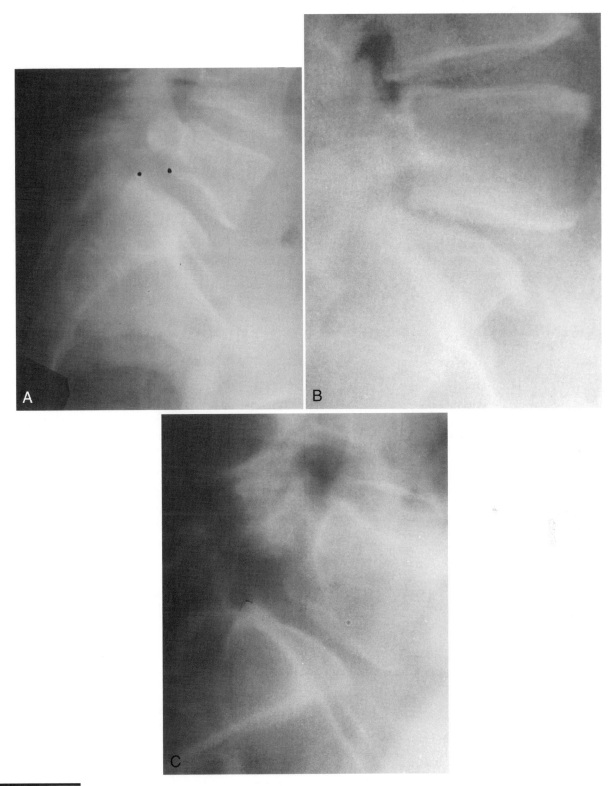

Figure 19.16.   A. Spondylolisthesis of L5 with parallel end-plate lines. B. Spondylolisthesis of L5 with posterior thinning of the disc. C. Spondylolisthesis of L5 with posterior widening of the disc space.

below. The Meyerding grading system should be utilized to determine the extent of anterior slippage of the motion segment involved.

Pediatric and adolescent evaluation is necessary for the detection and management of spondylolisthesis. Because spondylolisthesis has an abnormal mechanical association, it can predispose the individual to subluxation. Screening of subjects known to have spondylolisthesis is necessary in order to prevent the development of signs of subluxation. This preemptive evaluation, and treatment when indicated, may reduce the risk for the patient developing symptomatic disease.

Several methods of surgical treatment have been recommended for symptomatic spondylolysis and spondylolisthesis, ranging from repair of the defect to segmental fusion or a combination of both. Considering the much higher morbidity/mortality rate of general anesthesia and surgery when compared to conservative measures, chiropractic should be given adequate trial prior to the performance of more invasive procedures.

EXAMINATION

The patient was treated in an emergency room immediately following the accident. He spent the night in the hospital and was released the next day. The patient was treated for lacerations and a fractured left clavicle.

At a parent's request, the patient was to undergo chiropractic evaluation. The patient was reluctant and uncooperative during most phases of the examination. The patient presented for chiropractic evaluation four days following the initial trauma. He had a complaint of left and right sided low back pain. The low back pain was more pronounced on the left side and extended into the left leg and foot. The pain was worse in the morning.

The patient also complained of left-sided neck pain and pain at the anterior and posterior aspect of the left shoulder. His low-back pain is exacerbated by coughing. The neck pain was aggravated with right lateral flexion.

The patient had taken anti-inflammatory medication (ibuprofen) twice daily for three days prior to the chiropractic examination from a prescription he received from the hospital.

CLINICAL ASSESSMENTS

The patient's fractured left clavicle limited some examination strategies of the upper extremities and neck, such as grip strength.

The following orthopedic tests were positive:

1. Straight leg raise (left) at 90°
2. Braggard's (left)
3. Double leg raising and leg lowering were positive with pain at the upper and lower back
4. Soto-Hall
5. Linder's sign (bilateral)
6. Foraminal compression (right)

7. Shoulder depression (left)
8. Trendelenburg (left)

Neurological testing revealed the following:

1. Brachioradialis reflex diminished on the right (+1)
2. Achilles reflex decreased on the left (+1)

Posture analysis demonstrated an elevated iliac crest on the right and a high shoulder on the right.

Range of motion evaluation revealed the following:

Cervical Motion

Flexion: 55°
Extension: 70°
L. Rot.:   60°
R. Rot.:   60°
L. Lat. Flex: 35°
R. Lat. Flex: 30° with pain

Thoraco-Lumbar Motion:

Flexion: 85°
Extension: 25°
L. Lat. Flex: 20°
R. Lat. Flex: 15°

Left and right rotation of the thoraco-lumbar spine was not evaluated.

Dynamometer tests were not performed due to the fractured left clavicle.

Specific palpatory tenderness was noted at L5, T10, T4 and C7 although the entire cervical spine became tender during right or left lateral flexion of the neck.

Skin temperature instrumentation findings were present at L5, T10, T4 and C7.

Motion palpation revealed restriction in motion during bilateral lateral flexion and extension at L5, T10, T4 and C7.

RADIOLOGICAL ASSESSMENTS

There is a grade 1 spondylolisthesis of L5 which may or may not have been traumatically induced (Fig. 19.17A). A bone scan would have disclosed whether the fracture was of recent origin, however this was not obtained on this patient. The radiograph demonstrates a wedge-compression fracture of C5 (Fig. 19.17B). Flexion-extension of the cervical spine is shown in Figure 19.17C,D. The lateral spinal radiograph also demonstrated some minor compression deformity at T6 and T12. However, since a bone scan was not performed it is impossible to determine whether these findings are of traumatic origin. The patient's mechanism of trauma could undoubtedly explain most of the radiological findings.

DIAGNOSIS

In addition to the fractures noted above, the patient was diagnosed as having subluxations at C7, T4, T8, the sacrum, and the left ilium.

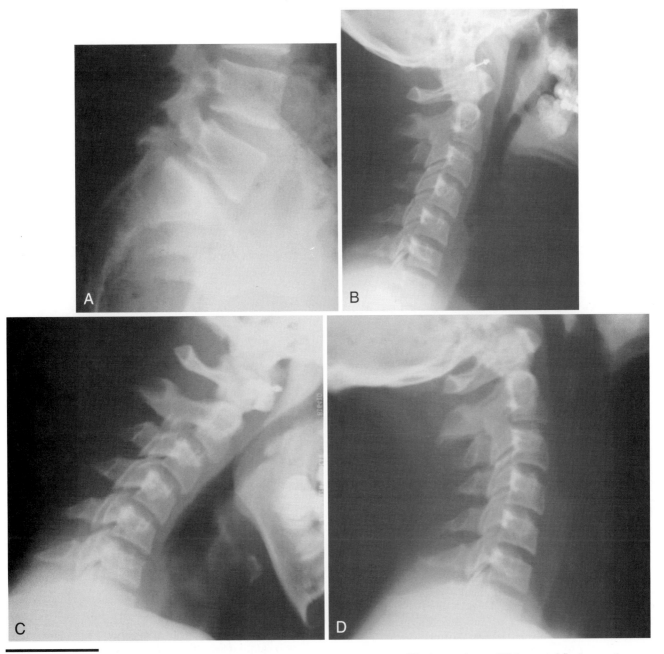

Figure 19.17. A. Grade 1 Spondylolisthesis of L5 from the chapter case presentation. B. Cervical portion from a lateral full spine radiograph. There is a slight compression deformity at the anterior aspect of C5. C. Flexion radiograph demonstrating restriction of flexion motion at C7. Increased flexion motion is noted at C5-C6. D. Extension radiograph demonstrating hypomobility at C4 through C6.

TREATMENT

Chiropractic treatment consisting of specific spinal adjustments at multiple levels of the spinal column was outlined for the patient's parent since the patient did not return for the report of findings. Conveyed through the parent, the patient did not believe that he was seriously injured and thought the pain medication would correct his problems. The patient was also under the care of a pediatrician and the patient related that he did not think it was necessary to be treated by a chiropractor. Therefore, the patient never underwent a chiropractic treatment program.

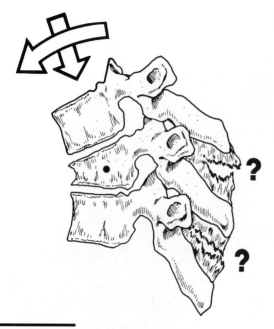

Figure 19.18.   Anterior compression fracture with ligamentous damage. The MIV has a flexion (+θX) as well as a compressive (-Y) component. These types of injuries are more likely to be unstable because of the damage to two columns.

FOLLOW-UP

Except for the follow-up visit with the patient's mother to provide the report of findings, there was no further evaluation of this patient.

Compression Fractures of the Thoracic Spine

INTRODUCTION

This 10-yr-old female was involved in an automobile accident on 11-12-89. On 11-24-89 she presented for chiropractic evaluation with complaints of difficulty in breathing, interscapular and lower thoracic pain, and left anterior costal pain. She was able to walk without difficulty. The patient was brought to the clinic by her mother, a former patient.

CLINICAL BIOMECHANICS

Study of this area has long been neglected since fractures of the thoracic spine constitute only a small percentage of spinal fractures (36). Fractures occur less often in the thoracic area than in other parts of the spine given the protection offered by the rib cage, the orientation of the facet planes and the fact that considerable force is required. Due to the architecture of the thoracic vertebrae, the neural canal is smallest in this area, thereby subjecting its contents (the spinal cord and nerve roots) to damage when a vertebra is either fractured or subluxated. The main causes of thoracic fractures are auto accidents, falls from excessive heights, and direct blows to the area (7).

Unstable fractures result in loss of anterior vertebral body height and progressive kyphotic deformity (i.e., Gibbus),

subluxation of the superior vertebra and disruption of the soft tissues, usually causing pain (Figs. 19.18 and 19.19). Stable compression fractures may also present a similar symptomatology and if not managed properly, instability can ensue when anterior column height exceeds 50% due to progressive stress at the posterior elements. Management includes comparative radiographic analyses to ensure there is no progression of kyphosis.

CLINICAL ASSESSMENTS

The patient walked with a slightly flexed forward antalgic lean. All movements were guarded especially rising from a seated position. While sitting, the patient had difficulty remaining erect and adopted a slightly flexed antalgic posture.

Subluxation findings, including restricted motion, skin temperature alterations, edema, and tenderness, were present at C1, C7, T4, T9 and the right sacroiliac joint. The primary site of subluxation was T9.

RADIOLOGICAL ASSESSMENTS

The lateral radiograph (Fig. 19.20) demonstrates compression fractures at T7 and T8. The AP radiograph reveals a slight decrease in the body height of the fractured vertebrae.

DIAGNOSIS

Subluxations were diagnosed at T9, T4, C7, C1 and the sacrum. The fractured vertebrae were not identified as exhibiting signs of subluxation.

TREATMENT

During the first two clinic visits, the T9 segment only was adjusted, and this was accomplished using a the prone patient

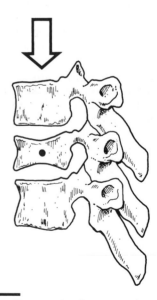

Figure 19.19.   Compression fracture with a more purely compressive (-Y) MIV. Posterior ligamentous damage is more unlikely with this injury.

position on a hi-lo table. Cervical adjustments were performed in the seated position and the sacrum was adjusted with the patient in the side posture position. Rotation of the spine was avoided during the side posture adjustment in order to minimize any strain to the thoracic spine. The patient was adjusted on 12 occasions over the course of the first five months post injury; at the sacrum (8X), T9 (4X), T4 (4X), C7 (1X) and C1 (3X).

FOLLOW-UP

Two weeks after beginning chiropractic care, the patient reported no symptomatology. Spinal palpatory tenderness and interstitial edema was absent after the third adjustment. Intersegmental ranges of motion were markedly improved after the sixth adjustment. The patient receives a check-up evaluation approximately every six to eight weeks and has been adjusted on 31 occasions over a five year period.

Burst Fracture of T7 with Transverse Process Fractures of the Lumbar Spine

INTRODUCTION

This 17-yr-old male sustained injuries during a truck accident. The patient was driving a small pick-up truck when he swerved to avoid hitting a dog. The vehicle left the roadway and hit a tree. The patient was not wearing any type of restraint device at the time of the collision. The patient stated that when he realized he was going to hit the tree, he laid on his side and protected his head with his arms before the actual impact. The impact was behind the door of the cab and in front of the bed of the truck on the driver's side. The vehicle did not roll or impact in any other area.

The patient was rendered unconscious immediately following the accident. He was transported to a local hospital for examination and treatment. The patient was admitted to the hospital where he was observed for a period of nine days. The medical diagnosis included an enlarged spleen, fractured ribs, transverse process fractures of L1-L3 on the left and vertebral body fractures at T7 and T8. The patient complained of stomach and digestive difficulties, pain in the mid-back referring into the ribs, leg pain, and neck soreness.

The parents of the patient consulted the chiropractor's office for an opinion on his case August 11, 1994 (seven days following the accident). The hospital radiographs were reviewed and it was decided to examine the patient in the hospital two days later. The chiropractor was able to evaluate the patient while he was in the hospital.

CLINICAL BIOMECHANICS

The burst fracture of the thoracic spine is produced through a compressive (-Y) force usually combined with forced flexion. The compressive force above pushes the nucleus through the endplate, bursting the vertebral body at right angles to the MIV. There is a sandwich effect as the injured vertebra is squeezed between the two adjacent vertebrae (7).

Fragments are often times driven posteriorward, damaging the posterior longitudinal ligament and compressing the

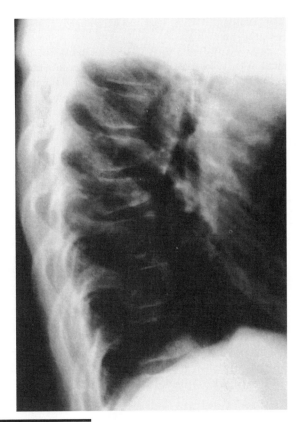

Figure 19.20.   Anterior compression fractures of T7 and T8. Reproduced with permission from Rowe DJ. Chiropractic management of spinal fractures and dislocations. In: Plaugher G, ed. Textbook of clinical chiropractic: a specific biomechanical approach. Baltimore: Williams & Wilkins, 1993:340.

anterior portion of the spinal cord (Fig. 19.21). A classic anterior spinal syndrome may ensue, causing immediate and complete motor paralysis, and cutaneous sensory nerve loss of pain and temperature below the level of nerve damage. Bilateral vibration and position sense are often left unaffected (7). Tuning fork evaluation can therefore still be used during the clinical examination.

The lateral radiograph demonstrates flattening of the comminuted vertebral body centrally. Anterior and posterior displacement of fragments can be visualized but do not necessarily give a clear indication of spinal stability (7,21).

The AP radiograph often demonstrates a vertical fracture line in the body of the vertebra. This radiographic sign is usually present in the burst fracture and absent in the simple compression fracture, making it useful as a differentiating factor (7,96).

The burst fracture is often missed, due to its tendency to reposition back to a more normal shape and position following the injury. This is due to the centering effect of the ligaments of the motion segment. This may leave the practitioner uncertain as to the level of neurological deficit if the radiograph shows no alterations (53). The CT scan is the best method of determining the level of communition and fracture (96). Due to the fact that the burst fracture involves the anterior and middle columns, it is always biomechanically and often neurologically unstable (7).

Transverse process fractures of the lumbar spine usually occur from excessive lateral flexion coupled with a hyperextension injury. The break usually occurs at L2 and L3 and is the second most frequently occurring lumbar fracture (96). It is often found at more than one level. Fifth lumbar transverse fractures commonly accompany pelvic fractures, such as the vertical sacral type (7).

Radiographically, transverse fractures appear as radiolucent lines that usually run vertically or obliquely. When, on occasion, they traverse horizontally, a Chance fracture should be suspected (See Chance Fracture Case Study). The transverse process fracture can be differentiated from developmental nonunion (ununited secondary growth centers) by evidence of the fracture's jagged irregular border and fracture line. A urinalysis and kidney exam should be performed since renal damage may be found concurrently with transverse process fractures (96). Transverse process fractures are usually stable unless accompanied by other fractures or ligamentous damage (7).

EXAMINATION

The patient was first seen for chiropractic evaluation while in the hospital. The radiographs were reviewed and a palpatory examination was performed on the patient.

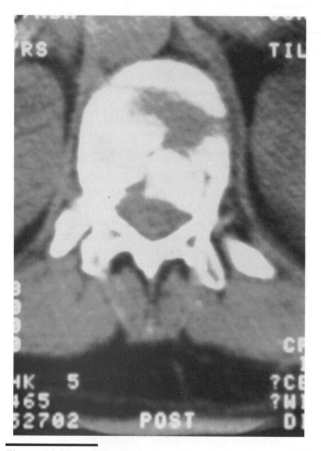

Figure 19.21.   CT scan of a lower thoracic burst fracture with moderate compromise of the spinal canal.

RADIOLOGICAL ASSESSMENTS

The radiographs disclosed a burst fracture at T7 (Fig. 19.22A,B). There is an increased anterior to posterior dimension of the vertebral body with retrodisplacement of the segment. These findings are consistent with that of a burst fracture (143). No CT examinations were obtained on the patient. The lateral lumbar radiograph demonstrates a retrolisthesis of L5 (Fig. 19.23).

The AP radiograph demonstrates the transverse process fractures of L1, L2 and L3 (Fig. 19.24).

CLINICAL ASSESSMENTS

Subluxation findings, including asymmetrical temperature patterns, edema, and tenderness, were present at T7, C7 and L5.

DIAGNOSIS

In addition to the patient's other injuries (i.e., fractured ribs, enlarged spleen, etc.), a fracture-subluxation was diagnosed at T7. Subluxations were also noted at C7 and L5.

TREATMENT

While the patient was in the hospital, the author was able to perform an adjustment in a posterior to anterior direction at the level of T7 using the spinous process as the contact point. The force was very light and a light preload was applied prior to the thrust. The patient's tolerance was evaluated constantly during the performance of the procedure. The patient was advised to apply ice to the area for 20 minutes at 3–4 hour intervals. A telephone conversation with the parents of the patient occurred the day following the adjustment. They reported that the patient was able to eat a normal meal for the first time since the accident and that the digestive process was normal. He was also able to sleep with more comfort. The patient was then released from the hospital and was able to be evaluated at the author's office three days following the first adjustment.

On August 15, 1994, full spine (AP and lateral) radiographs were obtained and reviewed (Fig. 19.25A,B). At this time the patient was adjusted at T7 on the hi-lo table using a single-hand spinous process contact. Using Elastikon tape, the region from T5 through T9 was secured with one strip directly over the spinous processes, followed by two strips in a criss-cross pattern with the crossing at the T7 and T8 region. The patient was advised to continue using the ice at home.

The patient was provided a brace before leaving the hospital, which he was instructed to wear at all times (Fig. 19.25C-E). The cost of the brace was $320.00. After a two week period (eight adjustments), the patient chose not to wear the brace except when riding in a car. After another eight adjustments (four weeks post injury), the patient ceased wearing the brace entirely.

FOLLOW-UP

The patient was able to perform all activities he had engaged in prior to the accident after eight adjustments. These activities included riding a four-wheeler, driving a tractor and attending school full-time. Nineteen adjustments were delivered at T7

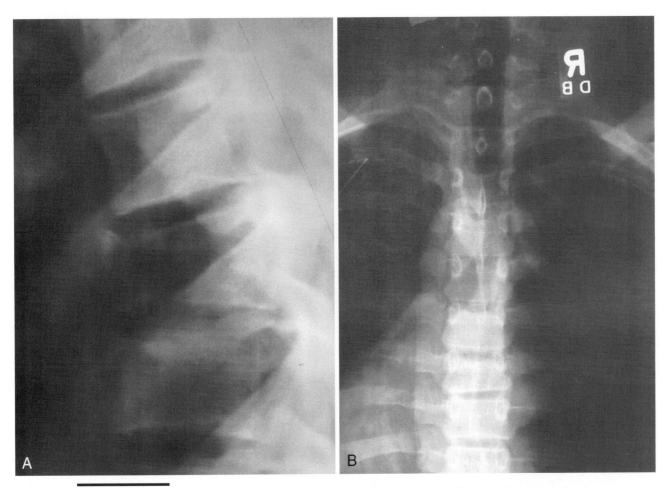

Figure 19.22.   A. Burst fracture of T7 with retrodisplacement of the vertebral body. B. AP radiograph demonstrating compression deformity of T7 with decreased body height.

over a three month period. During this same time period, 10 adjustments were provided at C7 and 15 at L5.

There was a total of 19 office visits from August 12, 1994 through November 22, 1994. The chiropractic costs for these visits was $416.00. The total hospital costs were approximately $15,000. At the time of this writing the patient was being seen every three weeks for chiropractic evaluation.

DISCUSSION

Knight et al. (33) have compared the results of operative versus conservative nonoperative treatment of lumbar burst fractures. Treatment complications, resumption of employment and quality of life measured through a simplified scale were used to evaluate 93 patients during a two-year study period. No significant difference in treatment outcome was established in the two groups. The authors recommend nonoperative interventions as a viable alternative to the medical treatment of these types of fractures.

The only other reported case of an adolescent with a compression-type fracture initially managed by a chiropractor is that presented by Guebert and Thompson (6). Their case management differs greatly from the protocol presented in the other cases in this chapter. Although the case by Guebert and Thompson is presented as a compression fracture, there is communition of the vertebral body with displacement of a portion of the vertebral body posteriorward into the spinal canal. This finding is more suggestive of a burst fracture. The patient was subsequently referred to an orthopedist where Harrington rods were placed. At the time of the case presentation by Guebert and Thompson, the patient was expected to have the rods removed about two years after placement. No long-term follow-up was presented on this patient.

Thoracolumbar burst fractures are commonly associated with other fractures (144). In a survey from Arthornthurasook and Thongmag (144), 36 patients with thoracolumbar burst fractures, presenting over a two year period, were analyzed for the presence of concomitant fractures. Nine of the patients or 25% had another spinal fracture. The case presented here, with fractures of transverse processes, is consistent with this finding. The additional fractures in the survey noted above consisted of burst or anterior compression fractures. One third were burst fractures, found at a distant level to the main burst fracture (144).

Anterolateral Compression Fracture of L1

INTRODUCTION

This 18-yr-old male patient presented for chiropractic evaluation on 7-24-94 with a complaint of intense midline and left sided low-back pain.

He stated that he had hurt his lower back earlier that day while riding a jet ski. During operation of the device he jumped a boat wave, propelling his watercraft 10 to 12 feet in the air. He landed stiff-legged and felt immediate, severe low-back pain which caused him to fall backwards into the wave.

CLINICAL BIOMECHANICS

The mechanism of injury for this fracture was sudden flexion with right lateral bending. The anterolateral compression fracture is more commonly associated with shoulder restraint types of seat belts. During head-on collisions, the unrestrained shoulder may move forward. This is known as the roll-out phenomenon and is responsible for creating the simultaneous forces of flexion and lateral bending. Miniaci et al. (145) have reviewed the histories and outcomes of four patients having suffered anterolateral compression fractures of the thoracolumbar spine. One patient had an additional distraction injury

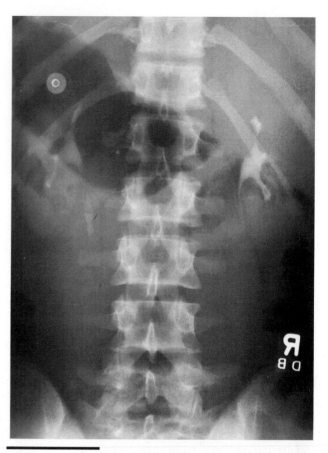

Figure 19.24. Left transverse process fractures of L1, L2 and L3.

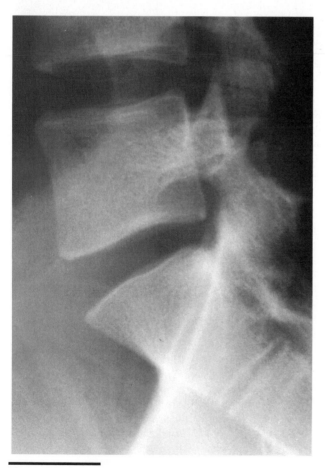

Figure 19.23. Retrolisthesis of L5.

involving a fractured transverse process at L3. All patients were medically treated non-operatively. Early mobilization (ambulation) by one patient increased pain and a mild deformity occurred. This patient was then treated with log-rolling and bed rest for six weeks. The patient ambulated with an orthosis for another six weeks. All of the patients returned to full activity levels. Three patients continued to suffer nondisabling back pain (145).

The finding of back pain following conservative interventions such as those described should alert the reader to the choice of chiropractic as a treatment, since spinal adjustments/manipulation are one of the few treatments that have been scientifically proven to reduce back pain.

Biomechanical studies with cadavers using flexion-rotation about a shoulder harness exhibited the exact same fracture with distraction, leading to the conclusion that flexion-rotation is the mechanism of injury (7,145) (Fig.19.26). Although none of the four patients in the study by Miniaci experienced any associated major injuries, due to the fact that both the anterior column and the contralateral posterior column were damaged, this injury must be considered biomechanically unstable (145). In all four cases there was no neurological deficit and all four fractures had healed at two years follow-up.

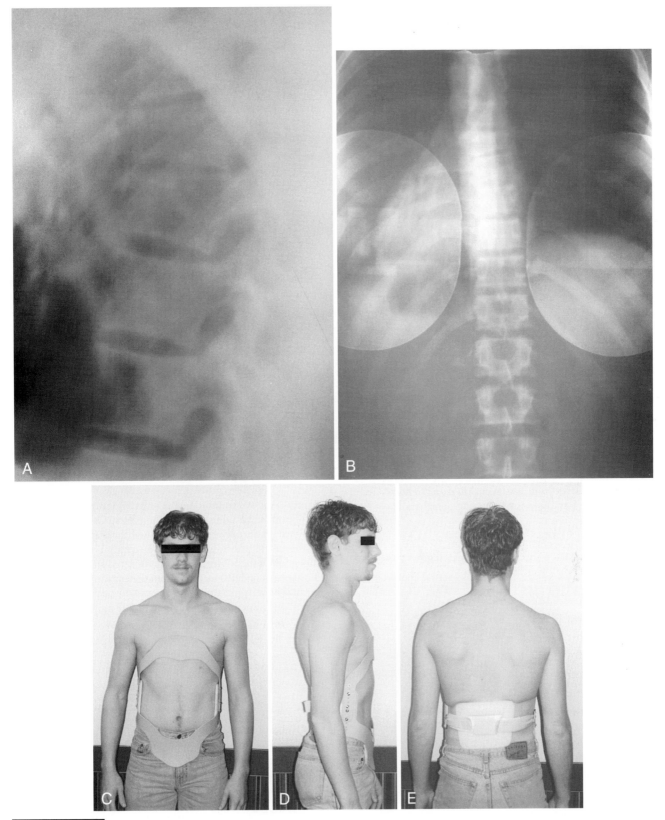

Figure 19.25.   A. Lateral view from a full spine radiograph demonstrates slight reduction of the retrodisplacement of the vertebral body of T7. Compare to Figure 19.22A. B. AP radiograph from a full spine radiograph showing the compression de-

formity at T7. C. Frontal view of the back brace used by the patient. D. Side view of the back brace. E. Posterior view of the back brace.

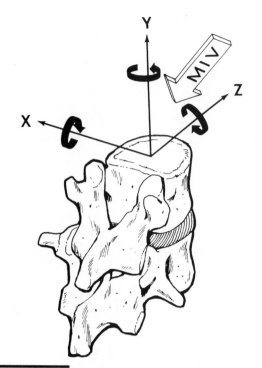

Figure 19.26.   Major injuring vector (MIV) for an anterolateral compression fracture.

EXAMINATION

The patient walks without assistance. His pain is reported to be confined to the low back not extending peripherally.

CLINICAL ASSESSMENTS

Ranges of motion of the dorsal-lumbar region were only mildly reduced. They were as follows:

Dorsal-Lumbar Flexion: 90/95

Dorsal-Lumbar Extension: 28/30

Dorsal Lumbar Lateral Flexion-Right: 25/30

Dorsal-Lumbar Lateral Flexion-Left: 25/30

Dorsal-Lumbar Rotation-Right: 30/30

Dorsal-Lumbar Rotation-Left: 30/30

The psoas test was positive bilaterally for muscle strength. Goldthwait, Lasegue, Braggard, FABERE-Patrick's, Leg-Drop test and Ely's were negative bilaterally. Patellar and achilles reflexes were normal. Palpation revealed tenderness at the level of T12 and L1 accompanied by left sided muscle spasm of the lumbar spine, most pronounced at the level of L2. The patient reported mild stiffness and soreness of the cervical spine and midback.

Skin temperature instrumentation disclosed findings at L5, L1, T8 and C7. These segments also exhibited motion restriction.

RADIOLOGICAL ASSESSMENTS

Anteroposterior and lateral full spine radiographs were obtained. They demonstrate an anterolateral compression fracture of L1 (Fig. 19.27A-C). There is greater than 50% loss of the anterior height of the vertebral body. Listings of intersegmental position of the motion segments derived from the radiographic analysis (See Chapter 7) demonstrated the following:

C1: ASLA (-θX,+θZ,-θY)

C7: PR (-Z,+θY)

T6: PRS (-Z,+θY,-θZ)

T8: P

T12: PLS (-Z,-θY,+θZ)

L5: PLI-m (-Z,-θY,-θZ)

Sacrum: Left: 64 mm; Right: 69 mm

Right Ilium: PI_2 In_{10}

DIAGNOSIS

The patient was diagnosed as having suffered an acute, traumatically induced anterolateral compression fracture of L1. There were findings of subluxation present at L5-S1, T8-T9 and C7-T1. Informed consent was obtained for this patient and the nature of the injury was explained to both the patient and his mother. The mother had been a patient at the clinic for 20 years and the patient had been seen by the author on an occasional basis since birth.

TREATMENT

The patient was adjusted beginning the day of the injury. The fifth lumbar was adjusted with the patient in the side-posture position on the pelvic bench. The eighth thoracic was adjusted in the prone position on the hi-lo table. The patient would flinch when the L5 vertebra was contacted for the adjustment. The patient had no reaction when the eighth thoracic vertebra was adjusted. The cervical chair was used to adjust C7 in the seated position. The patient was adjusted daily for six days and is currently on a three visit per week schedule. The cost of each clinic visit was $30.00.

FOLLOW-UP

At the time of this writing, the patient had been under care for approximately one month. The low-back pain had reduced markedly during this time, although there was considerable discomfort at the beginning of treatment. The student attends college classes without difficulty.

Chance Fracture of L3

INTRODUCTION

The patient is an 18-yr-old male, 5 ft. 9 in., and weighing 154 lbs. He was involved in a motor vehicle accident on 5-28-92. The patient was seated in the middle of the rear seat, wearing a lap belt. Sudden hyperflexion of the trunk of the patient was sustained due to an abrupt halting of the vehicle due to a collision with a tree. The patient was taken by ambulance to the nearest hospital, complaining of low-back pain and paresthesia in the lower extremities particularly on the medial aspect of the left calf. He was x-rayed and examined, then released 4 hours later, being advised that he had not suffered any injury.

CLINICAL BIOMECHANICS

In 1948, Chance (146) described a flexion distraction injury consisting of a horizontal splitting of the spine and neural arch ending in an upward curve which usually reaches the upper surface of the vertebral body just in front of the neural foramen.

Since children are often the passengers in rear seats, the use of lap seat belts has resulted in an increased incidence for the

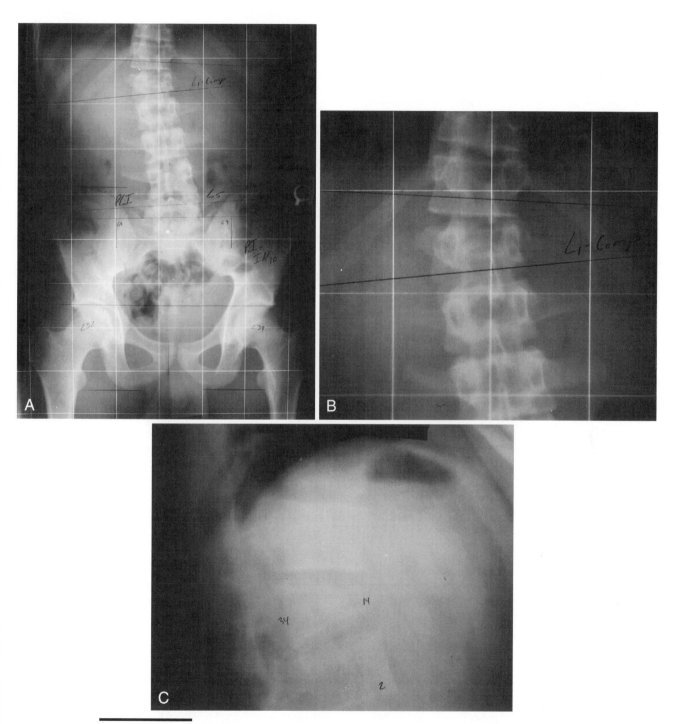

Figure 19.27.   A. AP radiograph of an anterolateral compression fracture of L1. B. Close-up of A. C. Lateral radiograph demonstrating anterior compression of the vertebral body.

Chance fracture in children (147). The Chance fracture, also known as a lap seat belt fracture, is a hyperflexion (+θX) injury with the center of rotation anterior to the body of the vertebra (7,57) (Fig. 19.28A). Since the center of rotation is anterior to that of a pure compression fracture, there is much greater tension put on the posterior bony elements. As the spinous processes separate to their physiological limits, the bone often fails before the posterior ligamentous structures, creating longitudinal fractures through the spinous process, posterior arch, the pedicles and often into the posterior aspects of the vertebral body itself (7) (Fig. 19.28B). The anterior portion of the vertebral body may suffer mild compression type fractures as well.

Although bone usually fails before the ligamentous structures, severe soft tissue injuries of the posterior ligaments, the posterior longitudinal ligament, and the disc itself are often associated with this injury due to the extreme tensile forces involved. These injuries are very rare. Within the medical community there are reports of treatment of Chance fractures with both non-operative and surgical methods (148).

There is currently no literature available that demonstrates whether one treatment is superior to another. This includes chiropractic methods, orthopedic bracing, surgery or the natural history of the injury.

Standard plain film lateral radiographs may show fractures in the spinous, lamina, pedicles, and posterior portion of the vertebral body. Since there is often soft tissue injury as well as splaying of spinous processes, an abnormally increased posterior disc height is often visualized (7,96).

A-P and lateral tomography can clearly demonstrate the fracture lines in a Chance fracture which are often poorly visualized in the axial view of CT. However, the reconstructed sagittal view of the CT scan can be quite helpful in visualizing and evaluating these horizontal fracture lines (57). The CT scan can also be useful in evaluating an associated burst fracture. In a group of Chance fractures described by Gertzbein (149), 70% had an accompanying vertebral body compression fracture. Fifteen percent had burst fractures and 15% had no vertebral body fracture. High force deceleration can cause the burst fracture due to increased -Y forces, while low velocity can lead to the posterior distraction (+θX) injury. Because the center of rotation is more anterior, it causes posterior element soft tissue damage combined with posterior body distraction fracture (7).

Flexion-distraction type injuries are extremely uncommon in children due to their greater flexibility. However, with the use of lap seat belts, the major focus of flexion with posterior element distraction is placed on the lumbar vertebrae at the level of the seat belt. With the belt functioning like a fulcrum, the forced flexion is concentrated in one spinal area as opposed to being dissipated over a greater area, thereby increasing the likelihood of damage (7,150).

Since the introduction of the lap seatbelt in the 1950s and 60s, the Chance fracture has occurred much more frequently (93). Approximately 50% of Chance fracture cases have associated intra-abdominal injuries (8,147).

EXAMINATION

Following the accident the patient was taken to a hospital and examined by a resident. The patient reported that the examination was performed in a very cursory fashion, although radiographs of the lumbar spine were obtained. The radiographs were interpreted as normal and the patient was prescribed some pain medication and then released.

Unsatisfied with his condition, the patient returned to the hospital three days later. The resident again advised him that everything was normal and that he should continue with the pain medication. As the patient was walking out of the hospital, an orthopedic surgeon came into the hallway. The resident then asked the surgeon to look at the radiographs to reassure the patient. The orthopedist identified a vertebral fracture at L3, ordered a CT examination and fitted the patient with a

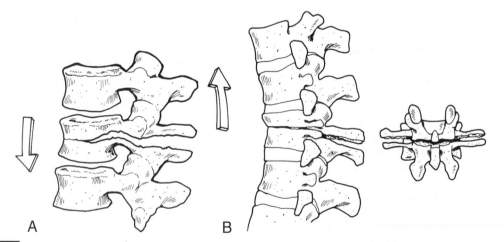

Figure 19.28. A. Major injuring vector (MIV) for the Chance fracture. Modified from Kaye JJ, Nance EP. Thoracic and lumbar spine trauma. Radiol Clin North Am 1990; 28:372. B. Vertebral injuries associated with the Chance fracture. Modified from

Smith WS, Kaufer H. A new pattern of spine injury associated with lap-type seatbelts: a preliminary report. Univ Michigan Medical Center J 1966; 33:247.

brace. The patient was told that he had sustained a nondisplaced fracture of L3 confined to the posterior ¼ of the vertebral body.

The patient's acute symptomatology did not improve under pain medications or the orthopedic brace and he was brought to a chiropractic clinic by his parents (who were also patients) 12 days following the accident. The patient presented with acute lumbar pain, severe paresthesia to the anterior left thigh, extending to the medial and posterior aspects of the left knee and upper margins of the gastrocnemius. He also described an intermittent inability to lock, at the knee, a fully extended leg. The knee occasionally "lets go" causing uncontrolled flexion.

CLINICAL ASSESSMENTS

The patient presented in obvious pain with a forward antalgic lean of the trunk and a hypolordotic lumbar spine. The hospital radiographs were reviewed prior to the examination.

All orthopedic and range of motion testing was performed very gently due to the presence of a fracture at the L3 level. There was severe reduction of global range of motion for lumbar right and left lateral flexion and lumbar extension. There was a positive Lasegue test for both lower extremities at less than 15°, although straight leg raising was more limited on the left. A modified Kemp's test (with limited extension and side bending) was performed to ascertain if symptoms were primarily arising from L3 or L5. The test was not performed as is typically done and only involved a mild degree of lateral flexion with extension. This test tended to demonstrate more facetal pain from the L3 than the lower lumbar levels. Provocation of the L3 level tended to reproduce the sensory changes in the lower leg of the left extremity. All deep tendon reflexes tested normally.

A large circular edematous area was observed extending from L1 to L4 with its center over the L3 spinous process. The spinous process of L3 was also extremely tender to palpation.

Skin temperature instrumentation (Nervo-scope) findings were present at C1-C2 and the L5-S1 levels. There were no positive findings detected by the temperature instrument at L3.

RADIOLOGICAL ASSESSMENTS

The chiropractic interpretation of the radiographic examination was found to be contradictory to the opinion verbally provided by the orthopedist at the hospital. Plain films demonstrated a Chance fracture of L3, extending from both laminae, through the pedicles, transverse processes and extending into the posterior-inferior portion of the vertebral body of L3, passing through the inferior endplate (Fig. 19.29A-C). It was clear that there existed a posterior displacement of the posterior-inferior aspect of the vertebral body with respect to the upper part of the L3 vertebra.

The computerized tomographic scans that were obtained during the second visit of the hospital demonstrated indentation into the anterior portion of the thecal sac (Fig. 19.30A-C).

Full spine radiographs were also obtained at the first visit to the chiropractic clinic, confirming the earlier plain films taken at the hospital.

An opinion was sought from a chiropractic radiologist. The films were sent by courier the same day to a Diplomate of the American Chiropractic Board of Radiology. The radiologist was requested to review the films immediately and get back to the chiropractor because the patient was in acute pain. After three weeks the radiological report was received by the attending chiropractor. The chiropractor received no phone call from the radiologist. The chiropractor elected to treat the patient the same day. The radiologist's findings, detailed in the late report, confirmed the diagnosis of a Chance fracture of L3. The radiologist also advised that "manipulation therapy is absolutely contraindicated. Orthopedic management of this condition is mandatory."

This advice, received nearly three weeks after the films were presented for review, was obviously not followed as is detailed below.

DIAGNOSIS

A fracture-subluxation was diagnosed at L3 and subluxation complex at the L5-S1 motion segment. There was retrolisthesis present at L5. The attending chiropractor reviewed the findings of the case with a colleague prior to initiating treatment.

INFORMED CONSENT

The patient and his parents had visited the hospital on two occasions. On the first visit, they were told that no injury was detected. The second time, the same information was conveyed; however a second opinion was obtained as they were walking out the door. This opinion led to a prescription for bed rest and an orthopedic appliance. These measures failed to satisfy the patient or his parents and he reported for chiropractic evaluation 10 days later. The patient and his parents were fully informed of the nature and seriousness of the injuries and a decision was made to attempt closed reduction of the lesion and place the patient under chiropractic care for his injuries.

TREATMENT

Following careful examination of the radiographs and considering the neurological signs, the attending chiropractor judged that the posterior-inferior structures of the L3 vertebra, including the lower portions of the vertebral body, the transverse processes, and the inferior articulating processes and spinous process were subluxated to the posterior relative to the more cephalad portion of the vertebra.

The patient was adjusted in the side-posture position on a pelvic bench. The L3 vertebra was adjusted as a retrolisthesis. The contact point was the inferior portion of the spinous process of L3. The L3 segment was adjusted on three occasions (with a push move) over eight days. Because of the patient's forward antalgic lean, an adjustment on the hi-lo table was deemed contraindicated. No axial rotation was applied with the patient in the side posture position. Had the patient not presented with a forward antalgic lean, a prone position such as on a hi-lo table would likely have been the initial position of choice.

Due to the extreme tenderness of the L3 spinous process, only an extremely light preload could be applied prior to the thrust. As the patient was slightly pretensioned for the adjustment, the doctor carefully assessed whether patient positioning was exacerbating symptomatology.

The first specific contact, high velocity adjustment felt as though the lower portion of L3 moved in relation to the upper portion. The audible could not be described as what is typically detected when coaptation of a facet joint occurs. Rather, the audible had a sound similar to what would be encountered when "crushing grapes."

Two subsequent adjustments at L3 were detected to move as a normal segment would (i.e., in relation to L4) with a normal audible and movement characteristics of a normal motion segment.

After the second adjustment to L3, all of the paresthesia to the left leg had disappeared and the low back pain had reduced considerably. The patient was adjusted on three occasions at L3 over the course of a week. The fifth lumbar was adjusted on five occasions during the next three weeks as a retrolisthesis (-Z). Approximately one month after beginning chiropractic care the patient reported that the leg symptomatology, including the uncontrollable flexion, was very much improved. The

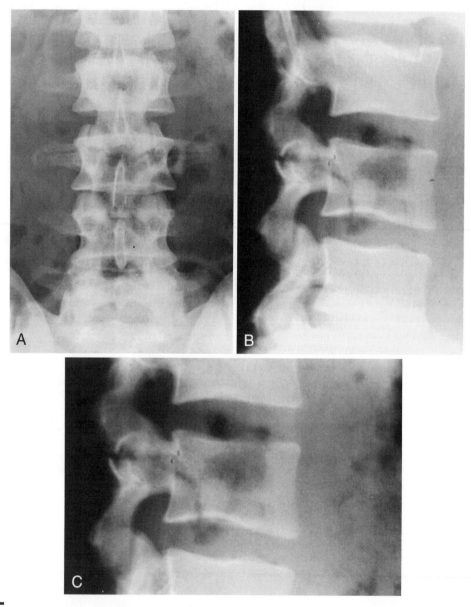

Figure 19.29.   A. AP radiograph demonstrating a Chance fracture at L3. B. Lateral radiograph of a Chance fracture at L3. Notice the separation at both the posterior and middle columns. There is a break in the continuity of the articular pillar and at the anterior portion of the spinal canal. C. Close-up of B.

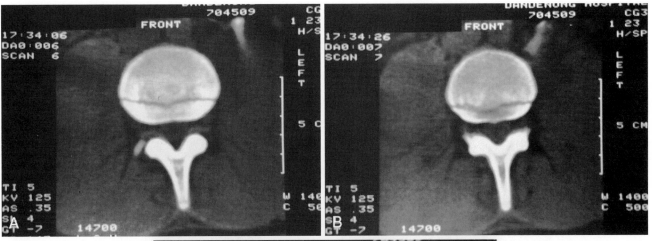

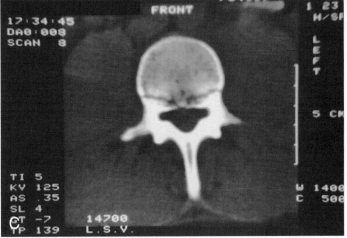

Figure 19.30.   A. CT scan of the Chance fracture at L3. Notice the indentation of the anterior thecal sac. B. More ceph-alad slice of vertebra depicted in A. C. More cephalad slice of vertebra depicted in B.

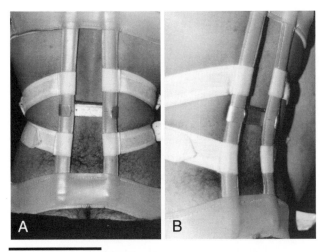

Figure 19.31.   A. A posterior view of the modified back brace with posterior to anterior pressure applied at the posterior-inferior portion of the spinous process of L3. B. Oblique close-up view of the modified back brace.

instability of the knee joint, although slightly better following adjustments to L3, did not measurably improve until the fifth lumbar subluxation was reduced.

The patient was fitted with a modified back brace (Fig. 19.31A,B) which had an additional padded cross-member, producing a straight anteriorly directed pressure at the posterior aspect of the L3 spinous process. A noticeable indentation of the subcutaneous tissues could be detected on subsequent visits to the clinic when the appliance was removed. This indentation confirmed that the brace was exerting anterior-ward pressure at the L3 vertebra. The patient was monitored over the course of three months and continued to wear the back brace when ambulatory throughout this period.

PROGNOSIS

The Chance fracture may or may not heal and return to being a stable motion segment. This is dependent on the tissues that are injured. A purely bony injury is most likely to heal. An injury with posterior supportive ligament or disc damage may never return to a stable situation. Regarding associated verte-

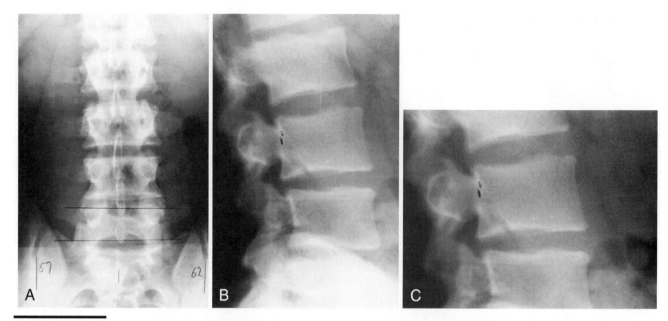

Figure 19.32.   A. Comparative AP radiograph at four months demonstrating union of the fracture at L3. B. Comparative lateral radiograph at four months demonstrating reduction of the fracture displacement at L3. Compare George's line at L3 and the articular pillar to B and C. C. Close-up view of B.

bral body fracture, the compression injury is much more likely to regain stability than the burst fracture (149). Neurological deficit occurs in 15% of all Chance fracture cases and the upper lumbar spine, especially L1-L3, is the most frequent site of occurrence (96).

FOLLOW-UP

Comparative radiographic examination was conducted approximately four months later (Fig. 19.32A-C). The radiographs demonstrated a considerable reduction in separation of the fracture segments.

The superior and inferior portions of the transverse processes have now been rejoined. The posterior margin of the vertebral body that had moved into the neural canal has been realigned. The separation within the vertebral body is close to acceptable limits. No comparative CT scans were obtained in this case.

Three months into care, the patient had a relapse of the uncontrolled leg flexion which then resolved after the L5 vertebra was adjusted.

At four months, the patient does not report any paresthesia to the left leg. The involuntary left knee flexion has ceased. The patient has occasional minor low-back pain which responds favorably to adjustments of L5. No further adjustments were made to L3 after the second week of care.

DISCUSSION

Regarding the patient's primary symptomatology of uncontrollable leg flexion and sensory changes in the lower left leg, these seemed to be arising from the injury sustained at L3. Although this was the primary etiological site for these symptoms, they did not measurably improve until the lower segment (i.e., L5 was adjusted). The authors interpret this as a case of a foundation problem leading to a lack of stabilization of the motion segment above.

Children are particularly susceptible to lap seatbelt injuries, including the Chance fracture, because they commonly ride in the rear seats of vehicles. The presence of lap seatbelt ecchymosis should prompt the clinician to conduct a careful search for related spine, bowel, and bladder injury (151,152). Glassman et al. (153) describe two patients with essentially bony injury, similar to the case presented in this chapter. The patients were initially braced (oyster shell brace in extension) because of a bowel injury that postponed surgery. They had satisfactory healing with the brace treatment alone. In their survey of 12 Chance fractures in patients less than 16 yrs-old, Glassman et al. (153) found that if the initial kyphotic deformity was less than 20 degrees, then the patients responded well to brace treatment.

REFERENCES

1. Cox JM. Low back pain. 5th ed. Baltimore: Williams & Wilkins, 1990.
2. Leach RA. The chiropractic theories. 3rd. ed. Baltimore: Williams & Wilkins, 1994.
3. Foreman SH, Croft AC. Whiplash injuries: the cervical acceleration/deceleration syndrome. 2nd. ed. Baltimore: Williams & Wilkins, 1995.
4. Nykoliation JW, Cassidy JD, Dupuis P, Yong-Hing K, Crnec M. Missed cervical spine fracture-dislocations prior to manipulation: a review of three cases. J Can Chiro Assoc 1986; 30:69–75.
5. Haldeman S, Rubinstein SM. Compression fractures in patients undergoing spinal manipulative therapy. J Manipulative Physiol Ther 1992; 15:450–454.
6. Guebert GM, Thompson JR. L1 compression fracture. ACA J Chiropractic 1986; 20(8):83–85.
7. Rowe DJ. Chiropractic management of spinal fractures and dislocations. In: Plaugher G, ed. Textbook of clinical chiropractic: a specific biomechanical approach. Baltimore: Williams & Wilkins, 1993:325–355.
8. Stedman's Medical Dictionary, 25th ed. Baltimore: Williams & Wilkins, 1989.
9. Anderson RT. Angulation of the basiocciput in three cranial series. Curr Anthropol 1983; 24;226–228.

10. Macmillan M, Stauffer ES. Transient neurologic deficits associated with thoracic and lumbar spine trauma without fracture or dislocation. Spine 1990; 15:466–469.
11. Ehara S, El-Khoury GK, Sato Y. Cervical spine injury in children: radiologic manifestations. Am J Radiol 1988; 151:1175–1178.
12. McGrory BJ, Klassen RA, Chao EYS, Staeheli JW, Weaver AL. Acute fractures and dislocations of the cervical spine in children and adolescents. J Bone Joint Surg 1993; 75A: 988–995.
13. Plaugher G, Cox DB, Thibodeau P. Chiropractic management of spinal fractures: a report of six cases. Proceedings: International Conference on Spinal Manipulation. Foundation for Chiropractic Education and Research, Arlington, VA, 1991:67–71.
14. Plaugher G, Rowe D, Gohl R. Chiropractic management of spinal fractures and dislocations. Proceedings: International Conference on Spinal Manipulation. Foundation for Chiropractic Education and Research, Arlington, VA, 1992:79–81.
15. Clements DS, Thiel HW, Cassidy JD, Mierau DR. Fractures of the thoracolumbar spine: a report of three cases. J Can Chiro Assoc 1991; 35:17–24.
16. Plaugher G. Letter to the Editor; re: fractures and spinal manipulative therapy. J Manipulative Physiol Ther 1993; 16:193–195.
17. Duke RFN, Spreadbury TH. Closed manipulation leading to immediate recovery from cervical spine dislocation with paraplegia. Lancet 1981; Sept. 12:577–578.
18. Winterstein JF. Diagnosis and management of stable thoracolumbar compression fractures. J Clin Chiro 1979; 3(2):43–54.
19. Post-graduate Continuing Education Instruction. Gonstead Seminar of Chiropractic. Mt. Horeb, WI.
20. Huelke DF, O'Day J, Mendelsohn RA. Cervical injuries suffered in automobile accidents. J Neurosurg 1981; 54:316–322.
21. Panjabi MM, Duranceau JS, Oxland TR, Bowen CE. Multidirectional instabilities of traumatic cervical spine injuries in a porcine model. Spine 1989; 14:111–115.
22. Tilton A, Warman J, MacEwen GD. Fracture rehabilitation. In: MacEwen GD, Kasser JR, Heinrich SD, eds. Pediatric fractures: a practical approach to assessment and treatment. Baltimore: Williams & Wilkins, 1993:405.
23. Cotler HB, Cotler JM, Alden ME, Sparks G, Biggs CA. The medical and economic impact of closed cervical spine fractures. Spine 1990; 15:448–452.
24. Roye WP, Dunn EL, Moody JA. Cervical spinal cord injury-a public catastrophe. J Trauma 1988; 28:1260–1264.
25. Reath DB, Kirby J, Lynch M, Maull KI. Injury and cost comparison of restrained and unrestrained motor vehicle crash victims. J Trauma 1989; 29:1173–1177.
26. Petrucelli E. Seat belt laws: The New York experience-preliminary data and some observations. J Trauma 1987; 27:706–710.
27. Wang SF, Tiu CM, Chou YH, Chang T. Obstructive intestinal herniation due to improper use of a seat belt: a case report. Pediatr Radiol 1993; 23:200–201.
28. Sato TB. Effects of seat belts and injuries resulting from improper use. J Trauma 1987; 27:754–758.
29. Raney EM, Bennett JT. Pediatric Chance fracture. Spine 1992; 17:1522–1524.
30. Scher AT. Cervical vertebral dislocation in a rugby player with congenital vertebral fusion. Br J Sports Med 1990; 24:167–168.
31. Scher AT. Spinal cord injuries in rugby players. J S Afr Sports Med 1988; 3(2):12–13.
32. Gaines RW, Humphreys WG. A plea for judgment in management of thoracolumbar fractures and fracture-dislocations. Clin Orthop 1984; 189:36–42.
33. Knight RQ, Stornelli DP, Chan DPK, Devanny JR, Jackson KV. Comparison of operative versus nonoperative treatment of lumbar burst fractures. Clin Orthop 1993; 293:112–121.
34. Chan DPK, Seng NK, Kaan KT. Nonoperative treatment in burst fractures of the lumbar spine (L2-L5) without neurologic deficits. Spine 1993; 18:320–325.
35. Nicoll EA. Fractures of the dorso-lumbar spine. J Bone Joint Surg 1949; 31B:376–394.
36. Hanley EN, Eskay ML. Thoracic spine fractures. Orthopedics 1989; 12:689–695.
37. Burke DC, Berryman D. The place of closed manipulation in the management of flexion-rotation dislocations of the cervical spine. J Bone Joint Surg 1971; 53B:165–82.
38. Mozes GC, Kollender Y, Sasson AA. Transpedicular screw-rod fixation in the treatment of unstable lower thoracic and lumbar fractures. Bull Hosp Joint Disease 1993; 53:37–44.
39. Jacobs RR, Asher MA, Snider RK. Thoracolumbar spinal injuries. Spine 1980; 5:463–477.
40. Hadley MN, Fitzpatrick BC, Sonntag VKH, Browner CM. Facet fracture-dislocation injuries of the cervical spine. Neurosurgery 1992; 31:661–666.
41. Doerr TE, Montesano PX, Burkus JK, Benson DR. Spinal canal decompression in traumatic thoracolumbar burst fractures: posterior distraction versus transpedicular screw fixation. J Orthop Trauma 1991; 5:403–411.
42. Krengel WF, Anderson PA, Henley MB. Early stabilization and decompression for incomplete paraplegia due to a thoracic-level spinal cord injury. Spine 1993; 14:2080–2087.
43. Albert TJ, Levine MJ, An HS, Cotler JM, Balderston RA. Concomitant noncontiguous thoracolumbar and sacral fractures. Spine 1993; 18:1285–1291.
44. Smith R. Where is the wisdom? The poverty of medical evidence. Br Med J 1991; 303:798–799.
45. Chang KW. Oligosegmental correction of post-traumatic thoracolumbar angular kyphosis. Spine 1993; 18:1909–1915.
46. Maiman DJ, Larson SJ, El-Ghatit AZ. Neurologic improvement associated with late decompression of the thoracolumbar spine. Neurosurgery 1984; 14:302–307.
47. Bohlman HH, Kirkpatrick JS, Delamarter RB, Leventhal M. Anterior decompression for late pain and paralysis after fractures of the thoracolumbar spine. Clin Orthop 1994; 300:24–29.
48. Donovan WH, Dwyer AP. An update on the early management of traumatic paraplegia (nonoperative and operative management). Clin Orthop 1984; 189: 12–21.
49. Place HM, Donaldson DH, Brown CW, Stringer EA. Stabilization of thoracic spine fractures resulting in complete paraplegia. Spine 1994; 19:1726–1730.
50. Vlach O, Bayer M. Sequelae of injuries of the thoracolumbar spine and indications for surgery. Acta Chir Orthop Traum 1991; 58:174–177.
51. Cook SD, Harding AF, Morgan EI, et al. Association of bone mineral density and pediatric fractures. J Pediatric Orthop 1987; 7:424–427.
52. Chan G, Hess M, Hollis J, Book L. Bone mineral status in childhood accidental fractures. Am J Dis Child 1984; 138:569–70.
53. White AA, Panjabi MM. Clinical biomechanics of the spine. 2nd. ed. Philadelphia: J.B. Lippincott Co., 1990.
54. Denis F. The three column spine and its significance in the classification of acute thoracolumbar spinal injuries. Spine 1983; 8:817–831.
55. Denis F. Spinal instability as defined by the three-column spine concept in acute spinal trauma. Clin Orthop 1984; 189:65–76.
56. Ferguson RL, Allen BL. A mechanistic classification of thoracolumbar spine fractures. Clin Orthop 1984; 189:77–88.
57. Kaye JJ, Nance EP. Thoracic and lumbar spine trauma. Orthopedics 1990; 28:361–377.
58. James KS, Wenger KH, Schlegel JD, Dunn HK. Biomechanical evaluation of the stability of thoracolumbar burst fractures. Spine 1994; 19:1731–1740.
59. Plaugher G, Lopes MA. Clinical anatomy and biomechanics of the spine. In: Plaugher G, ed. Textbook of clinical chiropractic: a specific biomechanical approach. Baltimore: Williams & Wilkins, 1993:38–41.
60. Andriacchi TP, Schultz AB, Belytschko TB, Galante JO. A model for studies of mechanical interactions between the human spine and rib cage. J Biomech 1974; 7:497–507.
61. Berg EE. The sternal-rib complex: a possible fourth column in thoracic spine fractures. Spine 1993; 18:1916–1919.
62. Brieg A. Adverse mechanical tension in the central nervous system. Stockholm: Almqvist & Wiksell International, 1978.
63. Towbin A. Spinal Injury related to the syndrome of sudden death ("crib death") in infants. Am J Clinical Pathology 1968; 49:562–567.
64. Leventhal HR. Birth injuries of the spinal cord. J Pediatrics 1960; 56:447–453.
65. Towbin A. Latent spinal cord and brain stem injury in newborn infants. Develop Med Child Neurol 1969; 11:54–68.
66. Aufdermaur M. Spinal injuries in juveniles. Necropsy findings in twelve cases. J Bone Joint Surg 1974; 56B:513–519.
67. Shulman ST, Madden JD, Esterly JR, Shanklin DR. Transection of spinal cord. A rare obstetrical complication of cephalic delivery. Arch Dis Child 1971; 291: 291–294.
68. Agerholm JS, Basse A, Arnbjerg J. Vertebral fractures in newborn calves. Acta Vet Scand 1993; 34:379–384.
69. Reid DC, Saboe L. Spine fractures in winter sports. Sports Med 1989; 7:393–399.
70. Swischuk LE. Spine and spinal cord trauma in the battered child syndrome. Radiology 1969; 92:733–738.
71. Ahmann PA, Smith SA, Schwartz JF, Clark DB. Spinal cord infarction due to minor trauma in children. Neurology 1975; 25:301–307.
72. Brown JK, Minns RA. Non-accidental head injury, with particular reference to whiplash shaking injury and medico-legal aspects. Develop Med Child Neurol 1993; 35:849–869.
73. Luerssen TG, Bruce DA, Humphreys RP. Position statement on identifying the infant with nonaccidental central nervous system injury (the whiplash-shake syndrome). Pediatric Neurosurg 1993; Jul/Aug:170.
74. Munger CE, Peiffer RL, Bouldin TW, Kylstra JA, Thompson RL. Ocular and associated neuropathologic observations in suspected whiplash shaken infant syndrome. A retrospective study of 12 cases. Am J Forensic Med Pathol 1993; 14:193–200.
75. Gatterman MI, Hansen DT. Development of chiropractic nomenclature through consensus. J Manipulative Physiol Ther 1994; 17:302–309.
76. Plaugher G. Skin temperature assessment for neuromusculoskeletal abnormalities of the spinal column. J Manipulative Physiol Ther 1992; 15:365–381.
77. Plaugher G, Lopes MA, Melch PE, Cremata EE. The inter- and intraexaminer reliability of a paraspinal skin temperature differential instrument. J Manipulative Physiol Ther 1991; 14:361–367.
78. Chang DG, Tencer AF, Ching RP, et al. Geometric changes in the cervical spinal canal during impact. Spine 1994; 19:973–980.
79. Keenen TL, Antony J, Benson DR. Non-contiguous spinal fractures. J Trauma 1990; 30:489–491.
80. Kewalramani LS, Taylor RG. Multiple non-contiguous injuries to the spine. Acta Orthop Scand 1976; 47:52–58.
81. Mahale YJ, Silver JR. Progressive paralysis after bilateral facet dislocation of the cervical spine. J Bone Joint Surg 1992; 74B; 219–23.
82. Gideon DE, Mulkey JC. Unilateral interfacetal dislocation in the lower cervical spine. J Am Osteopath Assoc 1988; 88:1223–1230.

83. Clark CR, Igram CM, El-Khoury GY, Ehara S. Radiographic evaluation of cervical spine injuries. Spine 1988; 13:742–747.

84. Acheson MB, Livingston RR, Richardson ML, Stimac GK. High-resolution CT scanning in the evaluation of cervical spine fractures: comparison with plain film examinations. Am J Radiol 1987; 148:1179–1185.

85. Crone-Munzebrock W, Jend HH, Heller M, Schottle H. Spinal fractures: results and experience with computer tomography. Arch Orthop Trauma Surg 1984; 103:36–41.

86. Angtuaco EJC, Binet EF. Radiology of thoracic and lumbar fractures. Clin Orthop 1984; 189:43–57.

87. Woodring JH, Lee C. The role and limitations of computed tomographic scanning in the evaluation of cervical trauma. J Trauma 1992; 33:698–708.

88. Goldberg AL, Rothfus WE, Deeb ZL, et al. The impact of magnetic resonance on the diagnostic evaluation of acute cervicothoracic spinal trauma. Skeletal Radiol 1988; 17:89–95.

89. Flanders AE, Schafer DM, Doan Ht, et al. Acute cervical spine trauma: correlation of MR imaging findings with degree of neurologic deficit. Radiol 1990; 177:25–33.

90. Glazer M, Sagar VV, Welck K. Radiograph of the month. Del Med Jrl 1994; 66:91–92.

91. Hildingsson C, Hietala SO, Toolanen G, Bjornebrink J. Negative scintigraphy despite spinal fractures in the multiply injured. Injury 1993; 24:467–470.

92. Silverman FN. Skeletal lesions in leukemia: clinical and roentgenographic observations in 103 infants and children, with review of literature. AJR 1948; 59:819–44.

93. Thomas LB, Forkner CE, Frei E, Besse BE, Stabenau JR. The skeletal lesions of acute leukemia. Cancer 1961; 14:608–21.

94. Oliveri MB, Mautalen CA, Rodriguez Fuchs CA, Carmen Romanelli M. Vertebral compression fractures at the onset of acute lymphoblastic leukemia in a child. Henry Ford Hosp Med J 1991; 39:45–48.

95. Vassilopoulou-Sellin R, Ramirez I. Severe osteopenia and vertebral compression fractures after complete remission in an adolescent with acute leukemia. Am J Hematol 1992; 39:142–143.

96. Yochum TR, Rowe LJ. Essentials of skeletal radiology. Baltimore: Williams & Wilkins, 1987.

97. Fredrickson BE, Edwards WT, Rauschning W, Bayley JC, Yuan HA. Vertebral burst fractures: an experimental, morphologic, and radiographic study. Spine 1992; 17:1012–1021.

98. Cremata EE, Plaugher G, Cox WA. Technique system application: the Gonstead approach. Chiropractic Technique 1991; 3:19–25.

99. Plaugher G, Cremata EE, Phillips RB. A retrospective consecutive case analysis of pre-treatment and comparative static radiological parameters following chiropractic adjustments. J Manipulative Physiol Ther 1990; 13:498–506.

100. Herbst, RW. Gonstead chiropractic science and art. Chicago: Sci-Chi Publications, 1968.

101. Rowe SH, Ray SG, Jakubowski AM, Picardi RJ. Plain film radiography in chiropractic. In: Plaugher G, ed. Textbook of clinical chiropractic: a specific biomechanical approach. Baltimore: Williams & Wilkins, 1993:112–149.

102. Plaugher G. The role of plain film radiography in chiropractic clinical practice. Chiropractic Journal of Australia 1992; 22:153–161.

103. Beyer CA, Cabanela ME. Unilateral facet dislocations and fracture-dislocations of the cervical spine: a review. Orthopedics 1992; 15:311–315.

104. Beatson TR. Fractures and dislocations of the cervical spine. J Bone Joint Surg 1963; 45B:21–35.

105. Papadopoulos SM. Discussion on traumatic quadriplegia with dislocation and central disc herniation. J Spinal Disorders 1991; 4:492.

106. Gerlock AJ, Kirchner SG, Heller RM, Kaye JJ. The cervical spine in trauma. Philadelphia: W. B. Saunders Co., 1978.

107. Braakman R, Vinken PJ. Unilateral facet interlocking in the lower cervical spine. J Bone Joint Surg 1967; 49B:249–257.

108. Rorabeck CH, Rock MG, Hawkins RJ, Bourne RB. Unilateral facet dislocation of the cervical spine: an analysis of the results of treatment in 26 patients. Spine 1987; 12:23–27.

109. Gideon DE, Mulkey JC. Unilateral interfacetal dislocation in the lower cervical spine. J Am Osteopath Assoc 1988; 88:1223–1230.

110. San Giorgi SM. Orthopedic aspects of the treatment of injuries of the lower cervical spine. Acta Neurochir 1970; 22:227–233.

111. Mahale YJ, Silver JR, Henderson NJ. Neurological complications of the reduction of cervical spine dislocations. J Bone Joint Surg 1993; 75B:403–409.

112. Robertson PA, Ryan MD. Neurological deterioration after reduction of cervical subluxation. J Bone Joint Surg 1992; 74B:224–7.

113. Harrington JF, Likavec MJ, Smith AS. Disc herniation in cervical fracture subluxation. Neurosurgery 1991; 29:374–379.

114. Hadley MN, Fitzpatrick BC, Sonntag VKH, Browner CM. Facet fracture-dislocation injuries of the cervical spine. Neurosurgery 1992; 31:661–666.

115. Willis BK, Greiner F, Orrison WW, Benzel EC. The incidence of vertebral artery injury after midcervical spine fracture or subluxation. Neurosurgery 1994; 34:435–442.

116. Louw JA, Mafoyane NA, Small B, Neser CP. Occlusion of the vertebral artery in cervical spine dislocations. J Bone Joint Surg 1990; 72B:679–681.

117. Quint DJ, Spickler EM. Magnetic resonance demonstration of vertebral artery dissection. J Neurosurg 1990; 72:964–967.

118. Meissner, Paun M, Johansen K. Duplex scanning for arterial trauma. Am J Surg 1991; 161:552–555.

119. Vernay D, Dubost JJ, Dordain G, Sauvezie B. Seizures and compression fracture. Neurology 1990; 40:725–726.

120. Wiltse LL, Newman P, MacNab H. Classification of spondylolysis and spondylolisthesis. Clin Orthop 1976; 117:23–29.

121. Mierau D, Cassidy JD, McGregor M, Kirkaldy-Willis WH. A comparison of the effectiveness of spinal manipulative therapy for low back pain patients with and without spondylolisthesis. J Manipulative Physiol The 1987; 10:49–55.

122. Sward LM, Hellstrom B, Jacobsson B, Peterson L. Spondylolysis and the sacro-horizontal angle in athletes. Acta Radiologica 1989; 30:359–64.

123. Eisenstein SM, Ashton IK, Roberts S, et al. Innervation of the spondylolysis "ligament." Spine 1994; 19:912–916.

124. Plaugher G, ed. Textbook of clinical chiropractic: a specific biomechanical approach. Baltimore: Williams and Wilkins, 1993.

125. Dandy DJ, Shannon MJ. Lumbo-sacral subluxation (group I spondylolisthesis). J Bone Joint Surg 1971; 53B:578–95.

126. Hensinger RN. Current concepts review: spondylolysis and spondylolisthesis in children and adolescents. J Bone Joint Surg 1989; 71A:1098–1107.

127. Cyron BM, Hutton WC. Variations in the amount and distribution of cortical bone across the partes interarticularis of L5: a predisposing factor in spondylolysis? Spine 1979; 4:163–167.

128. Batts M: The etiology of spondylolisthesis. J Bone Joint Surg 1939; 21A: 879–884.

129. Frederickson BE, Baker D, McHolick WJ, Yuan HA, Lubicky JP. The natural history of spondylolysis and spondylolisthesis. J Bone Joint Surg. 1984; 66A:699–707.

130. Rowe GG, Roche MB: The etiology of separate neural arch. J Bone Joint Surg 1953; 35A:102–110.

131. Wiltse LL. The effect of the common anomalies of the lumbar spine upon disc degeneration and low back pain. Orthop Clin North Am 1971; 2:569–582.

132. Szypryt EP, Twining P, Mulholland RC, Worthington BS. The prevalence of disc degeneration associated with neural arch defects of the lumbar spine assessed by magnetic resonance imaging. Spine 1989; 14:977–81.

133. Baker DR, McHollick W. Spondylolysis and spondylolisthesis. J Bone Joint Surg 1956; 38A:933–934.

134. Saha MM, Bhardwaj OP, Srivastava G, Pramanick A, Gupta A. Osteopetrosis with spondylolysis: four cases in one family. Br Radiol 1970; 43:738–740.

135. Stewart TD. The age incidence of neural arch defects in Alaskan natives, considered from the standpoint of etiology. J Bone Joint Surg 1953; 35A:937–950.

136. Wiltse LL, Widell EH, Jackson DW: Fatigue fracture. The basic lesion in isthmic spondylolisthesis. J Bone Joint Surg 1975; 57A:17–22.

137. Eisenstein S: Spondylolysis. A skeletal investigation of two population groups. J Bone Joint Surg 1978; 60B:488–494.

138. Turner RH, Bianco AJ. Spondylolysis and spondylolisthesis in children and teenagers. J Bone Joint Surg 1971; 53A:1298–1306.

139. Cyron BM, Hutton WC. The fatigue strength of the lumbar neural arch in spondylolysis. J Bone Joint Surg 1978; 60B:234–8.

140. Cyron BM, Hutton WC, Troup JDG. Spondylolytic fractures. J Bone Joint Surg 1976; 58B:462–466.

141. Jackson W, Douglas MD, Wiltse LL, Cirincione RJ. Spondylolysis in the female gymnast. Clin Orthop 1976; 117:68–73.

142. Gracovetsky S. The spinal engine. Wien: Springer-Verlag, 1988.

143. McGrory BJ, VanderWillde RS, Currier BL, Eismont FJ. Diagnosis of subtle thoracolumbar burst fractures: a new radiographic sign. Spine 1993; 18:2282–2285.

144. Arthornthurasook A, Thongmag P. Thoracolumbar burst fracture with another spinal fracture. J Med Assoc Thailand 1990; 73:279–82.

145. Miniaci A, McLaren AC. Anterolateral compression fracture of the thoracolumbar spine. Clin Orthop 1989; 240:153–156.

146. Chance GQ. Note on a type of flexion fracture of the spine. Br J Radiol 1948; 21:452–453.

147. Puno RM, Bhojraj SY, Glassman SD, Dimar JR, Johnson JR. Flexion-distraction injuries of the thoracolumbar and lumbar spine in the adult and pediatric patient. Spine: State of the Art Reviews 1993; 7:223–239.

148. Moskowitz, Blasier RD, Lamont RL. Chance fracture in a child: A case report with non-operative treatment. J Pediat Orthop 1985; 5:92–93.

149. Gertzbein SD, Court-Brown CM. Flexion-distraction injuries of the lumbar spine. Clin Orthop 1988; 227:52–59.

150. Moskowitz A. Lumbar seatbelt injury in a child: case report. J Trauma 1989; 29:1279–1282.

151. Sivit CJ, Taylor GA, Newman KD. Safety-belt injuries in children with lap-belt ecchymosis: CT findings in 61 patients. AJR 1991; 157:111–114.

152. Newman KD, Bowman LM, Eichelberger MR, et al. The lap belt complex: intestinal and lumbar spine injury in children. J Trauma 1990; 30:1133–1140.

153. Glassman SD, Johnson JR, Holt RT. Seatbelt injuries in children. J Trauma 1992; 33:882–886.

index

Page numbers in italic indicate figures; page numbers followed by t indicate tables.

A

Abdomen
    examination, 198-201
    examination of neonate, 133, *133*
    pain in children, 200t
Abdominal injuries, vehicle lap belts, 63, *63*
Abducens nerve, 494t
Aberrant posturing, 451, *451*
Abortion, spontaneous, 89-90
Acceleration injuries, inertial, 53
Accessory nerve, 495t
Acne, 188
Acoustic blink, infant reflex, 136, *136*
Acquired immunodeficiency syndrome (AIDS), 686
Acute lymphonodular pharyngitis, 683
Adam's test, scoliosis, 386, *386*
Adjustive thrust, 382-383
Adjustments
    acceleration-deceleration process, 329-331, *331*
    acute spinal fracture-subluxation, 741
        contraindications for, 741
    ASEX ilium, 408
    ASEX ilium (left) prone, 411, *411*
    ASEX ilium (left) side posture, 410, *410*
    ASEX ilium (right) prone, 408, *408,* 410, *410*
    ASEX ilium (right) side posture, 408, *408,* 409, *409, 412, 413*
    ASEX ilium (right) side posture pull, 409, *409, 410,* 411, *411*
    ASIN ilium, 405
    ASIN ilium (left) prone, *405,* 405-406, 406, *406*
    ASIN ilium (left) side posture, 406, *406,* 407
    ASIN ilium (right) prone, 407, *407*
    ASRS condyle supine, 337, *337*
    C1 AIL modified-toggle, 351-352, *352*
    C1 ASL seated, 348-349, *349,* 351, *352*
    C1 ASL side posture, 350, *350*
    C1 ASRA seated adjustment, 350, *350*
    C1 ASRP seated, 351, *351*
    C1 ASR seated, 351, *351*
    C1-C2, 347-348, *348*
    C2-C7, contact digit and stabilization, 357-358
    C2-C7 alternative procedures, 357t
    C2-C7 listings, 357t
    cerebral palsy, 700, *700-701*
    coccyx anterior and laterally flexed prone, 422, *422*
    coccyx anterior prone, 422, *422*
    AS condyle seated, 338-341, *338-341*
    AS condyle supine double thenar, 336, *336*
    AS condyle supine finger contact, 337, *337*
    C2 posterior prone, *358,* 358-359
    C2 posterior seated, 359, *359*
    C5 PRI-LA seated, 361, *361*
    C2 PR knee chest, 361, *361*
    C6 PR prone, 360, *360*
    C6 PR seated, 360, *360*
    C7 PR seated, *359,* 359-360
    EX ilium (right) prone, 414, *415*
    EX ilium (right) side posture pull, 414-415, *415-416*
    EX-IN ilia side posture pull/push, 416, *416,* 416-417, *417*
    IN and EX subluxation, 412
    AS ilium, 402
    AS ilium (left) prone, 402, *403*
    IN ilium (left) prone, 412, *412*
    AS ilium (left) side posture, 403-404, *403-404*
    IN ilium (left) side posture, 412-414, *413-414*
    IN ilium (left) side posture pull, 412, *413,* 413-414, *414*
    AS ilium right prone, 404, *404*
    AS ilium (right) side posture, 403, *403*
    In-EX ilium, 415-416
    L4 knee chest, 384, *384*
    long lever and non-specific, 327-328, *328-331*
    L4 PL, 379-380, *380*
    L3 PLI-M side posture, 380, *381*
    L3 PLS side posture, 380, *380*
    L5 PLS side posture, *378,* 379
    L5 posterior-inferior side posture, 378, *378*
    L1 posterior knee chest, 385, *385*
    L5 posterior knee chest, 383-384, *383-384*
    L5 posterior prone, 377, *377*
    L5 posterior prone posture, *377,* 377-378
    L5 posterior side posture, 378, *378*
    L2 PRI-M knee chest, 385, *385*
    L2 PRI-M side posture, 380-381, *381*
    L5 PR-M knee, 384, *384*
    L prone position, 374-375, *375*
    L5 PRS-INF side posture, 379, *379*
    L3 PRS knee chest, 384-385, *385*
    L5 PRS-M side posture, 379, *380*
    L side posture position, 376, *376*
    L5 spondylolisthesis side posture, 381, *382*
    lumbar, 374-386
    pelvic, 388-417
    P1EX ilium, 395
    P1EX ilium (left) prone, 395, *395,* 398, *399*
    P1EX ilium (left) side posture, 395-396, *396,* 398, *398*
    P1EX ilium (right) prone, 397, *397*
    P1EX ilium (right) side posture, 396, *396-397*
    P1EX ilium (right) side posture pull, 397-398, *397-398*
    PIIN ilium, 399
    PIIN ilium (left) prone, 399, *399,* 401, *401*
    PIIN ilium (left) side posture, 401, *401*
    PIIN ilium (left) side posture pull, 399-400, *400, 400, 401,* 402, *402*
    PIIN ilium (right) prone, 399, *400,* 402, 404, *402, 405*
    PIIN ilium (right) side posture, 400, *400*
    P1 ilium, 391
    P1 ilium (left) prone, 393, *393*
    P1 ilium (left) side posture, 393, *393, 394, 394*
    P1 ilium prone, 391, *392*
    P1 ilium (right) prone, 392, *393, 394, 395*
    P1 ilium side posture, 392, *392*
    in pregnancy
        Atlas ASLP, 108, *108*
        Atlas ASR, 107-108
        C5 PL, 110
        C6 PLI-la, 109
        C5 PRS, 108-109, *109*
        L3 PL-m thumb-pisiform, 118, *118*
        L5 PLS, 112, *112*

Adjustments—*Continued*
  in pregnancy—*Continued*
    L5 PRS, *117*, 117-118
    PIIn (left) side posture, 112-113, *113*
    P-L side posture, 113-114, *114*
    side posture sacral push, 113, *113*
    T1 PL, *110,* 110-111
    T3 PLI-t, 116, *116*
    T6 PLI-t prone, 115, *115*
    T11 posterior double-thenar, 117, *117*
    T8 posterior double-thumb, 116-117, *117*
    T2 PRI-t, 111, *111*
    T5 PRS prone, 114-115, *115*
  prone sacral push, 388-389, *389*
  PSLS condyle seated, 341-342, *342*
  PSLSLA condyle seated, 343, *343*
  PSRS, 342-343, *343*
  PSRSRP condyle seated, 344, *344*
  rotated sacrum (P-L) prone, 418-419, *418-419*
  rotated sacrum (P-L) side posture, 421, *421*
  sacral base posterior side posture, 381, *381*
  scoliosis, 659
  sitting assessment of axial rotation, 389
  sitting flexion, 389, *390*
  sitting lateral flexion, 389, *389*
  specific contact, short lever-art techniques, 327
  spinal dislocation-subluxation, 741
  S2 posterior prone, 418-419, *418-419*, 421, *421*
  S2 posterior side posture, 418-420, *419-420*
  standing flexion, 389, *390*
  standing hip flexion, 390, *391*
  thoracic, 365-366, *366*
  T5 PLI-T knee, 368-369, *369*
  T3 PLI-T seated, 372, *372*
  T8 PLS prone, 368, *368*
  T8 posterior knee chest, 369, *369*
  T8 posterior prone, *370,* 370-371
  T9 posterior prone, *363,* 363-364
  T1 PR seated, 371-372, *372*
  T4 PRS knee chest, *369,* 369-370
  T6 PRS prone, 371, *371*
Adolescence
  health maintenance in, 722-728
  stages of, 709-712, 710t, 711t, *712-713*
Adolescents
  acute spinal fractures, 730-774
    case presentations, 742-774
  chiropractic care, 707-728
  growth and development, 708-712
Adolescent scoliosis, 646-647, 655
Adrenergic receptors, 502t
Adult lap, child held during motor vehicle collision, 57-58, *58*
Adverse reactions
  diphtheria/tetanus vaccination, 41-42
  measles vaccine, 27-29
  mumps vaccine, 31-32
  polio vaccine, 35
  rubella vaccine, 32
Aerobics, during pregnancy, 167, *168*
Afferent impulses, large and small fiber, 505, 506t
Afferent nerve, convergent stimulation, 503
Air bags
  infants and, 65
  motor vehicle collisions, 54
Alcohol, maternal use of, 88-89
Alkaline phosphatase, skeletal maturity and, 654t
Allergies, history of, 181
Alopecia areata, 189
American Chiropractic Association (ACA), 2
  Council on Neurology, 2
American Chiropractic Pediatrics Association, 4
American College of Obstetrics and Gynecology, Home Exercise Program,
  162-164

Amniocentesis, prenatal diagnosis with, 83
Anaphylaxis, tetanus or diphtheria toxoid administration, 38
Aneurysmal bone cyst, 222, *223*
Ankylosing spondylitis, 225, 621-622
Antibiotics, otitis media, 610t
Apgar score, 127t, 127-128, 559t, 559-560
Apophysis injury, motor vehicle collision, 66
Appendicitis, 199
Arnold-Chiari malformation (ACM), 572
Arthritis, 638t, 638-639
  septic, 689
Arthrokinetic reflex, 475
Articular procedure descriptions, *327*
Ascending afferents/sensory tracts, 485
Asthma, 10, 197-198, 601-605
  in adolescence, 722-723
Astrocytoma, 223
Asymmetric tonic neck reflex, infant, 137
Atlanto-occipital hypermobility, sudden infant death syndrome and, 219, *220*
Attention deficit hyperactivity disorder (ADHD), 11, 459-460, 562-565, 564t, 702-703
Auditory screening, 191-192
AUDIT structured interview, 704t
Auscultation
  abdominal examination, 198
  heart and thorax examination, 196
Autism, 565-567, 566t
Autonomic afferent, unconscious small fiber input, 508
Autonomic nervous system, 488-501
  anatomy, 488, *488*
  central processes of, 488-489
  dysfunction, 513-520
  neurotransmitters of, 501-502, 502t
  parasympathetic and sympathetic divisions, 497, 498t-501t
  peripheral outflow of, 489, *490-491*
  synapses, 501
Axonotmesis, 474

B

Babinski response, *140*
Baby walkers, 614
Backpage, asymmetrical usage, spinal injury and, 326, *326*
Back pain, 10, 567-568
  disc herniation, 315
  infection, 315
  neoplasms, 314-315, *315*
  potential causes, *314*
  Scheuermann's disease, 315
  in scoliosis, 315, 650
  selection of imaging techniques for, 313-317, *316*
  spondylolisthesis, 315
Bacteremia, 688
Bacterial endocarditis, 195
Barlow's test, *152*
Basal ganglia, 482-483
Bend
  Chandler, 3
  Katherine, 3
Bilateral sagittal facets, 623
Birth process, 430-431
Birth trauma, 6-7, 152-160, 431-432, 438-439, *439*
  craniosacral therapy for, 424-453
  spinal problems and, 463-464, 617
Blink, infant reflex, 135, *135*
Blood pressure, 673
  heart examination, 194, 195t
Blood volume, maternal, *86,* 86-87
Bolin shielding, radiation exposure and, 210, *210*
Bone, biomechanics of, pediatric fractures and, 735
Bone and joint injuries, birth trauma, 158-159
Bone tumors, 637-638
Booster seat, *70*

Botulism, infant, 686
Brachial plexus, injury, 474-475, 568-593
Bracing, in scoliosis, 658-659
Brain
    abscess, 569
    blood supply, 486-487
    function, learning development and, 520t, 520-521
    structures, *481,* 481-486
Brain electrical activity mapping, 558
Brain hibernation, 520t, 520-521
Brain injury, motor vehicle collision, 66
Brain stem, 483
    level, 529, *529*
Brainstem auditory-evoked response, 558
Breastfeeding, 159-160, 455-459
    composition of human breast milk, 456-457
    contraindications, 456
    iron supplementation, 457
Breast self-examination, in adolescence, 722-723
Breech presentations, 100-102, *100-102,* 105-106, 324, *324*
Brown-Sequard syndrome, 596
Brucellosis, 686
Bubonic plague, 690
Bucket handle fracture, non-accidental trauma, 17
Bucky stand shielding, radiation exposure and, 210
Butterfly vertebra, radiology, 215

C

Cafe-au-lait spots, toddler skin, 187
Caffeine, maternal use of, 89
Caffey's syndrome, 678-679
CAGE instrument, 703t
Calcaneal apophysitis, 635
Calcaneovalgus foot, 635
Calcium, maternal, 88
Caloric requirements, pediatric nutrition, 457
Cancer, ionizing radiation and, 208
Caput succedaneum, 157, 157t
Cardiovascular disease, exercise during pregnancy and, 166
Cellulitis, 689
Center of gravity, pediatric motor vehicle collision injuries and, 56-57, *56-57*
Central cord syndrome, 596
Cephalhematoma, 157, 157t
Cerebellar function, older child, 539
Cerebellum, 483
Cerebral blood flow, disorders related to, 520t
Cerebral cortex, 481-482, *482*
Cerebral palsy, 569-572, 698-700, *698-700*
Cerebrospinal fluid
    flow, 487
    physiology, craniosacral therapy effects, 424
Cerebrum, 481, *481*
Cervical canal stenosis, 474
Cervical chair, use during pregnancy, 107, 371, *371*
Cervical collars, spinal injuries, 741
Cervical curve, *261*
Cervical disc injury, motor vehicle collision, 66
Cervical lordosis, 262-264, 352-362, *352-362*
Cervical ribs, radiology, 215, *217*
Cervical spine
    burst fracture of C7, 743-747, *745-747*
    compression fracture of C5, *755-761,* 755-762
    lower adjustment, biomechanical considerations in, 355-357, *356*
    problems, 619-620
    unilateral fracture-dislocation of C6, 747-754, *748-753*
Cervical spine injury, motor vehicle collision, 66-67, *67*
Cervicogenic headache, 578
C-fibers, excitation, local spinal cord reflexes and, 505
Challenged child, chiropractic management, 697-705
Chemicals
    maternal use of, 89
    neurotoxicity and, 586

Chest, examination of neonate, 133
Chickenpox. *see* Varicella
Child abuse, 14-22
    characteristics, 16-19, *17-18*
    chiropractors as primary health care providers, 21-22
    clinical indicators, 18-20
    emotional
        behavioral indicators, 19
        definition, 15
    history taking in, 20-21
    index of suspicion, 21
    intervention in, 21
    long-term effects, 14
    neglect
        behavioral indicators, 20
        definition, 15
        physical indicators, 20
    out-of-home placement in, 16
    physical
        behavioral indicators, 19
        definition, 15
        physical indicators, 19
    reports of, 14
    self-inflicted intentional injury, 16
    sexual, 14
        behavioral indicators, 19
        definition, 15
        non-specific indicators, 20
        physical indicators, 19
    signs and symptoms, 576t
    sociologic indicators, 16
    spinal problems and, 617
    spine and spinal cord trauma, 739
    statistics, 14
    suicide attempts and, 14
    third-world countries, 16
    unusual and bizarre forms, 15-16
Childhood illnesses and exposures, 181
Child on adult lap, pediatric motor vehicle collision and, 57-58, *58*
Child positioning in automobiles, guidelines, 60t, *61*
Children's Chiropractic Center, 3
Chip fracture, non-accidental trauma, 17
Chiropractic education, spinal fractures, 732-733
Chiropractic Home, 3, *3*
Chiropractic practice
    frequency of injury in, 732
    youth-oriented, 713-719
Chiropractic science, 8-9
Chiropractic scope and standards of practice, 732
Chiropractic specialties, 2-4
Chiropractic spinography, 202-203, 228
Chiropractor, role in child abuse cases, 21-22
Chlamydia pneumonia, 687
Cholera, 687
Chondromalacia patella, 631
Chorionic villus sampling, prenatal diagnosis with, 85
Chronic fatigue syndrome, in adolescence, 722-724, 724t
Clavicle fracture, 626
Clostridium tetani, 38
Cluster headache, 577-578
Cobb angle, measurement of scoliosis, 642, *643*
Coccyx, 421-422, 614
    first trimester of pregnancy, 76-77
Colic, 201
    infantile, 605-606
Collision time sequence, motor vehicle injury, 51
Color, examination of neonate, 132
Complementary foods, pediatric nutrition, 457
Compression injury, cancellous bone failure patterns, *737*
Computed tomography (CT), 307-308, 558
    magnetic resonance imaging comparison, 311-312
Condyle block, 335, *335*
    seated as, 336-337, *337*

Condyle block—*Continued*
supine as, 335, *335-336*
Congenital/developmental disorders, 572-573
Conjunctiva, examination, 190
Conjunctivitis, newborn inclusion, 687
Contact and stabilization, 328-329, *331*
Contact point, 742
Contraindications, vaccination, 30
Contralateral extension to stimulus, 528-529
Corneybacterium diphtheria, 37-38
Corticospinal tract, 484-485
Cosmetic deformity, in scoliosis, 650
Cow's milk feeding, 455-459
Cranial bones, motion patterns, 425
Cranial nerves, 494t-495t
auditory nerve (VIII), 542
examination, 540-543
examination of neonate, 134, *134*
facial nerve (VII), 542
glossopharyngeal and vagus nerves (IX, X), 543
hypoglossal nerve (XII), 543
oculomotor, trochlear, and abducens nerves (III, IV, VI), 540-542
olfactory nerve (I), 540
optic nerve (II), 540
spinal accessory nerve (XI), 543
testing, 524
trigeminal nerve (V), 542
Cranial parenchyma, influences, 493
Cranial restriction patterns, 424
Cranial rhythmic impulse, 425, *431*
Cranial suture mobility, 425
Craniosacral examination, findings, 425, 425t
Craniosacral procedures, 448-449, *449*
Craniosacral therapy, 424-453
case reports, 433-448
literature, 424-426
Craniovertebral junction, 426
Cranium, newborn, 427-430
Craven, John H., 2
Crawling, 614
Cry, examination of neonate, 132
Cuneatus, 485
Curve patterns, 644-646, *646*
Cycling, during pregnancy, 167, *167*

D

Deep tendon reflexes, 526
infant, 138-139, *139-140*
older child, 538-539
Dehydration, fever and, 677
Demographics, chiropractic care, 7
Dengue, 685
Dermatomyositis, 679
Dermatoses
inflammatory, newborn skin, 187
scaling, newborn skin, 187
Developmental history, 181-182
milestones, 183t-185t
Developmental milestones screening tests, 538
Developmental patterns and anomalies, 614-615
Development delay, screening protocol for, 698t
Diabetes
breast-fed infants, 456
exercise during pregnancy and, 166
Diaper dermatitis, 187
Diapering techniques, spinal injury and, 325, *325*
Diarrhea, breast-fed infants, 456
Diet supplementation in children, 463
Digital response, infant reflex, 138, *138*
Diphtheria, 687-688
tetanus toxoids and, 38
Diplomate for Chiropractic Sports Physicians, 2

Diplomate in neurology, 2
Diplomate in nutrition, 2
Diplomate of the American Board of Chiropractic Orthopedics, 2
Diplomate of the American Board of Chiropractic Radiology, 2
Discitis, 224, 636
Dislocations, spinal, etiology, 738-739
Doppler analysis, risk assessment in pregnancy, 119
Dorsal columns, 485
Dorsiflexion test, 534
Doscher, Dr. Bobby Callahan, 3, *4*
Down's syndrome, 573-575, 574t, 701-702
radiology, 214
Drug fever, 677
Drugs, neurotoxicity and, 586
Dubowitz neurodevelopmental protocol, neonatal behavior, 139-140, 141-147t
Dural membranes and septum, 426-427
Dvorak's maneuver, 345, *345*
Dynamic response, 353, *353-354*
Dysmenorrhea, 11, 201
adolescents, 720

E

Ear drum, structures, *192*
Ears, physical examination, 191-192
Eastern College of Chiropractic, 2
Eczema, 187
Eczema herpeticum, 684
Edmonston strain, measles, 26-27
Edmonston-Zagreb (EZ) vaccine, 27
Elbow, pulled or nursemaid's, *626,* 626-627
Electrical muscle stimulation, in scoliosis, 659
Electrodiagnosis, 557-558
Electromyography, 557
Emotional abuse. *see* Child abuse
Encephalitis, 684
Encephalopathy, diphtheria/tetanus vaccination and, 41
End-range position, active and passive, 742
Endurance competitions, sports nutrition, 463
Energy requirements, sports nutrition for children, 462-463
Enteric Escherichia coli, 692
Eosinophilic granuloma, 223
Epiglottis, 689
Epilepsy, 590-594
Epiphyseal disorders, 226
Epithalamus, 483
Erb's palsy, 627
Erysipelas, 693
Estriol excretion test, risk assessment in pregnancy, 120
Ewing's sarcoma, 223, 637-638
Exanthem subitum, 685
Exercise
postpartum period, 177
during pregnancy, 162-177
abdominal, 174-175, *174-175*
benefits, 166-168
cervical thoracic, 171-172, *171-172*
contraindications or cautions, 164
existing diseases and, 165-166
lumbopelvic and lower limb, 173-174, *173-174*
pelvic floor, 175, *175*
pelvic tilt, 176, *176-177*
precautions, 176-177
progression, 169
relaxation positions, 175-176, *175-176*
specific recommendations, 167-168
spinal, 169
warm-ups and cool-downs, 169-170, *170*
prenatal, 163-164
pre-pregnancy, 169
in scoliosis, 659
Extensor response to stimulus, 528, *528*
Extensor supporting reaction (negative), 530

Extensor supporting reaction (positive), 530
Extremities, craniosacral examination, 450
Extremity reaction to pelvic tilt stimulus, 533
Extremity response to head extension, 529
Extremity response to head flexion, 529
Extremity response to head rotation, 529, *529*
Eyelids, examination, 190
Eyes
    ears, nose and throat, fever related to, 673
    physical examination, 189-191

F

Face, physical examination, 189
Facet tropism, 217, *218,* 623
Facial asymmetry, 436-437, *437*
Facial fracture, motor vehicle collision, 66
Facial nerve, 494t
Facies, examination of neonate, 132
Falls, spinal problems and, 617
Falx cerebelli, 427
Falx cerebri, 426, *426,* 427
Family history, 182
Fasciculi gracilis, 485
Fast foods, 462
Feeding/nutritional history, 181
Fetal alcohol syndrome, 703t, 703-705, 704t
Fetal biophysical profile, risk assessment in pregnancy, 120
Fetal development
    external examination, 95-97, *95-99*
    first trimester, 80
    second trimester, 90
    skull, *92,* 92-93
    third trimester, 91
Fetal monitoring, electronic, risk assessment in pregnancy, 119
Fetopelvic relationships, 93, 93t
Fever, 671-695
    case management, 676-677
    chiropractic management, 673, *674*
    definition, 671-672
    infectious causes, 680-695
    laboratory and radiologic examinations, 675
    low-risk infants, definition, 675
    medical management, 675
    neoplastic disorders, 677-678
    noninfectious causes, 677
    parental considerations, 676
    pathophysiology, 671
    relapsing, 691
    role of, 671
    seizures and, 676
Fever of unknown origin (FUO), 676
Fiber irritations
    large, 508
    small, 506-508, *507*
Flat feet, 635
Flexion. *see* Adjustments
Folic acid, maternal, 88
Fontanelles, 428, *428*
Food allergies, 459
Football, injuries, 639
Formalin-killed vaccine
    measles, 25
    mumps, 31
Formula feeding, 455-459
Foundation for the Advancement of Chiropractic Tenets and Sciences, 4
Four-foot kneeling test, 534
Fractures, 624-625
    spinal
        accuracy of count, 740
        in adolescents, 730-774
        case presentations, 742-774
    clavicle, 626
        C7, burst fracture, 743-747, *745-747*

C5, compression fracture, *755-761,* 755-762
C6, unilateral fracture-dislocation, 747-754, *748-753*
etiology, 738-739
L3, 768-774, *768-774*
L5, anterolateral compression fracture of, 766-768, *766-768*
missed diagnosis, 740
    thoracic spine compression fracture, 762-765, *762-765*
Fruit juices, pediatric nutrition, 457
Fysh, Peter, 4

G

Gait, 373, 387
Galant's test, infant reflex, 136-137, *137*
Gastrointestinal system, fever related to, 674
Gastrointestinal tract, 522
Genetics, ionizing radiation and, 208
Genetic testing, 82-85
Genu valgus, 632-633, *632-633*
Genu varus, 632-633, *632-633*
Gestation, 429-430
Gilles de la Tourette syndrome, 600
Glandular involvement, fever, 681
Glasgow Coma Scale, 560, 560t
Glossopharyngeal nerve, 495t
Golden, Lorraine M., D.C., 3
Gonstead, Clarence S., D.C., 3
Gravidity, 80
Growing pains, 631
Growth, breast-fed infant nutrition and, 456
Growth abnormalities, exercise during pregnancy and, 166
Growth disorders, in adolescence, 725
Growth plate, injuries, 625, *625*
Growth rate, 615, *616*
Guillian Barré syndrome
    polio vaccination and, 35
    tetanus toxoid-induced, 38
Gymnastics and trampolene, injuries, 640

H

Haemophilus influenzae type B influenza (Hib), 36-37, 37t
Hand, foot, and mouth disease, toddlers, 188
Hand dominance, in scoliosis, 650
Handgrasp and foot or plantar grasp, 536-537, *537*
Hangman's fracture, 221, *221*
Harness, three-point, safety device, *70*
Head, examination of neonate, *130-131,* 130-132
Headache, 10, 577-580, 578t, 579t
    adolescents, 720
    classification, 578t
    diagnostic criteria, 579t
Head/hair, physical examination, 188-189
Head injury, 575-577, 577t
    birth trauma, *156,* 156-157, 157t
    non-accidental trauma, 17
Head restraints, motor vehicle collisions, 53
Head size, pediatric motor vehicle collision injuries and, 56
Head zones, 515t
Health care, chiropractors and, 8
Heart, examination, 193-195
Heart rate, at rest, 194t
Heavy metals, neurotoxicity and, 585-586
Hemangioma (vascular lesions), newborn skin, 187
Hemihypertrophy, congenital, 436-437, *437*
Hemivertebra, radiology, 215-216
Herpangina, 682
Herpes simplex, 193, 683-684
Herpes zoster, 684
Herpetic encephalitis, 684
Herpetic gingivostomatitis, 683-684
Herpetic keratoconjunctivitis, 684
Herpetic lesions
    recurrent, 684
    skin or mucosa, 684

Herpetic urethritis, 684
Herpetic vulvovaginitis, 684
Hib polysaccharide vaccine, 36-37, 37t
High fat and sugar diets, sports nutrition, 463
Hildebrandt, Roy, D.C., 4
Hi-lo table, 114, *114*, 366-367, *367*
Hip, congenital dislocation and dysplasia, 627-628, *628-629*
Hip dysplasia, congenital, 218
History, pediatric patient, 179-201
History of present illness, 180
History taking, techniques in suspected child abuse, 20-21
Hives, toddler skin, 187
Hodgkin lymphoma, fever and, 677
Hodgkin's disease, 637
Hopping test, 534
Hospitalizations, history of, 181
Houston Conference Motion Restriction Listings, 233
Houston Conference or Medicare Listings, 232, 233t
Human placental lactogen (HPL), 80
Humerus fracture, non-accidental trauma, 17
Hydration, sports nutrition, 463
Hydrocephalus, 572
Hydrotherapy, during pregnancy, 167
Hyperactive reflexes (hyperreflexia), 526-527
Hypermobility
    vs. hypomobility, 327
    spinal, 472-473
Hypoactive reflexes (hyporeflexia), 527
Hypoglossal nerve, 495t
Hypomobility
    spinal, 472
    vs. hypermobility, 327
Hypothalamus, 483
Hypotonic infant at rest, *526*

I

Iatrogenesis, 159, 159t
ICA Council on Chiropractic Pediatrics, 4
ICA Review, 4
Ice skating, during pregnancy, 168
Iliac spine, anterior superior, pediatric motor vehicle collision injuries
    and, 56
Ilium positional dyskinesia, 232
Imaging, 202-316
    advanced, spinal fractures, 740-741
    diagnostic, 558-559
Immunity, breast-fed infants, 455-456
Immunizations, history of, 181
Impact force, motor vehicle collision injury, 51
Impetigo, toddlers, 188
Index of suspicion, child abuse, 21
Inertia
    acceleration injuries, 53
    principle in motor vehicle collision injuries, 51-52
Infant adjusting table, 4-5, *5*
Infant botulism, 686
Infantile atopic dermatitis, 187
Infantile colic, 10
Infantile cortical hyperostosis, 678-679
Infantile coxa vara, 628
Infantile hypotonia (floppy baby), 580-581
Infantile scoliosis, 646, *646*
    case management, 654
Infant seats, 452, *452*
Infections
    bone and joint, 635-636
    spinal, 636
Infectious disorders, 606-607
Influenza, 680
Informed consent, for vaccination, 29
Injuries. *see also* Trauma
    history of, 181
    non-accidental, maltreatment and, 14-22

Innominate bones, first trimester of pregnancy, 76
Instrumentation, in pregnancy, 107
Integumentary system, fever related to, 674
Intellectual development, breast-fed infant nutrition and, 456
International Chiropractic Pediatrics Association (ICPA), 3-4
International Chiropractors Association, 4
International Listing System, 230, *230-232*, 232t
Intervention, initiation in child abuse, 21
Intervertebral disc, 612-613
    atlas, 613
    axis, 613
    cervical ribs, 613
    C3 to C7, 613
    lumbar spine, 613
    thoracic spine, 613
In-toeing, 633, *633*
In-utero constraint, 6, 97-106, 430
    chiropractic management, 102-105, *102-105*
    mechanism of injury, 324-325
    obstetric management, 105
In-utero malposition, *434*
Inversion analysis, 451, *451*
Inward (medial) femoral torsion, 634
Inward (medial) tibial torsion, 634
Iron, maternal, 87-88
Iron supplementation, breast-fed infants, 457
Ischemia, nerve fiber types, 508

J

Jacknifing, *57*
Janse, Joseph, 4
Jogging, during pregnancy, 167
Joint dysfunction, myopathology, 475
Joint sprains, 626, 626t
Journal of Clinical Chiropractic Pediatrics (JCCP), 4-5
Journal of Manipulative and Physiologic Therapeutics, 4
Juvenile rheumatoid arthritis, 224-225, 638-639
Juvenile scoliosis, 646, 655

K

Kawasaki's disease, 679
Kentuckiana Center for Health Education and Research, 3
Kernig's test, *154*
Kinesiopathology, *467*, 467-473
    spinal trauma, 204-205
KISS syndrome, 619
Klippel-Feil syndrome, 572, 620
    radiology, 215
Klumpke's paralysis, 627
Knee, 630-631
    acute injuries, 630
Knee-chest table, 116, *116*, 368, *368*, 382, *382*
Kneel-standing test, 534
Knife clasp deformity, 218, *218*
Kyphotic cervical curve, *262-264*

L

Labor education, 120-125
Labor preparation, *118*, 118-119
Laminae (Rexed), 511, *511-512*
Landau reflex, 534
Language, developmental screening tests, 538
Lap belt injuries, 62-65, *63-64*
Lateral flexion malposition, correction, 377
Lead poisoning, 227
Learning and behavior testing, 559
Learning problems, birth trauma and, 426
Legg-Calvé-Perthes disease (LCP), 226, 629-630
Leg length discrepancy, 205, 631
    scoliosis and, 655
Leptospirosis, 689
Leukemia, 637
    fever and, 678

Life Chiropractic College, 4
Ligamentous hyperflexion injury, non-accidental trauma, *17*
Lightening and engagement, pregnancy, 119
Limbic system, 483
Limping, 624
Listings for Fixation Dysfunction, 233, 233t
Lordosis angles, sacral base and lumbar, 205
Lordotic-kyphotic-lordotic cervical curve, *264*
Los Angeles College of Chiropractic, 2
Low-back pain, adolescents, 720
Lower extremity
    development, *631,* 631-635
    evaluation, 627-630
Lumbar puncture, 559
Lumbar spine, 372-385, 613
    anterolateral compression fracture of L1, 766-768, *766-768*
    problems, 622-623
    spondylolysis and spondylolisthesis of L5, *470, 755-761,* 755-762
Lumbar spine injuries
    motor vehicle collisions, 54
    pinching, *54*
Lumbosacral articulation, 428-429, *429-432*
Lumbosacral plexus neuropathy, 475
Lung disease, breast-fed infants, 456
Lungs, examination, 195-198
Lyme disease, 689
Lymphatic system, examination of neonate, 133

M

Magnetic resonance angiography (MRA), 558
Magnetic resonance imaging (MRI), 308-311, 309t-310t, 312t-313t, 558
    computed tomography comparison, 311-312
Major injuring vector
    analysis, 742
    definition, 735
Malignant lymphoma, 223
Maltreatment. *see* Child abuse
Mastoid, buckled, 441, *441*
Maternal anatomy
    first trimester of pregnancy, 75-76
    second trimester of pregnancy, 90
    third trimester of pregnancy, 90-91, *91*
        examination, 94-97, *95-97*
Maternal obstetric situations, 80
Maxillary manipulation, external, 425
Measles, 681, 685
    atypical, 27
Measles vaccination, 25-30
    adverse reactions, 27-29
    antigenic variability, 26-27
    efficacy, 25
    failures, 25-26
    side effects, 27
Measles virology, 24-25
Mechanoelectric measurements, 425
Medial longitudinal fasciculus, 485
Medical recommendations, for vaccination, 30
Meningitis, 581-583, 582t, 636
    aseptic, diphtheria/tetanus vaccination and, 41
    bacterial, 688
        Hib, 36-37, 37t
Meningococcal infections, 690
Meningoencephalitis, 681
Menstrual disorders, in adolescence, 725
Metaphyseal corner fracture, non-accidental trauma, *17*
Metatarsus adductus, 634, *634*
Midbrain, level, *530,* 530-531
Migliore, J. P., D.C., 4
Migraine headache, 577-580, 578t, 579t
Milia, newborn skin, 187
Minerals
    infant nutrition, 460
    sports nutrition, 463

Minnesota Chiropractic College, 2
Miscarriage, 89-90
MMR vaccine, 25
    thrombocytopenia and, 29
Monitoring System for Adverse Effects Following Immunization
        (MSAEFI), 35
Mononucleosis, infectious, 686
Moraten vaccine, 25
Moro reflex, 534, *534*
Moro response, infant reflex, 135, *136*
Motion palpation, *106,* 106-107, 332, *332,* 344, *350,* 352
    lumbar spine, 373, *373-374*
    pelvis, 387
    spinal fracture subluxation, 740
    thoracic spine, 362-363, *363-364*
Motor vehicle collisions
    children in adult restraints, 61, *61*
    children in restraints, 59-65
        injuries from, 61-62, *62*
        reduction in injuries, 59-60
    damage *versus* personal injury, 51
    injuries, 51-70
    litigation and outcome in, 55
    pediatric injuries, 55-70
        anthropometric and positioning variables, 56-65
        types, 65-70
    prognosis factors, 54, *54*
    spinal problems and, 617
Mouth
    craniosacral examination, 448, *450*
    examination, 193
Mucocutaneous lymph node syndrome, 679
Multiple myeloma, 223
Multiple sclerosis, 583
Mumps, 680
Mumps vaccination, 30-32
    efficacy, 31
    failure, 31
    recommendations, 32
    side effects and adverse reactions, 31-32
Mumps virology, 30-31
Murray valley encephalitis, 685
Muscle spindle function, overview, older child, 539
Muscular dystrophy, 583-585
    spinal, 596
Myesthesia gravis (MG), 585
Myocarditis, 683
Myopathology, 475
Myotonic dystrophy, 189

N

National Childhood Encephalopathy Study, diphtheria/tetanus vaccination
        and, 38, 41t
National Pediatric College, 2
National system, 232, 233t
National Vaccine Injury Compensation Program, 24
Neck, problems, 619-620
Neck righting reflex, *531*
    infant, 137
Neglect. *see* Child abuse
Neonatal death, spinal injury and, 463-464
Neonatal herpetic infections, 684
Neonate
    case history, 128-129
    clinical examination and assessment, 127
    color and position, 132, *132*
    cry, 132
    neurological examination, 133-134
    physical examination, 129-140, *130-140*
    skin, 132
Neonatology, 127-129
Neoplasms, 636-638
Nephroblastoma, 637

Nerve and nerve root traction and compression, 474
Nerve compression, 475
Nerve conduction velocity test (NCV), 557-558
Nerve injuries, birth trauma, 157-158
Nervoscope, 332-333, *333*
Nervous system
    blood supply, 486-487
    fever related to, 674
    postnatal development, 480-481
    primary structures, 481
    tumors, 599-600
Neuroanatomicophysiological regions, *510*
Neuroanatomy, functional, 480-486
    autonomic nervous system, 488-501
Neuroblastoma, 637
    fever and, 678
Neurological development, 522-523, *524*
    altered, 585-587
    breast-fed infant nutrition and, 456
Neurological evaluation, 522, *523, 524,* 524-525
    neonate, 133-134
    older child, 538-539
    responsibilities of the examiner, 525-526
    summary, 548-557
Neurologic reflexes, infant, 134-139
Neurologic symptoms, DTP vaccination, 41-42, 42t
Neurology, 479-611
Neuromusculoskeletal disorders, adolescents, 718-722, 719t
Neuromusculoskeletal trauma, 624-626
Neuron lesions, upper motor vs lower motor, 486
Neuropathology, 473-475
Neuropraxia, 474
Neurotmesis, 474
Neurotoxicity, 585-587
Niacin, 462
Nocturnal enuresis, 607-608
Non-accidental injury. *see* Injury, non-accidental
Non-Hodgkin lymphoma, fever and, 677
Non-segmentation (block vertebrae), 212-214, *212-215*
Non-tuberculosis vertebral osteomyelitis, 224
Northern California College of Chiropractic, 4
Northwestern College of Chiropractic, 4
Nose, examination, 192-193
Nutrition, 455-464
    in adolescence, 726, 727
    maternal, 85-88

O

Oaklahaven Children's Center, 3, *4*
Obesity, 460-462
Obstetric pelvis, *78-79, 78-80*
Occipital condyle listings, 334t
Occipito-atlantal (C0-C1), examination procedure, 331-332
Occiput and sacrum, synchronizing motion between, *450,* 450-451
Oculomotor nerve, 494t
Odontoid anomalies
    agenesis or hypoplasia, 620
    os odontoideum, 620
    os terminale, 620
Odontoid process variations, radiology, 215, *216*
Oophoritis, 681
Oral polio vaccine (OPV), 33-36
Orchitis, 681
Organ injuries, birth trauma, 159, 159t
Orthopedics, 612-640
Ortolani's test, *151-152*
Osgood-Schlatter's disease, 226, *226,* 298, *298,* 630-631, *631*
Os odontoideum, radiography, *216*
Osteoblastoma, 222
    benign, 638
Osteochondroma, 222
Osteogenic sarcoma, 637

Osteoid osteoma, 222, *223,* 638
Osteomyelitis, 635-636, 689
Osteosarcoma, 224
Otitis media, 11, 609-611, 610t
    breast-fed infants, 456
Otoscopic evaluation, 192, *192*
Outreach activity, youth-oriented chiropractic practice, 715
Out-toeing, 634-635, *635*

P

Palmar grasp, infant reflex, 138, *138*
Palmer, Daniel David, 2
Palmer-Evins Hylo table, *5*
Palmer-Gonstead-Firth, 231-232
Palmer School Lyceum, 2
Palmer School of Chiropractic, 2
Palmer West, 4
Palpation
    abdominal examination, 199
    heart and thorax examination, 195t, 195-196, *196*
    heart examination, 194
Pancarditis, 683
Pancreatitis, 681
Pap smear, in adolescence, 726
Parachute reflex, 537, *537*
    infant, 137, *137*
Parainfluenza viral infection, 680
Paralytic poliomyelitis, 682
Parasympathetic ganglia, plexi, and nerves, 490
Parasympathetic nuclei, 488
Parasympathetic outflow, 489, *490-491,* 496
Parietal bone, motion, 425
Parietal lift, *433*
Parietal manipulation, frontal, 425
Parotitis, 680
Parturition, 121-122
Passive cervical proprioceptive or neck right reflex, 535-536
Past medical history, 180
Patient consent form, *717*
Pauciarticular arthritis, 639
Pectus carinatum, 622
Pectus excavatum, 622
Pelvic bench, 111-112, *112,* 370, *370*
Pelvic height, pediatric motor vehicle collision injuries and, 56
Pelvic joints, first trimester of pregnancy, 77-78
Pelvic structures
    classifications, 80, 81-82t, *83-84*
    first trimester of pregnancy, 76, 77
Pelvis
    problems, 622-623
    specific adjustments, 385-422
Percussion
    abdominal examination, 198
    heart and thorax examination, 196
    heart examination, 194
Peripheral nerve fibers, classifications of, 504t
Peripheral nerve trauma, 627
Perks, Bill, 4
Permanent functional impairment, motor vehicle collision, 52
    chronicity of symptoms and, 53
Pertussis, tetanus or diphtheria toxoid administration, 38-39
Pertussis vaccination
    adverse reactions, 41
    development, 39
    infantile spasms, 40
    systemic reactions within first 24 hours, 40t
Pes planus, 635
Peter Pan Potential, Forrester and Anrig, 4
Pharyngitis, 193
Philosophical and scientific principles, 5, 6t
Physical abuse, spine injury from, 221
Physical assessment, pediatric patient, 179-201

Pityriasis rosea, 188
Placements, patient and doctor, 328
Placental function, 86
Placing response, *525*
    infant reflex, 137, *137*
Plague, 690
Pleurodynia, 682
Pneumonia, 688
Pneumonic plague, 690
Poliomyelitis, 587-588
Polio vaccination, 33-36
    contraindications, 35
    Guillain Barré syndrome, 35
    risk modifiers, 35
Polio virology, 33-36
Polyarteritis nodosa, 679
Polyarticular arthritis, 639
Polymyositis, 679
Ponee Table, 4
Port wine stains, newborn skin, 187
Positron emission tomography (PET), 558-559
Postnatal spinal development, 6
Post-polio syndrome, 588
Postural abnormalities, 615
Postural analysis, 386, *386*
Postural kyphosis, 622
Posture, 373
    adolescent, 718-791
    coronal plane spinal, 205
    in scoliosis, 652
    transverse plane, 205
Posture in horizontal or prone suspension, 536
Posture in upright or vertical suspension, 536, *536*
Pregnancy, 11
    exercise during, 162-177
    fetal position in, 93, 93t, *94*
    first trimester, 75-80
    induction and augmentation of labor, 124-125
    ionizing radiation and, 208
    labor education in, 120-125
    labor preparation, *118,* 118-119
    lightening and engagement, 119
    onset of labor, 121-122
        phenomena preliminary to, 122
    physiologic changes during, 164-165
    risk assessment, 119-120
    second trimester, 90
    stages of labor, 122
        chiropractic techniques, 123, *124*
        intravenous fluids, 123-124
        obstetrical procedures, 123
        physiologic process, 123, 125-127, *126*
    stimulation of labor, 121, 122t
Preload, 742
Prenatal diagnosis, 82-85
Prenatal spinal development, 5-6
Primary and automatic reactions, 525
Primitive reflexes, 534-535
Primum non nocere, 206
    adjustments, 327
Prone proprioceptive response (tonic), 529, *530*
Prone test, 534
Proprioceptive head raising response, 531, *531*
Proprioceptive head raising response (prone), 531, *531*
Proprioceptive head raising response (supine), 531, *531*
Protein, maternal, 88, 88t
Pseudosubluxation, 218
Psittacosis, 686-687
Psoriasis, 187, 188
Psychological injury, motor vehicle collision, 67
Psychological/psychiatric evaluation, 559
Psycho-social development, history, 182

Pulse, 673
Pyogenic septic arthritis, 635

R

Radial head dislocation, *626,* 626-627
Radiation, ionizing, 206
    general considerations, 209-210
    genetic effects, 208
    harmful effects and risks, 208-209
    risk assessment, 208-209
Radiography, 202
    AP lower cervical, 246-247, *249*
    AP lumbar, thoracic and cervical spine, 244, *244*
    AP lumbar spine, 240-244, *240-244*
    AP open mouth, 245, 248t
    AP pelvis and lumbar, 233-240, *233-240,* 234t
    AP thoracic, 244, 247t
    assessment of fetal development, 80
    atlas (C1-C2), 346-347, 347t
    automatic timers, 211
    bending or stress, 259-272, *260-272*
    Bucky stand shielding
    C5
        C6, and sacrum subluxation, 291, *292-293*
        C7 and S2 subluxation, 277, *278*
    C1, C7, S2, S3 subluxation, 273, *276-277*
    C6, L3, and ilium subluxation, 280, *281-282*
    C2, S2, and ilium subluxation, 282, *283*
    C1 and C2 subluxation, 284, *287-289,* 300, *301*
    C1 and C3 subluxation, 297, *297*
    C1 and C6 subluxation, 279, *280*
    C2 and C3 subluxation, 294, *295*
    C3 and C2 subluxation, 294, *295-296*
    C3 and C4 subluxation, 293, *294*
    C5 and C6 subluxation, 277-278, *278*
    C2 and ilium subluxation, 285, *290*
    C2 and L5 subluxation, 298, *298-299*
    C4 and S2 subluxation, 279-280, *281*
    C5 and S2 subluxation, 299, *301*
    C7 and T2 subluxation, 297, *297*
    C1-C2, 354-355
    C0-C1 alignment, 333-334, *334*
    collimation, 210
    C1 subluxation, 301-302, *302*
    C2 subluxation, 303, *304*
    C3 subluxation, 279, *279,* 284-285, *289,* 292, *293,* 298-299, *299,*
        305-306, *306*
    C4 subluxation, 292-293, *294*
    C5 subluxation, 284, *284-287,* 293, *294*
    C7 subluxation, 305, *306*
    C6 subluxation, 292, *293*
    C2 subluxation with upper cervical anomaly, 303, *303*
    film focal distance, 211
    film-screen speeds and sizes, 209
    filtration, 210
    grids, 210
    high frequency generators, 211
    ilium subluxation, 295-296, *296,* 306, *307*
    interpretation, systematic approach to, 227-228
    L3 and L5 subluxation, 275, *277*
    L5 and S2 subluxation, 300, *301-302*
    lateral cervical, 256, 257t
    lateral lumbar/sacrum, 249-250, 251t
    lateral thoracic, 245, 247t
    long wavelength filtration, 211
    lumbar oblique, 256, 256t
    nature of X-ray examination, 206-207
    normal developmental anatomy of spine, 212
    oblique, 250t
    occipital condyle and C1 subluxation, 296, *296,* 297
    Osgood-Schlatter's disease, 298, *298*
    patient positioning and equipment alignment, 211, *211*

Radiography—*Continued*
  plain film, spinal fracture subluxation, 740
  positioning, 210
  in pregnancy, 107
  processing, 211
  risk assessment in pregnancy, 120
  S1, S2, S3 subluxation, 273, *276*
  S2 and ilium subluxation, 299, *300, 304–305, 305*
  in scoliosis, 652
  shielding, 210, *210*
  split screens, 211
  S2 subluxation, 291, *291, 295, 296, 303–304, 304*
  thoracic spine, 363–365
  vertebral arch/pillar view, 249, 250t
Rat bite fever, 691
Reactive arthritis, 638–639
Reciprocal membrane tension, craniosacral examination, 450–451
Reciprocal reactions, 530
Reflexes, 524
  maturational, 535–537, 536t
  primitive, 534–535
Reflexive maturation (body rotation response), 530–531, *531*
Reflexive maturation (segmental torso response), 531, *531*
Reflex/referral relationships, 514, 515t
Reflex sympathetic dystrophy (RSD), 513–514, 517
  children, 518
  development and, 518–519
  mechanism, 518
  stages, 517–518
Reflex testing, 527, *527*
Regional enteritis, fever and, 677
Relaxation, during pregnancy, 168
Residual injury, motor vehicle collision, 52
Respiratory rates, 195t, 673
Respiratory syncytial virus (RSV) disease, 682
Respiratory system, fever related to, 673
Restraint misuse, motor vehicle collision, 68
Reticulospinal tract, 485
Retinoblastoma, 637
Retrolisthesis, lumbar, 205
  of L5, *253*
Rett syndrome, 589
Review of systems, history and physical assessment, 182, 186
Reye's syndrome, 590, 680
Rheumatic fever, 195, 694
Rib fracture, non-accidental trauma, 17
Rickets, 226–227, *227*
Ringworm. *see* Tinea corporis
Ritgen's maneuver, *428*
Roentgenometrics, 228–229, *228–229*
  AP lower cervical, 247
  APOM, 245, *248*
  AP pelvis, 234–240, *234–240*
  lateral cervical, 257, *257–259*
  L5 subluxation, *253–255*
  nomenclature, 230–232
  retrolisthesis of L5, *253*
  spondylolisthesis of L5, *251*
  S2 subluxation, *251–252*
  S3 subluxation, *251*
Roll-out phenomenon, motor vehicle collision, 68, *68*
Rooting, infant reflex, 134, *135, 527*
Roseola infantum, 685
Rubella, 681, 685
Rubella vaccination, 32–33
Rubella virology, 32–33
Rubrospinal tract, 485

S

Sacrum, 417–421, 614
  first trimester of pregnancy, 76
Safety pin cycle, *502*
Safety seat, child, *49, 69*

Salmonella infection, 691
Salter-Harris classification of physeal injuries, 625, *625*
Scabies, 188
Scarlet fever, 188, 693
Scheuermann's disease, 225, *225,* 315, 622
Schmorl's nodes, 221, *221*
School chairs, spinal injury and, 326, *326*
School lunches, 462
Scleroderma, 225
Scoliosis, 11, 225, 315, *469,* 621, 642–668
  Adam's test for, 386, *386*
  adolescent, 719t, 720, *721*
  adult, 654–660
  biomechanics, 655–656, *656*
  case reports, *648–649, 648–650, 661–667, 661–668*
  chiropractic adjustments, 659
  classification, 644–646
  clinical examination, 652
  identification and measurement, 642–644
  idiopathic, 646–647
  lumbar, 377
  morphometric changes to the vertebral body, 656–657, *657,* 658t
  neurophysiological and neuromuscular considerations, 655
  prediction progression of, 653–654, *653–654,* 654t
  progressive, 649–650
    treatment considerations, 657–658
  screening, 650–652
Scoliotic curves, measurements, 642–643, *643*
Screening procedures, special testing and, history of, 181
Scuba diving, during pregnancy, 168
Scurvy rickets, 227
Seat belts
  lap, child restraint, *56–57,* 62–65, *63–64*
  motor vehicle collisions, 53–54
Seat belt syndrome injuries, 67, *67–68*
Seborrheic dermatitis, 187–188
See-saw maneuver, 534
Seizures, 590–594
  febrile, 676
Sensory examination, 524
Sensory system, examination, 544
Septic arthritis, 689
Setting sun sign, *523*
Severs disease, 226, 635
Sexual abuse. *see* Child abuse
Shaken Baby syndrome, 576
Shaken impact syndrome, non-accidental trauma in infants, 18, *18*
Shaking, non-accidental trauma in infants, 17–18, *18*
Shigellosis, 692
Shingles, 684
Shoulder harness injuries, 65, *65*
Silent pain, 508
Simian position, 534
Single photon emission computed tomography (SPECT), 559
Sitting test, 534
Skeletal motor system, examination, 543
Skeletal trauma, child abuse, 16–18
Skiing
  injuries, 640
  during pregnancy, 168
Skin
  examination of neonate, 132
  physical examination, 186–188
Skin cancer, in adolescence, 726
Skin temperature instrumentation, spinal fracture subluxation, 739
Skull, clinical evaluation, 545
Skull fracture, non-accidental trauma, 17
Skull molding, excessive, 440, *440*
Skull pattern
  type C, 442–443, *443*
  type F, 443–444, *444*
Sleep apnea, 473
Sleep disorders, 595

Slipped capital femoral epiphysis, 218, 629, *629*
Slot table, 370, *370*
Smoking, neurotoxicity and, 586
Soft neurological signs, 544-545
Soft tissue injuries
  birth trauma, 159
  motor vehicle collision, 52
Somatic and visceral relationship, 516
Somatic pain, *vs.* visceral pain, 516
Somatic peripheral nerves, 485-486
Somatosensory-evoked potential, 558
Spears, Leo L., 3
Spears Free Clinic and Hospital for Poor Children, 3
Sphenobasilar articulation, 428-429, *429-432*
Spina bifida, 572, 624
Spina bifida occulta, 217, *217*
Spinal cord
  horizontal input, 503-504, 504t
  injuries, 595-596
  internuncial fields, *504,* 504-505
  level, 528, *528*
  local reflexes
    C-fiber excitation and, 505
    supraspinal influences on, 509
  patterns of impulse transmissions, 503
  referral processing, *502,* 502-503
  structures, 484, *484*
Spinal cord compression and traction, 473
Spinal cord concussion, 596
Spinal cord injury without radiographic abnormality (SCIWORA), 219,
    219t, 473-474
Spinal cord neurons, inherent properties, 503
Spinal cord shock, 595-596
Spinal cord trauma, 202-204
Spinal development and asymmetry
  postnatal, 6
  prenatal, 5-6
Spinal dura, 427, *427*
Spinal examination
  lower extremities, infant, 152, *152*
  neonate, 140, 148-149, *148-149*
  orthopedic, neonate, 149-152, *150-152*
Spinal nerves, 485
Spinal stability, 735-738, *738-739*
  fourth column, 735-738
  three column model, 735, *738*
Spinal tracts, 484, *484*
Spine
  adolescent, 718
  asymptomatic subluxation, 204
  blood supply, 487
  chiropractic education, 732-733
  chiropractic standards and practice, 732
  clinical examination, 204
  congenital anomalies, 623-624, 624t
  congenital variants, 212-214, *212-215*
  cord injury, society costs for, 733
  coronal plane posture, 205
  development, 612-615, *613*
  epidural abscess, 224, *225*
  examination and specific adjustments, 323-422
  fixation dysfunction
  fracture, *221,* 221-222. see also specific fracture
    accuracy of count, 740
    in adolescents, 730-774
    biomechanics of bone and, 735
    birth injury and neonatal death, 738-739
    case presentations, 742-774
    major injuring vector, 735
    missed diagnosis, 740
    prevention, 733
    surgical and non-surgical treatment, 733-735, *736*
  gunshot wound, *222*

histopathology and biochemical abnormalities, 475-476
hypomobility and hypermobility, 472-473
infections, 224
injury in chiropractic practice, 732
innervation of, 487
management of injury, 325-326
manipulation under anesthesia, 732
mechanism of injury, *324,* 324-325
motor vehicle accident injuries, 739
neoplasms, 222-224
normal developmental anatomy, radiography, 212
positional dyskinesia
postnatal abnormalities, 218-220
problems, 615-618, 617t
recreational and sports injuries, 739
sports injuries, 639-640
tuberculosis of, 224
vascular abnormalities, 476
Spinocerebellar tract
  anterior, 485
  posterior, 485
Spinography, chiropractic, 202-203, 228
Spinotectal tract, 485
Spinothalamic tract
  anterior, 485
  lateral, 485
Spinous process fracture, non-accidental trauma, *17*
Spondylolisthesis, 226, *227,* 622-623
  cause of back pain, 315
  L5, *251-252, 470*
  L5 side posture adjustment, 381-382, *382*
Spondylolysis, 226, *227,* 622
  spondylolisthesis and, L5, *755-761, 755-762*
Sports, during pregnancy, 168
Sports injuries, 639-640
  adolescents, 722
Sports nutrition, 462-463
Sprains, joint, 626, 626t
Sprengel's deformity, 627
  radiology, 215
Standard School of Chiropractic (New York), 2-3
Staphylococcal colonization and disease, 693
Static palpation, 106, 332, *332,* 344
  analysis, 742
  lumbar spine, 373
  pelvis, 387
  spinal fracture subluxation, 739
  thoracic spine, 362, *362*
Stevens Johnson syndrome, 679-680
Stierwalt, Dennis D., 4
Stillbirth, 473
Still's disease, 639
Stomatitis, 193
Strength, assessment of, 526
Streptococcal infections, 693
Stroke, 597
Structural and non-structural scoliosis, 644, 645t
Subcortical automatic movement reactions, *533,* 533-534
Subluxation. *see also* Radiography entries
  analysis and adjustment techniques, 106-118
  atlas (C1-C2), 344-347, *345-346*
  attention deficit hyperactivity disorder, 703
  case studies, 273-307, *274-307*
  cerebral palsy, 700, *700*
  AS condyle, 335, *335*
  Down's syndrome, 702
  fetal alcohol syndrome, 705
  in-utero constraint and, 97-106
  pediatric, 7
  spinal, 466-477
    etiology, 738-739
    historical perspective, 466
    motion palpation, 740

Subluxation—*Continued*
  spinal—*Continued*
    plain film radiography, 740
      skin temperature instrumentation, 739
      static palpation, 739
    spinal and pelvic, adjustments, 323-422
Subluxation injuries, 9
Submarining, pediatric motor vehicle collision and, 57
    infant in safety seat, 68, *68*
Subthalamus, 483
Sucking, infant reflex, 134-135, *135*
Sudden infant death syndrome (SIDS), 473, 597-598
    atlanto–occipital hypermobility and, 219, *220*
Suicide attempts, child abuse and, 14
Supine proprioceptive response (tonic), 529, *530*
Supine test, 533-534
Supraspinal autonomic influence, 509-510, *511-512*
Supraspinal compensation, 509, *510*
Surgery
    back pain in scoliosis, 650
    history of, 181
Swimming, during pregnancy, 167
Sympathetic nerve roots, 489-491, *492*
Sympathetic nervous system
    four regions of, 490-493, 493t, 494t-495t
    functional considerations, 496-497, 498t
    thoracic spine, *507*
Sympathetic nuclei, 489
Sympathetic outflow, 489, *490-491*
Sympathetic responses, fight or flight threat, 501t
Synovitis, transient, 630
Systemic immune system, 521-522
Systemic lupus erythematosus (SLE), 680

T

Talipes equinovarus, 635
Tectospinal tract, 485
Teething, fever and, 677
Temperature, body, control, 671
Temperature analysis
    C0-C1 scanning procedure, 332
    corresponding segmental levels for differentials, 332
    examination and adjustment instrumentation, 332
Temporals, external rotation, *434*
Temposcope, 332-333, *333*
Tension headache, 577
Tentorium cerebelli, 427
Testicular self-examination, in adolescence, 726
Tetanus, 38
Texas Chiropractic College, 2
Thalamic structures, 483
Thalamus, 483
The Chiropractor's Adjustor, 2, 5
Thermography, screening, for scoliosis, 651-652
Thoracic spine, 362-365, 613
    compression fracture, 762-765, *762-765*
    problems, 621-622
Thorax, examination, 195-198
Throat, examination, 193
Thrombocytopenia, caused by MMR vaccine, 29
Thrush, 193
Thrust, 742
Tinea capitis, 189
Tinea corporis, 188
Tissue injury, pediatric motor vehicle collision and, 57
Tissue receptor fields
    large afferent fibers, 506
    local, 505
    peripheral, 505
    small to large fiber afferent supply ratio from, 506
Tobacco, maternal use of, 89
Tonic neck reflex, 534, *534*

Tonsillitis, 193
Torso, craniosacral examination, 450
Torso balance, 643, *643*
Torticollis, 619
    acquired, 619-620
    congenital, 438-439, *439*, 444-448, *445-447*, 619
Toxic appearing infants and children, 675
Traction alopecia, 189
Traction response, 537
    infant reflex, 138
Transcranial Doppler imaging, 559
Transitional vertebrae, 218
Trauma
    acute spinal fractures, in adolescents, 730-774
    fever and, 677
    growth plate injuries, 625
    head injury, 575-577
    knee injuries, 630
    motor vehicle injuries, spinal problems and, 617
    neuromusculoskeletal, 624-626
    peripheral nerve, 627
    spinal, 595-596
      physical abuse and, 739
    sports injuries, 639-640
Trauma centers, chiropractors in, 731-732
Trichotillomania, 189
Trigeminal nerve, 494t
Trochlear nerve, 494t
Trunk
    growth, 614
    problems, 621-622
Trunk incurvation response, *523*
Tuberculosis, 695
Tularemia, 694

U

Ultrasonography
    assessment of fetal development, 80
    cranial, 559
    risk assessment in pregnancy, 119
Unicameral bone cyst, 223
Universal Spinographic Association, 2
Unrestrained children, pediatric motor vehicle collision and, 57-58, *58-59*
Upper cervical injury, motor vehicle collision, 66
Upper extremity, evaluation, 626-627
Urinary tract infection, 201
Urticaria, toddler skin, 187

V

Vaccination, issues, 24-44
    recommendations and contraindications, 29-30
Vaccination information pamphlets (VIPs), 24
Vaccine Adverse Reporting System (VAERS), 27
Vacuum extractor method, mechanism of spinal injury, *324*, 324-325
Vagal nerve, 495t
Vaginal birth, enhancing the probability, 120-121
Varicella, 684
    toddlers, 188
Vasotonic influences, general, 493
Vault and face, craniosacral examination, 448
Vault bones, 427-428, *428*
Vegetarian diet, 460
Ventricle system, cerebrospinal fluid flow, 487
Vertebral malposition, 468-470, *468-470*
Vertebral rotation, 643-644, *644*
Vertebral subluxation complex (VSC), 202-203, 466-477, *467*
    computed tomography, 307-308, *307-308*
    ligamentous injuries, 203
    low back problems, 203-204
    prevention of deformity and injury, 203
Vertebral wedging, 644, *644*
Vertebrogenic headache, 578

Vertical suspension, infant reflex, 138, *138*
Vesicular exanthem, 683
Vestibulospinal tract, 485
Victimization, 14–22
Visceral disorders, 601
Visceral pain, *vs.* somatic pain, 516
Visceral pathophysiology, 519–520
Vision, evaluation, 190–191, *191*
Visual-evoked response, 558
Visual righting reflexes (prone), 532, *532*
Visual righting reflexes (supine), 532, *533*
Visual righting reflexes (upright), 532, *533*
Vital signs, 673
Vitamin A, infant nutrition and, 457
Vitamin B12
    infant nutrition, 460
    maternal, 88
Vitamin D, infant nutrition and, 457
Vitamin K, infant nutrition and, 457

W
Walkers, baby, 614
Walking, 614
    developmental screening tests, 538
    during pregnancy, 167, *167*

Water consumption in children, 463–464
Water skiing, during pregnancy, 168
Water sports and diving, injuries, 639
Weakness, assessment of, 526
Webster, Larry, D.C., 3–4
Weight lifting, during pregnancy, 167, *168*
Weight-lifting, injuries, 640
West Coast Chiropractic College, 2
Whooping cough. *see* Pertussis
Wilm's tumor, 637
    fever and, 678
Withdrawal response to stimulus, 528, *528*
World Health Organization (WHO), Expanded Program on Immunization (EPI), 25

X
X-ray, 558

Y
Yellow fever, 685
Yoga, during pregnancy, 168

Z
Zinc, infant nutrition and, 457